QUALITY AND SAFETY EDUCAT
FOR NURSES (QSEN)

www.qsen.org

PATIENT-CENTERED CARE

Recognize the patient or designee as the source o.
in providing compassionate and coordinated care based c.
patient's preferences, values, and needs.

TEAMWORK AND COLLABORATION

Function effectively within nursing and interprofessional teams, fostering open communication, mutual respect, and shared decision making to achieve quality patient care.

EVIDENCE-BASED PRACTICE

Integrate best current evidence with clinical expertise and patient/family preferences and values for delivery of optimal health care.

QUALITY IMPROVEMENT

Use data to monitor the outcomes of care processes and use improvement methods to design and test changes to continuously improve the quality and safety of health care systems.

SAFETY

Minimize risk of harm to patients and providers through both system effectiveness and individual performance.

INFORMATICS

Use information and technology to communicate, manage knowledge, mitigate error, and support decision making.

Swearingen's

Manual of
Medical-Surgical

Swearingen's

Manual of Medical-Surgical Nursing: A Care Planning Resource

7th EDITION

Frances D. Monahan, PhD, RN, ANEF
Consultant in Nursing Education
Vero Beach, Florida

Marianne Neighbors, EdD, RN
Professor
Eleanor Mann School of Nursing;
Co-Director
Wally Cordes Teaching and Faculty Support Center
University of Arkansas
Fayetteville, Arkansas

Carol J. Green, PhD, MN, RN, CNE
Professor
School of Nursing
Graceland University
Independence, Missouri;
Captain, U.S. Navy Nurse Corps

ELSEVIER
MOSBY

3251 Riverport Lane
Maryland Heights, MO 63043

Swearingen's Manual of Medical-Surgical Nursing:
A Care Planning Resource

ISBN: 978-0-323-07254-0

Notices

Knowledge and best practice in this field are constantly changing. As new research and experience broaden our understanding, changes in research methods, professional practices, or medical treatment may become necessary.

Practitioners and researchers must always rely on their own experience and knowledge in evaluating and using any information, methods, compounds, or experiments described herein. In using such information or methods they should be mindful of their own safety and the safety of others, including parties for whom they have a professional responsibility.

With respect to any drug or pharmaceutical products identified, readers are advised to check the most current information provided (i) on procedures featured or (ii) by the manufacturer of each product to be administered, to verify the recommended dose or formula, the method and duration of administration, and contraindications. It is the responsibility of practitioners, relying on their own experience and knowledge of their patients, to make diagnoses, to determine dosages and the best treatment for each individual patient, and to take all appropriate safety precautions.

To the fullest extent of the law, neither the Publisher nor the authors, contributors, or editors, assume any liability for any injury and/or damage to persons or property as a matter of products liability, negligence or otherwise, or from any use or operation of any methods, products, instructions, or ideas contained in the material herein.

Nursing Diagnoses 5–Definitions and Classifications 2009-2011 © 2009, 2007, 2005, 2003, 2001, 1998, 1996, 1994 NANDA International. Used by arrangement with Wiley-Blackwell Publishing, a company of John Wiley and Sons, Inc.

Library of Congress Cataloging-in-Publication Data
Swearingen's manual of medical-surgical nursing : a care planning resource / [edited by] Frances D. Monahan, Marianne Neighbors, Carol J. Green.—7th ed.
    p. ; cm.
    Other title: Manual of medical-surgical nursing
    Rev. ed. of: Manual of medical-surgical nursing care. 6th ed. c2007.
    Includes bibliographical references.
    ISBN 978-0-323-07254-0 (pbk. : alk. paper)   1. Nursing–Handbooks, manuals, etc.   2. Surgical nursing–Handbooks, manuals, etc.   3. Nursing diagnosis–Handbooks, manuals, etc.   I. Swearingen, Pamela L.   II. Monahan, Frances Donovan. III. Neighbors, Marianne.   IV. Green, Carol J.   V. Manual of medical-surgical nursing care.   VI. Title: Manual of medical-surgical nursing.
    [DNLM: 1. Nursing Assessment–Handbooks.   2. Nursing Care–Handbooks.   3. Perioperative Nursing–Handbooks. WY 49 S974 2011]
    RT51.M365 2011
    617'.0231–dc22

2010024308

Executive Editor: Robin Carter
Managing Editor: Laurie K. Gower
Publishing Services Manager: Debbie Vogel
Senior Project Manager: Doug Turner
Project Manager: Bridget Healy
Design Direction: Teresa McBryan

Printed in the United States of America

Last digit is the print number: 9   8   7   6   5   4   3   2   1

Swearingen's Manual of Medical-Surgical Nursing: A Care Planning Resource is a thorough, clinically focused reference designed to enable both staff and student nurses to plan and evaluate care of the adult medical-surgical patient. The manual provides a focused review of pathophysiology, physical assessment, diagnostic testing, collaborative management, nursing interventions with expanded rationales, patient and family teaching, as well as discharge planning. The order of presentation of the information in each health alteration provides a hierarchy of data that enables the nurse to plan interventions specific to each patient. Generic information is found in Chapter 1: General Concepts in Caring for Medical-Surgical Patients, in which nursing diagnoses and interventions for perioperative care, pain, prolonged bedrest, cancer care, psychosocial support for patients, the patient's family and significant others, and older adult care are discussed. Additional generic information is found in Chapter 13: Care of the Patient with Special Needs and includes nutritional support, wound care, burns, and palliative/end-of-life care.

Staff and student nurses can use this reference to quickly access clinical information formerly found only in medical-surgical textbooks or large manuals. It is the first reference of its size to feature interventions for more than 125 health alterations. A consistent, easy-to-use format is incorporated to enhance the quick-reference feature of this book.

NEW TO THE SEVENTH EDITION

- New chapters include Chapter 11: Immunologic Disorders and Chapter 12: Cancer Care.
- Medical-surgical content throughout the manual has been thoroughly revised and updated by clinical experts.
- Newly expanded rationales for interventions with a focus on QSEN (Quality and Safety Education for Nurses) competencies.
- Content on burns added to Care for Patients with Special Needs (Chapter 13).
- The newest infection prevention and control guidelines issued by the Centers for Disease Control and Prevention (CDC) are included in the Appendix, and the text advocates use of the most recent CDC Precautions to reduce the risk of transmission of infectious diseases to patients and health care workers.
- A new patient teaching icon clearly delineates this information for each disorder.

FEATURES

- Bulleted format to provide content in concise manner without unnecessary repetition.
- Included with nursing diagnoses are outcome criteria—specific, positive statements that facilitate evaluation of care. Rationales have been added for most of the interventions.
- Where appropriate, information is summarized in tables and boxes to enhance the manual's clinical usefulness.
- Attractive and functional two-color design highlights key information for quick, easy reference.
- A variety of information resources, including links to websites, is included to facilitate the staff and student nurse in obtaining additional information and patient teaching services.

NOTES ABOUT THIS REFERENCE

- Throughout this text we use the phrase "health care provider" instead of the traditional "physician" or "doctor." This reflects the current trend of using Advanced Practice Nurses and Physician Assistants to provide care in the acute care setting.

- Health alterations included in this manual are those that are commonly seen as primary-admission diagnoses or, often, as secondary diagnoses in hospitalized patients. To control the number of pages and ensure a portable, handbook-size reference, we did not include discussions of pediatric, critical care, mental health, or other specialized areas.

Swearingen's Manual of Medical-Surgical Nursing: A Care Planning Resource is designed to help students and staff nurses care for patients in the "real world" of the acute care hospital. Reviewers indicate that it achieves this objective. The ultimate judgment rests with those nurses who read and use the manual on a daily basis. We welcome comments on how we could enhance its usefulness in subsequent editions.

Frances D. Monahan
Marianne Neighbors
Carol J. Green

Appendix 743

Selected Bibliography 764

Index 779

General Concepts in Caring for Medical-Surgical Patients

SECTION ONE **PERIOPERATIVE CARE**

NURSING DIAGNOSES AND INTERVENTIONS

Deficient knowledge related to surgical procedure, preoperative routine, and postoperative care

Desired outcome: Patient verbalizes knowledge about surgical procedure, including preoperative preparations and sensations and postoperative care and sensations, and demonstrates postoperative exercises and use of devices before surgical procedure or during immediate postoperative period for emergency surgery.

Nursing Interventions

Preoperatively

- Assess patient's facility with language, and engage an interpreter or provide language-appropriate written materials if necessary.
- Assess patient's understanding about the diagnosis, surgical procedure, preoperative routine, and postoperative regimen. Evaluate patient's desire for knowledge and readiness to learn about diagnosis and procedure (some individuals find detailed information helpful; others prefer very brief and simple explanations). Assess for limitations on ability to learn, such as blindness, decreased hearing, and limited reading ability, and obtain patient's self-assessment as to which modes of learning he or she finds most helpful, such as reading, listening, visual aids, and demonstration. Determine past surgical experiences and their positive or negative effect on patient. Assess the nature of any concerns or fears related to surgery. Document and communicate these assessment data to others involved in patient's care.
- Based on your assessment, clarify and explain diagnosis and surgical procedure accordingly. When possible, emphasize associated sensations (e.g., dry mouth, thirst, muscle weakness) to help reduce stress and anxiety. Use anatomic models, diagrams, and other audiovisual aids when possible. Provide written information appropriate to patient's language, reading ability, and culture to reinforce learning.
- Explain perioperative course of events. Review the following with patient and significant other:
  - Procedures for required preoperative assessment and testing and when and where they will be performed. Provide information regarding location of the preoperative testing center, parking arrangements, and expected length of time such testing will require. Issue written directions, phone numbers, and maps as indicated. Discuss location and proper arrival time for the surgery.

1

- Where patient will be before, during, and immediately after surgery (i.e., postanesthesia care unit [PACU], ICU, or other specialty unit). Clarify sounds and other sensations (e.g., sore throat, cool temperature, hard stretcher) patient may experience during immediate postoperative period. If possible, take patient to the new unit and introduce him or her to nursing staff.
- Preoperative medications and timing of surgery (scheduled time, expected duration).
- If indicated, preoperative bowel preparation.
- Pain management, including sensations to expect and methods of relief. If patient-controlled analgesia (PCA) or patient-controlled epidural anesthesia (PCEA) will be prescribed, have patient return demonstration of use of delivery device.
- Placement of tubes, catheters, drains, cooling systems (Cryo/Cuff), continuous passive motion (CPM) units, O_2 delivery devices, and similar devices routinely used for patient's surgery. Enable patient to see these devices when possible.
- Use of antiembolism stockings, sequential compression devices (SCDs), pneumatic foot pumps, or similar devices.
- Dietary alterations and progression, including NPO (nothing by mouth) status followed by clear liquids until return of full gastrointestinal (GI) function.
- Restrictions of activity and positions, as indicated by specific surgical procedure (e.g., total hip arthroplasty positional limitations).
- Need to refrain from smoking during perioperative period.
- Visiting hours and location of waiting room.

Postoperatively

◆ Explain postoperative activities, exercises, and precautions. Have patient return demonstration of the following devices and exercises, as appropriate:
  - Deep-breathing and coughing exercises (see **Ineffective airway clearance**, p. 3) unless increased intracranial, intrathoracic, or intraabdominal pressure contraindicates coughing.
  - Use of incentive spirometer and other respiratory devices.
  - Calf-pumping, ankle-circling, and footboard-pressing exercises *to promote circulation and prevent thrombophlebitis in the lower extremities* (see "Venous Thrombosis/Thrombophlebitis," p. 158, for more information).
  - Use of PCA/PCEA device.
  - Movement in, into, and out of bed.
◆ Before patient is discharged, teach prescribed activity precautions, such as getting maximum amounts of rest, increasing activities gradually to tolerance, avoiding heavy lifting (more than 10 lb), avoiding driving a car (often for as long as 4-6 wk). Include restrictions on sexual activity as indicated by the surgical procedure.
◆ Provide time for patient to ask questions and express feelings of anxiety; be reassuring and supportive. Be certain to address patient's main concerns.

Risk for injury related to exposure to pharmaceutical agents and other external factors during the perioperative period
Desired outcome: Patient does not experience injury or untoward effects of pharmacotherapy or other external factors.

Nursing Interventions

◆ Assess need for holding, administering, or adjusting patient's maintenance medications before or immediately after surgery. Some medications, such as anticonvulsants and cardiac medications, should be continued throughout the perioperative period. Sometimes patients need to be weaned from medications (e.g., baclofen) for the perioperative period. Other medications may require alternative routes or increased dosages during surgery (e.g., hydrocortisone in place of prednisone and with increased dosage for steroid-dependent patients). Consult health care provider as necessary.

♦ Reinforce importance of NPO status.

♦ Verify completion of preoperative activities and procedures, and document on preoperative checklist or nursing documentation.

♦ Be aware of the following: preoperative verification process must confirm the correct patient, procedure, and site of operation. This verification process should take place upon admission to the facility, before patient leaves the preoperative area, upon entry to the surgical room, and any time responsibility for patient care is transferred to another caregiver. The verification process should involve patient while he or she is still awake and aware if possible.

♦ Verify that an appropriate member of the surgical team has marked the operative site with a marker sufficiently permanent to remain visible after completion of skin prep. The marking should be unambiguous (i.e., initials or "YES" and/or a line representing proposed incision).

♦ Document allergies, any evidence of skin breakdown, bruises, rashes, or wounds, and presence of dressings, drains, or ostomy.

♦ Document presence of any ongoing pain problems. Include type, location, intensity, duration, onset, and precipitating and alleviating factors.

♦ Assess for and document patient's exposure to actual or potential abuse or neglect. All states require health care providers to report suspected abuse and neglect of children and vulnerable adults who are in their care.

♦ Document whether patient provides an advance directive (see p. 731). Laws about advance directives differ for each state.

♦ Document patient's access to care and transportation upon discharge.

♦ Ensure that consent has been signed and witnessed and patient appears to understand what the procedure involves. Answer questions or call health care provider to answer patient's questions. Ensure that patient's identification (ID) bracelet, blood transfusion bracelet, and allergy alert bracelet are in place. Review medical record to ensure that all appropriate documentation is present; report untoward findings (e.g., abnormal ECG, suspicious chest radiograph, abnormal laboratory findings) to health care provider.

♦ Prepare surgical site as prescribed (e.g., showering with antimicrobial agent and clipping of hair or use of depilatory agent [shaving is not usually recommended]). Accomplish additional presurgical procedures as indicated (e.g., douche, enemas, eyedrops).

♦ Administer preoperative analgesia, sedation, or other medications as prescribed. Give all medications, especially antibiotics, in a timely manner to ensure adequate serum levels. Make provisions for patient safety following administration (e.g., bed in lowest position, side rails up, and reminder to not to get out of bed without assistance).

♦ Be aware that once patient is in the location in which the procedure will be conducted and just before the procedure is started, a "time out" must be performed. The time out must involve the entire operative team and confirm correct patient identity, procedure, site, and position and availability of any special equipment, implants, and other requirements.

Ineffective airway clearance related to alterations in pulmonary physiology and function secondary to anesthetics, narcotics, mechanical ventilation, hypothermia and surgery; increased tracheobronchial secretions secondary to effects of anesthesia combined with ineffective coughing; and decreased function of the mucociliary clearance mechanism

Desired outcome: Patient's airway is clear as evidenced by normal breath sounds to auscultation, respiratory rate (RR) 12-20 breaths/min with normal depth and pattern (eupnea), normothermia, normal skin color, and O_2 saturation greater than 92% on room air.

Nursing Interventions

◆ Assess respiratory status, including breath sounds, q1-2h during immediate postoperative period and q8h during recovery. Note and report presence of rhonchi that do not clear with coughing, labored breathing, tachypnea (RR more than 20 breaths/min), mental status changes, restlessness, cyanosis, and presence of fever (temperature of 38.3° C [101° F] or higher).

◆ Use oximetry to assess O_2 saturation as indicated, such as for debilitated, obese, and older patients and those with COPD or other, respiratory or cardiovascular disease, and for patients undergoing cardiothoracic surgery, major surgery, prolonged general anesthesia, or surgery for a fractured pelvis or long bone. Report O_2 saturation of 92% or less.

◆ Encourage deep breathing and coughing q2h or more often for the first 72 hr postoperatively. In the presence of fine crackles (rales) and if not contraindicated, have patient cough to expectorate secretions. Facilitate deep breathing and coughing by demonstrating how to splint abdominal and thoracic incisions with hands or a pillow. If indicated, medicate ½ hr before deep breathing, coughing, or ambulation to promote adherence.

◆ If patient has a weak cough or poor reserve, try the "step-cough" technique. Coach patient to cough in rapid succession. *A few weak coughs in a row may stimulate a larger, productive cough at the end of the cycle.* Consider whether patient may be more motivated to perform pulmonary toilet with incentive spirometer or with positive expiratory pressure (PEP) device. Coughing after herniorrhaphy and some thoracic surgeries should be done in a controlled manner, with incision supported carefully. Vigorous coughing may be contraindicated for some individuals (e.g., those undergoing intracranial surgery, spinal fusion, eye and ear surgery, or similar procedures).

◆ Be certain that emergency airway equipment (i.e., intubation tray, endotracheal tubes, suctioning equipment, tracheostomy tray) is readily available in the event of sudden airway obstruction or ventilatory failure.

◆ Administer humidified O_2 as prescribed *to prevent further drying of respiratory passageways and secretions.*

Risk for aspiration related to entry of gastric secretions, food, or fluids into tracheobronchial passages secondary to central nervous system (CNS) depression, depressed cough and gag reflexes, decreased GI motility, abdominal distention, recumbent position, presence of gastric tube, diabetes, gastroesophageal reflux disease (GERD), obesity, and possible impaired swallowing in individuals with oral, facial, or neck surgery

Desired outcome: Patient's upper airway remains unobstructed as evidenced by clear breath sounds, RR 12-20 breaths/min with normal depth and pattern (eupnea), normal skin color, and a return to preoperative O_2 saturation

Nursing Interventions

◆ See first four interventions under **Ineffective airway clearance**, p. 3.

◆ If sedated patient experiences nausea or vomiting, turn immediately into a side-lying position. Fully alert patients may remain in an upright position. As necessary, suction oropharynx with Yankauer or similar suction device to remove vomitus.

◆ Check placement and patency of gastric tubes q8h and before instillation of feedings and medications. Consult health care provider before irrigating tubes for these individuals. Use caution when irrigating and otherwise manipulating GI tubes of patients with recent esophageal, gastric, or duodenal surgery *because the tube may be displaced or the surgical incision disrupted by such activity.*

- ◆ Assess abdomen q4-8h by inspection, auscultation, palpation, and percussion for evidence of distention (increasing size, firmness, increased tympany, decreased bowel sounds). Notify health care provider if distention is of rapid onset or if it is associated with pain.
- ◆ Encourage early and frequent ambulation *to improve GI motility and reduce abdominal distention caused by accumulated gases.*
- ◆ Introduce oral fluids cautiously, especially in patients with oral, facial, and neck surgery.
- ◆ Administer antiemetics, histamine H_2-receptor blocking agents, omeprazole, metoclopramide, and similar agents as prescribed.
- ◆ For additional information see "Providing Nutritional Support" for **Risk for aspiration**, p. 705.

Ineffective breathing pattern (or risk for same) related to decreased lung expansion secondary to CNS depression, pain, muscle splinting, recumbent position, obesity, narcotics, and effects of anesthesia
Desired outcome: Patient exhibits effective ventilation as evidenced by relaxed breathing, RR 12-20 breaths/min with normal depth and pattern (eupnea), clear breath sounds, normal color, return to preoperative O_2 saturation on room air, PaO_2 80 mm Hg or greater, pH 7.35-7.45, $PaCO_2$ 35-45 mm Hg, and bicarbonate (HCO_3^-) 22-26 mEq/L.

Nursing Interventions

- ◆ See interventions under **Ineffective airway clearance**, p. 3.
- ◆ Perform preoperative baseline assessment of patient's respiratory system, noting rate, rhythm, degree of chest expansion, quality of breath sounds, cough, and sputum production, as well as smoking history and current respiratory medications. Note preoperative O_2 saturation and arterial blood gas (ABG) values if available.
- ◆ If appropriate, encourage patient to refrain from smoking for at least 1 wk after surgery. Explain effects of smoking on the body.
- ◆ Monitor O_2 saturation continuously via oximetry in high-risk patients (e.g., patients who are heavily sedated, patients with preexisting lung disease, morbidly obese patients, patients having undergone upper airway surgery, or older patients) and at periodic intervals in other patients as indicated. Notify health care provider of O_2 saturation less than 92%.
- ◆ Evaluate ABG values, and notify health care provider of low or decreasing PaO_2 and high or increasing $PaCO_2$.
- ◆ Assist patient with turning and deep-breathing exercises q2h for the first 72 hr postoperatively *to promote lung expansion.* Be aware that opioid analgesics depress the respiratory system.
- ◆ If patient has an incentive spirometer or PEP device, provide instructions and ensure adherence to its use q2h or as prescribed.
- ◆ Unless contraindicated, assist patient with ambulation by second postoperative day *to enhance ventilation.*
- ◆ For other interventions, see "Atelectasis" for **Ineffective breathing pattern**, p. 58.

Risk for deficient fluid volume related to postoperative bleeding/hemorrhage
Desired outcomes: Patient is normovolemic as evidenced by BP 90/60 mm Hg or higher (or within patient's preoperative baseline), heart rate (HR) 60-100 bpm, RR 12-20 breaths/min with normal depth and pattern (eupnea), brisk capillary refill (less than 2 sec), warm extremities, amplitude of distal pulses greater than 2+ on a 0-4+ scale, urinary output 30 mL/hr or more, and urine specific gravity less than 1.030. Patient does not demonstrate significant mental status changes and verbalizes orientation to person, place, and time.

Nursing Interventions

◆ Monitor VS at frequent intervals during first 24 hr of postoperative period. Be alert to changes indicative of internal hemorrhage and impending shock, including decreasing pulse pressure (difference between SBP and DBP), decreasing BP, increasing HR, and increasing RR.

◆ Assess patient at frequent intervals during first 24 hr of postoperative period for indicators of internal hemorrhage and impending shock, including pallor, diaphoresis, cool extremities, delayed capillary refill, diminished intensity of distal pulses, restlessness, agitation, mental status changes, and disorientation. Also note subjective complaints of thirst, anxiety, or a sense of impending doom.

◆ Monitor and measure urinary output q4-8h during initial postoperative period. Report average hourly output less than 30 mL/hr. Assess urinary specific gravity, and report specific gravity less than 1.030.

◆ Inspect surgical dressing for evidence of frank bleeding (i.e., rapid saturation of dressing with bright red blood). Record saturated dressings and report significant findings to health care provider. If initial postoperative dressing becomes saturated, reinforce and notify health care provider because he or she may wish to perform initial dressing change.

◆ Monitor wound drains and drainage systems for excessive drainage (more than 50 mL/hr for 2-3 hr), and report findings to health care provider.

◆ Note amount and character of drainage from gastric and other tubes at least q8h. If drainage appears to contain blood (e.g., bright red, burgundy, or dark coffee ground appearance), perform an occult blood test. If test is newly or unexpectedly positive, report results to health care provider. Expect small amounts of bloody or blood-tinged drainage for the first 12-24 hr after gastric and some other GI surgeries. Be alert to large or increasing amounts of bloody drainage.

◆ Review CBC values for evidence of bleeding: decreases in hemoglobin (Hgb) from normal (male, 14-18 g/dL; female, 12-16 g/dL); decreases in hematocrit (Hct) from normal (male, 40%-54%; female, 37%-47%).

◆ Maintain patent 18-gauge or larger IV catheter for use if hemorrhagic shock develops. See "Cardiac and Noncardiac Shock," p. 136, for management.

Risk for deficient fluid volume related to active loss secondary to presence of indwelling drainage tubes, wound drainage, or vomiting; inadequate intake of fluids secondary to nausea, NPO status, CNS depression, or lack of access to fluids; or failure of regulatory mechanisms with third spacing of body fluids secondary to the effects of anesthesia, endogenous catecholamines, blood loss during surgery, and prolonged recumbency

Desired outcomes: Patient is normovolemic as evidenced by BP 90/60 mm Hg or higher (or within patient's preoperative baseline), HR 60-100 bpm, distal pulses greater than 2+ on a 0-4+ scale, urinary output 30 mL/hr or more, urine specific gravity 1.030 or less, stable or increasing weight, good skin turgor, warm skin, moist mucous membranes, and normothermia. Patient does not evidence significant mental status changes and verbalizes orientation to person, place, and time.

Nursing Interventions

◆ Monitor VS q4-8h during recovery phase. Be alert to changes consistent with dehydration, including decreasing BP, increasing HR, and slightly increased body temperature.

◆ Assess patient's physical status q4-8h. Be alert to indicators of dehydration, including dry skin, dry mucous membranes, excessive thirst, diminished intensity of peripheral pulses, and alteration in mental status. Assess skin turgor by gently pinching up a section of skin on the forehead, in the sternal area or beneath the clavicle. Release skin, and watch its return to original position. With good hydration, it will return quickly; with dehydration, skin will remain in lifted position (tenting) or return slowly.

- Monitor urinary output q4-8h. Be alert to increased concentration of urine (specific gravity more than 1.030) and low or decreasing output (average normal output is 60 mL/hr, or 1400-1500 mL/day).

- Measure, describe, and document any emesis. Be alert to and document excessive perspiration. Include your assessment of both with documentation of urinary, fecal, and other drainage for a total estimation of patient's fluid balance.

- Measure and record output from drains, ostomies, wounds, and other sources. Ensure patency of gastric and other drainage tubes. Record quality and quantity of output. Report and replace excessive losses.

- Monitor patient's weight daily, and use results as an indicator of patient's hydration and nutritional status. Always weigh patient at same time every day, and use same scale and same type and amount of bed clothing. Be aware that this method is not useful in detecting intravascular fluid loss due to third spacing.

- If nausea and vomiting are present, assess for potential causes, including administration of opioid analgesics, loss of gastric tube patency, and environmental factors (e.g., unpleasant odors or sights). Administer antiemetics, metoclopramide, or similar agents as prescribed to combat nausea and vomiting. Instruct patient to request medication before nausea becomes severe.

- Monitor serum electrolytes. Be alert to low K^+ levels (less than 3.5 mEq/L) and the following signs and symptoms of hypokalemia: lethargy, irritability, anorexia, vomiting, muscle weakness and cramping, paresthesias, weak and irregular pulse, and respiratory dysfunction.

- Also assess for low calcium (Ca^{++}) levels (less than 8.5 mg/dL) and the following signs and symptoms of hypocalcemia: tetany, muscle cramps, fatigue, irritability, personality changes, and Trousseau's or Chvostek's sign. Trousseau's sign is elicited by applying BP cuff to the arm, inflating it to slightly higher than SBP, and leaving it inflated for 1-4 min. Carpopedal spasms are indicative of hypocalcemia. Chvostek's sign is elicited by tapping the face just below the temple (where the facial nerve emerges). The sign consists of twitching occurs along side of nose, lip, or face.

- Administer and regulate IV fluids and electrolytes as prescribed until patient is able to resume oral intake. When IV fluids are discontinued, encourage intake of oral fluids, at least 2-3 L/day in nonrestricted patient. As possible, respect patient's preference in oral fluids, and keep them readily available in patient's room.

Excess fluid volume related to compromised regulatory mechanisms after major surgery

Desired outcome: Following intervention/treatment, patient becomes normovolemic as evidenced by BP within normal range of patient's preoperative baseline, distal pulses less than 4+ on a 0-4+ scale, presence of eupnea, clear breath sounds, absence of or barely detectable edema (1+ or less on a 0-4+ scale), urine specific gravity less than 1.010, and body weight near or at preoperative baseline.

Nursing Interventions

- Assess for and report any indicators of fluid overload, including elevated BP, bounding pulses, dyspnea, crackles (rales), and pretibial or sacral edema.

- Maintain record of 8-hr and 24-hr I&O. Note and report significant imbalance. Monitor urinary specific gravity and report consistently low (less than 1.010) findings. Remember that normal 24-hr output is 1400-1500 mL and normal 1-hr output is 60 mL.

- Weigh patient daily, and use same scale and same type and amount of bed clothing. Note significant weight gain. Remember that 1 L of fluid equals approximately 2.2 lb.
- Anticipate postoperative diuresis approximately 48-72 hr after surgery because of mobilization of third-space (interstitial) fluid.
- Administer furosemide as prescribed to mobilize interstitial fluid. Monitor for hypokalemia *because diuretic therapy may cause dangerous K^+ depletion.* See **Risk for deficient fluid volume**, p. 6, for signs and symptoms of hypokalemia.
- Be aware that older adults and individuals with cardiovascular disease are at risk for developing postoperative fluid volume excess.

Risk for infection related to inadequate primary defenses (e.g., broken skin, traumatized tissue, decrease in ciliary action, stasis of body fluids), invasive procedures, or chronic disease

Desired outcome: Patient is free of infection as evidenced by normothermia; HR 100 bpm or less; RR 20 breaths/min or less with normal depth and pattern (eupnea); negative cultures; clear and normal-smelling urine; clear and thin sputum; no significant mental status changes; orientation to person, place, and time; and absence of unusual tenderness, erythema, swelling, warmth, or drainage at the surgical incision.

Nursing Interventions

- Monitor VS for evidence of infection, such as elevated HR and RR and increased body temperature. Notify health care provider if these are new findings.
- Evaluate mental status, orientation, and level of consciousness (LOC) q8h. Consider infection if altered mental status or LOC is unexplained by other factors, such as age, medication, or disease process.
- Encourage and assist patient with coughing, deep breathing, incentive spirometry, and turning q2-4h, and note quality of breath sounds, cough, and sputum.
- Evaluate IV sites for evidence of infection: erythema, warmth, swelling, tenderness, unusual drainage. Change IV line and site if evidence of infection is present and according to agency protocol (q48-72h).
- Evaluate patency of all surgically placed tubes or drains. Monitor insertion sites for indications of infection (erythema, warmth, swelling, tenderness, unusual drainage). Irrigate, gently "milk," or attach to low-pressure suction as prescribed. Promptly report unrelieved loss of patency.
- Note color, character, and odor of all drainage. Report presence and amount of foul-smelling, purulent, or abnormal drainage.
- Evaluate incisions and wound sites for evidence of infection: unusual erythema, warmth, tenderness, induration, swelling, delayed healing, and purulent or excessive drainage.
- Change dressings as prescribed, using "no touch" and sterile techniques. Prevent cross-contamination of wounds in same patient by changing one dressing at a time and washing hands between dressing changes.
- Suspect evisceration if patient complains of a feeling of "letting go" or there is a sudden profusion of serous drainage on or a bulge in the dressing. If patient develops evisceration, do not reinsert tissue or organs. Place a sterile, saline-soaked gauze over eviscerated tissues and cover with a sterile towel until the wound can be evaluated by health care provider. Maintain patient on bed rest, usually in semi-Fowler's position with knees slightly bent *for comfort and to prevent further evisceration.* Begin to prepare patient for surgical repair: keep patient NPO and anticipate need for IV therapy.
- When appropriate, encourage use of intermittent catheterization q4-6h instead of indwelling catheter.

◆ Prevent reflux of urine into bladder by keeping drainage collection container below bladder level. Help prevent urinary stasis by avoiding kinks or obstructions in drainage tubing.

◆ Do not open closed urinary drainage system unless absolutely necessary, and irrigate catheter only with health care provider's prescription and when obstruction is the known cause.

◆ Assess for indicators of urinary tract infection (UTI), including chills; fever (temperature higher than 37.7° C [100° F]); dysuria; urgency; frequency; flank, low back, suprapubic, buttock, inner thigh, scrotal, or labial pain; and cloudy or foul-smelling urine.

◆ Encourage intake of 2-3 L/day in nonrestricted patients to minimize potential for UTI by diluting the urine and maximizing urinary flow.

◆ Ensure that perineum and meatus are cleansed during daily bath and perianal area is cleansed after bowel movements. Do not hesitate to remind patient of these hygiene measures. Be alert to indicators of meatal infection, including swelling, purulent drainage, and persistent meatal redness. Intervene if patient is unable to perform self-care.

◆ Change catheter according to established protocol or sooner if sandy particles can be felt in distal end of catheter or patient develops UTI. Change drainage collection container according to established protocol or sooner if it becomes foul smelling or leaks.

◆ Obtain cultures of suspicious drainage or secretions (e.g., sputum, urine, wound) as prescribed. For urine specimens, be certain to use sampling port, which is at proximal end of drainage tube. Cleanse area with an antimicrobial wipe and use a sterile syringe with 25-gauge needle to aspirate urine.

◆ Prevent transmission of infectious agents by washing hands well before and after caring for patient and by wearing gloves when contact with blood, drainage, or other body substance is likely.

◆ Use precautions (see Appendix 1, p. 743) for patients colonized with methicillin-resistant *Staphylococcus aureus* (MRSA), vancomycin-resistant *Enterococcus* (VRE), or other epidemiologically important organisms.

Constipation related to immobility, opioid analgesics and other medications, dehydration, lack of privacy, disruption of abdominal musculature, or manipulation of abdominal viscera during surgery

Desired outcome: Patient returns to his or her normal bowel elimination pattern as evidenced by return of active bowel sounds within 48-72 hr after most surgeries, absence of abdominal distention or sensation of fullness, and elimination of soft, formed stools.

Nursing Interventions

◆ Monitor for and document elimination of flatus or stool, *which signals returning intestinal motility.*

◆ Assess for evidence of decreased GI motility, including abdominal distention, tenderness, absent or hypoactive bowel sounds, and sensation of fullness. Report gross distention, extreme tenderness, and prolonged absence of bowel sounds.

◆ Encourage in-bed position changes, exercises, and ambulation to patient's tolerance unless contraindicated to stimulate peristalsis.

◆ If a nasogastric (NG) tube is in place, perform the following:
  • Check placement of tube after insertion, before any instillation, and q8h. For a larger-bore tube, aspirate gastric contents and assess for pH less than 5.0 for gastric tube placement. If the tube is in the trachea, patient may exhibit signs of respiratory distress or consistently low O_2 saturation levels, or there may be absence of drainage. Reposition tube immediately. Once assured of placement, mark tube to easily assess tube migration, and secure tubing in place. For smaller-bore tubes, check recent x-ray film to confirm position before instilling anything.

- Keep tube securely taped to patient's nose, and reinforce placement by attaching tube to patient's gown with safety pin or tape *to prevent tube migration.*
- Measure and record quantity and quality of output. Typically the color will be green. For patients who have undergone gastric surgery, output may be brownish initially because of small amounts of bloody drainage but should change to green after about 12 hr. Test reddish, brown, or black output for presence of blood, which *can signal GI bleeding.* Reposition tube as necessary unless patient has had gastric, esophageal, or duodenal surgery in which case the health care provider must be notified before the tube is manipulated.
- Maintain patency of NG tube with gentle instillation of normal saline as prescribed. Ensure low, intermittent suction of gastric sump tubes by maintaining patency of sump port (usually blue). If sump port becomes occluded by gastric contents, flush sump port with air until a "whoosh" sound is heard over epigastric area unless patient has had gastric, esophageal, or duodenal surgery in which case the health care provider must be notified before the tube is irrigated. Never clamp or otherwise occlude sump port because excessive pressure may accumulate and damage gastric mucosa.
- When tube is removed, monitor patient for abdominal distention, nausea, and vomiting.
- Monitor and document patient's response to diet advancement from clear liquids to a regular or other prescribed diet.
- Encourage oral fluid intake (more than 2500 mL/day), especially intake of prune juice.
- Administer stool softeners, mild laxatives, senna-based herbal teas, and enemas as prescribed. As appropriate, encourage high-bulk diet (fresh vegetables and fruits). Monitor and record results.
- Arrange periods of privacy during patient's attempts at bowel elimination.

Disturbed sleep pattern related to anxiety, stress, pain, noise, and altered environment

Desired outcome: Following intervention/treatment, patient relates minimal or no difficulty with falling asleep and describes a feeling of being well rested.

Nursing Interventions

- Administer sedative/hypnotic as prescribed. Be aware that these agents may cause CNS depression and contribute to respiratory depressant effects of opioid analgesics. Also be aware that active metabolites of many of the benzodiazepines may accumulate and result in greater physiologic effects or toxicity. Monitor respiratory function, including oximetry at frequent intervals, when administering sedative/hypnotic to patients with COPD because of the respiratory depressant effects of these drugs.
- After administering sedative/hypnotic, be certain to raise side rails, lower bed to its lowest position, and caution patient not to smoke in bed.
- Administer analgesics at bedtime to reduce pain and augment effects of hypnotic.
- Be certain that consent for surgery is signed before administering sedative/hypnotic.
- Use nonpharmacologic measures to promote sleep (**TABLE 1-1**).

Impaired physical mobility related to postoperative pain, decreased strength and endurance secondary to CNS effects of anesthesia or blood loss, musculoskeletal or neuromuscular impairment secondary to disease process or surgical procedure, perceptual impairment secondary to disease process or surgical

TABLE 1-1	NONPHARMACOLOGIC MEASURES TO PROMOTE SLEEP

ACTIVITY	EXAMPLES
Mask or eliminate environmental stimuli	Use eye shields or ear plugs; play soothing music; dim lights at bedtime; mask odors from dressings/drainage; change dressing or drainage container as indicated
Promote muscle relaxation	Encourage ambulation as tolerated throughout the day; teach and encourage in-bed exercises and position changes; perform back massage at bedtime; if not contraindicated, use heating pad
Reduce anxiety	Ensure adequate pain control; keep patient informed of progress and treatment measures; avoid overstimulation by visitors or other activities immediately before bedtime; avoid stimulant drugs (e.g., caffeine)
Promote comfort	Encourage patient to use own pillows and bed clothes if not contraindicated; adjust bed; rearrange linens; regulate room temperature
Promote usual presleep routine	Offer oral hygiene at bedtime; provide warm beverage at bedtime; encourage reading or other quiet activity
Minimize sleep disruption	Maintain quiet environment throughout the night; plan nursing activities to allow long periods (at least 90 min) of undisturbed sleep; use dim lights when checking on patient during the night

procedure (e.g., ocular surgery, neurosurgery), or cognitive deficit secondary to disease process or effects of opioid analgesics and anesthetics

Desired outcome: Optimally, by time of hospital discharge (depending on type of surgery), patient returns to preoperative baseline physical mobility as evidenced by ability to move in bed, transfer, and ambulate independently or with minimal assistance.

Nursing Interventions

◆ Assess patient's preoperative physical mobility by evaluating coordination and muscle strength, control, and mass. Be aware of medically imposed restrictions against movement, especially with conditions or surgeries that are orthopedic, neurosurgical, or ocular.

◆ Evaluate and correct factors limiting physical mobility, including oversedation with opioid analgesics, failure to achieve adequate pain control, and poorly arranged physical environment.

◆ Initiate movement from bed to chair and ambulation as soon as possible after surgery, depending on postoperative prescriptions, type of surgery, and patient's recovery from anesthetics. Assist patient to move slowly to a sitting position in bed and then stand at bedside before attempting ambulation *because many anesthetic agents depress normal vasoconstrictor mechanisms, which can result in sudden hypotension with quick changes in position.* For more information, see **Ineffective cerebral tissue perfusion**, p. 28.

◆ Encourage frequent movement and ambulation by postoperative patients. Provide assistance as indicated.

◆ Explain importance of movement in bed and ambulation in reducing postoperative complications, including atelectasis, pneumonia, thrombophlebitis, and depressed GI motility.

◆ Instruct patient in performance of in-bed exercises (e.g., gluteal and quadriceps muscle sets [isometrics], ankle circling, calf pumping).

- For additional information, see "Prolonged Bed Rest" for **Risk for activity intolerance**, p. 23, and **Risk for disuse syndrome**, p. 25.

Risk for trauma related to weakness, balancing difficulties, and reduced muscle coordination secondary to anesthetics and postoperative opioid analgesics
Desired outcome: Patient does not fall and remains free of trauma as evidenced by absence of bruises, wounds, or fractures.

Nursing Interventions

- Orient and reorient patient to person, place, and time during initial postoperative period. Inform patient that surgery is over. Repeat information until patient is fully awake and oriented (usually several hours but may be days in heavily sedated or otherwise obtunded individuals).
- Maintain side rails on stretchers and beds in upright and locked positions. Be aware that some individuals experience agitation and thrash about as they emerge from anesthesia.
- Secure all IV lines, drains, and tubing to prevent dislodgment.
- Maintain bed in its lowest position when leaving patient's room.
- Be certain call mechanism is within patient's reach; instruct patient in its use.
- Identify patients at risk for falling by assessing the following. Correct or compensate for risk factors.
  - Time of day: night shift, peak activity periods such as meals, bedtime.
  - Medications: opioid analgesics, sedatives, hypnotics, and anesthetics.
  - Impaired mobility: individuals requiring assistance with transfer and ambulation.
  - Sensory deficits: diminished visual acuity caused by disease process or environmental factors; changes in kinesthetic sense because of disease or trauma.
- Use restraints and protective devices if necessary and prescribed.

Risk for impaired skin integrity related to presence of secretions/excretions around percutaneous drains and tubes
Desired outcome: Patient's skin around percutaneous drains and tubes remains intact and nonerythematous.

Nursing Interventions

- Change dressings as soon as they become wet. The health care provider may prefer to perform the first dressing change for the surgical incision. Use sterile technique for all dressing changes.
- Keep area around drains as clean as possible (because intestinal secretions, bile, and similar drainage can lead quickly to skin excoriation). Sterile normal saline or a solution of saline and hydrogen peroxide or other prescribed solution may be used to clean around drain site.
- If some external drainage is present, position a pectin-wafer skin barrier around drain or tube. Ointments, such as zinc oxide, petrolatum, and aluminum paste, also may be used. Consult wound, ostomy, continence (WOC) enterostomal therapy (ET) nurse if drainage is excessive or skin excoriation develops. For additional information, see "Managing Wound Care," p. 716.

Impaired oral mucous membrane related to NPO status and/or presence of NG or endotracheal tube
Desired outcome: At time of hospital discharge, patient's oral mucosa is intact, without pain or evidence of bleeding.

Nursing Interventions

- Provide oral care and oral hygiene q4h and prn. Arrange for patient to gargle, brush teeth, and cleanse mouth with sponge-tipped applicators as necessary to prevent excoriation and excessive dryness.

- Use a moistened cotton-tipped applicator to remove encrustations. Carefully lubricate lips and nares with antimicrobial ointment, petroleum jelly, or emollient cream.
- If patient's throat is irritated from presence of NG tube, obtain a prescription for lidocaine gargling solution.
- For additional information, see "Stomatitis" for **Impaired oral mucous membrane**, p. 441.

❖ ❖ ❖

SECTION TWO **PAIN**

NURSING DIAGNOSES AND INTERVENTIONS

Acute pain or**Chronic pain** related to disease process, injury, or surgical procedure

Desired outcome: As reported by patient (subjective) or family pain is at an acceptable level, documented through use of a pain scale. Behavioral (**BOX 1-1**) and physiologic (**BOX 1-2**) indicators of pain are absent.

Nursing Interventions

- Assess for behavioral and physiologic indicators of pain (Boxes 1-1 and 1-2) at frequent intervals including during scheduled VS assessments.

BOX 1-1	BEHAVIORAL INDICATORS OF PAIN (SELECTED)	
Facial Expression	**Verbalization**	**Behaviors**
▪ Grimacing	▪ Praying	▪ Massaging
▪ Facial tension	▪ Counting	▪ Guarding
Vocalization	**Body Action**	▪ Short attention span
▪ Moaning	▪ Rocking	▪ Irritability
▪ Groaning	▪ Rubbing	▪ Sleep disturbances
▪ Sighing	▪ Restlessness	
▪ Crying		

BOX 1-2	PHYSIOLOGIC INDICATORS OF PAIN (SELECTED)

- ▪ Diaphoresis
- ▪ Vasoconstriction
- ▪ Increased systolic and diastolic blood pressure
- ▪ Increased pulse rate (more than 100 bpm)
- ▪ Pupillary dilation
- ▪ Change in respiratory rate (usually increased, more than 20 breaths/min)
- ▪ Muscle tension or spasm
- ▪ Decreased intestinal motility evidenced by nausea, vomiting, abdominal distention, and possibly ileus
- ▪ Endocrine imbalance, evidenced by sodium and water retention and mild hyperglycemia

bpm, Beats per minut.

BOX 1-3	HIERARCHY OF PAIN MEASUREMENT

- Self-report
- Report of family
- Behavioral indicators
- Physiologic indicators

- ◆ Obtain history about ongoing/previous pain experiences and previously used methods of pain control. Elicit what was/was not effective.
- ◆ Evaluate patient's health history for alcohol and drug (prescribed and nonprescribed) use, which could affect effective doses of analgesics (i.e., patient may require more or less). Ensure that surgeon, anesthesiologist, and other health care providers are aware of any significant findings. Consult a pain management team if available. All care providers must be consistent in setting limits while providing effective pain control through pharmacologic and nonpharmacologic methods. Psychiatric or clinical pharmacology consultation may be necessary.
- ◆ Teach patients that pain management is a part of their treatment inasmuch as they have the right to appropriate assessment and management of their pain (The Joint Commission, 2008).
- ◆ Develop a systematic and collaborative approach to pain management for each patient, using information gathered from pain history and the hierarchy of pain measurement (**BOX 1-3**) in which individual report of pain is recognized as the single most reliable indicator of pain (Goldman and Ausiello, 2008).
- ◆ Use a preventive approach: administer prn pain medications before pain becomes severe as well as before painful procedures, ambulation, and bedtime.
- ◆ Use a formal patient-specific method of assessing self-reported pain when possible, including description, location, intensity, and aggravating/alleviating factors.
- ◆ Select a Pain Intensity Rating Scale appropriate to patient and use it consistently to *ensure comparability of assessments.* Numeric rating scales (NRSs) of 0 (no pain) to 10 (worst possible pain) and descriptive scales (no pain, mild pain, moderate pain, severe pain, very severe pain, worst possible pain) are used commonly to assess intensity in adults who are cognitively intact. The Faces pain scale (Kim and Buschmann, 2006) is an alternative that may best meet the needs of older adults (Taylor and Herr, 2001). The Pain Assessment in Advanced Dementia (PAINAD) scale based on vocalizations, facial grimacing, bracing, rubbing, and restlessness has a pain intensity rating that can be converted to a numeric equivalent (D'Arcy, 2007). The Payen Behavioral Pain scale (BPS) contains an assessment of compliance with ventilation and is used for critically ill, intubated patients (D'Arcy, 2007).
- ◆ Reassess pain level
  - Routinely at scheduled intervals (e.g., q2-4h with VS).
  - With each report of pain.
  - Following administration of pain medication based on time to onset, time to peak effect, and duration of action.
- ◆ Remember that the right drug is the one that works with the fewest side effects. Selection of analgesic agent is based on three general considerations: (1) therapeutic goal, (2) patient's medical condition, and (3) drug cost. Additional considerations are patient's previous experience with a specific agent and recall of side effects experienced with a specific agent.
- ◆ Use at least two identifiers (e.g., patient's name, medical record number) before administering medications *to improve accuracy of patient*

BOX 1-4	WORLD HEALTH ORGANIZATION THREE-STEP ANALGESIA LADDER

- Level I: nonopioid ± adjuvant
- Level II: opioid for mild to moderate pain ± nonopioid ± adjuvant
- Level III: opioid for moderate to severe pain ± nonopioid ± adjuvant

Modified from World Health Organization: *Cancer pain relief*, ed. 2, Geneva, World Health Organization, 1996.

identification in keeping with Joint Commission National Patient Safety Goals (2008).

- Administer analgesics for pain according to the World Health Organization (WHO) three-step analgesic ladder (**BOX 1-4**).

- Titrate the dose to achieve the desired effect. *Initial effect and duration of action may differ vastly from very low in the elderly and acutely ill to very high in the young adult or chronic alcohol/drug user.* The goal is to develop a safe and effective pain management plan.

- Choice of route may be based on convenience, anticipated analgesic requirements, side effects, and cost. The preferred route is the one that is least invasive while achieving adequate relief (**TABLE 1-2**) *because aversion to painful routes of delivery (e.g., subcutaneous, intramuscular [IM]) may lead to underreporting of pain by patients and to undermedication by nurses.* Avoid the IM route whenever possible *because it provides inconsistent analgesia, is less titratable, and can cause complications such as hematoma, granuloma, infection, aseptic tissue necrosis, and nerve injury.*

- For relief of mild-moderate pain that may be associated with surgery, trauma, soft tissue injury, and inflammatory conditions, administer nonopioid agents such as salicylates, para-aminophenol derivatives, and non-steroidal antiinflammatory drugs (NSAIDs). Be certain that gastrointestinal (GI) function has returned (bowel sounds are present, vomiting is absent) before administering oral agents.

- The NSAID ketorolac may be given by the IM or IV route for patients unable to tolerate oral agents. Assess for undesirable side effects such as GI disturbances (epigastric pain, nausea, dyspepsia), platelet dysfunction, bleeding, and renal compromise.

- NSAIDs have peripheral effects and a different mechanism of action and thus are very effective when combined or used with centrally acting opioid analgesics. Unless contraindicated, use of nonopioid agents is beneficial even if pain is severe enough to require addition of an opioid *because of their dose-sparing effect and the potential for reduction of opioid side effects* (Goldman and Ausiello, 2008). *Another advantage of NSAIDs is their dual antipyretic and antiinflammatory actions.*

- Prescribers should consider emerging information when weighing benefits of NSAID use against risks for individual patients. Assess the individual patient's risk for cardiovascular events and other risks commonly associated with NSAIDs. See the most recent package labeling changes of these products for additional details.

- Use cyclooxygenase 2 (COX-2) selective NSAIDs with caution. Assess risks/benefits based on current information.

- Administer opioid analgesics (e.g., morphine) as prescribed for pain of greater severity (Box 1-4 and **TABLE 1-3**). Morphine is the standard of comparison for opioid analgesics, and morphine or related "mu" (μ) receptor agonists are preferred when possible.

TABLE 1-2	PHARMACOLOGIC INTERVENTIONS: ROUTES/SELECTED COMMONLY PRESCRIBED MEDICATIONS		
ROUTE	**COMMONLY PRESCRIBED MEDICATIONS**	**ADVANTAGES**	**DISADVANTAGES**
Oral	Codeine, oxycodone/acetaminophen (Percocet), morphine (MS Contin), hydromorphone (Dilaudid)	Useful for mild to moderate acute pain or chronic severe pain (large doses necessary)	Variable absorption Cannot be used until GI function returns; lengthy interval before onset of action
IV bolus	Morphine, fentanyl (Sublimaze), meperidine (Demerol)	Useful for severe, intermittent pain (i.e., for procedures, treatments) Rapid onset of action	Relatively short duration of pain relief Fluctuating levels Possibility of excessive sedation as drug levels peak
Continuous infusion	Morphine, fentanyl (Sublimaze), hydromorphone (Dilaudid)	Useful for severe, predictable pain or as a basal dose with bolus supplements for fluctuating pain Relieves pain with lower doses than IV bolus Avoids peaks and valleys of pain found with IV bolus and IM injections	Requires frequent observation to monitor sedation VS must be monitored based on time of onset and duration of action; weaning may be necessary
Patient-controlled analgesia (IV, subcutaneous, epidural)	Morphine, fentanyl, meperidine, hydromorphone	Useful for moderate to severe pain Enables titration by patient for effective analgesia without excessive sedation Relief of pain with lower dosages of medication Immediate delivery of medication	Specialized delivery system must be used Patient must have clear mental status Patient may underreport pain to avoid painful reinsertion

Route	Drugs	Advantages	Disadvantages/Comments
Neuraxial (epidural, caudal, intrathecal)	Morphine, fentanyl, hydromorphone	Very effective relief of moderate to severe pain Delivery close to opiate receptors provides pain control with small doses May be delivered with local anesthetic (e.g., bupivacaine) for increased effectiveness	Catheter must be inserted by anesthetist or anesthesiologist Specialized delivery system must be used Side effects include urinary incontinence, hypotension, respiratory depression, pruritus, nausea, vomiting; catheter complications include infections, epidural hematoma/abscess
Transdermal	Fentanyl (Duragesic)	Long duration of action (3 days) Useful when pain is moderate to severe and constant for prolonged periods	Delayed onset of action (up to 36 hr) Prolonged effects after removal Must be used with rapid-action supplement for variable pain Not usually appropriate for postoperative pain control unless patient using system preoperatively
IM injection	Meperidine, morphine, pentazocine (Talwin), nalbuphine (Nubain), butorphanol (Stadol), buprenorphine	Useful for moderate to severe pain Longer duration of action than with IV route	Variable absorption and fluctuating levels, especially in hypotensive and edematous patients Possibility of excessive sedation as drug levels peak Potential delay in administration

GI, Gastrointestinal; *IM*, intramuscular; *IV*, intravenous; *VS*, vital signs.

TABLE 1-3 COMMON ANALGESICS

COMMON NONOPIOID ANALGESICS	COMMON OPIOID ANALGESIC COMBINATIONS*	COMMON ANALGESIC ADJUVANTS/CO-ANALGESICS	OPIOIDS FOR MILD TO MODERATE PAIN	OPIOIDS FOR MODERATE TO SEVERE PAIN
Salicylates	**Hydrocodone/ Acetaminophen**	**Antiepileptics**	Tramadol	Morphine
Aspirin	Anexsia	Carbamazepine (Tegretol)	Codeine	Hydromorphone
Choline magnesium trisalicylate	Lorcet	Clonazepam (Klonopin)	Hydrocodone	Methadone
Para-aminophenol Derivatives	Lorcet Plus	Gabapentin (Neurontin)		Oxymorphone
Acetaminophen*	Lorcet HD	Valproate (Depacon)		Fentanyl
Nonsteroidal Antiinflammatory Agents	Lortab	**Tricyclic Antidepressants**		Oxycodone
	Norco	Amitriptyline (Elavil)		
Propionic Acids	Vicodin	Doxepin (Sinequan)		
Ibuprofen*	Vicodin ES	Imipramine (Tofranil)		
Ketorolac	Vicodin HP	Nortriptyline (Pamelor)		
Naproxen	Zydone	**Newer Antidepressants**		
Indoleacetic Acid	**Oxycodone/Acetaminophen**	Venlafaxine (Effexor)		
Indomethacin	Endocet	**Antihistamine**		
Cyclooxygenase-2 Inhibitor	Percocet	Diphenhydramine (Benadryl)		
Celecoxib	Roxicet	**Benzodiazepines**		
Oxicams	**Codeine/Acetaminophen**	Diazepam (Valium)		
Piroxicam	Tylenol No. 3	Lorazepam (Ativan)		
Meloxicam	Codeine/acetaminophen	Midazolam (Versed)		
Fenamates	**Hydrocodone/Ibuprofen**	**Local Anesthetics**		
Meclofenamate	Vicoprofen	Bupivacaine		
Mefenamic Acid		Eutectic mixture of local anesthetics (EMLA)		
Naphthylalkanones		Lidocaine		
Nambutone				
Pyranocacarbolic Acid				
Etodolac				

*Maximum adult acetaminophen dose per day is 4000 mg; maximum adult ibuprofen dose per day is 3200 mg; potential for excessive doses of acetaminophen or ibuprofen may be minimized by avoiding combination products.

- Use of meperidine (Demerol) should be avoided when possible. *Normeperidine, a metabolite of meperidine, is a central nervous system (CNS) excitotoxin, which with repetitive dosing may produce anxiety, muscle twitching, and seizures.* Patients with impaired renal function and those taking monoamine oxidase (MAO) inhibitors are particularly at risk. Naloxone does not reverse and may potentiate hyperexcitability.

- Mixed agonist-antagonist agents such as butorphanol (Stadol) and pentazocine (Talwin) produce analgesia by binding to opioid receptors, while blocking or remaining neutral to the μ receptors. Mixed agonist-antagonist agents may be useful in patients who are unable to tolerate other opioids. Do not administer mixed agonist-antagonist analgesics concurrently with morphine or other pure agonists *because reversal of analgesic effects may occur.*

- Assess patients receiving opioid analgesics for level of pain relief and potential side effects, including evidence of excessive sedation or respiratory depression (i.e., respiratory rate [RR] less than 10 breaths/min or functional O_2 saturation [SpO_2] less than 90%-92%). In the presence of respiratory depression, reduce amount or frequency of the dose as prescribed. Have naloxone (**BOX 1-5**) readily available *to reverse severe respiratory depression.* Monitor patients, especially older adults and individuals with COPD, asthma, and other respiratory disorders, closely for sedative effects because these effects precede respiratory depression. Consider need to use reduced doses and titrate carefully *to prevent respiratory depression.*

- Consult with prescriber to discuss converting to scheduled dosing with supplemental prn analgesics when pain exists for 12 of 24 hr. Experts recommend around-the-clock (ATC) dosing for patients with continuous pain *because it provides superior pain relief with fewer side effects* (Goldman and Ausiello, 2008). *Prolonged stimulation of pain receptors results in increased sensitivity to painful stimuli and increases amount of drug required to relieve pain.* Be aware that addiction to opioids occurs infrequently in hospitalized patients.

- Wean patient from opioid analgesics by decreasing dose or frequency. In general, doses should be reduced by no more that 10%-20% per day in order *to avoid withdrawal signs and symptoms.* Convert to oral therapy as soon as possible. When changing route of administration or medication, be certain to use equianalgesic doses (**TABLES 1-4** and **1-5**) of the new drug. Changing route of medication administration often results in inadequate pain relief because of ineffective equianalgesic conversion.

- Patient-controlled analgesia (PCA) is a patient-activated system for pain control that uses an infusion pump to deliver specified doses of analgesics with options of continuous infusions, bolus dosing, or both.

BOX 1-5   NALOXONE (NARCAN)

- Adult dosage range for respiratory depression secondary to opioid intoxication is 0.4-2 mg intravenously (preferred route), intramuscularly, or subcutaneously.
- Repeat dose every 2-3 minutes, depending on patient response.
- Maximum dose is 10 mg. If no response after 10 mg, another cause of respiratory depression is considered.

Caution: Continue close monitoring for recurrence of respiratory depression because the duration of action of naloxone is shorter (20-60 min) than that of most opioids and a repeat dose may be needed.

TABLE 1-4   EQUIANALGESIA: HOW TO CONVERT FROM ANOTHER OPIOID TO MORPHINE

Calculate the total amount of any opioid taken in a 24-hr period that **effectively** controls pain.

Multiply by the conversion factor (listed below) to convert to an approximate equivalent morphine dose. Adjust down by 20%-75% to allow for incomplete cross-tolerance between different opioids (may need to titrate up **liberally and rapidly** to achieve analgesic effect in first 24 hr).

Then divide by number of doses per day [e.g., 6 doses for immediate release PO morphine (q4h), or two doses for controlled-release morphine (q12h)] to determine the individual dose.

Example: If a patient has taken 5 doses of oral hydromorphone (Dilaudid) 4 mg in a day, this would be equivalent to 20 mg/24 hr. To convert to an equivalent dose of morphine, multiply by conversion factor of 4 (20 mg/day × 4 = 80 mg/day morphine equivalents). Adjust dose downward by 50% because of incomplete cross tolerance. An equivalent dose of morphine would be about 40 mg/day to begin with. Prescribe rapid-release (q4h) or sustained-release morphine (q12h) equivalent to 40 mg per 24-hr period. Allow prn morphine for breakthrough pain during titration. Reassess at least daily or as needed.

NOTE: Breakthrough or "rescue" doses are usually 10% of 24-hr dose.

Conversion Factors (Other Opioid to Morphine)

FROM ORAL	TO ORAL MORPHINE (MG)	FROM PARENTERAL	TO PARENTERAL MORPHINE (MG)
Methadone	4-14*	Methadone	4-12*
Hydromorphone	4	Hydromorphone	7
Codeine	0.1-0.15	Meperidine	0.13
Oxycodone	1-1.5	Fentanyl	100

*Both oral and parenteral methadone doses have great variability; conversion ratio of morphine to methadone is between 4:1 and 12:1.

IMPORTANT NOTE: These tables are for use as general guidelines in the pharmacologic management of acute and chronic pain. For complete prescribing considerations given a specific drug or clinical patient situation, please consult pain references or a pharmacology reference or pain medicine or palliative care consultants.

TABLE 1-5   METHADONE CONVERSION CHART

ORAL MORPHINE EQUIVALENT DAILY DOSE (mg/day)	INITIAL DOSE RATIO (ORAL MORPHINE:ORAL METHADONE)
30-90	4:1
90-300	8:1
More than 300	12:1

Data from Pereira J, Lawlor P, Vigano A et al: Equianalgesic dose ratios for opioids: a critical review and proposals for long-term dosing, *J Pain Symptom Manage* 22(2):672-687, 2001; and Anderson R, Saiers JH, Abram S, Schlicht C: Accuracy in equianalgesic dosing: conversion dilemmas, *J Pain Symptom Manage* 21(5):397-406, 2001.

- Patient selection is important because patients must be capable of understanding and activating the device and be willing to participate in their own treatment.
- Morphine, fentanyl, and hydromorphone are examples of opioids available for PCA use.

- Increase patient monitoring following initiation, during initial 24 hr, and at night *when patient may hypoventilate.* Monitoring involves pain, sedation, and respiratory assessments and may include SpO_2 and capnography.
- Implement strategies to reduce safety risks associated with PCA; keep up with current developments (Institute for Safe Medication Practices [ISMP] Medication Safety Alerts [ISMP, May 29, 2002; July 10 & 24, 2003; ISMP Nurse Advise-ERR, 2005, D'Arcy, 2008]).
- Do not assume pain is controlled; you still must assess patient to determine whether relief has been obtained.

◆ Neuraxial analgesia (spinal, epidural, and caudal) is a widely used option for regional analgesia. Characteristics of analgesia (extent and duration of action) are based on catheter placement, drug choice, and drug concentration and volume.
- Local anesthetics, opioids, steroids, and clonidine are examples of agents that may be used.
- Patient monitoring requirements are determined based on drug(s) being administered. Assessments may include sensory level and motor examination evaluations, level of pain intensity, sedation level, VS, and side effects. For local anesthetics, monitor pain intensity and motor examination/sensory level. Perform sensory assessments bilaterally along dermatomes. For opioids, monitor respiratory rate (RR), sedation level, and pain intensity.
- Potential side effects/complications include catheter migration, occlusion, hematoma, respiratory depression, hypotension, nausea/vomiting, urinary retention, and pruritus.

◆ Use analgesic adjuvants/co-analgesics (Box 1-4) as prescribed to prolong and enhance analgesia. Explain that these agents are being used to augment analgesia, not specifically to treat isolated incidents of anxiety or depression.

◆ Tricyclic antidepressant agents produce analgesia while improving mood and sleep. Amitriptyline has the best-documented analgesia but is the least well tolerated because of anticholinergic effects. Concomitant use with opioids may lead to sedation and orthostatic hypotension.

◆ Benzodiazepines are anxiolytic/sedatives with little to no analgesic effect. They are useful for decreasing recall, treating acute anxiety, and decreasing muscle spasm associated with acute pain. They may decrease opioid requirement by decreasing pain perception. If they are administered without an analgesic, patient's perception of pain may increase.

◆ Antiepileptics may be prescribed for pain associated with nerve injury from tumors or other destructive processes.

◆ Antihistamines potentiate the effect of opioid analgesics although promethazine (Phenergan) may increase perceived pain intensity and increase restlessness.

◆ Avoid substituting sedatives and tranquilizers for analgesics.

◆ Assess for and report analgesia side effects, which can include sedation, respiratory depression, nausea/vomiting, pruritus, constipation, and hypotension.

◆ Augment action of the medication by using nonpharmacologic methods of pain control (**BOX 1-6**). Many of these techniques may be taught to and implemented by patient and significant other.

◆ Maintain a quiet environment *to promote rest.* Plan nursing activities to enable long periods of uninterrupted rest at night.

◆ Evaluate for and correct coincidental sources of discomfort (e.g., position, full bladder, and infiltrated IV site).

◆ Position patient comfortably, and reposition at frequent intervals *to relieve discomfort caused by pressure and improve circulation.*

| BOX 1-6 | COMMON NONPHARMACOLOGIC METHODS OF PAIN CONTROL* |

Sensory/Cutaneous Stimulations

Touch
- Reflexology
- Acupressure
- Reiki

Cold/Heat
- Cold used initially to diminish tissue injury response and alter pain threshold
- Heat used to facilitate clearance of tissue toxins and mobilize fluids

Massage
- Used to relax muscular tension and increase local circulation (back and foot massages are especially relaxing)

ROM Exercises (Passive, Assisted, or Active)
- Used to relax muscles, improve circulation, and prevent pain related to stiffness and immobility

TENS
Battery-operated device used to send weak electrical impulses via electrodes placed on the body
Reduces sensation of pain during and sometimes after treatment

Cognitive Interventions
Cognitive Preparation
- Preparing patient by explaining what can be expected, thereby reducing stress and anxiety (e.g., preoperative teaching)

Patient Education
- Teaching methods for preventing or reducing pain (e.g., suggesting comfortable postoperative positions, methods of ambulation, and splinting of incisions when coughing)

Distraction
- Encouraging patient to focus on something unrelated to pain (e.g., conversing, reading, watching TV or videos, listening to music)
- Humor can be an excellent distraction and may help patient cope with stress

Relaxation
- Jaw relaxation
- Slow, rhythmic breathing (may be music assisted)

Guided Imagery
- A mental process that uses images to alter a physical or emotional state
- Promotes relaxation and reduces pain sensations

Behavioral
- Hypnosis
- Biofeedback
- Counseling

*Many of these techniques can be taught to and implemented by the patient and significant other.
ROM, range of motion; *TENS*, transcutaneous electrical nerve stimulation.

- Carefully evaluate patient and notify health care provider immediately if sudden or unexpected changes in pain intensity occur *because they can signal complications such as internal bleeding or leakage of visceral contents.*
- Document efficacy of analgesics and other pain control interventions using a pain scale or other formalized method.

❖ ❖ ❖

SECTION THREE **PROLONGED BED REST**

OVERVIEW/PATHOPHYSIOLOGY

Patients on prolonged bed rest face many potential physiologic problems. Some are short term and easily corrected. Others, such as joint contractures, may result in permanent disability. This section reviews the most common physiologic and psychosocial problems that may occur. With early discharge from the hospital, many of these problems now are seen when patient is transferred to a long-term care facility or when discharged to home.

NURSING DIAGNOSES AND INTERVENTIONS

Risk for activity intolerance related to deconditioned status (**BOX 1-7**)
Desired outcomes: Within 48 hr of discontinuing bed rest, patient exhibits cardiac tolerance to activity or exercise as evidenced by heart rate (HR) 20 beats per minute (bpm) or less over resting HR; SBP 20 mm Hg or less over or under resting SBP; RR 20 breaths/min or less with normal depth and pattern (eupnea); normal sinus rhythm; warm and dry skin; and absence of crackles (rales), new murmurs, new dysrhythmias, gallop, or chest pain. Patient rates perceived exertion (RPE) at 3 or less on a scale of 0 (none) to 10 (maximal).

Nursing Interventions

♦ Perform ROM exercises 2-4 ×/day on each extremity. Individualize the exercise plan based on the following guidelines.
  • Mode or type of exercise: Begin with passive exercises, moving the joints through the motions of abduction, adduction, flexion, and extension. Progress to active-assisted exercises in which you support the joints while patient initiates muscle contraction. When patient is able, supervise him or her in active isotonic exercises, during which patient contracts a selected muscle group, moves the extremity at a slow pace, and then relaxes the muscle group. Have patient repeat each exercise 3-10 ×.
  • Intensity: Begin with 3-5 repetitions as tolerated by patient. Measure HR and BP at rest, peak exercise, and 5 min after exercise to assess exercise

BOX 1-7	PHYSIOLOGIC EFFECTS OF PROLONGED BED REST

Cardiovascular (Deconditioning Effect)
▪ Increased heart rate and blood pressure for submaximal workload
▪ Decrease in functional capacity
▪ Decrease in circulating volume
▪ Increase in thromboemboli
▪ Orthostatic hypotension
▪ Reflex tachycardia

Pulmonary
▪ Modest decrease in pulmonary function
▪ Secretion stasis

Gastrointestinal
▪ Constipation
▪ Negative protein state
▪ Esophageal reflux and aspiration
▪ Negative N state

Musculoskeletal
▪ Loss of muscle mass
▪ Loss of muscle contractile strength
▪ Decreased periarticular tissue elasticity
▪ Joint contracture

tolerance. If HR or SBP increases more than 20 bpm or more than 20 mm Hg over resting level, decrease number of repetitions. If HR or SBP decreases more than 10 bpm or more than 10 mm Hg at peak exercise, this could be a sign of left ventricular failure, denoting that the heart cannot meet this workload. For other adverse signs and symptoms, see Assessment of exercise tolerance, following.

- Duration: Begin with 5 min or less of exercise. Gradually increase the exercise to 15 min as tolerated.
- Frequency: Begin with exercises 2-4 ×/day. As duration increases, the frequency can be reduced.
- Assessment of exercise tolerance: Be alert to signs and symptoms that the cardiovascular and respiratory systems are unable to meet the demands of the low-level ROM exercises. Excessive shortness of breath may occur if (1) transient pulmonary congestion occurs secondary to ischemia or left ventricular dysfunction, (2) lung volumes are decreased, (3) O_2-carrying capacity of the blood is reduced, or (4) there is shunting of blood from the right to the left side of the heart without adequate oxygenation. If cardiac output does not increase to meet the body's needs during modest levels of exercise, SBP may fall; the skin may become cool, cyanotic, and diaphoretic; dysrhythmias may be noted; crackles (rales) may be auscultated; or a systolic murmur of mitral regurgitation may occur. If patient tolerates the exercise, increase intensity or number of repetitions each day.
- Stop any exercise that results in muscular or skeletal pain. Consult a physical therapist PT = prothrombin time later about necessary modifications. Avoid isometric exercises in cardiac patients.

◆ Ask patient for RPE experienced during exercise, based on the following scale developed by Borg (1982):

  0 = nothing at all
  1 = very weak effort
  2 = weak (light) effort
  3 = moderate effort
  4 = somewhat stronger effort
  5 = strong effort
  7 = very strong effort
  9 = very, very strong effort
  10 = maximal effort

◆ Patient should not experience RPE greater than 3 while performing ROM exercises. Reduce intensity of the exercise and increase frequency until RPE 3 or less is attained.

◆ As patient's condition improves, increase activity as soon as possible to include sitting in a chair. Prepare patient for this change by increasing amount of time spent in high Fowler's position and moving patient slowly and in stages because orthostatic hypotension can occur as a result of decreased plasma volume and difficulty in adjusting immediately to postural change. The following describes activity progression in hospitalized patients:

Level I: Bed rest
Flexion and extension of extremities 4 ×/day, 15 × each extremity
Deep breathing 4 ×/day, 15 breaths
Position change from side to side q2h

Level II: Out of bed to chair
As tolerated, 3 ×/day for 20-30 min
May perform ROM exercises 2 ×/day while sitting in chair

Level III: Ambulate in room
As tolerated, 3 ×/day for 3-5 min in room

Level IV: Ambulate in hall
Initially, 50-200 ft 2 ×/day, progressing to 600 ft 4 ×/day
May incorporate slow stair climbing in preparation for hospital discharge

Signs of activity intolerance
Decrease in BP more than 20 mm Hg
Increase in HR to more than 120 bpm (or more than 20 bpm above resting HR in patients receiving β-blocker therapy)

◆ Increase activity level by having patient perform self-care activities such as eating, mouth care, and bathing as tolerated.
◆ Teach significant other the purpose and interventions for preventing deconditioning. Involve him or her in patient's plan of care.
◆ Provide emotional support to patient and significant other as patient's activity level is increased *to help allay fears of failure, pain, or medical setbacks.*

Risk for disuse syndrome related to paralysis, mechanical immobilization, prescribed immobilization, severe pain, or altered level of consciousness (LOC)
Desired outcome: When bed rest is discontinued, patient exhibits complete ROM of all joints without pain, and limb girth measurements are congruent with or increased over baseline measurements.

Nursing Interventions

◆ Perform ROM exercises at least 2 ×/day for all immobilized patients with normal joints. Modification may be required for patients with flaccidity (e.g., immediately after stroke or spinal cord injury [SCI]) to prevent subluxation, or for patient with spasticity (e.g., during the recovery period for patient with stroke or SCI) to prevent an increase in spasticity. Consult physical or occupational therapist (OT) for assistance in modifying the exercise plan for these patients. Also, be aware that ROM exercises are restricted or contraindicated for patients with rheumatologic disease during the inflammatory phase and for joints that are dislocated or fractured.
◆ Be alert to the following areas that are especially susceptible to joint contracture: shoulder, which can become "frozen" limiting abduction and extension; wrist, which can "drop," prohibiting extension; fingers, which can develop flexion contractures that limit extension; hips, which can develop flexion contractures that affect the gait by shortening the limb or develop external rotation or adduction deformities that affect the gait; knees, in which flexion contractures can develop that limit extension and alter the gait; and feet, which can "drop" as a result of plantar flexion, which limits dorsiflexion and alters the gait.
◆ Ensure patient's position is changed at least q2h *to maintain correct body alignment and thereby reduce strain on the joints, prevent contractures, minimize pressure on bony prominences, decrease venostasis, and promote maximal chest expansion.* Post a turning schedule at patient's bedside *to promote compliance with the q2h schedule.*
  • Try to place patient in a position that achieves proper standing alignment: head neutral or slightly flexed on the neck, hips extended, knees extended or minimally flexed, and feet at right angles to the legs. Maintain this position with pillows, towels, or other positioning aids.
  • Ensure that patient is prone or side lying, with hips extended, for the same amount of time patient spends in the supine position or, at a minimum, 3 ×/day for 1 hr to prevent hip flexion contractures.
  • When head of bed (HOB) must be elevated 30 degrees, extend patient's shoulders and arms, using pillows to support the position, and allow fingertips to extend over pillow's edge *to maintain normal arching of the hands.* Ensure that patient spends time with hips in

extension because elevating HOB promotes hip flexion (see preceding intervention).

- When patient is in the side-lying position, extend lower leg from the hip *to help prevent hip flexion contracture.*
- When able to place patient in the prone position, move patient to end of bed and allow feet to rest between mattress and footboard. *This will prevent not only plantar flexion and hip rotation, but also injury to heels and toes.* Place thin pads under the angles of the axillae and lateral aspects of the clavicles *to prevent internal rotation of the shoulders and maintain anatomic position of the shoulder girdle.*

- ◆ To maintain joints in neutral position, use the following as indicated: pillows, rolled towels, blankets, sandbags, antirotation boots, splints, and orthotics. When using adjunctive devices, monitor involved skin at frequent intervals for alterations in integrity, and implement measures to prevent skin breakdown.
- ◆ Assess for footdrop by inspecting feet for plantar flexion and evaluating patient's ability to pull toes upward toward the head. Because feet lie naturally in plantar flexion, be particularly alert to patient's inability to pull toes up. Document this assessment daily.
- ◆ Teach patient and significant other the rationale and procedure for ROM exercises, and have patient return demonstrations. Ensure that patient does not exceed his or her activity tolerance. Provide passive exercises for patients unable to perform active or active-assisted exercises. In addition, incorporate movement patterns into care activities, such as position changes, bed baths, getting patient on and off the bedpan, or changing patient's gown. Ensure that joints especially prone to contracture are exercised more stringently. Provide patient with a handout that reviews exercises and lists repetitions for each. Instruct significant other to encourage patient to perform exercises as required.
- ◆ Perform and document limb girth measurements, dynamography, and ROM, and establish exercise baseline *limits to assess patient's existing muscle mass, strength, and joint motion.*
- ◆ Explain to patient that muscle atrophy occurs because of the disuse or failure to use the joint, which often is caused by immediate or anticipated pain. Eventually disuse may result in decreased muscle mass and blood supply and a loss of periarticular tissue elasticity, which in turn can lead to increased muscle fatigue and joint pain with use.
- ◆ Emphasize importance of maintaining or increasing muscle strength and periarticular tissue elasticity through exercise. If unsure about patient's complicating pathologic condition, consult health care provider about the appropriate form of exercise for patient.
- ◆ Explain need to participate maximally in self-care as tolerated *to help maintain muscle strength and promote a sense of participation and control.*
- ◆ For noncardiac patients needing greater help with muscle strength, assist with resistive exercises (e.g., moderate weight lifting to increase size, endurance, and strength of the muscles). For patients in beds with Balkan frames, provide means for resistive exercise by implementing a system of weights and pulleys. First, determine patient's baseline level of performance on a given set of exercises, then set realistic goals with patient for repetitions (e.g., if patient can do 5 repetitions of lifting a 5-lb weight with the biceps muscle, the goal may be to increase repetitions to 10 within 1 wk, to an ultimate goal of 20 within 3 wk, and then advance to 7.5-lb weights).
- ◆ If the joints require rest, isometric exercises can be used. With these exercises, teach patient to contract a muscle group and hold the contraction for a count of 5 or 10. The sequence is repeated for increasing counts or

repetitions until an adequate level of endurance has been achieved. Thereafter, maintenance levels are performed.

- Provide a chart to show patient's progress, and combine this with large amounts of positive reinforcement. Post exercise regimen at the bedside to ensure consistency by all health care personnel. Instruct significant other in the exercise regimen, and elicit his or her support and encouragement of patient's performance of the exercises.
- As appropriate, teach transfer or crutch-walking techniques and use of a walker, wheelchair, or cane so that patient can maintain the highest possible level of mobility. Include significant other in demonstrations, and stress importance of good body mechanics.
- Provide periods of uninterrupted rest between exercises/activities *to enable patient to replenish energy stores.*
- Seek referral for physical or occupational therapy as appropriate.

Ineffective peripheral tissue perfusion related to interrupted venous flow secondary to prolonged immobility
Desired outcomes: At least 24 hr before hospital discharge, patient has adequate peripheral perfusion as evidenced by normal skin color and temperature and adequate distal pulses (amplitude greater than 2+ on a 0-4+ scale) in peripheral extremities. Patient performs exercises independently, adheres to the prophylactic regimen, and maintains intake of 2-3 L/day of fluid unless contraindicated.

Nursing Interventions

- Teach patient that pain, redness, swelling, and warmth in the involved area and coolness, edema, unnatural color or pallor, and superficial venous dilation distal to the involved area are all indicators of deep vein thrombosis (DVT) and should be reported to staff member immediately if they occur *because prompt intervention is needed.*
- Monitor for previously mentioned indicators of DVT at time of routine VS checks. If patient is asymptomatic for DVT, assess for positive Homans' sign: flex knee 30 degrees and dorsiflex the foot. Pain elicited with dorsiflexion may be a sign of DVT, and so obtain further evaluation. Additional signs of DVT may include fever, tachycardia, and elevated erythrocyte sedimentation rate (ESR). Normal ESR (Westergren method) in male patients younger than 50 yr is 0-15 mm/hr and older than 50 yr is 0-20 mm/hr; normal ESR in female patients younger than 50 yr is 0-20 mm/hr and older than 50 yr is 0-30 mm/hr.
- Teach patient calf-pumping (ankle dorsiflexion–plantar flexion) and ankle-circling exercises *to promote circulation.* Instruct patient to repeat each movement 10×, performing each exercise hourly during extended periods of immobility, provided that patient is free of symptoms of DVT. Perform passive ROM or encourage active ROM exercises *to promote circulation.*
- Encourage deep breathing, which increases negative pressure in the lungs and thorax, *to promote emptying of large veins.*
- When not contraindicated by peripheral vascular disease (PVD), ensure that patient wears antiembolism hose, pneumatic foot pump devices, or pneumatic sequential compression stockings. Remove them for 10-20 min q8h, and inspect underlying skin for evidence of irritation or breakdown. Reapply hose after elevating patient's legs at least 10 degrees for 10 min *to promote venous emptying.*
- Instruct patient not to cross feet at the ankles or knees while in bed to avoid contributing to venous stasis. If patient is at risk for DVT, elevate foot of the bed 10 degrees *to increase venous return.*
- In nonrestricted patient, increase fluid intake to at least 2-3 L/day *to reduce hemoconcentration, which can contribute to development of DVT.* Educate

patient about need to drink large amounts of fluid (9-14 8-oz glasses) daily. Monitor I&O *to ensure adherence.*

◆ Patients at risk for DVT, including those with chronic infection and history of PVD and smoking, as well as older, obese, and anemic patients, may require pharmacologic interventions such as aspirin, sodium warfarin, phenindione derivatives, heparin, or low-molecular-weight heparin (LMWH). Administer medication as prescribed, and monitor appropriate laboratory values (e.g., prothrombin time [PT], partial thromboplastin time [PTT]). Educate patient to self-monitor for and report bleeding (epistaxis, bleeding gums, hematemesis, hemoptysis, melena, hematuria, hematochezia, menometrorrhagia, ecchymoses). Many patients are taught how to self-administer LMWH injections after hospital discharge.

◆ Teach medication and food interactions that can affect warfarin.

◆ In patients prone to DVT, acquire bilateral baseline measurements of midcalf, knee, and midthigh circumferences, and enter them on patient's medical record. Monitor these measurements daily and compare them with baseline measurements *to rule out extremity enlargement caused by DVT.*

Ineffective cerebral tissue perfusion (orthostatic hypotension) related to interrupted arterial flow to the brain secondary to prolonged bed rest
Desired outcomes: When getting out of bed, patient has adequate cerebral perfusion as evidenced by HR less than 120 bpm and BP 90/60 mm Hg or greater (or within 20 mm Hg of patient's normal range) immediately after position change, dry skin, normal skin color, and absence of vertigo and syncope, with return of HR and BP to resting levels within 3 min of position change.

Nursing Interventions

◆ Assess patient for factors that increase risk of orthostatic hypotension as a result of fluid volume changes (recent diuresis, diaphoresis, or change in vasodilator therapy), altered autonomic control (diabetic cardiac neuropathy, denervation after heart transplant, or advanced age), or severe left ventricular dysfunction.

◆ Explain cause of orthostatic hypotension and measures for preventing it.

◆ Application of antiembolism hose, which are used to prevent DVT, may be useful in preventing orthostatic hypotension once patient is mobilized. For patients who continue to have difficulty with orthostatic hypotension, it may be necessary to supplement hose with elastic wraps to the groin to prevent venous pooling when patient is out of bed. Ensure that these wraps encompass entire leg surface.

◆ When patient is in bed, provide instructions for leg exercises as described under **Risk for activity intolerance**, p. 23. Encourage patient to perform leg exercises immediately before mobilization *to facilitate venous return.*

◆ Prepare patient for getting out of bed by encouraging position changes within necessary confines. It is sometimes possible and advisable to use a tilt table *to reacclimate patient to upright positions.*

◆ Follow these guidelines for mobilization:
   • Check BP in any high-risk patient for whom this will be the first time out of bed. Instruct patient to report immediately symptoms of lightheadedness or dizziness.
   • Have patient dangle legs at bedside. Be alert to indicators of orthostatic hypotension, including diaphoresis, pallor, tachycardia, hypotension, and syncope. Question patient about presence of lightheadedness or dizziness. Again, encourage performance of leg exercises.
   • If indicators of orthostatic hypotension occur, check VS. A drop in SBP of 20 mm Hg or greater and an increased pulse rate, combined with

symptoms of vertigo and impending syncope, signal need for return to supine position.

- If leg dangling is tolerated, have patient stand at the bedside with two staff members in attendance. If no adverse signs or symptoms occur, have patient progress to ambulation as tolerated.

Constipation related to less than adequate fluid or dietary intake and bulk, immobility, lack of privacy, positional restrictions, and use of opioid analgesics
Desired outcomes: Within 24 hr of this diagnosis, patient verbalizes knowledge of measures that promote bowel elimination. Patient reports return of normal pattern and character of bowel elimination within 3-5 days of this diagnosis.

Nursing Interventions

- ◆ Assess patient's bowel history to determine normal bowel habits and interventions that are used successfully at home.
- ◆ Monitor and document patient's bowel movements, diet, and I&O. Be alert to the following indications of constipation: fewer than usual number of bowel movements, abdominal discomfort or distention, straining at stool, and complaints of rectal pressure or fullness. Fecal impaction may be manifested by oozing of liquid stool and confirmed via digital examination.
- ◆ Auscultate each abdominal quadrant for at least 1 min *to determine presence of bowel sounds.* Normal sounds are gurgles occurring at a rate of 5-34/min. Bowel sounds are decreased or absent with paralytic ileus. High-pitched rushing sounds or "tinkles" may be heard during abdominal cramping, and they indicate intestinal obstruction.
- ◆ If rectal impaction is suspected, use a gloved, lubricated finger to remove stool from the rectum. This stimulation may be adequate to cause bowel movement. Oil retention enemas may soften impacted stool.
- ◆ Teach patient importance of a high-fiber diet and fluid intake of at least 2-3 L/day (unless this is contraindicated by a renal, hepatic, or cardiac disorder). High-fiber foods include bran, whole grains, nuts, and raw and coarse vegetables and fruits with skins.
- ◆ Maintain patient's normal bowel habits whenever possible by offering bedpan; ensuring privacy; and timing medications, enemas, or suppositories so that they take effect at the time of day patient normally has a bowel movement. Provide warm fluids before breakfast, and encourage toileting to take advantage of gastrocolic or duodenocolic reflexes.
- ◆ Maximize patient's activity level within limitations of endurance, therapy, and pain *to promote peristalsis.*
- ◆ Request pharmacologic interventions from health care provider when necessary. Make a priority list of interventions to *ensure minimal disruption of patient's normal bowel habits and to help prevent rebound constipation.* The following is a suggested hierarchy of interventions:
  - Bulk-building additives (psyllium), bran
  - Mild laxatives (apple or prune juice, Milk of Magnesia)
  - Stool softeners
  - Potent laxatives and cathartics
  - Medicated suppositories
  - Enemas
- ◆ Discuss the role that opioid agents and other medications play in causing constipation. Teach nonpharmacologic methods of pain control (Box 1-6).

Deficient diversional activity related to prolonged illness and hospitalization
Desired outcome: Within 24 hr of intervention, patient engages in diversional activities and relates absence of boredom.

Nursing Interventions

◆ Be alert to patient indicators of boredom, including wishing for something to read or do, daytime napping, and expressed inability to perform usual hobbies because of hospitalization.

◆ Assess patient's activity tolerance as described on p. 24.

◆ Collect a database by assessing patient's normal support systems and relationship patterns with significant other. Question patient and significant other about patient's interests, and explore diversional activities that may be suitable for the hospital setting and patient's level of activity tolerance.

◆ Personalize patient's environment with favorite objects and photographs of significant others.

◆ Provide low-level activities commensurate with patient's tolerance (e.g., books or magazines pertaining to patient's recreational or other interests, computer games, television, writing for short intervals).

◆ Initiate activities that require little concentration, and proceed to more complicated tasks as patient's condition allows (e.g., if reading requires more energy or concentration than patient is capable of, suggest that significant other read to patient or bring audiotapes of books).

◆ Encourage discussion of past activities or reminiscence as a substitute for performing favorite activities during convalescence.

◆ As patient's endurance improves, obtain appropriate diversional activities such as puzzles, model kits, handicrafts, and computerized games and activities; encourage patient to use them.

◆ Encourage significant other to visit within limits of patient's endurance and to involve patient in activities that are of interest to him or her, such as playing cards or backgammon. Encourage significant other to stagger visits throughout the day.

◆ Spend extra time with patient.

◆ Suggest that significant other bring in a radio or, if appropriate, rent a television or radio from the hospital if not part of the standard room charge.

◆ If appropriate for patient, arrange for hospital volunteers to visit, play cards, read books, or play board games.

◆ As appropriate for patient who desires social interaction, consider relocation to a room in an area of high traffic.

◆ As patient's condition improves, assist him or her with sitting in a chair near a window so that outside activities can be viewed. When patient is able, provide opportunities to sit in a solarium so that he or she can visit with other patients. If physical condition and weather permit, take patient outside for brief periods.

◆ Request consultation from social services, OT, pastoral services, and psychiatric nurse for interventions as appropriate.

◆ Increase patient's involvement in self-care *to provide a sense of purpose, accomplishment, and control.* Performing in-bed exercises (e.g., deep breathing, ankle circling, calf pumping), keeping track of I&O, and similar activities can and should be accomplished routinely by these patients.

Ineffective sexuality patterns related to actual or perceived physiologic limitations on sexual performance secondary to disease, therapy, or prolonged hospitalization

Desired outcome: Within 72 hr of this diagnosis, patient reports satisfaction with sexuality and/or understanding of ability to resume sexual activity.

Nursing Interventions

◆ Assess patient's normal sexual function, including importance placed on sex in the relationship, frequency of interaction, normal positions used, and the couple's ability to adapt or change to meet requirements of patient's limitations.

- Identify patient's problem diplomatically, and clarify it with patient. Indicators of sexual dysfunction can include regression, acting out with inappropriate behavior such as grabbing or pinching, sexual overtures toward hospital staff, self-enforced isolation, and similar behaviors.
- Encourage patient and significant other to verbalize feelings and anxieties about sexual abstinence, having sexual relations in the hospital, hurting patient, or having to use new or alternative methods for sexual gratification. Develop strategies in collaboration with patient and significant other.
- Encourage acceptable expressions of sexuality by patient (e.g., in a woman this could involve wearing makeup and jewelry).
- Inform patient and significant other that it is possible to have time alone together for intimacy. Provide that time accordingly by putting a "do not disturb" sign on the door, enforcing privacy by restricting staff and visitors to the room, or arranging for temporary private quarters.
- Encourage patient and significant other to seek alternate methods of sexual expression when necessary. This may include mutual masturbation, altered positions, use of a vibrator, and identification of other erotic areas for the partner.
- Refer patient and significant other to professional sexual counseling as necessary.

Ineffective role performance related to dependence vs. independence
Desired outcome: Within 48 hr of this diagnosis, patient collaborates with caregivers in planning realistic goals for independence, participates in own care, and takes responsibility for self-care.

Nursing Interventions

- Encourage patient to be as independent as possible within limitations of endurance, therapy, and pain. Be aware, however, that temporary periods of dependence are appropriate because they enable the individual *to restore energy reserves needed for recovery.*
- Ensure that all health care providers are consistent in conveying expectations of eventual independence.
- Alert patient to areas of excessive dependence, and involve him or her in collaborative goal setting to achieve independence.
- Do not minimize patient's expressed feelings of depression. Allow patient to express emotions, but provide support, understanding, and realistic hope for a positive role change.
- If indicated, provide self-help devices *to increase patient's independence with self-care.*

SECTION FOUR   **PSYCHOSOCIAL SUPPORT**

NURSING DIAGNOSES AND INTERVENTIONS

Deficient knowledge related to current health status and prescribed therapies
Desired outcome: Before procedures, or hospital discharge (as appropriate), patient verbalizes understanding regarding current health status and therapies.

Nursing Interventions

- Assess patient's facility with language, and engage an interpreter or provide language-appropriate written materials if necessary.
- Assess patient's current level of knowledge regarding health status.
- Assess cognitive and emotional readiness to learn.
- Recognize barriers to learning, such as ineffective communication, educational deficit, language barrier, neurologic deficit, sensory alterations, fear, anxiety, and lack of motivation.

◆ Assess learning needs and establish short-term and long-term goals.
◆ Use individualized verbal or written information *to promote learning and enhance understanding.* Give simple, direct instructions. As indicated, use audiovisual tools as supplemental information.
◆ Include caregiver in all patient teaching, and encourage reinforcement of correct information regarding diagnosis and treatments.
◆ Plan care collaboratively with patient *to encourage his or her involvement in care.* Explain rationale for care and therapies.
◆ Communicate often with patient to evaluate comprehension of information given. Request feedback regarding what has been taught. Individuals in crisis often need repeated explanations before information can be understood. Many individuals may not understand seemingly simple medical terms. Provide written information appropriate to patient's comprehension level *to reinforce teaching.*
◆ As appropriate, assess understanding of informed consent. Assist patient to use information received to make informed decisions regarding care.

Anxiety related to actual or perceived threat of death, change in health status, threat to self-concept or role, unfamiliar people and environment, medications, preexisting anxiety disorder, or the unknown
Desired outcome: Within 1-2 hr of intervention, patient's anxiety has resolved or decreased as evidenced by patient's verbalization of same, heart rate (HR) 100 beats per minute (bpm) or less, respiratory rate (RR) 20 breaths/min or less, and absence of or decrease in irritability and restlessness.

Nursing Interventions

◆ Engage in honest communication with patient, and provide empathetic understanding. Listen closely, and establish an atmosphere that allows free expression.
◆ Assess patient's level of anxiety. Be alert to verbal and nonverbal cues.
  • *Mild:* Restlessness, irritability, increased questions, focusing on the environment.
  • *Moderate:* Inattentiveness, expressions of concern, narrowed perceptions, insomnia, increased HR.
  • *Severe:* Expressions of feelings of doom, rapid speech, tremors, poor eye contact. Patient may be preoccupied with the past; may be unable to understand the present; and may have tachycardia, nausea, and hyperventilation.
  • *Panic:* Inability to concentrate or communicate, distortion of reality, increased motor activity, vomiting, tachypnea.
◆ For patients with severe anxiety or panic state, refer to psychiatric clinical nurse specialist, case manager, or other health care team members as appropriate.
◆ Approach patient with a calm, reassuring demeanor. Show concern and focused attention while listening to patient's concerns. Provide a safe environment and stay with patient during periods of intense anxiety.
◆ Restrict intake of caffeine, nicotine, and alcohol and avoid abrupt discontinuation of anxiolytics.
◆ If patient is hyperventilating, have him or her concentrate on a focal point and mimic your deliberately slow and deep breathing pattern.
◆ Validate assessment of anxiety with patient (e.g., "You seem distressed; are you feeling uncomfortable now?").
◆ After an episode of anxiety, review and discuss with patient the thoughts and feelings that led to the episode.
◆ Identify patient's current coping behaviors (e.g., denial; anger; repression; withdrawal; daydreaming; or dependence on tobacco products, alcohol, prescription medications, or illegal drugs). Review coping behaviors patient has used in the past. Assist patient with using adaptive coping to

manage anxiety (e.g., "I understand that your wife reads to you to help you relax—Would you like to spend a part of each day alone with her?").

◆ Encourage patient to express fears, concerns, and questions (e.g., "I know this room looks like a maze of wires and tubes; please let me know when you have any questions").

◆ Reduce sensory overload by providing an organized, quiet environment (see **Disturbed sensory perception**, p. 33).

◆ Introduce self and other health care team members; explain each individual's role as it relates to patient's care.

◆ Teach patient relaxation and imagery techniques. See **Health-seeking behaviors:** Relaxation technique effective for stress reduction, p. 106.

◆ Enable support persons to be in attendance whenever possible.

Impaired verbal communication related to neurologic or anatomic deficit, psychologic or physical barriers (e.g., tracheostomy, intubation), or cultural or developmental differences

Desired outcome: At the time of intervention, patient communicates needs and feelings and reports decreased or absent feelings of frustration over communication barriers.

Nursing Interventions

◆ Assess cause of impaired communication (e.g., tracheostomy, stroke, cerebral tumor, Guillain-Barré syndrome).

◆ Assess patient's ability to read, write, and understand English. If patient speaks a language other than English, collaborate with an interpreter or English-speaking family member to establish effective communication.

◆ When communicating with patient, face patient; make direct eye contact; and speak in a clear, normal tone of voice.

◆ When communicating with a deaf person about the treatment plan, arrange to have an interpreter present if possible.

◆ If patient cannot speak because of a physical barrier (e.g., tracheostomy, wired mandibles), provide reassurance and acknowledge his or her frustration (e.g., "I know this is frustrating for you, but please do not give up. I want to understand you.").

◆ Provide slate, word cards, pencil and paper, alphabet board, pictures, or other device to assist patient with communication. Adapt call system to meet patient's needs. Document meaning of signals used by patient to communicate.

◆ Explain source of patient's communication impairment to caregiver; teach caregiver effective communication alternatives.

◆ Be alert to nonverbal messages such as facial expressions, hand movements, and nodding of the head. Validate their meaning with patient.

◆ Recognize that the inability to speak may foster maladaptive behaviors. Encourage patient to communicate needs; reinforce independent behaviors.

◆ Be honest with patient; do not pretend to understand if you are unable to interpret patient's communication.

◆ If surgery is expected to create a physical condition that will interfere with communication, begin teaching preoperatively. Facilitate postoperative referrals for speech and swallowing.

◆ If appropriate, recommend patient support group that will provide patient with peer support.

Disturbed sensory perception related to therapeutically or socially restricted environment; psychologic stress; altered sensory reception, transmission, or integration; or chemical alteration

Desired outcome: At the time of intervention, patient verbalizes orientation to person, place, and time; reports the ability to concentrate; and expresses satisfaction with degree and type of sensory stimulation being received.

Nursing Interventions

◆ Assess factors contributing to patient's sensory-perceptual alteration.
- Environmental: Excessive noise in the environment; constant, monotonous noise; restricted environment (immobility, traction, isolation); social isolation (restricted visitors, impaired communication); therapies.
- Physiologic: Altered organ function, sleep or rest pattern disturbance, medication, history of altered sensory perception.

◆ Manage factors that contribute to environmental overload (e.g., avoid constant lighting [maintain day/night patterns]; reduce noise whenever possible [decrease alarm volumes, avoid loud talking, keep room door closed, provide earplugs]).

◆ Maintain a regular schedule if possible.

◆ Determine sensory stimulation appropriate for patient and plan care accordingly. If appropriate, provide meaningful sensory stimulation.
- Display clocks, large calendars, and meaningful photographs and objects from home.
- Depending on patient preference, provide a radio, music, reading materials, and tape recordings of family and significant other. Earphones help to block out external stimuli.
- Position patient to look toward window when possible. Stimulate patient's vision with mirrors, colored decorations, and pictures.
- Discuss current events, time of day, holidays, and topics of interest during patient care activities (e.g., "Good morning, Mr. Smith. I'm Ms. Stone, your nurse for the afternoon and evening, 3 to 11 PM. It's sunny outside. Today is the first day of summer.").
- Stimulate patient's sense of taste with sweet, salty, and sour substances as allowed.
- As needed, orient patient to surroundings and reason for hospitalization. When providing information, use simple terminology and maintain eye contact. Always advise patient before initiating any procedures or personal contact.
- Establish personal contact by touch *to help promote and maintain patient's contact with the real environment.*
- Encourage significant other to communicate with patient often and in a normal tone of voice.
- Convey concern and respect for patient. Introduce yourself and call patient by name.
- Encourage use of eyeglasses and hearing aids.

◆ Encourage patient to participate in health care planning and decision making whenever possible. Allow for choice when possible.

◆ Ensure patient's safety by maintaining proper lighting, positioning call bell within reach, and maintaining bed in the lowest position with side rails up.

◆ Assess patient's sleep/rest pattern *to evaluate its contribution to the sensory/perceptual disorder.* Make sure that patient attains at least 90 min of uninterrupted sleep as often as possible. For more information, see next nursing diagnosis.

Disturbed sleep pattern related to environmental changes, illness, therapeutic regimen, pain, immobility, psychologic stress, altered mental status, or hypoxia

Desired outcomes: After discussion, patient identifies factors that promote sleep. Within 8 hr of intervention, patient attains 90-min periods of uninterrupted sleep and verbalizes satisfaction with ability to rest.

Nursing Interventions

◆ Assess patient's usual sleeping patterns (e.g., bedtime routine, hours of sleep per night, sleeping position, use of pillows and blankets, napping during the day, nocturia).

◆ Explore relaxation techniques that promote patient's rest/sleep (e.g., imagining relaxing scenes, listening to soothing music or taped stories, using muscle relaxation exercises).

◆ Administer sleep medications at a time appropriate to induce sleep, taking into consideration time to onset and half-life.

◆ Administer pain medications before sleep if pain is interfering with sleep.

◆ Identify causative factors and activities that contribute to patient's insomnia, awaken patient, or adversely affect sleep patterns (e.g., pain, anxiety, hypoxia, therapies, depression, hallucinations, medications, underlying illness, sleep apnea, respiratory disorder, caffeine, fear).

◆ Promote physical comfort via such measures as massage, back rubs, bathing, and fresh linens before sleep.

◆ Organize procedures and activities to allow for 90-min periods of uninterrupted rest/sleep. Limit visiting during these periods.

◆ Whenever possible, maintain a quiet environment by providing earplugs or reducing alarm volume. White noise (i.e., low-pitched, monotonous sounds: electric fan, soft music) may facilitate sleep. Dim the lights for a period each day by drawing the drapes or providing blindfolds.

◆ If appropriate, put limitations on patient's daytime sleeping. Attempt to establish regularly scheduled daytime activity (e.g., ambulation, sitting in chair, active ROM), *which may promote nighttime sleep.*

◆ Investigate and provide nonpharmacologic comfort measures that are known to promote patient's sleep (Table 1-1).

◆ See **Disturbed sleep pattern** in "Perioperative Care," p. 10.

Fear related to separation from support systems, unfamiliarity with environment or therapeutic regimen, loss of sense of control, or uncertainty about the future
Desired outcome: Following intervention, patient expresses fears and concerns and reports feeling greater psychologic and physical comfort.

Nursing Interventions

◆ Assess patient's perceptions of the environment and health status *to determine factors contributing to patient's feelings of fear.* Evaluate patient's verbal and nonverbal responses.

◆ Validate patient's fears and concerns and provide opportunities for patient to express them (e.g., "You seem very concerned about receiving more blood today"). Listen closely to patient. Recognize that anger, denial, occasional withdrawal, and demanding behaviors may be coping responses.

◆ Encourage patient to ask questions and gather information about the unknown. Provide information about equipment, therapies, and routines according to patient's ability to understand.

◆ Encourage patient to participate in and plan care whenever possible to promote an increased sense of control, Provide continuity of care by establishing a routine and arranging for consistent caregivers whenever possible. Appoint a case manager or primary nurse.

◆ Discuss with health care team members the appropriateness of medication therapy for patients with disabling fear or anxiety.

◆ Explore patient's desire for spiritual or psychologic counseling.

◆ Consult health care provider regarding a visit by another individual with the same disorder or situation who has experienced the same treatment.

Ineffective coping related to health crisis, sense of vulnerability, or inadequate support systems
Desired outcome: Before hospital discharge, patient verbalizes feelings, identifies strengths and coping behaviors, and does not demonstrate ineffective coping behaviors.

Nursing Interventions

- Assess patient's perceptions and ability to understand current health status. Discuss the meaning of disease and current treatment with patient, and actively listen with a nonjudgmental attitude.
- Establish honest communication with patient (e.g., "Please tell me what I can do to help you"). Help patient identify strengths, stressors, inappropriate behaviors, and personal needs.
- Support positive coping behaviors (e.g., "I see that reading that book seems to help you relax") and explore effective coping behaviors used in the past. Identify factors that inhibit patient's ability to cope (e.g., unsatisfactory support system, knowledge deficit, grief, fear).
- Help patient identify or develop a support system.
- Provide opportunities for patient to express concerns, and gather information from nurses and other support persons or systems. Provide patient with explanations about prescribed routine, therapies, and equipment. Acknowledge patient's feelings and assessment of current health status and environment.
- Recognize maladaptive coping behaviors (e.g., severe depression; dependence on narcotics, sedatives, or tranquilizers; hostility; violence; suicidal ideation). If appropriate, discuss these behaviors with patient (e.g., "You seem to be requiring more pain medication—are you having more physical pain, or does it help you cope with your situation?"). Refer patient to psychiatric liaison, clinical nurse specialist, case manager, or clergy as appropriate.
- As patient's condition allows, assist with reducing anxiety. See **Anxiety**, p. 32.
- Help reduce patient's sensory overload by maintaining an organized, quiet environment. See **Disturbed sensory perception**, p. 33.
- Encourage frequent visits by family and caregiver if visits appear to be supportive to patient. Encourage conversations with patient *to help minimize patient's emotional and social isolation.*
- As appropriate, explain to caregiver that increased dependency, anger, and denial may be adaptive coping behaviors used by patient in early stages of crisis until effective coping behaviors are learned.
- Arrange community referrals, as appropriate.

Ineffective coping related to depression

Desired outcome: Before hospital discharge, patient discusses personal risk factors for and signs and symptoms of depression and begins to participate in prescribed treatment plan.

Nursing Interventions

- Assist patient and family with evaluating goals and beliefs regarding patient's illness and expected outcomes.
- Assume all references to suicide to be serious and report them to health care provider immediately for appropriate referrals.
- Teach patient and caregiver side effect management of psychotropic medications. In addition, caution patient regarding abrupt discontinuation of medications.
- Assist patient with problem solving and decision making inasmuch as depression may interfere with the motivation and personal energy to do so.
- Assist patient with personal care such as bathing and feeding if depression limits activities and ability to care for self.
- See **Ineffective coping,** which immediately precedes this nursing diagnosis.

Anticipatory grieving related to actual or potential loss of physiologic well-being (e.g., expected loss of body function or body part, changes in self-concept or body image, illness, death)

BOX 1-8	STAGES OF GRIEVING

Protest
- Denial: "No, not me"
- Disbelief: "But I just saw her this morning"
- Anger
- Hostility
- Resentment
- Bargaining to postpone loss
- Appeal for help to recover loss
- Loud complaints
- Altered sleep and appetite

Disorganization
- Depression
- Withdrawal
- Social isolation
- Psychomotor retardation
- Silence

Reorganization
- Acceptance of loss
- Development of new interests and attachments
- Restructuring of lifestyle
- Return to pre-loss level of functioning

Desired outcome: Following intervention, patient and caregiver express grief, participate in decisions about the future, and discuss concerns with health care team members and each another.

Nursing Interventions

- Assess factors contributing to actual or anticipated loss.
- Assess and accept patient's behavioral response. Expect reactions such as disbelief, denial, guilt, anger, and depression. Determine patient's stage of grieving as described in **BOX 1-8**.
- Assess spiritual, religious, and sociocultural expectations related to loss (e.g., "From what source do you find meaning for events in your life?" "How do you and your family usually cope with serious health problems?"). Refer to clergy or community support groups as appropriate.
- Encourage patient and significant other to share their concerns (e.g., "Is there anything you'd like to talk about today?"). Also respect their desire not to speak.
- Demonstrate empathy (e.g., "This must be a very difficult time for you and your family").
- In selected circumstances, explain the grieving process. *This approach may help patient and family to better understand and acknowledge their feelings.*
- When appropriate, provide referral for bereavement care.
- Assess grief reactions of patient and significant other, and identify those individuals with potential for dysfunctional grieving reactions (e.g., absence of emotion, hostility, avoidance). If potential for dysfunctional grieving is present, refer the individual to psychiatric clinical nurse specialist, case manager, clergy, or other source of counseling as appropriate.

Dysfunctional grieving related to failure to adjust to loss of physiologic well-being or chronic illness resulting in somatic symptoms, loss of normal behavior patterns, prolonged denial, and maladaptive behavior
Desired outcomes: Before hospital discharge, patient and significant others begin to express grief, discuss meaning of the loss, and communicate concerns with one another. Patient completes necessary self-care activities.

Nursing Interventions

◆ Assess grief stage (Box 1-8) and previous coping abilities. Discuss feelings, meaning of the loss, and goals with patient and significant others (e.g., "How do you feel about your condition/illness? What do you hope to accomplish in these next few days/weeks?")

◆ Acknowledge and permit anger; set limits on the expression of anger to discourage destructive behavior (e.g., "I understand that you must feel very angry, but for the safety of others, you may not throw equipment").

◆ Identify suicidal behavior (e.g., severe depression, statements of intent, suicide plan, and history of suicide attempt). Ensure patient safety, and refer patient to psychiatric clinical nurse specialist, psychiatrist, clergy, or other support persons or system.

◆ Encourage patient and significant other to participate in activities of daily living (ADL) and diversional activities. Identify physiologic problems related to loss (e.g., eating or sleeping disorders), and intervene accordingly.

◆ See **Anticipatory grieving**, p. 36.

Powerlessness related to absence of a sense of control over events

Desired outcome: Before hospital discharge, patient begins to make decisions about care and therapies and reports onset of an attitude of realistic hope and sense of self-control.

Nursing Interventions

◆ Assess patient's personal preferences, needs, values, and attitudes.

◆ Before providing information, assess patient's knowledge and understanding of condition and care.

◆ Provide patient with information regarding illness, treatment plan, and anticipated outcomes that will enable appropriate decision making.

◆ Recognize patient's expressions of fear, lack of response to events, and lack of interest in information, any of which may signal patient's sense of powerlessness.

◆ Evaluate caregiver practices, and adjust them to support patient's sense of control (e.g., if patient always bathes in the evening to promote relaxation before bedtime, modify care plan to include an evening bath rather than following hospital routine of giving a morning bath).

◆ Ask patient to identify activities that may be performed independently.

◆ Whenever possible, offer alternatives related to routine hygiene, diet, diversional activities, visiting hours, and treatment times that will enable patient to express self-determination.

◆ Ensure patient's right to privacy.

◆ Discourage patient's dependency on staff. Avoid overprotection and parenting behaviors toward patient. Instead, act as an advocate for patient and significant other.

◆ Assess support systems; involve significant other in patient care whenever possible.

◆ Offer realistic hope for the future, realizing that within any situation there is always a reason to be hopeful, even if it is a "good" or peaceful death.

◆ Determine patient's wishes about end-of-life decisions, and document advance directives as appropriate.

◆ Refer to clergy and other support persons or systems as appropriate.

Spiritual distress related to disturbances in belief and value systems that give meaning and a sense of hope

Desired outcome: Before hospital discharge, patient begins to verbalize religious or spiritual beliefs, continues previous practices, and expresses less distress and feelings of anxiety and fear.

Nursing Interventions

◆ Assess patient's spiritual or religious beliefs, values, and practices (e.g., "Do you have a religious preference? How important is it to you? Are there any religious or spiritual practices you wish to participate in while in the hospital?").

◆ Inform patient of availability of spiritual resources, such as a chapel or chaplain.

◆ Display a nonjudgmental attitude toward patient's religious or spiritual beliefs and values. Attempt to create an environment conducive to free expression.

◆ Identify available support persons or systems that may assist in meeting patient's religious or spiritual needs (e.g., clergy, fellow church members, support groups).

◆ Be alert to comments related to spiritual concerns or conflicts (e.g., "I don't know why God is doing this to me" or "I'm being punished for my sins").

◆ Listen closely and ask questions to help patient resolve conflicts related to spiritual issues. Encourage patients to discuss meaning their current illness holds for them.

◆ Provide privacy and opportunities for spiritual practices such as prayer and meditation. Encourage visits with spiritual teacher/leader, if appropriate.

◆ If spiritual beliefs and therapeutic regimens are in conflict, provide patient with honest, concrete information to encourage informed decision making (e.g., "I understand your religion discourages receiving blood transfusions. We respect your position; however, it does not allow us to give you the best care possible.").

◆ Refer patient for help with decision making if he or she is struggling with treatment-related decisions. Many hospitals provide assistance in the form of educational materials and counseling in order to help resolve such dilemmas.

Social isolation related to altered health status, inability to engage in satisfying personal relationships, altered mental status, body image change, or altered physical appearance
Desired outcome: Before hospital discharge patient demonstrates movement toward interaction and communication with others.

Nursing Interventions

◆ Assess factors contributing to patient's social isolation.
  • Restricted visiting hours.
  • Absence of or inadequate support system.
  • Inability to communicate (e.g., presence of intubation/tracheostomy).
  • Physical changes that affect self-concept.
  • Denial or withdrawal.
  • Hospital environment.

◆ Recognize patients at risk for social isolation: older adults; disabled, chronically ill, or economically disadvantaged persons.

◆ Help patient identify feelings associated with loneliness and isolation (e.g., "You seem very sad when your family leaves the room. Can you tell me more about your feelings?").

◆ Determine patient's need for socialization, and identify available and potential support person or systems. Explore methods for increasing social contact (e.g., television, radio, tapes of loved ones, intercom system, more frequent visitations, scheduled interaction with nurse or support staff).

◆ Provide positive reinforcement for socialization that lessens patient's feelings of isolation and loneliness (e.g., "Please continue to call me when you need to talk to someone. Talking will help both of us to better understand your feelings.").

BOX 1-9   INDICATORS SUGGESTING DISTURBED
                BODY IMAGE

Nonverbal Indicators
- Missing body part—internal or external (e.g., hysterectomy, amputated extremity)
- Change in structure (e.g., open, draining wound)
- Change in function (e.g., colostomy)
- Avoidance of looking at or touching body part
- Hiding or exposing body part

Verbal Indicators
- Expression of negative feelings about body
- Expression of feelings of helplessness, hopelessness, or powerlessness
- Personalization or depersonalization of missing or mutilated part
- Refusal to acknowledge change in structure or function of body part

◆ Facilitate patient's ability to communicate with others. (see **Impaired verbal communication**, p. 33).

Disturbed body image related to loss or change in body parts or function or physical trauma
Desired outcomes: Within the 24-hr period before hospital discharge, patient begins to acknowledge bodily changes and demonstrates movement toward incorporating changes into self-concept. Patient does not demonstrate maladaptive response, such as severe depression.

Nursing Interventions

◆ Establish open, honest communication with patient and promote an environment conducive to free expression (e.g., "Please feel free to talk to me whenever you have any questions"). Give patient permission to grieve loss. Assess patient for indicators suggesting body image disturbance (**BOX 1-9**).

◆ When planning patient's care, be aware of therapies that may influence patient's body image, and educate patient accordingly before they are implemented (e.g., medications, surgery, invasive procedures, and monitoring).

◆ Assess patient's knowledge of the pathophysiologic process that has occurred and present health status. Clarify any misconceptions.

◆ Discuss the loss or change with patient. Recognize that what may seem to be a small change may be of great significance to patient (e.g., arm immobilizer, catheter, hair loss, ecchymoses, facial abrasions). Practice nonjudgmental acceptance of patient's reality.

◆ Explore with patient concerns, fears, and feelings of guilt (e.g., "I understand that you are frightened. Your face looks different now, but you will see changes and it will improve. Gradually you will begin to look more like yourself.").

◆ Encourage patient and family members to interact with one another. Help family to avoid reinforcement of their loved one's unhappiness over a changed body part or function (e.g., "I know your son looks very different to you now, but it would help him if you speak to and touch him as you would normally").

◆ Encourage patient to participate gradually in self-care activities as he or she becomes physically and emotionally able. Allow for some initial withdrawal and denial behaviors (e.g., when changing dressings over traumatized part, explain what you are doing but do not expect patient to watch or participate initially).

◆ Discuss opportunities for reconstruction or rehabilitation of the loss or change (e.g., surgery, prosthesis, grafting, PT, cosmetic therapies, modified clothing, organ transplant).

- Recognize manifestations of severe depression (e.g., sleep disturbances, change in affect, and change in communication pattern). As appropriate, refer to psychiatric clinical nurse specialist, case manager, clergy, or support group.
- Assist patient with attaining a sense of autonomy and control by offering choices and alternatives whenever possible. Emphasize patient's strengths, and encourage activities that interest patient.
- If possible, refer patient to a support group or another patient who has had a similar experience (e.g., Reach to Recovery volunteer for a breast surgery patient).
- Be aware that touch may enhance a patient's self-concept and reduce his or her sense of isolation.
- Offer realistic hope for the future.
- See **Disturbed body image,** p. 496, in "Fecal Diversions."

Risk for violence (other-directed or self-directed) related to sensory overload, suicidal behavior, rage reactions, temporal lobe epilepsy, perceived threats, or toxic reaction to medications
Desired outcome: Patient does not harm self or others.

Nursing Interventions

- Assess factors that may contribute to or precipitate violent behavior (e.g., medication reactions, inability to cope, suicidal behavior, confusion, hypoxia, postictal states, unrecognized pain).
- Attempt to eliminate or treat causative factors (e.g., provide patient teaching, reorient patient, ensure delivery of prescribed O_2 therapy, reduce or prevent sensory overload; see **Disturbed sensory perception,** p. 33).
- Assess for history of physical aggression or family violence as maladaptive coping behaviors.
- Monitor for early signs of increasing anxiety and agitation (e.g., restlessness, verbal aggressiveness, inability to concentrate). Assess for body language indicative of violent behavior: clenched fists, rigid posture, increased motor activity.
- Approach patient in a positive manner, and encourage verbalization of feelings and concerns.
- Offer patient as much personal and environmental control as the situation allows (e.g., "Let's discuss the care you will need today. What fluids would you like to drink? Would you prefer a bath in the morning or evening?").
- Help patient distinguish reality from altered perceptions. Orient to person, place, and time. Alter the environment to promote reality-based thought processes (e.g., provide clocks, calendars, pictures of loved ones, familiar objects).
- For patient with acute confusion who becomes aggressive, do not attempt to reorient patient and avoid arguing. Instead, state, "I can understand why you may [hear, think, see] that." Use nonthreatening mannerisms, facial expressions, and tone of voice.
- Initiate measures that prevent or reduce excessive agitation.
  - Reduce environmental stimuli (e.g., alarms, loud or unnecessary talking).
  - Before touching patient, explain procedures and care, and use short, concise statements.
  - Speak quietly (but firmly, as necessary) and project a caring attitude toward patient (e.g., "We are very concerned for your comfort and safety. Can we do anything to help you feel more relaxed?").
  - Avoid crowding (e.g., of equipment, visitors, health care personnel) in patient's personal environment.
  - Avoid direct confrontation.
- Explain and discuss patient's behavior with significant other. Acknowledge frustration, concerns, fears, and questions. Review safety precautions with significant other (see next intervention).

BOX 1-10   SAFETY PRECAUTIONS IN THE EVENT
                  OF VIOLENT BEHAVIOR

Patient Safety
- Remove harmful objects from the environment (e.g., heavy objects or scissors).
- Apply padding to side rails according to agency protocol.
- Use restraints as necessary and prescribed; monitor patient's neurovascular status at frequent intervals.
- Set limits on patient's behavior, and use clear and simple commands.
- As prescribed, consider chemical sedation when unable to control patient's behavior by other means.
- Explain safety precautions to patient and family.

Caregiver Safety
- Alert hospital security department when risk of violence is present.
- Do not approach violent patient without adequate assistance from others.
- Never turn your back on a violent patient.
- Maintain a calm, matter-of-fact tone of voice.
- Monitor security measures often.
- Remain alert.

◆ In the event of violent behavior, institute safety precautions as discussed in **BOX 1-10**.

Hopelessness related to prolonged isolation or activity restriction, failing or deteriorating physiologic condition, long-term stress, or loss of faith in God or belief system
Desired outcome: Before hospital discharge, patient demonstrates beginning acceptance of condition and begins to verbalize hopeful aspects of health status.

Nursing Interventions

◆ Develop open, honest communication with patient. Listen closely, provide empathetic understanding of fears and doubts, and promote an environment that is conducive to free expression.

◆ Assess patient's and significant other's understanding of patient's health status and prognosis; clarify any misperceptions.

◆ Assess for indicators of hopelessness: unwillingness to accept help, pessimism, withdrawal, lack of interest, silence, loss of gratification in roles, previous history of hopeless behavior, hypoactivity, inability to accomplish tasks, expressions of incompetence, closing eyes, and turning away.

◆ Provide opportunities for patient to feel cared for, needed, and valued by others (e.g., emphasize importance of relationships by saying, "Tell me about your grandchildren." "It seems that your family loves you very much").

◆ Support significant other who seems to spark or maintain patient's feelings of hope (e.g., "Your husband's mood seemed to improve after your visit.").

◆ Recognize discussions and factors that promote patient's sense of hope (e.g., discussions about family members, reminiscing about better times).

◆ Explore patient's coping mechanisms; assist patient in expanding positive coping behavior (see **Ineffective coping**, p. 35).

◆ Assess patient's spiritual state and needs (see **Spiritual distress**, p. 38).

◆ Promote anticipation of positive events (e.g., mealtime, grandchildren's visits, bath time, extubation, discontinuation of traction).

◆ Help patient recognize that although there may be no hope for returning to original lifestyle, there is hope for a new, different life.

◆ Avoid insisting that patient assume a positive attitude. Encourage hope for the future, even if it is hope for a peaceful death.

◆ Set realistic, attainable goals, and reward achievement.

Fatigue related to disease process, treatment, medications, depression, or stress

Desired outcome: Before hospital discharge, patient and caregivers describe interventions that conserve energy resources.

Nursing Interventions

- ◆ Assess patient's patterns of fatigue and times of maximum energy.
- ◆ Assess how fatigue is affecting patient's emotional status and ability to perform activities of daily living (ADL). Suggest activity schedules to maximize energy expenditures (e.g., "After you eat lunch, take a 15-minute rest before you go to x-ray").
- ◆ Help patient maintain a regular sleep pattern by allowing for uninterrupted periods of sleep. Encourage patient to rest when fatigued rather than attempting to continue activity. Encourage naps during the day.
- ◆ Reduce environmental stimulation overload (e.g., noise level, visitors for long periods of time, lack of personal quiet time).
- ◆ Discuss with patient how to delegate chores to family and friends who are offering to assist.
- ◆ Encourage patient to maintain a regular schedule once discharged while recognizing that attempting to continue previous activity levels will likely not be realistic.
- ◆ Encourage mild exercise such as short walks and stretching, which may begin in the hospital if not contraindicated.

SECTION FIVE
PSYCHOSOCIAL SUPPORT FOR THE PATIENT'S FAMILY AND SIGNIFICANT OTHERS

The Health Insurance Portability and Accountability Act of 1996 (HIPAA) restricts who may request and receive health care–related information about a patient, in order to protect confidentiality. Health care providers must be sensitive to and aware of expressed patient preferences before discussing patient with others, including family. This includes divulging information regarding patient's presence in the hospital.

NURSING DIAGNOSES AND INTERVENTIONS

Interrupted family processes related to situational crisis (patient's illness)

Desired outcome: Following intervention, family members demonstrate effective adaptation to change/traumatic situation as evidenced by seeking external support when necessary and sharing concerns within the family unit.

Nursing Interventions

- ◆ Assess family's character: social, environmental, ethnic, and cultural factors; relationships; and role patterns. Identify family's developmental stage (e.g., family may be dealing with other situational or maturational crises, such as an elderly parent or a teenager with a learning disability).
- ◆ Assess previous adaptive behaviors (e.g., "How does your family react in stressful situations?"). Discuss observed conflicts and communication breakdown (e.g., "I noticed that your brother would not visit your mother today. Is there a problem we should be aware of? Knowing about it may help us better care for your mother.").
- ◆ Acknowledge family's involvement in patient care, and promote strengths (e.g., "You were able to encourage your wife to turn and cough. That is very important to her recovery."). Encourage family to participate in

patient care conferences. Promote frequent, regular patient visits by family members.

- Provide family with information and guidance related to patient. Discuss the stresses of hospitalization, and encourage family to discuss feelings of anger, guilt, hostility, depression, fear, or sorrow (e.g., "You seem to have been upset ever since being told that your husband would not be leaving the hospital today"). Refer to clergy, clinical nurse specialist, or social services as appropriate.
- Evaluate patient and family responses to one another. Encourage family to reorganize roles and establish priorities as appropriate (e.g., "I know your husband is concerned about his insurance policy and seems to expect you to investigate it. I'll ask the financial counselor to talk with you.").
- Encourage family to schedule periods of rest and activity outside the hospital and to seek support when necessary (e.g., "Your neighbor volunteered to stay in the waiting room this afternoon. Would you like to rest at home? I'll call you if anything changes.").

Readiness for enhanced family coping related to use of support persons or systems, referrals, and choosing experiences that optimize wellness
Desired outcomes: Family members express intent to use support persons, systems, and resources and identify alternative behaviors that promote family communication and strengths. Family members express realistic expectations and do not demonstrate ineffective coping behaviors.

Nursing Interventions

- Assess family relationships, interactions, support persons or systems, and individual coping behaviors. Permit movement through stages of adaptation. Encourage further positive coping.
- Acknowledge expressions of hope, plans, and growth among family members.
- Encourage development of open, honest communication within the family. Provide opportunities in a private setting for family interactions, discussions, and questions (e.g., "I know the waiting room is very crowded. Would your family like some private time together?").
- Refer family to community or support groups (e.g., ostomy support group, head injury rehabilitation group).
- Encourage family to explore outlets that foster positive feelings (e.g., time spent outside the hospital area; meaningful communication with patient or support individuals; and relaxing activities).

Compromised family coping related to inadequate or incorrect information or misunderstanding, temporary family disorganization and role change, exhausted support persons or systems, unrealistic expectations, fear, or anxiety
Desired outcome: Following intervention, family members begin to verbalize feelings, identify ineffective coping patterns, identify strengths and positive coping behaviors, and seek information and support from nurse or other support persons or systems outside the family.

Nursing Interventions

- Establish open, honest communication within the family. Assist family members with identifying strengths, stressors, inappropriate behaviors, and personal needs (e.g., "I understand that your mother was very ill last year. How did you manage the situation?" "I know that your loved one is very ill. How can I help you?").
- Assess family members for ineffective coping (e.g., depression, chemical dependency, violence, withdrawal), and identify factors that inhibit effective coping (e.g., inadequate support system, grief, fear of disapproval by others, knowledge deficit). (e.g., "You seem to be unable to talk about your husband's illness. Is there anyone with whom you can talk about it?)"

- Assess family's knowledge about patient's current health status and treatment. Provide information often, and allow sufficient time for questions. Reassess family's understanding at frequent intervals.
- Provide opportunities in a private setting for family members to talk and share concerns with nurses. If appropriate, refer family to psychiatric clinical nurse specialist for therapy.
- Offer realistic hope. Help the family to develop realistic expectations for the future and to identify support persons or systems that will assist them.
- Assist family with reducing anxiety by encouraging diversional activities (e.g., time spent outside the hospital) and interaction with support persons or systems outside the family (e.g., "I know you want to be near your son, but if you would like to go home to rest, I will call you if any changes occur").

Disabled family coping related to unexpressed feelings, ambivalent family relationships, or disharmonious coping styles among family members
Desired outcome: Within the 24-hr period before hospital discharge, family members begin to verbalize feelings; identify sources of support, as well as sources of ineffective coping behaviors that create ambivalence and disharmony; and do not demonstrate destructive behaviors.

Nursing Interventions

- Establish open, honest communication and rapport with family members (e.g., "I am here to care for your mother and to help your family as well.").
- Identify ineffective coping behaviors, such as violence, depression, substance misuse, withdrawal (e.g., "You seem to be angry. Would you like to talk to me about your feelings?"). Refer to psychiatric clinical nurse specialist, case manager, clergy, or support group as appropriate.
- Identify perceived or actual conflicts (e.g., "Are you able to talk freely with your family members?" "Are your brothers and sisters able to help and support you during this time?").
- Assist family in search for healthy functioning within the family unit. For example, facilitate open communication among family members and encourage behaviors that support family cohesiveness (e.g., "Your mother enjoyed your last visit. Would you like to see her now?")
- Assess family's knowledge about patient's current health status. Provide opportunities for questions; reassess family's understanding at frequent intervals.
- Assist family members in developing realistic goals, plans, and actions. Refer them to clergy, psychiatric nurse, social services, financial counseling, and family therapy as appropriate.
- Encourage family members to spend time outside the hospital and to interact with support individuals. Respect family's need for occasional withdrawal.
- Include family members in patient's plan of care. Offer them opportunities to become involved in patient care (e.g., ROM exercises, patient hygiene, comfort measures such as back rub).

Fear related to patient's life-threatening condition and knowledge deficit
Desired outcome: Following intervention, significant others/family members report that fear has lessened.

Nursing Interventions

- Assess family's fears and their understanding of patient's clinical situation. Evaluate verbal and nonverbal responses.
- Acknowledge family's fear (e.g., "I understand that these tubes must frighten you, but they are necessary to help nourish your son").
- Assess family's history of coping behavior (e.g., "How does your family react to difficult situations?"). Determine resources and significant others

available for support (e.g., "Who usually helps your family during stressful times?").

◆ Provide opportunities for family members to express fears and concerns. Recognize that anger, denial, withdrawal, and demanding behavior may be adaptive coping responses during initial period of crisis.

◆ Provide information at frequent intervals about patient's status, treatments, and equipment used. Demonstrate a caring attitude.

◆ Encourage family to use positive coping behaviors by identifying fears, developing goals, identifying supportive resources, facilitating realistic perceptions, and promoting problem solving.

◆ Recognize anxiety, and encourage family members to describe their feelings (e.g., "You seem very uncomfortable tonight. Can you describe your feelings?").

◆ Be alert to maladaptive responses to fear: potential for violence, withdrawal, severe depression, hostility, and unrealistic expectations for staff or of patient's recovery. Provide referrals to psychiatric clinical nurse specialist or other staff member as appropriate.

◆ Offer realistic hope, even if it is hope for patient's peaceful death.

◆ Explore family's desire for spiritual or other counseling.

◆ Assess your own feelings about patient's life-threatening illness. Without personal awareness of one's beliefs, a health care provider's attitude and fears may be reflected inadvertently to the family.

◆ For other interventions, see **Interrupted family processes** and **Disabled family coping** listed earlier in this section.

Deficient knowledge related to patient's current health status or therapies
Desired outcome: Following intervention, family members/significant others begin to verbalize knowledge and understanding about patient's current health status and treatment.

Nursing Interventions

◆ Assess the family's facility with language, and engage an interpreter or provide language-appropriate written materials if necessary.

◆ At frequent intervals, inform family about patient's current health status, therapies, and prognosis. Use individualized verbal, written, and audiovisual strategies to promote family's understanding.

◆ At frequent intervals, evaluate family's comprehension of information provided. Assess factors for misunderstanding, and adjust teaching as appropriate. Some individuals in crisis need repeated explanations before comprehension can be assured (e.g., "I have explained many things to you today. Would you mind summarizing what I've told you so that I can be sure you understand your husband's status and what we are doing to care for him?").

◆ Encourage family to relay correct information to patient. This also will reinforce comprehension for family and patient.

◆ Inquire of family members whether their information needs are being met (e.g., "Do you have any questions about the care your mother is receiving or about her condition?").

◆ Promote family's active participation in patient care when appropriate. Encourage them to seek information and express feelings, concerns, and questions.

◆ Help family members use the information they receive to make health care decisions about patient (e.g., surgery, resuscitation, organ donation). All patients should be encouraged to designate a durable power of attorney (DPOA) for health care if they have not already done so. This person should be fully aware of patient's preferences regarding care and capable of articulating those preferences if patient is unable to do so.

❖ ❖ ❖

SECTION SIX **OLDER ADULT CARE**

NURSING DIAGNOSES AND INTERVENTIONS

Risk for aspiration related to decreased masticatory muscle function secondary to age-related changes

Desired outcomes: Patient swallows independently without choking. Patient's airway is patent and lungs are clear to auscultation both before and after meals.

Nursing Interventions

- Assess patient's level of consciousness (LOC) on admission and then routinely during hospital stay.
- Assess patient's ability to swallow by asking whether he or she has any difficulty swallowing or whether any foods or fluids are difficult to swallow or cause gagging. If patient is unable to answer, consult patient's caregiver or significant other. Document findings.
- Assess for the gag reflex by gently touching one side and then the other of the posterior pharynx. Document both findings.
- Place patient in an upright position while eating or drinking, and support this position with pillows on patient's sides.
- Monitor patient when he or she is swallowing. Watch for limited lip, tongue, or jaw movement as indicated by drooling of saliva or food or inability to close lips around a straw. Check for retention of food in sides of mouth, which is an indication of poor tongue movement.
- Monitor patient for coughing or choking before, during, or after swallowing. This may occur up to several minutes following placement of food or fluid in the mouth and signals aspiration of material into the airway.
- Elders have increased risk for silent aspiration. Monitor patient for signs of aspiration, including changes in lung auscultation (e.g., crackles [rales], wheezes, rhonchi), shortness of breath, dyspnea, decreasing LOC, increasing temperature, and cyanosis.
- Monitor patient for a wet or gurgling sound when talking after a swallow. This indicates aspiration into the airway and signals delayed or absent swallow and gag reflexes.
- For patients with poor swallowing reflex, tilt head forward 45 degrees during swallowing. *This will help prevent inadvertent aspiration by closing off the airway.* For patients with hemiplegia, tilt head toward unaffected side.
- As indicated, request evaluation by speech therapist for further assessment of gag and swallow reflexes.
- Anticipate swallowing video fluoroscopy *to evaluate patient's gag and swallow reflexes.* Using four consistencies of barium, the radiologist and speech therapist watch for the presence of reduced or ineffective tongue function, reduced peristalsis in the pharynx, delayed or absent swallow reflex, and poor or limited ability to close the epiglottis, which protects the airway. *This procedure is used to determine whether patient is aspirating, consistency of materials most likely to be aspirated, and aspiration cause.*
- Based on results of the swallowing video fluoroscopy, thickened fluids may be prescribed. Agents are added to fluid *to make it more viscous and easier for patient to swallow.* Similarly, mechanical soft, pureed, or liquid diets may be prescribed *to enable patient to ingest food with less potential for aspiration.*
- Provide adequate rest periods before meals *to avoid fatigue, which increases risk for aspiration.*
- Monitor intake of food. Document consistencies and amounts of food patient eats, where patient places food in the mouth, how patient manipulates or chews before swallowing, and length of time before patient swallows the bolus of food.

♦ Remind patients with dementia to chew and swallow with each bite. Check for retained food in sides of mouth.

♦ Ensure that patient has dentures in place, if appropriate, and that they fit correctly.

♦ Ensure that someone stays with patient during meals or fluid intake.

♦ Provide patient with adequate time to eat and drink. *Generally, patients with swallowing deficits require twice as much time for eating and drinking as those whose swallowing is adequate.*

♦ Be aware of location of suction equipment to be used in the event of aspiration. If patient is at increased risk for aspiration, suction equipment should be available at the bedside.

♦ If patient aspirates, implement the following:
  • Follow American Heart Association (AHA) standards if patient displays characteristics of complete airway obstruction (i.e., choking).
  • For partial airway obstruction, encourage patient to cough as needed.
  • For partial airway obstruction in unconscious or nonresponsive individual who is not coughing, suction airway with a large-bore catheter such as Yankauer or tonsil suction tip.
  • For either complete or partial aspiration, inform health care provider and obtain prescription for chest x-ray examination.
  • Protect patient by implementing nothing by mouth (NPO) status until diagnosis is confirmed.
  • Monitor breathing pattern and respiratory rate (RR) q1-2h after a suspected aspiration for alterations (i.e., increased RR) that signal a change in patient's condition.
  • Anticipate use of antibiotics *to prevent infection.*
  • Encourage patient to cough and breathe deeply q2h while awake and q4h during the night *to promote expansion of available lung tissue.*

Constipation related to changes in diet, activity, and psychosocial factors secondary to hospitalization
Desired outcomes: Patient reports that bowel habit has returned to normal pattern within 3-4 days of this diagnosis. Stool appears soft, and patient does not strain in passing stools.

Nursing Interventions

♦ On admission, assess and document patient's normal bowel elimination pattern. Include frequency, time of day, associated habits, and successful methods used to correct constipation in the past. Consult patient's caregiver or significant other if patient is unable to provide this information.

♦ Inform patient that changes occurring with hospitalization may increase potential for constipation. Urge patient to institute successful nonpharmacologic methods used at home as soon as this problem is noticed or prophylactically as needed.

♦ Teach patient the relationship between fluid intake and constipation. Unless otherwise contraindicated, encourage fluid intake that exceeds 2500 mL/day. Monitor and record bowel movements (date, time, consistency, amount).

♦ Teach patient the relationship between types of foods consumed and constipation. Encourage patient to include roughage (e.g., raw fruits and vegetables, whole grains, nuts, fruits with skins) as a part of each meal when possible. For patients unable to tolerate raw foods, encourage intake of bran in cereals, muffins, and breads. Titrate amount of roughage to the degree of constipation.

♦ Teach patient the relationship between constipation and activity level. Encourage optimum activity for all patients. Establish and post an activity program to enhance participation; include devices necessary to enable independence.

- Advise patient about need to maintain normal bowel elimination pattern. Provide any materials or support environments patient normally uses (e.g., cup of coffee on arising, privacy, short walk).
- Ask patient if toilet seat height seems the same as at home. If the hospital toilet seat is too high, provide a footstool to raise patient's feet comfortably off the floor. A high-rise toilet seat may be used to increase height if necessary.
- Schedule interventions to coincide with patient's habit. If patient's bowel movement occurs in the early morning, use patient's gastrocolic or duodenocolic reflex to promote colonic emptying. If patient's bowel movement occurs in the evening, ambulate patient just before the appropriate time. Digital stimulation of the inner anal sphincter also may facilitate bowel movement.
- Attempt to use methods patient has used successfully in the past. Follow the maxim "go low, go slow" (i.e., use lowest level of nonnatural intervention and advance to more powerful interventions slowly). Older persons tend to focus on the loss of habit as an indicator of constipation rather than on the number of stools. Do not intervene pharmacologically until the older adult has not had a stool for 3 days.
- When requesting a pharmacologic intervention, use the more benign, oral methods first. The following hierarchy is suggested:
  1. Bulk-building additives such as psyllium or bran.
  2. Mild laxatives (apple or prune juice, Milk of Magnesia).
  3. Stool softeners (docusate sodium, docusate calcium).
  4. Potent laxatives or cathartics (bisacodyl, cascara sagrada).
  5. Medicated suppositories (glycerin, bisacodyl).
  6. Enema (tap water, saline, sodium biphosphate/phosphate).
- After diagnostic imaging of the gastrointestinal (GI) tract with barium, ensure that patient receives a postexamination laxative *to facilitate removal of the barium.* After any procedure involving a bowel clean-out, there may be rebound constipation from the severe disruption of bowel habit. Monitor hydration status for signs of dehydration, which can occur from osmotic agents used. Emphasize diet, fluid, activity, and resumption of routines. If no bowel movement occurs in 3 days, begin with mild laxatives *to try to regain normal pattern.*
- See "Prolonged Bed Rest," for **Constipation,** p. 29.

Risk for deficient fluid volume related to inability to obtain fluids by self secondary to illness, placement of fluid, or presence of chronic illness; or related to use of osmotic agents during radiologic tests
Desired outcomes: Patient's mental status; VS; and urine specific gravity, color, consistency, and concentration remain within normal limits for patient. Patient's mucous membranes remain moist, and there is no "tenting" of skin. Patient's intake equals output.

Nursing Interventions

- Monitor fluid intake. In nonrestricted individuals, encourage fluid intake of 2-3 L/day. Specify intake goals for day, evening, and night shifts.
- Assess and document skin turgor. Check hydration status by pinching skin over sternum or forehead. Skin that remains in the lifted position (tenting) and returns slowly to its original position indicates dehydration. A furrowed tongue is a signal of severe dehydration.
- Assess and document color, amount, and frequency of any fluid output, including emesis, urine, diarrhea, or other drainage.
- Monitor patient's orientation, ability to follow commands, and behavior. Loss of ability to follow commands, decrease in orientation, and confused behavior can signal a dehydrated state.

- Weigh patient daily at the same time of day (preferably before breakfast) using same scale and bed clothing. Be alert to wide variations in weight (e.g., 2.5 kg [5 lb] or greater).
- In patient who is dehydrated, anticipate elevation in serum Na^+, BUN, and serum creatinine levels.
- If patient is receiving IV therapy, monitor cardiac and respiratory systems for signs of overload, which could precipitate heart failure or pulmonary edema. Assess apical pulse and listen to lung fields during every VS assessment. A rising heart rate (HR) and crackles and bronchial wheezes in the lungs can be signals of heart failure or pulmonary edema.
- Carefully monitor I&O when patient is receiving tube feedings or dyes for contrast. These agents act osmotically to pull fluid into interstitial tissue. Watch for evidence of third spacing of fluids, including increasing peripheral edema, especially sacral; output significantly less than intake (1:2); and urine output less than 30 mL/hr.
- Whenever in the room, offer patient fluid. *Older persons have a decreased sense of thirst and need encouragement to drink.* Offer a variety of drinks patient likes, but limit caffeine *because it tends to act as a diuretic.*
- Assess patient's ability to obtain and drink fluids by himself or herself. Place fluids within easy reach. Use cups with tops *to minimize concern over spilling.*
- Ensure access to toilet, urinal, commode, or bedpan at least q2h when patient is awake and q4h at night. Answer call light quickly. The time between recognition of the need to void and urination decreases with age.

Impaired gas exchange or **Risk for impaired gas exchange** related to decreased functional lung tissue secondary to age-related changes
Desired outcomes: Patient's respiratory pattern and mental status remain normal for patient. Patient's arterial blood gas (ABG) or pulse oximetry values are within patient's normal limits.

Nursing Interventions

- Assess and document the following upon admission and routinely thereafter: RR and pattern and depth of respirations; breath sounds; cough; sputum; and sensorium.
- Assess patient for subtle changes in mentation such as increased restlessness, anxiety, disorientation, and presence of hostility. If equipment is available, monitor oxygenation status via ABG findings (optimally Pao_2 80%-95% or greater) or pulse oximetry (optimally greater than 92%).
- Assess lungs for presence of adventitious sounds. The aging lung has decreased elasticity. The lower part of the lungs is no longer adequately aerated. As a result, crackles commonly are heard in individuals 75 yr of age and older. This sign alone does not mean that a pathologic condition is present. Crackles (rales) that do not clear with coughing in an individual with no other clinical signs (e.g., fever, increasing anxiety, changes in mental status, increasing respiratory depth) are considered benign.
- Encourage patient to cough and breathe deeply *to promote alveolar expansion and clear secretions from the bronchial tree.* When appropriate, instruct patient in use of incentive spirometry. Encourage fluid intake to greater than 2.5 L/day *to ensure less viscous pulmonary secretions that are more easily mobilized.*
- Reduce potential for patient's increased O_2 consumption by treating fevers promptly, decreasing pain, minimizing pacing activity, and lessening anxiety.
- Instruct patient in use of support equipment such as O_2 masks or cannulas.
- Schedule and pace patient's activities according to tolerance. Document patient's ability to accomplish activities of daily living (ADL).

Hopelessness related to slow recovery from illness or surgery secondary to decreased physiologic reserve

Desired outcome: Within 2-4 days of interventions, patient verbalizes knowledge of his or her strengths, feelings about health, and the understanding of a potentially long recovery.

Nursing Interventions

♦ Monitor patient for signs of depression, such as refusal to participate in own care; refusal to answer questions; and statements such as "I don't care," "Leave me alone," and "Let me die."

♦ Encourage patient to verbalize feelings of despair, frustration, fear, and anger and concerns regarding hospitalization and health. Reassure patient and significant other that such feelings and concerns are normal.

♦ Discuss normal age-related changes with patient. Inform patient and significant other that recovery periods are longer for older adults than others because of decreased physiologic reserve. More energy is spent in maintaining normal status, and thus the body has less capacity to rebuild strength and endurance.

♦ Encourage short-term goals and praise small steps, such as participation in own care.

♦ Arrange a care conference to discuss discharge requirements specific to patient. Involve patient and significant other in the conference. Set realistic goals with patient based on patient's condition and desires.

Hypothermia related to age-related changes in thermoregulation and/or environmental exposure

Desired outcome: Patient's temperature and mental status remain within patient's normal limits, or they return to within normal limits with temperature rising at a rate of 1° F/hr, after interventions.

Nursing Interventions

♦ Monitor patient's temperature, using a low-range thermometer if possible. Be aware that older adults can have a normal temperature of 35.5° C (96° F).

♦ Assess patient's temperature orally by placing thermometer far back in patient's mouth. This will provide the most accurate assessment of patient's core temperature. If necessary, assess temperature rectally. Do not take axillary temperature in the older adult *because older persons have decreased peripheral circulation and loss of subcutaneous fat in the axillary area that result in formation of a pocket of air, which may make readings inaccurate.* If unable to measure patient's temperature orally, measure temperature via ear but note that reliability of electronic tympanic thermometers may be inconsistent because of improper use.

♦ Assess and document patient's mental status. Increasing disorientation, mental status changes, or presence of atypical behavior can signal hypothermia.

♦ Be alert to patients taking sedatives, hypnotics (including anesthetics), and muscle relaxants. These drugs decrease shivering and therefore place patients at risk for environmental hypothermia. In addition, all older adults are at risk for environmental hypothermia at ambient temperatures of 22.22°-23.89° C (72°-75° F).

♦ Ensure that patients going for testing or x-ray examination are sent with enough blankets to keep warm.

♦ If patient is mildly hypothermic, initiate slow rewarming using external methods, such as raising room temperature to at least 23.89° C (75° F). Other methods of external warming include use of warm blankets, head covers, and warm circulating air blankets.

♦ If patient's temperature falls to less than 35° C (95° F), warm patient internally by administering warm oral or IV fluids. Also anticipate use of warmed saline gastric or rectal irrigations or introduction of warmed humidified air into the airway.

◆ Be alert to signs of too rapid rewarming: irregular HR, dysrhythmias, and very warm extremities produced by vasodilation in the periphery, which causes heat loss from the core.

◆ If patient's temperature fails to rise 1° F/hr using these techniques, suspect a cause other than environmental. In this event, anticipate laboratory tests, including WBC count for possible sepsis, thyroid test for hypothyroidism, and glucose level for hypoglycemia.

◆ As prescribed, administer antibiotics for sepsis, initiate thyroid therapy, or administer glucose for hypoglycemia. Patient's temperature will not return to normal unless the underlying condition has been treated.

Risk for infection related to age-related changes in immune and integumentary systems, suppressed inflammatory response secondary to long-term medication use (e.g., antiinflammatory agents, steroids, analgesics), slowed ciliary response, or poor nutrition

Desired outcome: Patient remains free of infection as evidenced by orientation to person, place, and time and behavior within patient's normal limits; RR and pattern within patient's normal limits; urine that is straw colored, clear, and of characteristic odor; core temperature and HR within patient's normal limits; sputum that is clear to whitish; and skin that is intact and of normal color and temperature for patient. WBC count 11,000/mm^3 or higher can be a late sign of infection in older patients because the immune system is slow to respond to insult.

Nursing Interventions

◆ Assess patient's baseline VS, including LOC and orientation. A change in mentation is a leading sign of infection in older patients. Also be alert to HR greater than 100 beats per minute (bpm) and RR greater than 24 breaths/min. Auscultate lung fields for adventitious sounds. Be aware, however, that crackles (rales) may be a normal finding when heard in the lung bases.

◆ Monitor patient's temperature, using a low-range thermometer if possible. Be aware that a temperature of 35.5° C (96° F) may be normal for the patient. In that case, a patient with a temperature of 36.67°-37.22° C (98°-99° F) may be considered febrile.

◆ To ensure that patient's core temperature is being accurately determined, obtain temperature readings rectally if the oral reading does not match the clinical picture (i.e., patient's skin is very warm, patient is restless, mentation is depressed), or if the temperature reads 36.11° C (97° F) or higher. If temperature measurement is done using a tympanic thermometer, note that reliability of this thermometer may be inconsistent because of improper use.

◆ Assess patient's skin for tears, breaks, redness, or ulcers. Document condition of patient's skin on admission and as an ongoing assessment. (refer to **Risk for impaired skin integrity**, p. 723.)

◆ Assess quality and color of patient's urine. Urinary tract infection (UTI), as manifested by cloudy, foul-smelling urine without painful urination, is the most common infection in older adults. Document changes when noted, and report findings to health care provider. Also be alert to urinary incontinence, which *can signal UTI.*

◆ Avoid insertion of urinary catheters when possible *because of increased risk of infection.*

◆ Obtain drug history in reference to use of antiinflammatory or immunosuppressive drugs or long-term use of analgesics or steroids *because these drugs mask fever.*

◆ If infection is suspected, anticipate initiation of IV fluid therapy *for maintenance of fluid balance*; blood cultures, urinalysis, and urine culture *to isolate bacteria type*; and WBC count *to determine immune response.*

Expect a chest x-ray examination *to rule out pneumonia* if patient's chest sounds are not clear. If infection is present, prepare for initiation of broad-spectrum antibiotic therapy, O$_2$ therapy *to maintain adequate oxygenation to the brain*, and use of acetaminophen *to decrease temperature and cardiac output and thereby decrease cardiac load.*

Powerlessness related to hospital environment
Desired outcome: Within 2-4 days after interventions, patient participates in care and verbalizes feelings of control over his or her environment.

Nursing Interventions

- Encourage patient to verbalize feelings about hospitalization and illness.
- Assist patient in identifying factors that contribute to feelings of powerlessness.
- Encourage patient to participate in ADL as much as possible. Provide adequate time for patient to complete ADL.
- As often as possible, enable patient to participate in scheduling of activities.
- Discuss with patient and significant other realistic goals of care, and encourage patient's participation in care planning.
- Explain procedures and routines to patient. Inform patient when changes in the plan of care are necessary.
- Provide flexibility in patient's plan of care when possible (e.g., if patient wants to wear his or her own clothes, enable patient to do so).

Risk for impaired skin integrity related to decreased subcutaneous fat and decreased peripheral capillary networks secondary to age-related changes in the integumentary system
Desired outcome: Patient's skin remains nonerythemic and intact.

Nursing Interventions

- Assess patient's skin on admission and routinely thereafter. Note any areas of redness or any breaks in the skin surface.
- Ensure that patient turns frequently (at least q2h). Lift or roll patient across sheets when repositioning. *Pulling, dragging, or sliding patient across sheets can lead to shear injury of the cutaneous or subcutaneous tissue.*
- Monitor skin over bony prominences (i.e., sacrum, scapulae, heels, spine, hips, pelvis, greater trochanter, knees, ankles, costal margins, occiput) for erythema. Use pillows or pads around bony prominences to protect overlying skin, even when patient is up in a wheelchair or sits for long periods. *The skin over the ischial tuberosities is prone to breakdown when patient is in the seated position. Gel pads for chair or wheelchair seats aid in distributing pressure.*
- Use lotions on dry skin *to promote moisture and suppleness.* Lanolin-containing lotions are especially useful.
- *To protect skin from injury caused by prolonged pressure,* use alternating-pressure mattress, air-fluidized mattress, water bed, air bed, or other pressure-sensitive mattress for older patients who are on bed rest or unable to get out of bed.
- Avoid placing tubes under patient's limbs or head. *Excess pressure from tubes can create a pressure ulcer.* Place pillow or pad between patient and tube *for cushioning.*
- Optimize patient mobility; get patient out of bed as often as possible. Liberally use mechanical lifting devices *to aid in safe patient transfers.* If patient is unable to get out of bed, assist with position changes q2h. Establish and post a turning schedule on the patient care plan and at the bedside.
- At a minimum, ensure that patient's face, axillae, and genital areas are cleansed daily. Complete baths dry out older adults' skin and should be

given every other day instead. Use tepid water (90°-105° F [32.2°-40.5° C]) and super-fatted, nonperfumed soap *to help decrease dry skin*. Avoid hot water, *which can burn older adults, who have decreased pain sensitivity and decreased sensation to temperature.*

◆ Minimize use of plastic protective pads under patient. *These pads trap moisture and heat, which can lead to skin breakdown.* When plastic pads are used, place at least one layer of cloth (drawsheet) between patient and pad *to absorb moisture.*

◆ Document percentage of food intake with meals. Encourage significant other to provide patient's favorite foods. Suggest snacks high in protein and vitamin C if patient's diet is not restricted.

◆ Obtain nutritional consultation with dietitian as needed.

◆ Monitor serum albumin for evidence of protein status (normal value is 3.0 g/dL for older adults).

◆ For more information, see "Providing Nutritional Support," p. 692, and "Pressure Ulcers," p. 722.

Disturbed sleep pattern related to unfamiliar surroundings and hospital routines
Desired outcomes: Within 24 hr of interventions, patient reports attainment of adequate rest. Mental status remains normal for patient.

Nursing Interventions

◆ Assess and document patient's sleeping pattern, obtaining information from patient or patient's caregiver or significant other. Ask questions about naps and activity levels. Individuals who take naps and have a low level of activity often sleep only 4-5 hr/night.

◆ Determine patient's usual nighttime routine and attempt to emulate it.

◆ Inform patient of necessary interruptions during hospitalization.

◆ Attempt to group together activities such as medications, VS, and toileting to reduce the number of interruptions.

◆ Provide comfort measures at bedtime, such as pain medications, back rub, and conversation.

◆ Provide patient with compatible roommate when possible.

◆ Monitor patient's activity level. If patient complains of being tired after activities or displays behaviors such as irritability, yelling, or shouting, encourage napping after lunch or early in the afternoon. Otherwise, discourage daytime napping by involving patient in care or activities.

◆ Avoid stimulants such as caffeinated coffee, cola, and tea after 6 PM.

◆ Provide a quiet environment by avoiding loud noises and use of overhead lights and minimizing interruptions during sleep hours.

Disturbed thought processes related to decreased cerebral perfusion secondary to age-related decreased physiologic reserve or cardiac dysfunction, electrolyte imbalance secondary to age-related decreased renal function, altered sensory/perceptual reception secondary to poor vision or hearing, or decreased brain oxygenation secondary to illness state and decreased functional lung tissue
Desired outcomes: Patient's mental status returns to normal for patient within 3 days of treatment. Patient sustains no evidence of injury or harm as a result of mental status.

Nursing Interventions

◆ Assess patient's baseline LOC and mental status on admission. Ask patient to perform a three-step task (e.g., "Raise your right hand, place it on your left shoulder, and then place the right hand by your right side"). Test short-term memory by showing patient how to use call light, having patient return the demonstration, and then waiting at least 5 min before having patient demonstrate use of call light again. Inability to remember beyond 5 min indicates poor short-term memory. Document patient's response.

♦ Document patient's actions in behavioral terms. Describe the "confused" behavior.

♦ Obtain preconfusion functional and mental status abilities from significant other.

♦ Identify cause of acute confusion (e.g., consult health care provider regarding oximetry or ABG values *to assess oxygenation levels,* serum glucose or finger stick glucose *to determine glucose level,* and electrolytes and CBC to *ascertain imbalances and/or presence of elevated WBC count as a determinant of infection).* Pinch skin over sternum or forehead for turgor and check for dry mucous membranes and furrowed tongue *to assess hydration status.*

♦ Acute confusion can be a sign of pain. Assess for pain using a patient-appropriate rating scale. If patient is unable to use a scale, assess for behavioral cues such as grimacing, clenched fists, frowning, and hitting. Ask family/significant other to assist in identifying pain behaviors. Treat patient for pain, as indicated, and monitor behaviors. If pain caused the confusion, patient's behavior should change accordingly.

♦ Review cardiac status. Assess apical pulse and notify health care provider of an irregular pulse that is new to patient. If patient is on a cardiac monitor or telemetry, watch for dysrhythmias; notify health care provider accordingly.

♦ Review current medications, including over-the-counter (OTC) drugs, with pharmacist. Toxic levels of certain medications, such as digoxin or theophylline, cause acute confusion. Drugs that are anticholinergic also can cause confusion, as can drug interactions.

♦ Monitor I&O at least q8h. Output should match intake. Anticipate/encourage a creatinine clearance test to assess renal function. BUN and serum creatinine are affected by hydration status. Serum creatinine is affected by the aging process because lower muscle mass produces lower creatinine levels. Normal serum creatinine levels in a well-hydrated older adult can therefore signal renal insufficiency.

♦ Have patient wear glasses and hearing aid, or keep them close to the bedside and within easy reach for patient use.

♦ Keep patient's urinal and other routinely used items within easy reach for patient. If patient has short-term memory problems, do not expect him or her to use call light. Toilet or offer patient urinal or bedpan q2h while awake and q4h during the night. Establish a toileting schedule and post it on patient care plan and, inconspicuously, at the bedside.

♦ Check on patient at least q30min and every time you pass the room.

♦ Place patient close to nurses' station if possible. Provide an environment that is nonstimulating and safe. Provide music but not television (patients who are confused regarding place and time often think the action on television is happening in the room).

♦ Attempt to reorient patient to surroundings as needed. Keep a clock with large numerals and a large print calendar at the bedside; verbally remind patient of date and day as needed.

♦ Tell patient in simple terms what is occurring (e.g., "It's time to eat breakfast." "This medicine is for your heart." "I'm going to help you get out of bed.").

♦ Encourage patient's significant other to bring items familiar to patient, including blanket, bedspread, pictures of family and pets.

♦ If patient becomes belligerent, angry, or argumentative while you are attempting to reorient, stop this approach. Do not argue with patient or patient's interpretation of the environment. State, "I can understand why you may [hear, think, see] that."

♦ If patient displays hostile behavior or misperceives your role (e.g., nurse becomes thief, jailer), leave the room. Return in 15 min. Introduce yourself to patient as though you had never met. Begin dialogue anew. *Patients who are acutely confused have poor short-term memory and may not remember the previous encounter or that you were involved in that encounter.* When you return, enable patient to share feelings about the previous encounter as appropriate.

◆ If patient attempts to leave the hospital, walk with patient and attempt distraction. Ask patient to tell you about the destination (e.g., "That sounds like a wonderful place! Tell me about it."). Keep tone pleasant and conversational. Continue walking with patient away from exits and doors around the unit. After a few minutes, attempt to guide patient back to the room. Offer refreshments and a rest (e.g., "We've been walking for a while and I'm a little tired. Why don't we sit and have some juice while we talk?").

◆ If patient has a permanent or severe cognitive impairment, check on her or him at least q30min and reorient to baseline mental status as indicated; however, do not argue with patient about his or her perception of reality. *This can cause the cognitively impaired person to become aggressive and combative.* Individuals with severe cognitive impairment (e.g., Alzheimer's disease or dementia) also can experience acute confusional states (i.e., delirium) and can be returned to their baseline mental state.

◆ If patient tries to climb out of bed, he or she may need to use the toilet; offer urinal or bedpan, or assist to the commode. Alternately, if patient is not on bed rest, place him or her in chair or wheelchair at nurses' station for added supervision.

◆ Bargain with patient. Try to establish an agreement to stay for a defined period, such as until health care provider, meal, or significant other arrives.

◆ Have patient's significant other talk with patient by phone or come in and sit with patient if patient's behavior requires checking more often than q30min.

◆ If patient is attempting to pull out tubes, hide the tubes (e.g., under blankets). Put stockinette mesh dressing over IV lines. Tape feeding tubes to side of the face using paper tape, and drape the tube behind patient's ear. Remember: Out of sight, out of mind.

◆ Evaluate continued need for therapy that may have become an irritating stimulus (e.g., if patient is now drinking, discontinue IV line; if patient is eating, discontinue feeding tube; if patient has an indwelling urethral catheter, discontinue catheter and begin toileting routine).

◆ Use restraints with caution. *Patients can become more agitated when wrist and arm restraints are used.*

◆ Use medications cautiously for controlling behavior. Neuroleptics, such as haloperidol, can be used successfully in calming patients with dementia or psychiatric illness but are contraindicated for individuals with parkinsonism. However, if patient is experiencing acute confusion or delirium, short-acting benzodiazepines (e.g., lorazepam) are more effective in reducing anxiety and fear. Anxiety or fear usually triggers destructive or dangerous behaviors in acutely confused older patients. A short-acting benzodiazepine, such as lorazepam, will decrease feelings of anxiety and calm patient after one or two doses. Neuroleptics can cause akathisia, an adverse drug reaction evidenced by increased restlessness.

Respiratory Disorders

SECTION ONE **ACUTE RESPIRATORY DISORDERS**

Acute respiratory disorders are short-term diseases or acute complications of chronic conditions. They can occur once and respond to treatment or recur to further complicate an underlying disease process.

❖ ATELECTASIS

OVERVIEW/PATHOPHYSIOLOGY

Atelectasis is a spontaneous collapse of alveolar lung tissue secondary to persistent hypoinflation. It is most common following major abdominal or thoracic surgery and results from hypoventilation of dependent portions of the lungs or inadequate clearing of secretions. Atelectasis can be an acute or a chronic condition and occurs most often in individuals with COPD. Postoperatively, atelectasis can be precipitated by the effects of anesthesia, sedation, and decreased mobility. Other precipitating factors include mucus plugs, foreign objects in the airways, pleural effusion, bronchogenic carcinoma, history of smoking, and obesity. Atelectasis can lead to pulmonary infection.

ASSESSMENT

The clinical picture is determined by the site of collapse, rate of development, and size of the affected area.

Signs and symptoms/physical findings: Pleuritic chest pain, tachypnea, shortness of breath, fever, dyspnea, decreased chest wall movement on affected side, dullness to percussion, decreased or absent breath sounds, crackles (rales) persisting after deep inspiration or cough, restlessness, agitation, change in level of consciousness (LOC), cyanosis.

DIAGNOSTIC TESTS

Oximetry: Bedside oximetry may demonstrate decreased O_2 saturation (92% or less).

Chest x-ray examination: Reveals higher density in affected lung, elevation of the hemidiaphragm on affected side, and compensatory hyperinflation of adjacent lobes on the opposite side.

Arterial blood gas (ABG) values: May reveal acute respiratory acidosis, with pH less than 7.35 and $PaCO_2$ greater than 45 mm Hg. PaO_2 may be less than 80 mm Hg, which is consistent with hypoxemia.

COLLABORATIVE MANAGEMENT

Management is aimed at preventing this condition in all patients. If atelectasis occurs and is left untreated, the affected lung area eventually may become infected, fibrotic, and functionless.

Deep-breathing and coughing exercises: Expand alveoli deep in the lungs and mobilize/clear secretions.

Chest physiotherapy: Mobilizes secretions.

Hyperinflation therapy: Expands partially collapsed lung areas and thereby improve gas exchange. Incentive spirometry may be used at the bedside.

Analgesics: Reduce pain and thereby facilitate production of an effective cough.

Bronchoscopy: Patient is intubated and a fiberoptic scope is passed into the bronchi to visualize the area and remove mucous plugs, retained secretions, or foreign objects.

O_2 therapy: Maintains PaO_2 greater than 80 mm Hg or within patient's normal baseline range.

Chest tube insertion: Provides reinflation of collapsed areas of the lung through a small-bore (8F-14F) tube connected to a one-way flutter valve or to a closed chest-drainage system if drainage of fluid is significant.

NURSING DIAGNOSES AND INTERVENTIONS
For Patients at Risk for Atelectasis

Ineffective breathing pattern related to decreased lung expansion secondary to inactivity or omission of deep breathing

Desired outcomes: Patient demonstrates deep breathing and effective coughing at least hourly and is eupneic (respiratory rate [RR] 12-20 breaths/min with normal depth and pattern) at all other times. Auscultation of patient's lungs reveals no adventitious sounds.

Nursing Interventions

- Auscultate breath sounds at least q2-4h (or as indicated by patient's condition) and during hyperinflation therapy. Report any decrease in breath sounds or presence of/increase in adventitious breath sounds.
- Instruct patient in use of hyperinflation device (e.g., incentive spirometer) to expand the lungs maximally.
  - Inhale slowly and deeply 2 × normal tidal volume.
  - Hold breath at least 5 sec at the end of inspiration.
  - Do this 10 × per hr to maintain adequate alveolar inflation.

Deep breathing expands the alveoli and aids in mobilizing secretions to the airways, and coughing further mobilizes and clears the secretions. Monitor patient's progress and document in nurses' notes.

- Administer analgesics as prescribed *to reduce pain and thereby facilitate coughing and deep-breathing exercises.*
- When appropriate, teach methods of splinting wounds or painful areas *to enable coughing and deep breathing.*
- Instruct patients who are unable to cough effectively in technique of cascade cough (i.e., succession of short and more forceful exhalations).
- Encourage frequent position changes and other activity as prescribed *to help mobilize secretions and promote effective airway clearance.* Use upright sitting position if permitted to promote good chest expansion.
- When not contraindicated, instruct patient to increase fluid intake (to more than 2.5 L/day) *to decrease viscosity of pulmonary secretions and facilitate their mobilization.*
- When appropriate, coordinate deep-breathing and coughing exercises with peak effectiveness of bronchodilator therapy *to maximize potential for mobilization of secretions.*

Patient-Family Teaching and Discharge Planning

Provide verbal and written information about the following:

♦ Use of hyperinflation device if patient is to continue this therapy at home. Conduct a predischarge check of patient's technique and document assessment in progress notes.

♦ Importance of maintaining activity level as prescribed.

♦ Importance of maintaining fluid intake of more than 2.5 L/day.

♦ Medications, including drug name, purpose, dosage, schedule, precautions, and potential side effects. Also discuss drug/drug, herb/drug, and food/drug interactions.

♦ Pain management techniques, such as medications and splinting.

♦ Precipitating factors in the development of atelectasis.

♦ Importance of notifying health care provider if signs and symptoms recur.

♦ Importance of medical follow-up. Review date and time of next appointment.

❖ PNEUMONIA

OVERVIEW/PATHOPHYSIOLOGY

Pneumonia is an acute bacterial or viral infection that causes inflammation of the lung parenchyma (alveolar spaces and interstitial tissue). As a result of the inflammation, involved lung tissue becomes edematous and air spaces fill with exudate (consolidation), gas exchange cannot occur, and nonoxygenated blood is shunted into the vascular system, with resulting hypoxemia. Bacterial pneumonias involve all or part of a lobe, whereas viral pneumonias appear diffusely throughout the lungs.

Influenza, which can cause pneumonia, is the most serious viral airway infection for adults. Patients more than 65 yr old, residents of extended care facilities, and individuals with chronic health conditions have the highest mortality from influenza.

Pneumonias usually are classified into two general types: community acquired and hospital associated (nosocomial). A third type now recognized is pneumonia in the immunocompromised individual.

Community acquired: Individuals with community-acquired pneumonia, the most common type, generally do not require hospitalization unless an underlying medical condition, such as chronic obstructive pulmonary disease (COPD), cardiac disease, or diabetes mellitus, or an immunocompromised state complicates the illness.

Hospital associated (nosocomial): Nosocomial pneumonias usually occur following aspiration of oropharyngeal flora or stomach contents in an individual whose resistance is altered or whose coughing mechanisms are impaired (e.g., a patient who has decreased level of consciousness (LOC), dysphagia, diminished gag reflex, or a nasogastric tube or who has undergone thoracoabdominal surgery or is on mechanical ventilation). Bacteria invade the lower respiratory tract via three routes: (1) gastric acid aspiration (the most common route), which causes toxic injury to the lung and makes it susceptible to bacterial growth; (2) partial obstruction of airway by a foreign body or fluids contaminated with bacteria; and (3) outright infection (rare occurrence). Gram-negative pneumonias are associated with a high mortality rate, even with appropriate antibiotic therapy. If the alveolar-capillary membrane is affected, acute respiratory distress syndrome (ARDS) (formerly known as adult respiratory distress syndrome) may develop.

Pneumonia in the immunocompromised individual: Immunosuppression and neutropenia are predisposing factors in the development of nosocomial pneumonias from both common and unusual pathogens. Severely immunocompromised patients are affected not only by bacteria but also by fungi

(Candida, Aspergillus), viruses (cytomegalovirus), and protozoa (*Pneumocystis jiroveci*, formerly known as *P. carinii*). Most commonly, *P. jiroveci* is seen in persons with human immunodeficiency virus (HIV) disease or in persons who are immunosuppressed therapeutically following organ transplants.

ASSESSMENT

Findings are influenced by patient's age, extent of the disease process, underlying medical condition, and pathogen involved. Generally, any factor that alters integrity of the lower airways, thereby inhibiting ciliary activity, increases the likelihood of developing pneumonia (**TABLE 2-1**).

Signs and symptoms/physical findings: Cough (productive and nonproductive), increased sputum production (rust colored, discolored, purulent, bloody, or mucoid), fever, pleuritic chest pain (more common in community-acquired bacterial pneumonias), dyspnea, chills, headache, myalgia, restlessness; anxiety; decreased skin turgor and dry mucous membranes secondary to dehydration; presence of nasal flaring and expiratory grunt; use of accessory muscles of respiration (scalene, sternocleidomastoid, external intercostals); decreased chest expansion caused by pleuritic pain; dullness on percussion over affected (consolidated) areas; tachypnea (respiratory rate [RR] more than 20 breaths/min); tachycardia (heart rate [HR] more than 90 beats per minute [bpm]); increased vocal fremitus; egophony ("e" to "a" change) over area of consolidation; decreased breath sounds; high-pitched and inspiratory crackles (rales) (increased by or heard only after coughing); low-pitched inspiratory crackles (rales) caused by airway secretions; and circumoral cyanosis (a late finding). Older adults may be confused or disoriented and have low-grade fevers but may present with few other signs and symptoms.

DIAGNOSTIC TESTS

Chest x-ray examination: Confirms presence of pneumonia (i.e., infiltrate appearing on the film).

Sputum for Gram stain and culture and sensitivity tests: Sputum is obtained from lower respiratory tract by endotracheal aspiration, protected catheter brush, or bronchoalveolar lavage (BAL) before initiation or change of antibiotic therapy to identify causative organism in cases of hospital-acquired pneumonia. For community-acquired pneumonias, this approach is recommended only if organism resistant to usual antibiotic therapy is suspected.

WBC count: Increased (more than 12,000/mm^3) in the presence of bacterial pneumonias. Normal or low WBC (less than 4000/mm^3) count may be seen with viral or mycoplasma pneumonias.

Chemistry panel: Detects presence of hypernatremia and/or hyperglycemia.

Blood culture and sensitivity: Determine presence of bacteremia and aid in identification of causative organism. Used in cases of hospital-acquired pneumonia and in seriously ill patients with community-acquired pneumonia.

Oximetry: May reveal decreased O_2 saturation (92% or less).

Arterial blood gas (ABG) values: May vary, depending on presence of underlying pulmonary or other debilitating disease. May demonstrate hypoxemia (PaO_2 less than 80 mm Hg) and hypocarbia ($PaCO_2$ less than 32-35 mm Hg), with resultant respiratory alkalosis (pH more than 7.45), in the absence of underlying pulmonary disease.

Serologic studies: Acute and convalescent antibody titers drawn to diagnose viral pneumonia. A relative rise in antibody titers suggests viral infection.

Acid-fast stains and cultures: Rule out tuberculosis (TB).

COLLABORATIVE MANAGEMENT

O_2 therapy: Administered when O_2 saturation or ABG results demonstrate hypoxemia. Goal is to maintain PaO_2 at 60 mm Hg or higher. Special consideration must be given to patients with chronic CO_2 retention because their

TABLE 2-1   ASSESSMENT GUIDELINES BY PNEUMONIA TYPE

TYPE/ PATHOGEN	RISK GROUPS	ONSET	DEFINING CHARACTERISTICS	COMPLICATIONS/COMMENTS
Community-Acquired				
Pneumococcal (*Streptococcus pneumoniae*)	Persons older than 40 yr, especially men; risk increased with alcoholism and debilitating diseases (e.g., COPD, heart failure, multiple myeloma, sickle cell disease); often preceded by viral URIs	Abrupt	Single shaking chill, fever, pleuritic chest pain, severe cough, shortness of breath, rust-colored sputum, diaphoresis; many patients also have herpes labialis; abdominal pain and distention, and paralytic ileus	Pleural effusions, empyema, impaired liver function, bacteremia, meningitis; incidence of pneumococcal pneumonia peaks in winter and early spring; mortality increases if more than one lobe involved
Mycoplasma (*Mycoplasma pneumoniae*)	School-aged children to young adults (5-30 yr); intrafamilial spread common	Gradual	Cough, sore throat, fever, headache, chills, malaise, anorexia, nausea, vomiting, diarrhea; in children arthralgias involving large joints common	Persistent cough and sinusitis possible; pulse-temperature dissociation common; Occurrence rare
Legionnaires' (*Legionella pneumophila*)	Middle-aged, elderly populations (men at increased risk); smokers; individuals with malignant disease, immunosuppression, or chronic renal failure; exposure to contaminated construction site	Abrupt	Malaise, headache within 24 hr, fever with normal HR, shaking chills, progressive dyspnea, cough that may become productive; GI symptoms, including anorexia, vomiting, diarrhea; arthralgias, myalgias	Respiratory failure, hypotension, shock, acute renal failure
Viral influenza A	Elderly persons with chronic diseases (e.g., COPD, diabetes mellitus, heart failure); pregnant women	1 wk after onset of influenza symptoms	Severe dyspnea; cyanosis; scant sputum, occasionally with blood; fever; persistent and dry cough	Rapid course leading frequently to acute respiratory failure; develops as secondary bacterial pneumonia
Haemophilus influenzae	Adults (especially 50 yr of age or older) with chronic diseases (e.g., diabetes mellitus, COPD, chronic alcohol ingestion)	2-6 wk after URI	Fever, chills, dyspnea, cough, nausea, vomiting, pain	Fever may be minimal or absent; HR and RR may be normal

Continued

TABLE 2-1	ASSESSMENT GUIDELINES BY PNEUMONIA TYPE—cont'd			
TYPE/ PATHOGEN	RISK GROUPS	ONSET	DEFINING CHARACTERISTICS	COMPLICATIONS/COMMENTS
Nosocomial *Klebsiella (Klebsiella pneumoniae)*; also may be acquired in the community	Men older than 40 yr, alcoholic patients; patients with diabetes mellitus, COPD, or heart disease; those previously treated with antibiotics or ET intubation	Abrupt	Chills, fever, productive cough (copious purulent green or "currant jelly" sputum), severe pleuritic chest pain, dyspnea, cyanosis, jaundice, vomiting, diarrhea	Lung abscess and empyema, necrotizing pneumonitis with cavitation, acute respiratory failure; high mortality (greater than 50%); aspiration of oropharyngeal flora is responsible for both nosocomial and community-acquired cases
Pseudomonas; also may be acquired in the community	Patients who are neutropenic from chemotherapy or immunosuppressed secondary to cortisone therapy or other illnesses	Gradual	Fever, chills, confusion, delirium, bradycardia, purulent sputum (green, foul smelling)	Rare in previously healthy adults; high mortality
Proteus	Older adults with debilitating underlying diseases	Abrupt	High fever, chills, pleuritic chest pain	Occurrence rare; localizes to areas already damaged; occurs as a mixed infection; associated with four pathogenic species with differing antibiotic susceptibilities
Staphylococcus aureus	Patients with debilitating diseases (e.g., diabetes mellitus, renal failure, liver disease, COPD); those with a prior viral or influenza infection; injecting drug users	Abrupt with community acquired; insidious with hospital associated	Cough, chills, high fever, pleuritic pain, progressive dyspnea, cyanosis, bloody sputum	Pulmonary abscesses, empyema, pleural effusions; slow response to antibiotics

Aspiration of gastric contents	Patients with impaired gag/cough reflexes; general anesthesia; presence of NG/ET tube	Gradual; latent period between aspiration and onset of symptoms	Fever, wheezes, crackles (rales), rhonchi, dyspnea, cyanosis	Physiologic response depends on pH contents of material aspirated: 2.5 or higher, little necrosis occurs; less than 2.5, atelectasis, pulmonary edema, hemorrhage, and necrosis can occur
Immunocompromised Patient				
Pneumocystis (*Pneumocystis jiroveci*; formerly known as *P. carinii*)	Patients with AIDS or organ transplants	Insidious	Several weeks of fever, nonproductive cough, night sweats, dyspnea; hypoxemia with few auscultatory signs	Bronchoscopy with transbronchial biopsy usually required for diagnosis
Aspergillosis (*Aspergillus*)	Patients with AIDS, COPD, and transplants (especially autologous bone marrow transplant); also those receiving cytotoxic agents or steroids	Abrupt with immunosuppression; insidious with COPD	High fever; fungal ball within lung cyst or cavity; nonproductive cough; pleuritic chest pain	Cavitation frequent; hematogenous spread common in immunocompromised patient

NOTE: *Enterobacter* and *Serratia* are enteric organisms that cause pneumonia with the same clinical pattern as *Klebsiella* organisms.

AIDS, Acquired immunodeficiency syndrome; *COPD,* chronic obstructive pulmonary disease; *ET,* endotracheal; *GI,* gastrointestinal; *HR,* heart rate; *NG,* nasogastric; *RR,* respiratory rate; *URI,* upper respiratory infection.

respiratory drive is stimulated by low/decreasing PaO_2 levels and not by increasing $PaCO_2$ levels as is normal. Therefore high concentrations of O_2 can depress respiration in these patients so O_2 is delivered in low concentrations initially, and O_2 saturations or ABG levels are monitored closely. If O_2 saturation or PaO_2 does not rise to acceptable levels (greater than 92% or 60 mm Hg or more, respectively), fraction of inspired O_2 (FIO_2) is increased in small increments, with concomitant checks of ABG values or O_2 saturations.

Antibiotic agents: Prescribed empirically based on presenting signs and symptoms, clinical findings, and chest x-ray results until sputum or blood culture results are available. Many organisms responsible for nosocomial pneumonias are resistant to multiple antibiotics. Proper identification of the organism and determination of sensitivity to specific antibiotics are critical for determining appropriate therapy.

A macrolide or levofloxacin is used for empirical out-patient treatment of community-acquired pneumonia; cephalosporins plus a macrolide and doxycycline are used for patients who are not in the ICU; IV beta-lactam and an IV quinolone or IV azithromycin are used for ICU patients.

Hospital-acquired pneumonia is empirically treated with IV ceftriaxone, or levofloxacin, or ampicillin/sulbactam or ertapenem if it is early onset and the patient has no risk factors for multidrug-resistant (MDR) disease; all other cases are treated initially with multiagent regimens. Vancomycin is added if risk of methicillin-resistant *Staphylococcus aureus* (MRSA) exists.

Hydration: IV fluids may be necessary to replace fluids lost from insensible sources (e.g., tachypnea, diaphoresis, fever) and decreased oral intake.

Percussion and postural drainage: Indicated if deep breathing and coughing are ineffective in mobilizing secretions.

Hyperinflation therapy: Prescribed for patients with inadequate inspiratory effort. (See p. 58)

Antitussives: Given in the absence of sputum production if coughing is continuous and exhausting to the patient.

Antipyretics and analgesics: Prescribed to reduce fever and provide relief from pleuritic pain or pain from coughing.

Vaccines

Pneumococcal vaccine: Administered to patients who have chronic health conditions and to those who are more than 65 yr old and/or are residents of an extended care facility and who have not received the vaccine within the last 5 yr. Vaccine history should be assessed on admission, and vaccine should be given to patients who meet criteria without contraindications (allergy).

Influenza vaccine: Administered to patients with chronic health conditions and to those who are more than 50 yr old and/or are residents of an extended care facility and who have not received the vaccine within the year. Influenza vaccines are routinely administered from October through March. Vaccine history should be assessed on admission, and vaccine should be given to patients who meet criteria without contraindications (e.g., allergy, history of Guillain-Barré syndrome).

Infection control: See discussion in Appendix 1, p. 743.

NURSING DIAGNOSES AND INTERVENTIONS
For Patients with Pneumonia

Impaired gas exchange related to altered O_2 supply and alveolar-capillary membrane changes secondary to inflammatory process in the lungs

Desired outcomes: Hospital discharge based on patient exhibiting at least five of the following indicators: temperature 37.8° C or less, HR 100 bpm or less, RR 24 breaths/min or less, SBP 90 mm Hg or more, O_2 saturation 90% or more, and ability to maintain oral intake.

Nursing Interventions

- Administer antibiotics within 4 hr of hospital admission *to reduce risk of death.*
- Observe for restlessness, anxiety, mental status changes, shortness of breath, tachypnea, and use of accessory muscles of respiration, all of *which are indicators of respiratory distress.* Remember that cyanosis of the lips and nail beds may be a late indicator of hypoxia.
- Monitor and document VS q2-4h. Be alert to a rising temperature and other changes in VS that *may indicate infection* (e.g., increased HR, increased RR).
- Auscultate breath sounds at least q2-4h or as indicated by patient's condition. Monitor for decreased or adventitious sounds (e.g., crackles, wheezes).
- Monitor oximetry readings; report O_2 saturation 92% or less *because this can indicate a need for O_2 therapy.*
- Monitor ABG results. A decreasing PaO_2 often indicates need for O_2 therapy.
- Position patient for comfort (usually semi-Fowler's position) *to promote diaphragmatic descent, maximize inhalation, and decrease work of breathing (WOB).* In patients with unilateral pneumonia, positioning on unaffected side (i.e., "good side down") *promotes ventilation/perfusion matching.*
- Deliver O_2 with humidity as prescribed; monitor oximetry or inspired concentration of oxygen (FIO_2) *to ensure that oxygen is within prescribed concentrations.* Be aware that patients with COPD may not tolerate O_2 at a delivery greater than 2 L/min, which can suppress the centrally mediated respiratory drive.
- Facilitate coordination among health care providers to provide rest periods between care activities *to decrease O_2 demand.* Allow 90 min for undisturbed rest.

Ineffective airway clearance related to presence of tracheobronchial secretions secondary to infection or related to pain and fatigue secondary to lung consolidation

Desired outcomes: Patient demonstrates effective cough. Following intervention, patient's airway is free of adventitious breath sounds.

Nursing Interventions

- Maintain a patent airway and ensure that secretions are removed. Suction as indicated/prescribed.
- Auscultate breath sounds q2-4h (or as indicated by patient's condition), and report changes in patient's ability to clear pulmonary secretions.
- Inspect sputum for quantity, odor, color, and consistency; document findings. As patient's condition worsens, sputum can change in color from clear → white → yellow → green, or it may show other discoloration characteristic of underlying bacterial infection (e.g., rust colored, "currant jelly").
- Ensure that patient performs deep-breathing with coughing exercises at least q2h. Assist patient into position of comfort, usually semi-Fowler's position, *to facilitate effectiveness and ease of these exercises.*
- Assess need for hyperinflation therapy (i.e., patient's inability to take deep breaths). Report complications of hyperinflation therapy to health care provider, including hyperventilation, gastric distention, headache, hypotension, and signs and symptoms of pneumothorax (shortness of breath, sharp chest pain, unilateral diminished breath sounds, dyspnea, cough).
- Teach patient to splint chest with pillow, folded blanket, or crossed arms when coughing, *to reduce pain.*
- Ensure that patient receives prescribed chest physiotherapy. Document patient's response to treatment.

◆ Assist patient with position changes q2h to help mobilize secretions. If the patient is ambulatory, encourage ambulation to patient's tolerance.
◆ When not contraindicated, encourage fluid intake (2.5 L/day or more) *to decrease sputum viscosity.*
◆ For other interventions, see "Atelectasis" for **Ineffective breathing pattern,** p. 58.

Deficient fluid volume related to increased insensible loss secondary to tachypnea, fever, or diaphoresis
Desired outcomes: At least 24 hr before hospital discharge, patient is normovolemic as evidenced by urine output 30 mL/hr or more, stable weight, HR less than 100 bpm, SBP greater than 90 mm Hg, fluid intake approximating fluid output, moist mucous membranes, and normal skin turgor.

Nursing Interventions

◆ Monitor I&O. Consider insensible losses if patient is diaphoretic and tachypneic. Be alert to urinary output less than 30 mL/hr or 0.5 mL/kg/hr; report urinary output less than 30 mL/hr.
◆ Weigh patient daily at the same time of day and on the same scale; record weight. Report weight decreases of 1-1.5 kg/day.
◆ Encourage fluid intake (at least 2.5 L/day in the unrestricted patient) *to ensure adequate hydration.*
◆ Maintain IV fluid therapy as prescribed.
◆ Promote oral hygiene, including lip and tongue care, *to moisten dried tissues and mucous membranes.*
◆ Provide humidity for O_2 therapy to decrease convective losses of moisture.

For Patients at Risk for Developing Pneumonia

Risk for infection (nosocomial pneumonia) related to inadequate primary defenses (e.g., decreased ciliary action), invasive procedures (e.g., intubation), and/or chronic disease
Desired outcome: Patient is free of infection as evidenced by normothermia, WBC count 12,000/mm^3 or less, and sputum clear to whitish.

Nursing Interventions

◆ Perform good handwashing technique before and after contact with patient (even though gloves are worn).
◆ Identify presurgical candidate who is at increased risk for nosocomial pneumonia because of the following: older adult (more than 70 yr), obesity, COPD, other chronic pulmonary conditions (e.g., asthma), history of smoking, abnormal pulmonary function tests (PFTs; especially decreased forced expiratory flow rate), intubation, and upper abdominal/thoracic surgery.
◆ Provide preoperative teaching; explain and demonstrate the following pulmonary activities that will be used postoperatively to prevent respiratory infection: deep breathing, coughing, turning in bed, splinting wounds, ambulating, maintaining adequate oral fluid intake, and using hyperinflation device. Make sure that patient verbalizes knowledge of the exercises and their rationale and returns demonstrations appropriately.
◆ Advise patients who smoke to discontinue smoking, especially during preoperative and postoperative periods. Refer to a community-based smoking cessation program as needed. When appropriate, discuss possibility of health care provider's prescription of transdermal nicotine patches to facilitate smoking cessation.
◆ Administer analgesics $\frac{1}{2}$ hr before deep-breathing exercises *to control pain, which interferes with lung expansion.* Scheduled analgesics also promote

pain control. Support (splint) surgical wound with hands, pillows, or folded blanket placed firmly across site of incision.

◆ Identify patients who are at increased risk for aspiration: individuals with depressed LOC, dysphagia, or nasogastric (NG) or enteral tube in place. Maintain head of bead (HOB) at 30-45-degree elevation, and turn patient onto side rather than back. When patient receives enteral alimentation, recommend continuous rather than bolus feedings. Hold feedings when patient is lying flat.

◆ Recognize risk factors for patients with tracheostomy: presence of underlying lung disease or other serious illness, increased colonization of oropharynx or trachea by aerobic gram-negative bacteria, greater access of bacteria to lower respiratory tract, and cross-contamination caused by manipulation of tracheostomy tube.

- Wear gloves on both hands until tracheostomy wound has healed or formed granulation tissue around the tube or when handling mechanical ventilation tubing.
- Suction prn rather than on a routine basis because frequent suctioning increases risk of trauma and cross-contamination.
- Use sterile catheter for each suctioning procedure. Consider use of closed suction system *to further minimize risk of contamination*; replace closed suction system if soiled, for mechanical failure, or per agency policy. Always avoid reusing a suction system for subsequent patients. Avoid saline instillation during suctioning. If patient has tenacious secretions, increase heat and humidity *to loosen them.*
- Always wear gloves on both hands to suction.
- Recognize the ways in which nebulizer reservoirs can contaminate patient: introduction of nonsterile fluids or air, manipulation of nebulizer cup, or backflow of condensate from delivery tubing into reservoir or into patient when tubing is manipulated.
- Use only sterile fluids and dispense them using sterile technique.
- Replace (rather than replenish) solutions and equipment at frequent intervals. For example, empty reservoir completely and refill with sterile solution q8-24h, per agency protocol.
- Change breathing circuits every week unless circuits are soiled, mechanical failure occurs, or agency policy states otherwise.
- Fill fluid reservoirs immediately before use (not far in advance).
- Discard any fluid that has condensed in tubing; do not allow fluid to drain back into reservoir or into patient.

 ## Patient-Family Teaching and Discharge Planning

Provide verbal and written information about the following:

◆ Techniques that mobilize secretions and promote gas.

◆ Medications, including drug names, purpose, dosage, frequency or schedule, precautions, and potential side effects, particularly of antibiotics. Also discuss drug/drug, herb/drug, and food/drug interactions. Instruct patient to complete full regimen of antibiotics to prevent reinfection and subsequent readmission.

◆ Signs and symptoms of pneumonia and importance of reporting them promptly if they recur. Teach patient's significant others that changes in mental status may be the only indicator of pneumonia if patient is elderly.

◆ Importance of preventing fatigue by pacing activities and allowing frequent rest periods.

◆ Importance of avoiding exposure to individuals known to have flu and colds. Recommend that patient receive pneumococcal vaccination and annual influenza vaccination.

- Minimizing factors that can cause reinfection, including close living conditions, poor nutrition, and poorly ventilated living quarters or work environment.
- Importance of smoking cessation education and community resources to assist in cessation.
- Phone numbers to call if questions or concerns arise about therapy or disease after discharge. Additional general information can be obtained from the American Lung Association at www.lungusa.org.
- Information about the free brochures that discuss ways to stop smoking such as the following:
  How to Help Your Patients Stop Using Tobacco: A National Cancer Institute Manual for the Oral Health Team, from the Smoking and Tobacco Control Program of the National Cancer Institute; call (800) 4-CANCER.

❖ PLEURAL EFFUSION

OVERVIEW/PATHOPHYSIOLOGY

A pleural effusion is an accumulation of fluid (blood, pus, chyle, serous fluid) in the pleural space. Generally, fluid gravitates to the most dependent area of the thorax, and the adjacent lung becomes compressed. Pleural effusion is rarely a disease in itself, but rather it is caused by a number of inflammatory, circulatory, or neoplastic diseases. Transudate effusion results from changes in hydrodynamic forces in the circulation and usually is caused by heart failure (increased hydrostatic pressure) or cirrhosis (decreased colloidal osmotic pressure). Exudate effusion results from irritation of the pleural membranes secondary to inflammatory, infective, or malignant processes. More exact nomenclature can be used once the nature of the fluid in the pleural effusion has been identified, that is, hydrothorax (a transudate or exudate of serous fluid), pyothorax or empyema (collection of purulent material), hemothorax (bloody fluid), or chylothorax (effused chyle).

ASSESSMENT

Clinical indicators of pleural effusion are related to the underlying disease. Patients with a small effusion (less than 300 mL) may be asymptomatic.

Signs and symptoms/physical findings: Pleuritic chest or shoulder pain, diaphoresis, cough, fever, dyspnea, orthopnea, decreased breath sounds, dullness to percussion, decreased tactile fremitus, egophony ("e" to "a" change) over effusion site, tracheal deviation away from affected side, and pleural friction rub.

DIAGNOSTIC TESTS

Chest x-ray examination: Shows evidence of effusion if more than 300 mL of fluid is in the pleural space. With effusion greater than 1000 mL, the x-ray film may show mediastinal shift away from the affected lung.

Chest computed tomography (CT): Enables imaging of the entire pleural space, pulmonary parenchyma, and mediastinum simultaneously. CT assists in differentiation between lung consolidation and pleural effusion.

Thoracentesis: Removal of fluid from the pleural space for examination to provide definitive diagnosis and determine type of effusion.

Percutaneous pleural biopsy: Aids in diagnosing cause of effusion especially when tuberculosis (TB) or malignant disease is suspected.

COLLABORATIVE MANAGEMENT

Therapeutic thoracentesis: Removes fluid and thereby allows lung to reexpand. Rate of recurrence and time span for return of symptoms are recorded.

Chest tube insertion: Provides continuous drainage of larger effusions through 26F-30F catheter connected to closed chest-drainage system.

Sclerosing pleurodesis: Produces pleural fibrosis and symphysis (line of fusion between visceral and parietal pleural layers) by instillation of sclerosing agent (tetracycline, bleomycin, or nitrogen mustard) via chest tube.

NURSING DIAGNOSES AND INTERVENTIONS

Ineffective breathing pattern related to decreased lung expansion secondary to fluid accumulation in the pleural space

Desired outcome: Following intervention, patient's breathing pattern moves toward eupnea.

Nursing Interventions

- Auscultate breath sounds q2-4h (or as indicated by patient's condition), and monitor for decreasing breath sounds or presence of pleural friction rub.
- Monitor oximetry readings; report O_2 saturation 92% or less *because this can indicate need for O_2 therapy.*
- Ensure patency of chest drainage system (see guidelines, p. 79, in "Pneumothorax/Hemothorax").
- Position patient for maximum chest expansion, generally semi-Fowler's position.
- If hyperinflation therapy is prescribed, instruct patient in its use and document patient's progress.
- For patients with gross pleural effusion, provide the following instructions for apical expansion breathing exercise:
  - Sit upright.
  - Position fingers just below the clavicles.
  - Inhale and attempt to push upper chest wall against pressure of the fingers.
  - Hold breath for a few seconds, and then exhale passively.
  - When performed at frequent intervals, this exercise will help expand the involved lung tissues, minimize flattening of the upper chest, and mobilize secretions.

 Patient-Family Teaching and Discharge Planning

Provide verbal and written information about the following:

- Importance of smoking cessation. Provide patient with resources related to community smoking cessation programs. When appropriate, discuss possibility of health care provider's prescription of transdermal nicotine patches to facilitate smoking cessation.
- Signs of respiratory distress, such as restlessness, mental status changes, agitation, changes in behavior, and complaints of shortness of breath or dyspnea, and importance of rapidly notifying health care provider if these signs occur.
- Use of equipment at home (e.g., hyperinflation device, nebulizer, O_2).
- Medications, including drug names, dosage, purpose, schedule, precautions, and potential side effects. Also discuss drug/drug, herb/drug, and food/drug interactions.

❖ PULMONARY EMBOLISM

OVERVIEW/PATHOPHYSIOLOGY

The most common pulmonary perfusion abnormality is pulmonary embolism (PE). PE is caused by passage of a foreign substance (blood clot, fat, air, or amniotic fluid) into the pulmonary artery or its branches, with resulting obstruction of the blood supply to lung tissue and subsequent collapse. The most common source is a dislodged blood clot from the systemic circulation, typically the deep veins of the legs or pelvis. Thrombus formation is the result of the following factors: blood stasis, alterations in clotting factors, and injury to vessel walls. A fat embolus is the most common nonthrombotic cause of pulmonary perfusion disorders (see p. 74).

Total obstruction leading to pulmonary infarction is rare because the pulmonary circulation has multiple sources of blood supply. Early diagnosis and appropriate treatment reduce mortality to less than 10%. Although most cases of PE resolve completely with no residual deficits, some patients may be left with chronic pulmonary hypertension.

ASSESSMENT

Signs and symptoms/physical findings: Often nonspecific and variable, depending on extent of obstruction and whether patient has infarction as a result of the obstruction.

Sudden onset of dyspnea and sharp chest pain, restlessness, anxiety, nonproductive cough or hemoptysis, palpitations, nausea, syncope, tachypnea, tachycardia, hypotension, crackles (rales), decreased chest wall excursion secondary to splinting, S_3 and S_4 gallop rhythms, transient pleural friction rub, jugular venous distention, diaphoresis, edema, and cyanosis.

If infarction has occurred, fever, pleuritic chest pain, and hemoptysis are common.

History and risk factors

Immobility: Especially significant when it coexists with surgical or nonsurgical trauma, carcinoma, or cardiopulmonary disease. Risk increases as duration of immobility increases.

Cardiac disorders: Atrial fibrillation, heart failure, myocardial infarction, rheumatic heart disease.

Surgery: Risk increases in postoperative period, especially for patients with orthopedic, pelvic, thoracic, or abdominal surgery and for those with extensive burns or musculoskeletal injuries of the hip or knee.

Pregnancy: Especially during postpartum period.

Chronic pulmonary and infectious diseases

Trauma: Especially lower extremity fractures and burns. Degree of risk is related to severity, site, and extent of trauma.

Mechanical ventilation: Risk increases because of immobility and inflammatory processes.

Carcinoma: Particularly neoplasms involving the breast, lung, pancreas, and genitourinary and alimentary tracts.

Obesity: A 20% increase in ideal body weight is associated with increased incidence of PE.

Varicose veins or prior thromboembolic disease

Age: Risk of thromboembolism is greatest for patients 55-65 yr of age.

DIAGNOSTIC TESTS

Arterial blood gas (ABG) values: Hypoxemia (PaO_2 less than 80 mm Hg), hypocarbia ($PaCO_2$ less than 35 mm Hg), and respiratory alkalosis (pH more than 7.45) usually are present. Normal values do not rule out PE.

D-dimer: A degradation product produced by plasmin-mediated proteolysis of cross-linked fibrin and measured by enzyme-linked immunosorbent assay (ELISA). The higher the result (with less than 250 ng/mL considered negative in most laboratories), the more likely it is patient has PE. This test is not sensitive or specific enough to diagnose PE, but it may be used in conjunction with other diagnostic tests.

Cardiac troponin level: Elevated in PE as a result of right ventricular dilation and myocardial injury.

Chest x-ray examination: Initially findings are usually normal, or elevated hemidiaphragm may be present. After 24 hr, x-ray examination may reveal small infiltrates secondary to atelectasis that result from the decrease in surfactant. If pulmonary infarction is present, infiltrates and pleural effusions may be seen within 12-36 hr.

ECG results: Abnormal in 85% of patients with PE.

Spiral or helical computed tomography (CT): Images pulmonary arteries (PAs) during a single breath. Spiral CT is rapidly becoming the test of choice in diagnosing PE because of its higher specificity and sensitivity.

Pulmonary ventilation/perfusion scan: Used to detect abnormalities of ventilation or perfusion in the pulmonary system. Radiopaque agents are inhaled and injected peripherally. Images of distribution of both agents throughout the lung are scanned. If the scan shows a mismatch of ventilation and perfusion (i.e., pattern of normal ventilation with decreased perfusion), vascular obstruction is suggested.

Pulmonary angiography: Definitive study for PE: An invasive procedure that involves catheterization of right side of the heart and injection of dye into the PA to visualize pulmonary vessels. Abrupt vessel "cutoff" may be seen at the site of embolization. Usually, filling defects are seen. More specific findings are abnormal blood vessel diameters (i.e., obstruction of right PA would cause dilation of left PA) and abnormal blood vessel shapes (i.e., affected blood vessel may taper to a sharp point and disappear).

COLLABORATIVE MANAGEMENT

The three goals of therapy are (1) prophylaxis for individuals at risk for development of PE, (2) treatment during acute embolic event, and (3) prevention of future embolic events in individuals who have experienced PE.

O_2 therapy: Delivered at appropriate concentration to maintain a PaO_2 of more than 60 mm Hg or O_2 saturation greater than 90%.

Anticoagulation

Low molecular weight heparin (LMWH) or unfractionated heparin (UFH) therapy: Started immediately in patients without bleeding or clotting disorders and in whom PE is strongly suspected with the aim of inhibiting further thrombus growth, promoting resolution of the formed thrombus, and preventing further embolus formation. Continued for at least 5 days to allow for depletion of thrombin.

LMWH: Preferred to UFH because of more predictable dosing, fewer side effects, once- or twice-daily subcutaneous administration, and lack of need to monitor activated partial thromboplastin time. Dose is weight based and differs for various LMWH preparations. Dose must be adjusted for individuals with renal impairment because most LMWH is excreted by the kidneys. LMWH has been shown to be safe if given during pregnancy.

UFH: Has shorter half-life than LMWH and effect is completely reversible with protamine. Ideally, dosage is weight based (e.g., IV bolus of 80 units/kg followed by a maintenance dose of 18 units/kg/hr). Alternatively, an initial IV bolus of 5000-10,000 units followed by continuous infusion of 1000 units/hr may be given. Effect is monitored by activated partial thromboplastin time (aPTT) measurements every 6 hr after initial dose until the goal of 1.5 to 2.5 × control value is consistently established.

Oral anticoagulant (warfarin sodium) therapy: Begun on initiation of heparin therapy and given simultaneously to allow time for warfarin to inhibit vitamin K–dependent clotting factors before heparin or LMWH is discontinued. Used long term (3-6 mo, longer if significant risk factors are present). Initial dose, usually 10 mg/day, is based on prothrombin time (PT) with the goal of 1.25-1.50 × normal or international normalized ratio (INR) of 2.0-3.0. When an INR of 2.0-3.0 is obtained, UFH or LMWH can be discontinued. PT measurements are monitored daily.

Vitamin K (vitamin K_1, [phytonadione]or K_3 [menadione]): Reverses effects of warfarin in 24-36 hr. Fresh frozen plasma may be required in cases of serious bleeding. Warfarin crosses the placental barrier and can cause spontaneous abortion and birth defects.

Thrombolytic therapy: May be given in the first 24-48 hr after diagnosis of PE to speed the process of clot lysis via conversion of plasminogen to plasmin. Thrombolytic therapy may be preferred for initial treatment of PE in patients with hemodynamic compromise, with greater than 30% occlusion of pulmonary vasculature, and in whom therapy has been initiated no later than 3 days after onset of PE. Thrombin time is measured q4h during therapy to ensure adequate response, which should be 2-5 × normal. Partial thromboplastin time (PTT) can be used instead of thrombin time and should be 2-5 × control. Once thrombolytic therapy is stopped, thrombin time or PTT should be checked frequently until values fall to less than 2 × normal. When this occurs, heparin therapy is started and continued as described earlier. As many as 33% of patients receiving thrombolytic therapy have hemorrhagic complications.

Contraindications to thrombolytic therapy include active internal bleeding, recent stroke, intracranial bleeding within 2 mo of PE, intraspinal surgery, trauma, arteriovenous malformation, aneurysm, uncontrolled hypertension (DBP higher than 110 mm Hg or SBP higher than 185 mm Hg), pregnancy, and status less than 10 days post partum.

Surgical interventions: Used only in select cases because anticoagulant therapy is usually successful.

VENA CAVAL INTERRUPTION: Uses a filter approved by the U.S. Food and Drug Administration (FDA) to prevent passage of venous thrombi through the inferior vena cava. The following FDA-approved filters may be used: Greenfield, Venatech, Simon Nitinol, and Bird's Nest.

PULMONARY EMBOLECTOMY: Removes clots from the pulmonary circulation. Generally, use of thrombolytic agents eliminates need for this procedure.

NURSING DIAGNOSES AND INTERVENTIONS

Impaired gas exchange related to altered O_2 supply secondary to ventilation/perfusion mismatch

Desired outcomes: Following intervention/treatment, patient exhibits adequate gas exchange and ventilatory function as evidenced by respiratory rate (RR) of 12-20 breaths/min with normal pattern and depth (eupnea); no significant changes in mental status; and orientation to person, place, and time. At least 24 hr before hospital discharge, patient has O_2 saturation greater than 90% or PaO_2 80 mm Hg or higher, $PaCO_2$ 35-45 mm Hg, and pH 7.35-7.45 (or values consistent with patient's acceptable baseline parameters).

Nursing Interventions

◆ Monitor for signs and symptoms of increasing respiratory distress: RR increased from baseline; increasing dyspnea, anxiety, restlessness, confusion, and cyanosis.

◆ As indicated, monitor oximetry readings; report O_2 saturation 90% or less *because this can indicate need for O_2 therapy.*

◆ Position patient for comfort and optimal gas exchange. Ensure that area of the lung affected by embolus is not dependent when patient is in lateral decubitus position. Elevate head of bed (HOB) 30 degrees *to improve ventilation.*

◆ Avoid positioning patient with knees bent (i.e., gatching bed) *because this impedes venous return from legs and can increase risk of PE.* Instruct patient not to cross legs when lying in bed or sitting in a chair.

◆ Limit or pace patient's activities and procedures *to decrease metabolic demands for O_2.*

◆ Ensure that patient performs deep-breathing and coughing exercises 3-5 × q2h to maximize ventilation.

- Ensure delivery of prescribed concentrations and humidity of O_2.
- Monitor serial ABG values and assess for desired response to treatment. Report lack of response to treatment or worsening ABG values.

Ineffective protection related to risk of prolonged bleeding or hemorrhage secondary to anticoagulation therapy
Desired outcomes: Patient is free of frank or occult bleeding; body secretions/excretions test negative for blood.

Nursing Interventions

- Monitor VS for indicators of profuse bleeding or hemorrhage resulting from anticoagulant therapy: hypotension, tachycardia, tachypnea.
- At least once each shift inspect wounds, oral mucous membranes, any entry site of an invasive procedure, and nares for evidence of bleeding.
- At least once each shift inspect torso and extremities for petechiae or ecchymoses.
- *To prevent hematoma formation,* do not give intramuscular (IM) injection unless it is unavoidable. If parenteral medications are mandatory, attempt to administer subcutaneously using a small-gauge needle.
- Apply pressure to all venipuncture or arterial puncture sites until bleeding stops completely.
- Ensure easy access to the following antidotes for prescribed treatment:
  - *Protamine sulfate:* 1 mg counteracts 100 units of heparin, so 1 mg of protamine sulfate is administered for every 100 units of heparin in the body.
  - *Vitamin K (vitamin K_1 [phytonadione] or K_3 [menadione]):* Low doses— 2.5 mg PO or 0.5-1 mg IV—are generally used to control bleeding without hindering restoration of anticoagulation.
  - Fresh frozen plasma.
- If patient is receiving heparin therapy, monitor serial aPTT (desired range is 1.5-2.5 × control). If patient is receiving warfarin therapy, monitor serial PT (desired range is 1.25-1.5 × control, or INR value of 2.0-3.0). Report values outside desired range.
- *To prevent negative interactions with anticoagulants or thrombolytic therapy,* establish compatibility of all drugs before administering them.
  - *Heparin:* Digitalis, tetracycline, nicotine, and antihistamines decrease the effect of heparin therapy. Consult pharmacist about compatibility before infusing other IV drugs through heparin IV line.
  - *Warfarin sodium:* Numerous drugs decrease or increase response to treatment with warfarin. Consult pharmacist to obtain specific information about patient's medication profile. Antibiotics routinely increase INR levels, check with the pharmacist for drug interactions.
  - *Thrombolytic therapy:* Consult pharmacist before infusing any other medication through the same IV line.
- *Because aspirin and nonsteroidal antiinflammatory drugs (NSAIDs) are platelet aggregation inhibitors and can prolong episodes of bleeding,* use these medications cautiously.
- Discuss with patient and significant others the importance of reporting promptly the presence of bleeding from any of the following sources: hematuria, melena, frank bleeding from the mouth, epistaxis, hemoptysis, excessive vaginal bleeding (menometrorrhagia).
- Teach necessity of using sponge-tipped applicators and mouthwash for oral care *to minimize risk of gum bleeding.* Instruct patient to shave with electric rather than straight or safety razor.
- If patient is restless and combative, provide a safe environment. Use extreme care when moving patient *to avoid bumping patient's extremities into side rails and causing bleeding.*

Deficient knowledge related to oral anticoagulant therapy, potential side effects, and foods and medications to avoid during therapy
Desired outcome: Before hospital discharge, patient verbalizes knowledge of prescribed anticoagulant drug, potential side effects, and foods and medications to avoid while receiving oral anticoagulant therapy.

Nursing Interventions

◆ Assess patient's facility with language; engage an interpreter or language-appropriate written materials if necessary.
◆ Determine patient's knowledge of oral anticoagulant therapy. As appropriate, discuss drug name, purpose, dose, schedule, precautions, and potential side effects. Also discuss food/drug, herb/drug, and drug/drug interactions.
◆ Teach potential side effects/complications of anticoagulant therapy: easy bruising, prolonged bleeding from cuts, spontaneous nosebleeds, bleeding gums, black and tarry or bloody stools, vaginal bleeding, and blood in urine and sputum.
◆ Discuss importance of laboratory testing and follow-up visits with health care provider.
◆ Explain importance of informing all health care providers (including dentist) that patient is taking an anticoagulant. Suggest that patient wear a MedicAlert tag or otherwise carry identification *to alert health care providers about the anticoagulant therapy.*
◆ Teach patient to notify doctor if diet contains large amounts of foods high in vitamin K (e.g., fish, bananas, dark-green vegetables, tomatoes, cauliflower), *which can interfere with anticoagulation.*
◆ Caution patient that soft-bristled rather than hard-bristled toothbrush and electric rather than straight or safety razor should be used during anticoagulant therapy *to minimize risk of injury that could cause bleeding.*
◆ Instruct patient to consult health care provider before taking over-the-counter (OTC) or prescribed drugs that were used before initiating anticoagulant therapy. Aspirin, cimetidine, trimethaphan, and macrolides are among the many drugs that enhance response to warfarin. Drugs that decrease response include antacids, diuretics, oral contraceptives, and barbiturates.

Patient-Family Teaching and Discharge Planning

Reinforce patient teaching about oral anticoagulant therapy (see **Deficient knowledge**). Also provide verbal and written information about the following:
◆ Risk factors related to development of thrombi and embolization and preventive measures to reduce the risk.
◆ Signs and symptoms of thrombophlebitis: calf swelling; tenderness or warmth in the involved area; possible presence of pain in affected calf when ankle is dorsiflexed; slight fever; and distention of distal veins, coolness, edema, and pale color in the distal affected leg.
◆ Signs and symptoms of PE: sudden onset of dyspnea, anxiety, nonproductive cough or hemoptysis, palpitations, nausea, syncope.
◆ Importance of preventing impairment of venous return from the lower extremities by avoiding prolonged sitting, crossing legs, and wearing constrictive clothing.

FAT EMBOLISM

Fat embolism is the most common type of nonthrombotic PE. Free fatty acids cause toxic vasculitis, followed by thrombosis and obstruction of small pulmonary arteries by fat.

Assessment

Signs and symptoms/physical findings: Typically, patient is asymptomatic for 12-24 hr following embolization. This period ends with sudden cardiopulmonary and neurologic deterioration: apprehension, restlessness,

mental status changes, confusion, delirium, coma, dyspnea, tachypnea, tachycardia, and hypertension; fever; petechiae, especially of conjunctivae, neck,
upper torso, axillae, and proximal arms; inspiratory crowing; pulmonary
edema; profuse tracheobronchial secretions; fat globules in sputum; and
expiratory wheezes.

History and risk factors: Multiple long bone fractures, especially fractures
of the femur and pelvis; trauma to adipose tissue or liver; burns; osteomyelitis;
sickle cell crisis.

Diagnostic Tests

ABG values: Should be determined in patients at risk for fat embolus for the
first 48 hr following injury because early hypoxemia indicative of fat embolus
is apparent only with laboratory assessment. Hypoxemia (PaO_2 less than
80 mm Hg) and hypercarbia ($PaCO_2$ more than 45 mm Hg) are present with
respiratory acidosis (pH less than 7.35).

Chest x-ray examination: Pattern similar to that in acute respiratory distress
syndrome (ARDS) is seen: diffuse, extensive bilateral interstitial and alveolar
infiltrates.

Complete blood count (CBC): May reveal decreased hemoglobin (Hgb) and
hematocrit (Hct) secondary to hemorrhage into the lung. In addition, thrombocytopenia (platelets $150,000/mm^3$ or less) is indicative of fat embolism.

Serum lipase: Value rises with fat embolism.

Urinalysis: May reveal fat globules following fat embolus.

Collaborative Management

O_2: Concentration of O_2 is based on clinical picture, ABG results, and
patient's prior respiratory status. Intubation and mechanical ventilation may
be required.

Diuretics: Approximately 30% of patients with fat emboli develop pulmonary edema that necessitates use of diuretics.

Nursing Diagnoses and Interventions

See **Impaired gas exchange** on p. 72.

❖ PNEUMOTHORAX/HEMOTHORAX

OVERVIEW/PATHOPHYSIOLOGY OF PNEUMOTHORAX

Pneumothorax is an accumulation of air in the pleural space that leads to
increased intrapleural pressure. Risk factors include blunt or penetrating chest
injury, chronic obstructive pulmonary disease (COPD), previous pneumothorax, and positive-pressure ventilation. The three types of pneumothorax are
as follows:

Spontaneous: Also referred to as closed pneumothorax because the chest
wall remains intact with no leak to the atmosphere. It results from rupture of
a bleb or bulla on the visceral pleural surface, usually near the apex. Generally,
the cause of the rupture is unknown, although it may result from a weakness
related to a respiratory infection or from an underlying pulmonary disease
(e.g., COPD, tuberculosis (TB), malignant neoplasm). The affected individual
is usually young (20-40 yr), previously healthy, and male. Onset of symptoms
usually occurs at rest rather than with vigorous exercise or coughing. Potential
for recurrence is great; the second pneumothorax occurs an average of 2-3 yr
after the first.

Traumatic: Can be open or closed. An open pneumothorax occurs when air
enters the pleural space from the atmosphere through an opening in the chest
wall, such as with a gunshot wound, stab wound, or invasive medical procedure (e.g., thoracentesis or placement of a central line into a subclavian vein).
A sucking sound may be heard over the area of penetration during inspiration,
a feature that accounts for the classic wound description as a "sucking chest

wound." A closed traumatic pneumothorax occurs when the visceral pleura is penetrated but the chest wall remains intact with no atmospheric leak. This usually occurs following blunt trauma that results in rib fracture and dislocation. It also may occur from use of positive end-expiratory pressure (PEEP) or after cardiopulmonary resuscitation (CPR).

Tension: Generally occurs with closed pneumothorax; also can occur with open pneumothorax when a flap of tissue acts as a one-way valve. Air enters the pleural space through the pleural tear when the individual inhales, and it continues to accumulate but cannot escape during expiration because the tissue flap closes. With tension pneumothorax, as pressure in the thorax and mediastinum increases, it produces a shift in the affected lung and mediastinum toward the unaffected side that further impairs ventilatory efforts. The increase in pressure also compresses the vena cava. This compression impedes venous return and leads to a decrease in cardiac output and ultimately to circulatory collapse if the condition is not diagnosed and treated quickly. Tension pneumothorax is a life-threatening medical emergency.

OVERVIEW/PATHOPHYSIOLOGY OF HEMOTHORAX

Hemothorax is an accumulation of blood in the pleural space. Hemothorax generally results from blunt trauma to the chest wall, but it also can occur following thoracic surgery, after penetrating gunshot or stab wounds, as a result of anticoagulant therapy, after insertion of a central venous catheter, or following various thoracoabdominal organ biopsies. Mediastinal shift, ventilatory compromise, and lung collapse can occur, depending on the amount of blood accumulated.

ASSESSMENT

Signs and symptoms/physical findings vary, depending on type and size of the pneumothorax or hemothorax (**TABLE 2-2**).

DIAGNOSTIC TESTS

Chest x-ray examination: Reveals presence of air or blood in the pleural space on the affected side, pneumothorax/hemothorax size, and any shift in the trachea and mediastinum.

Arterial blood gas (ABG) values: Hypoxemia (PaO_2 less than 80 mm Hg) may be accompanied by hypercarbia ($PaCO_2$ greater than 45 mm Hg) with resultant respiratory acidosis (pH less than 7.35). Arterial O_2 saturation may be decreased initially but usually returns to normal within 24 hr.

Oximetry: Reveals decreased O_2 saturation (90% or less).

CBC: May reveal decreased Hgb proportionate to amount of blood lost in the hemothorax.

COLLABORATIVE MANAGEMENT

Management is determined by signs and symptoms. A small pneumothorax (less than 20%) may heal itself via reabsorption of the free air and may thereby render invasive procedures unnecessary unless an underlying disease process or injury is present. Hemothorax nearly always requires intervention.

O_2 therapy: Administered when ABG values or oximetry demonstrates presence of hypoxemia, which usually occurs when the pneumothorax/hemothorax is large. 100% O_2 may be administered to speed reabsorption of a pneumothorax.

Thoracentesis/air aspiration: Used for hemothorax to remove blood from the pleural space. For cases of tension pneumothorax, thoracentesis/air aspiration is performed immediately to remove air from the pleural space. A large-bore needle is inserted in the second intercostal space, midclavicular line, which correlates to the superior portion of the anterior axillary lobe. A sudden rushing out of air confirms the diagnosis of tension pneumothorax. Following release of entrapped air, chest tubes are inserted. Air aspiration may be done

TABLE 2-2		SIGNS AND SYMPTOMS/PHYSICAL FINDINGS WITH PNEUMOTHORAX OR HEMOTHORAX	
SPONTANEOUS OR TRAUMATIC PNEUMOTHORAX			
CLOSED	**OPEN**	**TENSION PNEUMOTHORAX**	**HEMOTHORAX**
Signs and Symptoms			
Shortness of breath, cough, chest tightness, chest pain	Shortness of breath, sharp chest pain	Dyspnea, chest pain	Dyspnea, chest pain
Physical Assessment			
Tachypnea, decreased thoracic movement, cyanosis, subcutaneous emphysema, hyperresonance over affected area, diminished breath sounds, paradoxical movement of chest wall (may signal flail chest), change in mental status	Agitation, restlessness, tachypnea, cyanosis, presence of chest wound, hyperresonance over affected area, sucking sound on inspiration, diminished breath sounds, change in mental status	Anxiety, tachycardia, cyanosis, jugular vein distention, tracheal deviation toward the unaffected side, absent breath sounds on affected side, distant heart sounds, hypotension, change in mental status	Tachypnea, pallor, cyanosis, dullness over affected side, tachycardia, hypotension, diminished or absent breath sounds, change mental status

when a pneumothorax is large enough to allow lung reexpansion; if only partial reexpansion occurs, a one-way valve may be attached to the thoracentesis catheter to allow for outpatient management.

Chest tube placement (tube thoracostomy): A chest tube (thoracic catheter) may be inserted in any patient who is symptomatic. During insertion the patient should be in an upright position so that the lung falls away from the chest wall. Thoracic catheter positioning depends on whether air, fluid, or both are to be drained. The thoracic catheter must be connected to an underwaterseal drainage system, dry suction system, or one-way flutter valve device. Suction may be used, depending on size of the pneumothorax or hemothorax, patient's condition, and amount of drainage. If drainage is minimal and no suction is required, a one-way flutter valve may be used instead of an underwaterseal drainage system or dry suction. After chest tube insertion and removal of air or fluid from the pleural space, the lung begins to reexpand. A chest tube may produce pleural inflammation, causing pleuritic pain, slight temperature elevation, and pleural friction rub.

Thoracotomy: Often indicated in patients who have had two or more spontaneous pneumothoraces on one side because of risk of continuous recurrence or if pneumothorax does not resolve within 7 days. With hemothorax, thoracotomy is performed to locate the source and control bleeding if blood loss is excessive. Thoracotomy may include mechanical abrasion of the pleural surfaces with a dry sterile sponge or chemical abrasion via an agent such as tetracycline solution or talc, which results in pleural adhesions (pleurodesis) that help prevent recurrence of pneumothorax. Partial pleurectomy may be performed instead of mechanical or chemical abrasion.

Video-assisted thoracic surgery (VATS): Performed in the operating room while patient is under general anesthesia. A small thoracoscope is inserted through a small chest incision. Pleural fluid is removed and pleural biopsy samples may be obtained. A chest tube is inserted and connected to suction for further drainage.

Chemical pleurodesis: Instillation of a sclerosing agent (e.g., tetracycline, talc) into the pleural cavity to produce adhesions and a line of fusion between visceral and parietal pleural layers.

IV therapy: Administered if significant loss of fluids or blood occurs.

Analgesia: Because of rich innervation of the pleura, chest tube placement or pleurodesis is painful, and significant analgesia is usually required.

NURSING DIAGNOSES AND INTERVENTIONS

Impaired gas exchange related to altered O_2 supply secondary to ventilation/perfusion mismatch

Desired outcomes: Following treatment/intervention, patient exhibits adequate gas exchange and ventilatory function as evidenced by respiratory rate (RR) 20 breaths/min or less with normal depth and pattern (eupnea); no significant mental status changes; and orientation to person, place, and time. At a minimum of 24 hr before hospital discharge, patient's ABG values are as follows: Pao_2 80 mm Hg or more and $Paco_2$ 35-45 mm Hg (or values within patient's acceptable baseline parameters), or oximetry readings demonstrate O_2 saturation greater than 90%.

Nursing Interventions

- Monitor serial ABG results to detect decreasing Pao_2 and increasing $Paco_2$, *which can signal impending respiratory compromise,* or monitor oximetry readings for O_2 saturation 90% or less. Report significant findings.
- Observe for increased restlessness, anxiety, tachycardia, and changes in mental status. Cyanosis may be a late sign. These signs indicate hypoxia.
- Assess VS and breath sounds q2h or as indicated by patient's condition.
- Following tube or exploratory thoracotomy, check q15min until stable for increased RR, diminished or absent movement of chest wall on affected side, paradoxical movement of the chest wall, increased work of breathing (WOB), use of accessory muscles of respiration, complaints of increased dyspnea, unilateral diminished breath sounds, and cyanosis, which indicates respiratory distress. Evaluate heart rate (HR) and BP for indications of shock (i.e., tachycardia and hypotension).
- Position patient to allow for full expansion of unaffected lung. Semi-Fowler's position usually provides comfort and allows adequate expansion of chest wall and descent of diaphragm.
- Change patient's position q2h to promote drainage and lung reexpansion and facilitate alveolar perfusion.
- Encourage patient to take deep breaths and provide necessary analgesia *to decrease discomfort during deep-breathing exercises.* Instruct patient in splinting thoracotomy site with arms, pillow, or folded blanket. Deep breathing *promotes full lung expansion and decreases risk of atelectasis.* Coughing *facilitates mobilization of tracheobronchial secretions, if present.*
- Deliver and monitor O_2 and humidity as indicated.

Ineffective breathing pattern (or risk for same) related to decreased lung expansion secondary to malfunction of chest drainage system

Desired outcome: Following intervention, patient becomes eupneic.

Nursing Interventions

- Monitor patient at frequent intervals (q2-4h, as appropriate) to assess breathing pattern while chest-drainage system is in place. Auscultate breath sounds, reporting diminished sounds; be alert for and report signs of respiratory distress, including tachycardia, restlessness, anxiety, and changes in mental status.

◆ Assess and maintain closed chest-drainage system as follows:
  • Tape all connections and secure chest tube to thorax with tape. Avoid all tubing kinks, and ensure that the bed and equipment are not compressing any component of the system.
  • Eliminate all dependent loops in tubing. These may impede removal of air and fluid from the pleural space.
  • Maintain fluid in underwater-seal chamber and suction chamber at appropriate levels.

◆ Be aware that the suction apparatus does not regulate amount of suction applied to closed chest-drainage system. The amount of suction is determined by water level in the suction control chamber. Minimal bubbling in this chamber is acceptable and desirable. Dial the level of dry suction per health care provider's recommendation. Suction aids in lung reexpansion, but removing suction for short periods, such as for transporting, will not be detrimental or disrupt the closed chest-drainage system.

◆ Avoid stripping of chest tubes. This mechanism for maintaining chest-tube patency is controversial and has been associated with creating high negative pressures in the pleural space, which can damage fragile lung tissue. Squeezing alternately hand over hand along the drainage tube may generate sufficient pressure to move fluid along the tube. Use of mechanical or handheld tube-stripping devices should be avoided.

◆ Be aware that fluctuations in the underwater-seal chamber are characteristic of a patent chest tube. Fluctuations stop when either the lung has reexpanded or there is a kink or obstruction in the chest tube as follows:
  • Bubbling in the underwater-seal chamber occurs on expiration and is a sign that air is leaving the pleural space. Continuous bubbling in the underwater-seal chamber may be a signal that air is leaking into the drainage system. Locate and seal the system's air leak, if possible.

◆ Keep the following necessary emergency supplies at the bedside:
  • Petrolatum gauze pad to apply over insertion site if the chest tube becomes dislodged; *use of this dressing provides an airtight seal to prevent recurrent pneumothorax.*
  • Bottle of sterile water in which to submerge the chest tube if it becomes disconnected from the underwater-seal system.

◆ Never clamp a chest tube without a specific directive from health care provider; clamping may lead to tension pneumothorax because air in the pleural space no longer can escape.

Acute pain related to impaired pleural integrity, inflammation, or presence of a chest tube

Desired outcomes: Within 1 hr of intervention, patient's subjective perception of pain decreases, as documented by pain scale. Objective indicators, such as grimacing, are absent or diminished.

Nursing Interventions

◆ At frequent intervals, assess patient's degree of discomfort by using an appropriate pain rating scale such as 0 (no pain) to 10 (worst pain), as well as patient's verbal and nonverbal cues.

◆ Medicate with analgesics as prescribed and use pain scale *to evaluate and document medication effectiveness.* Encourage patient to request analgesic before pain becomes severe.

◆ Premedicate patient 30 min before initiating coughing, exercising, or repositioning, *to minimize pain.*

◆ Teach patient to splint affected side when coughing, moving, or repositioning, *to minimize pain.*

- ◆ Facilitate coordination among health care providers to provide rest periods between care activities *to decrease O_2 demand.* Allow 90 min for undisturbed rest.
- ◆ Stabilize chest tube *to reduce pull or drag on latex connector tubing.* Tape chest tube securely to thorax. Position tube to ensure there are no dependent loops.
- ◆ For additional interventions, see "Pain," p. 13, in Chapter 1.

 Patient-Family Teaching and Discharge Planning

- ◆ Provide verbal and written information about the following:
  - Purpose of chest tube and its maintenance.
  - Potential for and symptoms of recurrence of spontaneous pneumothorax and importance of seeking medical care immediately.
  - Medications, including drug names, purpose, dosage, schedule, precautions, and potential side effects. Also discuss drug/drug, herb/drug, and food/drug interactions.

❖ PULMONARY TUBERCULOSIS

OVERVIEW/PATHOPHYSIOLOGY

Tuberculosis (TB) is an infectious disease caused primarily by *Mycobacterium tuberculosis.* In the United States an estimated 10 to 15 million persons are infected with this organism, most of whom have latent TB infection (LTBI) in which the bacteria are in the body (usually the lungs) in a dormant form that neither causes disease nor is communicable to other persons. A small proportion of persons (about 10%) with LTBI will develop active TB in their lifetimes.

For many years (from 1953 to 1984), reported cases of TB in the United States decreased by almost 6% each year, and the general perception was that TB was no longer a problem. This decline was due to many factors, including improved living conditions (less crowding and better ventilation), better nutrition, and antituberculosis drugs. As a result, the public health infrastructure to support TB control weakened as other diseases, for example, human immunodeficiency virus (HIV)/acquired immunodeficiency syndrome (HIV/AIDS), became more prominent. It was not until the late 1980s that a link between TB and HIV/AIDS became apparent, as was manifested partly by multidrug-resistant (MDR) TB outbreaks occurring in seven hospitals between 1990 and 1992 and resulting in many cases of LTBI, TB disease, and death. In addition, reported cases of TB increased 20% between 1985 and 1992. After the hospital outbreaks and other changes in administrative and legislative support to control TB, cases have steadily declined again in most areas of the country. In 2003, fewer than 15,000 cases of TB were reported in the United States, more than half of which were among foreign-born persons. Worldwide, TB remains a leading cause of death in developing countries; the World Health Organization (WHO) estimates that approximately one third of the world's population is infected with *M. tuberculosis.*

M. tuberculosis is transmitted by the airborne route via minute, invisible particles called droplet *nuclei.* When individuals with TB disease of the lungs or throat cough, sneeze, speak, or sing, TB organisms harboring in their respiratory secretions are expelled into the air and transform quickly into tiny droplet nuclei that can remain suspended in air for several hours, depending on the environment (especially within ventilation systems). To become infected, another person must breathe the air containing the droplet nuclei. A person's natural defenses of the nose and upper airway and immune system often prevent sufficient numbers of organisms from reaching the alveoli to cause infection. It generally takes 5 to 200 bacilli implanted in the alveoli to cause LTBI. When bacilli reach the alveoli, these organisms are ingested by macrophages. Some of these bacilli spread through the bloodstream when the macrophages die; however, the immune system response usually prevents the individual from developing TB disease. Although most TB cases are pulmonary (85%), TB can occur in almost any part of the body or as disseminated disease. About half the people with LTBI who develop active TB (5%) will do so within the first year or two after infection. The remainder (5%) will develop active TB within their lifetimes.

Close contacts of patients require identification so that they can undergo evaluation for the presence of LTBI. TB is reportable to the public health department.

ASSESSMENT

For an accurate diagnosis of TB, a complete medical and psychosocial history is needed along with a physical examination that includes a tuberculin skin test [TST], chest x-ray examination, and sputum examination (including acid-fast bacillus [AFB] smears, cultures, and drug sensitivity studies).

Signs and symptoms/physical findings: Productive prolonged cough, dyspnea, fever, night sweats, chest pain, hemoptysis, chills, loss of appetite, unintended weight loss over a short period of time, and tiredness.

History/risk factors for developing active TB: Immunocompromised state, especially HIV infection; injection drug use; radiographic evidence of prior, healed TB; weight loss of 10% or more of ideal body weight; and other medical conditions, including diabetes mellitus, silicosis, end-stage renal disease, some types of cancers, and certain immunosuppressive therapies. Persons who have emigrated from areas of the world with high rates of TB are also more likely to have LTBI than are persons born in the United States.

DIAGNOSTIC TESTS

Sputum culture: Three sputum cultures are obtained 8 to 24 hr apart and are sent for AFB smear and culture to ascertain presence of *M. tuberculosis.* Results of sputum culture are negative in persons with LTBI.

Acid-fast stain: Detection of AFB in stained smears examined under a microscope usually provides the first bacteriologic clue of TB. Smear results should be available within 24 hr of specimen collection. AFB in the smear may be mycobacteria other than *M. tuberculosis;* many patients can have TB and still have a negative smear. Specimens are generally collected by asking patient to expectorate sputum into a cup; however, tracheal washing, thoracentesis of pleural fluid, and lung biopsy are other options.

Chest x-ray examination: Involvement is most characteristically evident in the apex and posterior segments of the upper lobes. Although not diagnostically definitive, x-ray examination reveals calcification at original site, enlargement of hilar lymph nodes, parenchymal infiltrate, pleural effusion, and cavitation. Patients with HIV infection may have an atypical radiographic presentation of TB. Any abnormality on a chest x-ray film of a patient with AIDS should be considered possible TB until ruled out.

TST or intradermal injection of antigen: This test uses a purified protein derivative (PPD) of mycobacterial organisms that is administered intradermally and interpreted as positive or negative using measured millimeters of induration. The test is considered positive when an area of induration 10 mm or greater is present within 48-72 hr after injection. Tests in patients in high-risk categories such as HIV-infected and recently HIV-exposed patients are considered positive with 5 mm or greater induration. Those who are immunocompromised and some patients with active TB may have a negative PPD test, even in the presence of active TB disease. A positive PPD test indicates LTBI and is not diagnostic for active disease.

QuantiFERON-TB (QFT) blood test: Whole-blood interferon gamma assay that requires only one patient visit for a blood specimen to assess for

LTBI (rather than for active disease); use is currently limited because of laboratory requirements for specimen evaluation.

COLLABORATIVE MANAGEMENT

Common drug regimens for treatment of LTBI: For persons suspected of having LTBI, treatment should not begin until active TB disease has been excluded. The standard regimen (American Thoracic Society/Centers for Disease Control and Prevention [ATS/CDC]) for LTBI treatment is 6 to 9 mo of isoniazid (INH) or 4 mo of rifampin. Although these regimens are broadly applicable, modifications should be considered under special circumstances that include HIV infection, suspected drug resistance, pregnancy, and liver problems. Adequate LTBI treatment reduces risk for development of active TB by about 70% (i.e., from a lifetime risk of 10% to 3%).

Treatment for TB disease: For persons with TB disease, treatment with a single drug can lead to development of bacterial resistance to that drug; thus all TB disease treatment regimens must contain multiple drugs to which the organisms are susceptible. For most patients, the preferred regimen consists of initiation of a 2-mo phase of four drugs—rifampin, INH, pyrazinamide, and ethambutol (RIPE), followed by a continuation phase of INH and rifampin of at least 4 mo, for a minimal total treatment duration of 6 mo. TB treatment regimens may need to be altered for persons infected with HIV who are on antiretroviral therapy (ART), as well as when drug-susceptibility tests become available or when disease is severe and patient's response is less than adequate.

Directly observed therapy (DOT) adherence-enhancing strategy: Treatment success is often enhanced by using DOT for medication administration. DOT is achieved by having a trained health care worker or other specially trained person watch a patient swallow each dose of medication and record dates that the DOT was observed. In the United States DOT is the standard of care for all patients with TB disease and should be used for all doses during the course of therapy for TB disease and for LTBI whenever feasible.

Administrative, environmental, and respiratory controls for selected settings

Inpatient settings/patient rooms: Patient is placed in an airborne-infection isolation (AII) room until antimicrobial therapy is successful and patient is determined to be no longer infectious as indicated by AFB smear. AII requires a private room with special ventilation that dilutes and removes airborne contaminants and controls the direction of airflow so that air pressure inside the room is negative to the air pressure in the hallway. To enable adequate function of this negative airflow system, the door to the room should be closed as much as possible and the negative pressure monitored consistent with hospital policy. Persons entering the AII room should wear N-95 respirators designed to provide a tight face seal and filter particles in the 1- to 5-μm range. Patients should wear a standard surgical mask if it is necessary for them to leave the room.

Ambulatory care settings and medical offices: In these settings where patients with TB disease are treated, at least one room should meet requirements for an AII room. When a person with diagnosed or suspected TB enters the office, he/she should put on a surgical mask as soon as possible and shortly thereafter be placed in the AII room. When the person with TB leaves the AII room, sufficient time should elapse for adequate removal of air contaminated with *M. tuberculosis* (usually 30 min to 2 hr, depending on number of air changes and ventilation efficiency) before another patient is placed in the room. For staff and others entering the AII room with the TB patient and in the 30-120 min after patient leaves the room, an N-95 disposable respirator should be worn.

NURSING DIAGNOSES AND INTERVENTIONS

Deficient knowledge relate to the spread of TB and procedure for airborne-infection isolation

Desired outcome: Following instruction, patient and significant others verbalize how TB is spread and measures necessary to prevent the spread.

Nursing Interventions

♦ Assess patient's facility with language; engage an interpreter or language-appropriate written materials if necessary.

♦ Teach patient about TB and the mechanism by which it is spread (respiratory droplet nuclei).

♦ Explain AII to patient and significant others. Post appropriate notice of isolation/airborne precautions on patient's room door.

♦ Remind staff and visitors of need to keep door closed *to enable effective function of the ventilation system.*

♦ Explain to staff and visitors the importance of wearing N-95 or other high-efficiency respirators, including proper fit and use. Provide appropriate respirators at doorway or other convenient place.

♦ Teach patient importance of covering mouth and nose with tissue when sneezing or coughing and of disposing used tissue in appropriate waste container.

 Patient-Family Teaching and Discharge Planning

Provide verbal and written information about the following:

♦ Antituberculosis medications, including drug name, purpose, dosage, schedule, precautions, and potential side effects. Also discuss drug/drug, herb/drug, and food/drug interactions. Remind patient that medications are to be taken without interruption for the prescribed period. Remind patient of the need for continued laboratory monitoring for complications of pharmacotherapy. Describe DOT if that is the medication administration method selected.

♦ Importance of periodic reculturing of sputum.

♦ Importance of basic hygiene measures, including handwashing, covering cough with tissues, and proper disposal of contaminated items.

♦ Phone numbers to call if questions or concerns arise about therapy or disease after discharge.

♦ Additional general information can be obtained at the following websites:

Division of Tuberculosis Elimination at the Centers for Disease Control and Prevention, www.cdc.gov/tb

American Lung Association, www.lungusa.org

American Thoracic Society, www.thoracic.org

University of Medicine and Dentistry of New Jersey, New Jersey Medical School National Tuberculosis Center, www.umdnj.edu/ntbcweb

National Tuberculosis Curriculum Consortium at the University of California San Diego, http://NTCC.ucsd.edu

SECTION TWO # ACUTE RESPIRATORY FAILURE

OVERVIEW/PATHOPHYSIOLOGY

Acute respiratory failure (ARF) develops when the lungs are unable to exchange O_2 and CO_2 adequately. Clinically, respiratory failure exists when PaO_2 is less than 50 mm Hg with the patient at rest and breathing room air.

BOX 2-1 — DISEASE PROCESSES LEADING TO DEVELOPMENT OF RESPIRATORY FAILURE

Impaired Alveolar Ventilation
- Chronic obstructive pulmonary disease (emphysema, bronchitis, cystic fibrosis, obesity)
- Restrictive pulmonary disease (interstitial fibrosis, asthma, pleural effusion, pneumothorax, kyphoscoliosis, diaphragmatic paralysis)
- Neuromuscular defects (Guillain-Barré syndrome, myasthenia gravis, multiple sclerosis, muscular dystrophy, polio, brain/spinal cord injury)
- Depression of respiratory control centers (drug-induced cerebral infarction, acute or naïve narcotic use in large doses, drug/toxic agents)
- Chest trauma (rib fractures)

Ventilation or Perfusion Disturbances
- Pulmonary emboli
- Atelectasis
- Pneumonia
- Emphysema
- Chronic bronchitis
- Bronchiolitis
- Acute lung injury
- Acute respiratory distress syndrome (ARDS)—formerly known as adult respiratory distress syndrome

Diffusion Disturbances
- Pulmonary/interstitial fibrosis
- Pulmonary edema
- ARDS
- Acute lung injury*
- Anatomic loss of functioning lung tissue (tumor pneumonectomy)
- ARDS is characterized by all of the above criteria with a P/F ratio of less than 200. Acute lung injury is most often seen as part of a systemic inflammatory response, usually sepsis or other direct lung injury. The inflammatory response causes widespread destruction of alveolar capillary endothelia, extravasculation of protein-rich fluid, and interstitial edema in the alveoli. As a result, alveolar membranes become damaged by fluid filling the alveoli, with resulting destruction of surfactant production. This leads to refractory hypoxemia (increased O_2 requirements that necessitate a large amount of inspired oxygen), noncompliant lungs, and a profound ventilation/perfusion mismatch.
- Nursing management should be focused on monitoring and anticipation of intubation with mechanical ventilation.

From Bernard GR, Artigas A, Brigham KL et al: The American-European Consensus Conference on ARDS: definitions, mechanisms, relevant outcomes, and clinical trial coordination, *Am J Respir Crit Care Med* 149(3Pt1):818-824, 1994.
*Progression of respiratory failure in certain diagnoses can lead to acute lung injury and acute respiratory distress syndrome. Acute lung injury is characterized by bilateral pulmonary infiltrates on chest x-ray; noncardiogenic pulmonary edema; and a Pao_2/Fio_2 (P/F) ratio of less than 300. P/F ratio is the relationship of arterial blood gas (Pao_2) to inspired O_2 concentration (Fio_2). Normal P/F ratio is approximately 500 (100/0.20). In a patient with Pao_2 of 80 mm Hg and Fio_2 of 0.40, the P/F ratio would be 200 (80/0.40).

$Paco_2$ 50 mm Hg or more or pH less than 7.35 is significant for respiratory acidosis, which is the common precursor to ARF.

Although a variety of disease processes can lead to development of respiratory failure (**BOX 2-1**), four basic mechanisms are involved.

Alveolar hypoventilation: Occurs secondary to reduction in alveolar minute ventilation. Because differential indicators (cyanosis, somnolence) occur late in the process, the condition may go unnoticed until tissue hypoxia is severe.

Ventilation/perfusion mismatch: Considered the most common cause of hypoxemia. Normal alveolar ventilation occurs at a rate of 4 L/min, with normal pulmonary vascular blood flow occurring at a rate of 5 L/min. Normal ventilation/perfusion ratio is 0.8:1. Any disease process that interferes with either side of the equation upsets physiologic balance and can lead to respiratory failure as a result of reduction in arterial O_2 levels.

Diffusion disturbances: Processes that physically impair gas exchange across the alveolar-capillary membrane. Diffusion is impaired because of the increase in anatomic distance the gas must travel from alveoli to capillary and capillary to alveoli.

Right-to-left shunt: Occurs when the previously mentioned processes go untreated. Large amounts of blood pass from the right side of the heart to the left and out into the general circulation without adequate ventilation; therefore blood is poorly oxygenated. This mechanism occurs when alveoli are atelectatic or fluid filled, inasmuch as these conditions interfere with gas exchange. Unlike the first three responses, hypoxemia secondary to right-to-left shunting does not improve with O_2 administration because despite the increare in inspired oxygen concentration (FIO_2) the additional oxygen is unable to cross the alveolar-capillary membrane.

ASSESSMENT

Clinical indicators of ARF vary according to the underlying disease process and severity of the failure. ARF is one of the most common causes of impaired level of consciousness (LOC). Often it is misdiagnosed as heart failure, pneumonia, or stroke.

Signs and symptoms/physical findings

Early: Restlessness, changes in mental status, anxiety, headache, fatigue, cool and dry skin, increased BP, tachycardia, cardiac dysrhythmias.

Intermediate: Confusion, increased agitation, and increased O_2 requirements with decreased O_2 saturations. Patients who have hypoventilation respiratory failure often exhibit lethargy and bradypnea. Patients with ventilation/perfusion mismatch often exhibit tachypnea.

Late: Cyanosis, diaphoresis, coma, respiratory arrest.

DIAGNOSTIC TESTS

Arterial blood gas (ABG) analysis: Assesses adequacy of oxygenation and effectiveness of ventilation and is the most important diagnostic tool. Typical results are PaO_2 60 mm Hg or less, $PaCO_2$ 45 mm Hg or more, and pH less than 7.35, findings consistent with severe respiratory acidosis.

Chest x-ray examination: Ascertains presence of underlying pathophysiology or disease process that may be contributing to the failure.

COLLABORATIVE MANAGEMENT

Treatment is aimed at correcting the acid-base disturbance while treating underlying pathophysiology in an effort to prevent or correct ARF. Although the general rule is to bring the PaO_2 to greater than 60 mm Hg and the $PaCO_2$ to 35-45 mm Hg, patients with chronic obstructive pulmonary disease (COPD) may be clinically stable with $PaCO_2$ greater than 45 mm Hg; therefore determination of pH is critical in these individuals. For example, patients with chronically high $PaCO_2$ whose pH drops to less than baseline are at risk for ARF.

O_2 therapy: As determined by ABG values. O_2 therapy at an FIO_2 of 0.5 or less and pharmacotherapy (e.g., bronchodilators, steroids, antibiotics) often improve ABGs sufficiently to get patient out of danger, depending on ARF cause. Persistent respiratory acidosis following medical intervention may indicate need for intubation and mechanical ventilation.

Bronchodilator therapy: Delivered via nebulizer or noninvasive positive-pressure ventilation (NIPPV). It may eliminate necessity for intubation and mechanical ventilation.

Coughing/deep-breathing exercises: Mobilize secretions and promote full lung expansion. If cough is ineffective, suctioning may be necessary to stimulate cough reflex and clear secretions. Intermittent positive-pressure breathing (IPPB) may be used for patients who are unable to use incentive spirometer to assist with lung expansion.

Intubation and mechanical ventilation: Patient may require intubation and mechanical ventilation to provide adequate respiratory function and stabilize ABGs if ARF progresses. Mechanical support is used until underlying cause of the failure can be corrected and patient can resume ventilatory efforts independently.

Prophylaxis for gastric stress ulceration and deep vein thrombosis/pulmonary embolism (DVT/PE): Every patient with ARF is at risk for these complications.

NURSING DIAGNOSES AND INTERVENTIONS

See "Psychosocial Support," p. 31. See "Pneumonia" for **Impaired gas exchange,** p. 64, and **Deficient fluid volume,** p. 66. Also see "Pleural Effusion," p. 68; "Pulmonary Embolus," p. 69; "Pneumothorax/Hemothorax," p. 75; "Asthma," p. 91; "Multiple Sclerosis," p. 229; and "Guillain-Barré Syndrome," p. 238, because these disorders may be precursors to ARF.

 Patient-Family Teaching and Discharge Planning

ARF is an acute condition that is symptomatically treated during patient's hospitalization. Discharge planning and teaching should be directed at educating patient and significant others about underlying pathophysiology and treatment specific for that process. See sections in this chapter that relate specifically to the underlying pathophysiology contributing to development of ARF.

SECTION THREE   # CHRONIC OBSTRUCTIVE PULMONARY DISEASE

OVERVIEW/PATHOPHYSIOLOGY

COPD is the fourth leading cause of death in the United States. It is a disease state characterized by airflow limitation that is not fully reversible. Airflow limitation usually is progressive and associated with an abnormal inflammatory response of the lungs to noxious particles or gases and characterized by chronic inflammation throughout the airways, parenchyma, and pulmonary vasculature.

In the central airways, inflammatory cells infiltrate the surface epithelium. Enlarged mucus-secreting glands and an increased number of goblet cells lead to mucus hypersecretion. In smaller airways, chronic inflammation leads to repeated cycles of injury to the airway wall. Repair of the airway wall results in increased collagen content and scar tissue formation that narrow the lumen and produce fixed airway obstruction.

Destruction of lung parenchyma in patients with COPD typically occurs as emphysema, which involves dilation and destruction of the bronchioles. An imbalance of proteinases and antiproteinases in the lungs is believed to be a major mechanism causing these changes.

ASSESSMENT

Signs and symptoms/physical findings: Chronic cough (usually the first symptom) followed by dyspnea (usually reason for seeking health care) with a prolonged expiratory phase. As lung function deteriorates, perceived

BOX 2-2	INDICATORS FOR DIAGNOSING COPD

Chronic Cough
- Present intermittently or every day
- Often present throughout the day
- Seldom only nocturnal

Chronic Sputum
- Any pattern of sputum production

Dyspnea
- Progressive (worsens over time)
- Persistent (present every day)
- Described by patient as increased effort to breathe, heaviness, air hunger, or gasping
- Worse with exercise
- Worse during respiratory infections

History of Exposure to Risk Factors
- Tobacco smoke
- Occupational dust and chemicals
- Smoke from home cooking and heating fuels

increase in work of breathing (WOB), wheezing, chest tightness, use of accessory muscles of respiration, digital clubbing, decreased thoracic expansion, barrel chest appearance, dullness over areas of consolidation, adventitious breath sounds (especially coarse rhonchi and wheezing). Signs of COPD-related right-sided heart failure: include ankle edema, distended neck veins, hepatic congestion, and bloated appearance. See **BOX 2-2**.

History and risk factors: Cigarette smoking is the primary causative factor. Genetic factors (e.g., hereditary deficiency of alpha-1 antitrypsin) and exposure to outdoor/indoor air pollutants may also contribute.

DIAGNOSTIC TESTS

Chest x-ray: Rules out other causes of airway obstruction and lung cancer.

Computed tomography (CT) scan: Assesses for presence and extent of emphysema.

Arterial blood gas (ABG) values: Important in advanced COPD and should be obtained when there are signs of right-sided (diastolic) heart failure (e.g., jugular vein distention, peripheral edema) or respiratory failure (PaO_2 less than 60 mm Hg with or without $PaCO_2$ greater than 50 mm Hg).

Oximetry: Reveals decreased O_2 saturation (90% or less).

Alpha-1 antitrypsin deficiency screen: Performed in patients who develop COPD at a young age (less than 45 years) or who have a strong family history of the disease.

Spirometry: Confirms diagnosis of COPD. Clinical indicators and the forced expiratory volume in 1 sec (FEV_1) diagnose and classify severity of COPD. See **TABLE 2-3**. Should be monitored annually and during acute illness.

Sputum culture: May reveal presence of infective organisms. Sputum specimens are best collected when the patient first wakes in the morning.

Differential diagnosis: COPD may mimic many other diseases such as asthma, heart failure, bronchiectasis, tuberculosis (TB), obliterative bronchiolitis, and diffuse bronchiolitis.

COLLABORATIVE MANAGEMENT

O_2 therapy: To treat hypoxemia. It is used cautiously in patients with chronic CO_2 retention for whom hypoxemia, rather than hypercapnia, stimulates the respiratory drive. Long-term O_2 therapy has been shown to slow progression of COPD and reduce mortality.

TABLE 2-3	CLASSIFICATION OF COPD SEVERITY
STAGE	**CHARACTERISTICS**
0: At risk	Normal spirometry Chronic symptoms (cough, sputum production)
I: Mild	FEV_1/FVC less than 70% FEV_1 80% or more predicted With or without chronic symptoms (cough, sputum production)
II: Moderate	FEV_1/FVC less than 70% 50% FEV_1 less than 80% predicted With or without chronic symptoms (cough, sputum production)
III: Severe	FEV_1/FVC less than 70% 30% FEV_1 less than 50% predicted With or without chronic symptoms (cough, sputum production)
IV: Very severe	FEV_1/FVC less than 70% FEV_1 less than 30% predicted or FEV_1 less than 50% predicted plus chronic respiratory failure

FEV_1, Forced expiratory volume in 1 second; *FVC,* forced vital capacity.

Long-term O_2 therapy is generally introduced in patients with PaO_2 less than 60 mm Hg. O_2 delivered at 2 L/min via nasal cannula generally results in acceptable PaO_2 levels of 65-80 mm Hg.

Smoking cessation: Single most effective way of reducing risk of development and progression of COPD. Nicotine replacement therapy also should be considered to assist with withdrawal from tobacco.

Pulmonary rehabilitation: A comprehensive program includes exercise training, nutrition counseling, and education. Patients who have completed a pulmonary rehabilitation program have been shown to have improved quality of life and slowed progression of the disease.

Pharmacotherapy

Inhaled bronchodilators: Open airways by relaxing smooth muscles of the airways. The resultant increased airflow may help loosen mucus.

Inhaled steroids: Result in a small, one-time increase in FEV_1, decrease frequency and severity of exacerbations, and reduce mortality.

Oral steroids (prednisone): Used short term (10-14 days) for severe exacerbations to decrease inflammation and thereby increase airflow.

Antibiotics: Prescribed based on presence of infiltrate on chest x-ray film and other signs of infection.

IV or oral fluids: Administered to promote adequate hydration.

Diuretics or Na^+ restriction: Prescribed to reduce fluid overload in the presence of cardiac complications, such as heart failure.

NURSING DIAGNOSES AND INTERVENTIONS

Ineffective airway clearance related to decreased energy, which results in ineffective cough, or related to presence of increased tracheobronchial secretions

Desired outcomes: Following intervention, patient coughs appropriately and has effective airway clearance as evidenced by absence of adventitious breath sounds.

Nursing Interventions

◆ Auscultate breath sounds q2-4h (or as indicated by patient's condition) and after coughing. Be alert to and report changes in adventitious breath sounds.

◆ Teach patient the "double cough" technique to prevent small airway collapse, which can occur with forceful coughing.
- Sit upright with upper body flexed forward slightly.
- Take 2-3 breaths and exhale passively.

BOX 2-3	RECOMMENDED CALORIE SOURCES FOR PATIENTS WITH COPD

Foods High in Fat
- Cheese
- Cream
- Cream soups
- Custards
- Evaporated milk
- Fish
- Margarine
- Mayonnaise
- Meat
- Nuts
- Poultry
- Salad and cooking oils
- Whole milk

Foods to Avoid
- Cakes
- Cookies
- Jams
- Pastries
- Sugar-concentrated snacks

- Inhale again, but only to the midinspiratory point.
- Exhale by coughing quickly 2-3 ×.
◆ When not otherwise indicated, encourage fluid intake (2.5 L/day or more) *to decrease sputum viscosity.*

Imbalanced nutrition: less than body requirements related to decreased intake secondary to fatigue and anorexia
Desired outcome: For a minimum of 24 hr before hospital discharge, patient has adequate nutrition as evidenced by stable weight, positive N balance, and serum albumin 3.5-5.5 g/dL.

Nursing Interventions

◆ Monitor food and fluid intake. If indicated, obtain dietary consultation for calorie counts.
◆ Provide diet in small, frequent meals that are nutritious and easy to consume.
◆ Request consultation with dietitian so that patient can verbalize food likes and dislikes.
◆ Unless otherwise indicated, provide calories more from unsaturated fat sources (**BOX 2-3**) than from carbohydrate sources. *During the process of carbohydrate metabolism, the body uses O_2 and produces CO_2, which is then excreted by the lungs. Patients with COPD take in less O_2 and retain CO_2. A high-fat diet minimizes this problem because fat generates the least amount of CO_2 for a given amount of O_2 used, whereas carbohydrates generate the most.*
◆ Discuss with patient and significant others the importance of good nutrition in the treatment of COPD.

Ineffective breathing pattern related to decreased lung expansion secondary to chronic airflow limitations
Desired outcome: Following treatment/intervention, patient's breathing pattern improves as evidenced by reduction in or absence of dyspnea and movement toward a state of eupnea.

Nursing Interventions

- Assess respiratory status q2-4h and be alert for indicators of respiratory distress (i.e., agitation, restlessness, changes in mental status, decreased level of consciousness (LOC), use of accessory muscles of respiration). Auscultate breath sounds; report a decrease in breath sounds or an increase in adventitious breath sounds.
- Teach pursed-lip breathing, *which increases intraluminal air pressure and thus promotes internal stability of the airways and may prevent airway collapse during expiration.* Record patient's response to breathing technique.
  - Sit upright with hands on thighs, or lean forward with elbows propped on over-the-bed table.
  - Inhale slowly through nose with mouth closed.
  - Form lips in an O shape as though whistling.
  - Exhale slowly through pursed lips. Exhalation should take twice as long as inhalation (e.g., count to 5 on inhalation; count to 10 on exhalation).
- Administer bronchodilator therapy as prescribed. Monitor for side effects, including tachycardia and dysrhythmias.
- Monitor patient's response to prescribed O_2 therapy. Be aware that high concentrations of O_2 can depress the respiratory drive in individuals with chronic CO_2 retention.
- Monitor oximetry readings; report O_2 saturation 92% or less *because this can indicate need for O_2 therapy.*
- Monitor serial ABG values. Patients with chronic CO_2 retention may have chronically compensated respiratory acidosis with low normal pH (7.35-7.38) and $Paco_2$ greater than 45 mm Hg.

Activity intolerance related to imbalance between O_2 supply and demand secondary to inefficient work of breathing

Desired outcome: Patient reports decreasing dyspnea during activity or exercise and rates perceived exertion at 3 or less on a 0-10 scale.

Nursing Interventions

- Maintain prescribed activity levels and explain rationale to patient.
- Monitor patient's respiratory response to activity. *Activity intolerance is indicated by excessively increased respiratory rate (RR) (e.g., more than 10 breaths/min higher than baseline) and depth, dyspnea, and use of accessory muscles of respiration.* Ask patient to rate perceived exertion (see p. 90 for a description). If activity intolerance is noted, instruct patient to stop the activity and rest.
- Facilitate coordination among health care providers to ensure rest periods between care activities *to decrease O_2 demand.* Allow 90 min for undisturbed rest.
- Assist patient with active ROM exercises *to build stamina and prevent complications of decreased mobility.* For more information, see **Risk for activity intolerance** in "Prolonged Bed Rest," p. 23.

 Patient-Family Teaching and Discharge Planning

Provide verbal and written information about the following:

- Use of home O_2, including when to use it, importance of not increasing prescribed flow rate, precautions, and community resources for O_2 replacement when necessary. Request respiratory therapy consultation to assist with teaching related to O_2 therapy, if indicated.
- Medications, including drug names, route, purpose, dosage, schedule, precautions, and potential side effects. Also discuss drug/drug, herb/drug, and food/drug interactions. If patient will be taking oral corticosteroids while at home, provide instructions accordingly to ensure patient takes the correct amount, particularly during the period in which medication will be tapered.

- Signs and symptoms of heart failure that necessitate medical attention: increased dyspnea, fatigue, and coughing; changes in amount, color, or consistency of sputum; swelling of ankles and legs; fever; and sudden weight gain. For more information, see "Heart Failure," p. 107.
- Importance of avoiding contact with infectious individuals, especially those with respiratory infections.
- Recommendation that patient receive a pneumococcal vaccination and annual influenza vaccination.
- Review of Na$^+$-restricted diet (see Box 4-1, p. 165) and other dietary considerations as indicated.
- Importance of pacing activity level to conserve energy.
- Follow-up appointment with health care provider; confirm date and time of next appointment.
- Introduction to pulmonary rehabilitation programs.

SECTION FOUR ASTHMA

OVERVIEW/PATHOPHYSIOLOGY

Asthma is a chronic disorder characterized by an exaggerated bronchoconstrictive response to selective stimuli, recurrent and reversible obstruction of airflow in the bronchioles and smaller bronchi, and inflammation. Infiltration of the airways by inflammatory cells such as activated lymphocytes and eosinophils, denudation of the epithelium, deposition of collagen in the membrane, and presence of mast cells are often found in mild and moderate asthma. Severe asthma can lead to occlusion of the bronchial lumen by mucus, hyperplasia, and hypertrophy of the bronchial smooth muscles and hyperplasia of goblet cells. Over time, this inflammation can lead to remodeling and damage to the airways.

Approximately 12 million Americans have asthma. Mortality rates are estimated at around 4500 deaths/yr, an overall decline since 1995. Asthma mortality is nearly 3 × higher in black male than in white male patients and is 2.5 × higher in black female than in white female patients.

ASSESSMENT

Signs and symptoms/physical findings: Tachypnea, dyspnea, orthopnea, wheezing, coughing (often worse at night and in the morning), chest tightness, increased sputum production, tachycardia, anxiety, agitation, prolonged expiratory phase, use of accessory muscles of respiration, chest retractions (supraclavicular area, intercostal and suprasternal spaces), hyperexpansion of the thorax, hyperresonance, pulsus paradoxus, diaphoresis, and pallor.

Symptoms occur or worsen in the presence of exercise, viral infections, animals with fur or feathers, house-dust mites, mold, smoke (tobacco, wood), pollen, changes in weather, strong emotional expression (crying), airborne chemicals or dusts, and menses. If symptoms are left untreated, an acute asthmatic attack can progress to status asthmaticus (SA), a severe and unrelenting asthma attack. SA is an exhausting condition that results in respiratory insufficiency and hypoxia, and it may result in death if untreated.

DIAGNOSTIC TESTS

Oximetry: Reveals decreased O_2 saturation (90% or less).

Arterial blood gas (ABG) values: Acute respiratory acidosis ($Paco_2$ more than 45 mm Hg and pH less than 7.35) typically is present during an acute asthma attack.

Chest x-ray examination: Usually normal; lung hyperinflation may be seen with severe asthma.

CBC: May show increased WBCs with concurrent infection. Differential may show increased eosinophils, which indicates an allergic response.

Sputum: Gross examination may reveal increased viscosity or actual mucus plugs. Culture and sensitivity may reveal microorganisms if infection was the precipitating event.

Spirometry: Evaluates degree of airflow obstruction. Partially reversible obstruction (a more than 12% increase and 200 mL in FEV_1 after inhaling a short-acting bronchodilator or after receiving a short course of oral corticosteroids) is diagnostic.

Peak expiratory flow rate (PEFR): Provides objective measurement of lung function via a small handheld gauge called a peak flowmeter. Patient is instructed to inhale deeply and then forcibly exhale rapidly into the flowmeter, to provide a reading in L/min. The higher the number, the better the airflow. Normal peak flow rates vary across individuals and are based on gender, height, and age. Each patient should monitor daily morning PEFRs to determine normal values. A peak flowmeter is included in the asthma action plan to monitor therapy for asthmatic patients.

ECG results: Sinus tachycardia is an important baseline indicator because use of some bronchodilators may produce cardiac stimulant effects and dysrhythmias. Prominent P waves appear in chronic asthma.

COLLABORATIVE MANAGEMENT

Primarily, management is directed toward monitoring for and preventing acute asthma attacks.

Quick Relief or Symptomatic Therapy

O_2 therapy: Generally, these patients experience mild to moderate hypoxemia. Low-flow (1-3 L/min) O_2 is delivered via nasal cannula with humidity for O_2 saturation of less than 90%.

Pharmacotherapy: Initiated to relieve bronchospasm and continued until wheezing subsides and PFTs return to baseline.

Bronchodilators: Dilate smooth muscles of the airways. Nebulizer/aerosolized bronchodilators are used for acute exacerbation of symptoms.

Corticosteroids: Inhibit the inflammatory response. Acute adrenal insufficiency can develop in patients who take steroids routinely at home if these drugs are not given to the patient during hospitalization.

IV STEROIDS (METHYLPREDNISOLONE): Used to gain control of inflammation in severe attacks. Dosage varies according to severity of the episode and whether patient is currently taking steroids.

ORAL STEROIDS: Once stabilized, the patient in acute phase begins taking oral steroids. Steroids are used cautiously in patients with tuberculosis (TB), diabetes, and peptic ulcer.

Antibiotics: Initiated if there is concurrent fever, leukocytosis, purulent sputum, or unsuspected bacterial sinusitis.

Fluid replacement: Needed to maintain adequate hydration.

Long-Term Control

Nebulizer/aerosolized bronchodilators: Usually prescribed for short-term use for acute exacerbations of symptoms. However, some patients require maintenance doses to prevent recurrent attacks.

Steroids

Systemic corticosteroids (prednisone or methylprednisolone): Usually, patients are gradually weaned from steroids over 2-3 wk. Some patients may require low-dose steroids indefinitely.

Inhaled steroids: Mainstay of interim therapy to prevent or reduce the incidence of acute asthmatic attacks. Dosage is commonly 2-4 inhalations 2-4 ×/day. Some patients use inhalant bronchodilators simultaneously with steroid inhalers. To maximize effectiveness of the steroid inhaler, these patients should be taught to use the bronchodilator as prescribed, wait 10-15 min, and then use the steroid inhaler. Use of steroid inhalers may result in fungal overgrowth of the mouth or pharynx; patient should rinse mouth after each dose.

Nonsteroidal antiinflammatory inhalers (cromolyn, nedocromil sodium): These agents are believed to mediate endothelial response to allergens and thus prevent bronchospasm. Cromolyn is believed to inhibit secretion of the slow-reacting substance of anaphylaxis (SRS-A) from mast cells. Not all patients benefit from cromolyn. Usual dosage is 2-4 inhalations 2-4×/day.

Leukotriene modifiers (zafirlukast, zileuton): Inhibit effects of leukotrienes, which are potent inflammatory mediators that cause smooth muscle bronchoconstriction, increased vascular permeability, and mucus production. These modifiers are used in conjunction with antiinflammatory agents.

Methylxanthines (aminophylline, theophylline): Although methylxanthines were once first-line therapeutic agents, they are now considered third-line therapy. Methylxanthines have relatively weak bronchodilating properties and no effect on inflammatory response. When used, their dosage is carefully monitored by blood levels of theophylline.

NURSING DIAGNOSES AND INTERVENTIONS

Impaired gas exchange related to altered O_2 supply secondary to decreased alveolar ventilation as a result of narrowed airways

Desired outcomes: Following treatment/intervention, patient has adequate gas exchange as evidenced by a respiratory rate (RR) of 12-20 breaths/min (or values consistent with patient's baseline). Before hospital discharge, patient's ABG values are as follows: PaO_2 80 mm Hg or higher, $PaCO_2$ 35-40 mm Hg, and pH 7.35-7.45, or oximetry readings demonstrating O_2 saturation greater than 90%. Patient reports decreased dyspnea and diminished to no wheezes.

Nursing Interventions

- Observe for signs and symptoms of hypoxia (e.g., agitation, mental status changes, anxiety, restlessness, changes in mental status or level of consciousness (LOC)). Remember that cyanosis of the lips and nail beds is a late indicator of hypoxia.
- Position patient for comfort and to promote optimal gas exchange.
- Auscultate breath sounds q2-4h or more frequently as indicated by patient's condition. Monitor for decreased or adventitious sounds (e.g., crackles [rales], rhonchi, wheezes).
- Monitor oximetry readings; report O_2 saturation 90% or less *because this can indicate a need for O_2 therapy.*

 Patient-Family Teaching and Discharge Planning

The goal of asthma education is self-management to prevent unnecessary hospitalizations from acute exacerbations. Therefore teaching focuses on symptom control, an action plan for crisis management, and monitoring techniques. Verbal and written information should be provided about the following:

- Control of factors contributing to asthma severity: irritants or allergens that can precipitate an attack and importance of reducing exposure to these irritants from patient's environment.
- Need for regular exercise.
- Signs and symptoms of acute exacerbation (e.g., increased cough; increased dyspnea, especially at night or during activity; wheezing).
- Medications, including drug names, route, purpose, dosage, precautions, and potential side effects. Also discuss drug/drug, herb/drug, and food/drug interactions.
- Proper use of metered-dose inhalers, including use of a spacer (if indicated) to facilitate medication inhalation. Document adequate return

demonstration by the time of hospital discharge. Remind patient that over-the-counter (OTC) inhalers contain medications that can interfere with prescribed therapy. Instruct patient to contact health care provider before taking any OTC medications.

- If patient will take corticosteroids while at home, provide instructions accordingly to ensure that patient takes the correct amount, particularly during the period in which the medication will be tapered.
- Proper use of peak flowmeters; document return demonstration. Patient should measure and document PEFR, usually twice a day. Peak flowmeters should never be used alone to diagnose exacerbation. Peak flowmeter readings along with assessment of symptoms and use of inhalers will help determine severity.
- Development of an asthma action plan, which includes peak flow readings, symptoms, and use of rescue medications. An asthma action plan is a risk-stratified outline for steps to take if patient experiences an asthma attack. Many action plans also list emergency medications and contact information.
- Smoking cessation: the single most effective way to reduce asthma attacks. With every interaction, patients should be asked about their smoking status and advised of the importance of quitting, even if they have quit within the past year. A counseling session should include social support and scheduled follow-up visits. Nicotine replacement therapy also should be considered to assist with withdrawal from tobacco.
- Recommendation that patient receive a pneumococcal vaccination and annual influenza vaccination.
- Importance of follow-up care. Confirm date and time of next appointment.
- Phone numbers to call if questions or concerns arise about therapy or disease after discharge. Additional general information can be obtained from the following resource:

National Asthma Education and Prevention Program Expert Panel Report 2: Guidelines for the Diagnosis and Management of Asthma, National Heart, Lung, and Blood Institute, Department of Health and Human Services, National Institutes of Health. Available at www.nhlbi.nih.gov/guidelines/asthma/asthgdln.pdf

Cardiovascular Disorders

SECTION ONE DISEASES OF THE
CARDIOVASCULAR SYSTEM

❖ HYPERTENSION

OVERVIEW/PATHOPHYSIOLOGY

The incidence of hypertension among adults in the United States is 10%-15%, and the disease affects 50 million persons. One half of individuals over the age of 65 are affected by hypertension.

Complications of this disease include increased incidence of transient ischemic attack/stroke, retinopathy, coronary artery disease (CAD), heart failure (HF), aortic aneurysm, and renal failure.

ASSESSMENT

Signs and symptoms/physical findings: The Seventh Report of the Joint National Committee on Prevention, Detection, Evaluation, and Treatment of High Blood Pressure (JNC 7) of the National Institutes of Health (NIH) defines hypertension as follows:

Based upon the average of two or more properly measured readings at each of two or more visits after an initial screen, the following classification is used:

Normal BP: SBP less than 120 mm Hg and DBP less than 80 mm Hg
Prehypertension: SBP 120-139 mm Hg or DBP 80-89 mm Hg
Hypertension:
    Stage 1: SBP 140-159 mm Hg or DBP 90-99 mm Hg
    Stage 2: SBP 160 mm Hg or greater or DBP 100 mm Hg or greater

History and risk factors: Family history, race (incidence is higher in African-Americans), high salt intake, renal disease, obesity, excessive alcohol intake, smoking, and some endocrine disorders (i.e., Cushing's disease, pheochromocytoma).

COLLABORATIVE MANAGEMENT

The goal of treatment is a BP less than 140/90 mm Hg or less than 130/80 mm Hg if diabetes or renal disease is present. Treatment for this disease includes promotion of lifestyle modification: smoking cessation; weight loss; exercise; decreased intake of saturated fats, cholesterol, (Na^+), and alcohol; adequate dietary K^+.

The JNC 7 recommends initiating therapy in patients with uncomplicated stage 1 hypertension with a **low-dose thiazide diuretic** (such as hydrochlorothiazide, 12.5-25 mg). This drug improves outcomes, has few side effects, and is low in cost. **Second-line drug therapy** (needed for most patients with stage 2 hypertension) includes adding an angiotensin-converting enzyme (ACE) inhibitor, an angiotensin receptor blocker (ARB), a β-blocker, or a calcium channel blocker (CCB).

NURSING DIAGNOSES AND INTERVENTIONS

Deficient knowledge related to need for frequent BP checks and adherence to antihypertensive therapy and lifestyle changes

Desired outcome: Patient verbalizes knowledge of the importance of frequent BP checks and adhering to antihypertensive therapy and lifestyle changes.

Nursing Interventions

◆ Teach importance of getting BP checked at frequent intervals and adhering to prescribed medication therapy.

◆ Provide teaching guidelines on importance of exercise (aerobic, 30 min/day most days), weight loss (if appropriate), a diet containing less than 2.3 g/day Na^+, no more than 2 drinks (1 oz) per day for men and 1 drink (0.5 oz.) for women, and more than 3500 mg/day dietary K^+. Review with patient how to read food labels and choose appropriate foods.

◆ Caution patient about importance of seeking medical evaluation if BP reading is greater than 200/100 mm Hg or less than 90/60 mm Hg or if headache, dizziness, blurred vision, chest pain, dyspnea, or syncope occurs.

 Patient-Family Teaching and Discharge Planning

Reinforce patient teaching described under **Deficient knowledge**. Also provide verbal and written information about the following:

◆ Medications, including drug names, purpose, dosage, schedule, precautions, and potential side effects. Also discuss drug/drug, food/drug, and herb/drug interactions.

◆ Hypertension is a chronic disease requiring lifetime treatment.

◆ Need for physical support from family and outside agencies.

◆ Self-evaluation of BP if indicated: Monitoring machines are available in local department stores and pharmacies. Remind patient that evaluation of BP should be done while seated, ideally at the same time each day, and recorded.

◆ Availability of community and medical support from organizations such as the American Heart Association (website): *www.americanheart.org*

❖ CORONARY ARTERY DISEASE

OVERVIEW/PATHOPHYSIOLOGY

Coronary artery disease (CAD), the leading cause of death in the United States, affects almost 17 million Americans. More than 12 million have a history of angina or myocardial infarction (MI) or both. The coronary arteries supply the myocardial muscle with O_2 and the nutrients necessary for optimal function. In CAD, the arteries are narrowed or obstructed, potentially resulting in cardiac muscle death. Atherosclerotic lesions, arterial spasm, platelet aggregation, and thrombus formation all may cause obstruction. The most common symptom of CAD is angina, which is the result of decreased blood flow and insufficient O_2 supply to the heart muscle.

Acute coronary syndrome (ACS) refers to an imbalance between myocardial O_2 supply and demand secondary to an acute plaque disruption or erosion. ACS is an umbrella term that includes unstable angina (USA), non–ST-elevation myocardial infarction (NSTEMI), and ST-segment elevation myocardial infarction (STEMI).

USA is defined as an increase in severity, frequency, or intensity of anginal pain or a new onset of prolonged rest angina. This definition is based largely on clinical presentation. NSTEMI is defined by clinical presentation of chest pain with an elevation in cardiac biomarkers and changes on ECG that may include T-wave inversion or ST-segment depression but no ST-segment elevation. Diagnosis of STEMI is based on elevated cardiac biomarkers plus ST-segment elevation on ECG signifying ischemia. Of the three, STEMI is the most serious and life-threatening.

ASSESSMENT

Signs and symptoms/physical findings: Chest pain, substernal pressure and burning, and pain that radiates to the jaw, shoulder, or arm are the most common symptoms of CAD. Weakness, diaphoresis, nausea, vomiting, and acute anxiety also can occur. Heart rate (HR) may be abnormally slow (bradycardia), especially in right coronary artery (RCA) infarct, or may be rapid (tachycardia). Stable or progressively worsening angina occurs when myocardial demand for O_2 is more than the supply, such as during exercise. Pain usually is described as pressure or a crushing or burning substernal pain that radiates down one or both arms. It can be felt also in the neck, cheeks, and teeth. Usually it is relieved by discontinuation of exercise or administration of nitroglycerin (NTG).

Acute syndromes may have clinical manifestations of anxiety, hypertension, tachycardia, tachypnea, and dynamic changes on ECG. Severe hypotension may occur in shock states. Temperature elevations can occur secondary to the inflammatory process. Intensity of S_1 and S_2 heart sounds may be decreased. Pulmonary congestion may occur if ventricular failure is present, and S_3 and S_4 sounds may be auscultated.

History/risk factors: Family history, increasing age, male gender, smoking, oral contraceptive use, cocaine use, long-term use of nonsteroidal antiinflammatory drugs (NSAIDs), low high-density lipoprotein (HDL) values, hypercholesterolemia, diabetes mellitus (DM), hypertension. Obesity, glucose intolerance, low serum folate levels, exposure to air pollution from traffic, and a sedentary, stressful lifestyle also contribute to increased risk. Chest pain often occurs with exertion.

DIAGNOSTIC TESTS

ECG: Usually normal unless an MI has occurred or the individual is experiencing angina at the time of the test. If ECG is performed during chest pain, characteristic changes may include ST-segment elevation or depression greater than 0.05 mV in leads over the area of ischemia. The presence of a bundle branch block (BBB) also can be determined on ECG, as well as dysrhythmias. Serial ECGs are done in patients with ACS to identify area and extent of the infarct.

Cardiac biomarkers: Creatine kinase (CK), MB fraction of creatine kinase (CK-MB), and troponin are proteins released in response to ischemia or MI. Troponin may not be elevated on initial presentation. Serial enzymes q8h × 3 are recommended for accurate assessment of myocardial damage.

C-reactive protein: If elevated from normal range of 0.03-1.1 mg/dL, signals that coronary artery plaques are inflammatory and patient is at higher likelihood of an acute coronary event.

Echocardiogram: Assesses ventricular function, chamber size, valvular function, ejection fraction, wall motion, and hemodynamic measurements. Heart muscle damage may alter ventricular function, wall motion, and hemodynamic pressures.

Chest x-ray examination: Usually normal unless HF is present.

Total lipid panel: Obtained at some point during patient's evaluation and treatment to assess for hyperlipidemia, a risk factor in CAD. Low levels of HDL (value less than 40 mg/dL) and high levels of low-density lipoprotein

(LDL) (value greater than 100 mg/dL) are linked to atherosclerotic heart disease.

Stress tests: Over the past 2 decades, stress testing with concurrent imaging of the heart has become a standard means of evaluation. Stress tests typically are prescribed to assess coronary artery flow.

Exercise treadmill test: Determines amount of exercise-induced ischemia, hemodynamic response, and changes on ECG with exercise. Significant findings include 1 mm or more ST-segment depression or elevation, dysrhythmias, or a sudden decrease in BP.

Stress echocardiogram: Typically performed using either a treadmill or a bicycle. Echocardiograms are obtained before and immediately after exercise. A stress-induced imbalance in the myocardial supply/demand ratio will produce myocardial ischemia and regional wall motion abnormality. Stress echocardiography is particularly useful for identifying CAD in patients with multivessel disease.

Pharmacologic stress test: Pharmacologic agent used to stress heart for patients unable to exercise. Adenosine, dipyridamole, and the newly approved regadenoson are commonly used pharmacologic stress agents. Dobutamine is a second-line agent used when vasodilation stress in contraindicated.

Nuclear stress test: Radionuclide, such as thallium-201 or technetium-99m sestamibi, is injected and used to track myocardial perfusion and identify pattern of ischemia when the heart is stressed either by exercise or pharmacologic agent. Myocardial perfusion imaging detects CAD by documenting normal blood flow and normal tracer uptake in unobstructed coronary arteries and diminished flow and diminished tracer uptake in stenotic coronary arteries. A perfusion abnormality also is seen in an area of MI.

Cardiac nuclear imaging

Single photon emission computed tomography (SPECT): Myocardial imaging technique that provides three-dimensional views of cardiac processes and cellular level metabolism by viewing the heart from several different angles and using tomography methods to reconstruct the image. SPECT enables clearer resolution of myocardial ischemia and better quantification of cardiac damage.

Resting radionuclide angiography (RNA): Evaluates left ventricular ejection fraction (LVEF) and right ventricular ejection fraction (RVEF), LV volume, and regional wall motion. The first pass technique is a fast acquisition of myocardial images. Gated pool ejection or multiple-gated acquisition (MUGA) scan permits calculation of the amount of blood ejected with ventricular contraction and is used for risk stratification of patients after MI or with CAD.

Computed tomography (CT) scan: May be helpful in differentiating acute myocardial infarction (AMI) from aortic dissection in patients with severe, tearing back pain and associated dyspnea and/or syncope.

Ambulatory monitoring: A 24-hr monitoring by ECG (using a Holter monitor) can show activity-induced ST-segment changes or ischemia-induced dysrhythmias.

Coronary arteriography via cardiac catheterization: Gold standard of diagnostic testing for CAD. Arterial lesions (plaque) are located, and the amount of occlusion is determined. During this test, feasibility for coronary artery bypass grafting (CABG) or angioplasty is determined. For details, see "Cardiac Surgery," p. 139, and "Collaborative Management" (next major subsection).

Intravascular ultrasound (IVUS): Assesses degree of atherosclerosis during coronary angiogram. A flexible catheter with a miniature transducer at the tip is threaded from an arteriotomy (commonly femoral) retrograde to the coronary arteries to provide information on the interior of the coronary arteries. Ultrasound is used to create a cross-sectional image of the three layers of the arterial wall and its lumen.

COLLABORATIVE MANAGEMENT

Emergency department (ED) management: Aspirin is administered to all patients unless contraindicated. Time is of the essence in determining a treatment plan. All patients presenting to the ED with STEMI are considered high-priority triage cases. Primary angioplasty is widely viewed as therapy of choice for reperfusion in AMI. However, not all acute-care hospitals in the United States have availability for percutaneous coronary intervention (PCI). Because time is so critical in patients presenting with STEMI, a decision must be made by the ED physician to proceed with either fibrinolytic therapy or primary PCI within 10 min of presentation. The goal for door-to-needle time is within 30 min and door-to-balloon time within 90 min. Initiating thrombolysis within 70 min of symptom onset is key to reducing mortality and morbidity. If catheterization laboratory facilities for primary intervention are not available within this time frame, fibrinolytics are administered until transport can be arranged.

Relief of acute pain: Achieved with sublingual NTG, IV NTG, and/or morphine sulfate. IV NTG drip should be increased in increments of 10 mcg if pain persists, and SBP should be maintained at 90 mm Hg or higher until pain is relieved. IV morphine sulfate is added in small increments (2 mg).

O_2 therapy: Usually 2-4 L/min is given by nasal cannula. Hypoxia is common and adds stress to the compromised myocardium.

β-Blockers: Usually administered by IV route as initial treatment to slow the HR and decrease cardiac workload.

Treatment and prevention of dysrhythmias: Antidysrhythmic agents (e.g., lidocaine) for premature ventricular beats and atropine for bradydysrhythmias.

Antithrombins: Onset of unstable CAD is typically caused by rupture or erosion of an atherosclerotic plaque with development of a thrombus. Antithrombin drugs such as unfractionated heparin (UFH) or low-molecular-weight heparin (LMWH) are administered to halt further thrombus formation. UFH has been shown to have a low and variable bioavailability, which necessitates frequent hematologic evaluations. Patients receiving LMWHs do not require frequent blood testing.

Fibrinolytics (used with STEMI): In AMI, the goal of therapy is to restore patency and blood flow. One of the first-generation fibrinolytic drugs was streptokinase. Newer fibrinolytics have fewer side effects and are used more commonly. Alteplase, a second-generation fibrinolytic, is a weight-adjusted drug that must be given as a continuous infusion. Reteplase (Retavase, Rapilysin), a recombinant plasminogen activator (rPA) and one of the third-generation fibrinolytics, does not require continuous infusion and is a non–weight-based drug. Another third-generation fibrinolytic, tenecteplase (TNK), is administered as a single bolus and, like alteplase, is a weight-based drug. Intracranial hemorrhage is a risk with fibrinolytic drugs and should be monitored for.

Heparin therapy: LMWH or standard UFH is used along with or following fibrinolytic therapy to inhibit further clotting and prevent recurring coronary artery occlusion. Recombinant hirudin is a direct-action antithrombin agent for patients receiving fibrinolytic agents and is available for those who have heparin sensitivity.

Antiplatelet agents: Inhibit platelet aggregation and thrombus formation. They are used for adjunctive therapy in AMI, for MI prevention, or after PCI.
Oral: Aspirin, ticlopidine, clopidogrel.
IV: Glycoprotein IIb/IIIa receptor antagonists, abciximab, eptifibatide, and tirofiban.

Antihyperlipidemics
HMG-CoA reductase inhibitors (e.g., lovastatin, simvastatin, fluvastatin, pravastatin, atorvastatin): Reduce total cholesterol levels, including LDL and triglycerides, while increasing HDL.

Nicotinic acid (niacin): Vitamin that lowers triglyceride and LDL levels while raising HDL levels.

Fibric acid derivatives (e.g., gemfibrozil, fenofibrate): Lower triglycerides and raise HDL.

Bile acid sequestrant resin (e.g., cholestyramine, colestipol): Binds with bile acids in the intestine and removes LDL and cholesterol from the blood.

Management of fluid balance: Oral or IV fluids for dehydration; diuretics for fluid overload and/or treatment of ventricular failure.

Transfer to coronary care unit (CCU): May be necessary if patient is hemodynamically unstable.

PCI: A procedure that improves coronary blood flow by using a balloon inflation catheter to rupture plaque and dilate the artery. It is performed in the cardiac catheterization laboratory and uses local anesthesia and mild sedation, to enable patient to be awake and interact with the health care team. PCI is a common alternative to bypass surgery for individuals with discrete lesions. Balloon angioplasty traditionally is followed by stent placement. Following the procedure, patients routinely are placed on antiplatelet agents (i.e., acetyl-salicylic acid [aspirin, ASA] and clopidogrel [Plavix]) to reduce risk of in-stent restenosis after PCI. Additionally, drug-eluting stents are now available that further reduce risk of restenosis. An antirestenotic drug contained within the polymer of these stents is released over time to modify the healing response that would result in restenosis. Complications of PCI include bleeding, vascular injury, infection, MI, stroke, contrast-induced nephropathy, allergic reaction to medications or contrast, and death.

LONG-TERM MANAGEMENT OF ACS

Management of risk factors: Include eliminating tobacco, reducing BP, reducing serum lipid levels, controlling weight and stress, and initiating an exercise program.

O_2 therapy by nasal cannula: May be used during periods of angina.

Pharmacotherapy

Sublingual NTG: If pain is unrelieved within 5 min after one dose or returns very quickly, patient should seek emergency medical treatment. Two more doses may be taken 5 min apart for a total of three doses while treatment is awaited.

β-Blockers (e.g., metoprolol, atenolol, carvedilol): Decrease O_2 demand of the myocardium.

Angiotensin-converting enzyme (ACE) inhibitor (e.g., enalapril, captopril, quinapril, ramipril): Reduce O_2 demands by decreasing BP.

Long-acting nitrates (isosorbide preparations) or topical NTG: For anginal prophylaxis; they cause vasodilation and lower BP.

CCBs (e.g., nifedipine, diltiazem): Decrease coronary artery vasospasms.

Diet: Low in cholesterol (**TABLE 3-1**), saturated fat (**TABLE 3-2**), Na^+ (see Box 4-1, p. 165), calories, and triglycerides, as appropriate.

NURSING DIAGNOSES AND INTERVENTIONS

Acute pain (angina) related to decreased O_2 supply to the myocardium

Desired outcome: Within 30 min of onset of pain, patient's subjective perception of angina decreases, as documented by pain scale. Objective indicators, such as grimacing and diaphoresis, are absent.

Nursing Interventions

- Assess location, character, and severity of pain. Record severity on a subjective 0 (no pain) to 10 (worst pain) scale. Also record number of NTG tablets needed to relieve each episode, the factor or event that precipitated pain, and alleviating factors. Document angina relief obtained, using pain scale.
- Keep sublingual NTG within reach of patient, and explain that it is to be taken as soon as angina begins and the nurse notified.
- Obtain ECG as prescribed *to assess for ischemia*

TABLE 3-1	GUIDELINES FOR A DIET LOW IN CHOLESTEROL

FOODS TO AVOID	FOODS TO CHOOSE
Egg yolks (no more than 3/wk); foods made with many egg yolks (e.g., sponge cakes)	Egg whites, cholesterol-free egg substitutes
Fatty cuts of meat, fat on meats, luncheon meats or cold cuts, sausage, frankfurters	Lean, well-trimmed meats (minimize servings of beef, lamb, pork); dried peas and beans as meat substitutes
Shellfish (e.g., lobster, shrimp, crab); skin on chicken and turkey	Lean fish; skinless chicken and turkey
Whole milk, cream; whole milk cheese	Nonfat (skim) or low-fat (1% or 2%) milk; partially skim milk cheeses
Ice cream	Ice milk, sherbet, sorbet
Coconut and palm oils and products made with them (e.g., cream substitutes)	Polyunsaturated oils for cooking and food preparation: corn, safflower, cottonseed, sesame, sunflower
Commercially prepared foods with hydrogenated shortening (saturated fat)	Foods prepared from scratch with the suggested oils
Butter, lard, hydrogenated shortening	Margarines that list one of the polyunsaturated oils as their first ingredient
Fried meats and vegetables	Meats (in acceptable quantity) and vegetables prepared by broiling, steaming, or baking
Salad dressings containing cream, cheeses, or mayonnaise; sauces and gravies; seasonings containing large amounts of sugar and saturated fats	Spices, herbs, lemon juice, wine, flavored wine vinegars

TABLE 3-2	GUIDELINES FOR A DIET LOW IN SATURATED FAT

FOODS TO AVOID	FOODS TO CHOOSE
Red meat, especially when highly marbled; salami, sausage, bacon	Lean cuts of meat, fresh fish, poultry with skin removed before cooking, grilled meats
Whole milk, whipping cream	Nonfat (skim) or low-fat (1% or 2%) milk
Tropical oils (coconut, palm oils; cocoa butter)	Monounsaturated cooking oils (e.g., olive or canola oil)
Butter	Margarine (safflower oil listed as the first ingredient)
Salad dressing	Vinegar, lemon juice
Peanuts, peanut butter, hot dogs, potato chips	Unbuttered popcorn
Candy	Fresh fruits, vegetables
Ice cream	Nonfat yogurt, sherbet
Sweet rolls, donuts	Whole grain breads, cereals

- Stay with patient and provide reassurance during periods of angina.
- Monitor HR and BP during episodes of chest pain. Be alert to and report irregularities in HR and changes in SBP greater than 20 mm Hg from baseline.
- Monitor for presence of headache and hypotension after administering NTG. Keep patient recumbent during angina and NTG administration.
- Administer O_2 as prescribed to increase O_2 supply to the myocardium. Deliver O_2 with humidity *to help prevent its drying effects on oral and nasal mucosa.*

BOX 3-1   CLASSIFICATION OF ANGINA

- **Class I:** Angina occurs only with strenuous activity.
- **Class II:** Angina occurs with moderate activity such as walking quickly or climbing stairs rapidly, walking uphill, or walking at a normal pace for more than two blocks or up more than one flight of stairs.
- **Class III:** Angina occurs with mild activity such as climbing one flight of stairs or walking level for one to two blocks.
- **Class IV:** Angina occurs with any physical activity and may be present at rest.

- ◆ Emphasize to patient importance of immediately reporting angina to health care team.
- ◆ Instruct patient to avoid activities and factors known to cause stress and that may precipitate angina.
- ◆ Discuss value of relaxation techniques, including tapes, soothing music, biofeedback, meditation, or yoga. See **Health-seeking behaviors,** later.
- ◆ Administer β-blockers as prescribed to *decrease cardiac workload and O₂ demand.*
- ◆ Administer long-acting and/or topical nitrates *to decrease O₂ demand and likelihood of angina.*

Activity intolerance related to generalized weakness and imbalance between O₂ supply and demand secondary to tissue ischemia (MI)

Desired outcomes: During activity, patient rates perceived exertion at 3 or less on a 0-10 scale and exhibits cardiac tolerance to activity, as evidenced by respiratory rate (RR) 20 breaths/min or less, HR 120 beats per minute (bpm) or less (or within 20 bpm of resting HR), SBP within 20 mm Hg of patient's resting SBP, and absence of chest pain and new dysrhythmias.

Nursing Interventions

- ◆ Observe for and report increasing frequency of angina, angina that occurs at rest, angina that is unrelieved by NTG, or decreased exercise tolerance without angina. See **BOX 3-1** for classifications of angina.
- ◆ Assess patient's response to activity. Be alert to chest pain, increase in HR (greater than 20 bpm), change in SBP (20 mm Hg over or under resting BP), excessive fatigue, and shortness of breath. Ask patient to rate perceived exertion (see p. 90 for details).
- ◆ Assist patient with recognizing and limiting activities that increase O₂ demands, such as exercise and anxiety.
- ◆ Administer O₂ as prescribed for angina episodes. Deliver O₂ with humidity *to help prevent its drying effects on oral and nasal mucosa.*
  - ● Have patient perform ROM exercises, depending on tolerance and prescribed activity limitations. *Because cardiac intolerance to activity can be further aggravated by prolonged bed rest,* consult health care provider about in-bed exercises and activities that can be performed by patient as the condition improves.
- ◆ For further interventions, see "Prolonged Bed Rest," **Risk for activity intolerance,** p. 23, and **Risk for disuse syndrome,** p. 25.

Deficient knowledge related to catheterization procedure and postcatheterization regimen

Desired outcome: Before the procedure, patient verbalizes knowledge about cardiac catheterization and the postcatheterization plan of care.

Nursing Interventions

- ◆ Assess patient's facility with language; engage an interpreter or provide language-appropriate written materials if indicated.

- Assess patient's knowledge about catheterization procedure. As appropriate, reinforce health care provider's explanation, and answer any questions or concerns. If possible, arrange for an orientation visit to catheterization laboratory before the procedure.
- Before cardiac catheterization, have patient practice techniques (e.g., Valsalva maneuver, coughing, deep breathing) that will be used during procedure.
- Explain that after the procedure, bed rest will be required and VS, circulation, and insertion site will be checked at frequent intervals to ensure integrity. In addition, explain that flexion at insertion site (arm or groin) is contraindicated *to prevent bleeding.*
- Stress importance of promptly reporting signs and symptoms of concern, including groin, leg, or back pain; dizziness; chest pain; or shortness of breath. *Any of these symptoms may indicate hemorrhage or embolization of the stent.*

Ineffective cardiopulmonary, peripheral, and cerebral tissue perfusion related to interrupted arterial flow secondary to catheterization procedure
Desired outcomes: Within 1 hr after the procedure, patient has adequate perfusion, as evidenced by HR regular and within 20 bpm of baseline HR; apical/radial pulse equality; BP within 20 mm Hg of baseline BP; peripheral pulse amplitude greater than 2+ on a 0-4+ scale; warmth and normal color in the extremities; no significant change in mental status; and orientation to person, place, and time.

Nursing Interventions

- Monitor BP q15min until stable on three successive checks, q2h for the next 12 hr, and q4h for 24 hr unless otherwise indicated. If SBP drops 20 mm Hg or more below previous recordings, lower head of bed (HOB) and notify health care provider. If insertion site was the antecubital space, measure BP in unaffected arm.
- Be alert to and report indicators of decreased perfusion, including cool extremities, decreased amplitude of peripheral pulses, cyanosis, changes in mental status, decreased level of consciousness (LOC), and shortness of breath.
- Monitor HR, and notify health care provider if dysrhythmias occur. If patient is not on a cardiac monitor, auscultate apical and radial pulses with every BP check and report irregularities or apical/radial discrepancies.
- If the femoral artery was the insertion site, maintain HOB at no greater than a 30-degree elevation *to prevent acute hip joint flexion, which could compromise arterial flow.*

Risk for deficient fluid volume related to risk factors from hemorrhage or hematoma formation caused by arterial puncture and/or osmotic diuresis from the dye
Desired outcomes: Patient remains normovolemic, as evidenced by HR 100 bpm or less; BP 90/60 mm Hg or greater (or within 20 mm Hg of baseline range); no significant change in mental status; and orientation to person, place, and time. The dressing is dry, and there is no swelling at the puncture site.

Nursing Interventions

- Be alert to indicators of shock or hemorrhage, such as a decrease in BP, increase in HR, and decreasing LOC.
- Inspect dressing on groin or antecubital space for presence of frank bleeding, and check for hematoma formation (fluctuating swelling).
- Monitor peripheral perfusion, and be alert to decreased amplitude or absence of distal pulses, delayed capillary refill, coolness of the extremities, and pallor, *any of which can signal embolization or hemorrhagic shock.*

- Caution patient about flexing elbow or hip more than 30 degrees for 6-8 hr, or as prescribed, to minimize risk of bleeding and/or compromised circulation.
- If bleeding occurs, maintain pressure at insertion site as prescribed, usually 1 inch proximal to puncture site or introducer insertion site. Typically this is done with a pressure dressing or a $2\frac{1}{2}$- to 5-1b sandbag.

Ineffective peripheral (involved limb) tissue perfusion (or risk of same) related to interrupted arterial flow secondary to embolization
Desired outcome: Patient has adequate perfusion in the involved limb, as evidenced by peripheral pulse amplitude greater than 2+ on a 0-4+ scale; normal color, sensation, and temperature; and brisk capillary refill (refill time less than 2 sec).

Nursing Interventions

- Assess peripheral perfusion by palpating peripheral pulses q15min for 30 min, then q30min for 1 hr, then hourly for 2 hr, or per protocol.
- Monitor for and report any indicators of embolization in involved limb, such as faintness or absence of pulse; coolness of extremity; mottling; decreased capillary refill; cyanosis; and complaints of numbness, tingling, and pain at insertion site. Instruct patient to report any of these indicators promptly.
- If there is no evidence of embolus or thrombus formation, instruct patient to move fingers or toes and rotate wrist or ankle *to promote circulation.*
- Ensure that patient maintains bed rest for 4-6 hr or as prescribed.

Ineffective renal tissue perfusion (or risk for same) related to interrupted blood flow secondary to decreased cardiac output or reaction to contrast dye
Desired outcome: Patient has adequate renal perfusion as evidenced by urinary output of at least 30 mL/hr, specific gravity less than 1.030, good skin turgor, and moist mucous membranes.

Nursing Interventions

- Because contrast dye for cardiac catheterization may cause osmotic diuresis, monitor for indicators of dehydration, such as poor skin turgor, dry mucous membranes, and high urine specific gravity (1.030 or more).
- Monitor I&O. Notify health care provider if urinary output is less than 30 mL/hr in the presence of adequate intake.
- If urinary output is insufficient despite adequate intake, restrict fluids. Be alert to and report indicators of fluid overload, such as crackles (rales) on auscultation of lung fields, distended neck veins, and shortness of breath. Notify health care provider about significant findings.
- If patient does not exhibit signs of cardiac or renal failure, encourage daily intake of 2-3 L of fluids, or as prescribed, *to flush contrast dye out of the system.*

Imbalanced nutrition: more than body requirements related to excess intake of calories, Na^+, or fats
Desired outcome: Within the 24-hr period before hospital discharge, patient demonstrates knowledge of the dietary regimen by planning a 3-day menu that includes and excludes appropriate foods.

Nursing Interventions

- If patient is over ideal body weight, explain that a low-calorie diet is necessary.

- Discuss ways to decrease dietary intake of saturated (animal) fats and increase intake of polyunsaturated (vegetable oil) fats (Table 3-2).
- Teach patient to limit dietary intake of cholesterol to less than 300 mg/day (Table 3-1). Encourage use of food labels to determine cholesterol content of foods.
- Teach patient to limit dietary intake of refined/processed sugar.
- Teach patient to limit dietary intake of sodium chloride (NaCl) to less than 4 g/day (mild restriction). Encourage use of food labels to determine Na$^+$ content of foods (see Box 4-1, p. 165).
- Instruct patient and significant other in use of "Nutrition Facts" (federally mandated public information on all food product labels) to determine amount of calories, total fat, saturated fat, cholesterol, and Na$^+$ in foods. Teach them to be especially aware of the serving size listed for respective nutrients (i.e., a serving size listed as 4 oz on a package containing 12 oz would mean consumer would get 3 × the amount of each ingredient if he or she eats the entire contents of the container!).
- Encourage intake of fresh fruits, natural (unrefined or unprocessed) carbohydrates, fish, poultry, legumes, fresh vegetables, and grains for a healthy, balanced diet.

Deficient knowledge related to precautions and side effects of nitrates
Desired outcome: Within the 24-hr period before hospital discharge, patient verbalizes understanding of the precautions and side effects of prescribed medication.

Nursing Interventions

- Assess patient's facility with language; engage an interpreter or provide language-appropriate written materials if indicated.
- Instruct patient to report the presence of a headache associated with NTG *because the dose may need to be altered.*
- Teach patient to assume a recumbent position if a headache occurs. Explain that the drug's vasodilation effect can result in transient headache.
- Explain that vasodilation from nitrates also may decrease BP, which can result in orthostatic hypotension. Instruct patient to rise slowly from a sitting or lying position and to remain by chair or bed for 1 min after standing *to be assured he or she is not going to experience orthostatic changes.*
- Caution patient against using NTG more frequently than prescribed.

Deficient knowledge related to precautions and side effects of β-blockers
Desired outcome: Within the 24-hr period before hospital discharge, patient verbalizes understanding of the precautions and side effects of β-blockers.

Nursing Interventions

- Instruct patient to be alert to depression, fatigue, dizziness, erythematous rash, respiratory distress, and sexual dysfunction, which can occur as side effects of β-blockers. Explain importance of notifying health care provider promptly if these side effects occur.
- Explain that weight gain and peripheral and sacral edema can occur as side effects of β-blockers. Teach patient how to assess for edema and importance of reporting promptly if it occurs.
- Explain that BP and HR are assessed before administration of β-blockers *because these drugs can cause hypotension and excessive slowing of the heart.*
- Caution patient not to omit or abruptly stop taking β-blockers *because this may result in rebound tachycardia causing angina or MI.*

Deficient knowledge related to disease process and lifestyle implications of CAD

Desired outcome: Within the 24-hr period before hospital discharge, patient verbalizes knowledge about the disease process of CAD and concomitant lifestyle implications.

Nursing Interventions

◆ Teach patient about CAD, including pathophysiologic processes of cardiac ischemia, angina, and infarction.

◆ Assist with identifying risk factors for CAD and risk factor modification as follows:
  - Diet low in cholesterol and saturated fat.
  - Smoking cessation.
  - Regular activity/exercise programs.

◆ Discuss symptoms that necessitate medical attention, such as chest pain unrelieved by NTG, decreased exercise tolerance, increased shortness of breath, and loss of consciousness.

◆ Discuss guidelines for sexual activity, such as resting before intercourse, finding a comfortable position, taking prophylactic NTG, and postponing intercourse for 1-1½ hr after a heavy meal.

◆ Discuss procedures such as cardiac catheterization, PCI, and CABG, if appropriate.

Health-seeking behaviors related to relaxation technique effective for stress reduction

Desired outcome: Patient reports subjective relief of stress after using relaxation technique.

Nursing Interventions

◆ Discuss importance of relaxation *to decrease nervous system tone (sympathetic), energy requirements, and O₂ consumption.*

◆ Many techniques use breathing, concentration, or imagery *to promote relaxation and decrease energy requirements.* The following technique can be used easily by anyone. Speaking slowly and softly, give patient the following guidelines:
  - Find a comfortable position. Close your eyes.
  - Begin by concentrating on your feet and toes; tighten the muscles in your feet and toes, and hold this tightness for a count of three. Now slowly relax your feet and toes. Feel or imagine the tension flowing out of your feet and toes. Now concentrate on your lower legs. Tense the muscles of your lower legs for a count of three. Now slowly release this tightness and feel the tension drain from your lower legs. Continue with this purposeful tightening and relaxation with each successive major body part, moving up the body, until finally you reach your facial muscles. When you reach your face, tighten the muscles of your face for a count of three. When you relax the muscles in your face, take a deep breath and exhale. As you breathe out, imagine that you are blowing all the tension of your body out and away from you, leaving you totally relaxed and calm.
  - Now breathe through your nose. Concentrate on feeling the air move in and out. As you exhale, say the word "one" silently to yourself. Again continue feeling the air move in and out of your lungs. Continue for approximately 20 min.
  - Try to clear your mind of worries; be passive. Let relaxation occur. If distractions appear, gently push them away. Continue breathing through your nose, repeating "one" silently.

◆ Encourage patient to practice this technique 2-3 ×/day or whenever feeling stressed or tense. Acknowledge that this technique may feel strange at first but that it becomes easier and more effective with each practice.

◆ Explain that Baroque or New Age music, played softly, helps many individuals achieve an even greater state of relaxation.

Patient-Family Teaching and Discharge Planning

Reinforce previously taught information regarding prescribed nitrates, β-blockers, diet, exercise, relaxation, and symptoms requiring medical attention. Also provide verbal and written information about the following:

◆ Importance of reducing or eliminating intake of caffeine, which causes vasoconstriction and increases HR.

◆ Pulse monitoring: how to self-measure pulse, including parameters for target HRs and limits.

◆ Prescribed exercise program and importance of maintaining a regular exercise schedule, with referral to a cardiac rehabilitation program, in which individualized exercise programs are outlined for patient.

◆ Activity and dietary limitations as prescribed.

◆ Importance of follow-up with health care provider; confirm date and time of next appointment.

◆ Need for cessation of smoking: Refer patient to a "stop smoking" program as appropriate. The following free brochures outline ways to help patients stop smoking:

> *How to Help Your Patients Stop Using Tobacco: A National Cancer Institute Manual for the Oral Health Team,* from the Smoking and Tobacco Control Program of the National Cancer Institute, NIH Pub No. 93-3191.

> *Clinical Practice Guideline: A Quick Reference Guide for Smoking Cessation Specialists,* from the Agency for Healthcare Policy and Quality (AHRQ), US Department of Health and Human Services, Pub No. 96-0694.

◆ Importance of involvement and support of significant others in patient's lifestyle changes.

◆ Importance of getting BP checked at regular intervals (at least monthly if patient is hypertensive).

◆ Importance of avoiding strenuous activity for at least 1 hr after meals to help prevent excessive O_2 demands.

◆ Importance of reporting to health care provider any change in pattern or frequency of angina.

◆ Availability of community and medical support from organizations such as the American Heart Association (website): *www.americanheart.org*

❖ HEART FAILURE

OVERVIEW/PATHOPHYSIOLOGY

Heart failure (HF) is a complex clinical syndrome in which the heart is unable to pump sufficient blood to meet the body's metabolic demands. It is caused by any structural or functional cardiac disorder that impairs the ventricle's ability to fill with or eject blood. HF is a chronic condition that is prone to acute exacerbations (termed *acute decompensated heart failure* [ADHF]). In most cases of ADHF, severe volume overload and pulmonary edema are present. Acute pulmonary edema is an emergency situation in which hydrostatic pressure in the pulmonary vessels is greater than the vascular colloid osmotic pressure that holds fluid in the vessels. As a result, fluid floods the alveoli. When the alveoli contain fluid, their ability to participate in gas exchange is reduced, and hypoxia occurs. HF usually is a result of either systolic dysfunction (previously referred to as *left-sided failure)* or diastolic cardiac dysfunction (previously referred to as *right-sided failure)* or a combination of both. See **BOX 3-2**, Classifications of Heart Failure: Comparison of American College of Cardiology and American Heart Association (ACC/AHA) Heart Failure with New York Heart Association (NYHA) Functional Class, for more information.

BOX 3-2 CLASSIFICATIONS OF HEART FAILURE: COMPARISON OF AMERICAN COLLEGE OF CARDIOLOGY AND AMERICAN HEART ASSOCIATION HEART FAILURE STAGE WITH NEW YORK HEART ASSOCIATION FUNCTIONAL CLASS

ACC/AHA Heart Failure Stage*
- A At high risk for heart failure but without structural heart disease or symptoms of heart failure (e.g., patients with hypertension or coronary artery disease)
- B Structural heart disease but without symptoms of heart failure
- C Structural heart disease with prior or current symptoms of heart failure
- D Refractory heart failure requiring specialized interventions

NYHA Functional Class†
- I Asymptomatic
- II Symptomatic with moderate exertion
- III Symptomatic with minimal exertion
- IV Symptomatic at rest

Data from Hunt SA et al.: ACC/AHA 2005 guideline update for the diagnosis and management of chronic heart failure in the adult—summary article, *Circulation* 112:1-28, 2005.
Adapted from Farrell MH et al: Beta-blockers in heart failure: clinical applications, *JAMA* 287:890-897, 2002.
*The new American College of Cardiology and American Heart Association (ACC/AHA) classification guidelines were designed to complement the NYHA classification system. These new guidelines focus more on underlying disease and the need to treat early in the disease process, even before overt symptoms of heart failure are present.
†The New York Heart Association (NYHA) classification system is based largely on the assessment of symptoms.

Systolic dysfunction: Ventricular dilation and impaired ventricular contraction occur because of myocardial muscle injury or abnormality (see "Dilated cardiomyopathy (DCM)," later). The initial injury or stressor to the heart muscle results in impaired cardiac output. This triggers a cascade of compensatory mechanisms, which together contribute to development and progression of HF.

Increased neurohormonal activation: Activation of the sympathetic nervous system (SNS) and renin-angiotensin system (RAS) stimulates catecholamines and other neurohormones and causes increases in HR and BP, systemic vasoconstriction, decreased renal perfusion, and Na^+ and fluid retention in an effort to increase cardiac output.

Hemodynamic alterations: Increase in left ventricular (LV) end-diastolic volume/pressure (preload) and thickening and elongation of the myofibrils (stretch) initially result in increased force of contraction (Frank-Starling law). The rise in myocardial O_2 demand further stimulates the neurohormonal response. Increases in preload and afterload (because of increased systemic resistance) add to LV workload and cause excessive "stretch" of the myofibrils, thereby impairing ventricular contraction.

Remodeling: The foregoing mechanisms eventually lead to hypertrophy (enlargement and thickening of the LV wall). The heart becomes more spherical (dilated) in shape because of lengthening of the myofibrils, cell slippage, fibrosis, and myocyte death. These progressive changes in size, shape, and structure of the heart muscle are termed *remodeling*.

These structural, hemodynamic, and neurohormonal alterations cause progressive deterioration in systolic function associated with decreased left ventricular ejection fraction (LVEF), increased intracardiac pressures, impaired valvular function, decreased forward flow to vital organs and tissues, and increased pulmonary pressures. This process results in pulmonary (left-sided HF) and hepatic (right-sided HF) congestion, edema, renal impairment, and impaired oxygenation and metabolism. Ventricular and atrial dysrhythmias are common because of structural changes to the myocytes and increased myocardial O_2 demand and are a major cause of death in this population.

Diastolic dysfunction: The ventricle becomes noncompliant and unable to accommodate increased preload and afterload (or decreased preload). These patients may have symptoms of HF because of volume overload without a reduction in systolic function as seen in individuals with long-standing hypertension, coronary artery disease (CAD), and hypertrophic and restrictive cardiomyopathies (see later).

Cardiomyopathies: HF commonly occurs in the presence of an underlying cardiomyopathy (disorder of the heart muscle). Cardiomyopathies are classified according to underlying cause and abnormality in structure and function.

Dilated cardiomyopathy (DCM): Most prevalent type, characterized by enlargement of one (usually left) or both ventricles and impaired contraction (systolic dysfunction). The most common form is ischemic cardiomyopathy caused by severe coronary (ischemic) heart disease and/or myocardial infarction (MI). DCM also occurs secondary to hypertension, valvular heart disease, diabetes mellitus (DM), cardiotoxins, genetic causes, and metabolic, infectious, or systemic diseases. DCM is termed *idiopathic* when the cause cannot be identified. See "Systolic dysfunction," earlier, for additional information.

Hypertrophic cardiomyopathy: Characterized by an abnormally enlarged left ventricle but without a concomitant increase in cavity size. Filling is restricted and may be associated with LV outflow tract obstruction. Cardiac function can remain normal for varying periods before decompensation occurs. Symptoms are varied and may include HF symptoms, chest pain, palpitations, dizziness, near-syncope, syncope. Patients may be prone to ventricular dysrhythmias. Although it is theorized that hypertrophic cardiomyopathy has a strong hereditary link, etiology is unknown.

Restrictive cardiomyopathy: Least common in Western countries, it is characterized by inadequate compliance causing restriction of diastolic filling.

Other causes of heart failure

HF or acute pulmonary edema can occur secondary to other conditions that place excessive demands on cardiac output, such as hypertensive crisis, tachycardia due to hyperthyroidism, dysrhythmias, severe anemia, trauma, infection, volume overload (i.e., caused by IV fluids, postoperative fluid shifts), pregnancy, and conditions that affect capillary permeability. In these cases, treatment/correction of the underlying cause is essential and may result in normalization or improvement of cardiac function.

Severe pulmonary diseases, including COPD, pulmonary hypertension, and obstructive sleep apnea (OSA) can lead to diastolic HF (cor pulmonale). This condition is less likely to be reversible. Poorly compensated pulmonary disease, upper respiratory infection (URI), and pneumonia can exacerbate all types of HF and need to be treated aggressively.

ASSESSMENT

Signs and symptoms/physical findings

General: Dyspnea on exertion (DOE) or at rest, fatigue, decreased exercise tolerance, weakness, orthopnea (unable to lie flat; may need to sleep on pillows or sitting in a chair), paroxysmal nocturnal dyspnea, wheezing, cough, weight gain, lower extremity edema, abdominal distention, early satiety, and nocturia. Associated indicators include chest/anginal pains, palpitations, near-syncope, syncope, and falls. Low-output symptoms include positional light-headedness, weakness, mental status changes, and decreased urine output.

Physical findings include decreased or elevated BP, dysrhythmias, tachycardia, tachypnea, increased venous pulsations, pulsus alternans (alternating strong and weak heart beats), increased central venous pressure (CVP), jugular venous distention, crackles (rales), wheezes, decreased breath sounds, cardiac gallop and/or murmur, hepatomegaly, ascites, and pitting edema in dependent areas (lower extremities, sacrum).

ADHF: Typified by marked severity of HF symptoms and deterioration by one or more NYHA functional classes (Box 3-2). Pulmonary edema and cardiogenic shock (**TABLE 3-3**) may be present, and renal dysfunction may occur in more severe cases.

Acute pulmonary edema: Extreme dyspnea, anxiety, restlessness, frothy and blood-tinged sputum, severe orthopnea, paroxysmal nocturnal dyspnea, crackles (rales), wheezing, decreased breath sounds, tachycardia, tachypnea, engorged neck veins, and cardiac gallop/murmur. Patient exhibits "air hunger" and may thrash about and describe a sensation of drowning.

History and risk factors: CAD, hypertension, DM, OSA or other pulmonary disease, recent IV fluid infusions, surgery, pregnancy, recent/current infectious illness, pneumonia, nonadherence to medication or diet regimen, and recent use of nonsteroidal antiinflammatory drug (NSAID) or cyclooxygenase 2 (COX-2) selective agent. In addition, see "Other Causes of Heart Failure," earlier.

DIAGNOSTIC TESTS

Chest x-ray examination: May show cardiomegaly, engorged pulmonary vasculature, "Kerley B lines" suggestive of HF, and pleural or pericardial effusions.

ECG: Changes may indicate CAD, acute myocardial ischemia, LV hypertrophy (widened QRS complex), conduction defects, and dysrhythmias.

LVEF: Percentage of blood ejected from the left ventricle during systole. Normal LVEF is 50%-70%. In systolic dysfunction, it is reduced. LVEF less than 35% is associated with increased risk for fatal HF and dysrhythmias. In hypertrophic cardiomyopathy, LVEF may be greater than 70%. LVEF assessment can be measured during echocardiogram, LVgram, magnetic resonance imaging (MRI), or radionuclide studies (multiple-gated acquisition [MUGA] scan, nuclear stress test [see later]).

Echocardiography: Most commonly used means of evaluating ventricular function. It assesses left- and right-sided systolic function, LVEF, degree of ventricular dilation, wall thickness, abnormal wall and septal motion, valvular function, estimated pulmonary pressure, presence of thrombus, restriction, outflow tract obstruction, and pericardial effusion. Diastolic dysfunction may be evident. Tissue Doppler/three-dimensional echocardiography may reveal degree of ventricular synchrony and utility of cardiac resynchronization therapy (CRT) (see "Collaborative Management," later).

Cardiac catheterization: Rules out underlying ischemic heart disease and assesses hemodynamics (left- and right-sided filling pressures, cardiac output, and systemic and pulmonary vascular resistance).

Left ventriculography: Provides assessment of LV function and LVEF.

Endomyocardial biopsy: May be obtained during right-sided heart catheterization. Usually it is reserved for severe, refractory HF in nonelderly patients to assist in identifying pathologic agent and reversible causes.

Radionuclide stress test, stress echocardiogram: Assess for underlying ischemic heart disease and reversible or fixed ischemic defects.

Pulmonary function tests (PFTs): Useful in differentiating causes of shortness of breath and other HF symptoms. PFTs may reveal underlying COPD or reactive airways disease (asthma).

Oximetry/arterial blood gas (ABG) values: Reveals hypoxemia. Desaturations may be noted with activity. Overnight (sleep) oximetry may reveal underlying OSA.

TABLE 3-3 SYSTEMIC CLINICAL SIGNS OF SHOCK

	CARDIOGENIC	SEPTIC	HYPOVOLEMIC	NEUROGENIC	ANAPHYLACTIC
Cardiovascular	↓ BP ↑ HR ↓ Pulses	*Early:* ↑ BP ↑ Pulses *Late:* ↓ BP ↓ Pulses	↓ BP ↑ HR Flat neck veins	*Early:* vasodilation ↑ BP	↓ BP ↑ HR ↓ Pulses
Respiratory	Dyspnea, crackles	*Early:* ↑ RR *Late:* ↓ RR crackles(rales)	Lungs clear	Lungs clear	Dyspnea to air hunger; wheezes and complete obstruction
Neurologic	Confusion, lethargy, drowsiness	↓ LOC	↓ LOC	Normal or ↓ LOC	↓ LOC
Renal	↓ Urinary output	↓ Urinary output	↓ Urinary output	Normal or ↓ urinary output	↓ Urinary output
Cutaneous	Cool skin	*Early:* warm skin *Late:* cool skin	Cool skin	Warm skin (because of vasodilation)	Urticaria, angioedema

BP, Blood pressure; *HR,* heart rate; *LOC,* level of consciousness; *RR,* respiratory rate..

Blood urea nitrogen (BUN), serum creatinine: Elevated in renal insufficiency and chronic kidney disease due to low cardiac output and hypotension, possibly related to treatment with diuretics, angiotensin-converting enzyme (ACE) inhibitors, adrenergic receptor blockers (ARBs), or aldosterone antagonists.

Serum electrolytes: May reveal hyperkalemia due to renal dysfunction or ACE inhibitor/ARB or aldosterone antagonist use. Hypokalemia may occur as a result of diuretic use. The presence of hyponatremia is a poor prognostic indicator in advanced HF.

Serum enzymes: Mild elevations in cardiac troponins (with normal creatine kinase [CK]) are not uncommon in patients with chronic HF or chronic kidney disease. Cardiac troponin elevation in the presence of elevated CK may indicate acute coronary syndrome (ACS) (see p. 96).

Liver function tests, including serum aspartate aminotransferase (AST) and serum bilirubin assays: Levels may be elevated in patients with hepatic congestion.

Brain natriuretic peptide (BNP): Released from the ventricles in response to wall stress. This test is useful in differentiating HF from other causes of dyspnea, including pulmonary disease. Negative BNP test result (less than 100 pg/mL) suggests non-HF etiology. When used in conjunction with standard clinical assessment, elevated BNP may support diagnosis of HF and evaluate patient's response to treatment.

Digoxin level: The goal in HF is a level less than 1 ng/mL. Hypokalemia and impaired renal function can predispose patient to digoxin toxicity.

Complete blood count (CBC): May reveal decreased hemoglobin (Hgb) and hematocrit (Hct) in the presence of anemia.

Thyroid-stimulating hormone (TSH) level: Rules out hyperthyroidism or hypothyroidism, either of which may contribute to HF and dysrhythmias.

COLLABORATIVE MANAGEMENT

Identification and treatment of underlying causes: In the presence of active ischemia, patients may undergo coronary revascularization, that is, percutaneous coronary intervention (PCI) (see p. 100) or coronary artery bypass grafting (CABG) (see p. 139). Repair of valvular abnormalities also may be necessary.

Patient also may require aggressive treatment of coexisting hypertension (especially in diastolic dysfunction), DM, dysrhythmias, infection, anemia, and thyroid dysfunction. Assessment for nonadherence to medication regimen and Na$^+$-restricted diet as well as use of ethanol (ETOH) and inappropriate medications (see later) is important. Eighty percent of HF admissions are the result of preventable factors.

Low-Na$^+$ diet: A 2-g Na$^+$ diet is recommended for most patients. See Box 4-1, p. 165.

Daily morning weight monitoring: Assists in titration of diuretics and early identification of HF symptoms.

Heart transplantation: Option for select patients with end-stage (NYHA class IV) HF (Box 3-2).

Intraaortic balloon pump: Used in ADHF to increase coronary artery blood flow.

Mechanical ventricular assist devices: May be necessary for severe ADHF and patients in end-stage HF who are not eligible for transplantation.

Surgical techniques: May include LV reduction surgery (myomectomy), LV aneurysmectomy, cardiomyoplasty (investigational technique that involves transfer of the latissimus dorsi to the heart), and placement of Acorn CorCap Cardiac Support Device (a netted "cap" that supports the left ventricle).

Ultrafiltration (UF): Removes excess volume in ADHF patients with renal failure. UF requires central IV access and ICU monitoring. UF via peripheral access is being studied and may be accomplished without ICU monitoring.

Electrophysiology devices: CRT and implantable cardioverter defibrillators (ICDs) (see p. 146) may be used.

Correction of hypoxemia: In ADHF/pulmonary edema, high-flow O_2 may be given by nonrebreathing mask, positive airway pressure devices, or endotracheal intubation and mechanical ventilation. O_2 is delivered with humidity to help prevent its drying effects on oral and nasal mucosa. Once patient is stabilized, O_2 is titrated to keep pulse oximetry readings higher than 92%.

High Fowler's position (head of bed [HOB] up 90 degrees): Decreases venous return and eases work of breathing (WOB).

Continuous positive airway pressure (CPAP), bilevel positive airway pressure (BiPAP): May be necessary to treat OSA.

Pharmacotherapy

Loop diuretics: Promote excretion of water and Na^+, reduce preload, and prevent fluid retention. In ADHF, these diuretics are administered via IV bolus or drip form until stabilization occurs. These drugs can cause neurohormonal activation and aggravate preexisting renal dysfunction or hypokalemia.

Thiazide diuretics: Hydrochlorothiazide may be used for mild fluid retention. Metolazone is a potent drug that, when given $\frac{1}{2}$ hr before loop diuretics, markedly potentiates diuresis and therefore is reserved for more severe volume overload in ADHF or late-stage HF. Hyponatremia, hypokalemia, and worsening of renal function may occur and necessitate careful assessment.

IV vasodilators: Used in ADHF to decrease cardiac workload by reducing ventricular filling pressures and systemic vascular resistance (SVR) (afterload). These drugs are avoided in low-output HF and cardiogenic shock, and with SBP less than 90 mm Hg.

Nesiritide: Balanced arterial and venous vasodilator. This drug can alleviate acute dyspnea and reduce pulmonary capillary wedge pressure (PCWP) within the first 30 min of therapy. It promotes diuresis and natriuresis but does not replace need for diuretic therapy. It improves cardiac output by off-loading the heart and decreases neurohormonal activation. Use of nesiritide does not require CCU monitoring.

Nitroglycerin (NTG): Arterial and venous vasodilator. It also reduces PCWP and may require CCU monitoring. Because of tachyphylaxis (tolerance), patients may need escalating doses to achieve desired effect.

Nitroprusside: Potent arterial and venous vasodilator and afterload reducer. It must be administered in CCU because of the need for hemodynamic monitoring.

IV inotropic drugs: Increase strength of contractions. These drugs are reserved for use in ADHF-associated low cardiac output and cardiogenic shock until patient is stabilized. They may be used longer term in advanced-stage HF as a bridge to transplantation or for palliation of symptoms. Use may be associated with increased mortality and ventricular dysrhythmias. Administration of inotropic drugs may require transfer to CCU to monitor for hemodynamic effects and dysrhythmias.

Morphine sulfate: Coronary vasodilator. It may be given in ADHF or acute pulmonary edema to decrease anxiety and WOB and to relieve angina if ischemic heart disease is present.

Neurohormonal antagonists: Studies suggest ACE inhibitors, β-blockers, and aldosterone antagonists decrease mortality and hospitalizations and improve cardiac function and HF symptoms in patients with LV systolic dysfunction.

ACE inhibitors: Suppress effects of RAS by reducing angiotensin II and causing decreased aldosterone secretion. These drugs lower BP and reduce preload and afterload and thereby decrease work of the left ventricle.

ARBs: For patients who do not tolerate ACE inhibitors because of cough caused by bradykinin release.

β-Blockers and α/β-adrenergic blockers: Block effects of SNS and toxic effects of neurohormones on the myocardium. These drugs decrease heartrate (HR) and BP and thereby decrease cardiac workload.

Aldosterone antagonists: Block aldosterone, which causes Na^+ and fluid retention. These drugs have less potent diuretic properties than loop diuretics and thiazides. They may cause hyperkalemia and worsening of renal dysfunction.

Adjunct therapies

Digoxin: May improve HF symptoms and exercise tolerance and decrease hospitalizations, although mortality rate is not reduced. Levels are kept at less than 1 ng/mL.

Hydralazine: Oral vasodilator and afterload reducer. It is used in combination with nitrates in patients who are ACE inhibitor/ARB intolerant because of renal dysfunction. It decreases mortality and HF symptoms to a lesser degree than ACE inhibitors and can cause reflex tachycardia.

Nitrate: Coronary vasodilator, used in conjunction with hydralazine (see earlier); also used in ischemic heart disease as an antianginal drug.

Warfarin sodium (Coumadin): Given in the presence of thrombus formation, stasis of blood in the ventricle, LV aneurysm in severe LV dysfunction, or for other indications for anticoagulation, for example, atrial fibrillation.

Calcium channel blockers (CCBs): May be used in diastolic HF to assist with relaxation and filling and reduce outflow tract obstruction (hypertrophic cardiomyopathy). Except for amlodipine or felodipine, CCBs are avoided in LV systolic dysfunction inasmuch as they decrease cardiac contractility.

Amiodarone: Antidysrhythmic for patients with HF.

Epoetin alfa: Used in patients with HF and coexisting anemia and renal dysfunction.

NURSING DIAGNOSES AND INTERVENTIONS

Impaired gas exchange related to alveolar-capillary membrane changes secondary to fluid accumulation in the alveoli

Desired outcome: Within 30 min of treatment/intervention, patient has adequate gas exchange, as evidenced by normal breath sounds and skin color, presence of eupnea, HR 100 bpm or less, PaO_2 80 mm Hg or higher, and $PaCO_2$ 45 mm Hg or less.

Nursing Interventions

- Auscultate lung fields for breath sounds; be alert to crackles (rales), *which signal alveolar fluid congestion.*
- Assist patient into high Fowler's position (HOB up 90 degrees) *to decrease WOB and enhance gas exchange.*
- Teach patient to take slow, deep breaths *to increase oxygenation.*
- Administer O_2 as prescribed. Deliver with humidity *to help prevent its drying effects on oral and nasal mucosa.*
- Monitor oximetry and report findings of 92% or less. If ABGs are tested, monitor results for presence of hypoxemia (decreased PaO_2) and hypercapnia (increased $PaCO_2$).
- Be alert to signs of increasing respiratory distress: increased RR, mental status changes, gasping for air, cyanosis, or rapid HR.
- Administer diuretics as prescribed. Monitor K^+ levels *because of the potential for hypokalemia (K^+ less than 3.5 mEq/L) in patients taking certain diuretics.*
- Administer vasodilators such as nitrates as prescribed *to increase venous capacitance (venous dilation) and decrease pulmonary congestion.*
- As indicated, have emergency equipment (e.g., airway, manual resuscitation bag) available and functional.
- As indicated, prepare to transfer patient to ICU.

Excess fluid volume related to compromised regulatory mechanisms secondary to decreased cardiac output
Desired outcomes: Within 1 hr of intervention/treatment, patient demonstrates less shortness of breath and has output greater than intake on I&O monitoring. Within 1 day of treatment/intervention, edema is 1+ or less on a 0-4+ scale. Weight becomes stable within 2-3 days.

Nursing Interventions

- Closely monitor I&O, including insensible losses from diaphoresis and respirations.
- Record weight daily, and report steady gains.
- Assess for edema (interstitial fluids), especially in dependent areas such as ankles and sacrum.
- Assess respiratory system for crackles (rales) or pink-tinged, frothy sputum. These signs indicate fluid extravasation.
- Monitor for jugular vein distention, crackles (rales), elevated CVP, peripheral edema, and ascites. These signs indicate fluid overload.
- Monitor laboratory results for increased urinary specific gravity, decreased Hct, increased urine osmolality, hyponatremia, and hypochloremia. These findings indicate fluid retention.
- Monitor IV rate of flow *to prevent volume overload*. Use an infusion control device.
- Unless contraindicated, provide ice chips or Popsicles to help patient control thirst. Record amount on I&O record. Provide frequent mouth care *to reduce dry mucous membranes.*
- Administer diuretics as prescribed, and record patient's response.
- Administer morphine sulfate if prescribed *to induce vasodilation and decrease venous return to the heart.*

Ineffective cardiopulmonary, peripheral, and cerebral tissue perfusion related to interrupted blood flow secondary to decreased cardiac output
Desired outcomes: Within 2 hr of intervention/treatment, patient has adequate tissue perfusion, as evidenced by BP within 20 mm Hg of baseline BP; HR 100 beats per minute (bpm) or less with regular rhythm; RR 20 breaths/min or less with normal depth and pattern (eupnea); brisk capillary refill (less than 2 sec); and significant improvement in mental status or orientation to person, place, and time.

Nursing Interventions

- Monitor BP q15min or more frequently if unstable. Be alert to decreases greater than 20 mm Hg over patient's baseline or associated changes such as dizziness and altered mentation.
- Check pulse rate q15-30min. Monitor for irregularities, increased HR, or skipped beats, *which can signal decompensation and decreased function.*
- Monitor for cool extremities, pallor, and diaphoresis. These signs indicate peripheral vasoconstriction from SNS compensation. Evaluate capillary refill. Optimally, pink color should return within 1-2 sec after applying pressure to nail beds.
- Monitor for restlessness, anxiety, mental status changes, confusion, lethargy, stupor, and coma. These signs indicate decreased cerebral perfusion. Institute safety precautions accordingly.
- Administer inotropic drugs and vasodilators as prescribed. Monitor effects closely. Be alert to problems such as hypotension and irregular heartbeats.

Decreased cardiac output related to negative inotropic changes in the heart (decreased cardiac contractility) secondary to cardiac muscle changes
Desired outcomes: By at least 24 hr before hospital discharge, patient exhibits adequate cardiac output, as evidenced by SBP at least 90 mm Hg, HR 100 bpm

or less, urinary output at least 30 mL/hr, stable weight, eupnea, normal breath sounds, and edema 1+ or less on a 0-4+ scale. By at least 48 hr before hospital discharge, patient is free of new dysrhythmias, does not exhibit significant changes in mental status, and remains oriented to person, place, and time.

Nursing Interventions

- Assess for, document, and report evidence of decreased cardiac output, such as edema, jugular venous distention, adventitious breath sounds, shortness of breath, decreased urinary output, extra heart sound such as S_3, changes in mental status or level of consciousness (LOC), cool extremities, hypotension, tachycardia, and tachypnea.
- Keep accurate I&O records; weigh patient daily.
- Assist with activities of daily living (ADL) and facilitate coordination of health care providers *to ensure rest periods between care activities to decrease cardiac workload.* Allow 90 min for undisturbed rest. If necessary, limit visitors *to enable adequate rest.*
- Administer medications as prescribed, such as β-blockers, CCBs, and antidysrhythmic agents.
- Assist patient into position of comfort, usually semi-Fowler's position (HOB up 30-45 degrees).

Activity intolerance related to imbalance between O_2 supply and demand secondary to decrease in cardiac muscle contractility
Desired outcome: During activity, patient rates perceived exertion at 3 or less on a 0-10 scale and exhibits cardiac tolerance to activity, as evidenced by RR 20 breaths/min or less, SBP within 20 mm Hg of resting range, HR within 20 bpm of resting HR, and absence of chest pain and new dysrhythmias.

Nursing Interventions

- Monitor patient's physiologic response to activity. Report chest pain, new dysrhythmias, increased shortness of breath, HR increased greater than 20 bpm over resting HR, and SBP greater than 20 mm Hg over resting SBP. Ask patient to rate perceived exertion (see p. 24 for a description).
- Monitor BP and other VS q4h, and report changes such as irregular HR, HR greater than 100 bpm, or decreasing BP.
- Observe for and report oliguria, decreasing BP, decreased mentation, and dizziness. These signs indicate acute decreased cardiac output.
- Assess integrity of peripheral perfusion by monitoring peripheral pulses, distal extremity skin color, and urinary output. Report changes such as decreased amplitude of pulses, pallor or cyanosis, and decreased urinary output.
- In the presence of acute decreased cardiac output, ensure that patient's needs are met *so that activity can be avoided* (e.g., by keeping water at the bedside and urinal or commode nearby, maintaining a quiet environment, and limiting visitors as necessary to ensure adequate rest).
- Facilitate coordination of health care providers *to ensure rest periods between care activities to decrease cardiac workload. Allow 90 min for undisturbed rest.*
- Administer medications as prescribed.
- Assist with passive and some active or assistive ROM and other exercises, depending on patient's tolerance and prescribed limitations *to help prevent complications caused by immobility.*

Fear related to potentially life-threatening situation
Desired outcome: Within 24 hr of this diagnosis, patient communicates fears and concerns and reports increasing physical and psychological comfort.

Nursing Interventions

- Provide opportunity for patient and significant other to express feelings and fears. Be reassuring and supportive.
- Help make patient as comfortable as possible with prompt pain relief and positioning, typically high Fowler's position (HOB up 90 degrees).
- Keep environment as calm and quiet as possible to facilitate relaxation.
- Explain all treatment modalities, especially those that may be uncomfortable (e.g., O_2 face mask and rotating tourniquets).
- Remain with patient if possible, and provide emotional support for both patient and significant other.
- For further interventions, see "Psychosocial Support" for **Fear,** p. 35.

Deficient knowledge related to precautions and side effects of diuretic therapy
Desired outcome: Within the 24-hr period before hospital discharge, patient verbalizes knowledge of the precautions and side effects of diuretic therapy.

Nursing Interventions

- Assess patient's facility with language; engage an interpreter or provide language-appropriate materials if indicated.
- Depending on type of diuretic used, teach patient to report signs and symptoms of the following:
  - *Hypokalemia:* Anorexia, irregular pulse, nausea, apathy, and muscle cramps.
  - *Hyperkalemia:* Muscle weakness, hyporeflexia, and irregular HR, which can occur with K^+-sparing diuretics.
  - *Hyponatremia:* Fatigue, weakness, and edema (caused by fluid extravasation).
- For patients on long-term diuretic therapy, explain importance of follow-up monitoring of blood levels of Na^+ and K^+.
- For patients receiving K^+-wasting diuretics (e.g., furosemide), teach need to take in supplemental high-K^+ foods, such as apricots, bananas, oranges, raisins.
- As appropriate, instruct patient to use care when rising from a sitting or recumbent position *to prevent injury from orthostatic hypotension.*

Deficient knowledge related to precautions and side effects of digitalis therapy
Desired outcome: Within the 24-hr period before hospital discharge, patient verbalizes understanding of the precautions and side effects associated with digitalis therapy.

Nursing Interventions

- Assess patient's facility with language; engage an interpreter or provide language-appropriate materials if indicated.
- Teach technique and importance of assessing HR before taking digitalis. Explain that patient should obtain HR parameters from health care provider but that digitalis is usually withheld when HR is less than 60 bpm (unless patient's usual HR before digitalis administration is less than 60 bpm). Also instruct patient to hold dose if there is 20 bpm or greater change from his or her normal rate. Teach patient to notify health care provider if he or she has omitted a dose because of a slow or significantly changed HR.
- Explain that serum K^+ levels are monitored routinely *because low levels can potentiate digitalis toxicity.*
- Explain that apical HR and peripheral pulses are assessed for irregularity, *which is a sign of digitalis toxicity.*
- Teach patient to be alert to nausea, vomiting, anorexia, headache, diarrhea, blurred vision, yellow-haze vision, and mental confusion because these are

indicators of digitalis toxicity. Explain importance of reporting signs and symptoms promptly if they occur.

Deficient knowledge related to precautions and side effects of vasodilators
Desired outcome: Within the 24-hr period before hospital discharge, patient verbalizes knowledge of the precautions and side effects associated with vasodilators.

Nursing Interventions

- Assess patient's facility with language; engage an interpreter or provide language-appropriate materials if indicated.
- Explain that a headache can occur after administration of a vasodilator and that lying down will help alleviate pain.
- Teach importance of assessment for weight gain and signs of peripheral or sacral edema, any of which can occur as side effects of vasodilator therapy.
- For patients on long-term ACE inhibitor therapy, explain importance of follow-up monitoring of serum creatinine levels *because ACE inhibitors may decrease creatinine clearance.*
- For patients receiving ACE inhibitors, teach importance of using care when rising from a sitting or recumbent position *to prevent injury from orthostatic hypotension.*
- Teach patient receiving ACE inhibitors the technique for and importance of assessing BP before taking medication. It is possible to purchase automatic BP machines from local pharmacies. If necessary, seek information on reimbursement or funding from a social worker. Explain that patient should obtain BP parameters from health care provider but that ACE inhibitors are usually withheld when BP is less than 110/60 mm Hg. Teach patient to notify health care provider if he or she has omitted a dose because of low or significantly changed BP.
- Instruct patient to alert health care provider to side effects of this therapy.

Patient-Family Teaching and Discharge Planning

Reinforce previously taught informations about the disease, prescribed medications, and need for rest. In addition provide verbal and written information about the following:

- Medications, including drug names, purpose, dosage, schedule, precautions, and potential side effects. Also discuss drug/drug, food/drug, and herb/drug interactions.
- Signs and symptoms that necessitate immediate medical attention: dyspnea, decreased exercise tolerance, alterations in pulse rate/rhythm, loss of consciousness (caused by dysrhythmias or decreased cardiac output), oliguria, and steady weight gain (caused by HF).
- Reinforcement that cardiomyopathy is a chronic disease requiring lifetime treatment.
- Importance of abstaining from alcohol, which increases cardiac muscle deterioration.
- Need for physical support from family and outside agencies as disease progresses.
- Availability of community and medical support organizations such as the American Heart Association (website): *www.americanheart.org.*

❖ PULMONARY ARTERIAL HYPERTENSION

OVERVIEW/PATHOPHYSIOLOGY

As blood passes through the pulmonary vasculature, it exchanges CO_2 and particulate matter for O_2. Normally the pulmonary vascular bed offers little resistance to blood flow, but when resistance occurs, pulmonary pressures rise and pulmonary arterial hypertension (PAH) results. PAH can be primary or secondary (SPAH). Primary or idiopathic PAH is rare, has a poor prognosis, affects primarily young and middle-age women, and may be familial, linked to the bone morphogenetic protein receptor 2 (BMPR2). SPAH often responds to therapy and is found with a variety of medical conditions. The underlying cause of SPAH often is chronic hypoxia, which can result from increased pulmonary blood flow from a ventricular or atrial shunt, left ventricular (LV) failure, COPD or sleep apnea, pulmonary embolism (PE), interstitial lung disease, human immunodeficiency virus (HIV) infection, collagen vascular disorders such as scleroderma or lupus, portal hypertension due to liver disease, or any physiologic condition that increases pulmonary vascular resistance or constriction of the vessels in the pulmonary tree.

ASSESSMENT

Signs and symptoms/physical findings

Acute: Exertional dyspnea and fatigue (the most common presenting symptoms), eventually progressing to dyspnea at rest. Syncope, precordial chest pain, and palpitations can occur because of low cardiac output or hypoxia.

Chronic indicators: Signs of diastolic or systolic dysfunction (right ventricular [RV] or LV failure) as a result of RV enlargement and eventual fluid overload.

RV FAILURE: Peripheral edema, increased venous pressure and pulsations, liver engorgement, distended neck veins.

LV FAILURE: Dyspnea; shortness of breath, particularly on exertion; decreased BP; oliguria; orthopnea; anorexia.

Physical findings include cyanosis from decreased cardiac output with subsequent systemic vasoconstriction and ventilation/perfusion mismatch, systolic murmur caused by tricuspid regurgitation or pulmonary stenosis, diastolic murmur caused by pulmonary valvular incompetence, accentuated S_2 heart sound, possible S_3 or S_4, heart sound, and parasternal heave caused by RV enlargement.

DIAGNOSTIC TESTS

Chest x-ray examination: Shows enlargement of the pulmonary artery and right atrium and right ventricle (RV). Pulmonary vasculature may appear engorged.

Echocardiography: Valuable for showing increased RV dimension, thickened RV wall, and possible tricuspid or pulmonary valve dysfunction. This test indirectly measures pulmonary artery systolic pressure.

Radionuclide imaging: Assesses function of the right ventricle.

Computed tomography (CT): Evaluates diameter of the main pulmonary arteries, a feature helpful in evaluating severity of disease. High-resolution CT can confirm the presence of interstitial lung disease. Spiral CT is more specific in evaluating PE.

Right-sided heart catheterization: Necessary to confirm pulmonary hypertension; helps determine severity of disease and its prognosis. Pulmonary vascular resistance will be very high, and pulmonary artery and RV pressures can approach or equal systemic arterial pressures. Vasodilator challenge is often performed to assess reactivity and guide treatment. Adenosine, epoprostenol, and nitric oxide typically are used.

Pulmonary perfusion scintigraphy (perfusion scan): A noninvasive way to assess pulmonary blood flow. This study involves IV injection of serum albumin tagged with trace amounts of a radioisotope, most often technetium. The particles pass through the circulation and lodge in the pulmonary vascular bed. Subsequent scanning reveals concentrations of particles in areas of adequate pulmonary blood flow. Scan is normal in PAH. Abnormal scan suggests presence of thromboembolic PAH.

ECG: Shows evidence of right atrial enlargement and RV enlargement (evidenced by right axis deviation, right bundle branch block (BBB), tall and peaked P waves, and large R waves in V_1) secondary to the increased pressure needed to force blood through the hypertensive pulmonary vascular bed.

Pulmonary function tests (PFTs): Results are usually normal, although some individuals have increased residual volume, reduced maximum voluntary ventilation, and decreased vital capacity.

Sleep study: Confirms diagnosis of sleep apnea as cause of SPAH.

Exercise testing: Symptom-limited stress test or 6-min walk test can help assess severity of symptoms and guide response to treatment.

Arterial blood gas (ABG) analysis: May show low $Paco_2$ and high pH, which occur with hyperventilation, or increased $Paco_2$ with decreased gas exchange.

Oximetry: May show decreased O_2 (e.g., 92% or less).

Blood tests to rule out secondary causes of PAH: Antinuclear antibodies (ANA), rheumatoid agglutinin (RA), erythrocyte sedimentation rate (ESR) (tests for collagen vascular disorders), HIV, and thyroid-stimulating hormone (TSH) (thyroid abnormalities commonly coexist with PAH).

CBC: Polycythemia can occur in the presence of chronic hypoxemia as a result of compensation.

Liver function tests: Results may be abnormal if venous congestion is significant. Examples are increased aspartate aminotransferase (AST), alanine aminotransferase (ALT), and bilirubin.

COLLABORATIVE MANAGEMENT

O_2 therapy: Treats hypoxia. O_2 can be administered continuously or only at bedtime or with exercise when O_2 desaturation is most likely to occur. If hypoxia is severe, O_2 is administered by mask. Use care when administering O_2 to patients with a history of COPD.

Diet: Low in Na^+ (see Box 4-1, p. 165) if signs of HF are present. Encourage patient to use food labels to determine the Na^+ content of foods.

Pharmacotherapy

Diuretics: Used in the presence of right-sided (diastolic dysfunction) or left-sided (systolic dysfunction) heart failure (HF) and fluid overload.

Anticoagulant (warfarin sodium): Promotes improved long-term survival by preventing thromboembolic complications.

Vasodilators and calcium antagonists: Goal of medical therapy is to decrease pulmonary artery pressure by vasodilation. The following are all used in the management of PAH: prostanoid analog such as epoprostenol, which is a potent IV vasodilator that also inhibits platelet aggregation; endothelin receptor antagonists such as bosentan, which is an oral vasodilator; and phosphodiesterase 5 (PDE-5) inhibitors. Calcium channel blockers (CCBs) administered in higher doses than those used to treat hypertension are helpful in patients who demonstrate response to vasodilator challenge.

Treatment of causative factor, if possible: Examples are surgical closure of arteriovenous shunts; replacement of defective valves; and treatment of sleep apnea, PE, or COPD.

Heart-lung transplantation: May be considered for advanced (end-stage) pulmonary vascular disease that is not responsive to medical therapy.

NURSING DIAGNOSES AND INTERVENTIONS

Impaired gas exchange related to altered blood flow secondary to pulmonary capillary constriction

Desired outcome: Patient has improved gas exchange by at least 24 hr before hospital discharge, as evidenced by O_2 saturation greater than 92% (90% or greater for patients with COPD) and Pao_2 80 mm Hg or higher.

Nursing Interventions

Monitor oximetry for low O_2 saturation; report O_2 saturation 92% or less.

- Monitor ABG results for decreased PaO_2, increased $PaCO_2$, decreased pH, and hyperventilation (low $PaCO_2$ and high pH). These findings indicate hypoventilation. Report significant findings.
- Auscultate lung fields q4-8h, or more frequently as indicated, *to assess lung sounds*. Note and report the presence of adventitious sounds (especially crackles), which can occur with fluid overload.
- Assess respiratory rate (RR) and, pattern and depth of respirations; chest excursion; and use of accessory muscles of respiration q4h.
- Observe for and document presence of cyanosis or skin color change, *which can occur with decreased gas exchange.*
- Help patient into Fowler's position (head of bed [HOB] up 90 degrees), if possible, *to reduce work of breathing (WOB) and maximize chest excursion.*
- Teach patient to take slow, deep breaths *to promote gas exchange.*
- Administer prescribed low-flow O_2 as indicated. Deliver O_2 with humidity *to help prevent its drying effects on oral and nasal mucosa.*
- Monitor mental status and report changes in mental acuity or level of consciousness (LOC) *as indications of acid-base imbalance.*

Activity intolerance related to generalized weakness and imbalance between O_2 supply and demand secondary to RV and LV failure
Desired outcome: By at least 24 hr before hospital discharge, patient rates perceived exertion at 3 or less on a 0-10 scale and exhibits cardiac tolerance to activity, as evidenced by RR 20 breaths/min or less, heart rate 20 beats per minute (bpm) or less over resting HR, and SBP within 20 mm Hg of resting range.

Nursing Interventions

- Ask patient to rate perceived exertion during activity, and monitor for evidence of activity intolerance. For details, see **Risk for activity intolerance** in "Prolonged Bed Rest," p. 23. Notify health care provider of significant findings.
- Observe for and document any changes in VS. Monitor BP at least q4h. Report drops greater than 10-20 mm Hg, *which can signal decompensation of cardiac muscle.* Also be alert to other signs of LV failure, including dyspnea, shortness of breath, crackles (rales), and decreased O_2 saturation (92% or less) as determined by oximetry.
- Measure and document I&O and weight, reporting any steady gains or losses. Be alert for peripheral edema, both pedal and sacral; ascites; distended neck veins; and increased central venous pressure (CVP) (more than 12 cm H_2O) because they are signs of RV failure.
- Administer diuretics, vasodilators, and CCBs as prescribed.
- Facilitate coordination of health care providers to ensure rest periods between care activities *to decrease O_2 demand. Allow time for undisturbed rest.* If necessary, limit visitors *to enable adequate rest.*
- Keep frequently used items within patient's reach *so that exertion can be avoided as much as possible.*
- Assist with maintaining prescribed activity level and progress as tolerated. If activity intolerance is observed, stop the activity and have patient rest.
- Assist with ROM exercises at frequent intervals. *To help prevent complications caused by immobility*, plan progressive ambulation and exercise based on patient's tolerance and prescribed activity restrictions.

Deficient knowledge related to disease process and treatment
Desired outcome: Within 24 hr before hospital discharge, patient and significant other verbalize knowledge of the disease, its treatment, and measures that promote wellness.

Nursing Interventions

- Assess patient's facility with language; engage an interpreter or provide language-appropriate written materials if indicated.
- Assess patient's level of knowledge of the disease process and its treatment.
- Discuss purposes of the medications: to ease workload of the heart (vasodilators), "relax" the heart (calcium antagonists), and prevent fluid accumulation (diuretics).
- Provide emotional support to patient adapting to the concept of having a chronic disease.
- If the cause of PAH is known, reinforce explanations of the disease process and treatment.
- Discuss lifestyle changes that may be required to prevent future complications or control the disease process.
- Explain value of relaxation techniques, including tapes, soothing music, meditation, and biofeedback. See "Coronary Artery Disease," **Health-seeking behaviors:** Relaxation technique effective for stress reduction, p. 106.
- If patient smokes, explain that smoking increases workload of the heart by causing vasoconstriction. Provide materials that explain benefits of smoking cessation, such as pamphlets prepared by the American Heart Association, available at: *www.americanheart.org*
- Provide phone numbers for local smoking cessation programs.
- Confer with health care provider about type of exercise program that will benefit patient; provide patient teaching as indicated.
- If appropriate, involve dietitian to assist patient with planning low-Na^+ meals (see Table 4-1, p. 165).

 Patient-Family Teaching and Discharge Planning

Reinforce previous teaching about the disease and its treatment. Be sure to provide verbal and written information about the following:
- Indicators that necessitate medical attention: decreased exercise tolerance, increasing shortness of breath or dyspnea, swelling of ankles and legs, steady weight gain.
- Medications, including drug names, purpose, dosage, schedule, precautions, and potential side effects. Also discuss drug/drug, food/drug, and herb/drug interactions.
- Referral to a smoking cessation program.
- For additional information see **Deficient knowledge** on p. 121.

❖ ❖ ❖

SECTION TWO # INFLAMMATORY HEART DISORDERS

Inflammations or infections involving the heart muscle and its linings, the pericardium and endocardium, may be acute or chronic. Prognosis usually depends on extent of involvement, structures involved, and secondary disorders that occur.

❖ PERICARDITIS

OVERVIEW/PATHOPHYSIOLOGY

Pericarditis is an acute inflammation of the pericardium, the stiff, fibrous sac that surrounds, supports, and protects the heart. The pericardium is composed of a fibrous outer layer and a serous inner layer. The inflammatory condition produces friction between these layers during cardiac movement and causes exudate production and formation of chronic fibrinous adhesions. Pericardial effusions may develop that constrict the heart's ability to stretch and result in diastolic filling inability.

ASSESSMENT

Signs and symptoms/physical findings: Sharp chest pain is the primary symptom and may radiate to the back, neck, or left shoulder or arm. It is often increased with coughing or deep inspirations, movement, or lying down and is eased by sitting up and leaning forward. Other indicators include a characteristic pericardial friction rub (a scratching, grating, high-pitched sound) on auscultation, best heard with the diaphragm over lower to middle left sternal edge, dyspnea (resulting from thoracic pain, splinting the chest, or cardiac compression by fluid), tachycardia, fever, and pulsus paradoxus (decrease in pulse volume and an abnormal fall in SBP more than 10 mm Hg during inspiration as compared with exhalation).

Cardiac tamponade is a potentially life-threatening condition in which the heart is compromised by fluid accumulating in the pericardial sac. The presenting symptom is tachycardia, which occurs to maintain adequate cardiac output as the heart compensates for the ventricles' decreased ability to fill during diastole and provide adequate stroke volume. Additional symptoms may include anxiety, restlessness, dyspnea, feelings of fullness in the chest, distant heart sounds, narrowed pulse pressure, jugular venous distention, elevated central venous pressure (CVP), and changes in mental status progressing to loss of consciousness. As decompensation progresses, cardiac output, and thus BP, will fall, eventually creating a shocklike state. Treatment involves emergency pericardiocentesis (see "Collaborative Management").

History/risk factors: The most common etiologies are viral or bacterial infections, renal failure, immunologic disorders, AMI, radiation, drugs, neoplastic disease, and trauma.

DIAGNOSTIC TESTS

Serial ECGs: Typically show widespread ST-segment elevation in most leads, unlike localized ischemic ST-segment elevation, and PR segment depression.

CBC and other hematologic studies: Often show presence of increased WBCs (leukocytosis) and increased erythrocyte sedimentation rate (ESR) in the presence of inflammation. Blood cultures may be indicated to determine infection.

Cardiac enzymes: Troponin and MB fraction of creatine kinase (CK) may increase with inflammation.

Chest x-ray examination: Often normal, but with sufficient pericardial effusion, the heart appears more globe shaped. With chronic pericarditis, pericardial calcifications may be seen.

Echocardiogram: Reveals increase in pericardial fluid, which occurs with infection or irritation.

COLLABORATIVE MANAGEMENT
Treatment of Underlying Disorder

Bed rest: Until pain and fever are relieved, if severe.

Pharmacotherapy

Nonsteroidal antiinflammatory drugs (NSAIDs): Combat fever, reduce inflammation, and control pain.

Corticosteroids: (e.g., prednisone for 5-7 days and tapered thereafter) if symptoms are unrelieved by NSAIDs.

Antibiotics: Given only in the presence of purulent pericarditis.

Emergency pericardiocentesis: If cardiac tamponade (accumulation of fluid that restricts ventricular filling and reduces cardiac output) develops, needle aspiration of fluid in the pericardial sac may be performed to relieve pressure and allow for normal cardiac muscle contraction. Aspirated fluid may be sent for culture and sensitivity tests.

Partial or total pericardiectomy: Enables normal cardiac movement and function if pericarditis is recurrent and has produced scar tissue and constriction. This procedure involves removal of part (a pericardial "window") or all of the pericardium to prevent constriction by scar tissue, exudate, or bleeding.

NURSING DIAGNOSES AND INTERVENTIONS

Activity intolerance related to imbalance between O_2 supply and demand secondary to inflammation of the cardiac muscle and restriction of contraction

Desired outcomes: During activity, patient rates perceived exertion at 3 or less on a 0-10 scale and exhibits cardiac tolerance to activity, as evidenced by SBP within 20 mm Hg of resting SBP, respiratory rate (RR) 20 breaths/min or less, heart rate (HR) 20 beats per minute (bpm) or less above resting HR, and absence of chest pain or new dysrhythmias.

Nursing Interventions

◆ Ask patient to rate perceived exertion during activity, and monitor for evidence of activity intolerance. For details, see **Risk for activity intolerance** in "Prolonged Bed Rest," p. 23. Notify health care provider of significant findings.

◆ Ensure that patient maintains bed rest during febrile period and understands the rationale for doing so.

◆ Anticipate patient's needs by placing personal articles within easy reach.

◆ Advise patient about importance of frequent rest periods during convalescence to conserve energy.

◆ Monitor VS for changes indicative of cardiac or pulmonary decompensation, such as pallor, diaphoresis, dysrhythmias, decreasing BP, and increasing HR and RR.

◆ Assist with turning at least q2h, and provide passive ROM exercises at frequent intervals *to help prevent complications of immobility.* As patient's condition improves, consult health care provider about in-bed exercises that require more cardiac tolerance. Examples are found in "Prolonged Bed Rest," **Risk for activity intolerance,** p. 23, and **Risk for disuse syndrome,** p. 25.

Ineffective peripheral, cardiopulmonary, cerebral, and renal tissue perfusion (or risk for same) related to interrupted blood flow secondary to dysfunctional cardiac muscle

Desired outcomes: Within 24 hr of admission, patient has adequate tissue perfusion, as evidenced by amplitude of distal pulses more than 2+ on a 0-4+ scale; HR 100 bpm or less; BP at least 90/60 mm Hg; RR 20 breaths/min or less with normal depth and pattern (eupnea); normal heart sounds; absence of significant mental status changes; orientation to person, place, and time; and urinary output at least 30 mL/hr.

Nursing Interventions

◆ Observe for and report increasing restlessness or anxiety and changes in mentation, which can occur with decreased cerebral perfusion.

◆ Palpate distal pulses at least q2-4h *to assess peripheral perfusion and dysrhythmias.*

◆ Be alert to anxiety, restlessness, dyspnea, sensation of fullness in the chest, distant heart sounds, narrowed pulse pressure, jugular venous distention, elevated CVP, and changes in mental status progressing to loss of consciousness, because they are signs of cardiac tamponade. Report significant findings and prepare for emergency pericardiocentesis.

◆ Assess for pulsus paradoxus (decrease in pulse volume, and SBP 10 mm Hg higher during inhalation as compared with exhalation), which is produced by pericardial restriction and subsequent decreased ventricular filling. The assessment is performed as follows:

- Apply BP cuff to patient's arm; palpate the brachial pulse.
- Place stethoscope over the pulse point, and inflate cuff to above the level of patient's normal SBP.
- Slowly deflate cuff. Ask patient to exhale.
- Listen for the first sound that occurs after patient exhales. Note manometer reading, and tell patient to breathe normally.
- Continue to deflate BP cuff slowly until sounds are heard during inhalation and exhalation. Note the reading.
- Calculate the difference in mm Hg between the two readings. This is the measurement of pulsus paradoxus.

◆ Instruct patient to perform foot and leg exercises q4h *to promote venous circulation.* Consider use of antiembolism hose *to reduce venostasis* and sequential compression devices or pneumatic foot pumps *to further enhance venous return.* See "Prolonged Bed Rest," p. 23, for a description of exercises.

◆ If patient exhibits signs of decreased cerebral perfusion, reorient and institute safety precautions as necessary. Notify health care provider of significant or continued mental status changes.

◆ Monitor urinary output to determine renal perfusion. Be alert to output less than 30 mL/hr for 2 consecutive hr, and report findings if appropriate.

Acute pain (friction rub) related to inflammatory process
Desired outcome: Within 24 hr of initiation of antiinflammatory medication, patient's subjective perception of pain decreases, as documented by a pain scale. Objective indicators, such as grimacing, are absent.

Nursing Interventions

◆ Auscultate heart sounds for the presence of friction rub as an indicator of pericardial inflammation.

◆ Assess and document character, intensity, and duration of pain. Establish a pain scale with patient, rating pain from 0 (no pain) to 10 (worst pain). Administer pain medications as prescribed, and document effectiveness using the pain scale. Advise patient to request pain medication before pain becomes severe.

◆ Use the following interventions *to enhance medication effectiveness*: support patient in a side-lying position with pillows, or place patient in Fowler's position (head of bed [HOB] up 90 degrees); pad over-the-bed table with pillows or bath blankets to support patient; provide emotional support; and control environmental stimuli by limiting visitors (as necessary *to ensure adequate rest*), dimming lights, and maintaining quiet.

◆ Administer O_2 as prescribed, typically 2-3 L/min by nasal cannula. Deliver O_2 with humidity *to help prevent its drying effects on oral and nasal mucosa.*

◆ Administer NSAIDs, steroids, or antibiotics as prescribed *to manage the pericardial inflammation.*

Ineffective breathing pattern related to decreased lung expansion secondary to guarding because of pericardial pain
Desired outcomes: Within 1 hr of the intervention(s), patient's RR is 12-20 breaths/min with normal depth and pattern (eupnea), and O_2 saturation is greater than 92%.

Nursing Interventions

◆ Assess breath sounds and respirations at least q4h. Report presence of crackles (rales) or areas of diminished breath sounds because they *occur as a result of atelectasis caused by decreased depth of respirations (guarding).*

- Assess breathing effort for adequate depth at least q2h, and teach patient to breathe deeply. Teach use of an incentive spirometer.
- Monitor O_2 saturation; report saturation readings 92% or less to health care provider. Provide supplemental O_2 as prescribed, typically 2-3 L/min by nasal cannula. Deliver O_2 with *humidity to help prevent its drying effects on oral and nasal mucosa.*
- Teach cascade cough to reduce stressful coughing, which increases pain. Cascade cough is a series (2-5) of small forceful exhalations used *to mobilize secretions.*
- Place patient in semi-Fowler's (HOB up 30-45 degrees) or high Fowler's (HOB up 90 degrees) position *to ease pressure on the heart, which will help decrease effort of breathing.*

 Patient-Family Teaching and Discharge Planning

Provide verbal and written information about the following:

- Importance of frequent rest periods during convalescence.
- Importance of prompt treatment if symptoms of pericarditis recur.
- Procedure for measuring temperature, which can be an indicator of recurring inflammation.
- Importance of avoiding individuals with upper respiratory infections (URIs) and promptly seeking medical attention if influenza or cold symptoms occur.
- Medications, including drug names, purpose, dosage, schedule, precautions, and potential side effects. Also discuss drug/drug, food/drug, and herb/drug interactions.
- Importance of understanding that feelings of wellness do not necessarily mean inflammation has completely resolved.

❖ INFECTIVE ENDOCARDITIS

OVERVIEW/PATHOPHYSIOLOGY

Approximately 10,000 to 20,000 new cases of infective endocarditis (IE) occur each year in the United States. More than one-half of all cases occur in individuals over the age of 60, and men are infected twice as often as women. IE is a serious infection affecting the inner lining of the heart's chambers, septum, and, most commonly, the heart valves. Because the signs and symptoms of IE vary, practitioners need to maintain a high degree of suspicion in order to diagnose this potentially life-threatening condition swiftly and accurately.

For IE to develop, bacteria must enter the bloodstream, and endothelial injury must occur. Endothelial injury typically occurs where there is turbulence in blood flow, such as at the heart valves. Platelets collect at the site of injury and create a medium for bacteria to grow and develop into a vegetation.

There are four classifications of endocarditis:

Acute IE (short incubation period) with a rapid onset of symptoms from days to weeks. Symptoms are usually severe and patients decline in a short time.

Subacute IE (long incubation) with a gradual onset of symptoms from weeks to months, presenting a less dramatic picture. The causative agent is less virulent, such as *Streptococcus viridans*, commonly found in the mouth. Many of these patients have known cardiac defects, such as congenital or valvular disease.

Prosthetic valvular endocarditis, which develops in 2%-3% of patients within 1 yr of valve replacement.

Right-sided endocarditis, which involves the tricuspid valve. It commonly occurs from illicit IV drug use.

ASSESSMENT

Signs and symptoms/physical findings: Temperature elevation (may be low grade or as high as 104° F [40° C]), chills, headache, anemia, malaise, anorexia, weight loss, tachycardia, pallor, diaphoresis, night sweats, and muscle and joint pain. Murmurs occur with valve involvement (may be absent in right-sided IE) and if heart failure (HF) has developed as a result of valvular dysfunction, activity intolerance, dyspnea, crackles, edema, neck vein distention, splenomegaly, and hepatomegaly are presenting features. Skin manifestations include flat, painless red-to-blue lesions on palms and soles (Janeway lesions); small, tender nodules on pads of finger or toes (Osler's nodes); and splinter hemorrhages with pale centers on whites of the eyes, palate, chest, fingers, and toes (Roth's spots). Hematuria and proteinuria may be present if septic emboli affect the kidneys. If embolization has occurred, signs may include decreased cerebral and peripheral perfusion.

History and risk factors: IV drug use, prosthetic heart valves, recent heart surgery, prolonged IV therapy, structural heart disease, upper respiratory infection (URI), influenza, or other infectious process. Nosocomial infection from vascular access ports can cause bacteria or fungi in the bloodstream, as can infection from tattooing and body piercing.

DIAGNOSTIC TESTS

Blood cultures: At least three sets obtained from separate sites at different time periods to identify causative organism; should include aerobic and anaerobic cultures.

Erythrocyte sedimentation rate (ESR): Usually elevated because of inflammatory process.

WBC count: May be normal in subacute forms and can range from 15,000-20,000/mm^3 in acute disease.

Chest x-ray examination: May reveal early findings of HF (e.g., vascular engorgement, increased heart size).

Transthoracic two-dimensional echocardiography, combined with color-flow Doppler imaging: Gold standard for diagnosing IE. An echocardiogram can detect vegetations, valvular perforations, abscesses, and pericarditis and can assess ventricular function. Transesophageal echocardiogram may be used to improve sensitivity in detecting vegetations.

COLLABORATIVE MANAGEMENT

Before the availability of antimicrobial therapy, IE was invariably fatal. Approximately 80% of patients with IE now survive the infection.

Specific antibiotic therapy: Depends on causative organism and its susceptibility or sensitivity to drugs. In the subacute form of the disorder, it is satisfactory to wait until the organism is identified, but with acute IE, broad-spectrum antibiotic therapy is instituted immediately after blood cultures are drawn and then adjusted if necessary after organism identification. Intermittent IV antibiotics are given q4-6h. Duration of therapy usually is 4-6 wk. If patient is hemodynamically stable, IV antibiotics can be administered on an outpatient basis.

Bed rest

Well-balanced diet: Maintains resistance to infection.

Surgical repair or valve replacement: Performed when HF does not respond to medical management; the infection does not respond to antimicrobial therapy within 1 wk; repeated episodes of embolization occur, especially when vascular occlusions are found in the eyes, brain, coronary arteries, and kidneys; repeated infections occur (e.g., relapse after 3 mo); and fungal endocarditis is found. See discussion of mitral valve replacement in "Mitral Stenosis," p. 129.

Treatment of HF, if present: See "Heart Failure," p. 107.

NURSING DIAGNOSES AND INTERVENTIONS

Risk for infection related to risk factors associated with invasive procedures and inadequate secondary defenses (decreased immune response) resulting from prolonged antibiotic therapy

Desired outcome: Patient is free of infection, as evidenced by normothermia, normal skin temperature and color at IV sites, heart rate (HR) 100 beats per minute (bpm) or less, straw-colored and clear urine, and negative results on blood cultures × 2.

Nursing Interventions

- Use sterile technique when working with IV lines, urinary catheters, and wounds to minimize the risk for infection.
- Monitor patient's body temperature and WBC count for increases from baseline assessment. Both already may be increased as a result of the primary infection, but *unexplained increases may occur after resolution of the acute phase as a result of a secondary infection.*
- For patients with indwelling urinary catheters, monitor for cloudiness and foul odor because they are signs of infection. Cleanse the urethral meatus and surrounding area daily with soap and water.
- Rotate IV sites and change tubing and dressings q48-72h or per agency protocol to minimize the risk for IV infection.

Deficient knowledge related to disease process, therapeutic regimen, and assessment for infection

Desired outcome: Within the 24-hr period before hospital discharge, patient verbalizes understanding of the disease process and measures that prevent bacteremia.

Nursing Interventions

- Assess patient's facility with language; engage an interpreter or provide language-appropriate written materials if indicated.
- Assess patient's level of knowledge about the disease and therapy.
- As indicated, explain disease process and need for prolonged antibiotic therapy.
- Because of increased risk of bacteremia, discuss need for antibiotic prophylaxis before dental procedures and all major and minor surgical procedures and need of early treatment of common infections (e.g., urinary tract infection [UTI], URI, and wound infection).
- Teach early indicators of infection (see descriptions in "Care of the Renal Transplant Recipient," p. 193) and importance of reporting indicators to health care provider promptly. Teach patient how to measure body temperature and importance of monitoring temperature weekly if asymptomatic and more frequently if weakness, fatigue, or symptoms of a cold or influenza occur.

    Patient-Family Teaching and Discharge Planning

Reinforce previous teaching about IE, the need for prolonged and prophylactic antibiotic therapy, and signs and symptoms of infection requiring immediate treatment. Also provide verbal and written information about the following:

- Medications to be taken at home, including drug names, purpose, dosage, schedule, precautions, potential side effects. Also discuss drug/drug, food/drug, and herb/drug interactions. Patient may be required to self-administer IV antibiotics at home to decrease length of hospital stay; teach the technique if indicated.
- Importance of medical follow-up to check valve function; confirm date and time of next medical appointment.

♦ Informational booklet available from the American Heart Association entitled *Prevention of Endocarditis,* which summarizes preventive procedures. Available at *www.americanheart.org*

❖ ❖ ❖

SECTION THREE **VALVULAR HEART DISORDERS**

Cardiac valves maintain the forward flow of blood. Valvular disease interrupts this forward flow and creates a decrease in blood flow or regurgitation, which increases heart pressures and volume. The aortic and mitral valves are most commonly affected.

❖ MITRAL STENOSIS

OVERVIEW/PATHOPHYSIOLOGY

The mitral valve is composed of two leaflets. Stenosis occurs because of thickening of the leaflets and fusion of the commissures. Leaflet calcification and loss of leaflet mobility or fibrosis of the chordae tendineae and associated papillary muscles occur in late stages of the disease. Normal mitral valve area is 4-6 cm^2.

Because the mitral valve is located between the left atrium and ventricle, stenosis results in decreased left ventricular (LV) filling and increased left atrial and pulmonary pressures. As stenosis severity increases, maintenance of cardiac output becomes more difficult. In addition, high pulmonary pressures cause fluid extravasation into the alveoli that increases the diffusion gradient and result in pulmonary edema.

Individuals with valvular disorders may be predisposed to endocarditis. Bacteria in the bloodstream have a tendency to lodge in the malfunctioning valves because of calcium deposits or turbulent blood flow, so antibiotic prophylaxis should be initiated whenever a systemic infection is present or patient is undergoing major or minor surgical procedures, such as dental work. See also "Infective Endocarditis," p. 126.

ASSESSMENT

Signs and symptoms/physical findings: Symptoms often do not occur until late in the disease and include dyspnea, orthopnea, and paroxysmal nocturnal dyspnea. Even later, symptoms of diastolic dysfunction (right-sided heart failure (HF)) may occur, including elevated central venous pressure (CVP), ascites, peripheral edema, and hepatomegaly. LV impulse (the point of maximal impulse [PMI]) may be displaced by an enlarged right ventricle.
Mild mitral stenosis: Valve area of 1.6-2 cm^2. Mild dyspnea on exertion (DOE) is the most common symptom.
Moderate mitral stenosis: Valve area of 1-1.5 cm^2. Dyspnea, fatigue, paroxysmal nocturnal dyspnea, and atrial fibrillation may occur.
Severe mitral stenosis: Valve area less than 1 cm^2. Dyspnea at rest, cough, and hemoptysis may occur. As a result of pulmonary hypertension, symptoms may progress to those of right ventricular (RV) failure. Stagnation of left atrial blood flow and atrial fibrillation can cause thrombus formation with subsequent embolic events, including stroke. Chest pain can occur because of decreased myocardial perfusion.

A characteristic diastolic murmur, best heard while listening with the stethoscope bell when patient is in the left lateral position, commonly is audible at the cardiac apex. With increasing obstruction, a high-pitched "snap" and a loud first heart sound also may be heard as the mitral valve opens in the presence of increased atrial pressure.

History and risk factors: Rheumatic heart disease is the most common cause of mitral valve stenosis. Congenital deformities, valve vegetations, and malignancies, although rare, are other causes.

DIAGNOSTIC TESTS

Chest x-ray examination: Early in the disease, a normal cardiac silhouette is present. Later, evidence of an enlarged left atrium and right ventricle may appear. Symptomatic patients may show pulmonary congestion.

Echocardiography: Gold standard diagnostic tool for evaluating valvular disease. Mitral valve thickening may be seen along with abnormal leaflet motion. Disease severity is determined by measuring the valve area and gradient as well as the degree of mitral insufficiency. Left atrial enlargement and the degree of pulmonary hypertension also may be determined.

ECG: Although not useful for a definitive diagnosis, ECG demonstrates characteristic changes associated with left atrial and RV enlargement, such as tall, notched P waves and right axis deviation. Atrial fibrillation, a common complication, also may be seen.

Cardiac catheterization: Measures pulmonary vascular resistance and assesses the coronary arteries. See "Coronary Artery Disease," p. 98, for more information.

COLLABORATIVE MANAGEMENT

Medical management is aimed at preventing complications of the disease process, treating symptoms, and monitoring and treating disease progression.

Prevention of complications

Antibiotic prophylaxis for endocarditis: Before and after invasive procedures, including dental work. See "Infective Endocarditis," p. 126.

Preventing rheumatic fever: Treatment of streptococcal pharyngitis with appropriate antibiotic for adequate length of time.

Preventing embolic events: Restoration of sinus rhythm, ventricular response rate control, and anticoagulation in the presence of atrial fibrillation. Digoxin, β-blockers, or calcium channel blockers (CCBs) may be used for ventricular response rate control. Aspirin and warfarin are prescribed to prevent thrombus formation.

Treatment of symptoms

Decreased exercise tolerance: Restriction of physically strenuous activities.

Pulmonary congestion: Administration of diuretics and β-blockers.

Treatment as disease progresses

Percutaneous transvenous mitral valvotomy (PTMV): An alternative to surgery for some patients, PTMV is done in the cardiac catheterization laboratory, using local anesthetic. A balloon-dilating catheter is inserted into the valve and inflated across the area of stenosis.

Mitral valve replacement: Extensive calcification of mitral leaflets, patient's symptoms, and advanced degree of mitral insufficiency may make surgical repair necessary. Mechanical valves are recommended because of their longevity. Lifelong anticoagulation is necessary.

NURSING DIAGNOSES AND INTERVENTIONS

Activity intolerance related to generalized weakness and imbalance between O_2 supply and demand secondary to decreased cardiac output

Desired outcomes: By at least 24 hr before hospital discharge, patient rates perceived exertion at 3 or less on a 0-10 scale and exhibits cardiac tolerance to activity, as evidenced by HR 20 bpm or less over resting HR, SBP within 20 mm Hg of resting SBP, and RR 20 breaths/min or less with normal depth and pattern (eupnea).

Nursing Interventions

◆ Monitor VS with patient activity, and report significant (more than 20 mm Hg) decrease or increase in BP. Be alert to indicators of activity intolerance, including shortness of breath, dyspnea, and fatigue. Ask patient about perceived exertion (see description, p. 24).

◆ Assess for orthostatic changes in BP that occur when patient moves from supine to standing position.

◆ Assess peripheral pulses, capillary refill, and temperature and color of the extremities *as indicators of cardiac output.*

◆ Coordinate activities of health care providers to ensure rest periods between care activities *to decrease cardiac workload.* Ensure 90 min for undisturbed rest.

◆ Confer with health care provider about in-bed exercises that can be incorporated as patient's condition improves. Increase ambulation progressively and to patient's tolerance.

◆ For further interventions, see **Risk for activity intolerance,** p. 23, and **Risk for disuse syndrome,** p. 25, for examples of in-bed exercises.

Excess fluid volume related to compromised regulatory mechanisms secondary to right-sided HF

Desired outcomes: Within 24 hr of treatment, patient is normovolemic, as evidenced by CVP 5-12 cm H_2O, balanced I&O, stable weight, urine output at least 30 mL/hr, edema 1+ or less on a 0-4+ scale, flattened neck veins, and lungs clear on auscultation.

Nursing Interventions

◆ Observe for and report the following indicators of right-sided HF (diastolic dysfunction): increasing CVP (12 cm H_2O or more), peripheral edema, dyspnea, hepatic enlargement on palpation, and jugular vein distention.

◆ Monitor I&O and administer fluids only as prescribed *to ensure patient maintains adequate volume without overload.* Weigh patient daily, and report significant I&O imbalance.

◆ If fluids are limited, offer ice chips and Popsicles *to help patient control thirst.* Record amount of intake. Offer frequent oral hygiene *to reduce oral dryness.*

◆ As prescribed, administer inotropic drugs, such as digitalis, *to increase strength of cardiac contraction and decrease HR.*

◆ Administer diuretics as prescribed *to decrease volume load.*

Risk for infection (with concomitant endocarditis) related to risk factors from tissue destruction and increased exposure secondary to lodging of bacteria in the malfunctioning valve

Desired outcome: Patient is free of infection, as evidenced by normothermia, WBC count 11,000/mm^3 or less, and HR 100 bpm or less.

Nursing Interventions

◆ Maintain sterile technique for all invasive procedures to minimize risk for infection.

◆ Monitor temperature q4h, and report significant increases.

◆ Be alert to rising HR because it *can signal an infection.*

◆ Administer prescribed antibiotics on time *to maintain adequate blood levels.*

◆ Maintain hydration, as prescribed, through oral and prescribed intravenous (IV) fluids *to promote adequate volume without overload.*

Deficient knowledge related to disease process and treatments/management

Desired outcome: Within the 24-hr period before hospital discharge, patient verbalizes knowledge of valvular disorder, its treatment/management, and the potential for developing endocarditis.

Nursing Interventions

◆ Assess patient's facility with language; engage an interpreter or provide language-appropriate written materials if indicated.

- Discuss patient's valve disorder and associated physiologic effects and symptoms. As appropriate, describe treatment options, including commissurotomy, percutaneous balloon valvuloplasty, and valve replacement surgery.
- Assess patient's knowledge about the potential for endocarditis. As indicated, explain how endocarditis affects the heart and its valves and why individuals with valvular disorders are predisposed to developing this disorder.
- Teach the following indicators of endocarditis: temperature increases, malaise, anorexia, tachycardia, pallor. Explain importance of reporting symptoms early.
- Teach the indicators of commonly encountered infections (e.g., upper respiratory infection [URI], urinary tract infection [UTI], wound). Stress importance of reporting symptoms promptly if they occur because a systemic infection can lead to endocarditis.
- Discuss importance of antibiotic prophylaxis before and after any major or minor surgical procedures, including dental procedures.

 Patient-Family Teaching and Discharge Planning

Reinforce previous teaching about the disorder and its management. Also provide verbal and written information about the following:

- Medications, including drug names, purpose, dosage, schedule, precautions, and potential side effects. Also discuss drug/drug, food/drug, and herb/drug interactions. Emphasize importance of consulting health care provider before using over-the-counter (OTC) medications, especially aspirin products for individuals taking oral anticoagulants. Aspirin can prolong coagulation times.
- Gradually increasing exercise, avoiding heavy lifting (more than 10 lb), incorporating rest periods.
- Name and phone number of a resource person (e.g., health care provider, primary nurse) if questions arise after hospital discharge.
- Referral to cardiac rehabilitation program if appropriate.
- Resumption of sexual activity as directed by health care provider.
- Indicators that necessitate immediate medical attention: decreased exercise tolerance, signs of infection, shortness of breath, bleeding.
- Importance of follow-up care; confirm date and time of next medical appointment.

❖ MITRAL REGURGITATION

OVERVIEW/PATHOPHYSIOLOGY

Abnormalities of the mitral valve can cause mitral regurgitation (MR), or backward flow of blood through the left atrium during ventricular systole. Normally the mitral valve is closed during ventricular systole, but with MR the incompetent valve allows approximately half the ventricular volume back into the left atrium rather than forcing it forward into the aorta. The heart may be able to compensate for a period of time, but eventually cardiac output decreases and left ventricular (LV) hypertrophy occurs. In addition, the increased pulmonary vascular volume causes pulmonary hypertension (see p. 118). Acute MR may be caused by myocardial infarction (MI), chest trauma, or endocarditis. Chronic MR may be caused by rheumatic heart disease, ischemic damage to the papillary muscles, endocarditis, myxomatous degeneration, cardiomyopathy, or LV dilation.

ASSESSMENT

Signs and symptoms/physical findings: Fatigue, exhaustion, dyspnea, palpitations, dyspnea on exertion (DOE), paroxysmal nocturnal dyspnea, signs of heart failure (HF) (see p. 107) and pulmonary edema (see p. 69), holosystolic murmur heard at the apex and radiating toward the axilla, possible presence of S_3 heart sounds, and characteristic ejection click.

DIAGNOSTIC TESTS

ECG: Shows left atrial enlargement, possibly with atrial fibrillation. Results may reveal ischemic changes, especially with papillary muscle rupture.
Chest x-ray examination: May demonstrate cardiomegaly with LV and left atrial enlargement.
Echocardiography: Provides a definitive diagnosis and reveals severity of the disorder.
Radionuclide imaging: Often useful in follow-up; progressive increases in end-systolic or end-diastolic volumes can indicate a worsening condition.

COLLABORATIVE MANAGEMENT

Endocarditis prophylaxis with antibiotics: Initiated before major or minor surgical procedures, dental procedures, or any activity that may result in bacteremia.
Pharmacotherapy
Digitalis: Increases strength of contraction and slows ventricular response rate in atrial fibrillation.
Afterload reducing agents (e.g., angiotensin-converting enzyme [ACE] inhibitors, nitrates, or hydralazine): May be used to reduce afterload and promote forward flow.
Diuretics: Control fluid accumulation and prevent pulmonary edema.
Anticoagulants (heparin or warfarin): Prevent embolization.
Mitral valve replacement
Medical treatment for HF: As appropriate (see p. 112).

NURSING DIAGNOSES AND INTERVENTIONS

Activity intolerance related to generalized weakness and imbalance between O_2 supply and demand secondary to decreased cardiac output with valvular regurgitation
Desired outcomes: By a minimum of 24 hr before hospital discharge, patient rates perceived exertion at 3 or less on a 0-10 scale and exhibits cardiac tolerance to activity, as evidenced by heart rate (HR) of 20 beats per minute (bpm) or less over resting HR, SBP within 20 mm Hg of resting SBP, and respiratory rate (RR) 20 breaths/min or less with normal depth and pattern (eupnea).

Nursing Interventions

♦ Assess VS during activities, and be alert to HR more than 20 bpm over resting HR, SBP more than 20 mm Hg over or under resting SBP, and RR more than 20 breaths/min. Ask patient to rate perceived exertion (see p. 24 for description).
♦ Facilitate coordination of health care providers to ensure rest periods between care activities *to decrease cardiac workload.* Ensure 90 min for undisturbed rest.
♦ Encourage alternating activity and rest periods within patient's cardiopulmonary tolerance to prevent fatigue.
♦ As necessary, assist with activities of daily living (ADL) *to avoid shortness of breath.*
♦ Discuss ways to decrease energy output at home.
♦ Progressively increase ambulation to patient's tolerance. Be alert to dyspnea, fatigue, and shortness of breath with activity. Modify or restrict activities as indicated.

Patient-Family Teaching and Discharge Planning

See "Heart Failure," p. 107, or "Cardiac Surgery," p. 139, depending on patient's clinical course.

❖ AORTIC STENOSIS

OVERVIEW/PATHOPHYSIOLOGY

Aortic stenosis is a progressive disease in which patients remain asymptomatic for several years. This valvular condition obstructs outflow from the left ventricle into the ascending aorta. It is either congenital or acquired (most commonly from degenerative changes of aging or rheumatic fever). Aortic stenosis results from adhesions and fusion of the valve cusps. Initially, normal left ventricular (LV) output may be maintained by compensatory LV hypertrophy, but eventually progressive stenosis causes signs of low cardiac output. Aortic stenosis is graded in severity by valve area: aortic valve area greater than 1.5 cm^2 is graded mild, $1.1\text{-}1.5 \text{ cm}^2$ is graded moderate, and less than $0.8\text{-}1.0 \text{ cm}^2$ is graded severe.

ASSESSMENT

Signs and symptoms/physical findings: Often, patients with mild to moderate aortic stenosis are asymptomatic. As the disease progresses, patients report dyspnea on exertion (DOE) or fatigue. This may progress to symptoms of heart failure (HF) at rest. Exertional angina and lightheadedness or syncope may occur because of an increase in O_2 demand. A systolic ejection murmur (best heard at the base of the heart over the second intercostal space) is often the first diagnostic finding. Decreased SBP, decreased pulse pressure (the difference between systolic and diastolic pressures), increased LV impulse (point of maximal impulse [PMI], palpable at fifth intercostal space, midclavicular line, as a "lift" of the chest wall during ventricular systole), and S_4 usually are present. Acute drops in BP may occur secondary to inappropriate LV baroreceptor response. Sudden death, probably caused by ventricular fibrillation (VF), may be the presenting clinical manifestation.

DIAGNOSTIC TESTS

Brain natriuretic peptide (BNP) or N-terminal pro-BNP (NT-PROBNP): Evaluates severity of aortic stenosis, monitors early progression, and serves as a guide for timing of valve replacement.

ECG: LV hypertrophy may be evident; left axis deviation, left atrial enlargement, and left bundle branch block (BBB) may be present. ST-segment depression with exercise is common.

Chest x-ray examination: Most often normal until late in the disease when LV dilation and signs of HF are present.

Doppler echocardiography: Assesses stenosis severity, degree of aortic regurgitation, LV size and function, and estimation of pulmonary pressures.

Cardiac catheterization: More precise measure of gradient across valve and hence of valve area; also detects coexisting coronary artery disease (CAD). Indicated for patients reporting anginal symptoms or preoperative for aortic valve repair.

COLLABORATIVE MANAGEMENT

Antibiotics: As a prophylaxis against endocarditis.

Treatment of HF: If present. See this section in "Heart Failure," p. 112.

Aortic valve replacement: Appropriate for patients with LV dysfunction and symptoms of decreased cardiac output and functional disability. Aortic valve replacement is performed using heart-lung bypass, and patient is in ICU for 24 hr postoperatively. Artificial (prosthetic) mechanical valves, as well as those obtained from human donors (cadavers) and animals, may be used.

Patients with mechanical valves are maintained on lifetime anticoagulant therapy. Tissue valves do not require anticoagulation.

Percutaneous aortic valvotomy: Palliative alternative to surgery for some patients. The procedure uses a balloon-dilating catheter that is advanced to the stenotic valve and then inflated to dilate the valve. The procedure is performed using local anesthesia in the cardiac catheterization laboratory.

NURSING DIAGNOSES AND INTERVENTIONS

See sections on surgery (p. 139) and HF (p. 107).

❖ AORTIC REGURGITATION

OVERVIEW/PATHOPHYSIOLOGY

Aortic regurgitation is most commonly caused by rheumatic fever or an aneurysm of the ascending aorta or occurs as a result of degenerative changes of aging. Valve cusps become fibrotic and retract, preventing valve closure during diastole. Incompetence of this valve allows backward flow of blood from the aorta into the left ventricle. This situation results in large ventricular volume and decreased cardiac output.

ASSESSMENT

Signs and symptoms/physical findings: Patients may remain asymptomatic for years with chronic aortic insufficiency. Fatigue, dyspnea, orthopnea, changes in mentation, peripheral vasoconstriction, palpitations, and sensations of a forceful heartbeat (water-hammer or Corrigan's pulse), especially when lying on the left side, may occur as the disease progresses.

Widened aortic pulse pressure (difference between systolic and diastolic pressures), low DBP, high SBP until heart failure (HF) develops, low-pitched early diastolic murmur located in the second intercostal space to the right of the sternum, tachycardia, crackles (rales), and increased pulmonary arterial pressures occur. In chronic aortic regurgitation, the point of maximal impulse (PMI) is displaced laterally.

DIAGNOSTIC TESTS

Electrocardiogram (ECG): Demonstrates left axis deviation. Left ventricular (LV) conduction defects may be present with chronic aortic regurgitation. With acute regurgitation, nonspecific ST-segment changes or LV hypertrophy will be seen.

Chest x-ray examination: Results depend on severity and duration of the disorder, but it eventually demonstrates cardiac enlargement and LV dilation, along with subsequent signs of HF.

Echocardiography: May identify cause of regurgitation by revealing damaged cusps or vegetation caused by endocarditis. A transthoracic echocardiogram is especially useful in diagnosing dissection of the ascending and descending aorta.

Cardiac catheterization: Useful in determining severity of problem and identifying coexisting coronary artery disease (CAD).

COLLABORATIVE MANAGEMENT

Pharmacotherapy

Antibiotic prophylaxis: For all major and minor invasive procedures if LV function is depressed.

Treatment of HF: See "Heart Failure," p. 112.

Surgical interventions: Acute aortic regurgitation requires urgent aortic valve replacement. In the chronic form, the aortic valve should be replaced before irreversible LV dysfunction occurs (see "Mitral Valve Replacement," p. 130).

Balloon aortic valvotomy for palliation

NURSING DIAGNOSES AND INTERVENTIONS

 Patient-Family Teaching and Discharge Planning

See "Heart Failure," p. 107, and "Cardiac Surgery," p. 139, depending on patient's underlying diagnosis.

❖ ❖ ❖

SECTION FOUR   **CARDIOVASCULAR CONDITIONS SECONDARY TO OTHER DISEASE PROCESSES**

❖ CARDIAC AND NONCARDIAC SHOCK (CIRCULATORY FAILURE)

OVERVIEW/PATHOPHYSIOLOGY

A shock state exists when tissue perfusion decreases to the point of cellular metabolic dysfunction. Regardless of the cause, shock results in cellular hypoxia secondary to decreased perfusion and ultimately in cellular, tissue, and organ dysfunction. A prolonged shock state can result in death; therefore early recognition and intervention are essential. Shock is classified according to the causative event.

Hypovolemic shock: Occurs when volume in the intravascular space is inadequate and cannot meet the metabolic needs of tissues, as with severe hemorrhage or dehydration.

Cardiogenic shock: Occurs when cardiac failure results in decreased tissue perfusion, as in severe myocardial infarction (MI), in which more than 40% of heart muscle has been affected.

Distributive shock conditions: Characterized by displacement of a significant amount of vascular volume. The three types are neurogenic shock, anaphylactic shock, and septic shock.

Neurogenic shock: Occurs when a neurologic event (e.g., spinal cord injury) causes loss of sympathetic tone and results in massive vasodilation and decreased perfusion pressures.

Anaphylactic shock: Caused by a severe systemic response to an allergen (foreign protein) that results in massive vasodilation, increased capillary permeability, decreased perfusion, decreased venous return, and subsequent decreased cardiac output.

Septic shock: Occurs when bacterial toxins cause an overwhelming systemic infection.

ASSESSMENT

Signs and symptoms/physical findings

Early: Cool, pale, and clammy skin; rapid heart rate (HR) with decreased pulse strength; dry and pale mucous membranes; restlessness; hyperventilation; anxiety; nausea; thirst; weakness, decreased SBP and increased DBP secondary to catecholamine (sympathetic nervous system [SNS]) response.

Late: Decreased urinary output, hypothermia, drowsiness, diaphoresis, confusion, and lethargy, all of which can progress to a comatose state; thready, rapid HR; low or decreasing blood pressure (BP), usually with SBP less than 90 mm Hg; rapid and possibly irregular respiratory rate (RR).

Table 3-3 presents the signs and symptoms/physical findings listed by type of shock.

DIAGNOSTIC TESTS

Diagnosis is usually based on presenting symptoms and clinical signs.

Arterial blood gas (ABG) values: May reveal metabolic acidosis or respiratory alkalosis (bicarbonate [HCO_3^-] less than 22 mEq/L and pH less than 7.40) caused by anaerobic metabolism.

Serial measurement of urinary output: Output less than 30 mL/hr indicates decreased perfusion and decreased renal function.

Blood urea nitrogen (BUN) and serum creatinine: Increase with decreased renal perfusion.

Serum electrolyte levels: Identify renal complications and metabolic dysfunction as evidenced by hyperkalemia and hypernatremia.

For Septic Shock

Cultures of blood, sputum, wound, and urine: Identify causative organism.

WBC count: Elevated in the presence of infection.

For Hypovolemic Shock

CBC: Hematocrit (Hct) and hemoglobin (Hgb) are decreased because of decreased blood volume or falsely elevated in severe dehydration.

For Anaphylactic Shock

WBC count: Reveals increased eosinophils, a type of granulocyte that appears in the presence of allergic reaction.

COLLABORATIVE MANAGEMENT

Interventions are determined by clinical presentation and severity of the shock state. Patients are transferred to ICU for invasive hemodynamic monitoring with pulmonary artery catheter and use of vasoactive IV drips to improve tissue perfusion.

For Cardiogenic Shock

Vascular support: Reduces cardiac workload.

Intraaortic balloon counterpulsation: Augments perfusion pressures.

Ventricular assist devices: Bypasses or assists the ventricles, lowers myocardial O_2 requirements, reduces cardiac stress, and permits cardiac muscle rest.

Optimization of blood volume: Accomplished either with fluid administration or diuretics if there is evidence of fluid overload. An indwelling catheter should be inserted for accurate output measurement.

Pharmacotherapy

Inotropes (e.g., dopamine): Increase cardiac contractility.

Antidysrhythmics: Control irregular, rapid HR.

Vasodilators: Increase peripheral perfusion and reduce afterload vasoconstriction caused by vasopressors.

Osmotic diuretics: Increase renal blood flow.

O_2 support: Increases O_2 availability to the tissues.

Correction of acidosis and electrolyte imbalances

For Anaphylactic Shock

Pharmacotherapy

Epinephrine (0.5 mL, 1:1000 in 10 mL saline): Promotes vasoconstriction and decreases the allergic response by counteracting vasodilation caused by histamine release.

Bronchodilators: Relieve bronchospasm.

Antihistamines: Prevent relapse and relieve urticaria.

Hydrocortisone: Promotes antiinflammatory effects.

Vasopressors: May be necessary for reversing shock state.

O_2 and airway support: As needed.

For Hypovolemic Shock

Control of volume loss: If possible, depending on location and cause.
Blood transfusion: Increases O_2 delivery at the tissue level when more than 2 L of blood have been lost. Often a combination of packed RBCs and a crystalloid solution is administered.
Albumin: Sometimes used to increase vascular volume.
Ringer's solution: Often used as an isotonic solution to replace electrolytes and ions lost with bleeding.

For Septic Shock

Antibiotic therapy: Initial therapy is broad spectrum. Once the causative organism is identified, specific antibiotic therapy can be initiated.
Vasoactive drugs (e.g., norepinephrine, dopamine): May be required to reverse vasodilation and maintain perfusion.
Positive inotropic drugs: Augment cardiac contractility.
Fluid administration: Maintains adequate vascular volume.

NURSING DIAGNOSES AND INTERVENTIONS

Ineffective peripheral, cardiopulmonary, cerebral, and renal tissue perfusion related to decreased circulating blood volume
Desired outcomes: Within 1 hr of treatment, patient has adequate perfusion, as evidenced by peripheral pulse amplitude more than 2+ on a 0-4+ scale; brisk capillary refill (refill time less than 2 sec); BP within patient's normal range; central venous pressure (CVP) at least 5 cm H_2O; HR regular and 100 beats per minute (bpm) or less; no significant change in mental status; orientation to person, place, and time; and urine output at least 30 mL/hr.

Nursing Interventions

- Assess and document peripheral perfusion status. Report significant findings, such as coolness and pallor of the extremities, decreased amplitude of pulses, and delayed capillary refill.
- Monitor BP at frequent intervals; be alert to readings more than 20 mm Hg less than patient's normal range, dizziness, altered mentation, or decreased urinary output. These signs are indicators of hypotension.
- If hypotension is present, place patient in a supine position *to promote venous return.* Remember that BP must be at least 80/60 mm Hg for adequate coronary and renal artery perfusion.
- Monitor CVP (if line is inserted) *to determine adequacy of venous return and blood volume;* 5-10 cm H_2O usually is considered an adequate range. Values near zero can indicate hypovolemia, especially when associated with decreased urinary output, vasoconstriction, and increased HR, which are found with hypovolemia.
- Observe for indicators of decreased cerebral perfusion, such as restlessness, confusion, mental status changes, and decreased level of consciousness (LOC). If positive indicators are present, protect patient from injury by raising side rails and placing bed in its lowest position. Reorient patient as indicated.
- Monitor for chest pain and an irregular HR. These signs indicate decrease coronary artery perfusion.
- Monitor urinary output hourly. Notify health care provider if it is less than 30 mL/hr in the presence of adequate intake. Check weight daily for evidence of gain.
- Monitor laboratory results for elevated BUN (more than 20 mg/dL) and creatinine (more than 1.5 mg/dL) levels; report increases. These indicate renal compromise.
- Monitor serum electrolyte values for evidence of imbalances, particularly Na^+ (more than 147 mEq/L) and K^+ (more than 5.0 mEq/L). Be alert to signs of hyperkalemia, such as muscle weakness, hyporeflexia, and

irregular HR. Also monitor for signs of hypernatremia, such as fluid retention and edema.

♦ Administer fluids as prescribed *to increase vascular volume.* Type and amount of fluid depend on type of shock and patient's clinical situation. See Table 3-3 for a description of clinical signs associated with different types of shock.
- *Cardiogenic shock:* Fluids are probably limited to prevent overload, yet dehydration must be avoided to ensure support of vascular space and cardiac muscle.
- *Hypovolemic shock:* Amount lost is replaced. Ringer's solution, as much as 1000 mL/hr, may be administered if volume loss is severe. Most often this includes blood replacement.
- *Septic shock:* Ringer's solution, plasma, and blood are administered.

♦ Prepare for transfer of patient to ICU if appropriate.

Impaired gas exchange related to altered O_2 supply secondary to decreased respiratory muscle function occurring with altered metabolism
Desired outcomes: Within 1 hr of intervention, patient has adequate gas exchange, as evidenced by O_2 saturation greater than 92%; PaO_2 at least 80 mm Hg; $PaCO_2$ 45 mm Hg or less; pH at or near 7.35; presence of eupnea; and orientation to person, place, and time.

Nursing Interventions

♦ Monitor ABG results. Be alert to and report presence of hypoxemia (decreased O_2 saturation, decreased PaO_2), hypercapnia (increased $PaCO_2$), and acidosis (decreased pH, increased $PaCO_2$). Report significant findings.

♦ Monitor oximetry readings; be alert for readings 92% or less. Report significant findings.

♦ Monitor respirations q30min; note and report presence of tachypnea or dyspnea. Be alert to mental status changes, restlessness, irritability, and confusion, *which are indicators of hypoxia.*

♦ Teach patient to breathe slowly and deeply *to promote oxygenation.*

♦ Ensure patient has a patent airway; suction secretions as needed *to assist with gas exchange.*

♦ Administer O_2 as prescribed. Deliver O_2 with humidity *to help prevent drying of oral and nasal mucosa.*

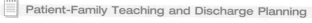

Patient-Family Teaching and Discharge Planning

For interventions, see discussion with patient's primary diagnosis.

❖ CARDIAC SURGERY

OVERVIEW/PATHOPHYSIOLOGY

Surgical intervention may be necessary to treat acquired or congenital heart disease. Coronary artery bypass grafting (CABG) is done to treat blocked coronary arteries. A portion of the saphenous vein, internal mammary artery, gastroepiploic artery, or radial artery is excised and anastomosed to coronary arteries, thereby revascularizing the affected myocardium. Valve replacement, another type of cardiac surgery, is performed for patients with valvular stenosis or valvular incompetence of the mitral, tricuspid, pulmonary, or aortic valve. Some patients may require replacement of the aortic arch and aortic valve because of an aortic aneurysm. Cardiac surgery is also performed to correct heart defects such as ventricular aneurysm, ventricular or atrial septal defects, transposition of the great vessels, and tetralogy of Fallot. Heart transplantation may be considered for some patients diagnosed with end-stage cardiac disease; however, the national shortage of acceptable donor organs remains a problem. Many patients waiting for heart transplants will undergo surgery to receive a ventricular assist device, which will serve as a bridge to transplantation. Combined heart-lung transplantation is performed for patients with end-stage disease affecting both organs. Immunosuppressive treatment to prevent organ rejection after heart transplantation is similar to that of patients who receive a renal transplant. See "Care of the Renal Transplant Recipient," p. 193.

Many patients undergoing cardiac surgery may have temporary epicardial pacing wires in place. These wires are placed on the heart at the time of surgery and pulled through the chest wall, where they can be attached to a temporary pacemaker. The wires are used for temporary postoperative pacing if needed for bradycardia. When the pacing wires are no longer needed, they are removed by nurses or other health care providers who have demonstrated technical proficiency.

Under normal circumstances, patients are admitted to the hospital the day of surgery. After surgery, most patients are in an ICU for 24 hr and then transferred to a step-down unit for 3-5 days.

NURSING DIAGNOSES AND INTERVENTIONS

Deficient knowledge related to diagnosis, surgical procedure, preoperative routine, and postoperative course
Desired outcome: Before surgery, patient verbalizes knowledge about the diagnosis, surgical procedure, and preoperative and postoperative regimens.

Nursing Interventions

◆ Assess patient's facility with language; provide an interpreter or language-appropriate written materials as indicated.
◆ Assess patient's level of knowledge about the diagnosis and surgical procedure, and provide information where necessary. Encourage questions, and allow time for verbalization of concerns and fears.
◆ When appropriate, provide orientation to the ICU and equipment that will be used postoperatively.
◆ Provide instructions for and demonstrate deep breathing and coughing, and ask that patient return the demonstration.
◆ Reassure patient that postoperative discomfort will be relieved with medication. Pain after a midline sternotomy (usual incision with cardiac surgery) most often is less than that with conventional thoracotomy because the somatic nerves are not divided by the surgical incision.
◆ Advise patient that speaking will be impossible in the immediate postoperative period because of the presence of an endotracheal tube, which will assist with breathing.
◆ Review sternal precautions. Demonstrate how to get in and out of bed and chair without using upper extremities. Advise patient not to lift, push, or pull more than 5-10 lb with either upper extremity for a period of 4-6 wk. Caution that driving a car is prohibited for 4-6 wk.

Activity intolerance related to generalized weakness and bed rest secondary to cardiac surgery
Desired outcomes: By a minimum of 24 hr before hospital discharge, patient rates perceived exertion at 3 or less on a 0-10 scale and exhibits cardiac tolerance to activity after cardiac surgery, as evidenced by heart rate (HR) 110 beats per minute (bpm) or less, SBP within 20 mm Hg of resting SBP, and respiratory rate (RR) 20 breaths/min or less with normal depth and pattern (eupnea).

Nursing Interventions

◆ Ask patient to rate perceived exertion during activity, and monitor for evidence of activity intolerance. Notify health care provider of significant findings.

- Monitor VS at frequent intervals, and be alert to indicators of cardiac complications, including hypotension, tachycardia, crackles (rales), tachypnea, and decreased amplitude of peripheral pulses. Notify health care provider of significant findings.
- Monitor BP and note a decrease greater than 20 mm Hg from resting SBP.
- Facilitate coordination of health care providers to ensure rest periods between care activities and thus *decrease cardiac workload*. Ensure 90 min for undisturbed rest.
- Assist with exercises, depending on tolerance and prescribed activity limitations. As prescribed, initiate physical therapy *to increase activity tolerance and provide teaching for home exercise program*. Reinforce sternal precautions.
- See **Risk for activity intolerance,** p. 23, and **Risk for disuse syndrome,** p. 25, for a discussion of in-bed exercises.

Patient-Family Teaching and Discharge Planning

Provide written information with verbal reinforcement and time for questions about the following:
- Medications, including drug names, dosage, schedule, purpose, precautions, and potential side effects. Also discuss drug/drug, herb/drug, and food/drug interactions.
- Untoward symptoms requiring medical attention for patients taking warfarin, such as bleeding from the nose (epistaxis) or gums, hemoptysis, hematemesis, hematuria, melena, hematochezia, menometrorrhagia, and excessive bruising. In addition, stress the following: take warfarin at the same time every day, notify health care provider if any signs of bleeding occur, avoid over-the-counter (OTC) and herbal medications unless approved by health care provider, wear/carry a MedicAlert bracelet or card, avoid constrictive or restrictive clothing, and use a soft-bristled toothbrush and electric razor.
- Maintenance of low-Na^+ and low-cholesterol diet. Encourage patients to use food labels to determine Na^+, fat, and cholesterol content of foods. See Box 4-1, p. 165, for high-Na^+ foods to avoid, Table 3-2 for low-fat foods, and Table 3-1 for low-cholesterol foods.
- Importance of pacing activities at home and allowing frequent rest periods.
- Technique for assessing radial pulse, temperature, and weight, if these indicators require monitoring at home, and reporting significant changes to health care provider.
- Phone number of nurse available to discuss concerns and questions or clarify unclear instructions.
- Importance of follow-up visits with health care provider; confirm date and time of next appointment.
- Signs and symptoms that necessitate immediate medical attention: edema, chest pain, dyspnea, shortness of breath, weight gain, and decrease in exercise tolerance.
- Activity restrictions (e.g., no heavy lifting, pushing, or pulling anything heavier than 5-10 lb with upper extremities for at least 4-6 wk); prescribed exercise program; and resumption of sexual activity, work, and driving a car, as directed.
- Care of incision site; importance of assessing for signs of infection, such as drainage, swelling, fever, persistent redness, and local warmth and tenderness.
- Referral to a cardiac rehabilitation program.
- Need for changes/adaptations of patient's home environment (e.g., too many steps to climb, activities of daily living (ADL) that are too strenuous).

◆ Introduction to local American Heart Association activities. Either provide the address or phone number for the local chapter or encourage patient to access the following:

American Heart Association: www.americanheart.org

◆ For patients awaiting heart transplantation, provide the following information, as appropriate:

The United Network for Organ Sharing: www.unos.org

❖ ❖ ❖

SECTION FIVE **DYSRHYTHMIAS**

❖ DYSRHYTHMIAS AND CONDUCTION DISTURBANCES

OVERVIEW/PATHOPHYSIOLOGY

Dysrhythmias are abnormal rhythms of the heart's electrical system. They can originate in any part of the conduction system, such as the sinus node, atrium, atrioventricular (A-V) node, His-Purkinje system, bundle branches, and ventricular tissue. Although a variety of diseases may cause dysrhythmias, the most common are coronary artery disease (CAD) and myocardial infarction (MI). Other causes may include electrolyte imbalance, changes in oxygenation, and drug toxicity. Cardiac dysrhythmias may result from the following mechanisms:

Disturbances in automaticity: May involve an increase or decrease in automaticity in the sinus node (i.e., sinus tachycardia or sinus bradycardia). Premature beats may arise via this mechanism from the atria, junction, or ventricles. Abnormal rhythms, such as atrial or ventricular tachycardia (VT), also may occur.

Disturbances in conductivity: Conduction may be too rapid, as in conditions caused by an accessory pathway (e.g., Wolff-Parkinson-White syndrome), or too slow (e.g., A-V block). Reentry is a situation in which a stimulus reexcites a conduction pathway through which it already has passed. Once started, this impulse may circulate repeatedly. For reentry to occur, there must be two different pathways for conduction: one with slowed conduction and one with unidirectional block.

Combinations of altered automaticity and conductivity: Observed when several dysrhythmias are noted, for example, a first-degree A-V block (disturbance in conductivity) and premature atrial contractions (PACs) (disturbance in automaticity).

ASSESSMENT

Signs and symptoms/physical findings: Can vary on a continuum from absence of symptoms to complete cardiopulmonary collapse. General indicators include alterations in level of consciousness (LOC), vertigo, syncope, seizures, weakness, fatigue, activity intolerance, shortness of breath, dysphea on exertion (DOE), chest pain, palpitations, sensation of "skipped beats," anxiety, and restlessness.

Physical findings include increases or decreases in heart rate (HR), BP, and respiratory rate (RR); dusky color or pallor; crackles (rales); cool skin; decreased urine output; and paradoxical pulse and abnormal heart sounds (e.g., paradoxical splitting of S_1 and S_2). Findings on ECG vary with the type of dysrhythmia and can involve abnormalities in rate such as sinus bradycardia or sinus tachycardia, irregular rhythm such as atrial fibrillation, extra beats such as PACs and premature junctional contractions (PJCs), wide and bizarre-looking beats such as premature ventricular contractions (PVCs) and VT, a fibrillating baseline such as in ventricular fibrillation (VF), and a straight line, as in asystole.

History and risk factors: CAD, recent MI, electrolyte disturbances, drug toxicity.

DIAGNOSTIC TESTS

12-lead ECG: Detects dysrhythmias and identify possible cause.

Serum electrolyte levels: Identify electrolyte abnormalities that can precipitate dysrhythmias; K^+ and magnesium abnormalities are most common.

Drug levels: Identify toxicities (e.g., of digoxin, quinidine, procainamide, aminophylline) that can precipitate dysrhythmias.

Ambulatory monitoring (e.g., Holter monitor or cardiac event recorder): Identifies subtle dysrhythmias, associates abnormal rhythms by means of patient's symptoms, and assesses response to exercise.

Electrophysiologic study: Invasive test in which 2-3 catheters are placed into the heart, to giving a pacing stimulus at varying sites and of varying voltages. The test determines origin of dysrhythmia, inducibility, and effectiveness of drug therapy in dysrhythmia suppression.

Exercise stress testing: Used in conjunction with Holter monitoring to detect advanced grades of PVCs (those caused by ischemia) and to guide therapy. During the test, ECGs and BP readings are taken while patient walks on a treadmill or pedals a stationary bicycle; response to a constant or increasing workload is observed. The test continues until patient reaches target HR or symptoms such as chest pain, severe fatigue, dysrhythmias, or abnormal BP occur.

Oximetry or arterial blood gas (ABG) values: Document trend of hypoxemia.

COLLABORATIVE MANAGEMENT

Antidysrhythmic drugs: See **BOX 3-3**.

Transthoracic cardioversion and defibrillation: Uses electric shock to terminate dysrhythmias; emergency procedure for VF; may be elective for VT, atrial fibrillation, or atrial flutter.

Pacemaker insertion: See "Pacemakers and Implantable Cardioverter Defibrillators," p. 146.

ICD (ICD): See "Pacemakers and Implantable Cardioverter Defibrillators," p. 146.

Dietary guidelines: Usually patients with recurrent dysrhythmias are placed on a diet that restricts or reduces caffeine and is low in cholesterol (Table 3-1) if multiple cardiac risk factors are present or if there is preexisting CAD.

Radiofrequency catheter ablation: Uses an electrode catheter inserted percutaneously to heat and destroy specific areas of tissue essential to maintaining the dysrhythmia; done simultaneously with electrophysiologic studies.

Left ventricular (LV) aneurysmectomy and infarctectomy: Surgical excision of possible focal spots of ventricular dysrhythmias.

NURSING DIAGNOSES AND INTERVENTIONS

Decreased cardiac output related to altered rate, rhythm, or conduction or negative inotropic changes secondary to cardiac disease

Desired outcome: Within 1 hr of treatment/intervention, patient has adequate cardiac output, as evidenced by BP 90/60 mm Hg or higher, HR 60-100 beats per minute (bpm), and normal sinus rhythm on ECG.

Nursing Interventions

◆ Monitor patient's heart rhythm continuously; note BP and if dysrhythmias occur or increase in occurrence.

BOX 3-3   ANTIDYSRHYTHMIC DRUGS

Class I
Local anesthetics and other drugs that decrease automaticity of ventricular
    conduction, delay ventricular repolarization, decrease conduction velocity,
    increase conduction via A-V node, and suppress ventricular automaticity.

Class IA
Decrease depolarization moderately and prolong repolarization.
- Disopyramide (PO)
- Procainamide (PO, IV, IM)
- Quinidine (PO, IV)

Class IB
Decrease depolarization and shorten repolarization.
- Mexiletine (PO)
- Phenytoin (PO)
- Tocainide (PO)

Class IC
Significantly decrease depolarization with minimal effect on repolarization.
- Encainide (PO)
- Flecainide (PO)
- Propafenone (PO)

Class II
β-Blockers that slow sinus automaticity, slow conduction via A-V node, control
    ventricular response to supraventricular tachycardias, and shorten the action
    potential of Purkinje fibers.
- Acebutolol (PO)
- Atenolol (PO)
- Metoprolol (PO, IV)
- Propranolol (PO, IV)

Class III
Increases the action potential and refractory period of Purkinje fibers, increase
    ventricular fibrillation threshold, restore injured myocardial cell electrophysiology
    toward normal, and suppress reentrant dysrhythmias.
- Amiodarone (PO, IV)
- Bretylium (IV, IM)
- Sotalol (PO)

Class IV
Calcium channel blockers that depress automaticity in the S-A and A-V nodes,
    block the slow calcium current in the A-V junctional tissue, reduce conduction
    via the A-V node, and are useful in treating tachydysrhythmias because of A-V
    junction reentry.
- Diltiazem (PO)
- Nifedipine (PO)
- Verapamil (IV)

A-V, Atrioventricular; *IV*, intravenous; *IM*, intramuscular; *PO*, by mouth; *S-A*, sinoatrial.

- If symptoms of decreased cardiac output occur, prepare to transfer patient
    to CCU.
- Document dysrhythmias with rhythm strip. Use a 12-lead ECG as neces-
    sary *to identify the dysrhythmia.*
- Monitor patient's laboratory data, particularly electrolyte and digoxin
    levels. Serum K^+ levels less than 3.5 mEq/L or more than 5.0 mEq/L. These
    values are associated with *dysrhythmias.*

♦ Administer antidysrhythmic agents as prescribed; note patient's response to therapy.

♦ Monitor corrected QT interval (QTc) when initiating drugs known to cause QT prolongation (i.e., sotalol, propafenone, dofetilide, flecainide). QTc equals QT (in seconds) divided by the square root of the RR interval (in seconds). *A prolonged QTc t can increase risk of dysrhythmias.*

♦ Provide O_2 as prescribed. O_2 *may be beneficial if dysrhythmias are related to ischemia.* Deliver O_2 with humidity *to help prevent drying of oral and nasal mucosa.*

♦ Maintain a quiet environment, and administer pain medications promptly. *Both stress and pain can increase sympathetic tone and cause dysrhythmias.*

♦ If life-threatening dysrhythmias occur, initiate emergency procedures and cardiopulmonary resuscitation (CPR) (as indicated by advanced cardiac life support [ACLS] protocol).

♦ When dysrhythmias occur, stay with patient; provide support and reassurance while performing assessments and administering treatment to decrease anxiety.

Deficient knowledge related to mechanism by which dysrhythmias occur and lifestyle implications
Desired outcome: Within the 24-hr period before hospital discharge, patient and significant other verbalize knowledge about causes of dysrhythmias and implications for patient's lifestyle modifications.

Nursing Interventions

♦ Assess patient's and significant other's facility with language; engage an interpreter or provide language-appropriate written materials if indicated.

♦ Discuss causal mechanisms for dysrhythmias, including resulting symptoms. Use a heart model or diagrams as necessary.

♦ Teach signs and symptoms of dysrhythmias that necessitate medical attention: unrelieved and prolonged palpitations, chest pain, shortness of breath, rapid pulse (more than 150 bpm), dizziness, and syncope.

♦ Teach patient and significant other how to check pulse rate for a full minute.

♦ Teach patient and significant other about medications that will be taken after hospital discharge, including drug names, purpose, dosage, schedule, precautions, and potential side effects. Also discuss drug/drug, food/drug, and herb/drug interactions. Stress that patient will be taking long-term antidysrhythmic therapy and that it could be life-threatening to stop or skip these medications without health care provider involvement because doing so may decrease blood levels effective for dysrhythmia suppression.

♦ Advise patient and significant other about availability of support groups and counseling; provide appropriate community referrals. Patients who survive sudden cardiac arrest may experience nightmares or other sleep disturbances at home. Explain that anxiety and fear, along with periodic feelings of denial, depression, anger, and confusion, are normal following this experience.

♦ Stress importance of leading a normal and productive life, even though patient may fear breakthrough of life-threatening dysrhythmias. If patient is going on vacation, advise taking along sufficient medication and investigating health care facilities in the vacation area.

♦ Advise patient and significant other to take CPR classes; provide addresses for community programs.

♦ Teach importance of follow-up care; confirm date and time of next appointment if known. Explain that outpatient Holter monitoring is performed periodically.

♦ Explain dietary restrictions that individuals with recurrent dysrhythmias should follow. Discuss need for reduced intake of products containing caffeine, including coffee, tea, chocolate, and colas. Because of the overlap between dysrhythmias and CAD, provide instruction for a general low-cholesterol diet (Table 3-1). Encourage patient to use food labels to determine cholesterol content of foods.

◆ As indicated, teach patient relaxation techniques, which will reduce stress and enable patient to decrease sympathetic tone (see p. 106).

 Patient-Family Teaching and Discharge Planning

See patient's primary diagnosis.

❖ PACEMAKERS AND IMPLANTABLE CARDIOVERTER DEFIBRILLATORS

Pacemakers
OVERVIEW/PATHOPHYSIOLOGY

In a normally functioning heart, the sinoatrial (S-A) node, or sinus node, is the natural pacemaker, and it dictates the intrinsic heart rate (HR). Impulses travel from the S-A node to the A-V node, which lies in the junction between the atrial and ventricular conduction systems. The His-Purkinje system lies below the A-V node and consists of the bundle of His and the right and left bundle branches. Impulses move from the A-V node to the bundle of His and onto the bundle branches.

A mechanical pacemaker delivers an electrical impulse to the heart to stimulate contraction when the heart's natural pacemakers fail to maintain normal rhythm. Patients for whom pacemakers are indicated have a history of syncopal episodes, dizziness, intolerance to exercise, or an episode of cardiac arrest. A newer indication includes ventricular dyssynchrony when it is associated with heart failure (HF) symptoms. A temporary pacemaker may be inserted when patients suffer from temporary or transient rhythm disturbances, such as severe bradycardia or a conduction block. Temporary pacemakers are seen most often in ICUs or telemetry units and on an emergency basis. The lead wire is inserted through a central vein to the right side of the heart, where it lodges in atrial and/or ventricular tissue to deliver the electrical impulse. An alternative method is transcutaneous pacing, which employs two large skin electrodes connected to a pulse generator. Generally this is an acute, short-term treatment option because significant patient discomfort occurs when a pacing stimulus is delivered transcutaneously.

Permanent pacemakers are indicated for patients with acquired A-V block (first, second, third degree), symptomatic bradycardia, other dysrhythmias, and other medical conditions that require drugs that result in symptomatic bradycardia and asystole (more than 3.0 sec) while awake, escape rhythm less than 40 beats per minute (bpm), neuromuscular disorders with A-V block, postoperative A-V block, chronic bifascicular and trifascicular block, post–myocardial infarction (MI) second-degree A-V block in the His-Purkinje system with bilateral bundle branch block (BBB), pause-dependent ventricular tachycardia (VT) with or without prolonged QT, congenital prolonged QT syndrome, recurrent syncope caused by carotid sinus stimulation in the absence of any medication that depresses sinus node or A-V conduction, post-transplant chronotropic/conduction incompetence, and postprocedure status after catheter ablation of the A-V junction, as well as for prevention and termination of tachydysrhythmias by pacing of symptomatic supraventricular tachycardia (SVT). Permanent pacemakers are implanted subcutaneously in the operating room (OR), catheterization laboratory, or electrophysiology laboratory using local anesthesia and, often, conscious sedation. Lead wires are inserted percutaneously via the subclavian vein, where they are passed into the right atrium and/or right ventricle. Lead wires also can be placed epicardially if vascular access is problematic. After implantation, patient is transferred to the telemetry unit for 24-48 hr of close monitoring. Patient is instructed not to raise the affected arm above the shoulder for 4-6 wk. Slings and other immobilizers have fallen out of favor because of risk of joint problems associated with prolonged immobility.

UNIVERSAL CODING

The increasing complexity of pacemakers led to the development in 1987 of a five-letter code known as the NASPE/BPEG Generic Pacemaker Code for Antibradycardia Pacing. This was revised and simplified in 2001.

First letter: Chamber that is paced.
V: Ventricle
A: Atrium
D: Dual (A and V)
S: Single (A or V)
O: None

Second letter: Chamber that is sensed.
V: Ventricle
A: Atrium
D: Dual (A and V)
S: Single (A or V)
O: None

Third letter: Mode of response to sensing.
T: Triggered by ventricular activity
I: Inhibited by ventricular activity
D: Dual—atrial triggered, ventricular inhibited
O: Neither (paces continuously)

Fourth letter: Rate modulation.
R: Rate response activated
O: Rate response not activated (See "Pacemaker Types" for details.)

Fifth letter: Multisite pacing.
A: Atrium
V: Ventricle
D: Dual (A and V)
O: None

PACEMAKER TYPES

Asynchronous or fixed rate: These pacemakers represent the original devices. They are coded VOO, AOO, or DOO. A pulse generator will revert to this mode with device malfunction or magnet application.

Demand: This type senses intrinsic cardiac function and discharges only when there is failure of the intrinsic system. These pacemakers are coded AAI, ADI, VVI, VDI, or DDI.

Sequential: Intrinsic activity is sensed in both the atrium and ventricle and stimulates sequentially as programmed. It is coded VDD or DDD.

Rate-adaptive (also called *rate-responsive*): This feature, if activated, permits the pacemaker to increase rate in response to activity. Current devices use (1) a piezoelectric sensor, which responds to vibration; (2) an accelerometer, which responds to body motion; and (3) minute ventilation, which responds to impedance changes during inspiration and expiration or in a combination of both items 2 and 3. It is coded AAIR, VVIR, DDDR, or DDIR.

Implantable Cardioverter Defibrillators
OVERVIEW/PATHOPHYSIOLOGY

An implantable cardioverter defibrillator (ICD) is a permanently implanted device used to treat lethal cardiac dysrhythmias. It is recommended for patients who have survived an episode of sudden cardiac death (cardiac arrest), those with coronary artery disease (CAD) who have had a cardiac arrest, and individuals with sustained ventricular dysrhythmias. In addition, patients who have CAD and left ventricular ejection fraction (LVEF) of 30% or less are recognized to be at high risk for sudden cardiac death and have been shown to benefit from prophylactic ICD placement. A pulse generator that is powered by lithium batteries is inserted much like a pacemaker (in the OR, electrophysiology laboratory, or catheterization laboratory; local anesthesia and conscious sedation are used) into a "pocket" formed in the pectoral area. Leads are inserted through the subclavian vein and advanced to the right atrium and right ventricle. The ICD is programmed to deliver the electrical stimulus at a predetermined rate after assessing morphology of the intracardiac electrogram stored by the ICD and/or after evaluating the relationship between the atrial and ventricular activity. First- and second-generation ICDs provided only for cardioversion or defibrillation. The newest ICDs provide overdrive pacing for atrial and ventricular dysrhythmias, low-energy cardioversion, high-energy shock, and dual-chamber pacing if indicated.

Postoperative complications following pacemaker or ICD insertion include atelectasis, pneumonia, hematoma at the generator "pocket," infection, pneumothorax, and venous thrombosis. Lead migration and lead fracture are the two most common structural problems. Interference from unipolar pacemakers, "myopotentials" (electrical interference), and lead fracture are common mechanical complications that can cause inappropriate ICD discharge. ICDs may need to be deactivated during surgical procedures when electrocautery is in use. This is simply done with an ICD programmer or placement of a donut magnet over the device. When the magnet is removed, the ICD will go back to preprogrammed parameters. If a device is deactivated for surgery, it should be checked by trained personnel afterward.

NURSING DIAGNOSES AND INTERVENTIONS

Deficient knowledge related to pacemaker/ICD insertion procedure, pacemaker/ICD function, and precautions to take after hospital discharge

Desired outcomes: Before the procedure, patient verbalizes knowledge about the insertion procedure and the function of the pacemaker/ICD. Before hospital discharge, patient describes precautions to take after hospital discharge.

Nursing Interventions

Before pacemaker/ICD insertion

- ◆ Assess patient's facility with language; provide an interpreter or language-appropriate written materials if indicated.
- ◆ Assess patient's knowledge about insertion procedure and pacemaker/ICD function. As appropriate, describe procedure and explain that the pacemaker stimulates patient's own heart to beat when the heart becomes "lazy" or slows down. An ICD can function as a pacemaker and, in addition, watches for abnormal heart rhythms that are then treated with overdrive pacing or shock.
- ◆ Begin a teaching program specific to patient's rhythm disorder and type of device inserted, including normal function of the heart, patient's rhythm disorder that requires a device, and how patient's device works.
- ◆ Reinforce explanation by health care provider about length of time of the procedure, use of local anesthetic or conscious sedation, and postprocedure care.
- ◆ Explain that after the procedure patient can expect the following: continuous monitoring by ECG, stiffness and soreness at insertion site, and no

vigorous activity. Explain that patient should request pain medication before pain becomes severe. Some health care providers prescribe that ice be placed on the wound for the first 24 hr postoperatively to prevent edema formation and reduce pain.

After pacemaker/ICD insertion

◆ Explain activity restrictions as directed by health care provider, such as no heavy lifting, and give instructions about amount and type of exercise allowed. Resumption of sexual activity probably will not be affected, but this will depend on patient's underlying condition. Driving may be restricted, depending on the reason for device implant.

◆ Teach signs and symptoms that necessitate medical attention, such as decreasing pulse rate, irregular pulse, dizziness, shortness of breath, ankle swelling, passing out, and signs of infection. Teach technique for measuring radial pulse.

◆ Stress necessity of follow-up care, usually at a device clinic; confirm date of next appointment. Telephonic monitoring of pacemakers is commonly used as a method of assessing patients between visits. Only select ICDs can be monitored via telephone. If this method is to be used, inform patient about this type of monitoring.

◆ Teach expected life of the device battery, which is approximate and can vary from 5-10 yr, depending on type of battery and individual usage. It is important to know manufacturer of the specific device.

◆ Advise need to carry device identification card and wear a MedicAlert bracelet. The card contains information for health care providers about type of device in the event of an emergency.

Ineffective cardiopulmonary and peripheral tissue perfusion (or risk for same) related to interrupted blood flow secondary to device malfunction
Desired outcome: On an ongoing basis, patient has adequate perfusion, as evidenced by BP within 20 mm Hg of baseline BP; peripheral pulse amplitude more than 2+ on a 0-4+ scale; and apical/radial pulses regular, equal, and at a rate equal to or greater than that established for pacemaker.

Nursing Interventions

◆ Monitor perfusion by assessing BP at frequent intervals.

◆ Assess rate and regularity of apical and radial pulses. At minimum, it should be the rate established for the pacemaker.

◆ Assess for apical/radial deficit, which, if present, indicates that the heart is mechanically contracting, but there is no peripheral perfusion (e.g., if apical pulse rate is 80 bpm with auscultation but palpable radial pulse is 42 bpm). Be alert to pulse irregularity because it *can signal device malfunction or change in heart rhythm.*

◆ Alert health care provider to significant findings.

Patient-Family Teaching and Discharge Planning

Reinforce previous teaching, including that about activity restriction, signs and symptoms that require medical attention, need for follow-up care, battery life expectancy, and need to carry medical alert information. Also include verbal and written information about the following:

◆ Technique for measuring radial pulse.

◆ Date and type (in-person or telephone monitoring) of follow-up appointment.

◆ Medications, including drug names, purpose, dosage, schedule, precautions, and potential side effects. Also discuss drug/drug, food/drug, and herb/drug interactions.

♦ Importance of using caution around strong magnetic fields, which can alter device function. Strong magnetic fields can convert some pacemakers to a fixed-rate mode. Once away from the magnetic field, the pacemaker will return to the normally programmed function.

SECTION SIX DISORDERS OF THE PERIPHERAL VASCULAR SYSTEM

❖ PERIPHERAL ARTERIAL DISEASE (PAD)/ATHEROSCLEROTIC ARTERIAL OCCLUSIVE DISEASE

OVERVIEW/PATHOPHYSIOLOGY

Inflammation is central to the pathogenesis of *atherosclerosis.* Injury to cell walls may occur secondary to hypertension, diabetes, infection, hyperlipidemia, nicotine use, or hereditary factors. Atherosclerotic lesions can develop from accumulation of plaque, hemorrhage, calcium deposits, or lipids. *Arteriosclerosis* generally defines any process that causes wall thickening.

Occlusive disease is diagnosed when 75% or more of a cross-section of artery has become blocked. In the presence of other comorbidities, such as myocardial infarction (MI), hypertension, chronic obstructive pulmonary disease (COPD), or diabetes mellitus (DM), loss of limb and life may be threatened.

ASSESSMENT

Signs and symptoms/physical findings: Intermittent claudication (severe cramping pain with exercise that is relieved by rest), feeling of heaviness in the legs, coolness of the legs to touch, bluish discoloration, decreased hair distribution, delayed healing, decreased sensory or motor function, leg ulcers, gangrene, and dependent rubor. Skin may appear shiny and the nails thickened. Audible bruits may be assessed with a stethoscope over partially occluded vessels. Delayed capillary filling of 2 or more sec, and decreased amplitude of peripheral pulses or pulses only detected by Doppler examination.

History and risk factors: Older age, hypertension, cigarette smoking, DM, family history of atherosclerotic disease, and dyslipidemia.

DIAGNOSTIC TESTS

Doppler flow studies: A transducer that emits sound waves through a probe is used to determine amount of blood flow through arteries in which palpable pulses are difficult to obtain. Waveforms also can be assessed similar to those of an ECG. The more normal or triphasic waveform looks like a regular heart rhythm. A flatter line with lengthening, called *monophasic,* indicates more severe disease. Pressures also can be obtained for determining the ankle-brachial index (ABI).

Duplex imaging: Ultrasound and Doppler are used to assess arteries for measuring flow and velocities. Originally used in carotid disease, duplex imaging is now useful for other arteries and veins in the body.

Exercise testing: Determines amount of exercise that precipitates claudication symptoms.

ABI: Reflects severity of arterial occlusion and subsequent ischemia. BP is determined at the ankle (using either posterior tibial or dorsalis pedis pulse) and at the brachial artery. The pressure obtained at the ankle is divided by that at the brachial artery. Normally ABI is greater than 1.0; resting pain occurs with an ABI of 0.3 or less.

Angiography of peripheral vasculature: Locates obstruction and reveals extent of vascular lesions by injecting dye into arteries and taking pictures of the arteries in a timed sequence. This imaging study is useful in patients in whom angioplasty or stenting may be possible.

Digital subtraction angiography (DSA): Arteriogram in which the computer subtracts early images from late images, to delete bone and soft tissue, so that only contrast-filled arteries appear.

Magnetic resonance angiography (MRA) and computed tomography (CT) angiography: Noninvasive tests that provide clear definition of arterial lesions and are used in planning revascularization.

COLLABORATIVE MANAGEMENT

Regular lower extremity exercise program: Walking is the best activity, and patients can be instructed to walk until they have pain, rest until recovery, and then resume walking. This approach is especially useful for patients with claudication and who have other risk factor modifications. Activity may be contraindicated for some patients with severe disease. See also **Impaired tissue integrity of extremity**, p. 152.

Cessation of cigarette smoking: Prevents increased vasoconstriction and severity of the circulation deficit, as well as alleviating the effects of nicotine on the lungs and other body organs.

Weight management

Control of hyperlipidemia and cholesterol levels: Prevents progression of atherosclerosis. This is accomplished through a low-fat (Table 3-2), low-cholesterol (Table 3-1) diet, weight loss, exercise, and/or lipid-lowering agents. There is increasing evidence, especially in individuals with DM, that a small amount of antihyperlipidemic agent is useful in preventing cardiac complications and stroke.

Control of hypertension: Administration of antihypertensive drugs, such as angiotensin-converting enzyme (ACE) inhibitors, β-blockers, diuretics, or calcium channel blockers (CCBs). Controlling both systolic hypertension and diastolic hypertension is important.

Diabetes management: Persons with DM should be encouraged to maintain strict control of their blood sugar by means of frequent monitoring of blood glucose levels and regular checking of their glycosylated hemoglobin (HbA$_{1C}$) values.

Pharmacotherapy

Mild analgesics: For relief of pain.

Opioid analgesics: May be given for postoperative pain control or rest pain before surgery. They may not be effective in some patients for rest pain, and they are used cautiously in older adults.

Antiplatelet agents: Most commonly, aspirin, clopidogrel, or ticlopidine is given to help prevent platelet adherence and thromboembolism.

Blood viscosity reducing/antiplatelet agent: Pentoxifylline or cilostazol may increase flexibility of erythrocytes and thereby enhance their movement through the microcirculation and prevent aggregation of RBCs and platelets. This therapy has the potential to increase circulation at the capillary level and to reduce or alleviate symptoms caused by lack of blood flow.

Lipid-lowering agents: Lovastatin, atorvastatin, simvastatin, and pravastatin reduce serum cholesterol levels and decrease inflammation in vessel walls.

Surgical management: For patients who have tissue loss, rest pain, or disabling claudication, endarterectomy or revascularization may be helpful.

Endarterectomy: Removal of the atheromatous obstruction via arterial incision.

Distal revascularization: Surgical bypass of the obstructed segment by suturing an autogenous vein or graft proximally and distally to the obstruction. In larger arteries, such as the aorta, graft material is either Dacron or Gore-Tex, whereas in the distal circulation, autogenous veins are best.

Percutaneous transluminal angioplasty (PTA or PTLA): May be used to treat focal arterial obstruction. This procedure works best in a large artery with a short lesion. A balloon-tipped catheter is inserted through the artery to the area of occlusion. The balloon is gradually inflated to ablate the obstruction.

Stent: During an arteriogram, a hollow tube is positioned and deployed within a stenosed vessel to stretch and improve blood flow. Various designs, materials, and deployment techniques have been developed. Combined with angioplasty, a stent may provide longer patency of the vessel. Stents are used in renal, mesenteric, carotid, and iliac arteries; they are not used for femoral, popliteal, or tibial arteries.

Amputation: See discussion in Chapter 9, p. 603.

NURSING DIAGNOSES AND INTERVENTIONS

Impaired tissue integrity of extremity (or risk for same) related to altered arterial circulation secondary to atherosclerotic process

Desired outcome: Patient's extremity tissue remains intact.

Nursing Interventions

- Assess legs and between toes for ulcerations that can occur with decreased arterial circulation.
- Teach patient that walking and ROM exercises for hip, knee, and ankle promote collateral circulation.
- Discuss an exercise program with health care provider, and describe routine to patient.
- Teach patient how to assess peripheral pulses, warmth, sensation, and color of lower extremities.
- Encourage smoking cessation and teach patient that smoking decreases both blood flow to the extremities and extremity temperature, particularly in fingers and toes. Provide smoking cessation literature. Discuss with health care provider use of medication for smoking cessation.
- Discuss importance of keeping feet warm and protected by wearing socks when walking or in bed. Caution patient about using heating pads, which increase metabolism and may promote ischemia if circulation is limited. Avoid pressure over areas of bony prominence.
- Discuss importance of night lights placed in bedrooms and bathrooms so patient can see *to avoid tissue trauma at night when getting up.*
- Encourage daily foot inspections by patient or by family members if patient's vision is compromised.
- Administer antiplatelet agents as prescribed *to help prevent platelet adherence.*

Chronic pain related to atherosclerotic obstructions and ischemia

Desired outcomes: By time of hospital discharge, patient's subjective perception of chronic pain decreases as documented by pain scale. Objective indicators, such as grimacing, are absent.

Nursing Interventions

- Assess for presence of pain, using a pain scale of from 0 (no pain) to 10 (worst pain). Administer pain medications as prescribed; document effectiveness using pain scale.

- Teach patient to rest and stop exercising before claudication (severe, cramping pain) occurs.
- Because the pain may be chronic and continuous, explore alternate methods of pain relief, such as visualization, guided imagery, biofeedback, meditation, and relaxation exercises or tapes. See "Coronary Artery Disease," **Health-seeking behaviors**, p. 106, for an example of a relaxation exercise.
- Institute measures to increase circulation to ischemic extremities, such as walking and use of medications as directed by health care provider (see **Impaired tissue integrity**, p. 152).
- Advise about possibility of "rest" pain, which occurs at night when recumbent and decreases when legs are in a dependent position.

Deficient knowledge related to risk for infection and impaired tissue integrity caused by decreased arterial circulation
Desired outcome: By time of hospital discharge, patient verbalizes knowledge about the potential for infection and impaired tissue integrity, as well as measures to prevent these problems.

Nursing Interventions

- Assess patient's facility with language; engage an interpreter or provide language-appropriate written materials if indicated.
- Teach how to assess for signs of infection or problems with skin integrity and to report significant findings to health care provider.
- Caution about increased potential for easily traumatizing skin (e.g., from bumping lower extremities).
- Instruct patient to inspect both feet each day for any open wounds or bruises. If necessary, suggest that patient use a long-handled mirror to see bottoms of feet. Advise patient to report any open areas to health care provider.
- Stress importance of wearing shoes or slippers that fit properly without areas of stress or friction.
- Instruct patient to cut toenails straight across *to prevent ingrown toenails.*
- Advise patient to cover corns or calluses with pads *to prevent further injury.*
- Encourage patient to keep feet clean and dry, to use mild soap and warm water for cleansing, and to apply mild lotion *to prevent dryness.*
- Advise patient not to scratch or rub feet *because this can result in abrasions that can easily become infected.*
- Suggest that patient keep feet warm with warm soaks and loose-fitting socks. Caution patient to check temperature of warm soaks and bath water carefully to protect skin from burns.

Ineffective peripheral tissue perfusion (or risk for same) related to interrupted arterial flow with postsurgical graft occlusion
Desired outcome: Patient has adequate peripheral perfusion, as evidenced by BP within 20 mm Hg of baseline BP and absence of the six Ps in the involved extremities: pain, pallor, pulselessness, paresthesia, polar (coolness), and paralysis.

Nursing Interventions

- Assess peripheral pulses and involved extremity for the six Ps. Sensory changes usually precede other symptoms of ischemia, that is, pain, loss of two-point discrimination, and paresthesias. Report significant findings.
- Monitor BP, another indicator of peripheral perfusion pressure. Report to health care provider any significant increase or decrease greater than 15-20 mm Hg, or as directed.

- If necessary, use Doppler ultrasonic probe to check pulses; hold probe to the skin at a 45-degree angle to the blood vessel. Optimally, pulsatile blood flow will be heard. Record presence or absence of pulsations, as well as rate, character, frequency, and intensity of sounds.
- *To prevent pressure on tissue,* use a foot cradle or foam protectors to keep sheets and blankets off legs and feet.
- For the first 48-72 hr after surgery (or as directed), prevent acute joint flexion in the presence of a *graft because it can occlude blood flow.* Mild foot elevation or light elastic (Ace) wrapping may help to ease hyperemia of the extremity.
- In the absence of acute cardiac or renal failure, encourage adequate fluid intake.

 Patient-Family Teaching and Discharge Planning

Reinforce previous teaching. Provide verbal and written information about the following:
- Exercise program as prescribed by health care provider; importance of rest periods if claudication occurs.
- Skin and foot care.
- Medications, including drug names, purpose, dosage, schedule, precautions, and potential side effects. Also discuss drug/drug, food/drug, and herb/drug interactions.
- Referral to a smoking cessation program in your area if appropriate.

❖ ANEURYSMS

OVERVIEW/PATHOPHYSIOLOGY

An aneurysm is a pathologic enlargement of a section of an artery. The most common cause is atherosclerosis; other causes include hereditary lack of elastin, vessel wall trauma, congenital defect, and infection. Undiagnosed and untreated aneurysms place affected individuals at risk for rupture and embolization. Although aneurysms can develop in any vessel, *abdominal aortic aneurysms (AAA)* are the most common.

Aneurysms in the thoracic aorta are a degenerative process of the aorta and are more prone to dissection. *Dissecting aneurysms* have atherosclerotic lesions and develop intimal tears. These tears allow bleeding into the layers of the vessel that causes false lumens to form that can obstruct or limit blood flow in the true lumen of the vessel and other vital organs. This pathology is distinctly different from that of AAAs.

Aneurysms are often referred to as "silent killers" because many times patients do not realize they have them, and acute rupture is life-threatening. However, there has been an increase in the detection of AAAs as a result of increased screening with ultrasound and CT scans of patients at risk.

ASSESSMENT

Signs and symptoms/physical findings

Abdominal aneurysm: A pulsatile, nontender mass may be palpated. Acute abdominal pain, often radiating to the back, of sudden onset, and severe in nature, is indicative of aneurysm rupture and must be treated emergently. AAAs occur most often in men and represent approximately 80% of all aneurysms.

Thoracic aneurysm: Patient may be asymptomatic for years. Pressure from the aneurysm on adjacent structures can result in dull pain in the upper back, dyspnea, cough, dysphagia, and hoarseness. If there is pain associated with these aneurysms, it is more likely to be nonradiating central chest pain.

Femoral aneurysm: Signs of decreased distal arterial blood flow occur. These aneurysms can rupture or thrombose. See indicators discussed under "Atherosclerotic Arterial Occlusive Disease," p. 150.

Acute indicators (rupture or dissection): Sudden onset of severe pain often described as tearing or ripping, pallor, diaphoresis, sudden loss of consciousness, decreased BP and peripheral pulses, tachycardia, cyanosis, and cool and clammy skin.

History and risk factors: Family history, male gender, age more than 60 yr, smoking, hypertension, dyslipidemia.

DIAGNOSTIC TESTS

Ultrasound: Sound waves may help determine aneurysm size, shape, and location. This is an inexpensive, noninvasive, quick, and simple screening examination.

Computed tomography (CT) scan: Preferred method of AAA diagnosis; three-dimensional CT scans are also available in many areas. These scans take a two-dimensional picture and, by looking at density, give a clear view of an aneurysm all the way around, thus making measurements more accurate for endograft repairs.

COLLABORATIVE MANAGEMENT

Management of BP: Important in chronic aneurysm disease management.

Decrease aortic pulsatile flow: Accomplished using medications that decrease myocardial contractility, such as propranolol.

Analgesics: Opioids may be necessary for pain relief in acute rupture.

Surgical interventions: Indicated if the aneurysm is symptomatic, increasing in size over time, larger than 4 cm in diameter; if peripheral embolization has occurred; if there is rupture (a surgical emergency); or if a stable aneurysm suddenly becomes tender or causes severe pain. The most common procedure is reconstructive and involves resection of the aneurysm and restoration of vascular flow with either a Dacron or Gore-Tex graft. Endovascular reconstruction using stent-anchored grafts inserted via the femoral artery while using local anesthesia is an alternative that is particularly useful in older adults or those otherwise at high risk for surgical or open repair.

NURSING DIAGNOSES AND INTERVENTIONS

Ineffective peripheral tissue perfusion (or risk for same) related to interrupted arterial flow secondary to rupture or embolization of artery

Desired outcomes: Patient has adequate peripheral perfusion, as evidenced by peripheral pulse amplitude greater than 2+ on a 0-4+ scale and brisk capillary refill (less than 2 sec), and exhibits baseline extremity sensation, motor function, color, and temperature.

Nursing Interventions

◆ Assess peripheral pulses at least hourly, and report decreases or absence of a pulse.

◆ Assess peripheral sensation and VS. Instruct patient to report impaired sensation promptly to staff members. Report significant findings.

◆ Ensure accurate I&O measurements, and pay special attention to urine output. Severe hypotension or renal artery occlusion can decrease renal perfusion.

◆ Report any changes in extremity color, capillary refill, temperature, and motor function.

◆ Maintain patient on bed rest until otherwise directed.

◆ Report any bloody diarrhea *because it may be a sign of bowel ischemia.*

◆ For further interventions, see "Perioperative Care," **Risk for deficient fluid volume** related to postoperative bleeding/hemorrhage, p. 5.

Patient-Family Teaching and Discharge Planning

Provide verbal and written information about the following:

◆ Importance of regular medical follow-up to ensure graft patency and prompt identification of the development of a new aneurysm.

◆ Prevention of recurrence of aneurysm by avoiding factors that accelerate atherosclerosis, such as cigarette smoking, obesity, and hypertension.

◆ Necessity of a regularly scheduled exercise program that alternates exercise with rest.

◆ Indicators of wound infection and thrombus or embolus formation and need to report them promptly if they occur.

◆ Medications, including drug names, purpose, dosage, schedule, precautions, and potential side effects. Also discuss drug/drug, herb/drug, and food/drug interactions. Caution patient about importance of antibiotic use similar to that for heart patients for any minor procedures or dental work.

◆ Phone number of nurse available to discuss concerns and questions or clarify unclear instructions.

◆ Importance of follow-up visits with health care provider; confirm date and time of next appointment.

◆ Potential for aneurysm rupture if surgery is not immediately planned.

◆ Importance of seeking immediate medical attention if aneurysm is not fixed and any signs and symptoms of rupture occur. Provide numbers of emergency services in the area.

◆ Potential need for ultrasound for other family members to rule out aneurysm.

❖ ARTERIAL EMBOLISM

OVERVIEW/PATHOPHYSIOLOGY

An arterial embolus is a fragment of thrombus, fat, atherosclerotic plaque, bacterial vegetation, or air that mobilizes within the arterial vessels and obstructs flow distal to the embolus. Most arterial emboli originate in the heart and may be caused by endocarditis, atrial fibrillation, rheumatic mitral stenosis, or wall motion abnormalities associated with a myocardial infarction (MI). Arterial emboli also can originate from an aneurysm or arteriosclerotic stenosis in an artery with secondary thrombosis formation. The arterial thrombus is a dry, friable mass composed of layers of platelets and fibrin.

ASSESSMENT

Signs and symptoms/physical findings: Typical presentation is with the six Ps: pain, pulselessness, pallor, polar (coolness), paresthesia, and paralysis. Differentiating between acute arterial thrombosis and embolism often is accomplished by analyzing clinical history.

Arterial embolism: Onset is sudden, with or without prior symptoms. Appearance of the affected limb is waxy and yellowish, and pain may be present. Often, there is history of atrial fibrillation. Inability to move the affected limb or decreased sensation, numbness, and/or tingling are serious symptoms of artery occlusion, requiring emergency evaluation and intervention.

Arterial thrombosis: Symptoms appear gradually with concomitant signs of arterial insufficiency, including decreased or absent pulse, coolness, and increased pain. Affected limb may appear pale and cool or mottled and cyanotic.

History/risk factors: Smoking, hypertension, hyperlipidemia, diabetes mellitus (DM), positive family history.

DIAGNOSTIC TESTS

Arterial Doppler studies: Helpful in diagnosis; however, definitive diagnosis requires arteriography. In an effort to save the extremity, patient may be taken immediately to the operating room to remove the clot and restore blood flow to the affected extremity.

Echocardiogram: Useful to determine whether the clot originated from the heart.

Computed tomography (CT) scans: May be needed to determine whether the embolus originated from the aorta, chest, abdomen, or pelvis.

COLLABORATIVE MANAGEMENT

Heparinization: Initiated immediately to prevent clot propagation.

Bed rest: Prevents further embolization.

Analgesics: Relieve pain caused by distal vasospasm and ischemia.

Embolectomy: Treatment of choice for acute arterial occlusion caused by an embolus. A small incision is made in the proximal artery, followed by insertion of a balloon catheter that is passed through the embolus. The balloon is inflated and gently withdrawn to remove the embolus without causing further damage to the vessel itself. The vessel is then irrigated with a heparinized saline solution. Thrombolytic agents such as tissue plasminogen activator (tPA) can be used to promote limb salvage. Heparin is used for 12-24 hr postoperatively to prevent recurrent embolization. Consideration of the cause of embolization is also important because many patients will require long-term anticoagulation therapy with warfarin.

NURSING DIAGNOSES AND INTERVENTIONS

Ineffective peripheral tissue perfusion related to interrupted arterial flow secondary to embolization (preoperative period)

Desired outcomes: Optimally, patient's peripheral perfusion is adequate, as evidenced by normal extremity color, temperature, sensation, and motor function. Capillary refill is less than 2 sec.

Nursing Interventions

♦ Monitor peripheral circulation. Keep extremities warm (room temperature). Advise patient to avoid chilled feet by wearing socks or slippers.

♦ Protect extremities from trauma. Provide a foot cradle or foam protectors *to keep weight of sheets and blankets off tissue that has decreased circulation.*

♦ Avoid pressure on vulnerable tissue *to prevent necrosis and ulcer formation.*

♦ Teach patient and significant other signs and symptoms of embolization that necessitate immediate medical attention: sudden onset of severe pain, gradual decrease in sensory and motor functioning, and presence of tingling, numbness, coolness, and cyanosis.

📝 Patient-Family Teaching and Discharge Planning

Provide verbal and written information about the following:

♦ Importance of walking to prevent peripheral stasis of the blood.

♦ Signs and symptoms that necessitate immediate medical attention: extremity pain, changes in sensation, coolness, pallor, cyanosis.

♦ Indicators of wound infection, if surgery was performed.

♦ Oral anticoagulant therapy: Need for regular medical checkups and immediate reporting of bleeding gums, epistaxis, ecchymosis, hemoptysis, hematemesis, hematochezia, melena, menometrorrhagia, or hematuria; administration at same time every day; not changing regular dietary habits (e.g., becoming a vegetarian without first consulting health care provider or nurse; many green, leafy vegetables are high in vitamin K, which reverses effect of warfarin; vegetarian diets may necessitate increase in warfarin dosage to achieve therapeutic anticoagulation); importance of consulting health care provider before taking any over-the-counter (OTC) or herbal medications or products containing aspirin, which affect platelet aggregation.

◆ Other medications, including drug names, purpose, dosage, schedule, precautions, and potential side effects. Also discuss drug/drug, food/drug, and herb/drug interactions.

◆ Risk factor modification, such as smoking cessation, control of hypertension, and dietary modifications to decrease potential for atherosclerosis and acute arterial occlusion.

❖ VENOUS THROMBOSIS/ THROMBOPHLEBITIS

OVERVIEW/PATHOPHYSIOLOGY

Although venous thrombosis and thrombophlebitis are different disorders, clinically the terms are used interchangeably to refer to development of a venous thrombus or thrombi, with associated inflammation. Disturbances in the venous system can have a variety of causes and precipitating factors, including stasis of blood, hemoconcentration, venous trauma, inflammation, or hypercoagulable states. Venous stasis can occur with heart failure (HF), shock states, immobility from prolonged bed rest, structural disorders of the veins, and immobility on the OR table or from abdominal, pelvic, or orthopedic operative procedures. Hemoconcentration most commonly occurs with dehydration or inadequate fluid resuscitation after surgery. Vessel trauma can result from chemical irritation caused by IV solutions, direct trauma, or positioning. Hypercoagulable states can occur because of malignancies, hereditary factors, or estrogen therapy (replacement or contraception). Venous thrombosis generally occurs in the deep venous system and thrombophlebitis in the superficial system. Both most often occur in the lower extremities, and the most serious complication is embolization from the deep system that causes a pulmonary embolism (PE).

ASSESSMENT

Signs and symptoms/physical findings: Signs and symptoms can be divided into those associated with inflammation that occur in the area of the thrombus and those associated with venous congestion distal to the thrombus. Pain, tenderness, erythema, local warmth, and increased limb circumference occur at the site of the thrombus. Distal to the area of thrombus the extremity is cool, pale or cyanotic, and edematous with prominent superficial veins. Additional findings include fever and tachycardia. Sometimes the condition is clinically "silent," and the presenting sign is a PE. See "Pulmonary Embolism," p. 69.

History and risk factors: Prolonged bed rest and immobility, leg trauma, recent surgery, use of oral contraceptives or hormone replacement therapy, hypercoagulable condition, obesity, varicose veins.

DIAGNOSTIC TESTS

Compression ultrasonography: Accurately detects thrombi in popliteal or more proximal veins; finding of a noncompressible section of vein is indicative of thrombosis.

Doppler ultrasound: Identifies changes in blood flow secondary to presence of a thrombus. Doppler venous sounds are similar to that of wind blowing and are respirophasic (wax and wane with patient's inspiration).

Duplex imaging: Use of ultrasound to assess veins for changes in flow and increased velocities when a clot is obstructing flow. Accuracy and sensitivity are good diagnostic measures for deep vein thrombosis (DVT).

Computed tomography (CT) or magnetic resonance imaging (MRI) scans
Plasma markers (D-dimer test): A positive plasma D-dimer test result is indicative of fibrin breakdown, and further evaluation is warranted. A negative D-dimer test is helpful in excluding deep vein thrombosis (DVT) if noninvasive testing also is negative.

COLLABORATIVE MANAGEMENT

Prevention: Involves identifying patients at risk, particularly those on bed rest or immobilized, and promoting leg exercises to prevent stasis, prescribing elastic stockings and early ambulation when possible, administering enoxaparin or heparin to prevent clot formation, and using sequential compression devices or pneumatic foot compression devices. A sequential compression device and pneumatic foot compression device is contraindicated in an extremity in which a known DVT is present. These devices may, however, be used on other extremities.

Therapeutic anticoagulation: Prevents propagation of a clot. Heparin (low-molecular-weight heparin [LMWH] preferred to unfractionated heparin [UFH] whenever feasible) is used during the acute phase, and long-term warfarin therapy is used after the acute phase. At least 3 months of anticoagulation is recommended for a first occurrence of DVT. LMWH heparin is administered subcutaneously, thus enabling outpatient management of DVT until warfarin levels are therapeutic.

Bed rest: Recommended during the acute phase, with light elastic (Ace) wrapping in graduated compression and leg elevation to decrease venous stasis.

Mild analgesics for pain: As indicated.

Below knee graduated compression stockings: Worn by all patients for 2 years after DVT or alternatively only if symptoms remain after the acute inflammatory process has subsided (up to 6 months).

Exercise regimen: Walking or leg exercises are encouraged after the acute phase.

Warm moist packs: May reduce discomfort and pain.

Thrombectomy: Usually unnecessary, but may be performed when danger of PE is extreme, patient cannot tolerate anticoagulation, or extremity damage from absence of venous drainage is imminent.

Vena caval filter: Placed transvenously to provide filtration of blood from distal sites to prevent PE: This approach is most often used when patients cannot be anticoagulated or have had PEs while being therapeutically anticoagulated.

NURSING DIAGNOSES AND INTERVENTIONS

Ineffective peripheral and cardiopulmonary tissue perfusion (or risk for same) related to interrupted blood flow secondary to embolization from thrombus formation

Desired outcomes: Patient has adequate peripheral and cardiopulmonary perfusion, as evidenced by normal extremity color, temperature, and sensation; respiratory rate (RR) 12-20 breaths/min with normal depth and pattern (eupnea); heart rate (HR) 100 beats per minute (bpm) or less; BP within 20 mm Hg of baseline BP; O_2 saturation greater than 92%; and normal breath sounds.

Nursing Interventions

♦ Be alert to and promptly report early indicators of peripheral thrombus formation: pain, erythema, increased limb girth, local warmth, distal pale skin, edema, and venous dilation. If indicators appear, maintain patient on bed rest and notify health care provider promptly.

♦ Monitor for and immediately report sudden onset of chest pain, dyspnea, tachypnea, tachycardia, hypotension, hemoptysis, shallow respirations, crackles (rales), O_2 saturation 92% or less, decreased breath sounds, and diaphoresis because they indicate PE. If they occur, prompt medical attention is crucial.

◆ Administer anticoagulants as prescribed. Double-check drip rates and doses with a colleague.

◆ Administer anticoagulants, provide ROM exercises, and apply support hose, sequential compression device, or pneumatic foot compression device as prescribed to minimize risk of PE.

◆ Maintain elevation of foot of bed *for promotion of venous drainage.*

Acute pain related to inflammatory process caused by thrombus formation
Desired outcome: Within 1 hr of intervention, patient's subjective perception of pain decreases, as documented by a pain scale. Objective indicators, such as grimacing, are absent.

Nursing Interventions

◆ Monitor patient for presence of pain. Document degree of pain, using a pain scale of from 0 (no pain) to 10 (worst pain). Administer analgesics as prescribed, and document pain relief obtained using pain scale.

◆ Ensure patient maintains bed rest during acute phase to minimize painful engorgement and potential for embolization.

◆ If prescribed, apply warm, moist packs. Be sure packs are warm (but not extremely so) and not allowed to cool. Continuous moist heat may be beneficial.

◆ *To promote venous drainage and reduce engorgement*, keep legs elevated when possible, and avoid flexion of hips or knees, which contributes to venous stasis.

Ineffective peripheral tissue perfusion (or risk for same) related to interrupted venous flow secondary to venous engorgement or edema
Desired outcome: Patient has adequate peripheral perfusion, as evidenced by absence of discomfort and presence of normal extremity temperature, color, sensation, and motor function.

Nursing Interventions

◆ Assess for signs of inadequate peripheral perfusion, such as pain and changes in skin temperature, color, and motor or sensory function. Be alert to venous engorgement (prominence) in lower extremities.

◆ Elevate patient's legs *to promote venous drainage.*

◆ As prescribed for patients without evidence of thrombus formation, apply antiembolic hose, which compresses superficial veins *to increase blood flow to the deeper veins*. Remove stockings for approximately 15 min q8h. Inspect skin for evidence of irritation.

◆ In the absence of known DVT, apply sequential compression device or pneumatic foot compression device as prescribed. Remove these devices for 15 min q8h, and inspect underlying skin for irritation. To reduce trapping of heat and moisture, place a cloth sleeve (stockinette) beneath plastic device.

◆ Encourage patient to perform ankle circling and active or assisted ROM exercises of the lower extremities to prevent venous stasis. Perform passive ROM exercises if patient cannot. If there are any signs of acute thrombus formation, such as calf hardness or tenderness, exercises are contraindicated because of risk of embolization. Notify health care provider.

◆ Encourage deep breathing, which creates increased negative pressure in the lungs and thorax, *to assist in emptying of large veins.*

◆ Arterial circulation usually will not be impaired unless there is arterial disease or severe edema compressing arterial flow. Assess pulses regularly, however, to confirm presence of good arterial flow.

Deficient knowledge related to disease process with venous thrombosis/thrombophlebitis and treatment/management measures after hospital discharge

Desired outcome: Before hospital discharge, patient verbalizes knowledge of the disease process and treatment/management measures that are to occur after hospital discharge.

Nursing Interventions

- Assess patient's facility with language; engage an interpreter or provide language-appropriate written materials if indicated.
- Discuss process of venous thrombosis/thrombophlebitis and ways to prevent thrombosis and discomfort, such as avoiding restrictive clothing, avoiding prolonged periods of standing, and elevating legs above heart level when sitting.
- Teach signs of venous stasis ulcers, such as redness and skin breakdown. Stress importance of avoiding trauma to extremities and keeping skin clean and dry.
- Instruct patient to inspect both feet each day for any open wounds or bruises. If necessary, suggest patient use a long-handled mirror to see bottoms of feet. Advise patient to report any open areas to health care provider.
- Discuss prescribed exercise program. Walking usually is considered the best exercise.
- Teach patient how to wear antiembolic hose if prescribed. The hose must fit properly without wrinkling and should be snug over the feet and progressively less snug as they reach the knee or thigh.
- Describe indicators that necessitate medical attention: persistent redness, swelling, tenderness, weak or absent pulses, and ulcerations in the extremities.
- Encourage long-term management with elastic stockings to prevent sequelae associated with postphlebitic syndrome and chronic venous insufficiency.

Patient-Family Teaching and Discharge Planning

When providing patient-family teaching, focus on sensory information, avoid giving excessive information, and initiate a visiting nurse referral for necessary follow-up teaching. Include verbal and written information about the following.

- See **Deficient knowledge** for topics to discuss, both verbally and through written information, with patient and significant other.
- If patient is discharged from hospital on warfarin therapy, provide the following information:
  - As directed, see health care provider for scheduled international normalized ratio (INR) checks.
  - Take warfarin at same time each day; do not skip days unless directed to by health care provider.
  - Wear a MedicAlert bracelet.
  - Avoid alcohol consumption and changes in diet (e.g., changing to a vegetarian diet), both of which can alter the body's response to warfarin.
  - When making appointments with other health care providers and dentists, inform them that warfarin is being taken.
  - Be alert to indicators that necessitate immediate medical attention: hematuria, hematemesis, menometrorrhagia, hematochezia, melena, epistaxis, bleeding gums, ecchymosis, hemoptysis, dizziness, and weakness.

- Avoid taking over-the-counter (OTC) medications (e.g., aspirin, which also prolongs coagulation time) without consulting health care provider or nurse.
- Avoid trauma to extremities.
- Stress importance of walking.
- Emphasize importance of attention to skin care and use of antiembolic stockings.

Renal-Urinary Disorders

SECTION ONE **RENAL DISORDERS**

❖ GLOMERULONEPHRITIS

OVERVIEW/PATHOPHYSIOLOGY

Glomerulonephritis (GN) refers to inflammation of and subsequent damage to the renal glomerular capillaries that lead to leakage of protein and RBCs into the urine. It is not an infection of the glomerulus, but rather is secondary to a systemic infection. GN may be acute or chronic. Most individuals with acute glomerulonephritis (AGN) improve dramatically within weeks and recover completely within 1-2 yr, but renal damage continues to progress for patients with chronic glomerulonephritis (CGN). CGN is one of the most common causes of chronic renal failure (CRF). Most forms of GN are the result of an immunologic response in which immune complexes, formed when antibodies attach to antigens, become entrapped in the glomerulus and produce inflammation (e.g., group A hemolytic streptococcal infection, systemic lupus erythematosus). Other risk factors for GN include metabolic disease, recent use of penicillin or sulfonamide antibiotics, or nephrotoxic drugs. See "Acute Renal Failure," p. 181, and "Chronic Kidney Disease," p. 174.

ASSESSMENT

Signs and symptoms/physical findings
AGN early indicators: Hematuria, proteinuria, oliguria, dull bilateral flank pain, headache, low-grade fever (less than 101° F).
AGN late indicators: Hypertension, edema. Clinical manifestations of AGN usually follow the initial source of inflammation by about 2 wk and can range from subtle to blatant, depending on patient's level of renal function.
CGN indicators: Bloody urine (hematuria; commonly reported as dark or rust-colored), fatigue, lethargy, malaise, anorexia, nausea, pruritus, metallic taste in mouth, nocturia, headache, weakness. CGN may go unrecognized until significant renal damage has occurred.
History and risk factors
AGN: History of recent upper respiratory infection (URI) or other infection, recent use of penicillin or sulfonamide antibiotics.
CGN: History of systemic lupus erythematosus or other autoimmune disease.

DIAGNOSTIC TESTS

Urinalysis and 24-hr urinary protein excretion: Hematuria with RBC casts and proteinuria are the cardinal features. Hyaline and granular casts also may be noted.

163

BUN/serum creatinine: May indicate decreased renal function if elevated.
Plasma complement, antinuclear antibody titer, antistreptolysin O titer, throat and blood cultures, hepatitis B antigen, and immunoelectrophoresis of serum and urine: Optional tests to determine cause of GN.
Renal biopsy: Indicated when tissue diagnosis is needed to direct therapy or provide prognostic data. Usually percutaneous (closed) renal biopsy is performed. Postbiopsy care includes keeping patient supine with a rolled towel under the biopsy site (to apply direct pressure) for 12 hr and frequent monitoring of VS (q15min initially). Bleeding and infection are possible complications of renal biopsy. Severe pain, hypotension, persistent gross hematuria, or fever should be reported to health care provider immediately. Samples of urine from the first several voidings may be saved to assess for hematuria.
WBC count: Indicated to rule out the presence of infection that may be contributing to formation of immune complexes.

COLLABORATIVE MANAGEMENT

Generally, treatment of AGN is supportive. Limited activity may be necessary for weeks to months. Management includes the following:
Pharmacotherapy
Corticosteroids and cytotoxic agents: Suppress the immune system and reduce antibody formation.
Anticoagulants: Reduce nonimmunologic mediators of glomerular damage.
Antibiotics: Prescribed if causative factor is bacterial.
Diuretics: Remove excess fluid.
Antihypertensives: Control BP. Angiotensin-converting enzyme (ACE) inhibitors or angiotensin II receptor antagonists may be used to decrease protein excretion.
Plasmapheresis: Removes immune complexes or antiglomerular basement antibodies. Used only in patients with Goodpasture's syndrome and rapidly progressing GN.
Diet: Na^+ and fluids are restricted if edema or hypertension is present. A high-carbohydrate diet is encouraged to maintain nutrition and prevent tissue catabolism that would further contribute to elevated BUN and creatinine. If renal function is markedly decreased, protein and phosphorus may be limited to prevent retention of excess nitrogenous wastes and hyperphosphatemia.
Peritoneal dialysis or hemodialysis: Maintains homeostasis or prevents uremic complications if renal function is markedly decreased (see "Renal Dialysis," p. 187).

NURSING DIAGNOSES AND INTERVENTIONS

Excess fluid volume related to compromised regulatory mechanisms secondary to decreased renal function
Desired outcomes: Following treatment/intervention, patient is normovolemic as evidenced by urine output of at least 30-60 mL/hr (or patient's normal range), stable weight, edema severity 1+ or less on a 0-4+ scale, and subjective statement that thirst is controlled. BP and heart rate (HR) are within patient's normal range, central venous pressure (CVP) is 5-12 cm H_2O, and respiratory rate (RR) is 12-20 breaths/min with normal depth and pattern (eupnea).

Nursing Interventions

- Assess/monitor for indicators of fluid overload: edema, hypertension, crackles (rales), tachycardia, lethargy, distended neck veins, shortness of breath, and increased CVP. *Edema occurs because of lowered serum colloidal osmotic pressure resulting from decreased serum albumin secondary to urinary losses.*
- Monitor I&O. Notify health care provider about sudden changes in output.
- Monitor weight daily. Weigh patient at same time each day; use same scale and have patient wear same amount of clothing. Report unusual or steady gains or losses (e.g., 0.5-1 kg/day).

◆ Offer ice chips or flavored ice pops. Record intake. *Helps minimizes thirst.*
◆ Provide frequent mouth care. *Helps minimize thirst.*

Deficient knowledge related to signs and symptoms of fluid and electrolyte imbalance (caused by decreased renal function or diuretic therapy)
Desired outcome: Within 36 hr of admission, patient verbalizes knowledge about signs and symptoms of fluid and electrolyte imbalance and importance of reporting them promptly to health care provider or staff if they occur.

Nursing Interventions

◆ Assess patient's facility with language, and engage an interpreter or provide language-appropriate written materials if necessary.
◆ Teach patient and significant others to report to health care provider or staff promptly if patient develops signs and symptoms of the following:
  ● *Hypokalemia:* Muscle weakness, lethargy, dysrhythmias, nausea, and vomiting.
  ● *Hyperkalemia:* Abdominal cramping, diarrhea, irritability, and muscle weakness (if severe).
  ● *Hypocalcemia:* Twitching, numbness and tingling of fingers and circumoral region, and muscle cramps.
  ● *Hyperphosphatemia:* May be asymptomatic; report joint or bone pain, rash, or painful or itchy skin lesions.
  ● *Uremia:* Anorexia, nausea, metallic taste in mouth, irritability, confusion, lethargy, restlessness, and pruritus (itching).
◆ Teach patient and significant other to read all labels carefully and avoid foods high in Na^+ (**BOX 4-1**) *because many over-the-counter (OTC) preparations are high in Na^+ (e.g., mouthwashes, antacids).*

Deficient knowledge related to disease process, treatment plan, and side effects of prescribed medications
Desired outcome: Before hospital discharge, patient verbalizes accurate information about disease process, dietary restrictions (if any), and side effects of prescribed medications that must be reported immediately.

Nursing Interventions

◆ Assess patient's facility with language, and engage an interpreter or provide language-appropriate written materials if necessary.

BOX 4-1	FOODS HIGH IN SODIUM

- Bouillon
- Celery
- Cheeses
- Dried fruits
- Frozen, canned, or packaged foods
- Mustard
- Olives
- Pickles
- Preserved meat
- Salad dressings and prepared sauces
- Sauerkraut
- Snack foods (e.g., crackers, chips, pretzels)
- Soups
- Soy sauce
- Any food or drink containing monosodium glutamate

◆ Teach patient and significant other:
- Need for reporting side effects of prescribed medications. Side effects are dependent on dose and duration of therapy and may include decreased resistance to infection, poor wound healing, increasing BP, mental changes, hyperglycemia, capillary fragility, and gastrointestinal (GI) bleeding.
- Need to avoid persons with known infections because *corticosteroids and cytotoxic agents suppress the immune system, reduce antibody formation, and thereby increase the risk for infections.*
- Need for avoiding the abrupt withdrawal from medication if corticosteroids are taken for 1 wk or longer. Therapy must be withdrawn, with gradual reductions in dosage. Signs and symptoms that can occur with abrupt medication withdrawal include fever, malaise, fatigue, anorexia, orthostatic hypotension, dyspnea, muscle and joint pain, and hypoglycemia. *Prevents adrenal insufficiency.*
- Potential for cystitis with hematuria, abnormal hair loss. See "Cancer Care," p. 657, for additional information about cytotoxic agents.
- Potential for development of Cushing's syndrome as a side effect of prolonged use of corticosteroids. Syndrome is manifested by edema, buffalo hump, hirsutism, moon face, skin striae and thinning, weight gain, peptic ulcer, headache, osteoporosis, aseptic necrosis, nervousness, insomnia, and metabolic acidosis. Notify health care provider or staff promptly if any of these symptoms occur. (See "Cushing's Disease," p. 400.) *Corticosteroids cause Na^+ and water retention and hypokalemia.*

Risk for infection related to immunosuppression from corticosteroid therapy, immobility, invasive techniques, and impaired skin integrity
Desired outcomes: Patient is free of infection as evidenced by normothermia and absence of adventitious breath sounds. Respiratory secretions are of normal color, consistency, and quantity.

Nursing Interventions

◆ Assess for signs of infection if patient is immunocompromised from prescribed corticosteroids or cytoxic agents. Signs of infection include increased body temperature; adventitious breath sounds; and increased, thickened, or colored airway secretions. Older adults and individuals who are uremic tend to have subnormal temperatures; therefore even slight fevers can be significant. *Corticosteroids and other immune suppressive agents may mask signs and symptoms of infection.*

◆ Encourage frequent deep breathing or coughing or provide suctioning at frequent intervals if respiratory secretions are noted, *to prevent atelectasis.* (See "Atelectasis," p. 57.)

◆ Use meticulous sterile technique when performing invasive procedures or manipulating urinary catheters, peripheral IV lines, or central venous catheters *to prevent the introduction of microorganisms.*

◆ Provide oral hygiene and skin care at frequent intervals. Edema, bed rest, and uremia all increase potential for skin breakdown. *Decreases risk for infection.*

Patient-Family Teaching and Discharge Planning

Include verbal and written information:

◆ Medications, including drug names, purpose, dosage, schedule, precautions, and potential side effects. Also discuss drug/drug, herb/drug, and food/drug interactions.

◆ Diet: include fact sheet listing foods that should be avoided or limited. Inform patient that diet and fluid restrictions may be altered as renal function changes. Provide sample menus with examples of how dietary restrictions may be incorporated into daily meals.

- Indicators that require medical attention: irregular pulse, fever, unusual shortness of breath or edema, sudden change in urine output, or unusual weakness.
- Technique for measuring temperature and pulse and recording I&O.
- Necessity for continued medical evaluation; confirm date and time of next health care provider appointment, if known.
- Importance of adjusting and gradually increasing activities to avoid fatigue.
- Necessity of avoiding infections and seeking treatment promptly if they occur. Teach signs and symptoms of URI, otitis media, urinary tract infection (UTI), and impetigo. (See "Urinary Tract Infection (Cystitis)," p. 197.)
- Phone numbers to call if questions or concerns arise about therapy or this condition after discharge. Additional general information can be obtained by accessing the following:

  National Institute of Diabetes and Digestive and Kidney Diseases: www.niddk. nih.gov

  National Kidney Foundation: www.kidney.org

- Available family and social service support if continued bed rest is indicated or activity is to be restricted at home. Consider such factors as meals, loss of income, housework, childcare, and transportation.

❖ PYELONEPHRITIS

OVERVIEW/PATHOPHYSIOLOGY

Acute pyelonephritis is an infection of the renal parenchyma and pelvis that usually occurs secondary to an ascending urinary tract infection (UTI). UTIs typically result from anatomic or functional obstruction to urine flow (e.g., from prostatic hypertrophy, renal calculi, or instrumentation such as catheterization or cystoscopy). Pathogenic organisms can ascend from the urinary bladder to the kidney via an incompetent ureterovesical junction, or they can reach the kidney via the bloodstream (hematogenous infection). *Acute pyelonephritis* refers to active infection. In the absence of anatomic obstruction or instrumentation, risk factors for acute pyelonephritis include female gender, increasing age, prostate disease in male patients, and chronic illness. The infecting organism may be a type of fecal flora, such as *Escherichia* or *Klebsiella,* or normal flora from periurethral skin (e.g., *Staphylococcus saprophyticus).* *Chronic pyelonephritis* refers to recurrent infections, which may be frequent in some patients. Chronic infections generally result from vesicoureteral reflux, obstructions, or urinary anomalies. Chronic kidney disease (CKD) is a rare complication.

ASSESSMENT

Signs and symptoms/physical findings: Fever, chills, flank pain (unilateral or bilateral), tender, enlarged kidney, costovertebral angle (CVA) tenderness, abdominal rigidity, nausea, vomiting, malaise, frequency and urgency of urination, dysuria, cloudy and foul-smelling urine, nocturia. Clinical indicators of acute pyelonephritis can be nonspecific, especially in older persons. Severe infection may produce peripheral vasoconstriction, hypotension, and acute renal failure (ARF).

History and risk factors: UTI or obstruction, recent urologic procedures, pregnancy.

DIAGNOSTIC TESTS

BUN/serum creatinine: Unless an anatomic or preexisting renal disease is present, renal function should remain normal.

Urine culture: Results are generally positive for the causative organism; however, asymptomatic bacteriuria is common in older persons.

Urinalysis: Reveals presence of WBCs, WBC casts, RBCs, and bacteria.

Blood culture: Results are positive for causative organism in hematogenous infection. Culture is obtained from patients who appear septic or are hypotensive.

CBC: Demonstrates leukocytosis.

Radiographic studies:

Kidney, ureter, bladder (KUB) (an abdominal flat plate film): May demonstrate renal or ureteral calculi.

Chest x-ray examination: May show pleural effusion.

Intravenous pyelogram (IVP) or retrograde pyelogram: May be performed if there are recurrent episodes or if obstruction is suspected.

COLLABORATIVE MANAGEMENT

The focus of collaborative management is on early recognition of infection, initiation of appropriate antibacterial therapy, and treatment of underlying cause.

Fluids: Oral fluids encouraged. IV fluids administered if oral fluids are not tolerated to replace losses and ensure adequate urinary output. Blueberry and cranberry juice may prevent bacterial adhesion to lining of urinary tract.

Pharmacotherapy

Antibiotics: Initially administered parenterally, then orally. Low-dose antimicrobial prophylaxis may be indicated for women with recurrent UTI.

Acetylsalicylic acid (ASA; aspirin) or acetaminophen: Controls fever and treats discomfort.

Surgical intervention: May be necessary if obstruction is present.

NURSING DIAGNOSES AND INTERVENTIONS

Acute pain related to tissue inflammation secondary to infection

Desired outcome: Within 1 hr of intervention, patient's subjective perception of discomfort decreases, as documented by pain scale. Objective indicators, such as grimacing, are absent or diminished.

Nursing Interventions

◆ Devise a pain scale with patient, rating pain from 0 (absent) to 10 (worst pain).

◆ Monitor for presence of CVA pain and tenderness, abdominal pain, and dysuria, all of which are *indicators of pyelonephritis.*

◆ Administer prescribed analgesics as needed and document their effectiveness using the pain scale. Encourage patient to request medication before discomfort becomes severe. Notify health care provider about unrelieved or increasing flank pain.

◆ Increase patient's fluid intake if not contraindicated *to help relieve dysuria.*

◆ Reposition if this approach is effective in relieving discomfort.

◆ Use nonpharmacologic interventions when possible (e.g., relaxation techniques, guided imagery, distraction). *Distraction may reduce patient's perception of pain.*

Impaired urinary elimination related to acute kidney infection and presence of risk factors

Desired outcomes: Patient is free of infection as evidenced by normothermia; urine clear and of normal odor; heart rate (HR) 100 beats per minute (bpm) or less; BP 90/60 mm Hg or greater (or within patient's normal range); absence of flank, CVA, low back, buttock, scrotal, or labial pain; and absence of dysuria, urgency, and frequency.

Nursing Interventions

◆ Assess/monitor for signs of infection: temperature of 38° C (100.4° F); flank, CVA, low back, buttock, scrotal, or labial pain; foul-smelling or cloudy urine; malaise; headache; and frequency and urgency of urination. *Establishes baseline for later comparisons to determine effectiveness of interventions.*

◆ Monitor BP, pulse, and for indications of peripheral vasoconstriction at least q4h. *Hypotension and tachycardia can indicate sepsis, which can lead to septic shock.*

◆ Monitor for indications of pulmonary infection. If secretions are noted, encourage frequent deep breathing or coughing or provide suctioning at frequent intervals. *CVA pain decreases patient's desire to cough and thereby increases the risk for atelectasis.* (See "Atelectasis," p. 57).

◆ Administer prescribed antibiotics as scheduled *to maintain effective antibiotic serum levels to assure eradication of infectious organism.*

◆ Avoid use of urinary catheters unless mandatory. Urinary catheterization is a significant source of pathogen introduction into the urinary system. *Intermittent catheterization carries less risk of UTI than does indwelling catheterization.*

◆ Use sterile technique when inserting or irrigating urinary catheters or obtaining specimens. Maintain unobstructed flow; always keep urinary collection container below level of patient's bladder to prevent reflux of urine; tape catheter to thigh or abdomen in male patients to decrease meatal irritation; and provide perineal care daily *to prevent infection or reinfection.*

◆ Send urine samples to the laboratory immediately after they are obtained, or refrigerate. Urine left at room temperature has greater potential for bacterial growth, turbidity, and alkalinity. Urine for culture should not be refrigerated. *Decreases risk for distorted test results.*

◆ Offer cranberry, plum, prune, or blueberry juice, or which leaves an acid ash in urine. *Decreases risk for UTI because it prevents adherence of pathogens to mucosal membranes of urinary tract.*

Deficient knowledge related to signs and symptoms of infection; prevention of infection/reinfection, need for adherence to antibiotic therapy and fluid intake; need for follow-up care

Desired outcome: Within a 24-hr period before hospital discharge, patient verbalizes understanding of the disorder, its treatment/management, and strategies for avoiding disease recurrence.

Nursing Interventions

◆ Assess patient's facility with language; engage an interpreter or provide language-appropriate written materials.

◆ Teach patient/significant other:
  • Disease process and risk factors for recurrent infections.
  • Indicators of kidney infection and the importance of reporting them promptly to health care provider or staff *to facilitate early treatment.*
  • Importance of emptying bladder at least q3-4h and once during the night *to help prevent UTI caused by residual urine, which can ascend into renal pelvis.*
  • Necessity of maintaining fluid intake of at least 2-3 L/day and drinking fruit juices (cranberry, plum, prune*)* that leave an acid ash in the urine. *Helps prevent pathogens from adhering to urinary bladder wall and ascending to the kidneys.*
  • Necessity for female patients to void before and immediately after sexual intercourse, wipe from front to back, and wear undergarments with cotton crotch, *to minimize the risk of introducing bacteria into the bladder and urinary tract.*

Patient-Family Teaching and Discharge Planning

Include verbal and written information about:

◆ Medications, including drug names, purpose, dosage, schedule, precautions, and potential side effects. Also discuss drug/drug, herb/drug, and food/drug interactions.

- Importance of taking medications for prescribed length of time, even if feeling "well."
- Necessity of reporting the following to their health care provider: chills; fever; hematuria; flank, CVA, suprapubic, low back, buttock, scrotal, or labial pain; cloudy and foul-smelling urine; increased frequency, urgency; dysuria; and increasing or recurring incontinence.
- Importance of continued medical follow-up because of high incidence of recurrence.

❖ HYDRONEPHROSIS

OVERVIEW/PATHOPHYSIOLOGY

Hydronephrosis is the dilation of the renal pelvis and calyces secondary to obstruction of urinary flow. It can occur in adults or children and results from any condition or abnormality that causes urinary tract obstruction. If the obstruction is not corrected, the affected kidney will eventually atrophy and fail. Obstruction of the urethra or bladder affects both kidneys, whereas obstruction of a single ureter or kidney affects only the involved kidney. Dramatic postobstructive diuresis can occur after release of the obstruction. Inappropriate loss of Na^+ and H_2O can in turn lead to volume depletion. Infection is a common complication of hydronephrosis.

ASSESSMENT

Signs and symptoms/physical findings
Kidney/ureteral obstruction: Flank tenderness, abdominal tenderness, gross hematuria.
Bladder neck/urethral obstruction: Distended bladder, urinary frequency, hesitancy, dribbling, incontinence, nocturia, suprapubic pain, anuria. Crackles (rales), renal insufficiency, and possibly hypertension and edema if patient has fluid overload from retention. Indicators are determined by the level, severity, and duration of obstruction. Onset of hydronephrosis usually is insidious.
History and risk factors: Urinary tract infection (UTI), nephrolithiasis, benign prostatic hypertrophy (BPH), neurogenic bladder, or other obstruction.

DIAGNOSTIC TESTS

BUN/serum creatinine: Determine level of renal function. Serum creatinine is a more sensitive indicator of kidney injury/disease than is BUN.
Urinalysis: Determines presence of stone formation or infection.
Renal ultrasound: Noninvasive technique that uses high-frequency sound waves to assess renal size, contour, and structural changes. Because it does not rely on dye uptake, it can be used to evaluate poorly functioning kidneys.
Abdominal x-ray examination, intravenous pyelogram (IVP), and retrograde pyelogram: Identify cause and location of obstruction.

COLLABORATIVE MANAGEMENT

Management of hydronephrosis focuses on the cause and duration of the urinary tract obstruction. Major causes of obstruction in the pelvis and ureter are calculi (see "Ureteral Calculi," p. 199) and neoplasms. Major causes of obstruction in the bladder and urethra are neoplasms, and neurogenic bladder (see "Neurogenic Bladder," p. 217), and benign prostatic hypertrophy (BPH) (see "Benign Prostatic Hypertrophy," p. 627).
Nephrostomy tube: Inserted into the renal pelvis to drain urine and relieve pressure. It is inserted percutaneously using local anesthesia, or it is inserted during an open surgical procedure. The tube may be permanent or temporary.
Ureteral stent: Tube inserted into ureter to drain urine into the bladder.

Pharmacotherapy

Antibiotics: Treats infection if present.
Corticosteroids: Reduces inflammation.

NURSING DIAGNOSES AND INTERVENTIONS

Risk for infection related to presence of risk factors and/or invasive proce-dure (insertion/presence of nephrostomy tube)
Desired outcome: Patient is free of infection as evidenced by normothermia, BP and heart rate (HR) within patient's normal range, urine that is clear and normal in odor and color, and absence of dysuria.

Nursing Interventions

◆ Maintain sterile technique when providing dressing changes and nephros-tomy tube care.
◆ Assess and monitor for indicators of infection, such as fever, pain, purulent drainage, and tachycardia. Document changes in color, odor, or clarity of urine *to establish a baseline for later comparison.*
◆ Do not change, clamp, or irrigate nephrostomy tube unless specifically prescribed by health care provider. Because the renal pelvis is small and holds little volume, never instill more than 5 mL at one time into the tube unless a larger amount has been specifically prescribed by health care provider.
◆ Avoid kinks in the tubing and keep urine collection container and tubing in a dependent position *to prevent reflux of tube contents into the renal pelvis.*
◆ Encourage fluid intake, unless contraindicated, to provide physiologic flushing of the system and tubing.

Risk for injury related to insertion/presence of nephrostomy tube
Desired outcome: Patient remains free of signs of nephrostomy tube complica-tions as evidenced by urine that is clear and of normal color after the first 24-48 hr, urine output of at least 30-60 mL/hr, and absence of discomfort/pain.
◆ Report gross hematuria (urine that is bright red, possibly with clots). Tran-sient hematuria can be expected for 24-48 hr after tube insertion.
◆ Notify health care provider of leakage around catheter, which can occur with blockage, or sudden decrease in urine output. *Signals a dislodged or blocked catheter.*
◆ Report sudden onset of or increase in pain. *Can indicate perforation of a body organ by the catheter.*
◆ Keep tube securely taped to patient's flank with elastic tape. If tube acci-dentally becomes dislodged, cover site with a sterile dressing; notify health care provider immediately. *Helps prevent tube from becoming dislodged.*
◆ Before removing nephrostomy tube, check with health care provider. Pro-vider may request that nephrostomy tube be clamped for several hours at a time to evaluate patient tolerance. While the tube is clamped, monitor patient for indications of ureteral obstruction: flank pain, diminished urinary output, and fever. *Signals excessive pressure within kidney.*

Patient-Family Teaching and Discharge Planning

Include verbal and written information about:
◆ Medications, including drug names, purpose, dosage, schedule, precau-tions, and potential side effects. Also discuss drug/drug, herb/drug, and food/drug interactions.
◆ Care of nephrostomy catheter, if catheter is in place upon discharge, and procedure to follow if the catheter becomes dislodged.
◆ Frequency of and procedure for dressing changes. Patient or significant others should demonstrate safe dressing-change technique before hospital discharge or receive a referral for home health follow-up.

- ◆ Need for continued medical follow-up; confirm date and time of next health care provider appointment, if known.
- ◆ Signs and symptoms that necessitate medical attention: fever; cloudy or foul-smelling urine; flank, costovertebral angle (CVA), low back, buttock, scrotal, or labial pain; increased catheter drainage; sudden decrease in catheter drainage; or drainage around catheter site.

❖ RENAL ARTERY STENOSIS

OVERVIEW/PATHOPHYSIOLOGY

Stenosis of the renal artery (renal artery stenosis) or one of its main branches usually is the result of fibromuscular dysplasia or arteriosclerotic changes. A reduction in the renal artery lumen causes a decrease in blood flow to the affected kidney, which in turn stimulates the renin-angiotensin system, causing systemic hypertension. The elevation in BP usually is proportional to the degree of ischemia in the affected kidney. If the hypertension is left untreated, the nonischemic kidney will develop arteriolar hyperplasia. Renal artery stenosis is an increasing recognized cause of renal insufficiency and renal failure, especially in older adults, when both kidneys are involved.

ASSESSMENT

Sign and symptoms/physical findings: Headache, nose bleeds, tinnitus, midepigastric area bruit, hypertensive retinopathy, and azotemia (elevated blood urea nitrogen [BUN] and serum creatinine). BP can be severely elevated.

History and risk factors: Accelerated hypertension with abrupt onset, dyslipidemia, diabetes mellitus (DM), cigarette smoking.

DIAGNOSTIC TESTS

Intravenous pyelogram (IVP): Visualizes kidneys via excretion of iodine-containing contrast medium; will demonstrate an ischemic kidney.

Renal arteriography: Injection of contrast medium into the renal arteries to visualize renal vasculature. The arteriogram can have false-positive results in older adults. Complications include allergic reaction to the contrast medium, contrast medium-induced acute renal failure (ARF), hemorrhage, embolus, and infection.

Radioisotope renogram: Demonstrates delayed transit time of the radioisotope through the affected kidney; may be performed in combination with the captopril test (see "Captopril test," following).

Renal vein renin levels: Show a difference between the two kidneys in unilateral disease; renin level from the ischemic kidney should be 1.5 times that of the nonischemic kidney.

Plasma renin level: Shows an increase because of stimulation of the renin-angiotensin system.

Captopril test: A significant increase in plasma renin levels after a dose of captopril suggests renovascular hypertension.

Captopril renal scan: Radioisotope scan performed before and after captopril administration. Decreased transit time after captopril suggests renal artery stenosis.

BUN/serum creatinine: May be normal or increased and renal artery stenosis level of renal function.

Serum K^+ levels: Often decreased secondary to increased secretion of aldosterone.

Urinalysis: To rule out the presence of protein, RBCs or RBC casts, which indicates glomerular damage. (See "Glomerulonephritis," p. 163.)

COLLABORATIVE MANAGEMENT

Renovascular hypertension can be treated (1) medically with angiotensin-converting enzyme (ACE) inhibitors, (2) invasively via percutaneous transluminal angioplasty with or without renal stent placement, or (3) surgically. Patients with diffuse arteriosclerotic vascular disease or bilateral renal artery lesions may be considered poor surgical risks. Medical treatment depends on the type and duration of the disease.

Percutaneous transluminal angioplasty: Invasive procedure performed if patient is a suitable candidate and necessary equipment and personnel are available. Angioplasty involves insertion of a balloon-tipped catheter to dilate the narrowed vessel. It can be performed using local anesthesia and requires minimal hospitalization.

Renal artery stent: After angioplasty is performed (see earlier), a small metal stent is placed in the narrowed portion of the renal artery to keep the artery open. Patients are often treated with ACE inhibitors after stent insertion because these drugs reduce intraglomerular hypertension.

Arterial endarterectomy: Surgical procedure with follow-up anticoagulant therapy.

Resection or bypass of the lesion (aortorenal bypass graft): Surgical procedure performed for patients who are unsuitable candidates for endarterectomy or angioplasty or when angioplasty has been unsuccessful or is unavailable. Revascularization may be achieved using patient's saphenous vein or internal iliac artery or a synthetic graft.

Pharmacotherapy

ACE inhibitor: Prevents conversion of angiotensin I to angiotensin II. These drugs are particularly useful after stent insertion (see later) because they offset the change in glomerular hydrostatic pressure caused by sudden reperfusion and thereby protect against poststent glomerulosclerosis.

NURSING DIAGNOSES AND INTERVENTIONS

Deficient knowledge related to technique for measuring BP; rationale for frequent assessments after aortorenal bypass graft, angioplasty, or endarterectomy

Desired outcomes: Patient verbalizes knowledge about the upcoming renal procedure and the rationale for frequent VS checks; patient demonstrates BP measurement technique before hospital discharge.

Nursing Interventions

- Assess patient's facility with language, and engage an interpreter or provide language-appropriate written materials if necessary.
- Teach patient/significant other:
  - Rationale for measuring VS q15min immediately after angioplasty. *Detects changes and determines integrity of pulses distal to angioplasty site.*
  - Rationale for monitoring for indications of bleeding and hematoma formation at angioplasty site. If a hematoma is noted, circle it with ink and note the time for later comparison, *to detect further bleeding.*
  - That BP may remain elevated after renal procedure and that antihypertensive medications still may be required, *to prevent patient from discontinuing medications without checking with provider.*
  - Care of incision or angioplasty site and importance of reporting erythema, purulent discharge, local warmth, or fever promptly to health care provider. These are *indicators of wound infection.*

 Patient-Family Teaching and Discharge Planning

Include verbal and written information about:

- Medications, including drug names, purpose, dosage, schedule, precautions, and potential side effects. Also discuss drug/drug, herb/drug, and food/drug interactions.

BOX 4-2	FOODS HIGH IN POTASSIUM
■ Apricots	■ Oranges, orange juice
■ Artichokes	■ Peanuts
■ Avocados	■ Potatoes
■ Bananas	■ Prune juice
■ Cantaloupe	■ Pumpkin
■ Carrots	■ Spinach
■ Cauliflower	■ Sweet potatoes
■ Chocolate	■ Swiss chard
■ Dried beans, peas	■ Tomatoes, tomato juice, tomato
■ Dried fruit	sauce
■ Mushrooms	■ Watermelon
■ Nuts	

- ◆ Diet: low in Na^+ (Box 4-1). Include list of foods high in K^+ (**BOX 4-2**) if patient is taking diuretics that cause hypokalemia. Consult renal dietitian if patient has elevated creatinine before suggesting increased K^+ intake. Provide sample menus and have patient demonstrate understanding of diet by planning meals for 3 days.
- ◆ Technique for measuring BP to patient and significant other before hospital discharge.
  - Monitor BP frequently during first 48 hr after aortorenal bypass graft. Hypertension during this period usually is temporary but may require treatment. When angioplasty is successful, hypertension should decrease within 4-6 hr after the procedure.
  - Measure BP under same conditions each day—sitting, standing, lying down—to ensure accuracy of BP readings.
- ◆ Need for continued medical follow-up to evaluate effectiveness of treatment.
- ◆ Importance of addressing or avoiding other risk factors for hypertension: obesity, smoking, stress, and poorly controlled DM.
- ◆ Phone numbers to call if questions or concerns arise about therapy or disease after discharge. Additional general information can be obtained by accessing the following:

  National Institute of Diabetes and Digestive and Kidney Diseases: www.niddk.nih.gov

  National Kidney Foundation: www.kidney.org

SECTION TWO   RENAL FAILURE

❖ ACUTE RENAL FAILURE

OVERVIEW/PATHOPHYSIOLOGY

Acute renal failure (ARF) is a sudden loss of renal function that may be accompanied by oliguria. The kidneys lose their ability to maintain biochemical homeostasis, with resulting retention of metabolic wastes and dramatic alterations in fluid, electrolyte, and acid-base balance. Although alteration in renal function usually is reversible, ARF may be associated with a mortality rate of 40%-80%. Mortality rate varies greatly with the cause of ARF, patient's age, and comorbid conditions.

Causes of ARF are classified according to the renal insult. Decreased renal function secondary to decreased renal perfusion but without parenchymal damage is called *prerenal failure*. Prerenal failure is caused by fluid volume deficit, shock, and decreased cardiac function. Restoration of renal perfusion restores normal renal function if hypoperfusion has not been prolonged. A reduction in urine output because of obstruction to urine flow is called *postrenal failure*. Neurogenic bladder, tumors, and urethral strictures are common causes of postrenal failure. Early detection of prerenal and postrenal failure is essential because, if prolonged, these conditions can lead to parenchymal damage.

Intrinsic renal failure, or renal failure that develops secondary to renal parenchymal damage, is caused by *acute tubular necrosis* (ATN). Although typically associated with prolonged ischemia (prerenal failure) or exposure to nephrotoxins (aminoglycoside antibiotics, heavy metals, radiographic contrast media), ATN also can occur after transfusion reactions, septic abortions, or crushing injuries. The clinical course of ATN can be divided into three phases: *oliguric* (lasting approximately 7-21 days), *diuretic* (7-14 days), and *recovery* (3-12 mo). Causes of intrinsic renal failure other than ATN include acute glomerulonephritis (AGN)), malignant hypertension, and hepatorenal syndrome. Medications associated with the development of ARF include nonsteroidal antiinflammatory drugs (NSAIDs), angiotensin-converting enzyme (ACE) inhibitors, immunosuppressants (e.g., cyclosporine), antineoplastics (e.g., cisplatin), and antifungals (e.g., amphotericin B).

ASSESSMENT

Signs and symptoms/physical findings: Pallor, edema (peripheral, periorbital, sacral), jugular vein distention, crackles (rales), elevated BP in patient who has fluid overload. Electrolyte disturbance (muscle weakness, dysrhythmias), oliguria, hypertension, pulmonary edema, metabolic acidosis (Kussmaul's respirations, hyperventilation, lethargy, headache). Uremia (retention of metabolic wastes): altered mental state, anorexia, nausea, diarrhea, constipation, gastrointestinal (GI) bleeding, abdominal distention, pale and sallow skin, purpura, decreased resistance to infection, anemia, fatigue. Uremia adversely affects all body systems.

History and risk factors: Exposure to nephrotoxic substances, recent blood transfusion, prolonged hypotensive episodes or decreased renal perfusion, sepsis, administration of radiolucent contrast media, or prostatic hypertrophy.

DIAGNOSTIC TESTS

BUN/serum creatinine: Provide information about the progression and management of ARF. Although both BUN and creatinine increase as renal function decreases, creatinine is a better indicator of renal function because it is not affected by diet, hydration, or tissue catabolism.

Creatinine clearance (CrCl): Measures kidney's ability to clear the blood of creatinine and approximates the glomerular filtration rate (GFR). It will decrease as renal function decreases. CrCl is normally decreased in older persons. Failure to collect all urine during the period of study can invalidate the test result.

Urinalysis: Provides information about cause and location of renal disease as reflected by abnormal urinary sediment (renal tubular cells and cell casts).

Urinary osmolality and urinary Na⁺ levels: Rule out renal perfusion compromise (prerenal). In ATN the kidney loses its ability to adjust urine concentration and conserve Na^+ and thus produces a urine Na^+ level greater than 40 mEq/L (in prerenal azotemia, urine Na^+ is less than 20 mEq/L).

Renal ultrasound: Provides information about renal anatomy and pelvic structures, evaluates renal masses, and detects obstruction and hydronephrosis.

Renal scan: Provides information about perfusion and function of the kidneys.

CT scan: Identifies dilation of renal calices in obstructive processes.

Retrograde urography: Assesses for postrenal causes (e.g., obstruction).

COLLABORATIVE MANAGEMENT

The goal of collaborative management is to remove the precipitating cause, maintain homeostatic balance, and prevent complications until the kidneys can resume function. Initially, prerenal or postrenal causes are ruled out or treated. A trial of fluid and diuretics may be used to rule out prerenal problems.

Fluids: Replace losses plus 400 mL/24 hr. Insensible fluid losses are only partially replaced to offset the water formed during metabolism of protein, carbohydrates, and fats.

Pharmacotherapy

Medications that are excreted primarily by the kidney **(BOX 4-3)** require modification of dosage or frequency to prevent medication toxicity. Renal failure also may decrease hepatic metabolism and protein binding of certain medications, with a resulting increase in medication effect.

Diuretics: For fluid removal during nonoliguric ARF. Furosemide (Lasix) (100-200 mg) or mannitol (12.5 g) may be given early in ARF to limit or prevent the development of oliguria.

Antihypertensives: Control BP.

ACE inhibitors: May be prescribed for their renal protective effects soon after renal disease is initially diagnosed. However, after chronic kidney disease (CKD) has developed, ACE inhibitors may be contraindicated because of risk of hyperkalemia and the potential of these drugs to increase rate of progression to end-stage renal disease (ESRD).

BOX 4-3	DRUG USAGE IN PATIENTS WITH RENAL FAILURE

Drugs handled primarily by the kidneys have an increased effect in patients with renal failure. Usually either the dosage or the scheduling of these drugs must be modified as a consequence.

Drugs That Require Modification of Dosage or Scheduling

Antibiotics
- Carbenicillin*
- Cefazolin*
- Gentamicin*
- Kanamycin*
- Tobramycin*
- Vancomycin

Histamine H₂-Receptor Blockers
- Cimetidine
- Famotidine
- Ranitidine

Antidysrhythmics
- Digoxin
- Procainamide*

Antihypertensives
- Angiotensin-converting enzyme inhibitors
- Atenolol*

Hypoglycemic Agent
- Insulin

Sedative
- Phenobarbital*

*Dialyzable drug that may require increased dosage after dialysis.

Phosphate binders (e.g., antacids, calcium carbonate, cationic polymer exchange medication, lanthanum carbonate, aluminum hydroxide): Control hyperphosphatemia. Use of aluminum-containing, phosphate-binding agents is limited because of increased risk of renal osteodystrophy and encephalopathy caused by elevated tissue aluminum levels.

Cation exchange resins (sodium polystyrene sulfonate [Kayexalate]): Control hyperkalemia. Severe hyperkalemia may be treated also with IV sodium bicarbonate, which shifts K^+ into the cells temporarily, or with glucose and insulin. Insulin helps move K^+ into the cells, and glucose helps prevent hypoglycemia, which can result from the insulin.

IV calcium: Reverses the cardiac effects of life-threatening hyperkalemia.

Calcium or vitamin D supplements: To control hypocalcemia if present.

Sodium bicarbonate: For treating metabolic acidosis when serum bicarbonate (HCO_3^-) level is less than 15 mmol/L. It is used cautiously in patients with hypocalcemia or fluid overload.

Vitamins B and C: Prescribed to replace inadvertent losses of these vitamins if patient is on dialysis.

Packed RBCs: Administered to counteract active bleeding or if anemia is poorly tolerated.

Diet: High-carbohydrate foods are increased to provide adequate calories and limit protein catabolism. Foods high in Na^+ (Box 4-1) are limited to prevent thirst and fluid retention. Foods high in K^+ (Box 4-2) and phosphorus (**BOX 4-4**) are limited because of the kidneys' decreased ability to excrete them. Protein is limited to minimize retention of nitrogenous wastes. K^+ intake may need to be increased during diuretic phase because of K^+ loss during that time. Total parenteral nutrition (TPN) may be necessary for patients unable to maintain adequate oral/enteral intake.

Peritoneal dialysis or hemodialysis: Dialysis is initiated early and done every 1-3 days, but may be done continuously in the ICU setting. Prophylactic use of dialysis has reduced incidence of complications and rate of death in patients with ARF (see "Renal Dialysis," p. 187).

NURSING DIAGNOSES AND INTERVENTIONS

Risk for infection related to uremia and loss of metabolic homeostasis. Sepsis is one of the primary causes of death in patients with ARF

Desired outcome: Patient is free of infection as evidenced by normothermia; WBC count 11,000/mm^3 or less; urine that is clear, with a normal odor; normal breath sounds; eupnea; and absence of erythema, warmth, tenderness, swelling, and drainage at the catheter or IV access site.

BOX 4-4	FOODS HIGH IN PHOSPHORUS

- Dried beans and peas
- Eggs and egg products (e.g., eggnog, soufflés)
- Fish
- Meats, especially organ meats (e.g., brain, liver, kidney)
- Milk and milk products (e.g., cheese, ice cream, cottage cheese)
- Nuts (e.g., Brazil nuts, peanuts)
- Poultry
- Seeds (e.g., pumpkin, sesame, sunflower)
- Whole grains (e.g., oatmeal, bran, barley)

From Heitz U, Horne MM, editors: *Pocket guide to fluid, electrolyte, and acid-base balance,* ed 5, St Louis, 2005, Mosby.

Nursing Interventions

♦ Monitor temperature and secretions for indicators of infection. Even minor increases in temperature can be significant *because uremia masks the febrile response and inhibits the body's ability to fight infection.*

♦ Use meticulous sterile technique when changing dressings or manipulating venous catheters, IV lines, or indwelling catheters, *to prevent contamination and increase risk for infection.*

♦ Avoid long-term use of indwelling urinary catheters. Whenever possible, use intermittent catheterization instead. *Indwelling urinary catheters are a common source of infection.*

♦ Provide oral hygiene and skin care at frequent intervals. Use emollients and gentle soap to avoid drying and cracking of skin, which can lead to breakdown and infection. Rinse off all soap when bathing patient *because soap residue may further irritate skin.*

Excess fluid volume related to compromised regulatory mechanisms secondary to renal dysfunction: oliguric phase
Desired outcomes: Patient adheres to prescribed fluid restrictions and becomes normovolemic as evidenced by decreasing or stable weight, normal breath sounds, edema severity 1+ or less on a 0-4+ scale, central venous pressure (CVP) 12 cm H_2O or less, and BP and HR within patient's normal range.

Nursing Interventions

♦ Monitor I&O closely and document same. *Increased urinary output in an oliguric patient indicates that patient is entering the diuretic phase of ARF.*

♦ Monitor weight daily. Patient should lose 0.5 kg/day if not eating; a sudden weight gain suggests excessive fluid volume. Weigh patient at the same time each day, with same scale and with patient wearing same amount of clothing. *Ensures weight accuracy.*

♦ Observe for indicators of fluid volume excess, including edema, hypertension, crackles (rales), tachycardia, distended neck veins, shortness of breath, and increased CVP. *Helps determine fluid needs and evaluates the effectiveness of treatment.*

♦ Restrict fluid intake during oliguric phase. Spread allotted fluids evenly over a 24-hr period, and record amount given. Instruct patient and significant others about need for fluid restriction. *Helps prevent fluid volume excess.*

♦ Provide oral hygiene at frequent intervals, and offer fluids in the form of ice chips or flavored ice pops *to minimize thirst. Hard candies also may be given to decrease thirst.*

Risk for deficient fluid volume related to excessive urinary output during diuretic phase
Desired outcome: Patient remains normovolemic as evidenced by stable weight, balanced I&O, good skin turgor, CVP 5 cm H_2O or greater, and BP and heart rate (HR) within patient's normal range.

Nursing Interventions

♦ Monitor I&O closely and document same. Urinary output may reach 3000 mL/day during the diuretic phase of ARF, and this places patient at risk for fluid volume deficit.

♦ Monitor weight daily. A weight loss of 0.5 kg/day or more may reflect excessive volume loss. Weigh patient at the same time each day, with same scale and with patient wearing same amount of clothing. *Ensures accuracy of weight.*

♦ Monitor for complaints of lightheadedness, poor skin turgor, hypotension, postural hypotension, tachycardia, and decreased CVP during the diuretic

phase of ARF. *These are indicators of volume depletion, which can occur during diuresis.*
- Encourage fluid intake if patient is dehydrated *to avoid fluid volume deficit in the presence of diuresis.*
- Report significant findings to health care provider so that early interventions can be employed *to prevent fluid volume deficit from diuresis.*

Imbalanced nutrition: less than body requirements related to uremia (nausea, vomiting, anorexia), and dietary restrictions
Desired outcomes: Within 2 days of admission, patient has stable weight and demonstrates normal intake of food within restrictions.

Nursing Interventions
- Monitor for signs of increased uremia (nausea, vomiting, anorexia, increased BUN and serum creatinine) and alert health care provider. BUN levels more than 80-100 mg/dL or serum creatinine levels that double indicate a 50% reduction in glomerular filtration rate (GFR), which generally requires dialytic therapy. *Facilitates early treatment to prevent fluid volume overload.*
- Provide frequent, small meals in a pleasant atmosphere, and especially control unpleasant odors *to prevent increased nausea.*
- Administer prescribed antiemetics (e.g., hydroxyzine, ondansetron, prochlorperazine, promethazine) as necessary. Instruct patient to request medication before discomfort becomes severe. *Controls nausea and vomiting.*
- Avoid giving patient foods high in K^+ (Box 4-2). Salt substitutes also contain K^+ and should be avoided t*o prevent hyperkalemia during oliguric phase.*
- Coordinate meal planning and dietary teaching with patient, significant others, and renal dietitian. Dietary restrictions may include reduced protein, Na^+, K^+, phosphorus, and fluid intake. Provide fact sheets that list foods to restrict. Demonstrate with sample menus examples of how dietary restrictions may be incorporated into daily meals. *Facilitates compliance with food and fluid restrictions.*

Ineffective protection related to neurosensory, musculoskeletal, and cardiac changes secondary to uremia, electrolyte imbalance, and metabolic acidosis
Desired outcomes: After treatment, patient verbalizes orientation to person, place, and time and is free of injury caused by neurosensory, musculoskeletal, or cardiac disturbances. Within the 24-hr period before hospital discharge, patient verbalizes signs and symptoms of electrolyte imbalance and metabolic acidosis and importance of reporting these signs promptly if they occur.

Nursing Interventions
- Minimize tissue catabolism by controlling fevers, maintaining adequate nutritional intake (especially calories), and preventing infections. If caloric intake is inadequate, body protein will be used for energy, with a resulting increase in end products of protein metabolism (i.e., nitrogenous wastes). A high-carbohydrate diet *helps minimize tissue catabolism and production of nitrogenous wastes.*
- Monitor for and report electrolyte abnormalities occurring during oliguric or diuretic phases of ARF *so that corrective interventions can be initiated early:*
  - *Hypokalemia:* Muscle weakness, lethargy, dysrhythmias; abdominal distention, nausea, and vomiting (secondary to ileus), especially during diuretic phase.
  - *Hyperkalemia:* Muscle cramps, dysrhythmias, muscle weakness, peaked T waves on ECG. A normal serum K^+ level is necessary for normal

cardiac function. Hyperkalemia is a common and potentially fatal complication of ARF during oliguric phase.

- *Hypocalcemia:* Neuromuscular irritability (e.g., Trousseau's sign [carpopedal spasm], Chvostek's sign [facial muscle spasm], and paresthesias).
- *Hyperphosphatemia:* Although usually asymptomatic, may cause bone or joint pain or painful/itchy skin lesions.
- *Uremia:* Anorexia, nausea, metallic taste in the mouth, irritability, confusion, lethargy, restlessness, and itching.
- *Metabolic acidosis:* Rapid, deep respirations; confusion.

◆ Monitor for and report signs of infection: urinary tract infection (UTI), septicemia, pulmonary infections during oliguric or diuretic phases of ARF. *Facilitates early treatment.*

◆ Avoid administering medications that may cause an increase in serum K^+ or use with caution (e.g., nonsteroidal antiinflammatory drugs (NSAIDs), ACE inhibitors, and K^+-sparing diuretics). For patients who exhibit signs of hyperkalemia, have emergency supplies (e.g., manual resuscitator bag, crash cart, emergency drug tray) available *to prevent or treat cardiac arrest or dysrhythmias.*

◆ Avoid medications that contain magnesium. Patients using magnesium-containing antacids such as Maalox typically are switched to aluminum hydroxide preparations such as ALternaGEL or Amphojel. Milk of Magnesia should be substituted with another (non–magnesium-containing) laxative, such as casanthranol, because these patients cannot excrete dietary magnesium. *Increased magnesium levels can alter cardiac function and lead to lethal dysrhythmias.*

◆ Administer aluminum hydroxide or calcium antacids as prescribed. Phosphate binders vary in their aluminum or calcium content. One may not be exchanged for another without first ensuring that patient is receiving the same amount of elemental aluminum or calcium. Aluminum-containing phosphate binders should not be used long term because of their potential to cause bone damage. *Controls hyperphosphatemia.*

◆ Assure patient and significant other that irritability, restlessness, and altered thinking are temporary. Use calendars, radios, familiar objects, and frequent reorientation *to facilitate orientation.*

◆ Ensure safety measures (e.g., padded side rails, airway) for patients who are confused or severely hypocalcemic *to prevent injury.*

Patient-Family Teaching and Discharge Planning

Include verbal and written information about:

◆ Medications, including drug names, purpose, dosage, schedule, precautions, and potential side effects. Also discuss drug/drug, herb/drug, and food/drug interactions.

◆ Diet: include fact sheets that list foods to restrict. Provide sample menus with examples of how dietary restrictions may be incorporated into daily meals.

◆ Care and observation of dialysis access if patient is discharged with such a device (see "Renal Dialysis," p. 187).

◆ Importance of continued medical follow-up of renal function.

◆ Signs and symptoms that must be reported. These should include excessive weight gain, swelling of extremities, irregular heart beat, lightheadedness, signs of infection or bleeding (especially from the GI tract for patients who are uremic).

◆ Coordination of dialysis treatments if patient requires dialysis after discharge.

◆ Phone numbers to call if questions or concerns arise about therapy or disease after discharge. Additional general information can be obtained by accessing the following:

National Kidney Disease Education Program (NKDEP): www.nkdep.nih.gov/
National Kidney Foundation: www.kidney.org

❖ CHRONIC KIDNEY DISEASE

OVERVIEW/PATHOPHYSIOLOGY

Chronic kidney disease (CKD) is a progressive, irreversible loss of kidney function that develops over days to years. Chronic renal failure (CRF) generally occurs in three stages. The first stage is known as *decreased renal reserve*. During this stage, renal compromise may go unnoticed unless significant demands are placed on the kidneys, such as surgery or illness. The second stage, which exists when at least 75% of functioning nephrons have been destroyed, is known as *renal insufficiency*. Individuals in this stage of CKD can lead a relatively normal life managed by diet and medications unless they become ill or dehydrated, although they will experience symptoms such as nocturia and polyuria that may go unnoticed. The final stage of CRF, which exists when at least 90% of nephrons have been destroyed, is known as *end-stage renal disease* (ESRD) or *uremia*. The length of time between decreased renal reserve and ESDR varies depending on the cause of renal disease and person's level of renal function at the time of diagnosis. Persons with ESRD require renal replacement therapy (dialysis or transplantation) to sustain life.

CRF adversely affects all body systems because of retention of metabolic end products and accompanying fluid and electrolyte imbalances. Alterations in neuromuscular, cardiovascular, and gastrointestinal (GI) function are common. Renal osteodystrophy and anemia are early and common complications, with alterations seen when the glomerular filtration rate (GFR) decreases to 60 mL/min. The collective manifestations of CKD are termed *uremia*.

ASSESSMENT

Signs and symptoms/physical findings: Regardless of the cause, the clinical presentation of CKD, particularly as the individual approaches development of ESRD, is similar. Signs and symptoms include the following: *fluid volume abnormalities*: crackles (rales), hypertension, edema (peripheral, periorbital, sacral), oliguria, anuria; *electrolyte disturbances:* muscle weakness, dysrhythmias, pruritus, neuromuscular irritability, tetany; *uremia* (retention of metabolic wastes): pallor, weakness, malaise, anorexia, dry and discolored skin, peripheral neuropathy, irritability, clouded thinking, ammonia odor to breath, metallic taste in mouth, nausea, vomiting; and *metabolic acidosis*: deep respirations, lethargy, headache.

History and risk factors: glomerulonephritis (GN); diabetes mellitus (DM); polycystic kidney disease; hypertension; systemic lupus erythematosus; chronic pyelonephritis; and analgesic abuse, especially the combination of phenacetin and aspirin.

DIAGNOSTIC TESTS

GFR: Measures kidney function and determines stage of renal disease. May be calculated using a mathematical formula. The MDRD (Modification of Diet in Renal Disease) GFR calculator is as follows:

$$\text{GFR} = 170 \times (\text{plasma creatinine in mg/dL})^{-0.999} \times (\text{age})^{-0.176}$$
$$\times (0.762 \text{ if female}) \times (1.180 \text{ if patient is black})$$
$$\times (\text{serum urea nitrogen in mg/dL})^{-0.170}$$
$$\times (\text{albumin in g/dL})^{0.318}$$

Creatinine clearance (CrCl): Measures kidney's ability to clear the blood of creatinine and approximates the GFR. CrCl decreases as renal function decreases. Dialysis is usually begun when the GFR is 12 mL/min if patient is symptomatic or the GFR is less than 6 mL/min. CrCl normally is decreased in older adults and may be measured through collection of a 24-hr urine sample or calculated using the Cockcroft-Gault equation:

$$Male\ patients: CrCl = \frac{(140 - age) \times weight\ (in\ kg)}{plasma\ creatinine\ (in\ mg/dL) \times 72}$$

$$Female\ patients: CrCl = \frac{(140 - age) \times weight\ (in\ kg)}{plasma\ creatinine\ (in\ mg/dL) \times 72 \times 85}$$

Failure to collect all urine specimens during the period of study will invalidate test results.

BUN/serum creatinine: Both are elevated. Nonrenal problems, such as dehydration or GI bleeding, also can cause BUN to increase, but no corresponding increase in creatinine occurs.

Kidney, ureter, bladder (KUB) x-ray examination: Documents presence of two kidneys, changes in size or shape, and some forms of obstruction.

Intravenous pyelogram (IVP), renal ultrasound, renal biopsy, renal scan (using radionuclides), and CT scan: Determine cause of renal insufficiency. Once patient has developed ESRD, these tests are not performed.

Serum chemistry studies, chest and hand x-ray examinations, and nerve conduction velocity test: Assess for development and progression of uremia and its complications.

COLLABORATIVE MANAGEMENT

Medical management is aimed at slowing the progression of CKD and avoiding complications. DM and hypertension (with target BP of less than 130/80 mm Hg) are treated aggressively (see also "Collaborative Management of Diabetes Mellitus," p. 415, and "Control of Hypertension," p. 95). Volume depletion, infection, and nephrotoxic agents must be rigorously avoided to prevent further deterioration of renal function. Once patient develops ESRD, management is aimed at alleviating uremic symptoms and providing dialysis or renal transplantation.

Diet: Protein and phosphorus (Box 4-4) are initially restricted to slow progression of CKD and prevent early development of renal osteodystrophy. Carbohydrates are increased for patients on protein-restricted diets to ensure adequate caloric intake to prevent tissue catabolism (contributing to buildup of nitrogenous wastes). As patient approaches ESRD, Na^+ intake is limited to reduce thirst and fluid retention (Box 4-1). K^+ intake is limited because of the kidneys' decreased ability to excrete this ion (Box 4-2), and protein may be further restricted to limit production of nitrogenous wastes. For patients on protein-restricted diets, protein intake should be primarily of high biologic value. Overrestriction of protein may lead to malnutrition; therefore, referral to a renal dietitian is recommended to ensure adequate intake.

Fluid restriction: For patients at risk for developing excess fluid volume. For patients on hemodialysis, interdialytic fluid weight gain should be limited to 3%-4% of an individual's "dry" weight (i.e., weight with stable fluid balance).

Pharmacotherapy: Medications that are excreted primarily by the kidney require modification of dosage or frequency. Of special concern are digitalis preparations, which are 85% excreted by the kidneys. Use of digitalis preparations in older adults with CKD requires careful dosage titration to allow adequate therapeutic effect while avoiding toxicity. Digitalis toxicity also may occur if K^+ levels fall too low during dialysis. Dialyzable medications may need to be increased or held and given after dialysis (Box 4-3). In addition, adjustment to standard analgesic doses may be required depending on patient's

TABLE 4-1	CONSIDERATIONS FOR ANALGESIA ADMINISTRATION IN PATIENTS WITH CHRONIC KIDNEY DISEASE

ANALGESIC	CONSIDERATIONS
Acetaminophen	Preferred analgesic for mild to moderate pain
Nonsteroidal antiinflammatory drugs	May cause hyperkalemia
	May cause reversible decrease in GFR for patients with CKD
	Limited to short-term use only with careful monitoring of K+ and GFR
	Use with caution in older adults
Opiates	Adverse effects (GI: nausea, vomiting, constipation), CNS depression, respiratory depression, hypotension, and pruritus more common in patients with CKD and ESRD; when prescribed, they should be used with caution, and patients should be monitored frequently for adverse effects
Codeine	Half-life is extended
	Normal doses may result in prolonged CNS depression
	Dose reduction based on GFR should be considered
Dihydrocodone	CNS depression has been reported
	Dose reduction based on GFR should be considered
Fentanyl	Clearance may be altered in patients with CKD
	Monitor patients with ESRD for sedation and respiratory depression
Hydromorphone	Reports indicate that this drug may be administered safely in patients with CKD and ESRD when doses have been reduced based on GFR
Meperidine	Metabolites lead to neurotoxicity, psychosis, and CNS and respiratory depression. **Caution:** *This drug should be avoided in patients with ESRD.*
Morphine	Half-life is extended in patients with CKD and ESRD
	Accumulation of morphine metabolites may lead to respiratory and CNS depression
	Dose adjustment based on GFR should be considered
Oxycodone	Half-life of this drug is prolonged
	Dose reduction based on GFR should be considered
	Caution: *Oxycodone is contraindicated when GFR is less than 10 mL/min.*
Propoxyphene	Metabolites are excreted by the kidney and therefore accumulate with use
	Accumulation of metabolites can lead to CNS and respiratory depression, cardiotoxicity, and hypoglycemia
	Caution: *Should be used with extreme caution in patients with ESRD.*

CKD, Chronic kidney disease; *CNS,* central nervous system; *ESRD,* end-stage renal disease. *GFR,* glomerular filtration rate; *GI,* gastrointestinal; *K+,* potassium.

GFR, and some analgesics are contraindicated in patients with ESRD (**TABLE 4-1**).

Phosphate binders (e.g., antacids, calcium carbonate, cationic polymer exchange medication, lanthanum carbonate, aluminum hydroxide): Control hyperphosphatemia. Use of aluminum-containing phosphate-binding agents is limited because of increased risk of renal osteodystrophy and encephalopathy caused by elevated tissue aluminum levels.

Antihypertensives: Control BP, slow progression of CKD, and/or reduce proteinuria/microalbuminuria. Angiotensin-converting enzyme (ACE) inhibitors and angiotensin receptor blockers (ARBs) are first-line drugs for management of patients with CKD and coexisting DM, proteinuria, and/or microalbuminuria. A diuretic and then a β-blocker or calcium channel blocker may also be added to achieve a target BP of less than 130/80 mm Hg. Patients may require up to four antihypertensives to control BP adequately. Because increased release of angiotensin may occur with renal pathology, some patients require bilateral nephrectomies to control excessive hypertension.

Multivitamins and folic acid: Prescribed for patients with dietary restrictions or who are on dialysis (water-soluble vitamins are lost during dialysis). Use of over-the-counter (OTC) multivitamins is contraindicated in patients undergoing dialysis because some vitamin levels may be toxic (e.g., vitamin A). Multivitamins for patients on dialysis are specially formulated (e.g., Nephro-Vite, Dialyvite). (See "Renal Dialysis," p. 187.)

Parenteral iron, ferrous sulfate, and recombinant human epoetin alfa (Epogen): Treat anemia. Epogen may be administered subcutaneously or intravenously.

Diphenhydramine: Treats pruritus.

Sodium bicarbonate: Treats acidosis.

Vitamin D preparations and calcium supplements: Treat hypocalcemia and prevent renal osteodystrophy. When the serum phosphorus level is near normal, calcitriol may be administered orally or intravenously to replace the lost ability of the kidneys to convert natural vitamin D and thus facilitate calcium absorption and prevent secondary hyperparathyroidism.

Deferoxamine: Treats iron or aluminum toxicity.

Packed RBCs: Treat severe or symptomatic anemia.

Maintenance of homeostasis and prevention of complications: Accomplished by avoiding the following: volume depletion, hypotension, use of radiopaque contrast medium, and nephrotoxic substances. Pregnancy is contraindicated.

Renal transplantation or dialysis: Patients with CKD with a GFR greater than 15 mL/min and a serum creatinine less than 6 mg/dL generally do not need maintenance dialysis. However, if the therapies listed are inadequate and GFR is less than 12 mL/min, intermittent dialysis is required (see "Renal Dialysis," p. 187).

NURSING DIAGNOSES AND INTERVENTIONS

Activity intolerance related to generalized weakness secondary to anemia and uremia

Desired outcomes: Following treatment, patient rates perceived exertion at 3 or less on a 0-10 scale and exhibits improving endurance to activity as evidenced by heart rate (HR) 20 beats per minute (bpm) or less over resting HR, SBP 20 mm Hg or less over or under resting SBP, and respiratory rate (RR) 20 breaths/min or less with normal depth and pattern (eupnea).

Nursing Interventions

♦ Administer epoetin alfa (Epogen) as prescribed. Anemia is usually proportional to the degree of azotemia, although anemia is better tolerated in uremic than in nonuremic patients. Current clinical practice guidelines recommend that epoetin alfa be started when hemoglobin (Hgb) decreases to less than 10 g/dL. Target Hgb for patients receiving epoetin alfa is 11.5 g/dL (or a range of 11.0-12.0 g/dL). Gently mix container (shaking may denature the glycoprotein); use only 1 dose per vial CG (do not reenter used vials; discard unused portions). *Prevents or corrects uremia-associated anemia.*

♦ Monitor for side effects of epoetin, which may include dyspnea, chest pain, seizures, and severe headache. Epoetin may be contraindicated in patients with uncontrolled hypertension or sensitivity to human albumin.

♦ Monitor patient during activity, and ask patient to rate perceived exertion. Patient should be allowed to rest when he or she feels the need to do so (see **Risk for activity intolerance,** p. 23, in "Prolonged Bed Rest," p. 23). *Patient's perception of fatigue/exertion may differ from nurse's perception.*

♦ Assist with identifying activities that increase fatigue and adjust activities accordingly. *Conserves energy and prevents fatigue or overexertion.*

♦ Assist with activities of daily living (ADL) while encouraging maximum independence to tolerance. *Conserves energy while allowing patient to feel a sense of control.*

♦ Establish realistic, progressive exercises and activity goals that are designed to increase endurance. Ensure that goals are within patient's prescribed limitations. *Realistic goals are more readily achieved.*

♦ Provide and encourage optimal nutrition. *Prevents nutritional deficits within fluid and dietary restrictions.*

♦ Observe for and report evidence of occult blood and blood loss. Notify health care provider of decreases in hematocrit (Hct). *Blood loss reduces Hgb and thereby increases anemia and resultant fatigue.*

♦ Avoid administering ferrous sulfate at same time as antacids. Antacids or calcium carbonate medications should be given at least 1 hr apart from ferrous sulfate. *Maximizes absorption of ferrous sulfate.*

♦ Administer parenteral iron if prescribed. *May help prevent anemia.*

♦ Provide emotional support and active listening. Fatigue is a common problem for patients with ESRD. Emotional support establishes trust and rapport and provides emotional relief when fatigue cannot be adequately relieved or controlled.

Impaired skin integrity related to pruritus and dry skin secondary to uremia and edema
Desired outcome: Patient's skin remains intact and free of erythema and abrasions.

Nursing Interventions

♦ Encourage use of prescribed phosphate binders when serum phosphorus level is elevated (Box 4-4). Excess phosphorus binds with free calcium in the serum. The resulting calcium-phosphate complex is deposited in soft tissues and can cause necrotic patches in the skin. In addition, elevation in calcium-phosphate product is associated with increased risk of death, aortic calcification, mitral valve calcification, and coronary artery calcification. *Phosphate binders help prevent elevation in calcium-phosphate product.*

♦ Administer antihistamines as prescribed if needed. Because accumulating nitrogenous wastes are excreted through the skin, pruritus is common in patients with uremia and causes frequent and intense scratching. Pruritus often decreases with a reduction in BUN and improved phosphorus control. *Decreases itching and subsequent scratching that can result in abrasions and/or infection.*

♦ Keep patient's fingernails cut short. *Prevents skin abrasions when scratching.*

♦ Teach patient to monitor scratches for evidence of infection and to seek medical attention early if signs and symptoms of infection appear. *Uremia retards wound healing and thus increases the risk for infection.*

♦ Encourage use of skin emollients and soaps with high fat content. Uremic skin is often dry and scaly because of reduction in oil gland activity. Skin emollients and soaps with high fat content replace oils and *help reduce itching from dryness.*

♦ Advise patient to bathe every other day and to apply skin lotion immediately upon exiting bath/shower. Patients should avoid harsh soaps, soaps or skin products containing alcohol, and excessive bathing, *to prevent skin dryness and itching.*

♦ Advise patient and significant others about increased risk for bruising. *Clotting abnormalities and capillary fragility place patient with uremia at increased risk for bruising.*

♦ Provide scheduled skin care and position changes for patients with edema. *Helps prevents skin breakdown from pressure.*

Deficient knowledge related to need for frequent BP checks and adherence to antihypertensive therapy and the potential for change in insulin requirements for individuals who have DM

Desired outcomes: Within the 24-hr period before hospital discharge, patient verbalizes knowledge about importance of frequent BP checks and adherence to antihypertensive therapy. Patients with DM verbalize knowledge about the potential for change in insulin requirements.

Nursing Interventions

♦ Assess patient's facility with language, and engage an interpreter or provide language-appropriate written materials if necessary.

♦ Teach patient/significant other:

  • Importance of getting BP checked at frequent intervals and adhering to prescribed antihypertensive therapy. *Control of hypertension may slow progression of chronic renal insufficiency and decrease risk of cardiovascular disease.*

  • Importance of a target BP of less than 130/80 mm Hg. Patients with CRF may experience hypertension because of fluid overload, excess renin secretion, or arteriosclerotic disease. *Maintaining target BP may slow disease progression.*

  • About antihypertensive medications, including drug names, purpose, dosage, schedule precautions, and potential side effects. Also discuss drug/drug, herb/drug, and food/drug interactions. *May slow disease progression.*

  • Importance of medical follow-up for monitoring of GFR, K^+ levels, hypotension, volume depletion, and electrolyte abnormalities.

  • Importance of limiting alcohol intake. Alcohol should be limited to less than 2 drinks/day for men and less than 1 drink/day for women *because of decreased ability to eliminate alcohol.*

  • Benefits of exercise and physical activity. Thirty minutes of physical activity of moderate intensity most days of the week is recommended for patients with CKD *to help prevent or manage hypertension.*

  • Patients with DM to be alert to indicators of hypoglycemia. Indicators of hypoglycemia include weakness, blurred vision, and headache. *Insulin requirements often decrease as renal function decreases because of decreased insulin excretion.* (See "Diabetes Mellitus," p. 411.)

♦ Consider referral to a dietitian. Patients with ESRD have many dietary restrictions, which can be confusing. Patients may need assistance with meal planning and to help them learn which foods, fluids, and supplements to avoid.

♦ Encourage weight loss if body mass index (BMI) is greater than 25 kg/m². Refer to a dietitian as indicated.

♦ Counsel patient on smoking cessation if applicable *to prevent further cardiovascular compromise.*

 Patient-Family Teaching and Discharge Planning

Include verbal and written information about:

♦ Medications, including drug names, purpose, dosage, schedule, precautions, and potential side effects. Also discuss drug/drug, herb/drug, and food/drug interactions.

- Subcutaneous administration of epoetin if prescribed. For patients not on dialysis but requiring epoetin, teach patient and/or significant other preparation of the medication and how to administer subcutaneous injections. Demonstrate how to gently mix the container (shaking may denature the glycoprotein); use only 1 dose per vial (do not reenter used vials, discard unused portions). Instruct patient and/or significant other to store epoetin in refrigerator but not to allow it to freeze. Teach importance of monitoring for and rapidly reporting to health care provider any of the following: dyspnea, chest pain, seizures, and severe headache.
- Diet: include fact sheet listing foods that are to be restricted or limited. Inform patient that diet and fluid restrictions may be altered as renal function decreases. Provide sample menus, and have patient demonstrate understanding by creating 3-day menus that incorporate dietary restrictions.
- Care and observation of dialysis access if patient has such a device (see "Renal Dialysis," p. 187).
- Signs and symptoms that necessitate medical attention: irregular pulse, fever, unusual shortness of breath or edema, sudden change in urine output, and unusual muscle weakness. Potential acute complications of uremia include the following: *heart failure*: crackles (rales), dyspnea, orthopnea; *pericarditis*: heart pain, elevated temperature, presence of pericardial friction or rub on auscultation; *cardiac tamponade*: hypotension, distant heart sounds, pulsus paradoxus (exaggerated inspiratory drop in SBP).
- Need for continued medical follow-up: confirm date and time of next health care provider appointment.
- Importance of avoiding infections and seeking treatment promptly if one develops. Teach indicators of frequently encountered infections, including upper respiratory infection (URI), urinary tract infection (UTI), impetigo, and otitis media.
- Provide information about various treatment options and support groups helpful to patients with or approaching ESRD. The local chapter of the National Kidney Foundation can be helpful in identifying support groups and organizations in the area. Patient and significant others should meet with renal dietitian and social worker before discharge.
- Coordinate discharge planning and teaching with dialysis unit or facility. If possible, have patient visit dialysis unit before discharge.
- Teach importance of coordinating all medical care for ESRD through the nephrologist and alerting all medical and dental personnel to patient's ESRD status because of increased risk of infection and need to adjust medication dosages. In addition, dentists may want to premedicate patients with ESRD with antibiotics before dental work and to avoid scheduling dental work on the day of dialysis because of heparinization that is used with dialytic therapy.
- Phone numbers to call if questions or concerns arise about therapy or disease after discharge. Additional general information can be obtained by accessing the following:

National Institute of Diabetes and Digestive and Kidney Diseases: www.niddk.nih.gov

National Kidney Foundation: www.kidney.org

❖ ❖ ❖

SECTION THREE **RENAL DIALYSIS**

OVERVIEW

Peritoneal dialysis and hemodialysis are lifesaving procedures used to treat patients with severely decreased or absent renal function. Dialysis can be either temporary, until the kidneys can resume adequate function, or permanent. *Dialysis* is defined as selective movement of water and solutes from one fluid compartment to another across a semipermeable membrane. The two fluid compartments are the patient's blood and the dialysate (electrolyte and glucose solution).

The care of patients undergoing dialysis can be complex, and the actual dialysis (especially hemodialysis) is generally accomplished by nurses with specialized education and guided experience. This section does not focus on specific patient care during dialysis but rather provides essential background data, especially regarding nursing care of patients who will undergo peritoneal dialysis and special issues related to patients who are receiving hemodialysis.

Indications for dialysis: Acute renal failura (ARF) or acute episodes of renal insufficiency that cannot be managed by diet, medications, and fluid restriction; end-stage renal disease (ESRD); drug overdose; hyperkalemia; fluid overload; and metabolic acidosis.

Functions of dialysis: Correction of electrolyte abnormalities, removal of excess fluid and metabolic wastes, and correction of acid-base abnormalities. Dialysis does not compensate completely for the lack of functioning kidneys. Medications and dietary and fluid restrictions are necessary to supplement dialysis.

Peritoneal dialysis: The peritoneum serves as a natural dialysis membrane; slower method; does not require heparinization; does require surgical placement of a peritoneal catheter; can be performed by trained medical-surgical nurses, patient, or significant other; requires a minimum of equipment.

Hemodialysis: The semipermeable membrane is an artificial dialysis membrane; faster method; requires heparinization, specially trained staff, expensive and complex equipment; patient must have adequate vasculature for access.

Continuous venovenous hemodiafiltration (CVVHDF): Use is currently limited to patients in critical care settings because it requires continuous monitoring. A double-lumen catheter is placed in a large vein, and blood is pumped from the vein through the dialysis circuit, passing through the hemofilter. It then returns to patient's circulation via venous access. Ultrafiltrate (fluid, metabolic wastes, and electrolytes) drains from the hemofilter into a collection device.

❖ CARE OF THE PATIENT UNDERGOING PERITONEAL DIALYSIS

OVERVIEW/PATHOPHYSIOLOGY

Peritoneal dialysis uses the peritoneum as the dialysis membrane. Dialysate is instilled into the peritoneal cavity via a catheter surgically placed through the abdominal wall. Once the dialysate is within the abdominal cavity, movement of solutes and fluid occurs between patient's capillary blood and the dialysate. At set intervals the peritoneal cavity is drained, and new dialysate is instilled.

COMPONENTS OF DIALYSIS

Catheter: Silastic tube that is implanted by surgical procedure with patient under general anesthesia (for patients who need long-term treatment) or is inserted at the bedside using local anesthetic (for patients who need short-term dialysis).

Dialysate: Sterile electrolyte solution similar in composition to normal plasma. The electrolyte composition of the dialysate is adjusted according to individual need. Glucose is added to the dialysate in varying concentrations to remove excess body fluid via osmosis. Some glucose crosses the peritoneal membrane and enters patient's blood. Patients with diabetes mellitus (DM) may require additional insulin. Observe for and report indicators of hyperglycemia (e.g., complaints of thirst, changes in sensorium). Medications (antibiotics: cefazolin sodium, tobramycin, vancomycin; other: heparin, insulin, K^+) may be added directly to the dialysate by dialysis nurses.

TYPES OF DIALYSIS

Intermittent peritoneal dialysis (IPD): Patient is dialyzed for periods of 8-10 hr, 4-5 ×/wk. A predetermined amount of dialysate (usually 2 L) is instilled for a set length of time (usually 20-30 min). It is then allowed to drain by gravity, and the process is repeated. IPD can be performed manually with individual bags or mechanically using a proportioning machine or cycler. Patient is restricted to chair or bed. IPD also can be performed as an acute, temporary procedure, in which case continuous hourly exchanges are performed for 48-72 hr. Patient is restricted to bed.

Continuous ambulatory peritoneal dialysis (CAPD): Using sterile technique, patient attaches a new bag of dialysate to the peritoneal catheter, allows the dialysate to drain out, and then allows new dialysate to drain in. Patient then clamps the catheter and places a new cap on the tubing using sterile technique. This process is repeated q4-6h (q8h at night), 7 days/wk. CAPD is used primarily to treat end-stage renal disease (ESRD).

Continuous cycling peritoneal dialysis (CCPD): This is a combination of IPD and CAPD. A cycler performs three dialysate exchanges at night. In the morning a fourth exchange is instilled and left in the peritoneal cavity for the entire day. At the end of the day, the fourth exchange is allowed to drain out, and the process is repeated. Patient is ambulatory by day and restricted to bed at night. CCPD is commonly done every night.

NURSING DIAGNOSES AND INTERVENTIONS

Risk for infection related to invasive procedure (direct access of the catheter to the peritoneum)

Desired outcomes: Patient is free of infection as evidenced by normothermia and absence of the following: abdominal pain, cloudy outflow, nausea, malaise, erythema, edema, increased local warmth, drainage, and tenderness at the exit site. Before hospital discharge, patient verbalizes signs and symptoms of infection and need for sterile technique for bag, tubing, and dressing changes.

Nursing Interventions

- Monitor for and report indications of peritonitis, including fever, abdominal pain, distention, abdominal wall rigidity, rebound tenderness, cloudy outflow, nausea, and malaise. The most common complication of peritoneal dialysis is peritonitis. It is essential that sterile technique be used when connecting and disconnecting catheter from dialysis system, *to prevent peritonitis.*
- Maintain sterile technique when adding medications to dialysate because it is instilled directly into the body. *Helps prevent peritonitis.*
- Follow agency policy for care of catheter exit site. *Decreases risk for infection.*
- Observe for and report redness, local warmth, edema, drainage, or tenderness at catheter exit site. Culture any exudate, and report results to health care provider. *Early intervention reduces the risk for extension of infection into peritoneal cavity.*
- Monitor for dialysate leakage around catheter exit site and report to health care provider. This can indicate an obstruction or need for another purse-string suture around catheter site. *Continued leakage at the site can lead to peritonitis.*
- Instruct patient in the preceding interventions and observations if peritoneal dialysis will be performed after hospital discharge. *Helps reduce risk for infection.*

Risk for imbalanced fluid volume related to hypertonicity of the dialysate or inadequate exchange

Desired outcomes: After dialysis, patient is normovolemic as evidenced by balanced I&O, stable weight, good skin turgor, central venous pressure (CVP) 5-12 cm H_2O, respiratory rate (RR) 12-20 breaths/min with normal depth and pattern (eupnea), and BP and heart rate (HR) within patient's normal range. The volume of dialysate outflow equals or exceeds inflow.

Nursing Interventions

- Observe for and report indicators of fluid overload, such as hypertension, dyspnea, tachycardia, distended neck veins, or increased CVP. Fluid retention can occur because of catheter complications that prevent adequate outflow or because of a severely scarred peritoneum that prevents adequate exchange. Accurate measurement and recording of outflow are essential *to determine amount of urine eliminated in dialysate.*
- Monitor for incomplete dialysate return. Outflow problems can occur because of:
  - *Full colon:* Use stool softeners, high-fiber diet, laxatives, or enemas if necessary.
  - *Catheter occlusion by fibrin* (usually occurs soon after insertion): Obtain prescription to irrigate with heparinized saline.
  - *Catheter obstruction by omentum:* Turn patient from side to side, elevate head of bed (HOB) or foot of bed, or apply firm pressure to the abdomen. Notify health care provider for unresolved outflow problems.
- Monitor I&O and weight daily. Weigh patient at same time each day, with same scale and with patient wearing same amount of clothing (or with same items on the bed if using a bed scale). *Steady weight gain indicates fluid retention.*
- Monitor for respiratory distress. If this occurs, elevate HOB, drain the dialysate, and notify health care provider. *Respiratory distress indicates compression of the diaphragm by the dialysate.*
- Monitor for and report gross bloody outflow. Bloody outflow may appear with initial exchanges but should subside. Report continued bloody outflow *because it may indicate puncture of an organ or bowel.*
- Observe for and report indicators of volume depletion, including poor skin turgor, hypotension, tachycardia, and decreased CVP. *Volume depletion can occur because dialysate is a hypertonic solution.*

Imbalanced nutrition: less than body requirements related to protein loss in the dialysate
Desired outcomes: At a minimum of 24 hr before hospital discharge, patient exhibits adequate nutrition as evidenced by stable weight and serum albumin 3.5-5.5 g/dL. Patient's protein intake is 1.2-1.5 g/kg/day.

Nursing Interventions

- Ensure adequate dietary intake of protein: 1.2-1.3 g/kg/day. Protein crosses the peritoneum, and a significant amount is lost in the dialysate. An increased intake of protein is necessary to prevent excessive tissue catabolism. *Protein loss increases with peritonitis.*
- Ensure that a dietary evaluation is performed and teaching program is initiated when patient changes from one type of dialysis to the other. Patients undergoing peritoneal dialysis typically have fewer dietary restrictions than those on hemodialysis.
- Have patient plan a 3-day menu that incorporates appropriate foods and restrictions, after providing lists of foods that are restricted and encouraged. *Validates patient's understanding of dietary requirements.*

❖ CARE OF THE PATIENT UNDERGOING HEMODIALYSIS

OVERVIEW/PATHOPHYSIOLOGY

During hemodialysis, blood is removed via a special vascular access, heparinized, pumped through an artificial kidney (dialyzer), and then returned to patient's circulation. Hemodialysis is a temporary, acute procedure performed as needed, or it is performed long term 2-4 ×/wk for 3-5 hr each treatment.

COMPONENTS OF HEMODIALYSIS

Artificial kidney (dialyzer): Composed of a blood compartment and dialysate compartment, separated by a semipermeable membrane that allows diffusion of solutes and filtration of water. Protein and bacteria do not cross the artificial membrane.

Dialysate: Electrolyte solution similar in composition to normal plasma. Each of the constituents may be varied according to patient's need. The most commonly altered components are K^+ and HCO_3^-. Glucose may be added to prevent sudden drops in serum osmolality and serum glucose during dialysis.

Vascular access: Provides a blood flow rate of 300-500 mL/min for effective dialysis. Vascular access sites may include *arteriovenous fistula, arteriovenous graft, internal jugular catheters* (right side preferred), *femoral vein catheters*, or *subclavian catheters*.

NURSING DIAGNOSES AND INTERVENTIONS

Risk for imbalanced fluid volume related to excessive fluid removal by hemodialysis, related to compromised regulatory mechanism resulting in fluid retention secondary to renal failure, or related to bleeding/hemorrhage occurring from vascular access puncture or disconnection

Desired outcomes: After dialysis, patient is normovolemic as evidenced by stable weight, respiratory rate (RR) 12-20 breaths/min with normal depth and pattern (eupnea), central venous pressure (CVP) 5-12 cm H_2O, heart rate (HR) and BP within patient's normal range, and absence of abnormal breath sounds and abnormal bleeding. After instruction, patient relates signs and symptoms of fluid volume excess and deficit.

Nursing Interventions

◆ Monitor I&O and daily weight as indicators of fluid status. Patient's weight is an important guideline for determining quantity of fluid that needs to be removed during dialysis. Weigh patient at the same time each day, with same scale and with patient wearing same amount of clothing (or with same items on the bed if using a bed scale). *A steady weight gain indicates retained fluid.*

◆ Observe for and report indications of fluid volume excess and instruct patient to do the same: edema, hypertension, crackles (rales), tachycardia, distended neck veins, shortness of breath, and increased CVP. Patient may be the first to recognize signs of fluid volume overload. *Early recognition of fluid volume excess allows for early implementation of corrective action to prevent cardiac and respiratory compromise.*

◆ Clarify with health care provider which medications should be held before hemodialysis treatment. Antihypertensive medications usually are held before and during dialysis *to help prevent hypotension during dialysis.*

◆ Observe for and report indication of fluid volume deficit following hemodialysis, including hypotension, decreased CVP, tachycardia, and complaints of dizziness or lightheadedness. Describe signs and symptoms to patient, and explain importance of reporting them promptly if they occur. Be aware that because of autonomic neuropathy, patient with uremia may not develop compensatory tachycardia when hypovolemic. *Helps ensure early reporting of possible complication.*

◆ Monitor for postdialysis bleeding (needle sites, incisions). Bleeding can occur because of heparin use during dialysis. Alert patient to potential for bleeding from these areas *to ensure early treatment.*

◆ Do not give intramuscular (IM) injections for at least 1 hr after dialysis. *Prevents hematoma formation.*

◆ Test all stools for presence of blood. Report significant findings. Gastrointestinal (GI) bleeding is common in patients with renal failure, *as a result of heparinization during procedure.*

Risk for ineffective peripheral tissue perfusion related to interrupted blood flow that can occur with clotting in the vascular access

Desired outcomes: Patient's vascular access remains intact and connected, and patient is normovolemic (see description in preceding nursing diagnosis, **Risk for imbalanced fluid volume**). Patient has adequate tissue perfusion as evidenced by normal skin temperature and color and brisk capillary refill (less than 2 sec) distal to the vascular access. Patient's access is patent as evidenced by presence of thrill with palpation and bruit with auscultation of fistula or graft.

Nursing Interventions

◆ Assess for vascular patency, auscultate for bruits, and palpate for thrills. *Detects adequacy of peripheral circulation following surgical creation of the vascular access.*

◆ Monitor for and report: complaints of severe or unrelieved pain, numbness, or tingling of the area of vascular access or extremity distal to the access; swelling, coolness, discoloration, or increased capillary refill time in the extremity distal to the vascular access. Any of these can signal impaired tissue perfusion or hypoxia as a result of reduced blood supply to the extremity (called *steal syndrome*). Some postoperative swelling along graft or fistula or area around the shunt is expected; elevate extremity accordingly. *Ensures early treatment to prevent tissue hypoxia.*

◆ Explain monitoring and care procedures to patient. Remember that the vascular access is patient's lifeline. *Patients are generally the first to recognize problems with their access sites.*

◆ Do not use hemodialysis lines for instillation of IV medications or blood drawing. These lines are heparinized with 1000-5000 units of heparin after dialysis use (variation is a result of dialysis unit policy), and improper withdrawal of heparin may inadvertently lead to heparinization of patient that results in bleeding. Inadequate heparinization following use may lead to clotting of the dialysis catheter, and access increases risk of infection. Hemodialysis lines must be closely monitored and handled with care *to prevent bleeding or clotting.*

◆ Follow the three principles of nursing care common to all types of vascular access: (1) prevent bleeding, (2) prevent clotting, and (3) prevent infection (see **Risk for infection,** immediately following).

  • *Fistula or graft:* Internal, permanent connection between an artery and a vein, or the insertion of an internal graft that is joined to an artery and vein. Grafts can be straight or U-shaped. Grafts and fistulas are most commonly located in the arm but may be placed in the thigh.

    • *Prevent bleeding:* Inspect needle puncture sites for postdialysis bleeding. If bleeding occurs, apply just enough pressure over the site to stop it. Release the pressure, and check for bleeding q5-10min.

    • *Prevent clotting:* A sign should be placed above head of bed (HOB) indicating extremity in which the fistula or graft has been placed and stating not to take BP, start IV line, or draw blood from affected limb. This information also should be clearly documented on patient's plan of care. Caution patient to avoid tight clothing, jewelry, name bands, or restraint on affected extremity. Palpate for thrill and auscultate for bruit at least every shift and after hypotensive episodes. Notify health care provider stat if bruit or thrill has changed significantly or is absent.

  • *Subclavian or femoral lines:* External, temporary catheters inserted into a large vein. These lines should not be used for instillation of IV medications or blood drawing *because these procedures increase risk of bleeding, clotting of the catheter, and line infection.*

    • *Prevent bleeding:* Anchor catheter securely if not sutured into place. Tape all connections. Keep clamps at bedside in case line becomes disconnected. If the line is removed or accidentally pulled out, apply firm pressure to site for at least 10 min.

- *Prevent air embolus*, which can occur if a subclavian line accidentally becomes pulled out or disconnected. If this occurs, immediately clamp the line. Turn patient onto a left side-lying position to help prevent air from blocking the pulmonary artery. Lower HOB to Trendelenburg position to increase intrathoracic pressure and decrease the flow of inspiratory air into the vein. Administer 100% oxygen by mask, and obtain VS. Notify health care provider stat.
- *Prevent clotting:* Only dialysis staff should access the line because improper heparin flushing increases risk of clotting.

Risk for infection related to invasive procedure (creation of vascular access for hemodialysis)
Desired outcome: Patient is free of infection as evidenced by normothermia and absence of erythema, local warmth, exudate, swelling, and tenderness at access site.

Nursing Interventions

- Prevent infection: Dressing changes and cultures of any drainage should be performed only by dialysis staff. If a dressing loosens, it needs to be reinforced; request that dialysis unit staff perform the dressing change *to decrease risk for infection.*
- Monitor for and report presence of erythema, local warmth, exudate, swelling, and tenderness at graft, fistula, or shunt site. These are indications of localized infection. *Early detection allows for early intervention.*
- Monitor VS. Elevated temperature and chills may be the first sign of infection. *Tachycardia and decreased BP are related to the vasodilator effect of increased body temperature and increased metabolic rate in response to infection.*
- Monitor laboratory data, especially complete blood count (CBC), differential, erythrocyte sedimentation rate (ESR), and culture reports. Evaluate presence and course of infection. Be alert to abnormal results and notify health care provider of significant findings.
- Maintain strict sterile technique for all invasive procedures. *Prevents introduction of pathogens, which may lead to infection.*
- Enforce good handwashing before contact with patient. Inadequate handwashing and contamination of access sites or invasive lines are common sources of infection. Good handwashing remains the single most important intervention *to minimize the risk of transmitting microorganisms to patient.*

SECTION FOUR   # CARE OF THE RENAL TRANSPLANT RECIPIENT

OVERVIEW/PATHOPHYSIOLOGY

Individuals with ESRD may choose from end-stage renal disease (ESRD) several treatment modalities—hemodialysis, peritoneal dialysis, no treatment, and renal transplantation. Diabetes mellitus (DM) is the leading cause of renal failure in the United States, and increasing numbers of simultaneous kidney-pancreas transplants are being performed as a consequence. Renal transplantation is not a cure for renal failure, and it can be done only in Medicare-approved facilities. Several types of donors are options for patients needing renal transplant: deceased (formerly referred to as cadaveric), living related, living unrelated, voluntary nondirected, and kidney-paired donors. Postoperatively, patients are sent to specialized units where nephrology nurses monitor them on an hourly basis for the first 24-36 hr. Subsequent admissions may occur at any hospital for treatment of a rejection episode, infection, medication complication, or unrelated illness. Rejection is the major complication of renal transplantation. Long-term complications secondary to use of immunosuppressive agents may include infection, hypertension, cardiovascular disease, chronic liver disease, bone demineralization, cataracts, gastrointestinal (GI) hemorrhage, and cancer.

IMMUNOSUPPRESSION

With the exception of identical twin donors, all transplant recipients must take drugs that suppress their immune system for the life of the graft to prevent rejection.

Immunosuppressive medication management: Each transplant center has a drug protocol outlining which combination of medications will be given to each patient. See **TABLE 4-2** for drug classifications, common names, and side effects. A complete list of patient's medications, including herbal remedies, should be included on patient's chart. Some herbs interfere with absorption of immunosuppressive medications, cause patients to have lower levels of medications in their systems, and potentially result in episodes of graft rejection and/or loss of the graft. Check the *PDR (Physicians' Desk Reference) for Herbal Medicines* if unsure about interactions.

Azathioprine: Dosage is adjusted or held based on patient's WBC count.

Prednisone: May produce steroid-induced DM.

Cyclosporine: Grapefruit juice has been known to potentiate medication and could cause nephrotoxicity and/or loss of graft function. Although cyclosporine is most commonly given as a capsule, if liquid oral form is required, use a glass container and metal spoon; mix with orange juice or chocolate milk to make it more palatable; do not allow solution to stand; and never mix with grapefruit juice.

ORGAN REJECTION

Acute: May begin weeks to 1 yr after surgery; potentially reversible; treated with increased immunosuppression.

Chronic: Usually classified as starting 1 yr after transplantation; irreversible; managed conservatively with diet and antihypertensive agents until dialysis is required.

Indicators of rejection: Oliguria, tenderness over graft site (located in iliac fossa), sudden weight gain (2-3 lb/day), fever, malaise, hypertension, and increased blood urea nitrogen (BUN) and serum creatinine. In addition, hyperglycemia develops with combined kidney-pancreas transplantation.

Management of acute rejection

Antithymocyte globulin (ATG): Immediate side effects include chills, fever, rash, hypertension, headache, hyperkalemia, joint pain, and anaphylaxis. This drug is contraindicated in patients with history of allergy to rabbit proteins or acute viral illness. Premedicate with corticosteroid, antihistamine, and acetaminophen as prescribed. Monitor WBC, platelet, and T-cell counts.

Monoclonal antibody muromonab-CD3 (Orthoclone OKT-3): Immediate side effects include fever, chills, rigors, tremor, headache, vomiting, nausea, dyspnea and bronchospasm, pulmonary edema, and cardiac arrest. Patients should be monitored closely during initial doses because there is a high incidence of side effects. Contraindicated in patients with history of allergy to mouse proteins. Patients usually develop high fevers (temperatures of 102°-107° F) approximately 4 hr after dose. Have a cooling blanket and ice packs available and ensure a prescription for acetaminophen is on the medication record. Pulmonary edema is most likely to occur if patient has excess fluid volume. A chest x-ray film should be taken before the first dose to confirm clear lung fields.

TABLE 4-2	CLASSIFICATIONS AND SIDE EFFECTS OF IMMUNOSUPPRESSIVE AGENTS	

CLASSIFICATION	AGENT	COMMON SIDE EFFECTS
Antiinflammatory	Prednisone, methylprednisolone (Medrol)	Altered fat deposition, cataracts, glaucoma, diabetes, hypertension, fluid retention, bone and muscle wasting, joint disease
Antiproliferative	Azathioprine (Imuran), mycophenolate (CellCept, Myfortic)	Neutropenia, thrombocytopenia *Mycophenolate:* diarrhea, gastrointestinal (GI) intolerance
Early activation inhibitors	Tacrolimus (Prograf), cyclosporine (Gengraf, Neoral)	Nephrotoxicity, diabetes, hypertension, hyperkalemia, tremors, neuropathies
Calcineurin inhibitors	*Cyclosporine modified* (Neoral)	*Cyclosporine modified:* hirsutism, gingival hyperplasia
Antiantigen recognition agents	*Polyclonal antibody therapy* (Thymoglobulin, Atgam)	*Polyclonal antibodies:* neutropenia, thrombocytopenia, bone marrow suppression
	Monoclonal antibodies: OKT3 *(murine),* basiliximab (Simulect) *(chimeric),* daclizumab (Zenapax) *(humanized)*	*Murine monoclonal:* pyrexia, dyspnea, cytokine release *Humanized and chimeric monoclonals:* well-tolerated
mTOR inhibitor	Sirolimus (Rapamune)	Hyperlipidemia, diarrhea, thrombocytopenia

Reprinted with permission of the American Nephrology Nurses' Association, publisher. *Transplantation Fact Sheet,* 2004. Retrieved from www.annanurse.org.
National Kidney Foundation. Dietary protein intake for chronic peritoneal dialysis. K/DOQI Update 2000. Accessed January 2010 from http://www.kidney.org/Professionals/kdoqi/guidelines_updates/nut_a16.html

Prednisone: Patients are usually taken off their oral dose and put on IV therapy, then weaned back to oral medication as rejection resolves. Patients may develop steroid-induced DM; therefore careful monitoring of their glucose levels is important.

NURSING DIAGNOSES AND INTERVENTIONS

Risk for infection related to invasive procedures, exposure to infected individuals, and immunosuppression

Desired outcomes: Patient is free of infection as evidenced by normothermia; heart rate (HR) 100 beats per minute (bpm) or less (or within patient's normal range); respiratory rate (RR) 12-20 breaths/min with normal depth and pattern; and absence of erythema, edema, increased local warmth, tenderness, or purulent drainage at wounds or catheter exit sites. Patient is free of signs and symptoms of oral, esophageal, respiratory, GI, genitourinary, and cutaneous infections. Patient verbalizes indicators of infection and importance of reporting them promptly to health care provider or staff.

Nursing Interventions

◆ Assess frequently for any indicator of infection. Patients are taking large doses of immunosuppressive agents; therefore, their immune response and their response to infectious agents are muted. Be especially sensitive to low-grade fever, and unexplained tachycardia, *to detect early signs of infection.*

◆ Instruct patient to be alert to signs and symptoms of commonly encountered infections and importance of reporting them promptly. These include the following:
  • *Urinary tract infection (UTI):* Cloudy and malodorous urine; dysuria, frequency, and urgency; pain in suprapubic area, buttock, thighs, labia, or scrotum (see "Urinary Tract Infection," p. 197).
  • *Upper respiratory infection (URI):* Productive cough; malodorous, purulent, colored, and copious secretions; chest pain or heaviness.
  • *Pharyngitis*: Painful swallowing.
  • *Otitis media*: Malaise; earache.
  • *Impetigo:* Inflamed or draining areas on the skin.

◆ Monitor for signs and symptoms of cytomegalovirus (CMV) infection, including fever, malaise, fatigue, and muscle aches. CMV is a common infectious agent in renal transplant recipients. Other infectious complications include *Legionella* pneumonia; cutaneous herpes simplex (shingles); varicella-zoster (chickenpox); Epstein-Barr virus (EBV); oral, esophageal, deep fungal, or mycotic pseudoaneurysm caused by *Candida;* and *Pneumocystis jiroveci* (formerly known as *P. carinii)* infection.

◆ Teach patient to avoid exposure to individuals known to have infections. *Patients who are immunosuppressed are at significantly increased risk for infection.*

◆ Consult with health care providers about the need for prophylactic antibiotics for any minor invasive procedures, including dental cleaning. *These procedures are associated with an increased risk for infection.*

◆ Use sterile technique with all invasive procedures and dressing changes. *Prevents contamination and minimizes risk for infection.*

◆ Teach patient to avoid eating undercooked meats and changing cat litter. *Decreases the risk for toxoplasmosis.*

Deficient knowledge related to signs and symptoms of rejection, side effects of immunosuppressive agents, transplantation complications, and importance of protecting existing hemodialysis vascular access
Desired outcome: Within the 24-hr period before hospital discharge, patient verbalizes knowledge of signs and symptoms of rejection, side effects of immunosuppressive therapy, complications of transplantation, and importance of protecting hemodialysis vascular access.

Nursing Interventions

◆ Assess patient's facility with language; engage an interpreter or provide language-appropriate written materials if necessary.

◆ Monitor renal function studies: I&O, daily weight, and BUN and serum creatinine values. *Increases in BUN, serum creatinine, and weight indicate decreased renal function.*

◆ Teach patients signs and symptoms of rejection and the need to report them immediately. Oliguria, tenderness over transplanted kidney (located in iliac fossa), sudden weight gain (2-3 lb), fever, malaise, hypertension, and increased BUN (greater than 20 mg/dL) and serum creatinine (greater than 1.5 mg/dL) may indicate rejection. *Rejection must be treated early to prevent loss of the graft.*

◆ Provide patients with a notebook in which to record daily VS and weight measurements. Instruct patients to weigh themselves at same time each day, with same scale and wearing same amount of clothing. Remind patients to bring the notebook to all outpatient visits and to report abnormal values promptly if they occur.

◆ Teach patient the reason for frequent monitoring of WBC and platelet counts. Significant decreases in WBC and platelet counts can be a side effect of immunosuppressive agents, and therefore serial monitoring is essential.

- Teach patient signs and symptoms of GI bleeding (e.g., tarry stools, "coffee-ground" emesis, orthostatic changes, dizziness, tachycardia, increasing fatigue and weakness) and importance of reporting them promptly if they occur. *GI bleeding is a potential side effect of immunosuppressive agents.*
- Teach patient and/or significant others how to measure BP, and provide guidelines for values that would necessitate notification of health care provider or staff member. In patient who has undergone renal transplantation, hypertension may develop for a variety of reasons, including cyclosporine or steroid use, rejection, and renal artery stenosis.
- Reinforce the need to continue caring for vascular access. For patients with a patent fistula or graft (hemodialysis vascular access), access will still be needed if they have to return to dialysis. Reinforce that taking BP, drawing blood, and starting an IV line are contraindicated in the vascular access arm, and therefore patient should warn others about these contraindications, *to prevent clotting or loss of access site.*
- Stress need for continued medical evaluation of the transplant. *Graft rejection is possible at any time, hence the need for continued monitoring.*
- Verify patient's knowledge of immunosuppressive medications and dosage. Patient will be self-administering own medications. It is essential that patient or caregiver clearly understand medication dosages, contraindications, and side effects.

❖ ❖ ❖

SECTION FIVE **DISORDERS OF THE URINARY TRACT**

❖ URINARY TRACT INFECTION (CYSTITIS)

OVERVIEW/PATHOPHYSIOLOGY

Cystitis, infection of the urinary bladder, is one of several upper and lower urinary tract infections (UTIs). It is caused when pathogenic microorganisms enter the urethra and urinary bladder and produce inflammation. Girls and women are especially prone to cystitis because of a short urethra. Although not common in men, cystitis, like other UTIs, can be a very serious disease when it does occur. Sexual intercourse (female patients), fecal contamination of the urethra, sexually transmitted diseases, chronic diseases (diabetes mellitus [DM], immune compromise, neurogenic bladder), and urinary catheterization are risk factors for cystitis. Indwelling urinary catheters are the most significant sources of nosocomial lower UTIs in hospitalized patients. Recurrence of cystitis is not uncommon, especially in older adults and pregnant women. Untreated cystitis can lead to pyelonephritis, sepsis, or kidney failure.

ASSESSMENT

Clinical indicators of cystitis can be nonspecific, especially in older persons. Assess for history of bladder infections, the presence of pain on urination (dysuria), urinary frequency and urgency, foul-smelling or cloudy urine, hematuria, suprapubic pressure or discomfort, and fatigue. Fever and chills may occur with severe infections but are usually an indication that the infection has ascended into the kidneys.

Interstitial cystitis refers to urinary bladder pain in the absence of infection. It differs from bacterial cystitis in that it does not respond to antibiotics. The cause is unknown, but hereditary predisposition is appears to be a factor. Symptoms are similar to those of bacterial cystitis.

DIAGNOSTIC TESTS

Urine culture: Confirms the presence of a causative organism. Not routinely performed for patients with isolated cases of cystitis, but indicated when patients have recurrent infections.

Urinalysis: Reveals presence of WBCs, WBC casts, RBCs, and bacteria.

Cystoscopy: Allows visualization of urinary bladder and biopsy of tissues when urinary infections are recurring.

CBC: Demonstrates leukocytosis related to inflammation and infection.

COLLABORATIVE MANGEMENT

The focus of collaborative management is similar to that of acute pyelonephritis and involves early recognition of infection, initiation of appropriate antibacterial therapy, and prevention of recurrent infections. Isolated episodes of lower UTI rarely require hospitalization; however, they commonly occur in hospitalized patients, especially among older adults (see "Pyelonephritis," p. 167).

Pharmacotherapy

Antibiotics: Short-term (1-7 days) antibiotic therapy eradicates most uncomplicated lower UTIs. Low-dose antimicrobial prophylaxis may be indicated for some patients with frequently recurring cystitis.

Acetylsalicylic acid (ASA), acetaminophen, or ibuprofen: Treats discomfort.

Fluids: Oral fluids, including blueberry, plum, prane, or cranberry juice, are encouraged to ensure adequate urinary output and flush microorganisms out of the urinary bladder and urethra. These juices may prevent bacterial adhesion to the urinary tract and help prevent UTIs.

Diet: Limit the intake of spicy or irritating foods (tomatoes, caffeine, alcohol) to prevent increased inflammation and decrease discomfort.

NURSING DIAGNOSES AND IMPLEMENTATION

Impaired urinary elimination related to bladder irritation and inflammation

Desired outcome: Patient is free of infection as evidenced by clear, nonmalodorous urine, and absence of pain, urgency, and frequency.

Nursing Interventions

◆ Assess/monitor for signs of infection: foul-smelling or cloudy urine; malaise; urinary frequency and urgency. *Establishes baseline for later comparisons to determine effectiveness of interventions.*

◆ Administer prescribed antibiotics as scheduled *to maintain effective antibiotic serum levels to ensure eradication of pathogenic organisms.*

◆ Avoid use of indwelling urinary catheters unless mandatory and remove them as early as possible. *Urinary catheterization is a significant source of pathogen introduction into the urinary system. Intermittent catheterization carries less risk of UTI than does indwelling catheterization. Indwelling urinary catheters are the most common cause of lower UTIs, especially in older adults.*

◆ Offer juices such as cranberry, plum, blueberry, or prune, *which leave an acid ash in urine that inhibits pathogens from adhering to mucosa of urinary tract.*

Acute pain (dysuria) related to bladder inflammation secondary to infection

Desired outcomes: Within 1 hr of intervention, patient reports relief of bladder discomfort.

Nursing Interventions

◆ Monitor for suprapubic tenderness and complaints of dysuria, frequency, and urgency.

◆ Administer analgesics as prescribed *to relieve pain.*

♦ Encourage oral fluid intake *to dilute urine and promote comfort by decreasing irritation of bladder mucosa.*

Deficient Knowledge related to prevention of infection/reinfection, need for adherence to antibiotic therapy and fluid intake; follow-up care
Desired outcomes: Within a 24 hr-hr period, patient verbalizes understanding of medication schedule and strategies for avoiding recurrence.

Nursing Interventions

♦ Assess patient's facility with language; engage an interpreter or provide language-appropriate written materials.
♦ Teach patient/significant other:
  • Risk factors for recurrent infections.
  • Necessity of maintaining fluid intake of at least 2-3 L/day and drinking fruit juices (cranberry, plum, blueberry, and prune) *to help prevent future lower UTIs.*
  • Signs and symptoms that indicate recurring infection and need to be reported.
  • Necessity for emptying bladder at least q3-4h and once during the night, *to help prevent UTI caused by residual urine, which can ascend into renal pelvis and cause infection of the kidney.*
  • Necessity for female patients to void before and immediately after sexual intercourse, wipe from front to back, and wear undergarments with a cotton crotch, *to minimize the risk of introducing bacteria into the bladder and urinary tract.*

📝 Patient-Family Teaching and Discharge Planning

When providing patient-family teaching, avoid giving excessive information, and provide oral and written information about:
♦ Medications, including drug names, purpose, dosage, schedule, precautions, and potential side effects. Also discuss drug/drug, herb/drug, and food/drug interactions.
♦ Importance of taking medications for prescribed length of time, even if feeling well, *to ensure that pathogenic organisms are eradicated and to prevent bacterial regrowth and later reinfection.*
♦ Importance of perineal hygiene for female patients (see **Deficient Knowledge**, earlier) *to minimize risk of introducing bacteria into the urinary tract.*
♦ Need for maintaining adequate fluid intake (see **Deficient Knowledge**, earlier).
♦ Importance of reporting recurring signs and symptoms early *so that therapy can be implemented, chronic bladder infections can be prevented, and kidney infections can be avoided.*

❖ URETERAL CALCULI

OVERVIEW/PATHOPHYSIOLOGY

Ureteral calculus (kidney stone) is the third most common urologic condition after urinary tract infection (UTI) and pathologic conditions of the prostate. Although the cause of stones is unknown in 50% of reported cases, it is believed that they originate in the kidney and are passed through the kidney to the ureter. About 90% of all stones pass from the ureter into the bladder and out of the urinary system spontaneously.

ASSESSMENT

Signs and symptoms/physical findings: Presents suddenly and may be sharp and intense or dull and aching. It is located in the flank area and often radiates toward the groin. Pain may be intermittent (colic) as the stone moves along the ureter and may subside when it enters the bladder. Patient is restless and unable to find a position of comfort. Assess for hypertension, pallor, diaphoresis, tachycardia, tachypnea, costovertebral angle (CVA) tenderness and guarding, nausea, vomiting, diarrhea, and abdominal pain. Bowel sounds may be absent if paralytic ileus occurs, and the abdomen may be distended and tympanic. Patients may experience urinary urgency and frequency, void in small amounts, and have hematuria. Fever may indicate infection secondary to tearing of the ureter mucosa as the stone migrates toward the bladder or may be secondary to UTI.

History and risk factors: Sedentary lifestyle; residence in geographic area in which water supply is high in stone-forming minerals; vitamin A deficiency; vitamin D excess; hereditary cystinuria; treatment with acetazolamide, which is given for glaucoma; inflammatory bowel disease; recurrent UTIs; prolonged periods of immobilization; gout or prophylactic therapy with allopurinol; decreased fluid intake; hyperparathyroidism; Paget's disease; sarcoidosis; and familial history of calculi or renal disease such as renal tubular acidosis.

DIAGNOSTIC TESTS

Serum tests: Calcium levels greater than 5.3 mEq/L, phosphorus levels greater than 2.6 mEq/L, and uric acid levels greater than 7.5 mg/dL have been implicated in stone formation.

BUN/serum creatinine: High BUN and serum creatinine levels with low urine creatinine levels indicate compromised kidney function. BUN levels are affected by fluid volume excess and deficit. Volume excess reduces BUN levels, whereas volume deficit increases levels. For the older adult, serum creatinine level may not be a reliable measure of renal function because of reduced muscle mass and decreased glomerular filtration rate (GFR). These tests must be evaluated based on adjustment for patient's age and hydration status and in comparison with other renal-urinary tests.

Urinalysis: Detects urinary system function, metabolic disease, and presence of UTI. Signs of UTI include the following: cloudy or hazy appearance; foul odor; pH greater than 8.0; and presence of RBCs, leukocyte esterase, WBCs, and WBC casts. A pH less than 5 is associated with uric acid calculi, whereas a pH of 7.5 or greater may signal presence of urea-splitting organisms (responsible for magnesium-ammonium-phosphate or struvite calculi).

Urine culture: Determines type of bacteria in the genitourinary tract if infection is present. A midstream specimen should be collected to avoid contamination. Deliver specimens to laboratory as quickly as possible after collecting. Urine left at room temperature has greater potential for bacterial growth, turbidity, and alkaline pH, any of which can distort the reading. Specimens for culture are not refrigerated.

24-hr urine collection: Tests for levels of uric acid, cystine, oxalate, calcium, phosphorus, or creatinine to determine stone composition. All urine samples should be sent to the laboratory immediately after they are obtained or refrigerated. If refrigeration is not possible, store according to instructions from laboratory personnel.

Kidney, ureter, bladder (KUB) x-ray examination: Outlines gross structural changes in the kidneys and urinary system. Typically, calcified calculi are seen (90% of urinary calculi are radiopaque [i.e., calcium or cystine]), but not all calculi are radiopaque. Serial radiography monitors progressive movement of the stone. Plain x-ray examination of the skeletal system may reveal Paget's disease, sarcoidosis, or changes associated with prolonged immobilization.

Excretory urogram/intravenous pyelogram (IVP): Used to visualize kidneys, renal pelvis, ureters, and bladder. This test also outlines nonradiopaque stones within the ureters. Nonradiopaque stones (e.g., uric acid calculi) are seen as radiolucent defects in the contrast media.

Renal ultrasound: Identifies ureteral dilation and presence of stones in the ureters.

CT scan with or without injection of contrast medium: Distinguishes cysts, tumors, calculi, and other masses and determines presence of ureteral dilation and bladder distention.

COLLABORATIVE MANAGEMENT

The focus of collaborative management is on pain control, prevention of infection, and maintenance of urinary function.

Pharmacotherapy

Opioid and antispasmodic agents: Relieve pain and ureteral spasms. Morphine increases ureteral peristalsis, which aids in passage of the stone but also can increase pain. Conservative therapy may consist of a trial of analgesiics, dissolution agents, and normal fluid intake to 1500-2000 mL/day. Dissolution agents such as orange juice alkalinize urine, which may shrink stones so that they can pass through the ureter.

Antiemetics (e.g., hydroxyzine, ondansetron, prochlorperazine, promethazine): For nausea and vomiting.

Antibiotics: For infection if present.

Prophylactic pharmacotherapy

URIC ACID STONES: Allopurinol or sodium bicarbonate will reduce uric acid production or alkalinize urine to keep pH at 6.5 or higher, respectively.

STRUVITE STONES: Antibiotics are indicated to eradicate infection and urease inhibitors (acetohydroxamic acid) are prescribed to decrease stone recurrence in patients with persistent urinary infections.

CALCIUM STONES: Sodium cellulose phosphate, when used with a calcium-restricted diet, reduces risk of stone formation. Sodium cellulose phosphate should be taken before meals, not be taken at bedtime, and should be used with caution in postmenopausal women at risk for osteoporosis. Orthophosphates (potassium acid phosphate and disodium and dipotassium phosphates) are given to decrease urinary excretion of citrate and pyrophosphate and thus inhibit stone formation. Thiazides also reduce excretion of citrate and reduce urinary calcium.

CYSTINE STONES: Sodium bicarbonate or sodium-potassium citrate solution is given to increase urinary pH to 7.5 or higher. Penicillamine or tiopronin can be given to lower urine cystine levels.

Fluids: For patients who are dehydrated or for IV alkalinization. IV fluids administered if oral fluids are not tolerated to ensure adequate urinary output and promote stone movement toward the urinary bladder.

Diet: Specific to patient's stone type.

Endoscopic removal of calculi via cystoscope: An invasive procedure in which a basket catheter is placed beyond the stone and rotated in a downward movement to capture and remove the stone.

Ureteral catheters (stents): Stent positioned above the stone to promote ureteral dilation and to allow the calculus to pass. These catheters also can be used for intermittent or continuous irrigation with an acidic solution to combat alkalinity. They may be placed temporarily after stone removal to allow for healing and promote ureteral patency in the presence of edema.

Extracorporeal shock wave lithotripsy (ESWL): Affected area is positioned under a membrane coupling device to generate shock waves that shatter the calculi. ESWL may be done using general, regional, or, in selected patients, local anesthesia. Usually 1000-2000 shock waves over a period of 30-45 min are adequate to break the calculi into fine particles. The fragments pass naturally in patient's urine within a few days.

Ureterolithotomy: Surgical removal of calculi that cannot pass through the ureter. The ureter is surgically incised, and the stone is manually removed.

Chemolysis: Instillation of solutions (acids, alkaline agents, chelate, thiol) via nephrostomy and ureteral catheters to dissolve stones or stone fragments left by other treatments.

NURSING DIAGNOSES AND INTERVENTIONS

Acute pain related to presence of calculus or the surgical procedure to remove it

Desired outcome: Patient's subjective perception of pain decreases within 1 hr of intervention, as documented by a pain scale. Objective indicators, such as grimacing, are absent or diminished.

Nursing Interventions

- Assess and document quality, location, intensity, and duration of pain. Devise a pain scale with patient that ranges from 0 (no pain) to 10 (worst pain). Notify health care provider of sudden and/or severe pain.
- Medicate patient with prescribed analgesics, narcotics, and antispasmodics; evaluate and document response based on pain scale. Encourage patient to request medication before discomfort becomes severe *to achieve maximum pain control.*
- Provide warm blankets, heating pad to affected area, or warm baths *to increase regional circulation and relax tense muscles.*
- Notify health care provider of a sudden cessation of pain, which *can signal passage of the stone.*

Impaired urinary elimination (dysuria, urgency, or frequency) related to obstruction caused by ureteral calculus, obstruction, or positional problems in presence of ureteral catheter

Desired outcomes: Patient reports return of a normal voiding pattern within 2 days. Patient demonstrates ability to record I&O and strain urine for stones. Patient has output from the ureteral catheter (if present) and is free of spasms or flank pain, which could signal obstruction or displacement.

Nursing Interventions

- Assess for and document patient's normal voiding pattern.
- Monitor quality and color of urine. Optimally, urine is straw colored and clear and has a characteristic urine odor. Dark urine is often indicative of dehydration, and blood-tinged urine can result from rupture of ureteral capillaries as the calculus passes through the ureter.
- Encourage fluid intake of at least 2-3 L/day (in patients for whom fluids are not restricted) *to help flush calculus through the ureter, into the bladder, and out through the urinary meatus.*
- Record accurate I&O; teach patient how to record I&O *to verify adequacy of urine output.*
- Strain all urine for evidence of solid matter; teach patient the procedure. Send any solid matter to the laboratory for analysis.
- Monitor output from ureteral catheter. If patient has more than one catheter, label one right and the other left, as appropriate; keep all drainage records separate. Amount will vary with each patient and depend on catheter dimension. If drainage is scant or absent, milk catheter and tubing gently to try to dislodge the obstruction. If this fails, notify health care provider. Never irrigate catheter without specific health care provider instructions to do so. If irrigation is prescribed, use gentle pressure and sterile technique. Always aspirate with sterile syringe before instillation *to prevent ureteral damage from overdistention.* Use another sterile syringe to instill irrigant amounts of 3 mL or less.
- Explain to patient that bed rest is required when ureteral catheter is indwelling. Semi-Fowler's and side-lying positions are acceptable. Fowler's position should be avoided, however, because sutures are seldom used and gravity can cause catheter to move into the bladder. Urinary bladder (ureteral) catheters are often attached to the urethral catheter after placement in the ureters. Carefully monitor urethral catheter for movement *to ensure that it is securely attached to patient.*

◆ Monitor for indicators of ureteral obstruction, including flank pain, CVA tenderness, nausea, and vomiting after ureteral catheters have been removed. Ureteral catheters are usually removed simultaneously with the urethral catheter.

Risk for impaired skin integrity related to wound drainage after ureterolithotomy or procedures that enter the ureter
Desired outcome: Patient's skin surrounding wound site remains nonerythemic and intact.

Nursing Interventions

◆ Monitor incisional dressings frequently during first 24 hr, and change or reinforce as needed. Flank incisional approaches to the ureter require muscle splitting and result in significant postoperative oozing of blood and urine leaking from the entered ureter. *Excoriation can result from prolonged contact of urine with the skin.*
◆ Assess and document odor, consistency, and color of drainage. Immediately after surgery, drainage may be red.
◆ Use Montgomery straps or net wraps rather than tape to secure dressing *to facilitate frequent dressing changes.*
◆ Apply wound drainage or ostomy pouch with a skin barrier over the incision if drainage is copious after drain removal *to prevent skin irritation from urine.* Use a pouch with an antireflux valve *to prevent contamination from reflux.*

Health-seeking behaviors related to dietary regimen and its relationship to calculus formation
Desired outcome: Within the 24-hr period before hospital discharge, patient verbalizes knowledge about foods and liquids to limit in order to prevent stone formation and demonstrates this knowledge by planning a 3-day menu that excludes or limits these foods.

Nursing Interventions

◆ Assess patient's knowledge about diet and its relationship to stone formation.
◆ Teach patient:
  - Importance of maintaining daily fluid intake of at least 2-3 L/day. Increasing urine output reduces saturation of stone-forming solutes. Hydrating after meals and exercise is especially important because solute load is highest at these times. Patients with cardiac, liver, or renal disease require special fluid intake instructions from their health care provider.
  - Dietary changes as specified by health care provider: Include fact sheets that list foods to restrict or add to the diet; provide sample menus with examples of how dietary restrictions and requirements may be incorporated into daily meals.
  - **Uric acid stones:** Limit intake of foods high in purines, such as lean meat, legumes, whole grains. Limit animal protein intake to 1 g/kg/day *to help decrease uric acid and new stone formation.*
  - **Calcium stones:** Limit intake of foods high in calcium, such as milk, cheese, green leafy vegetables, yogurt. Limit Na^+ intake (see Box 4-1 for foods high in Na^+). A low-Na^+ diet helps reduce intestinal absorption of calcium. Limit intake of refined carbohydrates and animal proteins, which cause hypercalciuria. Eat foods high in natural fiber content (e.g., bran, prunes, apples) because they provide phytic acid, which binds dietary calcium. Sodium cellulose phosphate, 5 g three ×/day, may be given *to bind with intestinal calcium and increase excretion of calcium.*
  - **Oxalate stones:** Limit intake of foods high in oxalate, such as chocolate, caffeine-containing drinks (including instant and decaffeinated

coffees), beets, spinach, rhubarb, berries, draft beer, and nuts such as almonds, walnuts, pecans, and cashews. Large doses of pyridoxine may help with certain types of oxalate stones, and cholestyramine, 4 g four ×/day, may be prescribed to bind with oxalate enterally. Vitamin C supplements should be avoided *because as much as half of the vitamin C is converted to oxalic acid.*

- Technique for measuring urine specific gravity via a hydrometer. Specific gravity should remain less than 1.010 to minimize stone formation.
- Technique for using phenaphthazine (Nitrazine) paper to assess pH of urine: desired pH will be determined by type of stone formation to which patient is prone. Instructions for use are on Nitrazine container.

Patient-Family Teaching and Discharge Planning

Include verbal and written information about:

- Medications, including drug names, purpose, dosage, schedule, precautions, and potential side effects. Also discuss drug/drug, herb/drug, and food/drug interactions.
- Indicators of UTI that necessitate medical attention: chills; fever; hematuria; flank, CVA, suprapubic, low back, buttock, scrotal, or labial pain; cloudy and foul-smelling urine; increased frequency, urgency; dysuria; and increasing or recurring incontinence.
- Care of incision or lithotripsy site (if excoriated), including cleansing and dressing; teach patient signs and symptoms of local infection, including redness, swelling, local warmth, tenderness, and purulent drainage.
- Care of drains or catheters if present on discharge.
- Activity restrictions as directed following surgical procedure: avoid lifting heavy objects (nothing greater than 10 lb) for the first 6 wk, be alert to fatigue, get maximum rest, increase activities gradually to tolerance.
- Importance of walking or other exercise to decrease risk of stone formation.

❖ URINARY TRACT OBSTRUCTION

OVERVIEW/PATHOPHYSIOLOGY

Urinary tract obstruction usually is the result of blockage from pelvic tumors, calculi, and urethral strictures. Additional causes include neoplasms, benign prostatic hypertrophy (BPH), ureteral or urethral trauma, inflammation of the urinary tract, pregnancy, and pelvic or colonic surgery in which ureteral damage has occurred. Obstructions can occur suddenly or slowly, over weeks to months. They can occur anywhere along the urinary tract, but the most common sites are the ureteropelvic and ureterovesical junctions, bladder neck, and urethral meatus. The obstruction acts like a dam, blocking passage of urine. Muscles in the area contract to push urine around the obstruction, and structures behind the obstruction begin to dilate. The smaller the site of obstruction, the greater the damage. Obstructions in the lower urinary structures, such as the bladder neck or urethra, can lead to urinary retention and urinary tract infection (UTI). Obstructions in the upper urinary tract can lead to bilateral involvement of the ureters and kidneys that can result in hydronephrosis, renal insufficiency, and kidney destruction. Hydrostatic pressure increases, and filtration and concentration processes in the tubules and glomerulus are compromised.

ASSESSMENT

Signs and symptoms/physical findings: Anuria, nausea, vomiting, local abdominal tenderness, hesitancy, straining to start a stream, dribbling, decreased caliber and force of urinary stream, hematuria, oliguria, and uremia. Pain may be sharp and intense or dull and aching, localized or referred (e.g., flank, low back, buttock, scrotal, labial pain); bladder distention and "kettle drum" sound over bladder with percussion (absent if obstruction is above the bladder); and mass in flank area, abdomen, pelvis, or rectum.

History and risk factors: Recent fever (possibly caused by the obstruction) or hypertensive episodes caused by increased renin production from the body's attempt to increase renal blood flow.

DIAGNOSTIC TESTS

Serum K^+ and Na^+ levels: Determine renal function. Normal range for K^+ is 3.5-5.0 mEq/L; normal range for Na^+ is 137-147 mEq/L.

BUN/creatinine: Evaluate renal-urinary status. Normally, values are elevated in patients with decreased renal-urinary function. These values must be considered based on patient's age and hydration status. For the older adult, serum creatinine level may not be a reliable indicator because of decreased muscle mass and decreased glomerular filtration rate (GFR). Hydration status can affect BUN: fluid volume excess can result in reduced values, whereas volume deficit can cause higher values.

Urinalysis: Provides baseline data on functioning of the urinary system, detects metabolic disease, and assesses for presence of UTI. The following are signals of UTI: cloudy, hazy appearance; foul odor; pH greater than 8.0; and presence of RBCs, leukocyte esterase, WBCs, and WBC casts.

Urine culture: Determines type of bacteria present in the genitourinary tract. The sample should be obtained from midstream collection to minimize contamination.

Hemoglobin (Hgb) and Hematocrit (Hct): Assess for anemia, which may be related to decreased renal secretion or erythropoietin.

Kidney, ureter, bladder (KUB) radiography: Identifies size, shape, and position of the kidneys, ureters, and bladder and abnormalities such as tumors, calculi, or malformations.

Imaging studies: A variety of imaging studies may be used to identify area and cause of obstruction.

Excretory urography/intravenous pyelogram (IVP): Evaluates cause of urinary dysfunction by visualizing the kidneys, renal pelvis, ureters, and bladder.

Antegrade urography: Percutaneous needle or nephrostomy tube is placed after which radiopaque contrast is injected. Antegrade urography is indicated when the kidney does not concentrate or excrete IV dye.

Retrograde urography: Radiopaque dye is injected through ureteral catheters placed during cystoscopy.

Cystogram: Radiopaque dye is instilled via cystoscope or catheter to enable visualization of the bladder and evaluation of the vesicoureteral reflex.

CT scans: Identify degree and location of obstruction, as well as cause in many situations.

Maximal urinary flow rate (MUFR): Less than 15 mL/sec indicates significant obstruction to urine flow.

Postvoid residual (PVR) volume: Normal is less than 12 mL. Higher volume signals obstructive process.

Cystoscopy: Determines degree of bladder outlet obstruction and facilitates visualization of any tumors or masses.

Ultrasonography: Reveals areas of ureteral dilation or distention from retained urine.

COLLABORATIVE MANAGEMENT

The emphasis of collaborative management is on early recognition and relief of the obstruction.

Catheterization: Establishes drainage of urine; may include urethral, ureteral, suprapubic, or percutaneous catheters placed in the renal pelvis.

Pharmacotherapy
Opioids: Relieve pain.

Antispasmodics: Relieve spasms.
Antibiotics: Treat bacterial infections.
Corticosteroids: Reduce local swelling.
IV fluid therapy: For acutely ill or dehydrated patient or to increase fluids in patient with calculi.
Surgically establish drainage: Catheters or drains (ureteral, urethral, suprapubic, or percutaneous) are placed above the point of obstruction.
Surgical removal of obstruction or dilation of strictures: Recurrent strictures may require dilation and placement of a stent or resection with end-to-end anastomosis.

NURSING DIAGNOSES AND INTERVENTIONS

Risk for deficient fluid volume related to postobstructive diuresis
Desired outcomes: Patient is normovolemic as evidenced by heart rate (HR) 100 beats per minute (bpm) or less (or within patient's normal range), BP 90/60 mm Hg or greater (or within patient's normal range), respiratory rate (RR) 20 breaths/min or less; no significant changes in mental status; and orientation to person, place, and time (within patient's normal range). Within 2 days after bladder decompression, output approximates input, patient's urinary output is normal for patient (or 30-60 mL/hr or greater), and weight becomes stable.

Nursing Interventions

♦ Place urinary catheter using sterile technique. *Drains patient's bladder.* Monitor patient carefully during catheterization; clamp the catheter if patient complains of abdominal pain or has a symptomatic drop in SBP of 20 mm Hg or greater. Research has demonstrated that rapid bladder decompression of greater than 750-1000 mL does not result in shock syndrome as previously believed, but it does produce discomfort for patient.
♦ Monitor I&O hourly for 4 hr and then q2h for 4 hr after bladder decompression. Notify health care provider if output exceeds 200 mL/hr or 2 L over an 8-hr period. If this occurs, anticipate initiation of IV infusion. *This can signal postobstructive diuresis, which can lead to major electrolyte imbalance.*
♦ Anticipate need for urine specimens for analysis of electrolytes and osmolality and blood specimens for analysis of electrolytes, *to determine need for replacement or to implement treatments to enhance electrolyte excretion (e.g., K^+).*
♦ Observe for and report indicators of the following:
  • *Hypokalemia:* Abdominal cramps, lethargy, dysrhythmias.
  • *Hyperkalemia:* Diarrhea, colic, irritability, nausea, muscle cramps, weakness, irregular apical or radial pulses.
  • *Hypocalcemia:* Muscle weakness and cramps, complaints of tingling in fingers, Trousseau's and Chvostek's signs.
  • *Hyperphosphatemia:* Excessive itching.
♦ Monitor mentation, noting signs of disorientation. *May indicate electrolyte disturbance.*
♦ Weigh patient daily using same scale and at same time of day (e.g., before breakfast). Weight fluctuations of 2-4 lb (0.9-1.8 kg) normally occur in a patient who is undergoing diuresis.

Acute pain related to bladder spasms
Desired outcome: Within 1 hr of intervention, patient's subjective perception of discomfort decreases, as documented by a pain scale. Objective indicators, such as grimacing, are absent or diminished.

Nursing Interventions

♦ Assess for and document complaints of pain in suprapubic or urethral area. Devise a pain scale with patient, and rate pain from 0 (no pain) to 10 (worst pain). Reassure patient that spasms are normal with obstruction. *Determines pain pattern and extent of pain.*

- Medicate with antispasmodics or analgesics as prescribed. Belladonna and opium (B&O) suppositories may be specifically prescribed *to decrease and/or control bladder spasms.*
- Check catheter and drainage tubing for evidence of obstruction if patient is losing urine around the catheter and has a distended bladder (with or without bladder spasms). Inspect for kinks and obstructions in drainage tubing, compress and roll catheter gently between fingers to assess for gritty matter within catheter, milk drainage tubing to release obstructions, or instruct patient to turn from side to side. Obtain prescription for catheter irrigation if these measures fail *to relieve the obstruction.*
- Encourage intake of fluids to at least 2-3 L/day in nonrestricted patients. *Helps reduce frequency of spasms.*
- Teach nonpharmacologic methods of pain relief. Guided imagery, relaxation techniques, and distraction may be used effectively *to reduce or relieve pain.*

 Patient-Family Teaching and Discharge Planning

When providing patient-family teaching, focus on sensory information, avoid giving excessive information, and initiate a visiting nurse referral for necessary follow-up teaching. Include verbal and written information about the following:

- Medications, including drug names, dosage, purpose, schedule, precautions, and potential side effects. Also discuss drug/drug, herb/drug, and food/drug interactions.
- Indicators that signal recurrent obstruction and require prompt medical attention: pain, fever, decreased urinary output.
- Activity restrictions as directed for patient who has had surgery: avoid lifting heavy objects (nothing greater than 10 lb) for first 6 wk, be alert to fatigue, get maximum rest, increase activities gradually to tolerance.
- Care of drains or catheters if patient is discharged with them; care of surgical incision if present.
- Indicators of wound infection: persistent redness, local warmth, tenderness, drainage, swelling, and fever.
- Indicators of UTI that necessitate medical attention: chills; fever; hematuria; flank, costovertebral angle (CVA), suprapubic, low back, buttock, scrotal, or labial pain; cloudy and foul-smelling urine; increased frequency, urgency; dysuria; and increasing or recurring incontinence.

❖ ❖ ❖

SECTION SIX **URINARY DISORDERS SECONDARY TO OTHER DISEASE PROCESSES**

❖ **URINARY INCONTINENCE**

OVERVIEW/PATHOPHYSIOLOGY

Urinary incontinence is the involuntary loss of urine. The ability to urinate requires complex interactions among the nerve pathways, detrusor muscle, internal sphincter, and external sphincter and a urethral pressure higher than bladder pressure. Urinary incontinence can be short term, caused by an acute illness, or it can be chronic. General causes can be classified as interference with neural control (as in stroke or spinal cord injury [SCI]), interference with bladder function (as in inflammatory states or loss of or increased contractility, constipation or impaction), interference with urethral sphincter mechanism (as in stress incontinence in women or incontinence in men after transurethral resection of the prostate [TURP]), and environmental interferences (such as from radiation therapy or medications such as diuretics or anticholinergics). These conditions manifest as stress, urge, overflow, or functional incontinence or as combinations of two factors.

ASSESSMENT

Signs and symptoms/physical findings: Polyuria; dysuria; low back or flank pain; loss of urine with increased intraabdominal pressure, such as during laughing, sneezing, coughing, lifting; involuntary urination occurring soon after the urge to void is sensed; involuntary passage of urine occurring at predictable intervals; inability to reach commode in time when environmental barriers exist or disorientation occurs; nocturia. Assess for cognitive ability and ability to identify need for toileting and desire to self-toilet, manual dexterity (ability to handle clothing fasteners), mobility (ability to get to a toilet), ability to perform toileting behaviors unaided, living and working conditions, and ability of caregiver to provide care for patient.

History and risk factors: Incontinence occurs when bladder pressure exceeds urethral resistance as a result of structural or musculature weakness or damage. Thus the bladder acts in response to bladder pressure, which becomes higher than that in the urethra. Neurologic dysfunctions, such as Parkinson's disease, stroke, brain injury, normal-pressure hydrocephalus, SCI or spinal cord lesions (a spinal cord lesion above S2 through S4 may result in loss of sensation or awareness of bladder filling because of interruption of the nerve pathways); multiple sclerosis (MS); acute or chronic impairment of cerebral functioning; abdominal or bladder surgery; radiation therapy for bladder cancer; meningitis; impaired mobility; diabetes mellitus (DM) (as a result of autonomic neuropathy and decreased detrusor contractility); multiparity; fecal impaction; low back syndrome; use of caffeine or alcohol; medications such as diuretics, anticholinergics and adrenergic agents, psychotropics, antidepressants, antiparkinsonian agents, phenothiazines, antispasmodics, opioid analgesics, sedatives, hypnotics, and central nervous system (CNS) depressants. Low fluid intake can lead to acidic urine that irritates the bladder, leading to causes bladder spasm and loss of urine.

DIAGNOSTIC TESTS

Urinalysis: Provides baseline data on the functioning of the urinary system, detects metabolic disease, and assesses for the presence of urinary tract infection (UTI). Indicators of UTI are as follows: cloudy or hazy appearance; foul odor; pH greater than 8.0; and presence of RBCs, leukocyte esterase, WBCs, and WBC casts. Obtain urine sample before rectal or genital examination. Urine collected after either examination may be contaminated by vaginal or prostatic secretions. Intermittent catheterization may be required to obtain sample.

Urine culture: Determines type of bacteria present in the genitourinary tract. To minimize risk of contamination, a specimen should be obtained from a midstream collection.

Urodynamic studies: Evaluate cause and extent of the incontinence.

Uroflowmetry: Provides information about bladder strength and opening ability of the urethral sphincter. If detrusor muscle contraction is adequately coordinated with sphincter relaxation, resistance to outlet flow will decrease as pressure within the bladder increases. Normal flow rate in male patients is 20-25 mL/sec, whereas in female patients normal flow rate is 20-30 mL/sec. A flow rate of 15 mL/sec or less indicates voiding dysfunction. Force of the urine stream is tested using a specially designed commode.

Cystometry: Measures pressure-volume relationship of the bladder and provides information on bladder capacity, ability of the bladder to accommodate fluid, patient's ability to sense bladder filling (and temperature of fluid instilled), and presence of an appropriate detrusor muscle contraction. The bladder is filled at a rate of 50 mL/min to its maximum capacity. Normally the bladder fills smoothly without contractions and empties when the individual desires.

Urethral pressure profile: Most helpful in detecting stress incontinence, this test identifies amount of closing pressure the urethra can produce via a dual-tip, microtip, pressure-sensitive catheter, which enables simultaneous measurement of intraurethral and intravesical pressures. The urethral pressure profile identifies either weakness or excessive response in either the internal or the external voluntary sphincter.

Electromyography EMG: Evaluates function of the striated pelvic floor. Results of this test are compared with results of cystometry to identify abnormalities in coordination between bladder and sphincter function.

Postvoid residual (PVR): Measures amount of urine in the bladder after normal voiding. Amounts greater than 100 mL signal retention problems.

BUN/creatinine: Serum values increase as renal-urinary function declines. These values can be affected by hydration status and age. Fluid volume deficit can falsely increase values, whereas fluid volume excess can decrease values. Creatinine values may be misleading in older adults because of loss of muscle mass and decreased glomerular filtration rate (GFR).

COLLABORATIVE MANAGEMENT

The therapy recommended depends on the type and severity of urinary incontinence and may include behavioral interventions, medications, or surgery. The goal of therapy is the promotion of more normal bladder function.

Bladder training: Behavioral therapy that incorporates progressively increased time intervals between voidings. Patient is taught to resist the urge to void and thus delay voiding until a set time. Intervals are set close together initially and then farther apart. Fluid intake also is adjusted. The goal with bladder training is reduction of small voidings.

Habit training: Behavioral therapy in which patient voids according to a set schedule on a planned basis. The schedule is set according to patient's voiding habits. The goal is for patient to remain dry. Habit training differs from bladder training in that there is no attempt to encourage patient to resist or delay voiding, and the caregiver takes the initiative in maintaining the schedule and toileting.

Prompted voidings: Behavioral therapy used in addition to habit training. The caregiver checks patient regularly, asks whether he or she is wet or dry, then requests that patient use the toilet. If successful, positive feedback about maintaining continence is given; if unsuccessful, the caregiver gives no feedback. This technique is used with cognitively impaired or dependent individuals. The goal is to have patient recognize incontinent status and learn to ask for assistance when needed.

Catheter drainage of urine: Either intermittent or continuous.

Vaginal cones: Cone-shaped devices of various weights used to improve pelvic muscle tone and strength in female patients. The cones are inserted intravaginally (light ones first), and patient retains the device using muscle contraction for 15 min twice daily. The cone's weight may provide heightened proprioceptive information to help patient achieve desired pelvic muscle contraction and increase pelvic muscle strength.

Pelvic muscle (Kegel) exercise program: Increases strength of voluntary periurethral and pelvic muscles via exercise of the pubococcygeus muscle. These exercises, which must be performed frequently during the day (e.g., 100 times), are done by tightening paravaginal muscles and anal sphincter as though controlling urination or defecation.

Fluid intake: At least 2-3 L/day in nonrestricted patients.

External (condom) catheter: For male patients, if appropriate.

Surgical procedures to restore bladder-urethral structure: Many surgical procedures may be employed to reestablish normal vesicourethral structure. The most common procedures are as follows:

Urethral suspension (Marshall-Marchetti-Krantz; Stamey) procedure: For stress incontinence. A retropubic urethrovesical resuspension is accomplished via suprapubic transverse incision to lengthen the urethra and thereby create resistance in the urethral lumen. The Pereyra procedure uses both vaginal and suprapubic approaches. Use of Teflon paste injected into periurethral tissues to increase urethral resistance is also being tried.

Pubovaginal sling urethropexy: After a small strip of rectus fascia is harvested through a small suprapubic incision, a transvaginal approach is used. The rectus fascia may be harvested from a cadaver or made of artificial material such as transvaginal tape (TVT). The area lateral to the urethra is joined to the junction of the pelvic floor and overlying symphysis pubis.

Artificial urinary sphincter: See "Neurogenic Bladder" p. 217.

Pharmacotherapy

Anticholinergics or smooth muscle relaxants and tricyclic antidepressants (e.g., oxybutynin, imipramine): May be prescribed for urge incontinence to inhibit uncontrolled bladder contractions and enhance functional bladder capacity. Anticholinergics must be used cautiously in older adults because they can increase occurrences of acute confusion.

Adrenergic drugs (e.g., such as pseudoephedrine, ephedrine, or phenylpropanolamine): Used for stress incontinence. They assist smooth muscle contraction of the bladder neck.

Estrogen therapy: Decreases muscle atrophy and is given for stress incontinence to improve urgency and frequency.

NURSING DIAGNOSES AND INTERVENTIONS

Patients with urinary incontinence may have overlapping conditions. For example, they may experience functional incontinence, which is made more severe by UTI superimposed on urge incontinence.

Stress urinary incontinence related to degenerative changes or weakness in pelvic muscles and structural supports secondary to menopause, childbirth, obesity, or surgical procedure interfering with normal vesicourethral structure

Desired outcome: Patient experiences continence after implementation of bladder training program.

Nursing Interventions

◆ Implement **bladder training program**. *Reduces frequent voiding of small void volumes and fosters a normal urinary elimination pattern.*

◆ Assess and document voiding pattern: time, amount voided, amount of fluid intake, timing of fluid intake followed by voiding, and related information such as degree of wetness experienced (e.g., number of incontinence pads used in a day; degree of underwear dampness) and exertion factor causing the wetness (e.g., laughing, sneezing, bending, lifting). Teach patient to keep a voiding diary that incorporates this information *to obtain information about the type and severity of incontinence.*

◆ Determine amount of time between voidings. Establish a voiding schedule that does not exceed this time period. *Estimates length of time patient can hold urine.*

◆ Assist patient with scheduling times for emptying bladder, such as (initially) q1-2h when awake and q4h at night. If successful, attempt to lengthen time intervals between voidings. Provide patient and significant other with written copy of the schedule. Individuals need to empty their bladders at least q4h *to reduce risk of UTI caused by urinary stasis.*

◆ Estimate and document urinary output when patient is incontinent in clothes or bed linens. A wet spot approximately 2 inches in diameter is equal to approximately 5 mL of urine.

♦ Teach patient to:
- Use techniques that strengthen sphincter and structural supports of the bladder, such as Kegel exercises (see **Deficient knowledge,** p. 213).
- Maintain fluid intake of at least 2-3 L/day if patients is not fluid restricted. Patients with urinary incontinence often reduce their fluid intake to avoid incontinence at the risk of dehydration and UTI.
- Avoid intake of bladder irritants. Caffeine and alcoholic beverages may increase stress incontinence *because they are natural diuretics and irritate the lining of the urinary bladder.*

Urge urinary incontinence related to bladder irritation or reduced bladder capacity secondary to radiation treatment for bladder cancer, UTI, increased urine concentration, use of caffeine or alcohol, or enlarged prostate
Desired outcome: After implementation of the toileting program, patient experiences continence.

Nursing Interventions

♦ Implement **bladder training program**. *Reduces frequent voidings of small amounts and fosters a normal urinary elimination pattern.*
♦ Assess and document usual pattern of voiding, including frequency and timing of incontinent episodes. *Determines type and extent of urinary incontinence.*
♦ Adhere to toileting program (see interventions for **Stress urinary incontinence,** p. 210, earlier).
♦ Teach patient to:
- Increase fluid intake to 2-3 L/day or more if patients not fluid restricted. *Prevents dehydration and UTI in patients who restrict their fluid intake to prevent or control urinary incontinence.*
- Avoid intake of natural diuretics and bladder irritants *to help decrease incontinence from bladder irritation.*
- Minimize occurrence of UTIs. Encourage intake of cranberry, blueberry, prunes, or plum juice. *They leave an acid ash in the urine and decrease microbial adherence to the bladder wall.*
- Decrease fluid intake a few hours before bedtime and void before sleep. *Prevents sleep disruption.*
- Take deep, slow breaths *to decrease urge to void when it occurs prematurely.*
♦ Keep urinal or bedpan at the bedside and instruct patient in its use. *Allows patient easy access to toileting.*
♦ Label bathroom door with signs that denote toilet to patient, such as a picture of a commode for patients who are ambulatory but have cognitive impairment. Adhere closely to toileting program and remind patient to void at scheduled intervals. *Serves as toileting cue.*
♦ Administer prescribed anticholinergics or smooth muscle relaxants. *Inhibits detrusor contractions and decreases detrusor instability.*

Functional urinary incontinence related to sensory, cognitive, or mobility deficits or related to environmental changes
Desired outcome: After implementation of habit training program, patient becomes continent.

Nursing Interventions

♦ Implement **habit training program**. Establishes a planned schedule for voiding *to reduce episodes of incontinence.*
♦ Assess and document pattern of voiding: time, amount voided, amount of fluid intake, and timing of fluid intake followed by voiding and other related factors. *Determines extent of functional incontinence.*
♦ Offer bedpan, urinal, or assistance to the bathroom at least q2h *to facilitate continence.*

◆ Maintain planned schedule for voiding. Note time of any incontinent episode that occurs between scheduled voidings. If patient's incontinence pattern consistently does not match voiding schedule, change the voiding schedule *to facilitate continence.*

◆ Determine environmental obstacles that prevent patient from toileting appropriately, and intervene accordingly. Remove obstacles between bed and bathroom, leave a light on in bathroom, and attach call light to bed sheet *to facilitate toileting and continence.*

◆ Monitor for increased need to void after taking medications such as diuretics. *These drugs increase urine production or sensation of urgency.*

◆ Administer diuretics in the morning or early afternoon. *Reduces the risk of nighttime incontinence.*

◆ Consult with health care provider about advisability of reducing infusion rate at night for patients with IV infusions. *Reduces risk of nighttime incontinence.*

◆ Keep call light within reach and answer call quickly for bedridden patients. *Reduces risk of incontinence.*

◆ Keep a clock and calendar in room and remind patient of the time and date as appropriate when patient is bedridden. *Toilet patient as described to reduce risk of incontinence.*

◆ Reorient to baseline and toilet patient as described previously if patient has permanent or severe cognitive impairment. *Reduces risk of incontinence.*

◆ Monitor patient's bowel function and status. *Constipation or impaction can cause symptoms of incontinence (e.g., dribbling).*

Risk for impaired skin integrity related to incontinence of urine
Desired outcome: Patient's perineal skin remains intact.

Nursing Interventions

◆ Assess for perineal area wetness at frequent intervals. Advise patient to alert staff as soon as wetness occurs. *Prolonged exposure to urine can cause skin breakdown.*

◆ Keep bed linen dry. As necessary, use and change absorbent materials such as protective underwear or underpads *to prevent urine contact with skin.*

◆ Keep perineum clean with mild soap and water; dry it well. Removes urine from skin and prevents moisture, *which helps reduce risk for skin breakdown.*

◆ Expose perineum to air whenever possible. Use a sheet draped over a bed cradle; ensure privacy. *Prevents skin irritation from excess moisture.*

◆ Use sealants and moisture-barrier ointments. *Protects skin.*

◆ Make sure plastic pads or sheet protectors do not contact patient's skin directly. Cover these pads with pillowcases, or place them under sheets *to reduce risk for maceration resulting from perspiration caused by plastic pads or sheets.*

◆ Educate patient in use of containment devices such as briefs with pads, adult absorptive briefs, and external catheters. *Protects skin from urine.*

Distorbed body image related to odor, discomfort, and embarrassment secondary to incontinence
Desired outcomes: After intervention(s), patient verbalizes feelings and frustrations without self-deprecating statements. Within the 24-hr period before hospital discharge, patient verbalizes knowledge about actions that will control either incontinence or odor and discomfort.

Nursing Interventions

◆ Encourage patient to discuss feelings and frustrations. *Helps patient recognize and resolve anxiety or negative feelings about changes in body image.*

◆ Offer reassurance and encouragement but be realistic with patient. *Provides information about treatment, especially about those activities that are within patient's own control.* If incontinence cannot be controlled, reassure that odor and discomfort can be controlled *to help reduce anxiety about incontinence.*

◆ Explore with patient methods for relief of discomfort and odor control. Methods include maintenance of good hygiene, frequent changes of undergarments, use and frequent changes of incontinence pads.

◆ Suggest that patient limit fluids when away from home environment and increase them on return. Although fluid intake of at least 2-3 L/day is essential for minimizing risk of UTI, fluid intake can be scheduled to reduce risk of incontinence. A decrease can also be incorporated into evening hours *to prevent nighttime incontinence.*

Deficient knowledge related to pelvic muscle (Kegel) exercise program to strengthen perineal muscles (effective for individuals with mild to moderate stress incontinence or for those with functional incontinence who are able to participate)
Desired outcome: Within the 24-hr period before hospital discharge, patient verbalizes and demonstrates knowledge about the pelvic muscle (Kegel) exercise program.

Nursing Interventions

◆ Assess patient's facility with language, and engage an interpreter or provide language-appropriate written materials if necessary.

◆ Teach patient Kegel exercises, and help patient identify the correct muscle group. A common error in attempting to identify the correct muscle group is contraction of the buttocks, quadriceps, and abdominal muscles. *Kegel exercises strengthen pelvic area muscles and thereby help patient regain bladder control.*
  - Proximal muscle: instruct patient to attempt to shut off urinary flow after beginning urination, hold for a few seconds, and then start the stream again. When this is accomplished, the correct muscle is being exercised.
  - Distal muscle: instruct patient to contract the muscle around the anus as though to stop a bowel movement.

◆ Teach patient to repeat Kegel exercises 10-20 times, 4×/day. These exercises may need to be done for 2-9 mo before any benefit is obtained.

◆ Use elastic mold to provide quantitative feedback on muscle strengthening process. For female patients it is possible to make a cast of the vagina from which an elastic mold can be created. This mold can be attached to a manometer, to allow patient visual evidence of her ability to contract muscles in the pelvic floor to compress the vagina and feedback on her progress in strengthening these muscles.

Deficient knowledge related to use of external (condom) catheter
Desired outcome: Within the 24-hr period before hospital discharge, patient or significant other successfully returns demonstration of condom catheter application and verbalizes knowledge about the rationale for its use.

Nursing Interventions

◆ Use external and internal catheters only if other methods of achieving urinary incontinence have failed. *The use of both catheter types is associated with increased frequency of UTI.*

◆ Assess patient's facility with language, and engage an interpreter or provide language-appropriate written materials if necessary.

◆ Teach male patient/significant other:
  - The procedure for application of a condom catheter. *Correct application prevents incontinence and skin compromise.*

- The importance of keeping pubic hair trimmed or moved away from penis. *Avoids contact between pubic hair and adhesive used with catheter.*
- To cleanse and dry penis thoroughly before and after every condom application. With uncircumcised patients, foreskin should be retracted to cleanse area under prepuce and then returned to its original position. *Drying the penis helps prevent skin breakdown.*

◆ Demonstrate, to ambulatory patients, connecting condom catheter to a leg drainage bag. For patients on bed rest, demonstrate connecting catheter to a bedside urinary collection container, such as that used with an indwelling catheter *to ensure dependent drainage of urine.*

◆ Advise patient to remove and replace catheter as directed. Most manufacturers recommend that external catheters be changed and replaced daily.

◆ Suggest that condom catheter be used only during the night if appropriate for patient. *Reduces the risk for nighttime incontinence.*

Patient-Family Teaching and Discharge Planning

When providing patient-family teaching, focus on sensory information, avoid giving excessive information, and initiate a visiting nurse referral for necessary follow-up teaching. Include verbal and written information about:

◆ Keeping a voiding record for at-home use, to document accurate information about frequency and timing of incontinent episodes.

◆ Medications, including drug names, dosage, purpose, schedule, precautions, and potential side effects. Also discuss drug/drug, herb/drug, and food/drug interactions.

◆ Diet: include importance of increasing dietary fiber to help prevent constipation and keep stools soft. Constipation leads to straining, which weakens sphincter tone. Provide fact sheet that lists foods high in fiber. Demonstrate with sample menus how dietary fiber may be incorporated into daily meals.

◆ Indicators of UTI that necessitate medical attention: chills; fever; hematuria; flank, costovertebral angle (CVA), low back, buttock, scrotal, or labial pain; cloudy and foul-smelling urine; increased frequency and urgency; dysuria; increasing or recurring incontinence.

◆ Care of catheters and drains if patient is discharged with them.

◆ Importance of maintaining fluid intake of at least 2-3 L/day and avoiding caffeine and alcohol, which act as bladder irritants and increase risk of urgency.

◆ Maintenance of schedule for bladder training program.

◆ Use of perineal muscle to improve bladder tone.

◆ Care of perineal skin.

◆ Care of incision, including cleansing and dressing, and indicators of infection: fever, tenderness, purulent drainage, persistent redness, swelling, warmth along incision line for surgical patients.

◆ Activity restrictions: no heavy lifting (nothing greater than 10 lb); resting when fatigued. Explain that prolonged periods of sitting can cause relaxation of bladder and sphincter musculature and can lead to incontinence. Encourage mild activity, such as walking, to improve muscle tone.

◆ Phone numbers to call if questions or concerns arise about therapy after discharge.

◆ Support groups (see **Body image disturbed:,** p. 212) or access:

National Association for Continence: www.nafc.org

The Simon Foundation for Continence: www.simonfoundation.org

❖ URINARY RETENTION

OVERVIEW/PATHOPHYSIOLOGY

Urinary retention occurs when urine is produced and accumulates in the bladder but is not released. In the acute care setting, urinary retention is most commonly seen as a postoperative complication after surgical procedures using general or spinal anesthesia.

ASSESSMENT

Signs and symptoms/physical findings: Sudden inability to void, intense suprapubic pain, restlessness, diaphoresis, voiding small amounts (20-50 mL) at frequent intervals. "Kettle drum" sound with bladder percussion, bladder distention, bladder displacement to one side of abdomen.

History and risk factors: urinary tract infection (UTI), obstruction (e.g., from benign prostatic hypertrophy (BPH), tumor, calculi, urethral stricture, fibrosis, meatal stenosis, or fecal impaction), cystocele, rectocele, decreased sensory stimulation to the bladder, anxiety or muscular tension, medications (e.g., opiates, sedatives, antihistamines, antispasmodics, major tranquilizers and antidepressants, and antidyskinetics).

DIAGNOSTIC TESTS

Urinalysis: Provides baseline data regarding urinary system function, detects metabolic disease, and detects presence of UTI. Signs of UTI are as follows: cloudy or hazy appearance; foul odor; pH greater than 8.0; and presence of RBCs, leukocyte esterase, WBCs, and WBC casts.

Urine culture: Determines type of bacteria present in the genitourinary tract. To minimize contamination, a midstream specimen should be collected. If patient is unable to urinate, a specimen can be obtained by intermittent catheterization.

BUN/creatinine: Evaluate renal-urinary function. *Generally, serum values increase in the presence of dysfunction.* BUN values are affected by patient's hydration status: fluid volume excess can result in decreased values, whereas volume deficit can result in increased values. Creatinine may not be a reliable indicator of renal function in the older adult because of decreased muscle mass and decreased glomerular filtration rate (GFR).

Cystoscopy: A lighted tubular scope is inserted into the bladder to allow visualization of potential sources of obstruction (e.g., strictures, calculi, malformations, or masses).

Cystogram: Radiopaque dye is instilled into the bladder via cystoscope or catheter to enable visualization of the bladder and evaluation of the vesicoureteral reflex.

Cystometrogram: Water or saline is instilled into the bladder via a catheter to create pressure against the bladder wall to evaluate bladder tone.

Kidney, ureter, bladder (KUB) radiography: Identifies size, shape, and position of the kidneys, ureters, and bladder and abnormalities such as tumors, calculi, or malformations.

Excretory urograms/intravenous pyelogram (IVP): Visualize kidney, renal pelvis, ureters, and bladder to assess for the cause of urinary dysfunction.

COLLABORATIVE MANAGEMENT

The focus of collaborative management is on catheterization to drain urine and treatment of the underlying cause.

Pharmacotherapy

Cholinergics: Stimulate bladder contractions.

Analgesics: Relieve pain.

Antibiotics: For infection if present.

IV therapy: Provide hydration of the acutely ill patient.

Surgery: Performed if obstruction is the cause of the retention (see "Urinary Tract Obstruction," p. 204).

NURSING DIAGNOSES AND INTERVENTIONS

Urinary retention related to weak detrusor muscle, blockage, inhibition of reflex arc, or strong sphincter

Desired outcomes: Patient reports a normal voiding pattern within 2 days or, if appropriate, patient demonstrates self-catheterization before hospital discharge.

Nursing Interventions

◆ Assess bladder for distention by inspection, percussion, and palpation . *Helps detect urine retention.*

◆ Measure and document I&O. *Determines effectiveness of treatment.*

◆ Implement noninvasive measures to aid patient in voiding when appropriate: position patient in a normal position for voiding; have patient listen to sound of running water or place hands in a basin of warm water; pour warm water over the perineum after measuring water if patient's I&O are documented. *Facilitates urination.*

◆ Avoid use of Credé's method (application of pressure from umbilicus to pubis). Credé's method *increases potential for reflux up the ureter that can lead to renal compromise.*

◆ Maintain privacy for patient who is trying to use commode, bedpan, or urinal; use a plastic or warmed bedpan; and encourage relaxation such as deep breathing or visualization. *Cold bedpans can cause muscle tension. Relaxation facilitates voiding.*

◆ Provide adequate amount of time (up to 10 min) for patient's urge to void to occur. *Rushing produces anxiety, which inhibits patient's ability to urinate.*

◆ Notify health care provider of inability to void, bladder distention, or suprapubic or urethral pain. *These findings indicate urinary retention.*

◆ Monitor patient's bowel function and status. *Constipation and impaction can cause urinary retention.*

◆ Perform urinary catheterization as needed. *Decompresses patient's urinary bladder and relieves retention.*

◆ Clamp catheter if patient complains of abdominal pain or has a symptomatic drop in SBP greater than 20 mm Hg during catheterization procedure. Leave catheter clamped until patient's SBP returns to within normal limits. Research has demonstrated that rapid bladder decompression of greater than 750-1000 mL does not result in shock syndrome, as previously believed.

◆ Use a coudé (bent tip) catheter instead of a straight catheter for men suspected of having BPH or in those over 65 yr of age. The tip of the coudé catheter is stiff and is easier to insert through the prostate gland. Lubricate catheter tip generously with a minimum of 5 mL of lubricating jelly before insertion. Insert catheter with bent tip pointing up to aid its movement through the urethra, *to facilitate catheterization.*

Patient-Family Teaching and Discharge Planning

Include verbal and written information about:

◆ Medications, including drug names, purpose, dosage, schedule, precautions, and potential side effects. Also discuss drug/drug, herb/drug, and food/drug interactions.

◆ Indicators of UTI and recurrent retention that necessitate medical attention: chills; fever; hematuria; flank, costovertebral angle (CVA), suprapubic, low back, buttock, scrotal, or labial pain; cloudy and foul-smelling urine; increased frequency, urgency; dysuria; increasing or recurring incontinence; increasing or recurring difficulty in voiding; and inability to urinate when feeling urge.

◆ Clean technique for self-catheterization technique, if appropriate.

❖ NEUROGENIC BLADDER

OVERVIEW/PATHOPHYSIOLOGY

Neurogenic bladder, also known as neuromuscular bladder dysfunction, neurologic bladder dysfunction, and neuropathic bladder disorder, is a complex phenomenon resulting from disruption of nerve impulse transmission from the bladder to the brain. Caused by a myriad of diseases, injuries, or lesions, interruption of transmission occurs in the central nervous system (CNS) within the brain or spinal cord. Certain conditions leave the sacral reflex intact while affecting the ability of the brain to receive or interpret the signal.

Conditions such as multiple sclerosis (MS), stroke, dementia, tumors, and spinal cord lesions above level T12 lead to reflex or uninhibited bladder control. Signal interruption at the spinal level leads to an autonomic neurogenic bladder, from which patient has no sensation of the need to void and no micturition reflex. Voiding occurs irregularly, and patient has no voluntary control of voiding. Lack of nerve impulse transmission for muscle control results in loss of bladder contraction and leads to overflow incontinence.

Conditions leading to overflow incontinence include sacral cord trauma, tumors, transection of pelvic parasympathetic nerves during abdominal surgery, and herniated intervertebral disk disease. Loss of the sensation to void results in atonic bladder as evidenced by dribbling, voiding in small amounts, or complaints of loss of sensation of bladder fullness. Atonic bladder occurs with damage to posterior (sensory) nerve roots or neuropathy associated with diabetes mellitus (DM).

ASSESSMENT

Signs and symptoms/physical findings
Upper motor neuron disturbance (spastic bladder): Urinary frequency, residual urine, urinary retention, recurrent urinary tract infections (UTIs), spontaneous loss of urine, urge incontinence, and lack of urinary control.
Lower motor neuron disturbance (flaccid bladder): Urinary retention, recurrent UTIs, inability to perceive need to void.
History and risk factors: spinal cord injury (SCI), spinal tumor, MS, DM, stroke, Parkinson's disease, Alzheimer's disease, herpes zoster.

DIAGNOSTIC TESTS

Urinalysis: Provides baseline data on urinary system functioning, detects metabolic disease, and assesses for presence of UTI, which further irritates the bladder. (See "Urinary Tract Infection (Cystitis)," p. 197.)
Urine culture: Determines type of bacteria present in the genitourinary tract.
Urodynamic studies: Evaluate cause and extent of incontinence.
Uroflowmetry: Provides information about bladder strength and opening ability of urethral sphincter. If detrusor muscle contraction is adequately coordinated with sphincter relaxation, resistance to outlet flow will decrease as pressure within the bladder increases. Normal flow rate in male patients is 20-25 mL/sec, whereas in female patients normal flow rate is 20-30 mL/sec. A flow rate of 15 mL/sec or less indicates voiding dysfunction. Urine stream force is tested using a specially designed commode.
Cystometry: Measures the bladder's pressure-volume relationship. The bladder is filled at a rate of 50 mL/min to its maximum capacity. Normally the bladder will fill smoothly without contractions and empty when the individual desires. Cystometry provides information on bladder capacity, ability of the bladder to accommodate fluid, patient's ability to sense bladder filling (and temperature of fluid instilled), and presence of appropriate detrusor muscle contraction.
Urethral pressure profile: Most helpful in detecting stress incontinence, this test identifies amount of closing urethral sphincteric pressure. Urethral

pressure profile identifies either weakness or excessive response in either the internal or external voluntary sphincter. (See "Urinary Incontinence," p. 207).
Electromyography (EMG): Evaluates function of striated pelvic floor. Results of this test are compared with results from cystometry to identify abnormalities in coordination between the bladder and sphincter function.
Postvoid residual (PVR): Patient is catheterized 15-20 min after voiding to assess for residual urine (amounts greater than 100 mL signal urinary retention).
Cystoscopy: Determines loss of muscle fibers and elastic tissue.
Pad test: Documents urine loss. Dye is administered (intravesical methylene blue [Urised] or oral phenazopyridine [Pyridium]). Patient wears perineal pad during normal activities. Blue or orange staining of pad indicates urine loss.

COLLABORATIVE MANAGEMENT

Pharmacotherapy
Parasympatholytics or anticholinergics: Commonly used drugs are oxybutynin, dicyclomine, methantheline bromide, and tolterodine. May not be well tolerated over time because of side effects, which can be reduced if drugs are alternated.
Parasympathomimetics (e.g., bethanechol chloride): Treats hypotonic bladders by increasing bladder tone.
Antispasmodics (e.g., trospium, solifenacin succinate, darifenacin, oxybutynin chloride): Relax smooth muscles of bladder and may decrease incontinences. May not be well tolerated because of sedative effects.
Antibiotics: Treat infection, if present.
Catheterization: Either intermittent or continuous.
Increased fluid intake: Prevents infection, minimizes calcium concentration in urine, and prevents formation of urinary calculi (optimal intake is 3 L/day).
Increased mobility: Augments renal blood flow and minimizes urinary stasis.
Low-calcium diet: Prevents calculus formation.
Neuroprosthetics (bladder pacemaker): Electrodes are implanted on ventral (motor) nerve roots of the sacral nerves that will produce detrusor contraction when stimulated. These electrodes are then connected to a subcutaneous receiver that can be controlled from outside the body. The bladder can be controlled selectively by the external transmitter.
Continent vesicostomy: Surgical closure of the bladder's urethral neck to form an internal reservoir for urine and to create an opening or valve in the bladder wall so that patient can insert a catheter intermittently to remove urine.
Artificial urinary sphincter implantation: Surgical placement of a hydraulically activated sphincter mechanism around the bladder neck or urethra. To empty the bladder, patient activates the device by squeezing the bulbs, which are implanted under the labia or in the scrotum.
Urethral occlusive devices: Artificial device used to block urethra. Must be frequently removed and are easily dislodged into the bladder or toilet.

NURSING DIAGNOSES AND INTERVENTIONS

Reflex urinary incontinence related to neurologic impairment secondary to injury or disease
Desired outcomes: Patient or significant other participates in a habit training program. Patient experiences a decrease in or absence of incontinent episodes.

Nursing Interventions
- Implement habit training program. (See "Urinary Incontinence," p. 207.)
- Monitor for bladder retention by assessing I&O, inspecting suprapubic area, and percussing and palpating the bladder. Be alert to presence of swelling proximal to symphysis pubis, a "kettle drum" sound (like tapping

on the side of a plastic gallon container of milk) with percussion of lower abdomen, and dribbling of urine.

- Teach patient techniques that stimulate voiding reflex, if appropriate. Examples are tapping suprapubic area with fingers, pulling pubic hair, and digitally stretching anal sphincter. The last technique is effective because rectal nerves follow basically the same path as for the urethral nerves; however, this maneuver is contraindicated in patients with SCI at or above T6 because it can cause autonomic dysreflexia (AD) (see "Autonomic dysreflexia," immediately following). Valsalva's maneuver also can be used to stimulate voiding: patient bears down as though having a bowel movement *to increase intrathoracic and intraabdominal pressure and to stimulate voiding.*

- Instruct patient to deflate valve q4h when artificial inflatable sphincter is used. Remind patient to wear a MedicAlert tag or bracelet to alert emergency personnel to presence and use of the device. *Allows the bladder to empty.*

- Provide condom care when condom catheter is used. See **Deficient knowledge**: related to external (condom) catheter in "Urinary Incontinence," p. 207, for appropriate nursing interventions.

- Teach care of penile clamp when male patient has extensive sphincter damage and penile clamp is prescribed. Before and after use, instruct patient (or significant other) to cleanse penis with soap and water, dry it thoroughly, and sprinkle powder along shaft. Explain that the clamp is placed horizontally behind the glans after voiding and is removed q3h. Stress importance of inspecting skin for redness along area where clamp presses. If breakdown occurs (i.e., redness does not disappear after massage), use of clamp must be discontinued. If swelling appears along the glans, advise patient to set clamp at a looser setting. Penile clamp must be alternated with condom catheter to minimize injury.

- Teach intermittent catheterization procedure to patient or significant other if prescribed. Emphasize need to follow a routine (e.g., q4h) *to minimize potential for UTI caused by stasis and bladder distention.*

- Encourage fluid intake of at least 2-3 L/day for nonrestricted patients. *Dilutes urine and increases output, thereby minimizing risk of developing infection and calculi.*

- Encourage as much mobility as patient can tolerate. *Helps prevent urinary stasis, which can lead to UTI. Also increases cardiac output, which nourishes the kidneys.*

- Administer diuretics, if prescribed, in the morning or early afternoon. *Reduces risk for nighttime incontinence.*

- For patients requiring IV infusions, consult with health care provider about advisability of reducing infusion rate at night. *Minimizes risk of nighttime incontinence.*

- Use visual toileting clues for patients with cognitive impairment. Cues, such as a sign on bathroom door that says "Toilet" or shows a picture of a toilet, *may facilitate continence.*

Autonomic dysreflexia (or risk for same) related to distended bladder
Desired outcomes: Patient is free of the indicators of AD. Patient and significant other verbalize understanding of indicators, prevention, and treatment of AD.

Nursing Interventions

Monitor for signs of AD. AD is a life-threatening condition that can occur in patients with neurogenic bladder, especially those with SCI at or above level T8. Signs of AD include headache, bradycardia, excessively high BP, blurred vision, flushing and sweating above level of injury, piloerection and pallor below level of injury, and nausea, and nasal congestion.

◆ Treat AD immediately. *Raise head of bed (HOB) immediately to help lower BP, and assess for bladder distention. Have patient empty bladder in accustomed manner, or check for patency of indwelling catheter.*

◆ Avoid catheter irrigation. Irrigation of urinary catheter can increase bladder pressure and intensify AD. If catheter is obstructed, either recatheterize patient using liberal amounts of anesthetic jelly or irrigate catheter gently, using 30 mL or less of normal saline in accordance with agency policy.

◆ Monitor BP for trends. Continuing increases in BP can be life-threatening and can lead to stroke, status epilepticus, and death.

◆ Administer appropriate medications as prescribed. Phenoxybenzamine hydrochloride is a long-acting vasodilator that increases blood flow to skin, mucosa, and abdominal viscera and lowers both standing and supine BP. Notify health care provider if symptoms do not disappear after bladder is emptied, if bladder is full and cannot be emptied, or if medication does not relieve symptoms.

◆ Encourage fluid intake of at least 2-3 L/day. *Dilutes urine and increases output and thereby minimizes risk of developing AD, infection, or calculi.*

◆ Encourage as much mobility as patient can tolerate. *Helps prevent urinary stasis, which can lead to UTI and consequently to AD.*

◆ Monitor bowel elimination pattern. *Reduces risk of impaction; fecal impaction can either cause AD itself or contribute to urinary retention leading to AD.*

◆ Teach patient and significant others indicators, prevention, and treatment of AD. Patient/significant other needs to understand the importance of seeking help immediately *to facilitate the prompt implementation of treatment.* (See **Autonomic dysreflexia** (or risk for same) in "Spinal Cord Injury," p. 294.)

Total urinary incontinence related to neuropathy preventing transmission of reflex indicating bladder fullness or related to lower motor neuron disturbance secondary to SCI below S3-S4
Desired outcomes: Patient or significant other follows habit training program; incontinent episodes decrease to less than 3/wk.

Nursing Interventions

◆ Implement habit training. (See "Urinary Incontinence," p. 207.)

◆ Administer diuretics in the morning or early afternoon. *Reduces risk for nighttime incontinence.*

◆ If patient has an IV infusion, consult with health care provider about advisability of reducing infusion rate at night. *Reduces risk for nighttime incontinence.*

◆ Provide information about incontinence aids. Aids such as incontinence pads and easy-to-remove clothing *facilitate dryness and may protect the skin.*

◆ Demonstrate use of external (condom) catheters to male patients for nighttime use (see "Urinary Incontinence," p. 207).

◆ Implement skin protection measures. *Protects skin from excoriation from long-term exposure to urine.* (See "Urinary Incontinence," p. 207.)

Deficient knowledge related to function and care of long-term indwelling catheters after continent vesicostomy (continent urinary reservoir)
Desired outcomes: Before continent vesicostomy, patient verbalizes rationale for use of a suprapubic catheter and vesicostomy tube, including approximate amount of time the devices will be indwelling. Within the 24-hr period before hospital discharge, patient or significant other demonstrates proficiency with intermittent catheterization, tube irrigation, and dressing changes.

Nursing Interventions

♦ Assess patient's facility with language. Engage an interpreter or provide language-appropriate written materials if necessary.

♦ Preoperatively, explain what patient should expect following surgery. Patient will return from surgery with a suprapubic catheter and vesicostomy tube in place. *Helps eliminate anxiety and fear.*

♦ Explain that patient will be discharged with catheter and readmitted for catheter removal in approximately 6 wk. After removal of indwelling catheter, intermittent catheterization will be performed hourly, progressing to 2-4 hr and ultimately to 4-6 hr. Continuous drainage will be used overnight. After removing indwelling catheter, ensure that patient or significant other demonstrates proficiency with:

  • Washing hands with soap and water before catheterization.
  • Selecting a clean catheter and placing it on a clean paper towel.
  • Cleaning stoma site with warm water and removing mucus that has drained from stoma.
  • Inserting catheter carefully into stoma and draining bladder of urine. Lubricants usually are not necessary. However, if lubrication is needed, teach patient to use a product that is water soluble—*never* products made from petroleum jelly, *which can damage the catheter.*
  • If mucus clogs catheter, removing catheter from stoma, rinsing it with hot water, and reinserting catheter to continue drainage.

♦ Encourage patient's participation in care, including tube irrigation, which removes mucus from the pouch, and dressing changes. *Facilitates evaluation of patient learning.*

♦ Demonstrate procedure for irrigation when prescribed. Typically, sterile normal saline (30-50 mL) is used for irrigation. Instruct patient to wash hands before handling catheters and to cleanse around catheter site daily with warm water *to prevent contamination.*

 Patient-Family Teaching and Discharge Planning

Include verbal and written information.

♦ Teach patients with artificial sphincters indicators of UTI and erosion: pain, fever, swelling, urinary retention, or incontinence.

♦ Teach patients with indwelling catheters how to care for drainage bags.

♦ Teach patients who require intermittent catheterization how to clean catheters for reuse.

♦ Provide phone numbers to call if questions or concerns arise about therapy or condition after discharge.

♦ Provide information about additional resources such as:

National Kidney Disease Education Program (NKDEP): www.nkdep.nih.gov/

National Kidney Foundation: www.kidney.org

SECTION SEVEN **URINARY DIVERSIONS**

OVERVIEW/PATHOPHYSIOLOGY

A urinary diversion is created when the bladder must be bypassed or is removed. Bladder cancer is the most common reason for creating a urinary diversion. However, malignancies of the prostate, urethra, vagina, uterus, or cervix may require creation of a urinary diversion if anterior, posterior, or total pelvic exenteration must be done. Individuals with severe, nonmalignant urinary problems, such as radiation damage to the bladder, vesicovaginal fistula, urethrovaginal fistula, neurogenic bladder, radiation or interstitial cystitis, or urinary incontinence that cannot be managed conservatively, also are candidates for urinary diversion. A radical cystectomy may or may not accompany placement of a urinary diversion. Although most urinary diversions are permanent, some act as a temporary bypass of urine, and reversal (undiversion) can be performed if patient's condition changes.

The urinary stream may be diverted at multiple points: the renal pelvis (pyelostomy or nephrostomy), the ureter (ureterostomy), the bladder (vesicostomy), or via an intestinal "conduit." Cutaneous ureterostomy was the diversion most commonly performed in the past; however, construction of a small bowel pouch (Kock procedure) or ileocolonic pouch (Indiana or Mainz procedure) is now the most common type of urinary diversion. These procedures reconstruct a new bladder from intestinal segments, and result in a more normal urinary pattern. Vesicostomies are most commonly performed in children as a temporary diversion.

Intestinal (ileal) conduit: Any segment of bowel may be used to create a passageway for urine, but the ileum conduit is most commonly used. A 15- to 20-cm section of the ileum is resected from the intestine to form a passageway for the urine. The proximal end is closed, and the distal end is brought out through the abdomen, to form a stoma. The ureters are resected from the bladder and anastomosed to the ileal segment. The intestine is reanastomosed, and therefore bowel function is unaffected. Occasionally, the jejunum is used for the conduit. However, jejunal-conduit syndrome (hyperkalemia, hyponatremia, hypochloremia) often occurs.

Cutaneous ureterostomy: The ureters are resected from the bladder and are brought out through the surface of the abdomen, either separately or with one attached to the other inside the body, thus resulting in only one abdominal stoma. Typically, the stoma is flush with the abdomen rather than protruding. Stenosis and ascending urinary tract infections (UTIs) are common problems with this diversion.

Continent urinary diversion (reservoir): There are several different continent procedures, but the two most commonly performed are the Indiana reservoir and the Kock continent urostomy. All continent urinary diversions are constructed with the following three components: a reservoir or reconstructed bladder, a continence mechanism, and an antireflux mechanism. For example, the Indiana reservoir uses 15-18 cm of the distal ileum and 20-24 cm of the cecum sutured together to create the pouch, which eventually stores up to 800 mL of urine. The antireflux mechanism is established via use of the ileocecal valve, which acts as a one-way valve keeping urine in the reservoir until a catheter is passed through the skin-level stoma. The presence of a tapered ileal segment further strengthens the continence mechanism by creating increased resistance to urine outflow pressures. The ureters are attached at an angle to the wall of the cecum, to prevent reflux of urine to the kidneys. Because male patients have an external urinary sphincter that can be left in place when the bladder is removed, men may undergo attachment of a reconstructed bladder to the urethra, which permits urination without use of catheterization. However, there is a 5%-10% risk of urethral recurrence of neoplasm with this procedure.

Orthotopic urinary diversion: Creates a pseudobladder from the ileum to which the urethra is attached to reestablish lower urinary tract function. Because this procedure requires an intact and functional external urethral sphincter, it is possible more often in male than female patients.

NURSING DIAGNOSES AND INTERVENTIONS

Anxiety related to threat to self-concept and/or interaction patterns, or fears regarding health status secondary to urinary diversion surgery

Desired outcomes: Before surgery, patient communicates fears and concerns, relates attainment of increased psychologic and physical comfort, and exhibits effective coping mechanisms.

Nursing Interventions

- Assess patient's perceptions of the impending surgery and resulting body function changes *to identify misconceptions that may increase fear or anxiety.*
- Provide opportunities for patient to express fears and concerns (e.g., "You seem very concerned about next week's surgery"). *Allows patient to identify factors that are causing anxiety or fear, and allows for early intervention to alleviate fears/anxiety.*
- Listen actively and acknowledge patient's fears and concerns. Recognize that anger, denial, withdrawal, and demanding behaviors may be coping responses.
- Provide brief, basic information regarding physiology of the procedure and equipment that will be used after surgery, including tubes and drains. Anxiety decreases patient's ability to remember, hence the need for repeating information. Providing information about what patient can expect *decreases fear of the unknown.*
- Show patient pouches that will be used after surgery. Assure patient that the pouch usually cannot be seen through clothing and that it is odor resistant, *to decrease anxiety and fears.*
- Explain that a pouching system may be needed for a short time after surgery if continent urostomy is being performed. Assure patient that teaching about accessing the continent urostomy will be done before hospital discharge, *to alleviate fear about permanence of urinary diversion.*
- Inquire about information that has been relayed by the surgeon about sexual implications of the surgery. Some male patients undergoing radical cystectomy with urinary diversion may become impotent, but more recent surgical advances have enabled preservation of potency for others. The pelvic plexus, which innervates the corpora cavernosa (and allows penile erection), may be damaged permanently. Autonomic nerve damage results in loss of erection and ejaculation; however, because sensation and orgasm are mediated by the pudendal nerve (sensorimotor), they are not affected. *Helps establish an open patient-nurse relationship and provides feedback about whether or not the information provided was understood.*
- Arrange for a preoperative visit by the enterostomal therapy (ET) nurse. The ET nurse will collaborate with the patient and surgeon to identify and mark the most appropriate site for the stoma. Showing patient the actual spot for placement may *help alleviate anxiety by reinforcing that impact on lifestyle and body image will be minimal.*

Risk for impaired skin integrity related to presence of urine or sensitivity to appliance material
Desired outcome: Patient's peristomal skin remains nonerythematous and intact.

Nursing Interventions

- For patient with significant allergy history, patch test skin for a 24-hr period, at least 24 hr before ostomy surgery, to assess for allergies to different tapes that may be used on the postoperative appliance. If erythema, swelling, bleb formation, itching, weeping, or other indicators of tape allergy occurs, document type of tape that caused the reaction and note on cover of chart "Allergic to _____ tape." *Prevents allergic reaction.*
- Inspect peristomal skin for integrity, inflamed hair follicles (folliculitis), or reaction to tape with each pouch change to detect changes. Question patient about presence of itching or burning, which can signal leakage. Change pouch routinely (per agency or surgeon preference) or immediately if leakage is suspected. Report folliculitis or rash *because it may indicate the presence of a yeast infection, which will require topical medication.*

◆ Assess stoma, pouch, and skin for crystalline deposits, which are signals of alkaline urine that must be addressed *to prevent skin irritation.*
◆ Teach patient to:
- Monitor urine pH every week and to *maintain pH less than 6.0.*
- Decrease urine pH by drinking fluids that leave acid ash in the urine, such as cranberry or orange juice, or taking ascorbic acid in a dose consistent with patient's size.
- Monitor for nausea, vomiting, heartburn, diarrhea, flushing, and insomnia, *which are signs of ascorbic acid toxicity.*
◆ Teach pouch care to patient:
- Wash peristomal skin with water or a special cleansing solution marketed by ostomy supply companies. Dry skin thoroughly before applying skin barrier and pouch.
- Change pouch: Instruct patient to hold a gauze pad on (but not in) stoma to absorb urine and keep skin dry. Measure stoma with a measuring guide and ensure that skin barrier opening is cut to exact size of the stoma to protect peristomal skin *to protect skin from maceration caused by pooling of urine on skin.*
- Two-piece system or pouch with a barrier: Size the barrier to fit snugly around stoma. If using a barrier and attaching an adhesive pouch, size barrier to fit snugly around stoma and size pouch to clear stoma by at least $\frac{1}{8}$ inch *to protect skin.*
- One-piece "adhesive-only" pouch: If pouch has an antireflux valve, size the pouch to clear stoma and any peristomal creases so that pouch adheres to a flat, dry surface. An antireflux valve prevents pooling of urine on skin. If pouch does not have an antireflux valve, size pouch so that it clears the stoma by $\frac{1}{8}$ inch to prevent stomal trauma while minimizing amount of exposed skin. Use a copolymer film sealant wipe on peristomal skin before applying adhesive-only pouch. *Provides a moisture barrier and reduces epidermal trauma when pouch is removed.*
- Following pouch application: Connect pouch to bedside drainage system if patient is on bed rest. When patient is no longer on bed rest, empty pouch when it is one-third to one-half full by opening spigot at bottom of pouch and draining urine into patient's measuring container. Do not allow pouch to become too full. *Prevents breaking the seal of the appliance and exposing skin to urine.*
◆ Change incisional dressing as often as it becomes wet, and use sterile technique *to reduce risk for infection.*
◆ Teach patient care of stoma, pouch, and peristomal skin before discharge. (See "Patient-Family Teaching and Discharge Planning," p. 228.)

Impaired urinary elimination (risk for) related to postoperative use of ureteral stents, catheters, or drains and/or urinary diversion surgery
Desired outcome: Patient's urinary output is 30 mL/hr or greater; urine is clear and straw colored with normal, characteristic odor.

Nursing Interventions

◆ Monitor color, clarity, and volume of urine output via stoma, stents, and/or catheter *to ensure early detection of urinary compromise so that corrective actions can be implemented.*
- *Ureterostomy:* Urine drains via stoma and/or ureteral stents.
- *Intestinal conduit:* Urine drains via stoma. Patient also may have ureteral stents and/or conduit catheter/stent in the early postoperative period to stabilize ureterointestinal anastomoses and maintain drainage from the conduit during early postoperative edema.
- *Continent urinary diversions or reservoirs*: Kock urostomy usually has a reservoir catheter and also may have ureteral stents. The Indiana

(ileocecal) reservoir usually has ureteral stents exiting from the stoma, through which most of the urine drains, and may have a reservoir catheter exiting from a stab wound, which serves as an overflow catheter. If urethral anastomosis was completed, a urethral catheter will be in place to drain urine, which initially will be light red to pink with mucus but should clear in 24-48 hr. This catheter generally remains in place for 21 days to ensure adequate healing of the anastomosis.

♦ Monitor functioning of ureteral stents, which exit from the stoma into the pouch. These stents maintain patency of the ureters and assist in healing of the anastomosis. Right stents usually are cut at a 90-degree angle, and left stents are cut at a 45-degree angle. Each usually produces approximately the same amount of urine, although the amount produced by each is not important as long as each drains adequately and total drainage from all sources is 30 mL/hr or greater. Urine is usually red to pink for the first 24-48 hr and becomes straw colored by the third postoperative day. Absence of urine or decrease in amount may indicate a blocked stent or problems with the ureter. Stents may become blocked with mucus. Urine should drain around stent, and output volume should be adequate if the stent is working properly.

♦ Monitor functioning of stoma catheters. In continent urinary diversions, a catheter is placed in the reservoir to prevent distention and promote healing of suture lines. This new reservoir (i.e., resected intestine) exudes large amounts of mucus, necessitating catheter irrigation with 30-50 mL of normal saline, which is instilled gently and allowed to empty via gravity. Expect output to include pink or light red urine with mucus and small red clots for the first 24 hr. Urine should become amber colored with occasional clots within 3 postoperative days. Mucus production will continue but should decrease in volume.

♦ Monitor functioning of drains. Any urinary diversion may have Penrose drains or closed drainage systems in place to facilitate healing of the ureterointestinal anastomosis. Excessive lymph fluid and urine can be removed via these drains to reduce pressure on anastomotic suture lines. Drainage from drainage systems may be light red to pink for the first 24 hr and then lighten to amber color and decrease in amount. In a continent urinary diversion, an increase in drainage after amounts have been low might signal an anastomotic leak. Notify health care provider if this occurs.

♦ Monitor I&O, and record total amount of urine output from urinary diversion for the first 24 hr postoperatively. Differentiate and record separately amounts from all drains, stents, and catheters. Notify health care provider of an output less than 60 mL during a 2-hr period because in the presence of adequate intake this can indicate a ureteral obstruction, a leak in one of the anastomotic sites, or impending renal failure.

♦ Assess for other indicators of ureteral obstruction—flank pain, costovertebral angle (CVA) tenderness, nausea, vomiting, and anuria—*to facilitate early corrective interventions.*

♦ Monitor drainage from Foley catheter or urethral drain (if present). Patients who have had a cystectomy may have a urethral drain, whereas those with a partial cystectomy will have a Foley catheter in place. Note color, consistency, and volume of drainage, which may be red to pink with mucus. Report sudden increase (which would occur with hemorrhage) or decrease (which can signal blockage that can lead to infection or, with partial cystectomy, hydronephrosis). Report significant findings to health care provider.

♦ Advise patient who has had a cystectomy that after removal of urethral catheter or drain, mucus drainage will continue from the urethral meatus for several months, *to relieve anxiety.*

♦ Encourage an intake of at least 2-3 L/day in the nonrestricted patient, *to keep the urinary tract well irrigated.*

Risk for infection related to an invasive surgical procedure and risk of ascending bacteriuria with urinary diversion

Desired outcome: Patient is free of infection as evidenced by normothermia; WBC count $11,000/mm^3$ or less; and absence of purulent or excessive drainage, erythema, edema, warmth, and tenderness along the incision.

Nursing Interventions

◆ Monitor patient's temperature q4h during first 24-48 hr after surgery. Notify health care provider of fever (greater than 101° F). *Fever may indicate infection.*

◆ Inspect dressing frequently for presence of purulent or excessive drainage. Infection is most likely to become evident after the first 72 hr. Change dressing when it becomes wet, and use sterile technique. Use extra care to prevent disruption of drains *to prevent contamination and subsequent infection.*

◆ Inspect incision for erythema, tenderness, local warmth, edema, and purulent or excessive drainage, *which are indicators of infection.*

◆ Monitor and record character of urine at least q8h. Mucus particles are normal in urine of patients with ileal conduits and continent urinary diversions because of the nature of the bowel segment used. Cloudy urine, however, is abnormal and can signal infection. Urine should be yellow or pink tinged during the first 24-48 hr after surgery.

◆ Assess for other indicators of UTI, including flank or CVA pain, malodorous urine, chills, and fever.

◆ Note position of the stoma relative to the incision. If they are close together, apply pouch first to avoid overlap of the pouch with the suture line, which can increase risk of infection. If necessary, cut pouch down on one side or place it at an angle *to avoid contact with drainage, which may loosen adhesive.*

◆ Assess indwelling urethral catheter if present. Patients with cystectomies without anastomosis to the urethra may have an indwelling urethral catheter to drain serosanguineous fluid from the peritoneal cavity. *Do not irrigate this catheter because irrigation can result in peritonitis.*

◆ Encourage fluid intake of at least 2-3 L/day *to help flush urine through the urinary tract, remove mucus shreds, and prevent stasis.*

Potential complications of urinary diversion (collaborative diagnosis): hyperchloremic metabolic acidosis with hypokalemia, which can occur secondary to reabsorption of Na^+ and chloride (Cl^-) from the urine in the ileal segment, which results in compensatory loss of K^+ and HCO_3^-); stomal compromise/necrosis; anastomotic breakdown/intraabdominal urine leakage.

Desired outcomes: Patient verbalizes orientation to person, place, and time (within patient's normal range); electrolytes remain within normal limits; stoma remains pink or bright red and shiny. The stoma of a cutaneous urostomy is raised, moist, and red; signs of intraabdominal urine leakage are absent.

Nursing Interventions

◆ Monitor serum electrolyte studies. For patients with ileal conduits, assess for indicators of hypokalemia and metabolic acidosis, including nausea and changes in level of consciousness (LOC) (ranging from sleepiness to combativeness), muscle tone (ranging from convulsions to flaccidity), and irregular heart rate (HR). Notify health provider of significant findings.

◆ Monitor for confusion or signs of motor dysfunction. If signs occur, keep bed in lowest position and raise side rails. If convulsions appear imminent, pad side rails. Notify health care provider of significant findings.

◆ Encourage oral intake as directed, and assess for need for IV management. Health care provider may prescribe IV fluids with K^+ supplements.

- Encourage foods high in K⁺ such as bananas, cantaloupes, and apricots if patient is allowed to eat, *to correct or prevent hypokalemia.* See Box 4-2 for other foods that are high in K⁺.
- Encourage patient to ambulate by second or third day after surgery. *Mobility will help prevent urinary stasis, which increases risk of electrolyte problems.*
- Inspect stoma at least q8h and as indicated. The stoma of an ileal conduit will be edematous and should be pink or red with a shiny appearance. *A stoma that is dusky or cyanotic in color is indicative of insufficient blood supply and impending necrosis* and must be reported to health care provider immediately.
- Evaluate stomal height in patients with ileal conduit. The stoma formed by a cutaneous ureterostomy is usually raised during the first few weeks after surgery, red, and moist. Report changes immediately.
- Monitor for evidence of anastomotic breakdown/intraabdominal urine leakage, which may occur in an individual with intestinal conduit or continent diversion: decreasing urinary output from stoma or stents, flank or abdominal pain, increasing abdominal distention, and increasing drainage from wound drains. Report abnormalities immediately.

Deficient knowledge related to self-care regarding urinary diversion
Desired outcomes: Patient or significant other demonstrates proper care of stoma and urinary diversion before hospital discharge.

Nursing Interventions

- Assess patient's facility with language, and engage an interpreter or provide language-appropriate written materials if necessary.
- Assess patient's or significant other's readiness to participate in care.
- Involve enterostomal therapy (ET) nurse in patient teaching if available.
- Assist patient with organizing the equipment and materials that are needed to accomplish home care. Usually patient is discharged with disposable pouching systems. Most patients continue using disposable systems for the long term. Those who will use reusable systems usually are not fitted until 6-8 wk after surgery.
- Teach patient/significant other:
  - How to remove and reapply pouch; how to empty it; and how to use gravity drainage system at night, including procedures for rinsing and cleansing drainage system.
  - Signs and symptoms of UTI, peristomal skin breakdown, and maintenance of acidic urine (if not contraindicated), importance of adequate fluid intake, and techniques for checking urine pH (which should be assessed weekly).
  - To keep urine pH should at 6.0 or less. Persons with urinary diversions have a higher incidence of UTI than that in the general public; therefore it is important to keep their urinary pH acidic. If it is greater than 6.0, advise patient to increase fluid intake and, with health care provider approval, to increase vitamin C intake to 500-1000 mg/day, *which will increase urine acidity.*
  - Technique for reservoir catheter irrigation if patient has a continent urinary diversion.
  - Signals of the urge to void and procedure to void to patients who have continent urinary diversions with urethral anastomosis. Vague feelings of abdominal discomfort, abdominal pressure, or abdominal cramping are signals to void. To void, relax perineal muscles and employ Valsalva maneuver.
  - Emphasize importance of follow-up visits, particularly for patients with continent urinary diversions, who will be taught how to catheterize the reservoir and use a small dressing over the stoma rather than an appliance.

- ◆ Provide a list of ostomy support groups and ET nurses in the area for referral and assistance.
- ◆ Provide patient with enough equipment and materials for the first week after hospital discharge. Remind patient that proper cleansing of ostomy appliances will reduce risk of bacterial growth and UTI.

 Patient-Family Teaching and Discharge Planning

When providing patient-family teaching, focus on sensory information, avoid giving excessive information, and initiate a visiting nurse referral for necessary follow-up teaching. Include verbal and written information about:

- ◆ Medications, including drug names, dosage, schedule, precautions, and potential side effects. Also discuss drug/drug, herb/drug, and food/drug interactions.
- ◆ Indicators that necessitate medical intervention: fever or chills; nausea or vomiting; abdominal pain, cramping, or distention; cloudy or malodorous urine; incisional drainage, edema, local warmth, pain, or redness; peristomal skin irritation; or abnormal changes in stoma shape or color from the normal bright and shiny red.
- ◆ Maintenance of fluid intake of at least 2-3 L/day *to maintain adequate kidney function.*
- ◆ Monitoring of urine pH, which should be checked weekly (See **Deficient knowledge**, immediately preceding).
- ◆ Care of stoma and application of urostomy appliances. Patient should be proficient in application technique before hospital discharge.
- ◆ Care of urostomy appliances. Remind patient that proper cleansing will reduce risk of bacterial growth, which contaminates urine and increases risk of UTI.
- ◆ Treatment of peristomal skin irritation:
  - Dry skin with a hairdryer on cool setting.
  - Dust peristomal skin with absorptive powder (e.g., karaya or Stomahesive).
  - If desired, blot skin with water or a sealant wipe to seal in the powder.
  - Use a porous tape to prevent moisture trapping.
  - Notify health care provider or ET nurse of any severe or nonresponsive skin problems.
- ◆ Activities of daily living (ADL): Discuss ADL with patient. Inform patient that showers, baths, and swimming can continue and that diet is not affected after the early postoperative period.
- ◆ Stoma: Inform patient that the stoma will shrink considerably over the first 6-8 wk and less significantly over the next year.
- ◆ Importance of follow-up care with health care provider and ET nurse. Confirm date and time of next appointment.
- ◆ Phone numbers to call if questions or concerns arise about therapy after discharge. In addition, many cities have local support groups. Information for these patients can be obtained by accessing the following:

United Ostomy Association: www.uoa.org

American Cancer Society: www.cancer.org

National Cancer Institute/Cancer Information Service (CIS): www.cancer.gov/ cancertopics/factsheet/

Neurologic Disorders

INFLAMMATORY DISORDERS
OF THE NERVOUS SYSTEM

❖ MULTIPLE SCLEROSIS

OVERVIEW/PATHOPHYSIOLOGY

Multiple sclerosis (MS) is an inflammatory autoimmune disorder causing scattered and sporadic demyelinization of the central nervous system (CNS). Myelin permits nerve impulses to travel quickly through the nerve pathways of the CNS. In response to the inflammation, the myelin nerve sheaths scar, degenerate, or separate from the axon cylinders. This demyelinization interrupts electrical nerve transmission and causes the wide variety of symptoms associated with MS. As less severe inflammation resolves, myelin function may regenerate, thereby enabling electrical nerve impulse transmission to be restored. When the inflammation is severe and causes irreversible destruction of myelin or axon degeneration, involved areas are replaced by dense glial scar tissue that forms patchy areas of sclerotic plaque that permanently damage conductive pathways of the CNS. Axon nerve fibers may degenerate. Deficits present after 3 mo usually are permanent.

The course of MS is highly variable, with several general categories of progression. Motor or coordination symptoms at onset and/or frequent attacks during the first 2 yr of the disease usually indicate a poor outlook. In the *benign* form of MS (10% of patients), attacks are few and mild. Complete or nearly complete clearing of symptoms occurs with little or no disability. At least initially, most patients (70%-80%) have the *relapsing-remitting* form characterized by episodes of neurologic impairment ("attacks," exacerbations), followed by complete or nearly complete recovery and stability with no disease progression (remission). Typically, increasing numbers of symptoms occur with each exacerbation, with less complete clearing of symptoms and with deficits becoming cumulative. Over time the relapsing-remitting form usually undergoes transition to the *secondary progressive* form, in which neurologic impairment progresses continuously with or without superimposed relapses. A small proportion of patients (10%-20%) will initially begin with the *primary progressive* form, characterized by gradual ongoing accumulation of symptoms and deficits, with absence of clear-cut exacerbations and remissions. The *progressive relapsing* form (5%) is characterized by a progressive disease course from onset, with clear acute exacerbations. Progression continues during the periods between disease exacerbations. In the most severe cases of acute MS, significant disability may occur in weeks or months.

ASSESSMENT

Signs and symptoms/physical findings: Onset of MS can be extremely rapid, or it can be insidious with exacerbations and remissions. Signs and symptoms vary widely, depending on site and extent of demyelinization, and can change from day to day. Usually early symptoms are mild, including fatigue, weakness, heaviness, clumsiness, numbness, and tingling. Optic neuritis and visual problems often are the first symptoms. Lhermitte's sign may be present, in which an electrical sensation runs down the back and legs during neck flexion. Ophthalmoscopic inspection may reveal temporal pallor of optic disks. Reflex assessment may show increased deep tendon reflexes (DTRs) and diminished abdominal skin and cremasteric reflexes.

Damage to motor nerve tracts: Weakness, paralysis, and spasticity. Fatigue is common. Diplopia may occur secondary to ocular muscle involvement.

Damage to cerebellar or brainstem regions: Intention tremor, nystagmus, or other tremors; incoordination, ataxia; and weakness of facial and throat muscles resulting in difficulty chewing, dysphagia, and dysarthria. Slurred speech often occurs early, whereas scanning speech (slow speech with pauses between syllables) is usually seen in later stages.

Damage to sensory nerve tracts: Often, only sensory symptoms occur in the beginning and may include decreased perception of pain, touch, and temperature; paresthesias such as numbness and tingling or "pins and needles"; decrease or loss of proprioception; and decrease or loss of vibratory sense. Optic neuritis is a common early symptom, potentially causing partial or total loss of vision, visual clouding or shimmering, and pain with eye movement.

Damage to cerebral cortex (especially frontal lobes): Mood swings, inappropriate affect, euphoria, apathy, irritability, depression, hyperexcitability, and poor memory, judgment, foresight and planning, and abstract reasoning. There is often trouble with word finding and difficulty with concentration, attention, and processing or learning new information.

Damage to motor and sensory control centers: Urinary frequency, urgency, or retention; urinary and fecal incontinence; constipation.

Sacral cord lesions: Impotence; diminished sensations that result in inhibited sexual response.

History and risk factors: Although the cause of MS is unknown, it is generally believed to result from an environmental insult to the body, such as an earlier viral infection that triggers an autoimmune response in a predisposed individual. MS is most common among people who have lived in cool, temperate climates before puberty. Incidence in African-Americans is half that in white Americans. More girls and women than boys and men are affected (not quite 2:1). Onset is usually 10-50 yr of age with peak onset at 20-40 yr of age. It is 15-20 × more common among siblings of individuals with the disease than in the general population, a finding suggesting a possible genetic susceptibility. Exacerbations may be fewer during pregnancy but increase immediately post partum. Heat and fever tend to aggravate symptoms.

DIAGNOSTIC TESTS

MS is sometimes called the "great masquerader." Diagnosis of MS usually is made after other neurologic disorders with similar symptoms have been ruled out (when the patient has experienced two or more exacerbations of neurologic symptoms) and when the patient has two or more areas of demyelinization or plaque formation throughout the CNS, as demonstrated by diagnostic tests such as magnetic resonance imaging (MRI) and evoked potential (EP) studies or by the patient's clinical symptoms.

MRI: Reveals presence of plaques and demyelinization in the CNS. This is the test of choice when MS is suspected, although it is not a definitive measure of MS. MRI technology is capable of identifying current sites of inflammation and demyelinization and showing changes associated with disease progression.

T1-weighted MRI sequences may show hypointense lesions (black holes), a finding that correlates with axonal loss and indicates old lesions. T2-weighted MRI sequences can show old and new lesions and is used to document response to treatment. Gadolinium (Gd) enhancement shows areas of active demyelinization. MRI diffusion tensor imaging and MR spectroscopy often reveal involvement of otherwise normal-appearing white matter. Magnetization transfer imaging may show indirect evidence of axonal loss. MR spectroscopy can measure decline in a brain chemical called N-acetylaspartate (NAA) as a marker of axonal damage and appears to predict disease severity. Functional MRI (fMRI) can show new lesions. Fluid-attenuated inversion recovery (FLAIR) is also used for detecting cerebral lesions, and short tau inversion recovery (STIR) is useful in detecting demyelinization.

EP studies: EPs may be slow or absent because of interference of nerve transmission from demyelinization or plaque formation. The tests include visual evoked potentials (VEPs), somatosensory evoked potentials (SSEPs), and brainstem auditory evoked potentials (BAEPs). VEPs are particularly useful because optic neuritis is so common.

Lumbar puncture (LP) and cerebrospinal fluid (CSF) analysis: Evaluates CSF levels of oligoclonal bands and free kappa chains of immunoglobulin G (IgG), protein, γ-globulin, myelin basic protein, and lymphocytes, any of which may be elevated in the presence of MS. During acute MS attacks, destruction of the myelin sheath releases myelin basic protein into the CSF. Oligoclonal bands of IgG are seen in 85%-95% of patients with MS. This and the finding of free kappa chains in the CSF support a diagnosis of MS. CSF analysis is the only test that can show the person has a chronic inflammatory disease.

CT scan: Demonstrates presence of plaques and rules out mass lesions. This scan is less effective than MRI in detecting areas of plaque and demyelinization.

EEG: Shows abnormal slowing in one-third of patients with MS because of altered nerve conduction.

Positron emission tomography (PET): May show altered locations and patterns of cerebral glucose metabolism.

COLLABORATIVE MANAGEMENT

Generally, treatment is symptomatic and supportive. Various treatments slow the rate of exacerbation or hasten recovery from an exacerbation, but the general course of the disease process has not been positively affected.

Activity: During acute exacerbations, patients should have adequate rest but be encouraged to keep mobile to their levels of tolerance. Immobile patients will require deep vein thrombosis (DVT) prevention therapy.

Pharmacotherapy

Glatiramer acetate: To reduce frequency of relapses in relapsing-remitting MS. This agent is a synthetic copy of myelin basic protein and is believed to act as a "decoy" to spare the patient's myelin from immune system attack.

Interferon beta-1a: For patients with relapsing-remitting MS, to aid in stabilizing clinical status. This biologic response modulator decreases the frequency of exacerbations.

Interferon beta-1b: For patients with relapsing-remitting MS and secondary progressive MS. It is also a biologic response modulator that decreases the frequency of exacerbations.

Mitoxantrone: For secondary progressive or worsening MS. In addition to being an immunosuppressive, this agent also may cause heart and liver toxicity. It is not indicated for treatment of primary progressive MS.

Steroidal antiinflammatory agents (e.g., methylprednisolone): For an exacerbation and for optic neuritis to reduce symptoms by decreasing inflammation and associated edema of the myelin and thereby hastening onset of remission. Antacids, histamine H_2-receptor blockers, insulin coverage, K^+ supplements, diuretics, BP medications, and psychotropic agents may be given to combat side effects of steroids.

IV immunoglobulin: For severe exacerbations, to reduce severity of attack and hasten remission.

Antispasmodics and muscle relaxants (e.g., baclofen, tizanidine, dantrolene sodium, and methocarbamol): To reduce spasticity. Severe spasticity may be treated with intramuscular (IM) injections of botulinum toxin or intrathecal baclofen administered continually via a surgically implanted pump. Intrathecal baclofen must not be stopped abruptly because doing so may cause seizures and hallucinations. Dantrolene, which causes muscle weakness, usually is reserved for nonambulatory patients. Cannabis medicinal extract taken by capsule or sublingually and titrated to effect is controversial but may help some spasticity.

Smooth muscle relaxants (e.g., tolterodine, oxybutynin, solifenacin, trospium): To decrease bladder spasms and urinary frequency and urgency. Intravesical injections of oxybutynine or botulinum toxin A into the detrusor muscle may be used to decrease detrusor overactivity that does not respond to oral agents.

Smooth muscle stimulants (e.g., bethanechol chloride): To help prevent urinary retention.

Desmopressin: To reduce nighttime incontinence, frequency, and enuresis.

Stool softeners (e.g., docusate), laxatives (e.g., bisacodyl), and suppositories: To prevent fecal impaction and minimize incontinence.

Antidepressants (e.g., fluoxetine, nortriptyline, and sertraline): For depression related to cerebral lesions. These agents also may reduce complaints of paresthesias.

Tranquilizers (e.g., diazepam): For anxiety reducing and muscle relaxant effects, which may help with spasms and tremors.

Antifatigue drugs (e.g., amantadine, fluoxetine): To relieve fatigue, which is the most common complaint in MS and does not correlate with level of disability.

Proton pump inhibitor (e.g., pantoprazole), histamine H_2-receptor blockers (e.g., famotidine), and sucralfate: To prevent stress ulcers.

Low-dose heparin, low-molecular-weight heparin (e.g., enoxaparin): For antithrombus prophylaxis.

Analgesics (e.g., acetaminophen), neuropathic pain medications (e.g., anticonvulsants such as carbamazepine, topiramate, and lamotrigine; tricyclic antidepressants such as amitriptyline and imipramine), and medications used for facial trigeminal pain or limb burning (e.g., amantadine, topical capsaicin, misoprostol, mexiletine, perphenazine): As needed for various types of pain.

Sexual medications (e.g., vardenafil, tadalafil, sildenafil): To enhance sexual functioning. Oral agents are contraindicated for people who are taking nitrates such as nitroglycerin because of the additive hypotensive effect. Patients with erections lasting longer than 4 hr should seek medical attention. Vaginal gels are used for lubrication in women.

Propranolol, clonazepam, or primidone: To decrease tremors.

Dextromethorphan-quinidine combination: To reduce inappropriate emotional episodes (e.g., laughing and crying).

Metoclopramide: For gastroparesis.

Meclizine: For nausea/vomiting and vertigo.

Physical medicine: Physical therapy (PT), occupational therapy (OT), and assistive devices or braces may be prescribed to maintain mobility and independence with activities of daily living (ADL). Muscle strengthening and conditioning exercises and gait training (to develop alternative muscle groups not yet weakened by demyelination), as well as stretching exercises, are also commonly indicated. Placing weights on affected limbs may help with mild tremors.

ROM exercises: Maintain or increase joint function and prevent contractures.

Bowel and bladder program: Prevents incontinence, constipation, and urinary retention. This program may include bowel and bladder training, pelvic floor exercises, intermittent catheterization, external drainage appliances, or urethral plugs. A bladder diary describing I&O, frequency of urgency, incontinent episodes, and postvoid residuals may help in evaluating bladder problems. Urodynamic studies may be done to determine specific physiologic deficits so a bladder program can be tailored to meet patient's individual needs. Bladder ultrasound scanning may be used for determining bladder fullness to help in retraining. Evaluate for urinary tract infection (UTI) if urgency or incontinent episodes increase. Functional electrical bladder and bowel stimulation also may be used, but these techniques require implanted sacral cord devices.

Nutrition: A low-fat diet generally is recommended. Vitamin C and cranberry juice are used to help prevent bladder infections, and fiber is used to reduce constipation.

Speech therapy: Improves speech deficits using accessory respiratory muscles, tongue, and facial muscles.

Counseling or psychotherapy: Helps patient and significant other adapt to the disability and deal with emotions and feelings that are direct or indirect results of the disease process. Sexual counseling also should be included.

Treatment of complications: Complications, such as respiratory infection or UTI, may require treatment with antibiotics or other measures.

Surgical interventions: Performed to treat complications such as contractures, spasticity, decreased mobility, and pain. Interventions may include peripheral nerve block with phenol, tenotomy, myotomy, peripheral neurectomy, rhizotomy, or stereotactic thalamotomy. A penile prosthesis may be implanted in men whose impotence occurs secondary to MS. Patients with recurrent or chronic UTIs may be candidates for urinary diversion. Patients with urge incontinence may be candidates for implanted sacral nerve stimulator or artificial urinary sphincter.

Controversial therapies

Immunosuppressive drug therapy (e.g., azathioprine, low-dose methotrexate, cyclophosphamide): These agents may decrease number and severity of exacerbations in patients who fail to gain relief from standard immunotherapy.

Monoclonal antibodies: Natalizumab, prescribed for patients with relapsing MS, was taken off the market voluntarily because of some episodes of progressive multifocal leukoencephalopathy, but clinical trials using the drug have been resumed. It is available to patients with relapsing MS who are enrolled in the TOUCH Prescribing Program. Other drugs in this class, such as daclizumab, which is used to prevent organ rejection in kidney transplant recipients, show promise in reducing relapses in clinical trials.

Plasmapheresis: Reduces patient's antibodies to CNS tissue by removing the plasma portion of the blood, which contains circulating antibodies. This therapy usually involves several exchanges that provide short-term improvement only. Typically it is used only in severe exacerbations of the primary progressive form of MS.

4-Aminopyridine (4-AP) (also known as fampridine): A K^+ channel blocker that may help relieve a number of symptoms, especially paresthesias.

NURSING DIAGNOSES AND INTERVENTIONS

Deficient knowledge related to factors that aggravate and exacerbate MS symptoms

Desired outcome: By day 3 (or before hospital discharge), patient and significant other verbalize factors that exacerbate, prevent, and ameliorate symptoms of MS.

Nursing Interventions

◆ Assess patient's facility with language; engage an interpreter or provide language-appropriate written materials if appropriate.

◆ Teach preventive measures, such as avoiding hot baths or showers and using acetaminophen or aspirin to reduce fever, if present. Inform patient and significant that heat, both external (hot weather, bath) and internal (fever), may be bothersome. *It tends to aggravate weakness and other symptoms of MS.* Also instruct patient in use of fans or air conditioning, chilled drinks, cool showers, and cool cloths to aid in reducing body temperature. High humidity with heat should be avoided.

◆ Caution patient to avoid exposure to persons known to have infections of any kind. Patients should receive immunizations and instructions in importance of and proper technique for handwashing. *Infection often precedes exacerbations,*

◆ Teach indicators of common infections and importance of seeking prompt medical treatment if they occur. Teach patient to monitor for increased frequency, urgency, or incontinence and to check urine for changes in odor or presence of cloudiness or blood. Instruct patient to check body temperature periodically for fever and indications that a UTI has reached the kidneys (e.g., costovertebral angle tenderness, chills, flank pain). *The patient with MS is susceptible to UTI because of urinary retention. Because of the disease process, patients may not feel any pain with urination.*

◆ Encourage patient to reduce factors that cause stress. Encourage use of stress reduction techniques such as progressive relaxation, self-coaching, and guided imagery. (See **Health-seeking behaviors:** Relaxation technique effective for stress reduction, p. 106.) *There is a relationship between stress and fatigue and the exacerbations.*

◆ Encourage patient to get sufficient rest, stop activity short of fatigue, and schedule activity and rest periods. Also teach how to conserve energy in ADL by sitting while getting dressed, rather than standing; sliding heavy objects along work surfaces, rather than lifting them; using a wheeled cart to transport items; having work surfaces at the proper height; and using assistive devices and delegating. Suggest that patient ask health care provider for medications, (e.g., amantadine, pemoline, modafinil) that combat fatigue.

◆ Identify priorities and eliminate nonessential activities. Encourage patient to plan each day, break projects into smaller tasks, distribute tasks throughout the day, rest before difficult tasks, and take planned recovery time after tasks. *Deconditioning can be reduced with a planned exercise program that can be incorporated into a scheduled activity/rest plan. Depression can contribute to sense of fatigue, and antidepressants may help.*

◆ Patients planning a pregnancy should consult and work with their health care providers before pregnancy. Provide information about birth control measures to female patients who desire counseling. *There may be a decreased relapse rate during pregnancy but increased exacerbations post partum.*

◆ As appropriate, reassure patient and significant other that most persons with MS do not become severely disabled. Optic neuritis is common and can be particularly frightening, but it usually remits. Encourage continued activity and normal lifestyle even when limitations are necessary.

Deficient knowledge related to precautions and potential side effects of prescribed medications
Desired outcome: By day 3 (or before hospital discharge), patient verbalizes accurate information about the prescribed medications.

Nursing Interventions

◆ Provide verbal instructions and language-appropriate written handouts that describe names, purpose, dose, and schedule of the prescribed medications. Also discuss drug/drug, herb/drug, and food/drug interactions.

◆ Give patients taking glatiramer injections these additional instructions:
  • *Common side effects:* self-limiting reaction of chest tightness, palpitation, flushing, panic, and anxiousness that may last 30 sec to 30 min after injection. Injection site reaction (redness, swelling, pain) is also common. Notify health care provider of injection site redness, ongoing chest pain, shortness of breath, or dizziness.
  • Refrigerate medication, administer it subcutaneously only, and rotate injection site daily.
◆ Give patients taking interferon injections these additional instructions:
  • Apply ice before injections and cortisone creams and rotate sites. *This intervention helps reduce skin inflammation, redness, and irritation from the injection.*
  • Flulike symptoms following each injection (fever, chills, headache, muscle aches and pains, malaise) are common and usually can be managed with analgesics such as acetaminophen and antihistamines such as diphenhydramine.
  • Other common side effects that may occur include fatigue, diarrhea, abdominal pain, nausea, vomiting, joint aches, back pain, and dizziness.
  • Report depression or suicidal thoughts and have periodic assessments of blood counts and liver function.
◆ Give patients taking steroids (e.g., methylprednisolone) these additional instructions:
  • *Common side effects:* Na^+ and fluid retention, hypertension, gastric ulcers, stomach upset, weakness, hypokalemia, mood changes, impaired wound healing, and masking of infections.
  • Monitor weight and BP for evidence of fluid retention. Advise patient to report symptoms of K^+ deficiency, such as anorexia, nausea, and muscle weakness, and to eat foods high in K^+ (see Box 4-2 p. 174). Encourage a diet low in Na^+ content (see Box 4-1, for high Na^{++} foods, p. 165). *This is to minimize the potential for fluid retention.*
  • Take the medication with food, milk, or buffering agents. *This helps prevent gastric irritation.* Avoid aspirin, indomethacin, caffeine, or other gastrointestinal (GI) irritants while taking this medication; and taper off rather than abruptly stopping the drug when it is discontinued. *This is to avoid adrenal crisis.*
  • Report black, tarry stools. *This may signal occult blood.*
  • Monitor glucose for hyperglycemia, report elevations, and as indicated, control glucose level with diet, oral agents, or insulin. Health care provider follow-up is important while the patient is taking these drugs.
◆ Give patients taking antispasmotics/muscle relaxants (e.g., baclofen or dantrolene) these additional instructions:
  • *Common side effects:* drowsiness, dizziness, fatigue, and nausea. In addition, dantrolene can cause diarrhea, muscle weakness, hepatitis, and photosensitivity.
  • Take the medication with food, milk, or a buffering agent. *This is to reduce gastric upset or nausea.*
  • Drowsiness is usually transient, so avoid activities that require alertness until the effect of the drug on the CNS is known. Avoid alcohol intake. *This is because of the additive CNS depression effects.*
  • Baclofen can lower the seizure threshold and should be used cautiously and never stopped abruptly. Baclofen also may raise blood glucose levels, and individuals with diabetes mellitus (DM) may need an insulin dose adjustment. Watch carefully during transfer and ambulation. *Some weak patients cannot tolerate the loss in spasticity that may be permitting them to bear weight.*
  • If taking dantrolene, monitor for and report fever, jaundice, dark urine, clay-colored stools, and itching. *These signs and symptoms may signal hepatitis or severe diarrhea.*

- Avoid exposure to the sun, and use sunscreens if exposure is unavoidable.
- If patient is on intrathecal baclofen, monitor for surgical complications such as CSF leak, wound dehiscence, catheter dislodgment, and meningitis (fevers, stiff neck, headache, altered mental status). Report pump catheter system failure (loss of effect) caused by catheter kink, breakage, or migration. Caution patient to avoid running out of medication. *It is important to ensure continuous operation because abrupt discontinuation of medication can result in seizures.*

◆ Give patients taking smooth muscle stimulants (e.g., bethanechol chloride) these additional instructions:
- *Common side effects:* hypotension, diarrhea, abdominal cramps, urinary urgency, and bronchoconstriction.
- Take the drug on an empty stomach. *This is to avoid nausea and vomiting.*
- Notify health care provider if lightheadedness occurs. *This can signal hypotension.*
- Seek medical attention if an asthmatic attack occurs.
- Caution patient to make position changes slowly and in stages. *This is to prevent fainting caused by orthostatic hypotension.*

◆ Give patients taking smooth muscle relaxants (e.g., tolterodine) these additional instructions:
- *Common side effects:* dryness of the mouth, blurred vision, constipation, palpitations, tachycardia, decreased sweating, and urinary retention or overflow incontinence.
- Measures that relieve constipation.
- Measures for remaining cool in hot or humid weather. *Heat stroke is more likely to develop while taking the medication.*
- Notify health care provider immediately if urinary retention or overflow incontinence occurs. In addition, if the patient can chew and swallow effectively, use sugarless gum, hard candy, or artificial saliva products. *These may reduce mouth dryness.*
- Encourage slow position changes and monitoring for dizziness. *Postural hypotension may occur when the drug is first started.*

◆ Give patients taking mitoxantrone these additional instructions:
- Patient will be evaluated for normal cardiac function before starting the drug and will need periodic cardiac monitoring. *This is to ensure that there are no toxic cardiac effects.*
- Report swelling of feet and lower legs, shortness of breath, mouth or lip sores, black tarry stools, jaundice, and stomach pains.
- Avoid people with infections or who have recently received live virus vaccinations. Report signs of infection to health care provider (e.g., fever, chills, cough, hoarseness, lower back or side pain, and painful or difficult urination). *Medication can decrease WBC counts, and thus risk of infection is increased.* Expect to have both WBC and liver function tests.
- Side effects that normally do not require medical attention include nausea, temporary hair loss, and menstrual changes. After taking medication, urine may be blue green for about 24 hr. The medication also may cause diarrhea, which should be reported if it continues.
- Medication has a lifetime cumulative dose restriction to limit toxicities.

Chronic pain and spasms related to motor and sensory nerve tract damage
Desired outcomes: Within 1-2 hr of intervention, patient's subjective evaluation of pain and spasms improves, as documented by pain scale. Objective indicators, such as grimacing, are absent or reduced.

Nursing Interventions

- Maintain a comfortable room temperature. Advise patient to keep environment cool in warm weather and avoid hot baths or showers. *This is because heat tends to aggravate MS symptoms.*
- Provide passive, assisted, or active ROM exercises q2h and periodic stretching exercises. Teach these exercises to patient and significant other, and encourage the performance of these exercises several times daily. *This is to reduce muscle tightness and spasms.* Tell patient to sleep in a prone position. *This may help decrease flexor spasm of the hips and knees.* Splints or cones for hands with elastic bands may help spasm. Ensure safety with transfers.
- Administer antispasmodics as prescribed.
- For other Nursing Interventions, see "General Care of Patients with Neurologic Deficits," **Acute pain**, p. 366.

Patient-Family Teaching and Discharge Planning

The patient with MS may have a wide variety of symptoms that cause disability, ranging from mild to severe. Include verbal and written information about the following:

- Remission/exacerbation aspects of the disease process and progression. Explain effects of demyelinization on sensory and motor function and factors that aggravate symptoms.
- Safety measures relative to decreased sensation, visual disturbances, and motor deficits, including fall prevention.
- Medications, including drug names, purpose, dosage, frequency, precautions, and potential side effects. Also discuss drug/drug, herb/drug, and food/drug interactions.
- Exercises that promote muscle strength and mobility, measures for preventing contractures and skin breakdown, transfer techniques and proper body mechanics, and use of assistive devices and other measures to minimize neurologic deficits.
- Measures for relieving pain, muscle spasms, or other discomfort and fatigue.
- Indications of constipation, urinary retention, or UTI; implementation of bowel and bladder training programs; and self-catheterization technique or care of indwelling urinary catheters.
- Indications of upper respiratory infection (URI); implementation of measures that help prevent regurgitation, aspiration, and respiratory infection.
- Dietary adjustments that may be appropriate for neurologic deficit (e.g., soft, semisolid foods for patients with chewing difficulties or a high-fiber diet for patients experiencing constipation).
- Importance of follow-up care, including visits to health care provider, PT, and OT, as well as speech, sexual, or psychologic counseling.
- Referrals to community resources, such as local and national Multiple Sclerosis Society chapters, public health nurse, visiting nurse association, community support groups, social workers, psychologists, vocational rehabilitation agencies, home health agencies, extended and skilled care facilities, and financial counseling. Additional general information can be obtained by accessing the following websites:

National Multiple Sclerosis Society: www.nationalmssociety.org

Multiple Sclerosis Foundation: www.msfacts.org

Multiple Sclerosis Association of America: www.msassociation.org

❖ GUILLAIN-BARRÉ SYNDROME

OVERVIEW/PATHOPHYSIOLOGY

Guillain-Barré syndrome (GBS) is a rapidly progressing acute idiopathic polyneuritis. It is an autoimmune disease triggered by a preceding infection that is commonly caused by *Campylobacter jejuni, Mycoplasma pneumoniae,* cytomegalovirus (CMV), or Epstein-Barr virus (EBV). An inflammatory process enables lymphocytes to enter perivascular spaces and destroy the myelin sheath covering peripheral or cranial nerves. Posterior (sensory) and anterior (motor) nerve roots can be affected because of this segmental demyelinization, and individuals may experience both sensory and motor losses. There is relative sparing of the axon, except in one form of the disease. Respiratory insufficiency may occur in as many as half of affected individuals. Life-threatening respiratory muscle weakness can develop as rapidly as 24-72 hr after onset of initial symptoms. In about 25% of cases, motor weakness progresses to total paralysis.

Peak severity of symptoms usually occurs within days to 3 wk after onset of symptoms. A plateau stage follows that usually lasts 1-2 wk. The recovery stage starts with a return of function as remyelinization occurs, but it may take months to years for a full recovery. Eighty to ninety percent of patients recover completely or have only minor residual weakness or abnormal sensations, such as numbness or tingling. Of patients with GBS, 5%-10% may have permanent severe disability. Deficits are the result of axonal nerve degeneration.

GBS has several variants defined by the symptoms, preceding infection, and severity. Variants of GBS include those with a rapid progressive phase (e.g., acute inflammatory demyelinating polyneuropathy, Miller-Fisher syndrome) and those with a slow progressive phase (e.g., recurrent GBS, multifocal motor neuropathy).

ASSESSMENT

Signs and symptoms/physical findings: Progressive weakness and areflexia are the most common indicators. Typically, numbness and weakness begin in the legs and ascend symmetrically upward, progressing to the arms and facial nerves. Ascending GBS is most common, but descending GBS, in which cranial nerves are affected first and weakness progresses downward with rapid respiratory involvement, also can occur. GBS does not affect level of consciousness (LOC), cognitive function, or pupillary function. Assess for symmetric motor weakness, impaired position and vibration sense, hypoactive or absent deep tendon reflexes (DTRs), hypotonia in affected muscles, and decreased ventilatory capacity.

Anterior (motor) nerve root involvement: Weakness or flaccid paralysis that can progress to tetraplegia. Respiratory muscle involvement can be life-threatening. There is loss of reflexes, muscle tension, and tone, but muscle atrophy usually does not occur.

Autonomic nervous system (ANS) involvement: Bradycardia, hypotension, cardiac dysrhythmias, tachycardia, hypertension, facial flushing, diaphoresis, inability to perspire, loss of sphincter control, urinary retention, adynamic ileus, syndrome of inappropriate antidiuretic hormone (SIADH), and increased pulmonary secretions are possible. ANS involvement may occur unexpectedly and can be life-threatening, but usually it does not persist for longer than 2 wk.

Cranial nerve involvement: Inability to chew, swallow, speak, or close the eyes.

Posterior (sensory) nerve root involvement: Presence of paresthesias, such as numbness and tingling, which usually are minor compared with the degree of motor loss. Ascending sensory loss often precedes motor loss. Muscle cramping, tenderness, or pain may occur.

DIAGNOSTIC TESTS

Diagnostic tests are performed to rule out other diseases, such as acute polio-myelitis. Diagnosis of GBS is based on clinical presentation, history of recent infectious illness, and CSF findings.

Lumbar puncture (LP) and cerebrospinal fluid (CSF) analysis: About 7 days after initial symptoms, elevated protein (especially immunoglobulin G IgG]) without an increase in WBC count is significant. Although CSF pressure usually is normal, in severe disease it may be elevated.

EMG: Reveals slowed nerve conduction velocities soon after paralysis appears because of demyelinization. Denervation potentials appear later.

CBC: Shows presence of leukocytosis early in illness, possibly as a result of the inflammatory process associated with demyelinization.

Evoked potential (EP) studies (auditory, visual, brainstem): May be used to distinguish GBS from other neuropathologic conditions.

COLLABORATIVE MANAGEMENT

Patients are likely to be in the ICU when the neurologic deficit is progressing and are at risk for respiratory failure and autonomic dysfunction. Treatment is focused on ventilatory support and administration of immunomodulating agents to shorten the course of the diseaase. Only plasma exchange therapy and IV immune serum globulin have proved to be effective.

Respiratory support: Serial vital capacity measurements (q2-4h), pulmo-nary function tests, pulse oximetry, and arterial blood gas (ABG) analysis to monitor for respiratory muscle weakness or paralysis. Endotracheal tube, tracheostomy, or mechanical ventilation is used as necessary, generally when vital capacity falls below a preset level, usually less than 800-1000 mL or less than $\frac{2}{3}$ vital capacity for weight. Head of bed (HOB) should be elevated, if BP permits, to aid respirations and prevent aspiration.

Pharmacotherapy

IV immunoglobulins: May be prescribed soon after symptom onset (ideally within 1-5 days) in an attempt to positively affect antibody response.

Analgesics (e.g., acetaminophen, codeine, morphine): May be prescribed for muscle pain. A continuous morphine drip may be needed. Other medica-tions that may be tried to relieve uncomfortable paresthesias include anticon-vulsants such as gabapentin and carbamazepine and tricyclic antidepressants such as amitriptyline.

Stool softeners (e.g., docusate), laxatives (e.g., bisacodyl), and suppositories: May be prescribed to prevent fecal impaction and minimize incontinence.

Proton pump inhibitor (e.g., pantoprazole), histamine H_2-receptor blockers (e.g., famotidine), and sucralfate: May be prescribed to prevent stress ulcers.

Low-dose heparin, low-molecular-weight heparin (e.g., enoxaparin): May be prescribed for antithrombus prophylaxis.

Plasmapheresis: Reduces antibodies to peripheral and cranial nerve tissue by removing the plasma portion of the blood, which contains circulating antibodies. If multiple treatments are performed within 7-14 days of symptom onset, removal of these autoantibodies appears to lessen disease duration and severity. Earlier treatment yields better results.

Immunoadsorption therapy: Alternative to plasmapheresis for antibody removal.

Exercise and activity: Passive ROM exercise during acute phase with a goal of preventing contractures, dislocations, or subluxations. Turning and meticu-lous skin care to prevent skin breakdown are important interventions. After patient stabilizes, active ROM or active-assistive ROM is implemented, and PT and a rehabilitation program are initiated with a goal of early mobilization. OT and assistive devices or braces are employed so that patient can maintain mobility and independence with activities of daily living (ADL). Muscle strengthening exercises, conditioning exercises, and gait training are commonly prescribed.

Antithrombus prophylaxis: May include antiembolism hose and pharmacotherapy.

Nutritional support: A high-fiber diet may be prescribed to help prevent constipation. If patient cannot chew or swallow effectively because of cranial nerve involvement, gastric, gastrostomy, or parenteral feedings may be initiated. Patient is advanced to a solid diet upon return of gag reflex and swallowing ability.

Management of bowel and bladder dysfunction: A regular bowel program is started to prevent fecal impaction. Indwelling urinary catheters, intermittent catheterizations, or external urinary collection devices may be needed until strength and mobility return.

Management of acute autonomic dysfunction: Short-acting antihypertensive agents for hypertension; intravascular volume expanders or vasopressors for hypotension; cardiac monitoring of dysrhythmias; gastric suction, nutrition, and parenteral fluids for adynamic ileus; and catheterization and medications for urinary retention. Phenoxybenzamine may be used to help with paroxysmal hypertension, headache, sweating, anxiety, and fever. Diabetes insipidus (DI) (see p. 404) and SIADH (see p. 409) have been reported; therefore urine output, state of hydration, and serum and urine electrolytes are monitored.

Treatment of complications: For example, antibiotic therapy for aspiration pneumonia or anticoagulant therapy for deep vein thrombosis (DVT) or emboli.

NURSING DIAGNOSES AND INTERVENTIONS

Ineffective breathing pattern related to neuromuscular weakness or paralysis of the facial, throat, and respiratory muscles

Desired outcome: Deterioration in patient's breathing pattern (e.g., PaO_2 less than 80 mm Hg, vital capacity less than 800-1000 mL [or less than 10-12 mL/kg], tidal volume less than 75% of predicted value, or O_2 saturation 92% or less via oximetry) is detected and reported promptly, resulting in immediate and effective medical treatment.

Nursing Interventions

♦ Test for ascending loss of sensation by touching patient lightly with a pin or fingers at frequent intervals (hourly or more frequently initially). Assess from the level of the iliac crest upward toward the shoulders. Measure the highest level at which decreased sensation occurs. *Decreased sensation often precedes motor weakness.* If it ascends to the level of the T8 dermatome, anticipate that intercostal muscles (used with respirations) soon will be impaired. Also monitor for upper arm and shoulder weakness by checking patient for the presence of arm drift and inability to shrug the shoulders. *This weakness precedes respiratory failure.* Arm drift is detected in the following way: have patient hold both arms out in front of the body, level with the shoulders and with palms up; instruct patient to close eyes while holding this position. Weakness is present if one arm pronates or drifts down or out from its original position. Alert health care provider to significant findings.

♦ Assist with oral intake to detect changes or difficulties. Assess patient q8h and before oral intake for cough reflexes, gag reflexes, and difficulty swallowing. *Deficiencies may indicate ascending paralysis.*

♦ Observe for changes in mental status, LOC, and orientation. *These may signal reduced oxygenation to the brain.* Monitor patient's respiratory rate (RR), rhythm, and depth. Watch for accessory muscle use, nasal flaring, dyspnea, shallow respirations, apnea, and loss of abdominal breathing. Auscultate for diminished breath sounds. Monitor patient for breathlessness while speaking. To assess for breathlessness, ask patient to take a deep breath and slowly count as high as possible on one breath. *A reduced ability to count to a higher number before breathlessness occurs may signal grossly reduced ventilatory function.*

♦ Check serial vital capacity results on pulmonary function tests. *This is to monitor effectiveness of breathing.* If vital capacity is less than 800-1000 mL or is rapidly trending downward or if patient exhibits signs of hypoxia such as tachycardia, increasing restlessness, mental dullness, cyanosis, decreased pulse oximetry readings, or difficulty handling secretions, report findings immediately to health care provider.

♦ Monitor ABG levels and pulse oximetry. *This is to detect hypoxia or hypercapnia.*

♦ Raise HOB and encourage coughing and deep breathing. *This will promote optimal chest excursion and reduce aspiration risk.*

♦ The patient may require tracheostomy, endotracheal intubation, or mechanical ventilation to support respiratory function. Prepare patient emotionally for such procedures or for the eventual transfer to ICU or transition care unit for closer monitoring.

♦ For other nursing interventions, see **Risk for aspiration** in "Older Adult Care," p. 47.

Acute pain related to muscle tenderness; hypersensitivity to touch; or discomfort in shoulders, thighs, and back
Desired outcomes: Within 1-2 hr of intervention, patient's subjective perception of discomfort decreases, as documented by pain scale. Objective indicators, such as grimacing, are absent or diminished.

Nursing Interventions

♦ For patients with muscle tenderness, consider use of massage, moist heat packs, cold application, or warm baths. *This is very soothing for the muscles.*

♦ For patients with hypersensitivity, assess amount of touch that can be tolerated and incorporate this information into patient's plan of care.

♦ Reposition patient at frequent intervals. Some individuals find that a supine "frog-leg" position is particularly comfortable. Provide passive ROM and gentle stretching. *This reduces muscle tension, joint stiffness, and fatigue.*

♦ Opioids are often the most effective means of pain control, and a continuous morphine drip may be needed. Other medications that may be tried to relieve uncomfortable paresthesias include anticonvulsants and tricyclic antidepressants.

♦ For other nursing interventions, see **Acute pain,** p. 366, in "General Care of Patients with Neurologic Deficits."

Ineffective (decreased) cardiac and cerebral tissue perfusion (or risk for same) related to interrupted sympathetic outflow with concomitant BP fluctuations secondary to autonomic dysfunction
Desired outcomes: Patient has optimal cardiopulmonary and cerebral tissue perfusion as evidenced by SBP at least 90 mm Hg and less than 160 mm Hg, no significant mental status changes, and orientation to person, place, and time. BP fluctuations, if they occur, are detected and reported promptly.

Nursing Interventions

♦ Monitor BP and note wide fluctuations; report significant findings to health care provider. Short-acting hypertensive agents may be required for persistent hypertension. Look for changes in heart rate (HR) and BP during activities such as coughing, suctioning, position changes, or straining at stool. Changes in BP that result in severe hypotension or hypertension may occur because of unopposed sympathetic outflow or loss of outflow to the peripheral nervous system that causes changes in vascular tone.

◆ For patients with hypotension or postural hypotension, see **Ineffective cerebral tissue perfusion and risk for decreased cardiac tissue perfusion,** p. 300, in "Spinal Cord Injury."

Imbalanced nutrition: less than body requirements related to adynamic ileus
Desired outcome: Patient has adequate nutrition as evidenced by maintenance of baseline body weight.

Nursing Interventions

◆ Auscultate abdominal sounds, and note presence, absence, or changes that may signal onset of ileus. Be alert to abdominal distention or tenderness, nausea and vomiting, and absence of stool output. Notify health care provider of significant findings.
◆ Patients with adynamic ileus generally require gastric decompression with a nasogastric (NG) tube. Because these patients are unable to take foods orally, parenteral nutrition may be required (see "Providing Nutritional Support," p. 692).
◆ For general nursing interventions, see **Imbalanced nutrition,** p. 357, in "General Care of Patients with Neurologic Deficits."

Anxiety related to threat to biologic integrity and loss of control
Desired outcome: Within 24 hr of this diagnosis, patient expresses concern regarding changes in life events, states anxiety is lessened or under control, and exhibits fewer symptoms of increased anxiety (e.g., less apprehension, decreased tension).

Nursing Interventions

◆ For patients with progressing neurologic deficit, transfer to a room close to nurses' station to help alleviate the anxiety of being suddenly incapacitated and helpless.
◆ Be sure call light is within easy reach, and frequently assess patient's ability to use it.
◆ Provide continuity of patient care through assignment of staff and use of care plan.
◆ Perform assessments at frequent intervals, and let patient know you are there. Provide care in a calm and reassuring manner.
◆ Allow time for patient to ventilate concerns and provide realistic feedback regarding what patient may experience. Determine past effective coping behaviors and problem solve for ways these behaviors, or others, may prove useful in current situation.
◆ For other nursing interventions, see **Anxiety,** p. 32, and **Fear,** p. 35, in "Psychosocial Support."

Deficient knowledge related to therapeutic plasma exchange procedure
Desired outcome: Before scheduled date of each procedure, patient verbalizes accurate information about the plasma exchange procedure.

Nursing Interventions

◆ Before the plasma exchange procedure, patient's health care provider explains the reason for the procedure, its risks, and anticipated benefits or outcome. Determine patient's level of understanding of health care provider's explanation, and clarify or reinforce information accordingly. Assess patient's facility with language; provide interpreter or language-appropriate written materials if indicated. Obtain signed permit.
◆ Notify health care provider if patient is taking angiotensin-converting enzyme (ACE) inhibitor medication. *ACE inhibitor use is associated with flushing, hypotension, abdominal cramping, and other gastrointestinal (GI)*

signs and symptoms during plasmapheresis. These medications usually are held for 24 hr before the procedure to avoid problems.

♦ Determine patient's experience with plasmapheresis, positive or negative effects, and nature of any fears or concerns. Document and communicate this information to other caregivers.

♦ Explain in words patient can understand that the goal of plasma exchange is to remove autoimmune factors from the blood to decrease or eliminate symptoms. These antibodies to patient's peripheral and cranial nerve tissue are reduced by removal of the blood's plasma portion, which contains the circulating antibodies. The procedure is similar to hemodialysis. Blood is removed from patient and separated into its components. The patient's plasma is discarded; other blood components (e.g., RBCs, WBCs, platelets) are saved and returned to patient with donor plasma or replacement fluid. If started within 1-2 wk of GBS symptoms, the exchange process seems to decrease disease duration and severity. Multiple exchanges over a period of weeks can be expected.

♦ Patient is at risk for the following complications during this procedure: deficient fluid volume, hypotension, fluid overload, hypokalemia (from dilution with albumin replacement), hypocalcemia (from free calcium binding to the citrate used during the procedure), cardiac dysrhythmias (from electrolyte shifts), clotting disorders (from decreased clotting factors with plasma removal), anemia, phlebitis, infection, hypothermia, and air embolism. Answer any questions regarding these complications accordingly.

♦ This procedure requires good blood flow. The antecubital vein may be accessed, but the health care provider may need to insert a central IV line or a femoral catheter. If the antecubital site is used, place a sign alerting others to avoid using this site for routine laboratory needle sticks.

♦ Explain that patient can expect the procedure to take 2-4 hr, although it may take considerably longer, depending on condition of patient's veins, blood flow, and hematocrit (Hct) level.

♦ Explain that patient can expect preprocedure and postprocedure blood work for clotting factors and electrolyte levels. Patient may be placed on cardiac monitoring. *This is to assess for electrolyte imbalance, particularly if taking prednisone or digitalis.* Weight and VS will be taken before and after the procedure, with frequent VS checks during the procedure. Calcium gluconate or KCl may be administered. *This is to correct electrolyte imbalances.*

♦ Encourage patient to report any unusual feelings or symptoms during plasma exchange—for example:
  • Chills, fever, hives, sweating, or lightheadedness. *This may signal reaction to donor plasma.*
  • Thirst, faintness, or dizziness. *This can occur with hypotension or hypovolemia.* Patients should take oral fluids during the procedure if possible.
  • Numbness or tingling around lips or in the hands, arms, and legs; muscle twitching; cramping; or tetany. *This can occur with hypocalcemia.* Fatigue, nausea, weakness, or cramping. *This may signal hypokalemia.*

♦ Inform patient that medications (e.g., plasma-bound drugs) may be held until after the procedure to prevent their removal from the blood.

♦ If the patient does not have a urinary catheter, remind the patient to void before and during the procedure. *This is done to avoid any mild hypotension caused by a full bladder.* I&O will be monitored closely. *Decreased urine output may signal hypovolemia.*

♦ Explain that patient's temperature will be checked during the procedure and warm blankets will be provided. *This is to prevent hypothermia.*

♦ Explain that patient probably will feel fatigued 1-2 days after the procedure. *This is caused by decreased plasma protein levels.* Encourage extra rest and a high-protein diet during this time. Encourage consumption of milk products.

- Teach patient to monitor IV access site for signs of infection, such as warmth, redness, swelling, or drainage, and to report significant findings.
- Teach patient to monitor for signs of bruising or bleeding. *The anticoagulant citrate dextrose is used in the extracorporeal machine circuitry to prevent clotting. This may cause excessive bleeding at the access site.* Inform patient to observe for black, tarry stools. *This finding usually signals presence of blood.* Tell patient that the presence of any of these signs should be reported.
- A pressure dressing may be kept in place over the access site for 2-4 hr after the procedure. Caution patient about avoiding cutting self or bumping into objects and to sustain pressure over cuts if they occur.

Patient-Family Teaching and Discharge Planning

Most patients with GBS eventually recover fully, but because the recovery period can be prolonged, the patient often goes home with some degree of neurologic deficit. Discharge planning and teaching will vary according to the degree of disability. Include verbal and written information about the following:

- Disease process, expected improvement, and importance of continuing in rehabilitation or PT program to promote as full a recovery as possible.
- Safety measures relative to decreased sensorimotor deficit.
- Exercises that promote muscle strength and mobility, measures for preventing contractures and skin breakdown, transfer techniques and proper body mechanics, and use of assistive devices.
- Indications of constipation, urinary retention, or UTI; implementation of bowel and bladder training programs; and if appropriate, care of indwelling catheters or self-catheterization technique.
- Indications of URI; measures for preventing regurgitation, aspiration, and respiratory infection.
- Medications, including drug names, purpose, dosage, schedule, precautions, and potential side effects. Also discuss drug/drug, herb/drug, and food/drug interactions.
- Importance of follow-up care, including visits to health care provider, PT, and OT.
- Referrals to community resources such as public health nurse, visiting nurse association, community support groups, social workers, psychologic therapy, home health agencies, and extended and skilled care facilities. Additional general information can be obtained by accessing the following website:

  GBS/CIDP Foundation International: www.gbs-cidp.org

❖ BACTERIAL MENINGITIS

OVERVIEW/PATHOPHYSIOLOGY

Bacterial meningitis is an infection that results in inflammation of the meningeal membranes covering the brain and spinal cord. Bacteria in the subarachnoid space multiply and cause an inflammatory reaction of the pia and arachnoid meninges. Purulent exudate is produced, and inflammation and infection spread quickly through the cerebrospinal fluid (CSF) that circulates around the brain and spinal cord. Bacteria and exudate can create vascular congestion, plugging the arachnoid villi. This obstruction of CSF flow and decreased reabsorption of CSF can lead to hydrocephalus, increased intracranial pressure (IICP), brain herniation, and death.

Meningitis generally is transmitted in one of four ways: (1) via airborne droplets or contact with oral secretions from infected individuals; (2) from direct contamination (e.g., from a penetrating skull wound; a skull fracture, often basilar, causing a tear in the dura; lumbar puncture (LP); ventricular shunt; or surgical procedure); (3) via the bloodstream (e.g., pneumonia, endocarditis); or (4) from direct contact with an infectious process that invades the meningeal membranes, as can occur with osteomyelitis, sinusitis, otitis media, mastoiditis, or brain abscess. In adults, pneumococcal meningitis, caused by *Streptococcus pneumoniae,* is the most common bacterial meningitis. Meningococcal meningitis, caused by *Neisseria meningitidis,* is next. Infection with *Haemophilus influenzae* type b has decreased significantly with the immunization of infants. *Listeria monocytogenes* infection is on the rise, especially in the immunocompromised or the extremely young or old. Outbreaks have been associated with consumption of contaminated dairy or undercooked fish, chicken, and meat. Any bacterium can cause meningitis, and some forms of meningitis, such as one caused by *Staphylococcus aureus,* can be difficult to treat because of their resistance to important antibiotics. Adhesions and fibrotic changes in the arachnoid layer and subspace may cause obstruction or reabsorption problems with CSF that result in hydrocephalus. Although the mortality rate is still high among untreated or delayed-treatment cases, prognosis for most patients with bacterial meningitis is generally good. Complete neurologic recovery is possible if the disorder is recognized early and antibiotic treatment is initiated promptly.

ASSESSMENT

Signs and symptoms/physical findings: Cardinal signs include headache, fever, stiff neck, change in mental status.
Infection: Fever, chills, malaise.
IICP and herniation: Decreased level of consciousness (LOC) (irritability, drowsiness, stupor, coma), nausea and vomiting, decreasing Glasgow Coma Scale (GCS) score (see p. 307), VS changes (increased BP, decreased heart rate [HR], widening pulse pressure), changes in respiratory pattern, decreased pupillary reaction to light, pupillary dilation or inequality, and severe headache.
Meningeal irritation: Back stiffness and pain, headache, nuchal rigidity.
Other: Generalized seizures and photophobia. In the presence of *H. influenzae* infection, deafness or joint pain may occur.

Physical Assessment

- Brudzinski's sign may be elicited because of meningeal irritation: when the neck is passively flexed forward, both legs flex involuntarily at the hip and knee.
- Kernig's sign also may be found: when the thigh is flexed 90 degrees at the hip, the individual cannot extend the leg completely without pain.
- Meningococcal rash pressure test: the rash fails to whiten under pressure. In the presence of meningococcal meningitis, the following may occur: a pink, macular rash; petechiae; ecchymoses; purpura; and increased deep tendon reflexes (DTRs). The rash signals septicemia and is associated with a 40% mortality rate, even with appropriate antibiotics. The rash can progress to gangrenous necrosis that may need debridement or even amputation. Myocarditis also occurs often.

DIAGNOSTIC TESTS

LP, CSF analysis, and Gram stain and culture: Identify causative organism. Glucose is generally decreased, and protein is increased. Increased total low-density lipoprotein (LDH) in CSF is a consistent finding. Presence or absence of C-reactive protein (CRP) in the CSF can differentiate between bacterial (positive for CRP) and nonbacterial (negative for CRP) meningitis. Typically, CSF is cloudy or milky because of increased white blood cells (WBCs); CSF pressure is increased because of the inflammation and exudate, causing an obstruction in outflow of CSF from the arachnoid villi. If performed (CFS analysis via LP) in the presence of IICP, LP can cause brain herniation. If CSF pressure is elevated, check neurologic LP status and VS at frequent intervals for signs of brain herniation (decreased LOC; pupillary changes such as dilation, inequality, or decreased reaction; irregular respirations; hemiparesis).

Culture and sensitivity testing of blood, sputum, urine, and other body secretions: Identifies infective organism and/or its source and determines appropriate antibiotic.

Coagglutination tests: Detect microbial antigens in CSF and enable identification of the causative organism. Generally coagglutination tests have replaced counterimmunoelectrophoresis (CIE) because results are obtainable much more rapidly.

Polymerase chain reaction (PCR) assay: Analyzes DNA in peripheral blood or CSF to identify causative infectious agents.

Radioimmunoassay (RIA), latex particle agglutination (LPA), or **enzyme-linked immunosorbent assay (ELISA):** Detects microbial antigens in the CSF to identify causative organism.

Xpert enteroviral [meningitis] (EV) test: Isolates and amplifies viral genetic material present in CSF and helps distinguish between viral and bacterial meningitis.

Petechial skin scraping: For Gram stain analysis of bacteria.

Sinus, skull, and chest x-ray examinations: Performed after treatment is started to rule out sinusitis, pneumonia, and cranial osteomyelitis.

CT scan with contrast: Rules out hydrocephalus or mass lesions such as brain abscess and detects exudate in CSF spaces.

MRI: Rules out hydrocephalus or mass lesion and detects exudate in CSF spaces.

COLLABORATIVE MANAGEMENT

Transmission-based precautions: droplet Patients infected with *N. meningitidis* or *H. influenzae,* or in whom the causative organism is in doubt, require observation with Transmission-Based Precautions: Droplet for 24 hr after initiation of appropriate antibiotic therapy. Patient should be placed in a private room if possible. If private room is not available, infected patient may be placed in a room with another patient who is at low risk for adverse outcome if transmission occurs, after ensuring that patients are physically separated (i.e., more than 3 ft) from each other. Infection may be spread by contact with respiratory droplets or oral secretions. Masks should be worn for close patient contact (e.g., within 3 ft), along with adherence to Standard Precautions (see p. 743).

Pharmacotherapy

Parenteral antibiotics: Because treatment cannot be delayed until culture results are known, high doses are started immediately, based on Gram stain results. The antibiotic must penetrate the blood-brain barrier into the CSF. Adjustments in therapy can be made after coagglutination test, CIE, and culture and sensitivity test results are available. Antibiotics may include the following (usually in combination): penicillin G, ampicillin, cefotaxime, ceftriaxone, ceftazidime, chloramphenicol, gentamicin, and vancomycin.

Prophylactic antibiotic treatment of significant other and close contacts: Usually, rifampin is administered. Other antibiotics, such as ciprofloxacin, ceftriaxone, chloramphenicol, sulfadiazine, or minocycline, may be used as well. It is important that all contacts be notified as soon as possible for treatment and known signs and symptoms to report to health care provider (e.g., headache, fever, stiff neck, change in mental status).

Glucocorticosteroids (e.g., dexamethasone): Ideally given before or at same time as first dose of antibiotics and then on an ongoing basis to reduce inflammation caused by toxic byproducts released by bacterial cells as they are killed by antibiotics. This therapy can reduce hearing loss in children that is caused by *H. influenzae.*

CRP replacement therapy (e.g., drotrecogin alfa [activated]): For septic meningococcal meningitis and purpura fulminans.

Osmotic diuretics (e.g., mannitol) and loop diuretics (e.g., furosemide): Decrease cerebral edema in the presence of impending IICP.

Antiepilepsy drugs (AEDs) (e.g., carbamazepine, diazepam, phenytoin, phenobarbital, fosphenytoin): Control seizures.

Analgesics (e.g., acetaminophen, codeine): Relieve headache, myalgia, and other pain.

Antipyretics (e.g., acetaminophen): For control of fever to reduce cerebral metabolism.

Mild sedatives (e.g., diphenhydramine): Promote rest.

Antacids and histamine H_2-receptor blockers (e.g., ranitidine) or proton pump inhibitor (pantoprazole): Reduce gastric acidity and prevent hemorrhage or ulcer formation.

Stool softeners and laxatives (e.g., docusate sodium, Milk of Magnesia): Prevent constipation and straining at stool, which would increase intracranial pressure (ICP).

Tranquilizers (e.g., chlorpromazine): Control shivering, which can increase ICP.

Low-dose heparin, low-molecular-weight heparin (e.g., enoxaparin): For antithrombus prophylaxis.

Respiratory support: Via O_2, pulse oximetry monitoring, suctioning, airway maintenance, or intubation with ventilatory assistance as necessary.

Bed rest with elevation of HOB and seizure precautions: Promotes venous drainage, helps reduce cerebral congestion and edema, and prevents injury from possible seizure activity.

Fluid management: Maintains normovolemia.

Nutritional support: Parenteral or enteral feedings or modified diet, depending on patient's LOC and ability to swallow.

Measures to reduce hyperthermia: Tepid sponges, cooling blankets, and convection blankets may assist in controlling hyperpyrexia.

Antithrombus therapy: Antiembolism hose, sequential compression devices (SCDs), or pneumatic foot pumps may be prescribed to prevent thrombophlebitis in legs from venous stasis.

Treatment of complications: Examples of complications include disseminated intravascular coagulation (DIC), hyponatremia, syndrome of inappropriate antidiuretic hormone (SIADH), IICP, respiratory or heart failure, and septic shock. External ventriculostomy or shunt may be needed if hydrocephalus from arachnoid adhesions and fibrotic changes persists. Meningococcal meningitis may cause adrenal hemorrhage and insufficiency leading to vascular collapse and death. See "Addisonian Crisis," p. 396.

Intrathecal antibiotics: Sometimes used if it is believed that systemic antibiotics alone will not be curative in the presence of particular bacteria (e.g., *Pseudomonas, Enterobacter, Staphylococcus*).

Physical medicine: Physical therapy and rehabilitation program may be needed, depending on neurologic deficits.

Vaccination: A pneumococcal vaccine is available to help protect against meningitis and other infections caused by *S. pneumoniae*. The American Academy of Pediatrics recommends that pneumococcal vaccine (PCV7) be given to all children ages 24-59 mo who are at high risk for the infection. *H. influenzae* type b vaccine should be incorporated as part of all routine childhood inoculations. *N. meningitidis* has several subgroup strains. For people at increased risk (e.g., travelers to countries with endemic infections), a meningococcal polysaccharide vaccine (protects against groups A, C, Y, (and W-135) is available, although it does not confer 100% protection. The Centers for Disease Control and Prevention (CDC) recommends this meningococcal vaccine for children 11-12 yr, adolescents at high school entry, and college freshmen living in dormitories. The PCV7 meningococcal vaccine is recommended for high-risk groups such as college students, military personnel, and travelers to foreign countries where there is a high incidence of *N. meningitidis* disease.

NURSING DIAGNOSES
AND INTERVENTIONS

Deficient knowledge related to side effects and precautions for prescribed antibiotics
Desired outcome: Before beginning medication regimen, patient and significant other verbalize knowledge about potential side effects and precautions for prescribed antibiotics.

Nursing Interventions

- Assess patient's and significant others' facility with language; provide interpreter or language-appropriate written materials as indicated.
- For close contacts taking prophylactic rifampin, explain prescribed dose and schedule. Rifampin should be taken 1 hr before meals. *This is for maximum absorption.* Emphasize importance of taking this drug as prescribed. *This regimen is a preventive measure against meningitis.* Describe potential side effects such as nausea, vomiting, diarrhea, orange urine, headache, and dizziness. Caution against wearing contact lenses. *The drug will permanently color them orange.* In addition, explain rifampin is contraindicated during pregnancy. *It reduces effectiveness of oral contraceptives.*
- Instruct close contacts who are taking rifampin to report onset of jaundice (yellow skin or sclera), allergic reactions, and persistence of gastrointestinal (GI) side effects.
- Teach, as appropriate, about other antibiotics that may be given.

Deficient knowledge related to rationale and procedure for Transmission-Based Precautions: Droplet
Desired outcome: Before visitation, patient and significant other verbalize knowledge about the rationale for Transmission-Based Precautions: Droplet and comply with prescribed restrictions and precautionary measures.

Nursing Interventions

- Patients with *N. meningitidis or H. influenzae* infection or meningitis caused by an unidentified organism will be placed in a private room, if possible, and will require Transmission-Based Precautions: Droplet for 24 hr after initiation of appropriate antibiotic therapy. Masks should be worn for contact (e.g., within 3 ft), and Standard Precautions procedures should be observed.
- For patients with meningitis caused by *H. influenzae* or *N. meningitidis,* explain method of disease transmission via respiratory droplets generated by patient when coughing, sneezing, or talking or during performance of cough-inducing procedures (e.g., suctioning) and by contact with oral secretions and rationale for private room and droplet precautions.
- Provide instructions for covering mouth before coughing or sneezing and properly disposing of tissue (Respiratory Hygiene/Cough Etiquette).
- Instruct patients with Transmission-Based Precautions: Droplet to stay in their rooms. If they must leave the room for a procedure or test, explain that a mask must be worn. *This is to protect others from contact with respiratory droplets.*
- For individuals in contact with patient, explain importance of wearing a surgical mask and using good handwashing technique. Gloves should be worn when handling any body fluid, especially oral secretions. For more information, see Appendix 1, "Infection Prevention and Control," p. 743.
- Reassure patient that Transmission-Based Precautions: Droplet are temporary and will be discontinued once patient has been taking appropriate antibiotic for at least 24 hr.
- Instruct individuals in contact with patient that if symptoms of meningitis develop (e.g., headache, fever, neck stiffness, photophobia, change in

mental status), they should report immediately to their health care providers. *Immediate treatment is essential to reduce risk of mortality.*

Acute pain related to headache, photophobia, and neck stiffness secondary to meningitis
Desired outcomes: Within 1-2 hr of intervention, patient's subjective perception of discomfort decreases, as documented by pain scale. Objective indicators, such as grimacing, are absent or diminished.

Nursing Interventions

◆ Provide a quiet environment and a darkened room. Promote bed rest and assist with activities of daily living (ADL) as needed to decrease movement. Restrict visitors as necessary. Suggest wearing sunglasses. *These interventions may prevent or reduce pain and photophobia.*

◆ Apply ice bag to head or cool cloth to eyes. *This is to to help diminish headache.*

◆ Support patient in a position of comfort. Many persons with meningitis are comforted in a position with head in extension and body slightly curled. Head of bed (HOB) elevated to 30 degrees also may help. Keep neck in alignment during position changes.

◆ Provide gentle passive ROM and massage to neck and shoulder joints and muscles. *This may help relieve stiffness.* If patient is afebrile, apply moist heat to neck and back. *This promotes muscle relaxation and may decrease pain.*

◆ Keep communication simple and direct, and use a soft, calm tone of voice. Even gentle touching may startle patient. Loosen constricting bed clothing. Avoid restraining patient. Reduce stimulation to the minimal amount needed to accomplish required activity. *Patients tend to be hyperirritable with hyperalgesia (increased sensitivity to pain).*

◆ For other nursing interventions see **Acute pain** in "General Care of Patients with Neurologic Deficits," p. 366.

Patient-Family Teaching and Discharge Planning

The extent of teaching and discharge planning will depend on whether the patient has any residual damage. Include verbal and written information about the following:

◆ Referrals to community resources, such as public health nurse, visiting nurses association, community support groups, social workers, psychologic therapy, vocational rehabilitation agency, home health agencies, and extended and skilled care facilities.

◆ Medications, including drug names, purpose, dosage, schedule, precautions, and potential side effects for patient's medications, as well as those for the prophylactic antibiotics taken by family and significant other. Also discuss drug/drug, herb/drug, and food/drug interactions. Close contacts taking prophylactic antibiotics should know signs and symptoms to report to health care provider (e.g., headache, fever, neck stiffness).

◆ For patients with residual neurologic deficits, teach the following as appropriate: exercises that promote muscle strength and mobility; measures for preventing contractures and skin breakdown; transfer techniques and proper body mechanics; safety measures if patient has decreased pain and sensation or visual disturbances; use of assistive devices; indications of constipation, urinary retention, or urinary tract infection (UTI); bowel and bladder training programs; self-catheterization technique or care of indwelling catheters; and seizure precautions if indicated.

◆ Obtain additional information by accessing the following website:
Meningitis Foundation of America, Inc.: www.musa.org

❖ ❖ ❖

SECTION TWO **DEGENERATIVE DISORDERS OF THE NERVOUS SYSTEM**

❖ PARKINSON'S DISEASE/PARKINSONISM

OVERVIEW/PATHOPHYSIOLOGY

Parkinson's disease (PD), also known as parkinsonism, is a slowly progressive degenerative disorder of the central nervous system (CNS) that affects the brain centers that regulate movement and balance. For unknown reasons, cell death occurs in the substantia nigra of the midbrain. When healthy, the substantia nigra projects dopaminergic neurons into the corpus striatum and releases the neurotransmitter dopamine in that area. Degeneration of these neurons leads to an abnormally low concentration of dopamine in the basal ganglia. The basal ganglia control muscle tone and voluntary motor movement via a balance between two main neurotransmitters, dopamine and acetylcholine. The deficit of dopamine, which has an inhibitory effect, allows the relative excess of acetylcholine. The excitatory effect of acetylcholine causes overactivity of the basal ganglia, which interferes with normal muscle tone and control of smooth, purposeful movement and causes the characteristic triad of symptoms of PD: muscle rigidity, tremors, and bradykinesia. Nerve cell loss in the substantia nigra and accumulation of Lewy bodies in the brainstem and pigmented areas of the brain are the pathologic hallmarks of PD. Lewy bodies are tiny abnormal spherical alpha-synuclein protein deposits that accumulate inside the damaged nerve cells and disrupt the brain's normal functioning. Symptoms start when cell loss reaches about 80%. PD is usually progressive, and death can result from aspiration pneumonia or choking. *Neuroleptic malignant syndrome,* a medical emergency, is usually precipitated by failure to take prescribed medications. *Acute akinesia,* sometimes referred to as *parkinsonian crisis,* is another medical emergency and seems associated with infections or surgical procedures.

ASSESSMENT

Signs and symptoms/physical findings: Initially, signs and symptoms are mild and include stiffness or slight hand tremors. Symptoms may be subtle and not be noticed for years. Typically, they begin on one side (may remain worse on that side) and then gradually increase. The symptoms may become disabling. Cardinal features are tremors, rigidity, and bradykinesia that start on one side and over time become bilateral. Clinical features most suggestive of idiopathic PD include unilateral onset, presence of resting tremor, and a clear-cut response to treatment with L-dopa. Assessment findings vary in degree and are highly individualized. PD is sometimes categorized as either tremor-dominant type or postural instability and gait disturbance (PIGD)–dominant type. Usually a positive blink reflex is elicited by tapping a finger between the patient's eyebrows. Blinking may occur 5-10 ×/min instead of the normal 20 ×/min. A positive palmomental (palm-chin) reflex can be elicited (muscles of the chin and corner of mouth contract when the patient's palm is stroked). Diminished postural reflexes are present on neurologic examination; however, there is risk of injury with postural reflex testing because patients may quickly lose balance and fall.

Tremors: Increase when the limb is at rest and completely supported against gravity and stop with voluntary movement and during sleep (nonintentional "resting" tremor). "Pill-rolling" tremor of the hands and "to-and-fro" tremor of the head are typical. Some people with PD do not have serious tremors.

Bradykinesia: Slowness, stiffness, and difficulty initiating movement. Patients may have a masklike, blank facial expression; unblinking stare; difficulty chewing and swallowing; drooling caused by decreased frequency of swallowing; and a high-pitched, monotone, weak voice. Speech may be slow and slurred. The patient also has loss of automatic associated movements, such as the normal arm-swing movement when walking unless making a conscious effort and episodes of "freezing." Handwriting becomes progressively smaller, cramped, and tremulous.

Increased muscle rigidity: Limb muscles become rigid on passive motion. Typically, this rigidity results in jerky ("cogwheel") motions or steady resistance to all movement ("lead pipe" rigidity). It may limit movement and cause pain.

Loss of postural reflexes: Causes the typical stooped, forward-leaning, shuffling, propulsive gait with short, rapidly accelerating steps; stumbling; and difficulty maintaining or regaining balance, which makes the individual prone to stumbling and falling. Abnormal gait in which the body is bent backward (retropulsion) also may be present.

Speech changes: Speech may be rapid or monotone with some slurring or repeating or hesitating with words.

Autonomic: Excessive diaphoresis, seborrhea, postural hypotension, decreased libido, hypomotility of the gastrointestinal (GI) tract (causing constipation), and urinary hesitancy. Vision may blur as a result of lost pupillary accommodation.

Mental health/psychiatric: Dementia (e.g., forgetfulness, irritability, paranoia, hallucinations) is commonly associated with PD. However, not all patients develop impaired intellectual and mental functioning. Mental status testing may be complicated by the patient's movement disorder. Some patients may experience akathisia, a condition of motor restlessness in which there is a compelling need to walk about constantly. Depression is common. Psychosis is often drug induced.

Neuroleptic malignant syndrome: Classic triad of symptoms includes fever (100%), rigidity (90%), and cognitive changes (e.g., drowsiness, confusion progressing to stupor and coma). Other signs and symptoms include tremor, tachypnea, diaphoresis, and occasionally dystonia and chorea. Symptoms reappear with discontinuation or reduction in dopaminergic medications. This sudden and severe increase in muscle rigidity can cause inability to swallow or maintain a patent airway.

Acute akinesia: This sudden decrease in motor performance or inability to move ("frozen" posture) lasts for more than 48 hr and is transiently unresponsive to dopaminergic rescue medication (e.g., apomorphine) or increases in dopaminergic medications. Triggering factors include infections, surgery, GI disease, and drug manipulations.

Oculogyric crisis: Fixation of eyes in one position, generally upward, sometimes for several hours. This is relatively rare.

History and risk factors: PD has many possible causes. Metabolic causes such as hypothyroidism need to be ruled out. Long-term therapy with large doses of medications, such as haloperidol, phenothiazines, metoclopramide, methyldopa, reserpine, or chlorpromazine, can produce extrapyramidal side effects known as *pseudoparkinsonism.* If the condition is caused by these medications, symptoms will disappear when the drug is discontinued. The recreational drug "ecstasy" and an improperly synthesized heroin-like substance, 1-methyl-4-phenyl-1,2,3,6-tetrahydropyridine (MPTP), also have induced parkinsonism. Other causes include toxins (e.g., heavy metals, pesticides, lacquer thinner, and carbon monoxide), cerebrovascular disease, head injury (especially repeated injury), and viral encephalitis. Living in a rural area is associated with increased PD risk, whereas nicotine intake is associated with decreased PD risk. Most cases of PD occur without an apparent or known cause, although genetic susceptibility is believed to play a role. Genetic factors appear to be more predominant when the disease begins before the age of 45-50 yr, with the most common known forms of hereditary parkinsonism caused by mutations in the parkin gene *(PARK2)* and the alpha-synuclein gene. Men are more likely to develop the disease.

BOX 5-1		STAGING OF PARKINSON'S DISEASE
Mild	I	Unilateral disease
	II	Bilateral disease without impairment of balance
Moderate	III	Mild to moderate bilateral disease with some postural instability; physically independent
	IV	Considerable disability; markedly impaired balance; still able to stand or walk unassisted
Severe	V	Wheelchair bound or bedridden unless aided

Modified from National Institute of Neurological Disorders and Stroke: *Hoehn and Yahr staging of Parkinson's disease. Parkinson's disease: hope through research.* Available at: www.ninds.nih.gov/disorders/parkinsons_disease/detail_parkinsons_disease.htm. Accessed March 2010.

Unified Parkinson's Disease rating scale (UPDRS): Often used as a standardized assessment tool. UPDRS is comprehensive but complicated and includes evaluation of mentation, behavior, and mood, ADL during both "on" and "off" periods, motor abilities, and recent complications of therapy.

Hoehn and Yahr stage scale: Simple scale that stages PD severity and disability. The different stages of disease are classified from I to V (**BOX 5-1**).

DIAGNOSTIC TESTS

There are no definitive tests for PD. Diagnosis usually is made on the basis of physical assessment and characteristic symptoms and after other neurologic conditions have been ruled out. The diagnosis is likely if the patient has the classic triad of symptoms, onset on one side of the body, greater tremor at rest, and a significant response to levodopa. However, the first serum diagnostic test for PD (and Alzheimer's disease [ALZ]), called NuroPro, is currently being tested in several clinical trials and shows promising results.

Positron emission tomography (PET) (e.g., 6-^{18}F-fluoro-L-dopa [FDOPA/PET], ^{18}F-fluorodeoxyglucose [FDG/PET]): May reveal areas of decreased dopamine metabolism via use of the labeled dopamine-transporter amino acids FDOPA, used for diagnosis in Europe, or FDG, used with PET imaging.

Urinalysis for dopamine metabolites: May reveal decreased dopamine level, which supports the diagnosis.

EEG: Often shows such abnormalities as diffuse, nonspecific slowing of theta (Θ)-waves, which are slow, high-amplitude waves present during sleep but abnormal in awake adults.

Lumbar puncture (LP) with CSF analysis: CSF fluid is analyzed for specific proteins and chemicals that are leaked from the brain in PD and that cannot be measured in blood. Abnormalities of a protein called alpha-synuclein are found in PD and may serve as a disease marker and be used to monitor disease progression.

Single photon emission computed tomography (SPECT): Reveals how a radioisotope-tagged drug accumulates in the brain; may be useful in detecting PD and gauging disease progress.

Tremor studies: Serial measurements of functional activity show decreased performance.

Cineradiographic study of swallowing: May show abnormal pattern and delayed relaxation of cricopharyngeal muscles.

COLLABORATIVE MANAGEMENT

Pharmacotherapy: Medications can help manage patients' symptoms. It is important to avoid medications that will make symptoms worse, such as phenothiazines, metoclopramide, methyldopas, and reserpine.

Dopamine replacements (e.g., levodopa, levodopa-carbidopa): Given in increasing amounts until symptoms are reduced or patient's tolerance to side effects is reached. These agents may be used for initial therapy or later when other medications can no longer control symptoms. They pass into the brain and are converted into dopamine. Levodopa combined with carbodopa prevents premature conversion to dopamine outside the brain. It also prevents nausea. Levodopa-benserazide combinations are available in Canada and Europe.

Antiviral agents (e.g., amantadine): Less effective than levodopa but with less severe side effects. Amantadine may be used as initial therapy or as an adjunct. Effects diminish in a few months; therefore, this drug may be used intermittently. It may help in late stages with involuntary movements.

Dopamine agonists (e.g., pramipexole, ropinirole, bromocriptine, rotigotime, cabergoline): Administered with a concomitant reduction of dopamine replacement dosage; may be used to reduce levodopa-induced dyskinesia, such as involuntary movements and the frequency of "on-off" responses. Apomorphine is a dopamine agonist given subcutaneously as a "rescue" drug for acute intermittent treatment of hypomobility ("off" episodes). It is given along with an antiemetic to reduce emesis and orthostatic hypotension.

Monoamine oxidase (MAO) type B inhibitors (e.g., selegiline, rasagiline): Used as an early intervention or as adjuncts with levodopa to inhibit the breakdown of naturally occuring dopamine and dopamine formed from levodopa; the result is less fluctuation in blood levels.

Catechol O-methyltransferase (COMT) inhibitor (e.g., entacapone, tolcapone): Reduces levodopa degradation in the GI tract, kidneys, and liver to minimize fluctuation in serum levels. Tolcapone is used only for people who do not respond to other therapies because of potential side effects, such as hepatotoxicity.

Anticholinergics (e.g., trihexyphenidyl, benztropine mesylate): Often used in conjunction with dopamine replacement therapy but may be used alone if patient's symptoms are mild or if patient cannot tolerate levodopa. Anticholinergics may improve tremor and rigidity but often do little for bradykinesia or balance problems.

Antihistamines (e.g., diphenhydramine): Usually given in conjunction with anticholinergic drugs but may be used alone if patient's symptoms are mild. Antihistamines have a central cholinergic blocking action, and they prolong dopamine action by inhibiting its uptake and storage.

Antidyskinetics (e.g., ethopropazine): Generally used in combination with other antiparkinson drugs to reduce rigidity, tremors, and spasms.

Laxatives and stool softeners (e.g., docusate sodium, Milk of Magnesia): Prevent constipation. A reduction in anticholinergic medications may help constipation.

Antitremor medications (e.g., propranolol, primidone, clonazepam): May be used to decrease tremors. Clonazepam also may help with restless leg syndrome.

Antidepressants (e.g., fluoxetine, sertraline, paroxetine, venlafaxine, amitriptyline): Treat depression, as well as some PD symptoms; help to block reabsorption of dopamine and have some anticholinergic properties.

Antiorthostatic hypotension agents (e.g., fludrocortisone, midodrine): Prevent orthostatic hypotension.

Atypical antipsychotics (e.g., quetiapine, olanzapine, clozapine): Decrease psychotic symptoms.

Anticholinergics (e.g., hyoscyamine, glycopyrrolate): Reduce volume of secretions to help prevent drooling.

Botulinum toxin A: Injected into the parotid salivary glands to reduce salivary secretion and treat drooling; also may be injected into the axilla to reduce excessive sweating. For GI symptoms, intrapyloric botulinun toxin injections may improve gastric emptying, whereas injection into the puborectalis muscle may correct anorectal dysfunction that causes constipation.

Cholinesterase inhibitors (e.g., donepezil, rivastigmine, galantamine): Off-label use to improve mild to moderate memory deficit, cognitive decline, and dementia.

Antiemetics (e.g., trimethobenzamide): For nausea.

Treatment of complications of dopamine replacement therapy: Many of the problems associated with dopamine replacement therapy are related to fluctuating blood levels. Use of medication preparations in extended-release forms, transdermal forms (as they are developed and become available), or continuous infusion forms should help prevent these problems.

Choreiform or involuntary, spasmodic, jerking movements, (e.g., facial grimacing, tongue protrusion, restlessness)
◆ Dose reduction or redistribution throughout the day and dopamine agonist or extended-release forms of levodopa-carbidopa.

Severe mental status changes (e.g., agitation, confusion, psychosis)
◆ Dose reduction.
◆ Clozapine, quetiapine, olanzapin, or risperidone for drug-related psychoses.

"End of dose" wearing-off phenomenon: Return of signs and symptoms (bradykinesis, tremors, rigidity) before next dose is due.
◆ Administer smaller, more frequent doses.
◆ Use slow-release medication preparations or transdermal dosing (if available).
◆ Increase dosing; add dopamine agonist or COMT inhibitor.
◆ Encourage redistributed protein diet (see discussion in "Diet," later).

Vivid dreaming
◆ Reduce last dose of levodopa given at night.

On-off response: This is a rapid fluctuation or change in patient's condition. The individual is "on" one moment, in a state of relative mobility, and "off" the next, in a state of complete or nearly complete immobility. Cause is uncertain but appears to be related to fluctuating drug levels in the brain as loss of striatal ability to store dopamine progresses. Usually this response occurs after patient has been on medication for several years and has not found relief through increasing levodopa dosages.
◆ Smaller, more frequent doses to titrate and space levodopa doses during the 24-hr day. Mix with water; do not give with food.
◆ Combining levodopa with anticholinergic medications, dopamine agonists, or amantadine may be helpful.
◆ Use of sustained-release forms of levodopa.
◆ Use of liquid preparations.
◆ Administration of subcutaneous apomorphine. This dopamine agonist can counter the on-off response. IV apomorphine can serve as a "rescue" drug if the on-off effect is severe enough to require going off levodopa for a few days. An antiemetic (e.g., trimethobenzamide) is given before apomorphine to reduce emesis and orthostatic hypotension.
◆ Continuous enteral infusion of levodopa or gel formulation of levodopa/carbidopa via gastric or jejunal (percutaneous endoscopic gastrostomy [PEG] or percutaneous endoscopic jejunostomy [PEJ]) tubes.

Treatment for neuroleptic malignant syndrome: The dopaminergic drug should be restarted as soon as possible to prevent rhabdomyolysis and renal failure. Therapy is supportive, with adequate hydration and electrolyte stabilization and with cooling blankets to reduce hyperthermia. Ventilatory assistance may be required, and occasionally renal dialysis is necessary.

Treatment for acute akinesia: This akinetic state lasts several days and does not respond to dopaminergic drugs. Treatment is supportive and may necessitate respiratory and cardiac support. A search for a triggering cause, such as systemic infection, recent surgery, fractures, or GI disorder should be initiated and treated when found.

Physical medicine and exercise program: Massage; muscle stretching; active/passive ROM, especially on hands and feet; walking and gait training exercises; suggestions for maintaining mobility and initiating movements; occupational therapy (OT) evaluation for assistive devices to help with self-care and ADL.

Speech/swallowing evaluation and therapy: For patients with verbal deficits and swallowing difficulties.

Antiembolism hose: Help prevent postural hypotension.

Counseling or psychotherapy: Helps patient and significant other adapt to the disability and cope with emotions and feelings, such as depression, that are either a direct or an indirect result of the disease process or drug therapy. Occasionally, electroconvulsive therapy is used for persistent and serious depression.

Diet: A controlled, "redistributed" protein diet to reduce the negative impact high protein content has on levodopa effectiveness. This diet restricts daytime protein intake to promote daytime motor performance and shifts a greater portion of the daily protein to the evening meal. Pyridoxine (vitamin B_6) also reduces effectiveness of levodopa. A high-fiber diet may be given to prevent constipation. Because use of caffeine may increase patient's symptoms, a caffeine-free diet helps some individuals. Giving medications 20-30 min before meals may help improve appetite and thereby aid nutrition. Thickened liquids or gastrostomy tube may be needed for patients at risk of aspiration.

Deep brain electrostimulation: Achieved by surgically implanting electrodes connected to a pacemaker-like device. It is now used preferentially over ablative procedures inasmuch as it has the same effect without destroying parts of the brain. Stimulation of the thalamus helps with tremors, whereas globus pallidus stimulation works better in controlling rigidity and balance and reduces medication side effects, thereby leading to better drug tolerance, but it does not reduce the amount of medication given. Stimulation of the subthalamic nucleus (STN) helps with all symptoms of PD and enables reduction in medication. STN is the preferred target for deep brain stimulation. The patient switches stimulation on and off with a magnet.

Stereotactic pallidotomy surgery: Involves use of electrical coagulation, freezing, radioactivity, or ultrasound to destroy portions of the globus pallidus or ventrolateral nucleus of the thalamus to prevent involuntary movement and help relieve tremors and rigidity of the extremities. Gamma knife radiosurgery of this region is also effective in reducing tremors, but final results take 6-8 wk to determine.

Collagen injections into vocal cord: Treat voice loss.

Neural gastric electrical stimulation: Treats gastroparesis.

NURSING DIAGNOSES AND INTERVENTIONS

Risk for falls related to unsteady gait secondary to bradykinesia, tremors, and rigidity

Desired outcome: Following instruction, patient demonstrates safe and effective ambulatory techniques and preventive measures against falls and remains free of trauma.

Nursing Interventions

- During ambulation, encourage patient to deliberately swing arms to assist gait and raise feet. *This will help prevent falls.* Advise patient to step over imaginary object or line and practice taking long steps to increase stride. *This will help raise feet higher and avoid shuffling.*
- Have patient practice movements that are especially difficult (e.g., turning). Teach patient to walk in a wide arc ("U-turn") rather than pivot when turning. *This is to avoid crossing one leg over the other.*
- Teach head and neck exercises to promote good posture. Remind patient repeatedly to maintain upright posture and look up, not down, especially

when walking. *This is particularly important for patients with bifocal glasses inasmuch as a stooped posture promotes looking down through the reading portion of the bifocal lens where distant items appear blurred.*

◆ Advise patient to stop occasionally to slow walking speed. Teach patient to concentrate on listening to feet as they touch the floor and count cadence. *This will prevent a too-fast gait.* Encourage patient to lift toes and to walk with heels touching floor first. Remind patient to maintain a wide-based gait.

◆ Provide a clear pathway while patient is walking. Teach patient to avoid crowds, scatter rugs, uneven surfaces, fast turns, narrow doorways, and obstructions. *This is to prevent falls and other injuries.*

◆ Advise patient to wear leather-soled or smooth-soled shoes but to test shoes first to ensure they are not too slippery. *Rubber-soled or crepe-soled shoes tend to catch on floors, especially carpeted floors, which may cause falls.*

◆ Encourage patient not to hurry or rush, but slowness of gait and inability to get to the bathroom fast enough may cause incontinence. Encourage male patients to keep a urinal at bedside and female patients to keep a commode at bedside. *This may prevent rushing and potential falls trying to get to the bathroom.*

◆ Encourage patient to perform ROM and stretching exercises daily and to exercise. This will help maintain flexibility, strength, gait, and balance. Emphasize that routine exercises, along with prescribed medications, may prevent or delay disability.

◆ Ask physical therapy department to suggest exercises that improve balance. Tai chi, for example, uses slow, graceful movements to relax and strengthen muscles and joints and may be encouraged as an option for some patients.

◆ For other nursing interventions, see **Risk for falls**, p. 355, in "General Care of Patients with Neurologic Deficits."

Impaired physical mobility related to difficulty initiating movement
Desired outcome: Following instruction, patient demonstrates measures that enhance ability to initiate desired movement.

Nursing Interventions

◆ Teach patient to rock from side to side or march in place a few steps before resuming forward motion. *This may may help initiate leg movement.* Other measures that may promote movement are relaxing back on heels and raising toes; tapping hip of the leg to be moved; bending at knees and straightening up; raising arms in a sudden, short motion; or humming a marching tune. If feet remain "glued" to the floor despite these measures, suggest that patient think of something else for a few moments and then try again. It may work to try changing directions (e.g., move sideways if going forward is impossible).

◆ Teach patient to get out of a chair by getting to edge of seat, placing hands on arm supports, bending forward slightly, moving feet back, and then rhythmically rocking in the chair a few times before trying to get up. Advise patient to sit in chairs with backs and arms and to purchase elevated toilet seats or sidebars in the bathroom to assist with rising. *This should reduce the chance of falling.*

◆ Teach measures that may help with getting out of bed: rocking to a sitting position, placing blocks under legs of head of bed (HOB) to elevate it, and tying a rope or sheet to foot of bed to help patient pull to a sitting position.

◆ "Freezing" is variable and can fluctuate with stress or emotional state. Teach patient and significant others to recognize situations that can cause freezing episodes so they can anticipate and plan to avoid them. For example, attempting two movements simultaneously, such as trying to change direction quickly while walking, can cause freezing. Distracting environmental, visual, or auditory stimuli also can precipitate a freezing episode. Doorways, narrow passages, or a change in floor color, texture, or slope can pose problems for many patients.

◆ Specially trained dogs (e.g., Canine Partners) can help patients walk and get up after a fall and are trained to help break a "freeze" by tapping on patient's foot.

◆ PD makes it more difficult to move, which can affect intimacy. Suggest that sexual relations be planned for when the prescribed drug is working to good effect and the person is rested. Being flexible about time; experimenting with positions; manual, oral, and vibrator stimulation; and use of sildenafil have proved beneficial.

Deficient knowledge related to side effects of and precautionary measures for taking antiparkinsonian medications
Desired outcome: Following instruction and before hospital discharge, patient and significant other verbalize knowledge about side effects of and necessary precautionary measures for taking antiparkinsonian medications.

Nursing Interventions

◆ Teach patient and significant other to report adverse side effects promptly, because many side effects are dose-related and can be controlled by a dosage adjustment.

◆ Stress importance of taking medication on schedule and not forgetting a dose. *Missing doses may adversely affect mobility.* Patient and health care provider can adjust dose schedule so that medication peaks at mealtime or at times when patient needs mobility most. Premeasure doses in segmented or separate containers labeled with date and time of dose. *This will assist patient having difficulty with self-medication.*

◆ Teach patient to take non–levodopa-containing medications with meals. Encourage patient with anorexia to eat frequent small, nutritious snacks and meals. *This will decrease the potential for nausea.*

◆ Advise patient to make position changes slowly and in stages, and elevate the HOB. Teach patient to dangle legs a few minutes before standing. Anti-embolism hose may help as well. *These measures will counteract orthostatic hypotension.* Tips for reducing morning orthostatic hypotension include not limiting late evening fluid intake and keeping a glass of water at the bedside at night so it is available to drink in the morning before getting up. Encourage male patients to urinate from a sitting rather than standing position if possible. Keep bedside urinal and walker available. Increasing dietary salt intake also may help, Teach patient to report dizziness to health care provider inasmuch as medication adjustment may be needed.

◆ Advise increasing fluid intake. *This will prevent dehydration in warm weather.*

◆ Teach use of sugarless chewing gum or hard candy, frequent mouth rinses with water, or artificial saliva products. *This will ease dry mouth and maintain integrity of oral mucous membrane.*

◆ Advise patient to report any urinary hesitancy or incontinence. *It may signal urinary retention.* Individuals taking anticholinergics may find that voiding before taking medication relieves this problem. See "Urinary Retention," p. 214, for additional measures.

◆ Constipation is a common problem with these medications. For nursing interventions, see **Constipation**, p. 29, in "Prolonged Bed Rest."

◆ Many of these drugs can cause or aggravate mental status changes such as confusion; mental slowness or dullness; and even agitation, paranoia, and hallucinations. Teach patient to report these signs to health care provider promptly for possible dose adjustment.

◆ For patient with blurred vision, orient to surroundings, teach others to identify themselves when entering room, keep walkways unobstructed, and encourage patient to ask for assistance when ambulating.

◆ See **TABLE 5-1** for the teaching interventions related to side effects common to specific antiparkinsonian medications.

Health-seeking behaviors related to facial and tongue exercises that enhance verbal communication and help prevent choking
Desired outcome: Following demonstration and within the 24-hr period before hospital discharge, patient demonstrates facial and tongue exercises and states the rationale for their use.

TABLE 5-1	ANTIPARKINSONIAN DRUGS AND SIDE EFFECTS WITH RELATED TEACHING INTERVENTIONS
MEDICATION	**SIDE EFFECTS WITH RELATED TEACHING INTERVENTIONS**
Dopamine Replacements Levodopa, carbidopa-levodopa	▪ Teach patient that levodopa should be taken with a full glass of water on an empty stomach to facilitate absorption. If nausea or GI upset occurs, suggest patient eat 10-15 min after taking medication. If patient continues to experience nausea or GI upset, the medication may be taken with food.
	▪ Teach patient to avoid vitamin preparations or fortified cereals that contain pyridoxine (vitamin B_6), which reduces effectiveness of levodopa. Intake of foods high in pyridoxine, such as wheat germ, whole grain cereals, legumes, and liver, may be limited.
	▪ Teach patient that a dietary intake high in protein may interfere with effectiveness of levodopa. Although diet should meet recommended daily allowance of protein (i.e., 0.8 g/kg body weight/day), patient should avoid excessive amounts of meat, eggs, dairy products, and legumes. If prescribed, dietary supplementation with L-tryptophan needs to be calculated into total protein allotment. If possible, protein intake should be shifted to evening meals to minimize interaction with levodopa.
	▪ Instruct patient to report muscle twitching or spasmodic winking because these are early signs of overdose.
	▪ Explain signs and symptoms of neuroleptic malignant syndrome and acute akinesia. Emphasize need for immediate medical intervention with these crises because respiratory and cardiac support may be necessary. Teach patient that to avoid neuroleptic malignant syndrome, it is necessary to take levodopa as scheduled and not to stop this medication abruptly.
	▪ Explain signs of on-off response, wearing off, other complications of therapy, and interventions (previously listed) and importance of working with health care provider on fine tuning medication regimen.
	▪ Monitor for behavioral changes. Severe depression with suicidal overtones can be caused by this drug and should be reported immediately. The health care provider may prescribe a dose reduction.
	▪ Explain that patient's medication may cause dark-colored urine and sweat.
	▪ Caution patient to avoid alcohol because it impairs effectiveness of levodopa.
	▪ Explain importance of medical follow-up while taking this drug to monitor for such problems as increased intraocular pressure and changes in glucose control.

| TABLE 5-1 | ANTIPARKINSONIAN DRUGS AND SIDE EFFECTS WITH RELATED TEACHING INTERVENTIONS—cont'd |

MEDICATION	SIDE EFFECTS WITH RELATED TEACHING INTERVENTIONS
Dopamine Antagonists Pramipexole, ropinirole, bromocriptine, rotigotine, cabergoline, apomorphine	▪ Caution patient to avoid alcohol when taking these medications because alcohol tolerance is lessened. ▪ Bromocriptine can cause digital vasospasm. Teach patient to avoid exposure to cold and to report onset of finger or toe pallor. ▪ Teach patient that bromocriptine and cabergoline have been associated with pulmonary fibrosis and require regular follow-up evaluation for monitoring of lungs. ▪ Dopamine agonist therapy has been associated with potentially reversible pathologic gambling. Teach patient that changing the medication should help this problem. ▪ Pramipexole is also associated with abrupt somnolence without premonition. Caution patient against driving or using machinery while on this drug, to avoid accidents. ▪ Explain that apomorphine does not contain morphine and is not addictive. Apomorphine often causes severe nausea and vomiting, and an antiemetic (e.g., trimethobenzamide) needs to be taken before taking apomorphine, ideally on a prophylactic basis 3 days before initiation of therapy. Tolerance to nausea and vomiting usually develops after about 8 wk. Dizziness or postural hypotension also occurs, and precautions should be taken accordingly. Injection site reactions include bruising, itching, and lumps that typically resolve on their own. Yawning, dyskinesia, somnolence, rhinorrhea, hallucination, and extremity edema also can occur. Erections in men can occur spontaneously and should be reported to health care provider if they last longer than 3-4 hr.
Antivirals Amantadine	▪ Teach that taking amantadine early in the day may prevent insomnia. ▪ Teach patient and significant other to monitor for and report any shortness of breath, peripheral edema, significant weight gain, or change in mental status because these signs often signal heart failure. ▪ Instruct patient not to stop taking this medication abruptly because doing so may precipitate parkinsonian crisis. ▪ A diffuse, rose-colored mottling of the skin, usually confined to lower extremities, may develop. The condition may subside with continued therapy and will disappear in a few weeks to months after the drug is discontinued. Exposure to cold or prolonged standing may make color more prominent. Teach patient to report this condition if it occurs, but reassure patient that the condition is more cosmetic than serious. ▪ Patient with history of seizures may have an increase in the number of seizures. Instruct patient to monitor and promptly report to health care provider a loss of seizure control. ▪ Caution patient to avoid alcohol and CNS depressants because these agents potentiate effects of amantadine. ▪ Explain that most side effects of amantadine are dose related.

Continued

| | TABLE 5-1 | ANTIPARKINSONIAN DRUGS AND SIDE EFFECTS WITH RELATED TEACHING INTERVENTIONS—cont'd |

MEDICATION	SIDE EFFECTS WITH RELATED TEACHING INTERVENTIONS
Anticholinergics Trihexyphenidyl, benztropine mesylate	■ Explain that this medication may decrease perspiration. Explain that patient should avoid strenuous exercise and keep cool during summer to avoid heat stroke. ■ Teach patient not to stop taking this medication abruptly because doing so can result in parkinsonian crisis. ■ Teach patient to monitor for tachycardia or palpitation and to report either condition. ■ Teach patient and significant others to monitor for memory dysfunction, confusion, and urinary hesitancy and retention (especially in older men) and to report symptoms to health care provider.
Monoamine Oxidase (MAO) Type B Inhibitors Selegiline, rasagiline	■ Stress importance of taking this medication only in prescribed dose. Selegiline is a selective MAO type B inhibitor and in the recommended dose of 10 mg or less per day does not cause the hypertensive crisis that can occur when tyramine-containing foods (e.g., cheese, red wine, beer, yogurt) are eaten. Dosages greater than 10 mg/day may result in hypertension if these foods are eaten. Usually, dietary modifications to reduce intake of tyramine-containing foods are recommended. ■ Although rasagiline is a MAO type B inhibitor, it is not yet proved that this drug is a selective MAO type B inhibitor like selegiline. It is commonly used in combination with levodopa. Caution patient that it should not be taken with any appetite stimulants. ■ Suggest avoidance of meperidine and other opioids. At recommended doses, no drug interactions have been noted. However, fatal drug interactions have occurred with patients taking other nonselective MAO inhibitors and such interactions could conceivably occur if higher-than-recommended doses are taken. ■ Teach patient that taking drug early in the day may prevent insomnia.
Catechol O-Methyltransferase (COMT) Inhibitor Entacapone	■ Teach patient that this medication may cause urine discoloration (brownish orange), but it is not clinically important. ■ Explain that the drug may be taken with or without food. ■ Teach patient that hallucinations, increased dyskinesia, or persistent nausea or diarrhea should be reported promptly.

CNS, Central nervous system; *GI,* gastrointestinal.

Nursing Interventions

◆ Explain that special exercises can help strengthen and control facial and tongue muscles. *This is to help improve verbal communication and help prevent choking.* Along with prescribed medications, the exercises may prevent or delay disability. Refer patient to a speech pathologist to design and individualize a speech program.

- Teach the following exercises, and have patient complete a return demonstration: hold a sound for 5 sec; sing the scale; recite alphabet and days of the week; practice vowel breaths (ah, oh, oo) and syllables (ma, me, mi, pull, pill, pie).
- Encourage patient to practice increasing voice volume: take a deep breath before speaking, open mouth to let sound come out more, use shorter sentences, exaggerate sound of every syllable, speak louder than others may think necessary, and use a tape recorder for feedback. Patient should practice reading or reciting out loud, focusing on breathing and using a strong voice. Suggest that patient read newspapers out loud and determine how many words can be said in one breath before volume decreases. Voice should vary from soft to loud. Teach patient to raise voice with a question and lower it with an answer.
- Teach tongue exercises: Stick tongue out as far as possible and hold; move tongue slowly from corner to corner; stretch tongue to nose and then chin and then cheek; stick out tongue and put it back in the mouth as quickly as possible; move tongue in circles as quickly as possible. *This may improve articulation.*
- Teach lip and jaw exercises: Open and close mouth slowly and then quickly; close lips and press tightly; stretch lips in a wide smile and hold; then pucker lips and hold. Advise patient to practice in front of a mirror to see and evaluate lip and tongue movement.
- Provide a written handout that lists and describes the preceding exercises. Encourage patient to perform them hourly while awake.
- Teach importance of stating feelings verbally. This is because monotone speech and lack of facial expression impede nonverbal communication. Encourage use of a mirror to practice expressing emotions such as happiness and displeasure. Advise patients to face the people to whom they are speaking and speak for themselves and not let others speak for them. *This helps maintain self-esteem and independence.*

Deficient knowledge related to deep brain stimulation
Desired outcome: Following the explanation, patient verbalizes accurate understanding of the deep brain stimulation procedure, including presurgical and postsurgical care.

Nursing Interventions

- After health care provider's explanation of the procedure, determine patient's level of understanding of purpose, risks, and anticipated benefits or outcome. Intervene accordingly, or reinforce health care provider's explanation as appropriate. Determine patient's facility with language; engage an interpreter or provide language-appropriate written materials if indicated.
- Explain that the neurostimulator is an implantable pulse generator powered by a small battery that is implanted subcutaneously near the clavicle. The stimulation parameter is set to optimize symptom management with minimum adverse effects. Adverse effects may include paresthesia, muscle contractions, double vision, and mood disturbances, all of which are usually transient. It is seldom possible to alleviate completely all PD symptoms with the stimulator alone. Therefore medication may be needed, with adjustments made as needed for the first few months. Health care provider follow-up is essential.
- Advise patients they will be monitored for dysphagia after surgery. Choreiform movements may occur initially. Generally patients will go home in about 2 days, but older individuals or those with postoperative confusion, hallucinations, agitation, or disorientation may be prescribed quetiapine and kept under observation longer.
- Instruct patient that activities usually are limited after surgery. *This promotes wound healing.* Light activities, including housework and sexual

activity, usually are restricted for the first 2 wk after surgery. More strenuous activities are restricted for 4-6 wk.

- Explain there is often immediate symptom reduction from surgical microlesions and edema. This effect will wear off with surgical healing, but stimulations will be started in 1-2 wk.

- Instruct patient in wound care, which includes not scratching or irritating wound areas. Quetiapine or other antippsychotic medication may be prescribed for compulsive picking at suture wounds, which would increase infection risk. Pin sites typically will be covered with adhesive bandages until they are dry. Washing the head with a damp cloth is acceptable as long as the surgical area is avoided. Gentle hair shampooing should only be done after stitches or staples are removed in 7-10 days.

- Caution patient to call health care provider for any of the following signs and symptom: severe and persistent headache, bleeding from the incision, redness or increased swelling in the area of the incision, sudden change or loss of vision, and persistent temperature of 101° F or higher.

- Advise that the sudden appearance of additional parkinsonian symptoms may be the only indicator of battery failure. There are handheld devices that enable determination of the on or off status of the neurostimulator as well as battery charge status. Turning the neurostimulator off at night to conserve the battery is not recommended. *This is because some symptoms, such as rigidity, respond only to continuous stimulation.*

- Explain that incorrect lead placement, poor anchoring, and drifting of leads (ineffective stimulation) may necessitate removal to accurately reposition the electrodes.

- Teach that adverse effects resulting from stimulation of nearby structures include tingling of head or hand, depression, slurred speech, loss of balance or muscle tone, and double vision, and these adverse effects are corrected by reducing the amount of stimulation.

- Explain that excessive STN stimulation may cause disabling dyskinesia and would be a reason to turn off the device until reprogramming can be performed.

- Caution patient that some devices, such as theft detectors and screening devices found in airports, department stores, and public libraries, can cause the neurostimulator to switch on or off. Usually, this only causes an uncomfortable sensation. However, symptoms could worsen suddenly. Patient always should carry the identification card given with the device and use it to request assistance to bypass those devices. Ultrasonic dental equipment and electrocautery also may affect the device. Patients should avoid activities that may result in blunt trauma to the implanted device area. Reassure patient that computers and cellular phone do not interfere with the device.

- Caution patients they cannot undergo chest or thoracic magnetic resonance imaging (MRI). *This is because of possible movement of the leads or diathermy (shortwave or microwave), which can heat up the wires and leads and can result in serious injury or death.*

- Instruct in use of magnet to activate and deactivate the stimulator. This magnet may damage televisions, credit cards, and computer disks and therefore should be kept at least one foot away from these items.

Patient-Family Teaching and Discharge Planning

Include verbal and written information about the following:

- Referrals to community resources, such as local and national PD organization chapters, public health nurse, visiting nurses association, community support groups, social workers, psychologic therapy, vocational rehabilitation agency, home health agencies, and extended and skilled care facilities.

- Speech therapy tips for communication related to dysarthria and for swallowing precautions.
- Related safety measures and fall prevention for patients with bradykinesia, muscle rigidity, and tremors.
- Emphasis that disability may be prevented or delayed through exercises and medications.
- Evaluation of home environment and tips for home accident prevention.
- Measures to prevent or lessen postural hypotension.
- Signs and symptoms of neuroleptic malignant and acute akinesia and the need for immediate medical attention.
- Additional general information, which can be obtained by accessing the websites of the following organizations:

American Parkinson Disease Association, Inc.: www.apdaparkinson.org

Parkinson's Disease Foundation, Inc.: www.pdf.org

National Parkinson Foundation, Inc.: www.parkinson.org

- For other nursing interventions, see "Patient-Family Teaching and Discharge Planning" (third through seventh entries only), in "Multiple Sclerosis," p. 237.

❖ ALZHEIMER'S DISEASE

OVERVIEW/PATHOPHYSIOLOGY

Alzheimer's disease (ALZ) is a progressive disorder of the brain that is among the most costly diseases to society in the United States. It is characterized by changes and degeneration of the cerebral cortical nerve cells and nerve endings that result in abnormal neurofibrillary tangles and neuritic amyloid beta plaque. Amyloid beta plaque is a toxic protein deposited between the nerve cells that affect nerve conduction; neurofibrillary tangles comprise a disorganized accumulation of twisted hyperphosphorylated tau protein fragments within the nerve cell. In addition, there is an acetylcholine neurotransmitter deficiency probably related to nerve cell loss. Other neurotransmitters also may be reduced but to a lesser degree.

This process causes irreversible impairment of memory, deterioration of intellectual functions, and dementia. Genetics plays a role in some patients with ALZ. Early onset (younger than 60 yr of age) is fairly rare and is linked to an autosomal dominant inheritance mechanism involving, thus far, three genes. Presenilin-1 *(PS1)* mutations account for a majority of the patients with early-onset familial ALZ. Late disease onset (older than 60 yr of age) appears to be linked with a genetic risk factor rather than a causative gene. For example, the gene called *ApoE4* increases the risk of developing late-onset ALZ, but carrying the gene does not mean a person inevitably will develop ALZ. Onset is insidious, and it can strike individuals as young as 40 yr of age. The disease progresses to total disability and eventually results in death from problems such as infection or aspiration, usually within 3-15 yr, with the average at 7-10 yr.

ASSESSMENT

Signs and symptoms/physical findings: The appearance and severity of signs and symptoms vary from individual to individual. ALZ is characterized by progressive memory failure, intellectual deterioration, and personality change. It is usually classified into four stages: early, middle, late, and terminal, depending on patient's degree of impairment. The 10 warning signs are memory loss, difficulty performing simple tasks, language difficulty, disorientation, poor judgment, difficulty with abstract thinking, misplacing objects or clothing, changes in behavior and moodiness, personality changes, and loss of purpose or initiative. Initial indicators are mild, but short-term memory loss is a cardinal early sign. In this early stage, forgetfulness, losing things, getting lost, and trouble with word-finding is typical, but patients still can function independently. It may take several years before a definite diagnosis can be made. Often a diagnosis is not made until the middle stage, when patients become more confused and disoriented and have trouble recognizing objects or things, carrying out previously performed skills or activities, or communicating. Assistance is needed with activities of daily living (ADL), and supervision is required inasmuch as wandering, increased confusion, paranoia, and agitation become a problem. By the late stage, memory and intellectual ability are mostly absent. Complete assistance is generally needed with ADL, and patient function will deteriorate with loss of ability to walk, stand, sit, talk, eat safely, or maintain bladder or bowel continence. In the terminal stage, the individual is in both a mental and physical vegetative condition. Patients cannot verbalize, do not recognize family, are incontinent, need to be fed, have difficulty eating and swallowing, and are bedridden.

Memory: Initially, slight memory loss, usually consisting of inability to retain recently acquired information, is the most common first sign. Individuals may lose things and forget dates and how to use common objects and tools while retaining the power and coordination necessary for performing these activities. Long-term memory eventually is lost. Patients become lost in the home or other familiar surroundings and gradually lose ability to recognize or name common objects and familiar people, including members of the immediate family.

Cognitive process: Decreasing ability to think through problems, poor decision-making ability, shortened attention span, lack of insight, inability to perform simple arithmetic calculations, and loss of reading and writing capabilities. Gradually the ability to manage familiar activities, such as shopping or cooking, fails. Individuals become hesitant and reluctant to carry out minor and familiar tasks. As ability to reason and abstract declines, they fail to recognize unsafe behaviors, with a resulting potential for injury. Hallucinations often occur because of misconceptions of the environment. Following even simple two- or three-step instructions is increasingly difficult. Eventually there is total loss of intellectual ability and comprehension, with inability to participate in any activities. In the last stages, there may be instinctual and emotional awareness of family voices, touching, or presence, but there is no intellectual or conscious awareness or conscious interaction with the environment.

Personality changes: Realization that memory and intellect are deteriorating may result in depression, frustration, bitterness, anxiety, and apathy. Difficulty with tasks that are beyond the individual's capacity leads to easy frustration. As insight declines, depression becomes less of a problem. Emotional lability, panic, fear, bewilderment, and perplexity are common. As awareness of the environment declines, apathy may become more prominent. Symptoms of paranoia, delusion, agitation, and hallucination may appear, resulting in suspiciousness and accusing others of stealing things that have been misplaced. Previous psychotic-like traits are exaggerated. As ability to communicate decreases and the world becomes more frightening, the potential for violence and agitation increases. Patients may have catastrophic reactions and emotional outbursts when they are faced with complex tasks.

Social behavior: Decreased ability to handle social interaction, loss of social graces, loss of inhibitions (resulting in inappropriate language or acts), helplessness, and dependency.

Communication patterns: Difficulty finding words, loss of spontaneity in speech, inability to express thoughts, incoherent speech. Individuals gradually lose all language ability and become unable to communicate other than with such behaviors as yelling, noisiness, or striking out. Eventually, this limited ability may be lost, and they may be able only to grunt or express pain by grimacing.

Sleep pattern: Restlessness, pacing, and wandering. Sleep/wake cycles are maintained, but need for sleep usually decreases. Nocturnal awakenings and reversals of normal sleep patterns are common. Toward the final stages, the individual often sleeps excessively.

Self-care: Progressive neglect of routine tasks and personal hygiene; weight loss owing to refusal to eat and lack of awareness of the importance of nutrition; increasing inability to dress, bathe, toilet, and self-feed or to recognize need to or where to urinate or defecate (resulting in incontinence). Eventually, patients become totally dependent on others for all self-care activities.

Mobility/posture: Stooped and shuffling gait; progressive balance and coordination problems; falling; inability to walk and use arms, hands, and legs for purposeful movement. Individuals become bedridden. Joint contractures and muscle rigidity are common in the final stages.

Other: In the last stages of ALZ, myoclonus and seizures can occur. Spontaneous involuntary movement occurs, but ability to open the eyes and track is maintained. Brainstem reflexes are present, and grasping, snout (evidenced by tapping the nose, which results in a marked facial grimace), and sucking reflexes can be elicited. Control of sphincter muscles is gone, and individuals may be incontinent of stool and urine. Chewing and swallowing incoordination develops, and death usually occurs as a result of aspiration pneumonia.

History and risk factors: People with a first-degree relative such as a parent or sibling with ALZ have a 10%-30% chance of developing the disorder. Male gender, higher education, nonsteroidal antiinflammatory drug (NSAID) use, regular exercise, and use of cholesterol-lowering drugs known as statins all have been associated with decreased incidence of ALZ. Endogenous toxins, such as glutamate, and trauma have been speculated as playing a role in the pathogenesis of ALZ. Patients with Down syndrome also are likely to get ALZ. The primary risk factor for ALZ is advancing age.

DIAGNOSTIC TESTS

Many disorders that can cause a progressive dementia syndrome (e.g., head injuries, brain tumors, depression, arteriosclerosis, drug toxicity, metabolic disorders such as hypothyroidism, alcoholism) need to be ruled out. This is especially important because some dementias are reversible. The only definitive test for ALZ is brain biopsy, but this is done only after death. Usually diagnosis is made on the basis of findings on neurologic and mental status examinations and after other causes have been ruled out.

Mental status examination (e.g., Mini-Mental State Exam [MMSE] or ALZ assessment scale): Tests orientation, memory, calculation, abstraction, judgment, and mood. Several other scales and tests are available, such as the Global Deterioration Scale, Blessed Dementia Scale, Word List Memory Recall and Recognition, and Clock Drawing Test.

Neurologic examination: Indicators that may signal ALZ include the following: release signs, such as snout, grasp, and sucking reflexes; olfactory deficits; impaired stereognosis (inability to recognize touch or smell of a familiar object when placed in the hand); short-stepped, bradykinetic gait; tremor; and abnormalities on cerebellar testing.

Positron emission tomography (PET): May show lower cerebral cortex metabolic rates for glucose, even in early stages of the disease. PET is now considered the most definitive diagnostic procedure for ALZ. Amyloid-imaging PET tracing may provide quantitative information on amyloid changes.

MRI: May reveal brain atrophy, symmetric bilateral ventricular enlargement, and a striking volume loss in the hippocampus, which help support diagnosis. Both functional MRI (fMRI) and magnetic resonance (MR) spectroscopy may identify ALZ at a very early stage because they can detect both biochemical and anatomic changes.

CT scan: May reveal brain atrophy and symmetric bilateral ventricular enlargement, which help support diagnosis; also helps rule out other neurologic problems, particularly mass lesions.

Single photon emission computed tomography (SPECT): May show a pattern of bilateral hypoperfusion in parietal and temporal regions of the brain that is suggestive of ALZ. Frontal lobe hypoperfusion occurs later in the illness.

EEG: May reveal generalized slowed brain wave activity and reduced voltage, which support diagnosis. Using new computer software that analyzes EEG data, physicians can determine whether the patient is showing early signs of ALZ or normal aging by looking at differences between the left and right sides of the brain.

Eye test: Researchers have developed a pair of optical tests that can determine the presence of amyloid beta proteins in the lens of the eye. These proteins are found in all patients with ALZ. An interior laser ophthalmoscope can pick up the presence of the amyloid protein.

CSF: May show reduced acetylcholinesterase or abnormal levels of amyloid beta, tau protein, and neural thread protein (hyperphosphorylated tau). Tau protein in CSF may predict progression. Testing for these proteins is very specialized and not often available in standard laboratories.

Brain biopsy: Demonstrates presence of neurofibrillary tangles and neuritic plaques; usually done only at autopsy.

Other tests: May be performed to rule out other causes of dementia. Examples are skull and chest x-ray examinations, lumbar puncture (LP), serum tests (e.g., liver, thyroid, syphilis, vitamin B_{12} deficiency), urinalysis, arteriograms, drug screen, and brain scan. Genotype testing, although not usually done, is an adjunct to diagnosis and early detection/prediction of the disease. The first serum diagnostic test for ALZ (and Parkinson's disease [PD]), called NuroPro, is currently being tested in several clinical trials and is showing promising results.

COLLABORATIVE MANAGEMENT

Generally, treatment is supportive only. No cure exists at this time.

Pharmacotherapy: The following medications, if prescribed, are used to treat symptoms or behavioral manifestations. Generally, medical or environmental triggers for the behavioral manifestation are treated specifically. If this approach fails to correct the problem, drug therapy is considered.

Early Stage

Cholinesterase inhibitors (e.g., donepezil, rivastigmine, galantamine): Improve mild to moderate memory deficit, although they do not alter the course of the underlying dementia. It is believed they work by blocking the enzyme that breaks down acetylcholine, thus correcting the deficiency. Monitor for nausea, diarrhea, fatigue, insomnia, anorexia, and muscle cramping, which are usually transient and generally mild.

Antidepressants of the selective serotonin reuptake inhibitor type (e.g., sertraline, citalopram, paroxetine, fluoxetine): May relieve depression and elevate mood. Monitor for fatigue, drowsiness, orthostatic hypotension.

Stimulants (e.g., methylphenidate, dextroamphetamine): For loss of spontaneity or inattention.

Hormone replacement therapy (e.g., estrogen): May play a role in slowing disease progression. Benefits in early studies have not been duplicated in more recent studies, so use is controversial.

Vitamin E and selegiline: Appear to slow disease progression and may delay but not change outcome. Vitamin E is preferred inasmuch as it is less expensive than selegiline.

Nonsteroidal antiinflammatory drugs (NSAIDs): May play a role in reducing risk of disease and in decreasing severity and progression of ALZ.

Other: Although most vitamins (e.g., niacin, folate, B$_{12}$), zinc, and lecithin treatments have not been proven effective in treating ALZ, they are relatively harmless, and the family may find some consolation in their use.

Middle Stage

N-methyl-D-aspartate (NMDA)-receptor antagonists (e.g., memantine): May reduce clinical deterioration in moderate to severe disease. These agents are contraindicated in patients with severe renal impairment. Adverse side effects include dizziness, headache, confusion, hallucinations, and tiredness.
Antianxiety agents (e.g., buspirone): Help reduce anxiety and restlessness.
Tranquilizers or sedatives (e.g., trazodone, lorazepam): Control hyperactivity, restlessness, and sleep disturbances. Trazodone is also an antidepressant.
Antipsychotic agents (e.g., quetiapine, clozapine): For agitated or combative patients. Carbamazepine also may be useful for agitated patients. Divalproex may be used for aggression. Haloperidol may be used as well, but it has more extrapyramidal side effects.

Late Stage

Antiepileptic drugs (AEDs) (e.g., carbamazepine, phenobarbital, phenytoin, diazepam, fosphenytoin): Control seizures.
Laxatives and stool softeners (e.g., psyllium, docusate): For constipation.

Terminal Stage

Narcotic pain relievers (e.g., oral morphine): May be given (in small doses) to patients who have developed restlessness or hypersensitivity to touch.
Anticholinergics (e.g., atropine or scopolamine): May be given to decrease respiratory secretions and need for frequent, uncomfortable suctioning.
Diet: A high-fiber diet may be given to prevent constipation. For restless, hyperactive patients, a high-calorie diet or supplements may be prescribed. Caffeine is avoided because of its stimulating effect. In later stages, tube feedings may be an option for some patients.
Activity: Exercise may delay disease progression and has a positive benefit on depression and other behaviors such as wandering.
Counseling or psychotherapy: Counseling is generally focused on significant others to help them deal with the depression, grief, guilt, and emotions caused by patient's progressive disability and behavior. In all but the early stages, patients with ALZ quickly lose the insight and intellectual ability that would make counseling beneficial to them.
Other treatments under investigation: Multiple clinical research trials are ongoing to test new drugs and treatments for ALZ, including a vaccine nasal spray. More information on the clinical trials can be found at the Food and Drug Administration website:
www.fda.gov

NURSING DIAGNOSES AND INTERVENTIONS

Risk for trauma related to lack of awareness of environmental hazards secondary to cognitive deficit
Desired outcomes: Patient is free of symptoms of physical trauma. At least 24 hr before patient's hospital discharge, significant other identifies and plans to eliminate or control potentially dangerous factors in patient's home environment.

Nursing Interventions

◆ Orient to new surroundings. Reorient as needed. Keep necessary items, including water, phone, and call light, within easy reach. Assess patient's ability to use these items. Keep bed in its lowest position. Side rail position (up or down) will vary with the patient. *This is because the patient may be at risk of falling from climbing over side rails.*

◆ Maintain uncluttered environment. *This is to minimize risk of environmental confusion and tripping.* Ensure adequate lighting to help prevent falls in the dark.

◆ Prevent exposure to hot food or equipment. Discourage use of heating pads. Check temperature of heating device and bath water before patient is exposed to them. *This will reduce the risk of burn injuries.*

◆ Encourage patient to use low-heel, nonskid shoes for walking. Teach wide-based gait. *This will give an unsteady patient a broader base of support.* Assess for ataxia, and assist with walking as necessary. Use gestures or turn patient's body in direction he or she is to go. The of canes and walkers may be too complicated for patients with ALZ.

◆ Request that significant other assist with watching restless patient. Provide attendant care if necessary. Avoid restraining patient. *This may increase agitation.* If restraints must be used, reassure patient that he or she is not being punished, that you are trying to help him or her regain control, and that restraints will be removed when staff is certain patient will not cause self-injury. Take the patient for a walk. *For many persons with ALZ, walking will reduce agitation.*

◆ Check patient at frequent intervals. If necessary, move patient closer to the nursing station, away from stairways or unit exits, or seat patient in a chair at nursing station. Consider obtaining picture of patient to assist in a search if necessary.

◆ Watch for nonverbal clues of pain or distress, such as restlessness, wincing, wrinkled brow, cautious breathing, rapid or shallow breathing, poor appetite, or crying. Provide scheduled bathroom breaks. Report significant findings.

◆ Try to make tubes as unobtrusive as possible to prevent their removal. Use fabric sleeve or netting to limit access to catheter dressing/IV tubing. Place IV tubing high on dominant arm. Dress patient in long-sleeved gown with cuff, with IV tubing going up sleeve and out neck opening of the gown. Place binders over dressing. *This will help prevent picking.* Position hand splints to eliminate pincer grasp.

Nursing Interventions for Home Safety

◆ Encourage significant other to evaluate home environment carefully for potential safety hazards. Caution him or her to remove harmful objects (e.g., matches, scissors) from bedside and to store medications and chemicals (e.g., insect spray, cleaning supplies, lighter fluid) in locked cabinets. *This is to prevent accidental ingestion because these patients tend to put objects in their mouth.* Remove toxic plants, plastic fruit, and toiletries. *This is because patient may attempt to eat them.* Temperature of home hot water heater should be turned down. *This will prevent accidental scalding.* Lock up hazardous power tools, lawn mowers, knives, and kitchen appliances. Place gates or guardrails on porches and stairways as needed. Safety plugs should be placed in electrical outlets. Handrails and grab bars also may be helpful. Remind significant other to check house carefully before leaving. It may be necessary to remove knobs from stove burners and oven or to disable appliance with an override turn-off valve or switch. *Because of the memory loss, patients may leave stove on or water running.*

◆ Advise significant other to dress patient according to physical environment and individual need. *Patient may not know or be able to communicate if he or she is too cold or too warm.*

◆ Advise significant other to keep patient's home environment simple, uncluttered, and familiar. *Rearranging furniture can increase patient's confusion and potential for falls.* Remove breakables. Encourage use of night-lights.

- If patient tends to wander, encourage significant other to have identification bracelet made with patient's name, phone number, and diagnosis. An identifying label can be sewn into clothes. Alert neighbors and local police to call if they notice patient wandering. Keep a clear, current picture of patient available. These tips will help if the patient becomes lost or is unable to speak a name or address, or to identify the patient in a search. Covering door handles with child-safe doorknobs or cloth hangings or covering door with a poster may be sufficient to prevent patient from exiting. Locks on doors to keep patient inside may be necessary but should not require a key because this may hamper escape in case of a fire. A childproof device mounted either high or very low on the door may be sufficient. Door or exit alarms can be installed on home doors; a mat alarm under a bedside rug or a motion detector may also help. Advise family to prepare a search plan and let neighbors know about it. If patient is lost, call for help, assign a search section to helpers, have someone stay home, and search all areas. Daily walks or exercise tends to decrease amount of wandering. Exercise areas should be safe and securely enclosed. Register patient with "Safe Return" program through local Alzheimer's Association chapter (see "Patient-Family Teaching and Discharge Planning," p. 277).
- Caution significant other that patient who is disoriented should be allowed to smoke only while being observed. Advise significant other to get a smoke detector and to take control of matches (i.e., lock up matches and lighters). Patient should cook only when being directly observed. *This is to prevent accidental self-injury and home fires.*
- Advise significant other that patient should be restricted from driving. Document this advice. Suggest that significant other hide car keys and store them in a locked cabinet, or disable car (e.g., remove distributor cap) if necessary.

Imbalanced nutrition: less than body requirements related to decreased intake secondary to cognitive and motor deficit and to increased nutritional needs secondary to constant pacing and restlessness
Desired outcome: Patient maintains baseline body weight.

Nursing Interventions

- Request that significant other assist with menu planning or bring in meals and dishes patient recognizes. Encourage significant other to attend meals to provide a more social environment. *This is because patient may not eat food that does not look familiar or is served in unfamilar surroundings.*
- Remind patient to close mouth, chew, and swallow, and be sure to watch for swallowing. Use touch, verbal cuing, and encouragement to provide guidance. Smile and praise patient. Keep suction equipment available. *This is because the patient may forget the voluntary steps of eating and swallowing.*
- Provide help with menu selection. *Patients with ALZ often are overwhelmed with choices.*
- When patient is no longer able to handle a fork, knife, and spoon, cut up food for patient and/or provide finger foods and privacy. Accept eating with hands and whimsical food mixtures.
- For patient who is in constant motion, provide small snacks around the clock and a high-calorie diet unless contraindicated.
- Tolerate spills without scolding, and obtain unbreakable plates and nonspill cups when needed.
- Try to limit number of foods on plate or serve foods in courses. *Too many foods can be overwhelming.*
- If patient clenches teeth and refuses to eat, stimulate oral suck reflex by stroking cheeks or stimulating mouth with a spoon. Use patient's forgetfulness to advantage by taking a short break from feeding and returning in a few moments when patient may be more receptive.

◆ For other nursing interventions, see **Imbalanced nutrition** in "General Care of Patients with Neurologic Deficits," p. 357.

Impaired environmental interpretation syndrome related to chronic confusional state secondary to degeneration of neuronal functioning
Desired outcome: After intervention and on an ongoing basis, patient interacts appropriately with the environment.

Nursing Interventions

◆ Monitor for and record short-term memory deficit. Once level of comprehension has been determined, avoid repeatedly asking whether patient knows who and where he or she is and what time it is. This may cause frustration and agitation. At frequent intervals, orient to reality, time, and place in the following ways: call patient by name; keep clocks and calendars in room; inform patient of day and time; correct patient gently; minimize disturbing noise; ensure good lighting to prevent shadows; request that significant other bring in familiar objects and family pictures; speak with patient about his or her interests, both present and past; allow patient to reminisce, and listen with tolerance to repeated stories; ensure that staff members show their name tags and identify themselves each time they encounter patient; explain upcoming events; set up regular schedules for hygiene, eating, and waste elimination; and do only one activity at a time, using simple step-by-step instructions, Be consistent and use repetition. Write down daily plan or schedule.
◆ Approach patient in a calm, slow, relaxed, nonthreatening, friendly manner. Treat patient with dignity and respect. Remain calm and patient when repeating questions. Be nonjudgmental and objective when confronted with inappropriate behavior.
◆ Keep patient's personal belongings where they can be used and seen.
◆ Evaluate cognitive impairment for any relation to medication use (e.g., sedatives, tranquilizers). Consult health care provider if necessary.
◆ Provide a quiet, calm, pleasant environment. Simple, minimally decorated rooms are best. The patient may not recognize self in a mirror. Cover or remove artwork and mirrors if patient misinterprets images. *Wallpaper patterns may be disturbing to some patients.* Turn off public address system in patient's room. *This prevents stimulation and misinterpretation of the sound.*
◆ Provide stimulation patient can handle. Soft music may be appropriate, but television may be too overwhelming. Interpret strange noises for patient.
◆ Limit visitors as appropriate. *Crowds and complex social interactions are often beyond patient's ability to tolerate.*
◆ Check to ensure that individuals who need eyeglasses or hearing aids wear them as appropriate. Eyeglasses should be clean and have current prescription. Hearing aids should be functioning.
◆ If patient becomes agitated, reduce environmental stimuli. Use a soft, reassuring voice and gentle touch. Avoid quick, unexpected movements.
◆ If patient leaves the ward for testing or other procedures, communicate patient's cognitive level to other caregivers (e.g., patient will wander).

Impaired environmental interpretation syndrome (urinating in inappropriate places) related to cognitive deficit
Desired outcome: Patient urinates in the toilet stool (commode) on an ongoing basis.

Nursing Interventions

◆ Make sure patient knows location of bathroom. If possible, locate patient within sight of bathroom, ensure a clear path, and provide adequate light at night. Take patient to the bathroom q1-2h; avoid a sense of hurry. Restrict fluids in evenings. *This minimizes the risk of enuresis.*

◆ Identify bathroom door with picture of a toilet. *This reminds patient how to locate the bathroom.*

◆ Assess for nonverbal clues (e.g., restlessness, holding himself or herself) that can signal need to void.

◆ As appropriate, provide disposable underpants rather than catheterize the patient. *Indwelling and external catheters may increase confusion.* Male patients may be able to accept condom catheters to help manage incontinence.

◆ Investigate cause of incontinence to determine whether it is treatable. *Incontinence may signal urinary tract infection (UTI).*

◆ After patient has voided, assess for cleanliness and dryness of perianal area; intervene accordingly to help ensure skin integrity.

◆ Bathroom door lock removal may be necessary. *This is to prevent patient from locking self in and not being able to get out.*

Impaired environmental interpretation syndrome (defecating in inappropriate places) related to inability to find bathroom or decreased awareness or loss of sphincter control secondary to cognitive deficit
Desired outcome: Following intervention(s), patient has no or fewer episodes of defecating in inappropriate places.

Nursing Interventions

◆ Identify bathroom door with picture of a toilet. *This reminds patient how to locate the bathroom.*

◆ Assess normal bowel habits. Take patient to bathroom at time of day patient normally has bowel movement (e.g., first thing in morning, following cup of coffee, or after meals).

◆ Evaluate for nonverbal indications of need to eliminate wastes (e.g., restlessness, picking at clothes, facial expressions or grunting sounds indicative of bearing down, passing flatus).

◆ As appropriate, provide disposable underpants.

◆ After bowel elimination, assess for cleanliness of perianal area. *This is to maintain skin integrity. The patient may forget to wipe perianal area or clean the area only partially.*

◆ Bathroom door lock removal may be necessary. *This prevents patient from locking self in and not being able to get out.*

◆ For other suggestions, see **Constipation,** p. 29, in "Prolonged Bed Rest."

Self-care deficit related to memory loss and coordination problems secondary to cognitive and motor deficits
Desired outcome: On an ongoing basis, patient's physical needs are met by self, staff, or significant other.

◆ Provide care for totally dependent patients, and assist those who are not totally dependent. Allow ample time to perform activities, and encourage independence. Ask patient to perform only one task at a time; go through each step separately. Do not hurry patient. Involve significant others with care activities if they wish to be involved. Ask significant others when patient normally bathes at home, and establish this as part of daily routine. Provide a consistent caregiver. Use simple visual and verbal cues and gestures for self-care.

◆ Place stool in the shower if sitting will enhance self-care. Use handheld showerhead. *This prevents water from hitting patient's head, which can be frightening.* Save shampooing for last. A partial or sponge bath may be better tolerated than a shower. Cover body parts not being bathed or bathe patient under a towel. *This promotes tolerance of bathing because the patient may be fearful while undressed.*

♦ Encourage significant other to buy shoes with elastic laces, without laces, or with self-stick (Velcro) fasteners and clothing that is loose fitting or has snaps, Velcro closures, or elastic waistbands. Offer clothing items one at a time, sequentially. Allow agitated patients for whom hygiene is not a problem to sleep in shoes and clothing, and attempt a clothes change later. Lay out clothes to wear. *This facilitates dressing and undressing, which can be quite difficult for the patient.*

♦ Provide a commode chair or elevated toilet seat as needed.

♦ If patient becomes combative or agitated, postpone ADL and try again a short time later. *The patient may forget reason for the resistance.*

Impaired verbal communication related to aphasia and altered sensory reception, transmission, and integration secondary to cognitive deficits
Desired outcome: Following the intervention(s), patient communicates needs to staff, follows instructions, and answers questions.

Nursing Interventions

♦ Provide a supportive and relaxed environment for patients who are unable to form words or sentences or who are unable to speak clearly or appropriately. Acknowledge patient's frustration about inability to communicate. Maintain a calm, positive attitude; eliminate distracting noises, such as radio or television. Observe for nonverbal communication cues, such as gestures. Consider discomfort such as pain, hunger, thirst, and need to urinate as possible causes of restlessness, moaning, guarding, and yelling; provide analgesia as needed. Avoid meperidine, if possible, because of its common side effect of restlessness. Anticipate patient's needs.

♦ Explain activities in short, easily understood sentences, and present only one idea at a time. Use simple gestures, point to objects, or use demonstration if possible. When giving directions, be sure to break tasks into small, understandable units, using simple terms. Ask patient to do only one task at a time. Give patient time to accomplish one task before progressing to the next. Explain each procedure or task before initiating it.

♦ If possible, ensure continuity of caregivers.

♦ Be sure you have the patient's attention. Only one staff member should speak at a time. *This prevents confusion.* Repeat patient's name or gently touch patient to get his or her attention. Use touch to communicate if patient is receptive to it. Speak slowly and calmly, and use a clear, low-pitched voice. Use short, simple words and sentences, but speak as though patient understands you. Ask only one question at a time, and formulate questions that can be answered by "yes" or "no." Wait for a response. If patient does not respond (within 15 sec), repeat question again, exactly as before, to help patient mentally process the question.

♦ Listen to and include patient in conversation.

Anxiety related to actual or perceived threats or changes (e.g., from bewildering hospital environment, multiple tests and procedures)
Desired outcome: Within 1 hr of intervention, patient's anxiety is absent or reduced as evidenced by heart rate (HR) 100 beats per minute (bpm) or less, respiratory rate (RR) 20 breaths/min or less with normal depth and pattern, and absence of or decrease in irritability and restlessness.

Nursing Interventions

♦ Remain calm with patient. Use slow, deliberate gestures. *Patients with ALZ often mirror emotions of others.* Use a low, soothing voice and gentle touch. Tone of voice is often more important than actual words used. Use long, slow-stroke massage or therapeutic touch. *This may help reduce anxiety and restlessness.*

♦ Provide time for patient to verbalize feelings of fear, concern, and anxiety. Listen with regard. *ALZ patients often have trouble finding correct words and may not be able to string more than a few words together.* Provide calm and realistic assurance, and stay with patient during periods of acute anxiety.

♦ Provide a consistent caregiver. Avoid changing patient's room. Ask caregiver about patient's normal routine and document this information. Attempt to incorporate patient's normal routine whenever possible. *This helps reduce anxiety and establishes an ongoing rapport with the patient.*

♦ Patient who still has reading capability may find reassurance with notes, orienting signs, or lists of names, phone numbers, or activities (e.g., the phone numbers of significant others or a written reminder of the reason they are in the hospital). *This may reassure patient that he or she is not lost or abandoned.*

♦ Encourage significant others to bring in familiar items. Address patient with preferred name.

♦ Permit patient to hoard inanimate objects. Enable patient to keep personal belongings (e.g., purse, wallet) in bed. *This may provide him or her with a sense of security.*

♦ Label drawers and belongings. *This assists with finding misplaced items, a common problem.*

♦ Refrain from forcing activities or giving patient too many choices.

♦ Encourage ambulation. *Walking helps reduce anxiety and agitation.*

♦ Encourage unlimited visiting hours for familiar significant others. A tape of familiar voices when family is unavailable may be comforting.

♦ Encourage patient to avoid caffeine. *It has a stimulating effect.*

♦ Encourage use of a behavior diary by significant other to document specific symptoms, frequency, severity, and possible causal relationships (e.g., occurred during bathing or with a meal). *This will help evaluate and problem solve situations.*

Risk for violence (self-directed or others) related to irritability, frustration, and disorientation secondary to degeneration of cognitive thinking
Desired outcome: Patient demonstrates control of his or her behavior with absence of violence.

Nursing Interventions

♦ Ask caregiver how patient usually acts when tired or overwhelmed, and ask what caregiver does to calm patient. Document this information.

♦ Monitor patient for signs of increasing anxiety, fright, or panic (e.g., inability to verbalize feelings, suspiciousness of others, fear of others or self, irritability, agitation). *These signs may precede a violent act.* Monitor what patient is saying (e.g., cursing), changes in patient's voice (e.g., louder, faster, tone), face, (expression, color), behavior (body language, tenseness, restless, pacing, clenched hands), and emotions. Remove potential weapons (e.g., scissors) from environment.

♦ Encourage verbalization of feelings rather than suppression. Suppression may cause frustration, which can lead to violence. Avoid asking why patient wants to do something. *This may be overwhelming and increase frustration.* Praise efforts at self-control.

♦ Try to identify what is immediately distressing to patient (e.g., full bladder, hunger, thirst, heat, cold, pain), and attempt to remedy it. Respond to the emotion rather than argue the facts (e.g., if patient repeatedly asks where his or her spouse is, ask whether patient is lonely rather than just replying the spouse isn't there). Respond to patient's questions in simple, concrete replies that relate directly to patient's questions, frustrations, or anger. Avoid making promises that cannot reasonably be kept. If the situation cannot be remedied by calming the patient, use distraction and try to defuse the situation by redirecting attention away from source of irritation. Talk about other topics, and vary topics periodically. Provide diversional activities, offer juice, or walk with patient until agitation has lessened. Use questions to interrupt repetitive or disturbing train of thought. Request the patient's help with tasks such as folding and unfolding towels or making a bed. *This may promote calm behavior by returning a sense of mastery or control.*

◆ Remain calm, and keep gestures slow and deliberate. Keep your hands open and below your waist where they can be seen. Approach patient slowly in a confident, relaxed, open manner. Avoid sudden changes or surprises. Keep your voice low and soft, and smile. Humor and gentle laughter may help change patient's mood. Some patients may respond positively to gentle touch (e.g., start with touching either a hand or arm because this is less threatening than touching other parts of the body).

◆ Reduce environmental stimuli, including people entering room. Provide a private room if possible. Reduce noise level by turning television volume down or off. *Too much stimulation can increase agitation for the patient.*

◆ Do not give routine care when patient is upset or agitated. Leave room briefly, and return when patient is calmer and more approachable. If patient cannot be left alone, sit quietly with no talking except gentle reassurance. Use patient's forgetfulness to your advantage.

◆ If patient is not combative unless approached, simply supervise from a safe distance. If you must approach patient, do so from the side rather than face-to-face. Stand off to one side, and maintain distance of at least one arm's length from patient.

◆ If patient is upset or agitated, avoid turning your back on him or her. Avoid cornering patient or being cornered. Think of escape routes for yourself, and be alert to potential weapons patient may use. Get help; protect yourself.

◆ Never attempt to deal with a physically aggressive patient by yourself. If other interventions fail, use physical or chemical restraints as necessary for your own or patient's safety.

◆ Document signs and symptoms, precipitating factor, time of onset, duration, and successful interventions. Prevent further episodes by controlling precipitating stressors (e.g., controlling pain, simplifying schedule, limiting visitors).

Disturbed sleep pattern related to restlessness and disorientation secondary to cognitive deficits
Desired outcome: Following intervention(s), patient sleeps at least 6 hr per night or an amount of time appropriate for patient.

Nursing Interventions

◆ Space activities with quiet periods. *This is so that patient does not become excessively tired and require a daytime nap.* Tiredness may contribute to catastrophic reactions.

◆ Prevent patient from falling asleep during the day through such measures as periodic short walks, planned activities, and keeping patient upright as much as possible. If patient does nap during the day but also sleeps well at night, there is no need to impose a specific sleep schedule.

◆ Patient who naps should do so in an easy chair, if possible, rather than in bed. *The easy chair may serve as a cue that patient is just napping.*

◆ Avoid continuous use of restraints. *Restraints often increase agitation and limit patient's ability to rest.*

◆ Adhere to regular bedtime schedules and rituals, such as a bedtime snack and toileting. Keep room lighted until patient is ready for sleep. Provide soft music, and tell patient that it is time for sleep.

◆ Administer tranquilizers and sedatives as prescribed to facilitate sleeping.

◆ Avoid turning on overhead light at night. *It may cue patient to think it is time to get up.*

◆ Try to schedule VS monitoring, medications, and treatments to allow uninterrupted sleep at night.

Interrupted family processes related to situational crisis (illness of family member)

Desired outcome: Within the 24-hr period before patient's hospital discharge, significant other verbalizes knowledge of measures that will assist with care of patient after hospital discharge.

Nursing Interventions

♦ Encourage significant other to interpret patient's behavior as a reflection of the disease process rather than a willful act. Advise significant other that generally another illness, surgery, or disease process will exaggerate patient's disorientation. Once these problems are corrected, patient usually returns to previous cognitive level. Caregivers will eventually need to reduce their expectations of patient's abilities as disease process progresses.

♦ Encourage major caregiver to have other family members or hired help take care of patient regularly. This is so caregiver can have scheduled respites. Caregiver should schedule rest breaks for himself or herself throughout the day. A neighbor looking in or a home health aide on a part-time, overnight, or live-in basis is another option. Local daycare or respite programs also are useful. If patient is a veteran, he or she may be eligible for some respite programs offered by the Department of Veterans Affairs. Advise caregiver that some home health agencies or daycare programs have sliding payment scales for their services. Short-stay respite care may be available for a caregiver "vacation." Refer to community sources that supply equipment for home use. Encourage use of other support services, such as homemakers, chore workers, home-delivered food, and volunteer drivers. Support significant other in asking for help. Encourage formation of a plan of care in the event that the caretaker becomes ill.

♦ If significant other is unaccustomed to handling finances, refer him or her to a place where help with financial management is available. *Patients with ALZ lose ability to manage finances and balance checkbooks and may give away money inappropriately.* Eventually the patient's checkbook and credit cards will have to be taken away. Phone use may require monitoring. *This is because these patients cannot differentiate between local and long-distance calls.* As appropriate, suggest that significant others post important phone numbers and secure long-distance numbers. *This may help prevent excessively high phone bills.* Families should locate and identify patient's various assets, sources of income, and liabilities and make arrangements for their security and daily management.

♦ Encourage early family legal planning and consultation. *This is especially important because an individual must have mental capacity and competence to sign documents.* Legal planning may involve wills, advance directives for health care, inter vivos trusts, subpayee assignment for Social Security, traditional and durable power of attorney or attorney in fact (AIF), guardianship, and conservatorship. Advise family that some free legal services are available to older persons in most areas.

♦ Explain to significant other that if patient refuses medication or is unable to swallow pills, obtaining a liquid form of the drug or crushing the pills and mixing them with soft food may help.

♦ Some individuals with this disease go through a phase in which, because of increased motor activity and lessening social inhibitions, they have increased sexual demands. This may result in increased sexual encounters. Be sure family is aware that this is a symptom of the disease process. Further, the patient eventually will lose ability to be intimate and tender. Sex will become a mindless act. Mates may feel rejected, frustrated, humiliated, or repulsed. Suggest that professional counseling be obtained. *This is to assist in dealing with these feelings that may become overwhelming.* Suggest that use of gentle dissuasion or distraction may be effective.

Remind patient that certain public behavior is unacceptable. Do not overreact. Move to a private place and leave patient alone for a while.

◆ Encourage caregivers to maintain their own friendships and attend social functions. *The patient's embarrassing behaviors and the demands of giving care can lead to withdrawal from society.*

◆ Encourage significant other to focus on specific problems as they occur and establish priorities (e.g., safety). Help him or her develop a plan of care and schedule of daily activities. Caregiver should focus on one difficult behavior at a time to target intervention strategies and prevent feeling overwhelmed. Note when behavior occurs and focus on stimuli that precede or trigger the behavior (e.g., overstimulation, noise). Consider other causes, such as a recent change in the environment.

◆ Encourage professional counseling and support so that significant other can work through feelings such as anger, guilt, embarrassment, and depression and can develop effective coping strategies and mechanisms. Each new and subtle loss of patient function brings another round of grieving. Decisions about institutionalization and extent of health care measures also are emotionally difficult. Behaviors such as hoarding, unjust accusations, angry outbursts, and clinging can precipitate burnout in caregiver. Caregiver must be reassessed continually for ability to care for patient at home. Keep information regarding institutionalizing available.

◆ Encourage participation in local or national support groups, such as Family-Caregiver Alliance (see "Patient-Family Teaching and Discharge Planning," immediately following).

◆ For other nursing interventions, see **Interrupted family processes** in "Psychosocial Support for the Patient's Family and Significant Others," p. 43.

Patient-Family Teaching and Discharge Planning

The degree and scope of discharge teaching and planning depend on severity of patient's condition. Include verbal and written information about the following:

◆ Referrals to community resources, local and national ALZ organization chapters, public health nurse, visiting nurses association, community support groups, social workers, counseling and psychologic therapy, home health agencies, in-home assistance, day care centers, and extended and skilled care facilities.

◆ Measures that assist in reorienting and communicating with patient in view of cognitive deficits and techniques for managing behavioral problems.

◆ Importance of scheduled respites and involvement in support groups for significant other.

◆ Medications, including drug names, purpose, dosage, frequency, precautions, and potential side effects. Also discuss drug/drug, herb/drug, and food/drug interactions.

◆ Exercises that promote muscle strength and mobility, measures for preventing contractures and skin breakdown, transfer techniques and proper body mechanics, and use of assistive devices if appropriate.

◆ Safety measures for preventing injury relative to cognitive deficits.

◆ Techniques for dealing with incontinence, indications of constipation or infection, implementation of bowel and bladder training programs, and indwelling catheter care if appropriate.

◆ Indications of upper respiratory infection (URI) and measures that prevent regurgitation, aspiration, and infection.

◆ Techniques for encouraging adequate food and fluid intake and performance of ADL.

◆ Importance of seeking financial and legal counseling and taking care of these issues early inasmuch as the disease is progressive and patient will lose ability to sign legal documents. Planning should anticipate nursing home placement and patient's eventual death.

◆ Additional general information, which can be obtained by accessing the following websites:

Alzheimer's Association: www.alz.org

Alzheimer's Disease Education and Referral Center: www.alzheimers.org

Eldercare Locator: www.eldercare.gov

Alzheimer's Caregiver Support Online: www.alzonline.net

Family Caregiver Alliance: www.caregiver.org

❖ ❖ ❖

SECTION THREE **TRAUMATIC DISORDERS OF THE NERVOUS SYSTEM**

❖ INTERVERTEBRAL DISK DISEASE

OVERVIEW/PATHOPHYSIOLOGY

The intervertebral disk is a semifluid-filled fibrous capsule that facilitates movement of the spine and acts as a shock absorber. The disk's ability to withstand stressors is not unlimited and diminishes with aging. Pressure on the disk eventually may force elastic material from the center of the disk, called the nucleus pulposus, to break (herniate) through the fibrous rim of the disk, called the annulus. Herniation usually occurs posteriorly because the posterior longitudinal ligament is inherently weaker than the anterior longitudinal ligament. The bulging or rupture (protrusion or extrusion) of an intervertebral disk causes its typical symptoms by pressing on and irritating the spinal nerve roots or spinal cord itself. Herniated nucleus pulposus usually is the result of injury or a series of insults to the vertebral column resulting from lifting or twisting. When the disk ruptures without a known discrete injury, it is believed to be caused by degenerative changes. Deterioration usually occurs suddenly with rupture, but it may happen gradually, with symptoms appearing months or years after the initial injury. Almost all herniated disks occur in the lumbar spine, with the majority of the problems occurring at L5-S1. This may be the result of thinning of the posterior longitudinal ligament at this point. The spinal cord ends around L1, so lumbar herniated disks impinge on spinal nerves, which are more resilient than actual spinal cord tissue. The spinal nerves usually bounce back and function normally once the problem is relieved. Terminology associated with lumbar disk disease includes the following: disk bulge (annular fibers still intact), disk protrusion (bulging with injury to some annular fibers), disk extrusion (bulge with loss of annular fibers but intact disk), and disk sequestration (piece of disk broken off from nucleus pulposus). Cervical disk problems most often occur at C5-6 and C6-7 and generally are caused by degenerative changes or trauma, such as whiplash or hyperextension. Cervical herniations may compress spinal nerves or impinge on the spinal cord itself. A genetic mutation (*COL 9 AZ* gene) also can cause some disk disease. Thoracic disk problems are rare because of the rigid structure of the thoracic spine.

Herniated disks account for about 4% of cases of back pain. Most back pain is related to muscle and ligament strain. Other causes of non-disk back pain include spondylolisthesis (slippage between two vertebrae) and degenerative changes such as stenosis; osteophyte (e.g., bone spur) formation, which can cause spinal nerve root compression; osteoporosis, which can lead to compression fractures; osteoarthritis of the facet joints; neoplasm; and infection.

ASSESSMENT

Signs and symptoms/physical findings: General indicators include an onset that can be sudden, with intense unilateral pain or with pain that is dull, diffuse, deep, and aching. Many patients cannot state the precise time the problem started because they may just have multiple episodes of minor low back pain. Symptoms vary according to level of injury and nerves involved. Because nerve roots exit the spine below the disks, the herniation affects the nerve root below the problem. Usually, pain is increased with movement or activities that increase intraabdominal or intrathoracic pressure, such as sneezing, coughing, and straining. Often pain is variably relieved by lying down. Immediate medical attention is essential if there is any weakness or paralysis, extreme sensory loss, or altered bowel or bladder function, which indicate spinal cord compression in the lumbar back (e.g., cauda equina syndrome) and need for emergency decompression surgery. Indicators of cervical spinal cord compression (and need for early surgical treatment) include balance problems, unsteadiness when standing with eyes closed (Romberg's sign), hyperreflexes, and generalized numbness in feet and legs.

Cervical disk disease: Pain or numbness in upper extremities, shoulders, thorax, occipital area, or back of the head or neck. Pain can radiate down the forearms and into hands and fingers. Interscapular aching or suboccipital headaches are commonly associated with cervical disk disease. Usually the neck has restricted mobility, and cervical muscle spasm and loss of normal cervical lordosis can occur. Patients may have upper extremity muscle weakness with diminished biceps or triceps reflexes.

Lumbar disk disease: Pain in the lumbosacral area with possible radiculopathy (sciatica) to the buttock, down the posterior surface of the thigh and calf, and to the lateral border of the foot and toes. Sensory distribution for the L5 nerve root is the medial portion of the foot and the great toe, whereas sensory distribution for S1 is the lateral aspect of the foot, fifth toe, and sole of the foot. Often mobility is altered, as evidenced by decreased ability to stand upright, listing to one side, asymmetric gait, limited ability to flex forward, and restricted side movement caused by pain and muscle spasms. The individual walks cautiously, bears little weight on the affected side, and often finds sitting or climbing stairs particularly painful. Reflex muscle spasms can cause bulging of the back with concomitant flattening of the lumbar curve and possible scoliosis at the level of the affected disk. Usually patellar and Achilles tendon reflexes are depressed because of nerve impingement. Sciatica usually is associated with intervertebral disk herniation.

Assessment findings may include depressed reflexes, muscle atrophy, decreased lumbar ROM, abnormal gait or posture, paresthesias (described as "pins and needles"), or anesthesia (numbness) in the dermatome of the involved nerves. The following tests are two of several that are performed to confirm presence of lumbar disk disease in the physical assessment.

Straight leg raise test: With the patient lying supine, examiner extends and raises patient's leg. The test is positive if patient has pain on the posterior aspect of the legwhen the leg is lifted 30-70 degrees. People without injury usually can have a leg raised to 90 degrees without significant discomfort.

Sciatic nerve test: Examiner extends and raises patient's leg until pain is elicited and then lowers the leg to a comfortable level. The examiner then dorsiflexes the foot to stretch the sciatic nerve. If this causes pain, the test is positive for sciatic nerve involvement. However, nerve stretch tests are often negative.

History and risk factors: Repetitive bending or lifting involving a twisting motion, continuous vibration, smoking, poor physical condition (especially weak abdominal muscles), poor posture, obesity, above-average height, osteoporosis, prolonged sitting, depression, severe scoliosis, spondylolisthesis, or genetic predisposition.

DIAGNOSTIC TESTS

In the absence of serious symptoms, diagnostic testing may not be done until 3 mo have passed and symptoms persist because in 90% of the cases, back pain resolves in less than 1 mo. Diagnostic testing should be done for pain that is constant, severe, unrelieved by rest or position, and not calmed by antiinflammatory medication inasmuch as these symptoms may indicate the presence of neoplasm or infection. Thoracic back pain also should be investigated because it may be caused by medical problems (e.g., aortic aneurysm).

MRI: May reveal a disk impinging on the spinal cord or nerve root or may show a related pathologic condition, such as a tumor or spondylosis. An MR neurogram helps to image nerves after they leave the spinal column and can show compressions as they travel through the spinal foramina. MR myelogram helps view the cerebral spinal fluid sac without having to use a needle puncture. MRI is now the standard imaging test.

CT scan of the spine: May be useful but is less sensitive than MRI. May reveal disk protrusion/prolapse or a related pathologic condition, such as a bone spur, tumor, spondylosis, or spinal stenosis.

Myelogram: May show characteristic deformity and filling defect or a related pathologic condition, but it is an invasive procedure requiring lumbar puncture (LP).

X-ray examination of the spine: May show narrowing of the vertebral interspaces in affected areas, loss of spine curvature, bone spur formation, and spondylosis. X-ray studies are usually not helpful in diagnosing disk disease but may help rule out other diseases.

Diskography: Identifies degenerated or extruded disks or annulus tear by means of contrast medium injected into disk space using fluoroscopy. Often it is done in combination with CT and may differentiate between disk infection and rupture.

EMG: May show denervation patterns of specific nerve roots to indicate level and site of injury.

Bone scan: May be used to rule out tumor, trauma, or infection.

Evoked potential (EP) studies (e.g., somatosensory [SSEP]): May show slowed conduction resulting from nerve root compromise and can localize specific nerve root.

Laboratory tests (serum alkaline and acid phosphatase, glucose, calcium, erythrocyte sedimentation rate [ESR], WBCs): Although not helpful to diagnose disk disease, they may rule out metabolic bone disease, metastatic tumors, diabetic mononeuritis, and disk space infection.

COLLABORATIVE MANAGEMENT

Activity: Prescribed to patient's tolerance, with general avoidance of lifting, twisting, and bending. Usually patients resume normal activity as soon as possible. Walking is recommended for overall toning of the body and spine. High-impact activities such as running may be limited until the injury is well healed.

Medium-firm to firm mattress: Supports normal lumbar spine curvature and minimizes spinal flexion.

Thermotherapy (heat, ice): Applying intermittent heat may reduce muscle spasm, whereas icing may prevent further inflammatory swelling and provide some topical anesthesia. Icing should be done frequently, especially for the first 24-48 hr, and is often recommended after exercise. Continuous low-level heat wrap therapy reduces pain and improves function.

Physical therapy (PT) and graded exercise program: Strengthen legs, back, and abdominal muscles and teach correct body mechanics, posture, and specific stretching exercises. Therapy is initiated once acute symptoms subside. Physical therapy (PT) has become the mainstay of therapy for low back pain.

Souchard's global postural reeducation (GPR): French physical therapy (PT) technique that has been effective in restoring function and relieving long-term chronic pain. It consists of a series of maneuvers in which patient is in supine, sitting, and standing positions and involves stretching the paraspinal muscles and those of the abdominal wall so that joints are relieved of the compression that is typically the source of pain.

Cervical traction: Helps a bulging cervical disk slip back into place and unloads the muscles and ligaments. Traditional method is a neck/head harness attached to a pulley and weight. An example of a home device is an inflatable collar that expands to push the head away from the shoulders.

Orthotics (e.g., splints, braces, girdles, cervical collars): Limit motion of the vertebral column. Generally, long-term use of braces is discouraged because it prohibits development of necessary supporting musculature. Soft or hard collars aid in immobilization of the cervical spine. Temporary use of a back brace or corset enables earlier return to activity with lumbar disk disease.

Sequential compression devices (SCDs), antiembolism hose: Prevent thrombophlebitis while patient is on bed rest. SCDs or hose should be worn until amount of time out of bed ambulating is equal to amount of time in bed. However, bed rest is not generally recommended and should not exceed more than 2 days.

Percutaneous electrical nerve stimulation: Uses acupuncture-like needle probes positioned in soft tissues and/or muscles to stimulate peripheral sensory nerves to relieve persistent back pain.

Other therapeutic modalities: Include hydrotherapy, aquatherapy, massage, acupressure, acupuncture, diathermy/ultrasound electrotherapy, transcutaneous electrical nerve stimulation (TENS), dorsal column stimulation, biofeedback, and stress reduction techniques. Whole-body vibration exercise and spinal manipulation may be considered for uncomplicated back problems with no radiculopathy.

Pharmacotherapy

Acute Phase

Analgesics (e.g., nonsteroidal antiinflammatory drugs [NSAIDs], and opiate combinations such as hydrocodone and acetaminophen or oxycodone and acetaminophen): Reduce inflammation and relieve pain. Ibuprofen is the usual drug of choice for mild to moderately severe pain. Dosing usually is scheduled initially to obtain a sustained antiinflammatory effect. Side effects include blood thinning and gastric irritation, and kidneys may be affected if these drugs are taken for a long time. Stomach protectants such as sucralfate or ranitidine may be considered to reduce gastric irritation.

Muscle relaxants (e.g., cyclobenzaprine, methocarbamol, benzodiazepines): Reduce muscle spasms and thereby reduce pain. Common side effects are drowsiness, fatigue, dizziness, dry mouth, and gastrointestinal (GI) upset. Clinical studies have proved positive effects of muscle relaxants.

Corticosteroids (e.g., dexamethasone): May be given for a short period to reduce spinal cord edema, if present, but use is controversial.

Stool softeners or laxatives (e.g., docusate): Prevent constipation or painful straining.

Proton pump inhibitor (e.g., pantoprazole), histamine H_2-receptor blocker (e.g., famotidine), and sucralfate: Prevent stress ulcers, especially if NSAIDs or corticosteroids are used.

Chronic Phase

Analgesics (e.g., NSAIDs, tramadol, gabapentin): NSAIDs are used in the chronic phase, but opioids are not recommended for chronic pain. Tramadol, a centrally acting analgesic, may be used long term, especially for older adults. Tricyclic antidepressants (e.g., amitriptyline, desipramine, doxepin) may help with chronic pain. Anticonvulsants such as gabapentin help with neuropathic pain caused by nerve injury.

Local injection of anesthetic (lidocaine or bupivacaine) and/or cortisone into epidural spaces, facet joints, sacroiliac joint, or trigger points: Reduces pain and muscle spasms and increases function.

Botulinum toxin injection into paravertebral regions: Relieves pain, probably through decreased muscle spasm, and improves function for 3-8 wk.

Surgery: Performed without delay if signs of spinal cord compression are present, such as significant motor or sensory loss or loss of sphincter control. Otherwise, surgery is considered only after symptoms fail to respond to conservative therapy and/or if the patient's ability to function in activities of daily living (ADL) is seriously limited. Patients must be monitored postoperatively for signs of spinal cord compression caused by bleeding and/or hematoma formation, which is a medical emergency.

Microdiskectomy: Herniated portion of the disk and small parts of the lamina are removed using microsurgical techniques. This surgery results in less tissue damage, less pain, fewer spasms, and increased postoperative spinal stability. Patient usually is out of bed the first day and may be released as an outpatient or discharged the next day. Diskectomy is an effective option in the short term for leg pain, but it is not accepted as a standard of care in isolation for chronic back pain.

Diskectomy with laminectomy: An incision is made, thus enabling removal of part of the vertebra (laminectomy) so that the disk's herniated portion can be removed (diskectomy). If multiple intervertebral disk spaces are explored, a wound drain may be present after surgery. Complications include paralytic ileus, urinary retention, cerebrospinal fluid (CSF) leakage, meningitis, hematoma at operative site, nerve root injury causing wrist drop or footdrop, arachnoiditis, and postural deformity.

Percutaneous lumbar disk removal: An ultrasonic nucleotome cannula or fiberoptic arthroscopic cannula can be inserted into the intervertebral space via fluoroscopy to allow fragmentation of the disk and its aspiration. A laser may be used to aid in disk excision. This is a relatively less invasive method of relieving pain from herniated disks. The procedure is done using local anesthesia and may be performed on an outpatient basis. Back stiffness, soreness, or spasm and transient syncope may occur after the procedure. Patients should be told to report immediately any numbness, weakness, or change in bowel or bladder function after hospital discharge.

Artificial disk replacement (ADR), also called total intervertebral disk replacement (TDR): Uses artificial disks such as the Charité or ProDisc to replace the degenerated disk. Helps reduce need for spinal fusions and avoid premature degeneration at adjacent levels of the spine.

Spinal fusion: Fusion may be indicated for patients with recurrent low back or neck pain, spondylolisthesis, subluxation of the vertebrae, or multilevel disease. Some health care providers promote primary use of fusion for patients who have not responded to conservative therapy. Bone chips are harvested from the iliac crest or tibia and are placed between vertebrae in the prepared area of the unstable spine to fuse and stabilize the area. Internal fixation (e.g., rods, wiring, pedicle screws, lateral mass screws, fusion cages, interbody implants, bone rings, plates) may be necessary to provide added stability until the fusion has healed fully. Intervertebral body fusion using a carbon fiber implant or cage or threaded titanium cage also relieves nerve root compression and stabilizes the spine. If the patient's own bone quality or quantity is inadequate, allograft (e.g., cadaver) bone or use of recombinant human osteogenic protein preparation ("bone putty") as a bone graft substitute or supplement may be considered. Bone stimulators, which emit low-voltage electrical current, may be used for patients who have a lower likelihood of obtaining a solid fusion, such as those with previously failed fusion or multilevel fusions or patients who smoke.

Usually the cervical and lumbar spine will require an anterior or posterior approach. Patients undergoing anterior cervical fusion may have difficulty swallowing or managing secretions because of postoperative edema and hematoma formation secondary to retraction of the trachea and esophagus during surgery. Hoarseness also can occur secondary to nerve irritation. Complaints of excessive pressure in the neck or severe, uncontrolled incisional pain may signal excessive bleeding.

Other surgical procedures: *Foraminotomy* involves surgical enlargement of the intravertebral foramen to reduce tension and make more room for the nerve root that exits and crosses this area. *Hemilaminectomy* removes part of the lamina of a vertebra to reduce pressure on an adjacent nerve. *Intradiskal electrothermal treatment (IDET)* uses a probe that uses electricity to heat and shrink collagen tissue within the annulus wall to seal up painful tears. After healing, the disk toughens and desensitizes. *Kyphoplasty* for compression fractures is a minimally invasive, percutaneous technique to reestablish the original height of a collapsed vertebra by using an inflated balloon to make a cavity within the vertebra, which is then filled with bone cement. *Vertebroplasty* is similar to kyphoplasty, except that bone cement is injected directly into the fractured vertebra (without use of the balloon) to seal and stabilize the fracture and relieve pain. *Diskoplasty* reduces or reshapes a bulging disk via a small puncture, which enables threading of a probe into the center of the disc and using a laser or radiofrequency to remove/evaporate the disk's center. *Implantable epidural spinal cord stimulators (SCSs)* have been placed to aid in control of chronic pain when all other measures have failed. Endoscopes, laparoscopes, surgical microscopes, percutaneous techniques, and computer-assisted imaging devices are expanding surgical options and are making surgery less invasive.

NURSING DIAGNOSES AND INTERVENTIONS

Health-seeking behaviors related to proper body mechanics and other measures that prevent back injury

Desired outcome: Within the treatment session (outpatient) or within the 24-hr period before hospital discharge, patient verbalizes knowledge of measures that prevent back injury and demonstrates proper body mechanics.

Nursing Interventions

♦ Teach proper body mechanics: Stand and sit straight with chin and head up and pelvis and back straight; bend at knees and hips (squat) rather than at the waist, and keep back straight (not stooping forward); when carrying objects, hold them close to the body, and avoid twisting when lifting or reaching. Spread feet when standing. *This provides a wider base of support.* Lift with the legs, not the back. Turn using entire body. Do not strain to reach things. If an object is overhead, raise yourself to its level, or move things out of the way if they are obstructing the object. Avoid lifting anything heavier than 10-20 lb. Encourage use of long-handled pickup sticks to pick up small objects. Have patient demonstrate proper body mechanics, if possible, before hospital discharge. *This ensures that the patient understood the instructions.*

♦ Teach patient to sit close to pedals when driving a car, and use a seat belt and firm back rest to support the back; support feet on a footstool when sitting so that knees are elevated to hip level or higher; obtain a firm mattress or bed board; use a flat pillow when sleeping to avoid strain on neck, arms, and shoulders; sleep in a side-lying position with knees bent or in a supine position with knees and legs supported on pillows; avoid sleeping in a prone position; avoid reaching or stretching to pick up objects; avoid sitting on furniture that does not support back. *These measures keep the body in alignment.*

♦ Encourage patient to achieve and/or maintain proper weight for age, height, and gender; continue exercise program prescribed by health care provider for strengthening abdominal, thoracic, and back muscles; use thoracic and abdominal muscles when lifting to keep a significant portion of weight off vertebral disks; when standing for any length of time, stand with one foot on a step stool; sit in a firm chair for support. *These measures relieve pressure on the back.*

- Instruct patient to wear supportive shoes with a low or moderate heel height for walking.
- Encourage smoking cessation inasmuch as smoking reduces circulation to disks.
- Teach the following technique for sitting up at the bedside from a supine position: Logroll to side, then raise to sitting position by pushing against mattress with hands while swinging legs over side of bed. Instruct patient to maintain alignment of the back during procedure.
- Teach rationale and procedure for back exercises if recommended. There are a variety of exercises that have been promoted over the past decade including Williams' flexion exercises and McKenzie's exercise protocol (which are somewhat contradictory to each other). Most recently, computerized exercise devices and strengthening of trunk muscles under controlled and reproducible conditions tend to be the norm. Encourage patient to continue with the prescribed regular exercise and stretching program. Walking and exercising in water can be included.
- Caution patient that pain is the signal to stop or change an activity or position. Teach patient that the following indicators necessitate medical attention: increased sensory loss, increased motor loss/weakness, and loss of bowel and bladder function.

Health-seeking behaviors related to pain control measures

Desired outcome: Following instruction within outpatient treatment session or within the 24-hr period before hospital discharge, patient verbalizes knowledge about pain control measures and demonstrates ability to initiate these measures when appropriate.

Nursing Interventions

- Teach patient about mechanisms of pain, as discussed earlier in this section.
- Teach methods of controlling pain and their individual applications. Methods include distraction, use of counterirritants, massage, hydrotherapy, dorsal column stimulation, use of TENS, behavior modification, relaxation techniques, hypnosis, music therapy, imagery, biofeedback, and diathermy. In addition, suggest application of local heat (e.g., warm/hot showers or heating pads) or cold massage to painful areas. The latter can be achieved by freezing water in a paper cup, tearing off top of cup to expose the ice, and massaging in a circular motion, using remaining portion of cup as a handle. A bag of frozen peas or corn may be used to apply continuous cold to lower back. A layer of cloth should be used so that ice does not touch the skin. A 20-min application of heat or cold × 4-6 times per day is recommended.
- Suggest patient use a stool to rest affected leg when standing.
- Advise patient to sit in a straight-back chair that is high enough to get out of easily. A raised toilet seat also may be useful. Straddling a straight-back chair and resting arms on the chair back is comfortable for many individuals.
- Encourage use of a moderately firm to firm mattress and extra pillows as needed for positioning. *This supports normal spinal curvature.* Some patients find the normal bed height too low and use blocks to raise it to a more comfortable level.
- Caution patient to avoid sudden twisting or turning movements. Explain importance of logrolling when moving from side to side. *This prevents exacerbations of pain.* The patient on bed rest should roll rather than lift off the bedpan and may find a fracture bedpan more comfortable than a regular bedpan.
- Advise patient to avoid staying in one position too long, fatigue, chilling, and anxiety. *These are factors that enhance spasms.*
- Suggest positions of comfort, such as lying on side with knees bent or lying supine with knees supported on pillows. Use a small pillow to support the

nape of the neck. *This may be helpful with cervical pain.* Teach patient to avoid prolonged periods of sitting. *This may increase stress on the back.*

- Suggest the patient apply a heating pad to the back for 15-30 min before getting out of bed in the morning. *This will help allay stiffness and discomfort.* Heating pads should be used only for short intervals and only if patient's temperature sensations are intact. Remind patient to place a towel or cloth between heating pad and skin. *This prevents burns.*
- Encourage patient to rest when tired or stressed and not to exercise when in pain.
- Encourage a high-bulk diet, adequate or increased fluids, and stool softeners. *These measures prevent constipation, which would cause straining and increased pain.*

Deficient knowledge related to diskectomy with laminectomy or fusion procedure

Desired outcomes: Before surgery, patient verbalizes knowledge about the surgical procedure, preoperative routine, and postoperative regimen. Patient demonstrates activities and exercises correctly.

Nursing Interventions

- For general nursing interventions, see this nursing diagnosis in "Perioperative Care," p. 1.
- Instruct patient to expect surgical team to confirm verbally and then mark the correct spinal level and correct side (e.g., anterior, posterior, right, left) of the surgical site to ensure an accurate surgery.
- Teach technique for deep breathing, which will be performed immediately after surgery (coughing may be contraindicated in immediate postoperative period to prevent disruption of fusion or surgical repair). Also teach patient use of incentive spirometry.
- Document baseline neurovascular checks, including color, capillary refill, pulse, warmth, muscle strength, movement, and sensation. Explain that VS and neurologic status will be evaluated at frequent intervals after surgery and compared with baseline. Reassure patient that this is normal and does not indicate that anything is wrong. Teach the following indicators of impairment, which necessitate immediate attention by health care staff: paresthesias, weakness, paralysis, radiculopathy, and changes in bowel or bladder function. Signs of hypovolemia, such as decreased BP, increased heart rate (HR), and thirst, may be present. Teach patient to report faintness or dizziness. *Patients undergoing fusion lose more blood during surgery than those undergoing laminectomy, but both can lose enough to become hypovolemic.*
- Explain that the surgical dressing will be inspected for excess drainage or oozing at frequent intervals. Bleeding with a laminectomy usually is minimal. Patients with fusion may have slight bloody oozing postoperatively. A closed wound drainage device may be present for 1-3 days postoperatively. Serous drainage usually is checked with a glucose reagent strip. *Presence of glucose is a signal of CSF leakage.* Bulging in the area of the wound should be reported. *This may also signal CSF leakage or hematoma formation.* Monitor dressing for increased drainage after patient has been up. Lumbar dressings will be checked after each bedpan use. *Wet or contaminated dressings require changing to prevent infection.* Inform patient undergoing fusions that he or she will have a second dressing at the donor site.
- Instruct patient to report any nausea or vomiting, which is not uncommon. *This is so that antiemetics can be given as soon as symptoms appear.* Explain that patient will be monitored for bowel and bladder dysfunction after the procedure. The abdomen will be checked for bowel sounds and distention. Patient may be asked to void within 8 hr of the procedure. *This is to check for urinary retention.* Caution patient to avoid straining at stool.
- Explain that fever may occur during first few days postoperatively but that this does not necessarily signal an infection. Patient will be assessed for

other indicators of infection, such as heat, redness, irritation, swelling, or drainage at wound site. Instruct patient to report headache, neck stiffness, or photophobia.

♦ Inform patient that postoperative pain or tingling (paresthesia) often is caused by nerve root irritation and edema. Spasms are common on the third or fourth postoperative day and should not discourage patient. Pain may take days or weeks to resolve and does not indicate that surgery was unsuccessful. The patient should request medication for pain as needed and not let pain get out of control. Patient-controlled analgesia (PCA) and NSAIDs also may be used for postoperative pain control. Patients who have had a fusion may expect significant pain from bone graft donor site (commonly the iliac crest). The donor site may have extra padding. Muscle relaxants may be prescribed. *This is to supplement pain control.*

♦ Explain that in the immediate postoperative period patient will follow the surgeon's activity restrictions, which will depend on techniques and stabilization devices used during surgery. Patients may be required to lie supine for several hours. *This is to minimize possibility of wound hematoma formation.* After this period, the head of bed (HOB) of laminectomy patients usually can be raised to 20 degrees. *This facilitates eating and bedpan use.* Patients undergoing spinal fusion may be kept flat and on bed rest longer than patients with laminectomies. *Activity progression for patients undergoing spinal fusion is usually more cautious and slower than for patients undergoing laminectomy.* Best practice regarding trapeze use is to restrict it during the initial 24-48 hr following lumbar and cervical procedures and avoid its use after thoracic procedures.

♦ Only the logroll method is used for turning. Teach patient the following technique: Position a pillow between legs, cross arms across chest while turning, and contract long back muscles. *This maintains shoulders and pelvis in straight alignment.* Explain that, initially, patient will be assisted in this procedure. Use a turning sheet and sufficient help when logrolling patient.

♦ Teach the following technique for getting out of bed: Logroll to side, splint back, and rise to a sitting position by pushing against mattress while swinging legs over side of bed. While in hospital with an electric bed, the HOB may be raised to facilitate a sitting position. Initially patient will be helped to a sitting position and should not push against mattress. Patients with cervical laminectomy should not pull themselves up with their arms. When assisting patients with cervical laminectomy to a sitting position, caution them not to put their arms on nurse's shoulders. Pillows can be used to support arms for comfort.

♦ Explain that antiembolism hose and possibly SCDs will be applied after surgery. *This is to prevent thrombus formation.* Teach techniques for ankle circling and calf pumping. *This promotes venous circulation in legs.* Teach patient to report calf pain, tenderness, or warmth. *These signs may indicate a thrombus or embolism.*

♦ Advise patient that health care provider will prescribe certain postoperative activity restrictions. Sitting is commonly restricted or allowed for only limited, prescribed periods in a straight-back chair. Teach patient not to sit for long periods on edge of mattress. *This does not provide enough support for the back.* Sitting and walking are done with hips and shoulders in good alignment. Explain that weakness, dizziness, and lightheadedness may occur on a first walk. Patient is encouraged to walk progressively longer distances.

♦ Instruct patient to avoid stretching, twisting, flexing, or jarring spine. *This is to prevent vertebral collapse, shifting of bone graft, or a bleeding episode.* Explain that the spine should be kept aligned and in a neutral position. Lifting and pulling/pushing objects is to be avoided.

♦ If patient is scheduled for cervical laminectomy or fusion, caution not to pull with arms on objects such as side rails and avoid twisting, flexion, and extensions of the neck. Explain that a cervical collar may be worn postoperatively. See "Spinal Cord Injury," p. 305, for cervical collar use.

◆ Teach use of braces or corsets if prescribed. Braces should be applied while in bed. Wearing cotton underwear under brace, powdering skin lightly with cornstarch, or providing additional padding is important. *This will help protect skin from irritation.* Skin should be inspected daily for signs of irritation or breakdown. Persons undergoing a fusion procedure often wear a supportive brace or corset for 3 mo or less. *This is done to keep operative site immobile so that the graft will heal and not dislodge.*

◆ Explain that health care provider will provide instructions for at-home activity restrictions, including driving or riding in car (may be restricted 6-8 wk up to several months), sexual activity, lifting and carrying objects, tub bathing (generally, soaking incision is avoided until about 1 wk after sutures are out), going up and down stairs, amount of time to spend in and out of bed, back exercises, and expected time away from work.

◆ Patient should call health care provider for symptoms such as increased weakness and numbness or change in bowel or bladder function.

◆ Teach the following symptoms of postoperative wound infection that require medical attention: swelling, discharge, drainage, persistent redness, local warmth, fever, and pain. The incision should be kept dry and open to the air.

Impaired swallowing (or risk for same) related to postoperative edema or hematoma formation secondary to anterior cervical fusion
Desired outcome: Patient regains uncompromised swallowing ability (usually by the third postoperative day) as evidenced by normal breath sounds and absence of food in the oral cavity or choking/coughing.

Nursing Interventions

◆ As part of preoperative teaching, instruct patient about potential for difficulty with swallowing after anterior cervical fusion. Caution patient of need to report promptly any significant postoperative difficulty with swallowing. A sore throat is not unexpected. A soft diet and throat lozenges may be prescribed for 2-3 days postoperatively.

◆ Monitor for edema of face or neck or tracheal compression or deviation. *These problems could compromise respiratory function.* Monitor and rapidly report stridor or respiratory distress.

◆ Listen for hoarseness. *It can indicate laryngeal nerve irritation and signal ineffective cough or swallowing difficulty in a particular patient.* For patients with hoarseness, the voice will usually return to normal as inflammation around laryngeal nerve subsides. Encourage voice rest and facilitate alternative communication (e.g., provide storyboards, pen and pencil, flash cards). Report immediately any respiratory distress, inability to speak, worsening hoarseness, or voice change.

◆ Monitor and report diminished breath sounds compared with patient's normal or preoperative status.

◆ As indicated, monitor oximetry as a quantitative measure of systemic oxygenation.

◆ Monitor for complaints of excessive pressure in neck or severe, uncontrolled incisional pain. *This may indicate excessive bleeding.* Monitor closed suction devices, and recharge suction device/chamber as indicated. *This will facilitate wound drainage.*

◆ Check gag and swallowing reflexes before oral intake. Begin postoperative diet with clear fluids, and progress to more solid foods only after patient demonstrates ability to ingest fluids safely.

◆ Position patient in Fowler's position, or semi-Fowler's position at minimum, when initiating fluid intake. If not prohibited by surgery, encourage use of chin tuck. *These measures will minimize risk of aspiration.*

◆ Also see **Risk for aspiration,** p. 47, in "Older Adult Care."

Patient-Family Teaching and Discharge Planning

Include verbal and written information about the following:

♦ Prescribed exercise regimen, including rationale for each exercise, technique for performing the exercise, number of repetitions of each, and frequency of exercise periods. If possible, ensure that patient demonstrates understanding of exercise regimen and proper body mechanics before hospital discharge.

♦ Wound incision care. Indicators of postoperative wound infection that necessitate medical attention include swelling, discharge, persistent redness, local warmth, fever, and pain.

♦ Review of use and application of cervical collar for patients who have had a cervical fusion (see "Spinal Cord Injury," p. 305).

♦ Use and care of a brace or immobilizer if appropriate.

♦ Medications, including drug names, rationale, dosage, schedule, precautions, and potential side effects. Also discuss drug/drug, herb/drug, and food/drug interactions.

♦ Anticonstipation routine, which should be initiated during hospitalization.

♦ Pain control measures.

♦ Phone number of a resource person in case questions arise after hospital discharge.

♦ Postsurgical activity restrictions as directed by health care provider. These may affect the following: driving and riding in a car, returning to work, sexual activity, lifting and carrying, tub bathing, going up and down steps, and amount of time spent in or out of bed.

♦ Signs and symptoms of worsening neurologic function and the importance of notifying health care provider immediately if they develop. These include numbness, weakness, paralysis, and bowel and bladder dysfunction.

♦ Additional general information, which can be obtained by accessing the following websites:

National Institutes of Health: www.nlm.nih.gov

Spine-Health: www.spine-health.com

❖ SPINAL CORD INJURY

OVERVIEW/PATHOPHYSIOLOGY

Spinal cord injuries (SCIs) are caused by vertebral fractures or dislocations that sever, lacerate, stretch, or compress the spinal cord and interrupt neuronal function and transmission of nerve impulses. Concussive trauma can cause damage from bruising, swelling, and inflammation. When blood supply to the spinal cord is interrupted, the spinal cord swells in response, and this, along with hemorrhage, can cause additional compression, ischemia, and compromised function. Neurologic deficits resulting from compression may be reversible if the resulting edema and ischemia do not lead to spinal cord degeneration and necrosis. Common causes of injury include motor vehicle accidents, diving or other sporting accidents, falls, and gunshot wounds. SCIs are classified in a number of different ways according to type (open, closed), cause (concussion, contusion, laceration, transection), site (level of spinal cord involved), mechanism of injury (compression, hyperflexion, hyperextension, rotational, penetrating), stability, and degree of spinal cord function loss (complete, incomplete), or syndromes (central cord, Brown-Séquard [lateral], anterior cord, conus medullaris, cauda equina, and posterior cord). A *spinal cord concussion* involves a transient loss of cord function caused by a traumatic event with immediate onset of flaccid paralysis that resolves completely in a matter of minutes or hours.

Prognosis: Any evidence of voluntary motor function, sensory function, or sacral sensation below the level of injury (lowest level in which motor function and sensation remain intact) indicates an incomplete SCI, with potential for partial or complete recovery. After an acute injury, the spinal cord usually goes into a condition called *spinal shock,* in which there can be total loss of spinal cord function below the level of injury. During spinal shock there is no reflex activity. Resolution of spinal shock with return of reflexes usually occurs within 1-2 wk but may take 6 mo or more. If there is no evidence of returning motor function after local reflexes have returned, the spinal cord is considered irreversibly damaged. Generally, SCI does not cause immediate death unless it is at C1 through C3, which results in respiratory muscle paralysis. Individuals who survive these injuries require a ventilator for the rest of their lives. If the injury occurs at C4, respiratory difficulties may result in death, although some individuals who have survived the initial injury have been successfully weaned from the ventilator. Injuries below C4 also can be life-threatening because of ascending spinal cord edema, which can cause respiratory muscle paralysis. Immediately after injury, common complications that require treatment include hypotension (systolic blood pressure [SBP] less than 80 mm Hg), bradycardia, paralytic ileus, urinary retention, pneumonia, and stress ulcers. Other long-term, life-threatening complications of SCI include autonomic dysreflexia (AD), pneumonia, decubitus ulcers, sepsis, urinary calculi, and urinary tract infection (UTI).

ASSESSMENT

Signs and symptoms/physical findings: There are a variety of neurologic assessment and functional outcome scales to assess for signs and symptoms of SCI, including the American Spinal Injury Association (ASIA) impairment scale, in which the following are described:

A *Complete:* No motor or sensory function is preserved in sacral segment S4-S5.

B *Incomplete:* Sensory but no motor function is preserved below the neurologic level and includes the sacral segment S4-S5.

C *Incomplete:* Motor function is preserved below the neurologic level, and more than half of key muscles below the neurologic level have a muscle grade less than 3 (unable to lift against gravity).

D *Incomplete:* Motor function is preserved below the neurologic level, and more than half of key muscles below the neurologic level have a muscle grade of 3 or more (can lift against gravity).

E *Normal:* Motor and sensory functions are normal.

Acute injury: Loss of sensation, weakness, or paralysis below level of injury, localized pain or tenderness over site of injury, headache, hypothermia or hyperthermia, and alterations in bowel and bladder function.

CERVICAL INJURY: Possible alterations in LOC; weakness or paralysis in all four extremities (tetraparesis or tetraplegia, previously termed quadriparesis or quadriplegia); and paralysis of respiratory muscles or signs of respiratory problems, such as flaring nostrils and use of accessory muscles for respirations. Any cervical injury can result in low body temperature (to 96° F [35.5° C]), slowed pulse rate (less than 60 beats per minute [bpm]) caused by vagal stimulation of the heart, hypotension (SBP less than 80 mm Hg) caused by vasodilation, and decreased peristalsis.

THORACIC AND LUMBAR INJURIES: Paraparesis/paraplegia or altered sensation in the legs; hand and arm involvement in upper thoracic injuries.

ACUTE SPINAL SHOCK: Absence of deep tendon reflexes (DTRs) below level of injury; absence of cremasteric reflex (scratching or light stroking of inner thigh for male patients causes testicle on that side to elevate) for T12 and L1 injuries; absence of penile or anal sphincter reflex. Can last from 2 days to 4-6 mo but usually resolves in 1-2 wk. Spinal shock results from loss of sympathetic nerve outflow and reflex function in all segments below level of injury. Indicators depend on injury severity and include total loss of spinal cord function, loss of skin sensation, flaccid paralysis or absence of reflexes below level of injury, paralytic ileus and constipation secondary to atonic bowel, bladder distention secondary to atonic bladder, bradycardia, low/falling BP secondary to loss of vasomotor tone and decreased venous return, and anhidrosis (absence of sweating and loss of temperature regulation) below level of injury. Autonomic instability is more dramatic in higher (e.g., cervical) lesions. Resolution of spinal shock is indicated by return of both the bulbocavernosus reflex (slight muscle contraction when glans penis is squeezed or urinary catheter is pulled, causing scrotal retraction) and the anal reflex (anal puckering on digital examination or gentle scratching around the anus). Remaining reflexes may take weeks to return.

Chronic injury: Generally, increased DTRs occur if the spinal cord lesion is of the upper motor neuron (UMN) type. As spinal shock resolves, muscle tone, reflexes, and some function may return, depending on severity and level of injury. Return of reflexes usually results in muscle spasticity. Chronic autonomic dysfunction may be manifested as fever; mild hypotension; anhidrosis; and alterations in bowel, bladder, and sexual function. Chronic neural pain may occur after SCI and tends to occur as either diffuse pain below level of injury or pain adjacent to level of injury. Injuries at or below L1 may result in permanent flaccid paralysis. Orthostatic hypotension is more typical of lesions above T7.

UMN INVOLVEMENT: UMNs are nerve cell bodies that originate in high levels of the CNS and transmit impulses from the brain down the spinal cord. Injury interrupts this impulse transmission and causes muscle or organ dysfunction below the level of injury. However, because the injury does not interrupt reflex arcs coming from those muscles or organs to the spinal cord, hypertonic reflexes, clonus paralysis, and spastic paralysis are seen. The patient will have a positive Babinski reflex.

LOWER MOTOR NEURON (LMN) INVOLVEMENT: LMNs are anterior horn cell bodies that originate in the spinal cord. LMNs transmit nerve impulses to muscles and organs and are involved in reflex arcs that control involuntary responses. Damage to LMNs abolishes voluntary and reflex responses of muscles and organs and results in flaccid paralysis, hypotonia, atrophy, and muscle fibrillations and fasciculations. The patient will have an absent Babinski reflex. The spinal cord ends at the T12-L1 level. Below that level, a bundle of nerve roots from the spinal cord, called the cauda equina, fills the spinal canal. Injuries at or below L1 that damage nerve fiber after it leaves the spinal cord result in flaccid paralysis because of interrupted reflex arc activity.

BOWEL AND BLADDER DYSFUNCTION: Usually, conscious sensation of the need to void or defecate is lost. UMN bowel and bladder involvement results in reflex incontinence. Flaccid LMN bladder involvement causes urinary retention with overflow incontinence. Flaccid LMN bowel involvement causes fecal retention/impaction.

SEXUAL DYSFUNCTION: Degree of dysfunction varies according to degree of completeness and whether injury is UMN or LMN. Male patients with complete UMN injuries have a loss of psychogenic erection but may have reflex erections. Ejaculation rates with complete UMN injuries are as quite low. Female patients have a loss of psychogenic lubrication but may have reflex lubrication. With complete LMN injuries, about one-fourth of male patients will have psychogenic erections but none will have reflex erections. Incomplete injuries will result in better sexual functioning that may include both erections and ejaculations.

AD (also known as autonomic hyperreflexia): Exaggerated and unopposed sympathetic response to noxious stimuli below the SCI lesion can be life-threatening as reflex activity returns. AD is seen most commonly in patients with injuries at or above T6, but it has been reported with injuries as low as T8. Signs and symptoms include gross hypertension (BP more than 20 mm Hg above baseline, but BP can be as high as 240-300/150 mm Hg), pounding headache, blurred vision, bradycardia, nausea, and nasal congestion. Above level of injury, flushing and sweating may occur. Below level of injury, pilo-erection (goose bumps) and skin pallor, which signal vasoconstriction, may be present. Seizures, subarachnoid hemorrhage (SAH), stroke, or retinal hemorrhage also may occur.

DIAGNOSTIC TESTS

X-ray examination of spine: Delineates fracture, deformity, displacement of vertebrae, and soft tissue masses such as hematomas.

CT scan: Reveals changes in the spinal cord, vertebrae, and soft tissue surrounding the spine.

Myelography: Shows blockage or disruption of the spinal canal; used if other diagnostic examinations are inconclusive. Allows visualization of spinal nerves more clearly. Radiopaque dye is injected into the subarachnoid space of the spine, by using LP or cervical puncture.

MRI: Reveals changes in spinal cord and surrounding soft tissue. MRI evaluation is preferred and is considered the standard for evaluation of degree of injury in patients who can tolerate it.

ABG (arterial blood gas)/pulmonary function tests: Assess effectiveness of respirations and detect need for O_2 or mechanical ventilation.

Pulmonary fluoroscopy: Evaluates degree of diaphragm movement and effectiveness in individuals with high cervical injuries.

Evoked potential (EP) studies (e.g., somatosensory [SSEP]): Help locate level of spinal cord lesion by evaluating integrity of anatomic pathways and connections of the nervous system. Stimulation of a peripheral nerve triggers a discrete electrical response along a neurologic pathway to the brain. Response or lack of response to stimulation is measured in this test.

Cystometry/urodynamic evaluation: Assesses bladder capacity and function after resolution of spinal shock for the best type of bladder training program.

Deep vein thrombosis (DVT) studies (e.g., venogram, duplex Doppler ultrasound): Monitor for development of DVT.

COLLABORATIVE MANAGEMENT

The goals of treatment and management are to stabilize the injury, decrease inflammation, increase blood flow, reduce degradation and cell death, and eventually, improve nerve regeneration.

Acute Care

Patient usually is in ICU for the first 7-14 days for cardiac, hemodynamic, and respiratory monitoring.

Immobilization/bed rest: Essential for preventing further damage. See "Surgery/immobilization," p. 291. This usually involves complete spine immobilization with rigid cervical collar and backboard or other firm surface until extent of injury is determined. Patient is continued on bed rest on a firm surface (e.g., Roto Rest Kinetic Treatment Table).

Pharmacotherapy

Corticosteroids (e.g., methylprednisolone): IV megadose is given within 8 hr of injury to reduce damage and improve functional recovery by protecting the neuromembrane from further destruction. However, harmful side effects (e.g., increased infection rate, hyperglycemia, gastrointestinal [GI] bleeding) may outweigh clinical benefits.

Osmotic diuretics (e.g., mannitol): Sometimes used for 10 days to reduce spinal cord edema after initial injury and to minimize ascending cord edema.

Analgesics (e.g., acetaminophen, codeine) and sedatives: Decrease pain and anxiety.

Antacids (e.g., Maalox), histamine H_2-receptor blockers (e.g., ranitidine), proton pump inhibitor (e.g., pantoprazole), and sucralfate: Prevent gastric ulceration, which may occur because of increased production of gastric secretions with SCI and steroid use.

Anticoagulants (e.g., heparin, enoxaparin, warfarin): Prevent thrombophlebitis and reduce potential for pulmonary embolism (PE).

Stool softeners (e.g., docusate sodium): Keep stool soft and prevent fecal impaction while the bowel is atonic.

Vasopressors (e.g., dopamine): Treat hypotension in the immediate postinjury stage caused by loss of vasomotor tone. Fluid therapy also may be given for hypotension, and atropine may be given for bradycardia. Typically, patient is on a cardiac monitor and in ICU during this stage.

Aggressive respiratory therapy: For all patients with SCIs. Patients with injuries above C5 are intubated and put on a ventilator. Nasal intubation or tracheostomy may be used to prevent neck extension (and thus further damage) during intubation. Intermittent positive-pressure breathing (IPPB) and chest physiotherapy are used to prevent and treat atelectasis. Respiratory therapy is ongoing past the acute stage. Noninvasive positive pressure ventilation may be used with some patients.

Nasogastric (NG) decompression during spinal shock phase: Prevents aspiration of gastric contents and treats paralytic ileus.

Continuous bladder drainage or intermittent catheterization: For bladder decompression during spinal shock phase.

Surgery/immobilization: May include traction, fusion, laminectomy, and closed or open reduction of fractures. Use of lamina hooks, pedicle screws, lateral mass screws, wiring, plates, and interbody fusion cages provides multiple fixative points and enables greater postoperative stability. The surgical goals are to realign, stabilize, and immobilize the spine and, if indicated, decompress the spinal cord or remove bone fragments as soon as possible after injury. Complete healing may take 3-4 mo. Surgical stabilization has reduced the need for traction in many cases.

Cervical spine: Immobilized with devices such as Crutchfield tongs, Vinke tongs, Gardner-Wells tongs, and halo traction. Halo traction does not need to be removed for surgery; it enables early mobilization, and some types can be used in MRI machines.

Thoracic spine: Immobilized with a variety of appliances such as a surgical corset; plaster Minerva jacket; Jewett brace; thoracolumbar standing orthosis brace; Cotrel and DuBousset rods; or spinal fusion with bone graft, pedicle screws, fusion cages, or lamina hooks. Braces may not actually prevent deformity or hardware failure postoperatively but are effective for reminding the patient to restrict activities.

Lumbar spine injuries: Usually treated with closed reduction and hyperextension or extension with traction techniques, followed by immobilization in a plastic jacket or spica cast. If these interventions are unsuccessful or if neurologic symptoms occur, laminectomy is usually performed. A halo type of device that provides femoral distraction has been developed for lumbar injuries.

Sacral (cauda equina) fracture: Usually treated with a laminectomy and spinal fusion.

Tracheostomy: If patient needs long-term ventilation.

Nutrition: Parenteral nutrition and fluids until the GI tract starts functioning and oral intake is possible. A diet high in protein and fiber usually is prescribed.

Bowel program during spinal shock: Usually consists of manual disimpaction and small-volume enemas while the bowel is atonic.

PT and occupational therapy (OT): Passive ROM is started on all joints. After the injury is stabilized, an aggressive rehabilitation program is initiated, including muscle strengthening and conditioning exercises to develop alternative muscle groups needed for independence; a sitting program; massage; instruction in adaptive devices, equipment, and transfer techniques as appropriate; and instruction in orthotics and braces or splints to prevent contractures. Patients with sacral injuries have the potential to walk and should be instructed in use of braces, crutches, or cane as appropriate. Functional electrical stimulation (FES) of paralyzed muscles assists some paraplegic patients with walking. A therapy program is ongoing throughout the patient's rehabilitation.

Antiembolism hose or sequential compression devices (SCDs): Prevent thrombophlebitis and reduce effects of orthostatic hypotension.

Counseling and psychotherapy: Help patient and significant other adjust to the disability. This is ongoing and should address sexual functioning and vocational rehabilitation.

Other: There are many investigational treatments on the horizon for SCI (e.g., moderate hypothermia, acupuncture) and drugs such as tirilizad and atorvastatin. Some of the drugs have proved effective in laboratory animals but not yet in humans.

Chronic Care

Pharmacotherapy

Muscle relaxants (e.g., diazepam): Decrease spasms and reduce anxiety.

Antispasmodics (e.g., baclofen, tizanidine, or dantrolene): Decrease spasms. More severe spasticity may be treated with intramuscular (IM) injections of botulinum toxin. Dantrolene causes muscle weakness, so it is generally reserved for patients on bed rest. Intrathecal baclofen involves use of a programmable implanted pump to deliver a continuous dose of baclofen into the spinal canal sheath to control spasticity. Intrathecal baclofen must not be abruptly stopped because doing so may cause seizures and hallucinations.

Antibiotics (e.g., methenamine mandelate): Prevent bladder infection.

Stool softeners (e.g., docusate sodium), laxatives (e.g., Milk of Magnesia,), contact irritants and stimulants (e.g., bisacodyl, senna), suppositories, and small-volume enemas (e.g., Enemeez): Maintain a bowel program that prevents fecal impaction and minimizes incontinence. Suppositories are avoided or used with caution in individuals at risk for AD. Liquid suppositories available in mini-enemas include docusate and glycerin, a liquid soap base.

Anticholinergics (e.g., oxybutynin, tolterodine, propantheline): Reduce uninhibited bladder contractions causing incontinence in the failure-to-store hyperreflexic bladder.

Intravesical injections of oxybutynin or botulinum toxin A into the detrusor muscle: Decrease detrusor overactivity that does not respond to oral agents.

Smooth muscle stimulant (e.g., bethanechol chloride): Helps prevent urinary retention in the failure-to-empty areflexic bladder.

Adrenergic antagonists (e.g., phenoxybenzamine): Help prevent urinary retention resulting from outlet obstruction (helps relax outlet).

Analgesics: Nonnarcotic analgesics (e.g., acetaminophen) and neuropathic pain medications.

Other medications: Include anticonvulsants such as carbamazepine, gabapentin, topiramate, and lamotrigine (see "Seizures and Epilepsy," p. 348, for side effects/precautions), and tricyclic antidepressants (e.g., amitriptyline or imipramine). Also review pharmacology discussion under "Acute care." Many of those medications are used on an ongoing basis.

Sexual enhancement medications: Oral agents include vardenafil, tadalafil, and sildenafil, which are taken orally to produce an erection but are contraindicated for people who are taking nitrates (e.g., nitroglycerin) because of the additive hypotensive effect. Patients with erections lasting longer than 4 hr should seek medical attention. Vaginal gels are used to help lubrication in women.

Osteoporosis prevention: Bisphosphonate derivatives (e.g., pamidronate, etidronate, clodronate) and calcium and vitamin D supplementation are used if diet is inadequate to prevent the demineralization that occurs following SCI. Monitor serum calcium levels, and encourage early mobilization and use of standing frames to obtain weight bearing. Bone density also may be monitored.

Orthostatic hypotension prevention: Salt tablets and fludrocortisone may be used if nonmedication methods (e.g., antiembolism hose, slow position changes) are ineffective.

Dietary management: Diet should include adequate calcium and vitamin D (for osteoporosis prevention), but excessive calcium should be avoided to minimize risk of renal calculi. Juices (e.g., cranberry, plum, prune) that leave an acid ash in the urine and decrease urinary pH are encouraged, to reduce the potential for infection. Vitamin C also may be used to acidify urine. Diet should have adequate fiber to promote soft stools. SCI causes an obligatory negative nitrogen balance, and therefore diet should have adequate to high protein content.

Prevention of heterotopic ossification (HO): HO is the abnormal formation of true bone within the extraskeletal soft tissues; it causes pain, swelling, redness, warmth, and decreased ROM and function. It occurs most commonly around the hips. Etidronate, NSAIDs such as indomethacin, ROM exercises, and external beam irradiation are prevention therapies. Once HO has formed, resection usually is necessary.

Skin care and turning: Necessary to prevent skin breakdown and pressure ulcers. Patients in wheelchairs need to lift themselves and shift their weight q15-30min and use gel cushions for extra padding. See "Pressure Ulcers," p. 722, for management.

Respiratory management: Pneumonia is a leading cause of death in individuals with SCI. Deep breathing and coughing, using assisted cough technique, are important interventions.

Insufflation-exsufflation cough machine: Used to deliver breaths to patient and produces a more effective mechanically assisted cough.

Glossopharyngeal and neck accessory muscle breathing: Involves a series of gulps using lips, tongue, pharynx, and larynx to pull air into the lungs. Cycles of 6-10 gulps are followed by passive exhalation. This technique improves forced vital capacity (80% of normal) and can provide time off ventilator, decrease dependency on ventilator in case of accidental disconnection, improve cough function, and increase volume of speaking voice.

Management of AD: AD is a medical emergency that can occur after spinal shock resolution for patients with SCIs at or above T6. The noxious stimulus (e.g., a distended bladder) must be found and alleviated as quickly as possible. The following may be administered during crisis to control hypertension: fast-acting calcium channel blockers, vasodilators, hypotensive nondiuretic thiazides, adrenergic blockers, and ganglionic blocking agents. Tetracaine or lidocaine may be instilled into the bladder to reduce bladder excitability. (For nursing interventions, see **Autonomic dysreflexia,** later).

Prevention of PE: Use of antiembolism hose or SCD to prevent thrombophlebitis. Subcutaneous heparin or enoxaparin also may be used. Placement of vena cava filters may be necessary to prevent emboli from reaching the lungs.

Bladder and bowel programs: See nursing diagnoses **Constipation,** p. 296, and **Urinary retention** or **Reflex urinary incontinence,** p. 300. Bladder ultrasound may be used to determine fullness and aid in retraining.

Body weight–supported treadmill training (BWSTT): With the body supported during therapy, the legs are moved along a treadmill in a repetitive up-and-down pattern that mimics walking. Patient progressively does more weight bearing. This therapy enhances ambulation and gait recovery in patients with incomplete SCI lesions. The mechanism is not totally understood but is attributed to activation of central pattern generators in the spinal cord below the area of injury. Central pattern generators are a complex circuit of neurons responsible for coordinated, rhythmic muscle activity such as locomotion. Repeated leg movements can teach the damaged spinal cord to adapt, reorganize, and respond more appropriately.

Functional magnetic stimulation: A special magnet placed over sacral nerves or suprapubic area appears to suppress detrusor hyperreflexia and improve bladder emptying and training. Peripheral repetitive magnetic stimulation can reduce spastic tone after application over the spinal cord.

FES using surface stimulators: Muscle groups are stimulated with surface electrodes to aid patient in standing, ambulating, and using stationary bicycle. This helps prevent deconditioning and muscle loss; weight bearing reduces risk of osteoporosis.

Surgical interventions

FES: Use of an implanted device to stimulate specific muscle groups to create contraction and relaxation for assisted function. One example is the diaphragm pacer a phrenic nerve stimulator that may enable selected patients on ventilators to be off the ventilator for short periods. Electrodes are implanted over the phrenic nerve and, when activated, cause the diaphragm to contract, thereby generating a breath. Other FES modalities are bladder stimulation, hand-grasping neuroprosthesis (for patients with C5-C6 injuries), and bowel stimulation. A spinal cord or peripheral nerve stimulator has been shown to be effective for pain control.

Tenotomies, myotomies, peripheral neurectomies, and rhizotomy: These are some of the surgical approaches that may be used to treat spasticity that cannot be managed by medications or more conservative measures such as stretching or ROM.

Tendon transfer, muscle transplants: Performed in tetraplegic patients with C6-C7 injury to improve hand function.

Peripheral nerve rerouting: Uses peripheral nerves from the area above the injury and connects them to nerves below the injury for selective restorations.

Urinary diversion: May be considered for patients whose bladders cannot be retrained.

Artificial urinary sphincter: May be used to promote bladder continence. The urethra is surgically closed at the bladder junction, and an artificial opening with a special valve to the outside enables self-catheterization. A continent vesicostomy allows self-catheterization via a stoma.

External sphincterectomy: Reduces sphincter resistance to produce continuous emptying.

Colostomy: For difficult bowel evacuation or incontinence that cannot be managed effectively.

Assistive devices/animals: Some powered wheelchairs can climb stairs, elevate a seated passenger to normal eye level to enable the patient to reach high places without help, elevate the seat to a standing position, and tilt patient every 10 min to promote circulation. There is also an "all-terrain" wheelchair. Computer devices interfaced with tools and gadgets can help with daily routines. Some assistive animals are trained to call for help or to fetch specific items the patient may need.

NURSING DIAGNOSES AND INTERVENTIONS

Autonomic dysreflexia (or risk for same) related to exaggerated unopposed autonomic response to noxious stimuli for individuals with SCI at or above T6 (could be as low as T8)

Desired outcomes: On an ongoing basis, patient is free of AD symptoms as evidenced by BP within patient's baseline range, heart rate (HR) 60-100 bpm, and absence of headache and other clinical indicators of AD. Following instruction, patient and significant other verbalize factors that cause AD, treatment and prevention, and when immediate emergency treatment is indicated.

Nursing Interventions

◆ Maintain a good bowel regimen and skin integrity program. *These are key factors in preventing the noxious stimuli that constipation or pressure areas may cause.* Prevention is the best way to deal with AD.

- Loosen clothing, bed sheets, and constricting bands and turn patient off side. Keep the bed free of sharp objects and wrinkles. Adhere to turning schedules. *This is to relieve other possible sources of pressure.*
- Institute measures to reduce the potential for UTI and urinary calculi, and teach patient self-inspection of skin and urinary catheter and importance of using anesthetic jelly for catheterization and disimpaction.
- Monitor for indicators of AD, including hypertension (BP more than 20 mm Hg above baseline, but may go as high as 240-300/150 mm Hg), pounding headache, bradycardia, blurred vision, nausea, nasal congestion, flushing and sweating above the level of injury, and piloerection (goose bumps) or pallor below level of injury. Remove antiembolism hose.
- If AD is suspected, raise head of bed (HOB) immediately to 90 degrees or assist patient into a sitting position. *This is to lower the BP.*
- Call for someone to notify health care provider; stay with patient, and systematically search to identify and relieve the noxious stimulus. Speed is essential. Monitor BP q3-5min during hypertensive episode. Remain calm and supportive of patient and significant other. Patient will be very anxious.
- Assess the following sites for causes, and implement measures for removing the noxious stimulus.

BLADDER (MOST LIKELY CAUSE): Distention, UTI, calculus and other obstructions, bladder spasms, catheterization, or bladder irrigations performed too quickly or with too cold a liquid.

- Do not use Credé's method for a distended bladder. *The increased bladder pressure could further stimulate the reflex and worsen the condition.* Catheterize patient (ideally using anesthetic jelly) if there is a possibility or question of bladder distention. Consult health care provider immediately. If a catheter is already in place, check tubing for kinks and lower drainage bag. For obstruction, such as sediment in tubing, slowly irrigate catheter as indicated, using 30 mL or less of normal saline. If catheter patency is uncertain, recatheterize patient using anesthetic jelly. If the bladder is not distended, check for signs of UTI and/or urinary calculi, including cloudy urine, hematuria, and positive laboratory or x-ray examination results. Obtain urine specimen for culture and sensitivity studies as indicated.

BOWEL (SECOND MOST LIKELY CAUSE): Constipation, impaction, insertion of suppository or enema, or rectal examination.

- Do not attempt rectal examination without first anesthetizing the rectal sphincter and anal canal with anesthetic jelly. Use large amounts of anesthetic jelly in anus and rectum before disimpacting bowel to remove potential stimulus. Allow 5 min for anesthetic jelly to work, as manifested by lower BP, before disimpacting.

SKIN: Pressure, infection, injury, heat, pain, or cold.

- Loosen clothing and remove antiembolism hose, leg bandages, abdominal binder, or constrictive sheets as appropriate. For male patients, check for pressure source on penis, scrotum, or testicles and remove pressure if present. Check skin surface below level of injury. Monitor for presence of a pressure area or sore, infection, laceration, rash, sunburn, ingrown toenail, or infected area, or check skin for contact with a hard object. If indicated, apply a topical anesthetic. Observe for and remove source of heat or cold (e.g., ice pack, heating pad). Spray any irritated areas with a topical anesthetic agent.

ADDITIONAL CAUSES: Surgical manipulation, incisional pain, sexual activity, menstrual cramps, labor, vaginal infection, or intraabdominal problems such as appendicitis.

- Administer antihypertensive agents as prescribed. Check for use of sildenafil, an erectile dysfunction medication, before giving nitroglycerin. Mecamylamine, prazosin, or clonidine may be used for recurrent AD. On resolution of the crisis, answer patient's and significant other's questions about AD. Discuss signs and symptoms, treatment, and methods of prevention. Encourage patient to wear a MedicAlert bracelet or tag. Encourage keeping an AD kit on hand that includes a glove, lubricant jelly, straight catheter, electronic BP machine, and alert card.

Constipation or fecal impaction related to immobility and decreased peristalsis, atonic bowel, and loss of sensation and voluntary sphincter control secondary to sensorimotor deficit
Desired outcome: Patient has bowel movements that are soft and formed every 1-3 days or within patient's preinjury pattern.

Nursing Interventions

◆ During acute phase of spinal shock, assess patient's bowel function by auscultating for bowel sounds; inspecting for presence of abdominal distention; and monitoring for nausea, vomiting, and fecal impaction. Notify health care provider of significant findings. In the presence of fecal impaction, gentle manual removal or a small cleansing enema may be prescribed. Administer small-volume enemas only. *This is because the atonic intestine distends easily.*

◆ Manage a flaccid bowel with increased intraabdominal pressure techniques, manual disimpaction, and small-volume enemas. *Lesions below the conus medullaris (T12) may injure S3, S4, and S5 nerve segments, with resulting disruption of the reflex arc, causing LMN flaccid bowel, and loss of anal tone.* Avoid long-term use of enemas.

◆ For UMN reflex bowel, once bowel activity returns, teach patient to attempt bowel movement 30 min after a meal or warm drink. This regimen will allow patient's gastrocolic and duodenocolic mass peristalsis reflexes to assist with evacuation. Increasing intraabdominal pressure by sitting, bearing down, bending forward, or applying manual pressure to the abdomen also will help promote bowel evacuation. An abdominal belt may be used if patient is unable to strain at stool. Massaging abdomen in a clockwise, circular motion may help. A prescribed, medicated suppository also may be used if necessary. If allowed, provide a bedside commode. Check patient's ability to maintain balance on a commode. If patient is bedridden, turn patient onto side and use a pad rather than a bedpan to catch bowel movement. *Lesions above the conus medullaris (located at the lower two levels of the thoracic region where the cord begins to taper) generally leave S3, S4, and S5 spinal cord nerve segments intact. If this spinal reflex arc is intact, patient will have UMN bowel and be capable of stimulating (training) reflex evacuation of the bowel.*

◆ For patients with injuries at T8 or above, promote adequate fluid intake (more than 2500 mL/day) and use of stool softeners and high-fiber diet. Use suppositories and enemas only when essential and with extreme caution. *This is because suppositories and enemas can precipitate AD.* Use anesthetic jelly liberally when performing a rectal examination or inserting a suppository or an enema.

◆ For patients with hand mobility (who are not at risk for AD), teach technique for suppository insertion and digital stimulation of the anus to promote reflex bowel evacuation. For digital stimulation, insert lubricated finger about $1\frac{1}{2}$-$2\frac{1}{2}$ inches into rectum and gently rotate in a slow circular motion, gently stretching sphincter, for about 30 sec (but no longer than 1 min at a time) until the internal sphincter relaxes. Restart circular motion if sphincter tightens and remove finger if bowel movement begins. Stop if sphincter spasms are felt or if signs of AD occur. Repeat q5-10min several times until adequate evacuation occurs. If unsuccessful after 20-30 min of stimulation, insert a suppository. Suppository inserters and rectal stimulation devices are available for patients with limited hand mobility. Teach patient to keep fingernails cut short.

◆ For other nursing interventions, see **Constipation** in "Prolonged Bed Rest," p. 29.

Ineffective airway clearance related to neuromuscular paralysis/weakness or restriction of chest expansion secondary to halo vest obstruction

Desired outcome: Following intervention, patient has a clear airway as evidenced by respiratory rate (RR) of 12-20 breaths/min with normal depth and pattern (eupnea) and absence of adventitious breath sounds.

Nursing Interventions

♦ Monitor ventilation capability by checking vital capacity, tidal volume, and pulmonary function tests. Monitor serial ABG values and/or pulse oximetry readings. If vital capacity is less than 1 L or if patient exhibits signs of hypoxia (PaO_2 less than 80 mm Hg, O_2 saturation 92% or less, tachycardia, increased restlessness, mental status changes or dullness, cyanosis), notify health care provider immediately. *This may indicate an impaired airway or other respiratory distress.*

♦ Monitor for ascending spinal cord edema, which may be signaled by increasing difficulty with secretions, coughing, respiratory difficulties, bradycardia, fluctuating BP, and increased motor and sensory losses at a higher level than baseline findings.

♦ Monitor for loss of previous ability to bend arms at the elbows (C5-C6) or shrug shoulders (C3-C4). If these findings are noted, notify health care provider immediately.

♦ Maintain patent airway. Keep patient's head in neutral position, and suction as necessary but be observent of the respiratory status. *Suctioning may cause severe bradycardia in the patient with AD.* If indicated, prepare patient for tracheostomy, endotracheal intubation, and/or mechanical ventilation. *This is to support respiratory function if needed.*

♦ If patient is wearing halo vest traction, assess respiratory status at least q4h or more frequently as indicated. Monitor ability to swallow. *This is to ensure that vest is not restricting chest expansion.* Teach use of incentive spirometry. Be alert to the following indicators of PE: shortness of breath, hemoptysis, tachycardia, and diminished breath sounds. Pain may or may not be present with PE. *It will depend on level of SCI. Sudden shoulder pain may be referred pain from PE.*

♦ If patient's cough is ineffective, implement the following technique, known as *assisted coughing:* Place the heel of your hand under patient's diaphragm (below xiphoid process and above navel). Have patient take several deep breaths, hold a deep breath, and then cough. As patient exhales forcibly, quickly push up into diaphragm to assist in producing a more forceful cough. Assisted coughing may be contraindicated in patients with spinal instability.

♦ Feed patients while they are in the prone position in special beds. Raise stable patients in halo traction to high Fowler's position if it is not contraindicated. *This is to minimize potential for aspiration.*

♦ For additional information, see **Risk for aspiration,** p. 47, in "Older Adult Care."

Risk for disuse syndrome related to paralysis, immobilization, or spasticity secondary to SCI

Desired outcomes: After stabilization of the injury, patient exhibits complete ROM of all joints. By time of discharge, patient demonstrates measures that enhance mobility, reduce spasms, and prevent complications.

Nursing Interventions

♦ Once injury is stabilized, assist patient with position changes. For example, change to a prone position, if not contraindicated. *This helps prevent sacral pressure sores and hip contractures.* Assist patient into this position on a regular schedule.

- For patients with spasticity, use hand splints or cones. *This helps with maintaining a functional grasp.* Fingers are kept extended.
- For patients with spasticity, it may be helpful to fit patient with splints or high-top tennis shoes that are cut off at the toes so that each shoe ends just proximal to the metatarsal head. *This helps prevent foot contractures. These shoes help keep feet dorsiflexed but prevent contact of balls of feet with a hard surface, which can cause spasticity.* Avoid footboards for these patients. *The hard surface may trigger spasticity and promote plantar flexion.*
- Teach patient that some factors that trigger spasms are cold, anxiety, fatigue, emotional distress, infections, bowel or bladder distention, ulcers, pain, tight clothing, and lying too long in one position. Controlling these factors is important. *That may reduce number of spasms experienced.*
- Teach patients with spasticity proper positioning, ROM, and daily sustained stretching exercises. *Steady, continuous, directional stretching several times daily is especially important because it may decrease amount of spasticity for several hours.* Cooling and icing techniques, heat, vibration therapy, and transcutaneous electrical nerve stimulation (TENS) of spastic muscles also may be helpful.
- Touch by caregivers should be limited. *This is because tactile stimulation may trigger spasms.* When touch is necessary, do it in a firm, gentle, steady manner.
- For additional nursing interventions, see **Risk for disuse syndrome,** p. 25, in "Prolonged Bed Rest."

Risk for injury related to incorrect neck position, irritation of cranial nerves or impaired lateral vision secondary to presence of halo vest traction, and lack of access for external cardiac compression
Desired outcomes: At time of discharge (and ongoing during use of halo traction), patient exhibits no adverse changes in motor, sensory, or cranial nerve function and is free of symptoms of injury caused by impaired vision.

Nursing Interventions

- Assess position of patient's neck in relation to the body. Alert health care provider to presence of flexion or hyperextension. Assess any difficulty with swallowing. *This may signal improper position of neck and chin.* Keep a torque screwdriver in a secure place. *This is so the health care provider can readily adjust tension on bars to return patient's neck position to neutral.*
- Evaluate degree of sensation and movement of upper extremities, and assess cranial nerve function. *Changes in cranial nerve function can occur if cranial pins compress or irritate a nerve.* Notify health care provider of sudden changes in motor, sensory, or cranial nerve function (e.g., weakness, paresthesias, ptosis, difficulty chewing or swallowing). Jaw pain may occur when chewing is attempted, and this needs to be differentiated from cranial nerve problems. A diet of soft foods, cut into small pieces, will help jaw pain.
- Assess pins, bolts, and vest structure for looseness at least daily. Clicking sounds may signal a loose pin. Never use superstructure of halo traction in turning or moving patient. Notify health care provider if pins or vest becomes loose or dislodged. Stabilize patient's head as necessary.
- Instruct patient to avoid pulling clothes over top of halo apparatus. *This may loosen pins.* Patient should instead step into clothes and pull them up over feet and legs. Advise patient to buy strapless bras, tube tops, or clothes that are several sizes too large, or to modify neck openings (e.g., with self-stick [Velcro] closures, ties). *This may prevent pulling on the device or dislodging it.*
- Avoid loosening a buckle without health care provider's directive. Buckle holes or straps should be marked. *This will ensure that they are always cinched correctly to appropriate snugness.*

- Ambulatory patients should walk initially with assistance of two people. Teach how to survey environment while walking, either by using a mirror, by turning eyes to their extreme lateral positions, or by turning entire body. A cane may help determine height of curbs and detect unseen objects or uneven walking surfaces. *Trunk flexibility is limited, and achieving balance can be difficult because of the top-heavy weight of the vest.* Ambulating with a walker initially may help patient learn to adjust. Teach abdominal and back strengthening exercises. *This may aid balance and walking.* Advise patient to walk only in low-heeled shoes. Extra space allowance may be needed when passing through doorways. *This is to keep the patient from bumping into objects.*
- Teach patient that bending over can be hazardous. *This is due to top heaviness.* A shower chair that rolls usually can fit over a toilet seat, providing an extra 3-6 inches in height. Slip-on shoes should be worn and long-handled assistive devices used to reach or pick up objects.
- To get out of bed, teach patient to roll onto his or her side at edge of bed and then drop legs over side of bed while pushing up trunk sideways.
- Recommend backing into car seat with body bent forward when getting into a car. Caution patient against driving. *At this time, the patient has a limited field of vision.*
- Teach patient that a high table will help bring objects into view and that a swivel chair at home is helpful. *This will permit easier visualization of the environment.*
- Explain that patient will need assistance of another person to shampoo hair safely. Shampooing a short haircut is easiest, and hair should be blown dry. *Toweling hair may loosen pins.*
- Encourage experimenting with side and prone positions for sleeping, but caution against placing pillows under support bars.
- Teach caregivers and significant other how to release vest in an emergency. *This is in case there is need for external cardiac compression.*

Risk for impaired skin integrity and/or **Impaired tissue integrity** related to altered circulation and mechanical factors secondary to presence of halo vest traction or tongs
Desired outcome: At time of discharge and on an ongoing basis, patient's skin is nonerythremic and unbroken; tissue underlying and surrounding the halo vest blanches appropriately.

Nursing Interventions

- Inspect skin around vest edges for erythema and other signs of irritation. Keep skin dry. Massage nonerythematous areas routinely. *This is to promote circulation and help prevent breakdown.* Teach skin inspection, which may require use of a mirror, flashlight, or another person. Teach patient to alert medical personnel if breakdown, sensitive spots, odor, dirty vest liner, or loose pins are present.
- Investigate complaints of discomfort or uncomfortable fit. A finger should be able to fit between vest and patient's skin. Weight loss or gain can affect fit. Pad vest as needed until it can be properly adjusted or trimmed by health care provider. Protect vest from moisture and soiling. Be alert to foul odor from in or around cast openings. *This may signal pressure necrosis beneath vest.* Check for serosanguineous drainage on a pillowcase slipped through the vest from one side to another. *This may indicate an area of skin breakdown.*
- Instruct/assist patient with changing body position q2h. Support vest while patient is in bed, and use logroll technique with sufficient help. Use pads to prevent pressure on prominent body areas such as forehead or shoulder. Use a small pillow under the head. *This is for comfort at sleep time.*

♦ Skin care should include cleansing with soap and warm water. Usually, releasing one vest belt at a time as patient is lying down is allowed for washing. Avoid use of lotion and powder. *These products can cake under vest.* Replace soiled linens promptly. Perspiration may be dried with hair dryer on a cool setting. Inspect for redness, swelling, bruising, or chafing. Close the open side and repeat on the opposite side.

♦ If a rash appears, consider that patient may be allergic to vest lining. A synthetic liner, knitted body stockinette, or T-shirt may correct this problem.

♦ Provide oral care. A flexible disposable straw can be used both to sip clear water for rinsing teeth and to expel rinse water into a sink or basin.

♦ In the event of skin breakdown, keep skin cleansed, dried, and covered with a transparent dressing. Notify health care provider and orthotist accordingly because skin breakdown requires a brace adjustment.

♦ Place rubber corks over tips of halo device. *This is to diminish annoying sound vibrations if the apparatus is bumped and to prevent lacerations from possible sharp edges.*

♦ Check tong placement at least daily. If slippage has occurred, immobilize patient's head with a sandbag and notify health care provider. Pain may signal erosion of bone and displacement into muscle. Check drainage for presence of cerebrospinal fluid (CSF) (see p. 266). Ensure that traction weights are hanging freely.

♦ Provide analgesia, as needed, for mild headache and discomfort. A soft diet may be indicated. *This is to ease jaw pain associated with chewing.*

♦ For a discussion of pin care, see "Fractures," p. 594, for **Deficient knowledge:** Function of external fixation, pin care, and signs and symptoms of pin site infection.

Urinary retention or Reflex urinary incontinence related to neurologic impairment (spasticity or flaccidity occurring with SCI)
Desired outcomes: Patient has urinary output without incontinence. Patient empties bladder with residual volumes of less than 50 mL by time of discharge. Following instruction, patient demonstrates triggering mechanism and gains some control over voiding.

Nursing Interventions

Bladder dysfunction is complicated and should be assessed by cystometric testing to determine the best type of bladder program. Lesions above the conus medullaris (located at the lower two levels of the thoracic region where the cord begins to taper) generally leave the S2, S3, and S4 spinal cord nerve segments intact. If this spinal reflex arc is intact, the patient will have UMN-involved bladder, resulting in a spastic bladder. This bladder has tone and occasional bladder contractions and periodically will empty on its own, resulting in reflex incontinence. The UMN-involved bladder is "trainable" with techniques that stimulate reflex voiding. Lesions below the conus medullaris (T12) may injure S2, S3, and S4 nerve segments, which will disrupt the reflex arc and cause LMN-involved flaccid bladder. This bladder has no tone and will distend until it overflows, resulting in overflow incontinence.

Bladder dysfunction care guidelines are listed in **BOX 5-2**.

Ineffective cerebral tissue perfusion and risk for decreased cardiac tissue perfusion related to relative hypovolemia secondary to decreased vasomotor tone with SCI
Desired outcomes: By at least 24 hr before hospital discharge (or as soon as vasomotor tone improves), patient has adequate cardiopulmonary and cerebral tissue perfusion as evidenced by SBP 90 mm Hg or higher and orientation to person, place, and time. For a minimum of 48 hr before hospital discharge, patient is free of dysrhythmias.

BOX 5-2   BLADDER DYSFUNCTION CARE GUIDELINES

Guidelines for Patients with Bladder Dysfunction

- Initially during acute spinal shock patient will have an indwelling urinary catheter or scheduled intermittent catheterizations. If intermittent catheterization is used and episodes of incontinence occur or more than 500 mL of urine is obtained, catheterize patient more often. As spinal reflexes return, intermittent catheterization or other bladder emptying technique is used, and indwelling catheters are avoided because of potential for UTI.
- Teach patient and significant other procedure for intermittent catheterization, care of indwelling catheters, and indicators of UTI (e.g., fever, chills, cloudy and/or foul-smelling urine, malaise, anorexia, restlessness, increased frequency or urgency, incontinence).
- Teach patient and significant other that habit/bladder scheduling program consists of gradually increasing time between catheterizations or periodically clamping indwelling catheters. The goal is a gradual increase in bladder tone. When the bladder can hold 300-400 mL of urine, measures to stimulate voiding are attempted. Bladder ultrasound may be used to determine fullness and aid in retraining.
- Make sure patient takes fluids at even intervals throughout the day. Restrict fluids before bedtime to prevent nighttime incontinence. Alcohol and caffeine-containing foods and beverages (e.g., cola, chocolate, coffee, tea) have a diuretic effect and may cause incontinence. In addition, caffeine-containing products may increase bladder spasms and reflex incontinence.
- Patients using bladder-emptying techniques should void at least q3h. A wristwatch with timer alarm or an alarm clock can help patient maintain this schedule. To obtain postvoid residual urine, catheterize patient after an attempt to empty bladder. Residual amounts greater than 100 mL usually indicate need for return to a scheduled intermittent catheterization program.

Guidelines for Patients with UMN-Involved Spastic Reflex Bladder

- Explain to these patients that eventually they may be able to empty the bladder automatically and therefore may not require catheterization.
- Teach techniques that stimulate voiding reflex, such as tapping the suprapubic area with fingers, gently pulling pubic hair, digitally stretching anal sphincter, stroking glans penis, stroking inner thigh, lightly punching abdominal area just proximal to inguinal ligaments, or using a handheld vibration device against the lower abdomen.
- Perform selected technique for 2-3 min or until a good urine stream has started. Wait 1 min before trying another stimulation technique.
- Bladder tapping: Position self in a half-sitting position. Tapping is performed over the suprapubic area, and the patient may shift the site of stimulation within that area to find the most effective site. Tapping is performed rapidly (7-8 ×/sec) with one hand for approximately 50 single taps. Continue tapping until a good stream starts. When stream stops, wait about 1 min and repeat tapping until bladder is empty. One or two tapping attempts without response indicate that no more urine will be expelled.

Continued

BOX 5-2	BLADDER DYSFUNCTION CARE GUIDELINES—cont'd

| Guidelines for Patients with LMN-Involved Flaccid Bladders | ■ Anal stretch technique (contraindicated in individuals with lesions at T8 or above because of the potential for AD): Position self on commode or toilet. Lean forward on thighs and insert one or two lubricated fingers into anus to anal sphincter. Spread anal sphincter gently by spreading fingers apart or pulling in a posterior direction. Maintain stretching position, take a deep breath, and hold breath while bearing down to void. Relax and repeat until bladder is empty.
■ Be aware that stimulating reflex trigger zones accidentally may result in incontinence. Incontinence briefs will help control accidents. Avoid plastic or rubber sheets because these trap heat and moisture, thereby promoting skin breakdown.
■ Increasing intraabdominal pressure can overcome sphincter pressure, which may empty the bladder. This may be contraindicated, however, depending on risk of ureteral reflux.
■ Explain that patient may be able to empty bladder manually well enough to avoid catheterization. Need for catheterization can be determined by checking residual urine volume.
■ Bladder-emptying techniques (e.g., straining, Valsalva's maneuver) to increase intraabdominal pressure are controversial and generally not encouraged because of potential for reflux past the vesicoureteral junction that increases potential for ascending UTIs. If Credé's method is prescribed, teach the following technique: Place ulnar surface of the hand horizontally along or just below umbilicus; while bearing down with abdominal muscles, press hand downward and toward bladder in a kneading motion until urination is initiated; continue 30 sec or until urination ceases. Wait a few minutes and repeat the procedure to ensure complete emptying of the bladder.
■ If patient's bladder cannot be trained to empty completely, intermittent catheterization or external collection devices usually are indicated, and patient may be a candidate for an artificial inflatable sphincter device or urinary diversion. |

AD, Autonomic dysreflexia; *LMN,* lower motor neuron; *UMN,* upper motor neuron; *UTI,* urinary tract infection.

Also see "Urinary Incontinence," p. 207; "Urinary Retention," p. 214; and "Neurogenic Bladder," p. 217.

Nursing Interventions

◆ Monitor for hypotension (drop in SBP more than 20 mm Hg, SBP less than 90 mm Hg), lightheadedness, dizziness, fainting, and confusion.

◆ Monitor HR and rhythm. *This is because sinus tachycardia/bradycardia may result from impaired sympathetic innervation or unopposed vagal stimulation.*

◆ Monitor I&O. Give prescribed IV fluids cautiously. *This is because impaired vascular tone can make patient sensitive to small increases in circulating volume.* Intravascular volume expanders or vasopressors may be required for hypotension.

◆ Change position slowly. Implement measures that prevent episodes of decreased cardiac output caused by postural hypotension.

◆ Perform ROM exercises q2h. *This is to prevent venous pooling.*

- Prevent patient's legs from crossing, especially when in a dependent position.
- Patients with SCI at higher levels, especially above T6, may require abdominal binder in addition to antiembolic hose, leg wraps, and SCDs or pneumatic foot pumps. *This is because these individuals are prone to more severe hypotensive reactions, even with minor changes such as raising HOB.*
- Work with physical therapist to implement a gradual sitting program. *This will help patient progress from a supine to an upright position. The goal is to increase patient's ability to sit upright while avoiding adverse effects, such as hypertension, dizziness, and fainting.* This may include a bed that can rotate gradually from a horizontal position to a vertical position or a chair that has multiple positions progressing from flat to sitting.
- For additional information, see **Ineffective cerebral tissue perfusion** in "Prolonged Bed Rest," p. 27.

Ineffective peripheral perfusion and risk for decreased cardiac tissue perfusion related to interrupted blood flow (venous stasis) with corresponding risk of thrombophlebitis and PE secondary to immobility and decreased vasomotor tone
Desired outcome: For at least 24 hr before hospital discharge and on an ongoing basis, patient has adequate peripheral and cardiopulmonary tissue perfusion as evidenced by absence of heat, erythema, and swelling in calves and thighs; HR 100 bpm or less, RR 20 breaths/min or less with normal depth and pattern (eupnea), and PaO_2 80 mm Hg or more or O_2 saturation greater than 92%.

Nursing Interventions

- Monitor for indicators of thrombophlebitis: erythema, warmth, decreased pulses, and swelling over area of inflammation and venous dilation; coolness, paleness, and edema distal to thrombus. Measure calves and thighs daily while patient is supine or before activity, and monitor for increased circumference. *An increase of 1.5 cm or more in 1 day is significant, as is calf diameter greater than 3 cm larger than opposite calf.* The presence of pain or tenderness depends on level of SCI. Monitor for low-grade fever. *This may also signal thrombophlebitis.* Notify health care provider about significant findings.
- Protect patient's legs from injury during transfers and turning and position them so they do not cross. Avoid IM injections in the legs, and do not massage the legs.
- Provide ROM to legs four ×/day. If not contraindicated, place patient in Trendelenburg's position for 15 min q2h. *This is to promote venous drainage, or elevate legs 10-15 degrees.*
- Monitor for indicators of PE: tachycardia, shortness of breath, hemoptysis, decrease in PaO_2, O_2 saturation 92% or less, and decreased or adventitious breath sounds. Presence of pain depends on level of injury. *Sudden shoulder pain may represent referred pain from PE.* Notify health care provider about significant findings.
- Consult health care provider about use of antiembolism hose, SCDs, pneumatic foot pumps, or prophylactic pharmacotherapy.
- Recognize that patient may need Doppler ultrasound, impedence plethysmography, or venogram if DVT is suspected. A vena cava filter may be needed if DVT or PE is confirmed.
- For other nursing interventions, see **Ineffective peripheral tissue perfusion** in "Prolonged Bed Rest," p. 27.

Sexual dysfunction related to altered body function secondary to SCI
Desired outcome: Within the 24-hr period before hospital discharge, patient discusses concerns about sexuality and verbalizes knowledge of alternative methods of sexual expression.

Nursing Interventions

◆ Evaluate your own feelings about sexuality. Refer patient to someone who can address patient's sexual concerns if you are uncomfortable discussing these issues.

◆ Provide a supportive, nonjudgmental environment that gives patient permission to have and express sexual concerns. Sexuality can be discussed as it relates to an erection that occurs during a bath or to objective findings noted during physical assessment. Elicit patient's knowledge, concerns, and questions. Expect acting-out behavior related to patient's sexuality. *This is a normal response to anxiety about sexual response and prognosis.* Such behaviors may include asking questions, sexual jokes or innuendoes, self-deprecating remarks, or flirting with staff.

◆ Provide information about normal sexual response and changes caused by SCI. Sexual functioning may be different but still possible with SCI. The general rule for men is the higher the lesion, the greater the chance of retaining the ability to have an erection (but with less chance of ejaculation). Women may have problems with lubrication, and orgasm may be difficult to achieve because of decreases sensation. Women also may have a transient loss of ovulation; however, ovulation usually returns, and women can become pregnant and deliver vaginally. Uterine contractions of labor in women with SCI lesion at T8 or above, however, may cause AD. Provide information about birth control and oral contraception for women who desire it. Oral contraceptives may be contraindicated because of risk of thrombophlebitis. Sperm quality decreases in men after SCI, but they may still be capable of fathering a child naturally. Electroejaculation via electrical stimulation in the area of the prostate to obtain sperm, in utero insemination, in vitro fertilization, and intracytoplasmic sperm injection have improved fertility.

◆ Sexual activity may seem impossible to the patient with SCI. Specific suggestions that may provide gratification include oral-genital sex, digital stimulation, vibrator stimulation, cuddling, mutual masturbation, anal eroticism, and massage. Erection assistive techniques and devices may help men with SCI to attain erections. Specific suggestions for managing common problems include decreasing fluid intake 2-3 hr before sexual encounter, emptying bladder and bowels (if necessary) before a sexual encounter, (for men) folding back indwelling catheter along the penis and holding it in place with a condom, (for women) taping catheter to the abdomen and leaving it in place, taking a warm bath before sexual activity to reduce spasticity, planning sexual activity for a time of day in which both partners are rested, experimenting with a variety of positions, and applying topical anesthetics to areas that are hypersensitive to touch. Explain that water-soluble lubricants are useful, if needed, but that petroleum-based lubricants should be avoided. This is because they can cause a UTI. Adductor spasms in women may pose a barrier but can be overcome if a rear entry is acceptable. Prolonged foreplay with stroking and light massage also may relax muscles. If AD occurs during sexual activity, suggest that patient consult health care provider about preventive measures.

◆ Suggest that patient's partner be included in discussion about sexual concerns. *Explaining the physical condition caused by SCI and preparing the partner for scars, lack of muscle tone, atrophy, and presence of a catheter are important and will provide the partner with an opportunity to discuss sexual concerns.*

◆ Nurses may not be able to answer all concerns and questions. When this occurs, acknowledge patient's concerns and refer to someone with more expertise.

◆ For additional nursing interventions, see **Ineffective sexuality pattern** in "Prolonged Bed Rest," p. 30.

Deficient knowledge related to cervical collar use and precautions
Desired outcome: Following explanation, patient and significant other/care-taker verbalize understanding about use of prescribed cervical collar, including purpose, precautions, skin care, and reportable conditions.

Nursing Interventions

♦ Before teaching begins, assess patient's facility with language; engage an interpreter or provide language-appropriate written materials as appropriate.

♦ Caution that the collar should not be removed before cervical spine injury has been ruled out by x-ray examination.

♦ Explain that the collar should be worn at all times until health care provider says otherwise. The collar should prevent patient from nodding head "yes" or "no". Chin should fit on chin shelf and not be able to move off the shelf. Patient should continue to be cautious. *This is because the collar does not prevent all movement.* Patient cannot drive while wearing the collar.

♦ Suction equipment should be available when possible. *This is because the collar may make swallowing harder and vomiting difficult.* Explain that facial droop or drooling may indicate pressure on the facial cranial nerve (CN) (i.e., CN VII) and that increased neurologic symptoms (weakness, numbness) should be reported.

♦ Teach importance of looking under jaw, shoulders, neck, back of head, and ears for pressure points and reporting redness and open areas to health care provider. *This may indicate the need for collar adjustments or padding.*

♦ Advise that the neck should be inspected and cleansed every 1-2 days, and patient always should have assistance for washing or shaving. Patient should lie flat on back and open front portion of collar; patient should keep head and neck still and straight while collar is open. Only mild soap should be used, and neck should be well rinsed and dried completely. *This is to prevent skin problems.* Caution patient to avoid moving the head up and down during shaving. After front portion of the collar is closed, patient then turns to side using small pillow for support. Side attachment is then opened, and back of neck is washed, rinsed, and dried as described. After side attachment is closed, patient turns to other side, and the process is repeated.

♦ Advise that a silk scarf can be worn beneath the collar and pulled smooth to avoid wrinkles. *This may decrease discomfort.* Cornstarch or powder can be used, but excessive amounts that could cake should be avoided. *This is to prevent maceration.* A small, thin pillow may be used. *This is to support the head and neck when the patient is turned.*

♦ Caution that patient should avoid watching wall-mounted television units. *This is because of risk of neck extension, rotation, and flexion.*

 Patient-Family Teaching and Discharge Planning

The degree and scope of discharge teaching and planning depend on severity of patient's condition. Include verbal and written information about the following:

♦ Spinal cord functioning and the effects trauma has on how the body works.

♦ Referrals to community resources, such as public health nurse, visiting nurses association, community support groups, social workers, psychologic therapy, vocational rehabilitation agency, home health agencies, and extended and skilled care facilities.

♦ Safety measures relative to decreased sensation, motor deficits, orthostatic hypotension and symptoms, preventive measures, and interventions for AD.

♦ Use and care of a brace or immobilizer, medical equipment, and mobility aids as appropriate.

♦ What patient can expect if transferred to rehabilitation center.

◆ Techniques and devices for performing activities of daily living (ADL). The patient may need home accessibility evaluation and driving evaluation and training.

◆ Indicators of ureteral calculi and dietary measures to prevent their formation.

◆ Indicators of DVT and measures to prevent it.

◆ Additional general information, which can be obtained by accessing the following websites:

American Spinal Injury Association (ASIA): www.asia-spinalinjury.org

Christopher Reeve Foundation: www.christopherreeve.org

Cure Paralysis: www.cureparalysis.org

disABILITY Information and Resources: www.makoa.org

National Spinal Cord Injury Association (NSCIA): www.spinalcord.org

Paralinks: Wheelchair Nation, the Electronic Directory for People with Spinal Cord Injury: www.wheelchairnation.com

Paralyzed Veterans of America (PVA): www.pva.org

◆ For additional information, see teaching and discharge planning nursing interventions (the fourth through seventh entries only) as appropriate in "Multiple Sclerosis," p. 237.

❖ TRAUMATIC BRAIN INJURY

OVERVIEW/PATHOPHYSIOLOGY

Traumatic brain injury (TBI) can cause various degrees of damage to the skull and brain tissue. Primary injuries occur at the time of impact and include skull fracture, concussion, contusion, scalp laceration, brain tissue laceration, and tear or rupture of cerebral vessels. Secondary problems that arise soon after and are the result of the primary injury include hemorrhage and hematoma formation from tear or rupture of vessels, ischemia from interrupted blood flow, cerebral swelling and edema, infection (e.g., meningitis or abscess), and increased intracranial pressure (IICP) or brain herniation, any of which can interrupt neuronal function. These secondary injuries or events increase the extent of initial injury and result in poorer recovery and higher risk of death. Cervical neck injuries are commonly associated with TBIs. Because of the potential for spinal cord injury (SCI), all patients with TBI should be assumed to have cervical neck injury until it is conclusively ruled out by cervical spine x-ray examination.

Most TBIs result from direct impact to the head. Depending on force and angle of impact, the brain may suffer injury directly under the point of impact (coup) or in the region opposite the point of impact (contrecoup) because of brain rebound action within the skull, or tissue tearing or shearing may occur elsewhere because of the rotational action of the brain within the cranial vault. TBI may be classified by location, severity, extent, or mechanism (contact, acceleration, deceleration, rotational). Common causes include motor vehicle accidents; falls; and sports-related injuries, such as those occurring in football or boxing. Acts of violence, such as gunshot or stab wounds, often result in missile or impalement TBIs.

ASSESSMENT

Signs and symptoms/physical findings: The Glasgow Coma Scale (GCS) (**BOX 5-3**) standardizes observations for objective assessment of a patient's level of consciousness (LOC). In the GCS, 13-15 is mild, 9-12 is moderate, and 3-8 is severe. This or some other objective scale should be used to prevent confusion with terminology and to quickly detect changes or trends in patient's LOC. LOC is the most sensitive indicator of overall brain function.

BOX 5-3 — GLASGOW COMA SCALE

PARAMETER	PATIENT RESPONSE	SCORE
Best eye opening response (record "C" if eyes closed because of swelling)	Spontaneously	4
	To speech	3
	To pain	2
	No response	1
Best motor response (record best upper limb response to painful stimuli)	Obeys verbal command	6
	Localizes pain	5
	Flexion—withdrawal, purposeless movement	4
	Flexion—abnormal	3
	Extension—abnormal	2
	No response (flaccid)	1
Best verbal response (record "E" if endotracheal tube is in place or "T" if tracheostomy tube is in place)	Conversation—oriented × 3	5
	Conversation—confused	4
	Speech—inappropriate	3
	Sounds—incomprehensible	2
	No response	1

**TOTAL SCORE INTERPRETATION
(SUM OF SCORES FOR EACH OF THE THREE GROUPS)**

15	Normal
13-15	Minor head injury
9-12	Moderate head injury
3-8	Severe head injury
≤7	Coma
3	Deep coma or brain death

Modified from Teasdale G, Jennett B: Assessment of coma and impaired consciousness. A practical scale. *The Lancet* 13;2(7872):81-84, 1974. Available at Internet Stroke Center website: www.stroke-center.org. Accessed May 2009.

BOX 5-4 — GRADING OF CONCUSSIONS RESULTING FROM TRAUMATIC BRAIN INJURY

Grade I	No loss of consciousness
	Transient confusion
	Symptoms resolve in less than 15 min
Grade II	No loss of consciousness
	Transient confusion
	Symptoms last more than 15 min
	If symptoms last more than 1 wk, imaging may be needed
Grade III	Any loss of consciousness

Concussion: Mild diffuse TBI in which there is temporary, reversible neurologic impairment may involve loss of consciousness and possible amnesia of the event. No damage to brain structure is visible on CT or MRI examination. TBI concussions are graded as noted in **BOX 5-4**.

After concussion, patients may have headache, dizziness, nausea, lethargy, difficulty focusing, and irritability, especially to bright lights or loud noises. Although full recovery usually occurs in a few days, a postconcussion syndrome may continue for several weeks or months, with headache; dizziness; irritability; emotional lability; lethargy; sleep disturbance; and decreased attention, judgment, concentration, and memory abilities.

Diffuse axonal injury (DAI): Diffuse brain injury caused by stretching and tearing of the neuronal projections because of a rotational, shearing type of injury. Diffuse microscopic damage occurs. No distinct focal lesion, such as infarction, ischemia, contusion, or intracerebral bleeding, is noted, but patients have an immediate and prolonged unconsciousness at least 6 hr in duration. CT scan may show small hemorrhagic areas in the corpus callosum, cerebral edema, and small midline ventricles. Brainstem injury may be associated with DAI and may result in autonomic dysfunction.

Mild DAI is coma lasting 6-24 hr, with patient beginning to follow commands by 24 hr. Full recovery is expected. Moderate DAI is coma lasting longer than 24 hr but without prominent brainstem signs. Severe DAI is prolonged coma with prominent brainstem signs, such as decortication or decerebration, and usually predicts severe disability, possible vegetative state, or death.

Contusion: Bruising of brain tissue, which produces a longer-lasting neurologic deficit than concussion. Size and severity of bruising vary widely, and the bruise or a small, diffuse venous hemorrhage usually is visible on computed tomography (CT) scan. Traumatic amnesia often occurs, causing loss of memory not only of the trauma, but also of events occurring before the incident. Loss of consciousness is common, and it is generally more prolonged than that with concussion. Changes in behavior, such as agitation or confusion, can last for several hours to days. Headache, nausea, lethargy, motor paralysis, paresis, and possibly seizures can occur as well. Depending on extent of damage, there is potential for either full recovery or permanent neurologic deficit, such as seizures, paralysis, paresis, or even coma and death.

Brain laceration: Actual tearing of the brain's cortical surface, resulting in direct mechanical disruption of neural function and causing focal deficits. Blood vessel tearing causes hemorrhage, resulting in contusion, edema, or hematoma formation. Seizures often occur as well. Brain lacerations usually result from depressed skull fractures, penetrating injuries, missile or impalement injuries, or rotational shearing injury within the skull. Shock waves from a bullet's high energy produce additional damage. A knife or other impalement object should be supported and left in the wound to control bleeding until it can be removed during surgery. Contusions and lacerations often are found together. The consequences of a laceration usually are more serious than those with a contusion because of the increased severity of trauma.

Skull fracture: Can be closed (simple, with skin intact) or open (compound), depending on whether the scalp is torn, thereby exposing the skull to the outside environment. Skull fractures are further classified as linear (hairline), comminuted (fragmented, splintered), or depressed (pushed inward toward the brain tissue). A blow forceful enough to break the skull is capable of causing significant brain tissue damage, and therefore close observation is essential. With a penetrating wound or basilar fracture (see next), there is potential for cerebrospinal fluid (CSF) leakage, meningitis, encephalitis, brain abscess, cellulitis, or osteomyelitis.

Basilar fractures: Fractures of the base of the skull do not show up easily on skull/cervical x-ray examination. Indicators include blood from the nose, throat, ears; serous or serosanguineous drainage from the nose (rhinorrhea), throat, ears (otorrhea), eyes; Battle's sign (bruising noted behind the ear); "raccoon's eyes" (bruising around eyes in the absence of eye injury); and bleeding behind the tympanum (eardrum) noted on otoscopic examination. Glucose in serous drainage signals the presence of CSF. CSF leakage indicates a tear in the dura, which makes the patient particularly susceptible to meningitis. Basilar fractures may damage the internal carotid artery and cranial nerves. Hearing loss also may occur.

Temporal fractures: May result in deafness or facial paralysis.

Occipital fractures: May cause visual field and gait disturbances.

Sphenoidal fractures: May disrupt the optic nerve, possibly causing blindness.

Rupture of cerebral blood vessels

Epidural (extradural) hematoma or hemorrhage: Usually, bleeding between the dura mater (outer meninges) and skull causes hematoma formation. This creates pressure on the underlying brain and produces a local mass effect, causing IICP and shifting of tissue, which leads to brainstem compression and herniation. Indicators are primarily those of IICP: altered LOC, headache, vomiting, unilateral pupil dilation (on same side as the lesion), and possibly hemiparesis. Although some individuals never regain consciousness, most patients lose consciousness for a short period immediately after injury, regain consciousness, and have a lucid period lasting a few hours or 1-2 days. However, because arterial bleeding causes a rapid rise in intracranial pressure (ICP), a rapid decrease in LOC often ensues. The bleeding site often is the middle meningeal artery or vein because of temporal bone fracture. These patients are at risk for brainstem herniation. A unilateral dilated fixed pupil is a sign of impending herniation and is a neurosurgical emergency. Patients should not be left alone because respiratory arrest may occur at any time.

Subdural hematoma or hemorrhage: Accumulation of venous blood between the dura mater (outer meninges) and arachnoid membrane (middle meninges) that is not reabsorbed. Hematoma formation creates pressure on the underlying brain and produces a local mass effect, causing IICP and shifting of tissue that leads to brainstem compression and herniation. This type of hematoma is classified as acute, subacute, or chronic depending on how quickly indicators arise. In acute subdural hematomas, indicators appear within 24-48 hr, resulting from focal neurologic deficit (hemiparesis, pupillary dilation) and IICP (decreased LOC, falling GCS score, nausea, vomiting, headache). When indicators occur 2-14 days later, the hematoma is considered subacute. When indicators occur more than 2 wk later, it is considered chronic. Early indicators can include headache, progressive personality changes, decreased intellectual functioning, slowness, confusion, and drowsiness. Later indicators may include unilateral weakness or paralysis, loss of consciousness, and occasionally seizures. Patients with cerebral atrophy (e.g., older persons, long-term alcohol users) are more prone to subdural hematoma formation.

Intracerebral hemorrhage: Arterial or venous bleeding into the brain's white matter. Signs of IICP may develop early if the bleeding causes a rapidly expanding space-occupying lesion. If the bleeding is slower, signs of IICP can take 36-72 hr to develop. Indicators depend on hematoma location and size and can include altered LOC, headache, aphasia, hemiparesis, hemiplegia, hemisensory deficits, pupillary changes, and loss of consciousness.

Subarachnoid hemorrhage (SAH): Bleeding into the subarachnoid space below the arachnoid membrane (middle meninges) and above the pia mater (inner meninges next to brain). The patient often has a severe headache. Other general indicators include vomiting, restlessness, seizures, and loss of consciousness. Signs of meningeal irritation include nuchal rigidity and Kernig's and Brudzinski's signs. This patient may be a candidate for a shunt because of hemorrhagic interference with CSF circulation and reabsorption and is at particular risk of cerebral vasospasm.

Indicators of IICP: ICP is the pressure exerted by brain tissue, CSF, and cerebral blood volume within the rigid, unyielding skull. An increase in any one of these components without a corresponding decrease in another will increase ICP. Normal ICP is 0-10 mm Hg; IICP is greater than 15 mm Hg. Cerebral perfusion pressure (CPP) is the difference between mean arterial pressure (MAP) and ICP. As ICP rises, CPP may decrease. Normal CPP is 70-100 mm Hg. If CPP falls below 40-60 mm Hg, ischemia occurs. When CPP falls to 0, cerebral blood flow (CBF) ceases. Cerebral edema and IICP usually peak 2-3 days after injury and then decrease over 1-2 wk.

Early indicators: The single most important early indicator of IICP is a change in LOC. Alteration in LOC may range from irritability, restlessness, and confusion to lethargy; possible onset or worsening of headache; beginning pupillary dysfunction, such as sluggishness of response onset of sensorimotor changes (or increase in them) such as; visual disturbances, such as diplopia or blurred vision; onset of or increase in sensorimotor changes or deficits, such as weakness; and onset or worsening of nausea.

Late indicators: Late indicators of IICP usually signal impending or occurring brainstem herniation. Signs generally are related to brainstem compression and disruption of cranial nerves and vital centers. Hypotension and tachycardia in the absence of explainable causes, such as hypovolemia, usually are seen as a terminal event in TBI. Continued deterioration of LOC leads to stupor and coma; projectile vomiting; hemiplegia; posturing; alterations in VS (typically increased SBP, widening pulse pressure, decreased pulse rate); respiratory irregularities, such as Cheyne-Stokes breathing; pupillary changes, such as inequality, dilation, and nonreactivity to light; papilledema; and impaired brainstem reflexes (corneal, gag, swallowing).

Brain herniation: Occurs when IICP causes displacement of brain tissue from one intracranial compartment to another and results in compression, destruction, and laceration of brain tissue. See "Late indicators of IICP" for signs of impending or initial herniation. In the presence of actual brain herniation, patient is in a deep coma, pupils become fixed and dilated bilaterally, posturing may progress to bilateral flaccidity, brainstem reflexes generally are lost, and respirations and VS deteriorate and may cease.

Brain death: Universal criteria for determining brain death are not universally agreed upon. Check state and institutional guidelines. General criteria include absent brainstem reflexes (e.g., apnea, pupils nonreactive to light, no corneal reflex, no oculovestibular reflex to ice water calorics), absent cortical activity (e.g., several flat electroencephalogram [EEG] tracings spaced over time), and coma irreversibility continued over a prescribed period (e.g., 24 hr). Brainstem auditory evoked responses and CBF studies (e.g., transcranial Doppler [TCD], angiography, brain scan with a cerebral perfusion agent) also may be used to help confirm brain death.

DIAGNOSTIC TESTS

Cervical spine and skull x-ray examinations: Performed to locate neck and skull fractures. Because of the close association between TBIs and spinal or vertebral injuries, cervical immobilization is essential until cervical x-ray examination rules out fracture and potential SCI.

CT scan: Used with acute injury to identify type, location, and extent of injury, such as accumulation of blood or a shift of midline structure caused by IICP.

MRI: Identifies type, location, and extent of injury. Often not performed in acute, unstable patients, but this test is the study of choice for subacute or chronic TBI. It is superior to CT scan for detecting isodense chronic subdural hematomas or evaluating contusions and shearing injuries, especially in the brainstem area. MRI techniques such as FLAIR are particularly sensitive to detecting DAI and small hemorrhages.

EEG: Reveals abnormal electrical activity indicating neuronal damage caused by ischemia or hemorrhage. EEG may be used to establish brain death in conjunction with other tests and may be done serially to assess development of pathologic waves.

CBF studies (TCD, xenon inhalation–enhanced CT): Determine focal areas of low blood flow or spasm, possibly indicating ischemic areas, by noninvasively measuring CBF velocities.

Positron emission tomography (PET): Evaluates tissue metabolism of glucose and O_2.

Single photon emission computed tomography (SPECT): Determines low CBF and areas at risk for ischemic tissue perfusion.

Evoked potential (EP) studies: Evaluate integrity of the anatomic pathways and connections of the brain. Stimulation of a sense organ, such as an ear, triggers a discrete electrical response (i.e., EP) along a neurologic pathway to the brain. Measurement of the brain's response to auditory, visual, and/or somatosensory stimulation also aids in predicting neurologic outcome.

Cerebral angiography: Reveals presence of a hematoma and status of blood vessels secondary to rupture or compression. Angiography usually is performed only if CT scan or MRI is unavailable or to evaluate possible carotid or vertebral artery dissection.

Infrared spectroscopy: Continuously and noninvasively assesses cerebral O_2 saturation.

Cisternogram: Identifies dural tear site with basilar skull fracture. It helps to detect problems with CSF circulation.

CSF analysis: Evaluates for presence of infection, if indicators are present.

COLLABORATIVE MANAGEMENT

Respiratory support: Airway maintenance, intubation, and ventilation as necessary. Monitor oximetry and arterial blood gas (ABG) values and provide O_2 to maintain saturation at 92% or greater. If indicated, O_2 is administered to prevent hypoxia. Preoxygenate before suctioning and limit suctioning to 10 sec. CO_2 retention and the resulting respiratory acidosis can cause vasodilation of the cerebral arteries that can lead to cerebral edema and is to be avoided. Lowering cerebral CO_2 results in alkalosis, which causes cerebral vasoconstriction resulting in decreased CBF and ICP. The vasoconstriction also may cause decreased cerebral O_2 delivery, which could increase injury. Blowing off CO_2 through hyperventilation resulting in $Paco_2$ less than 35 mm Hg generally is avoided and used only in cases of acute deterioration as a "quick fix" for IICP until other interventions such as mannitol can be instituted or in cases in which IICP is refractory and responds to nothing else. Ideally, CBF measurements, continuous jugular venous O_2 saturation (Sjo_2), and brain tissue oxygenation ($Pbto_2$) are considered to monitor for effectiveness (i.e., decreased IICP without decreased cerebral O_2 delivery) if hyperventilation is used as a treatment. Nasal intubation or cricothyroidotomy may be performed to prevent neck hyperextension in patients in whom cervical neck injury has not yet been ruled out.

Monitoring of VS/neurologic status: Baseline assessment is established, and patient is monitored frequently for changes.

Positioning: Bed rest with head of bed (HOB) at whichever level optimizes CPP or as prescribed. Without monitoring equipment, having HOB at 30 degrees is considered safe and effective in promoting venous drainage and helping reduce cerebral edema as long as patient is not hypovolemic, which could threaten CPP. If a subdural drain is placed, HOB may be flat while the drain is in place and for 24 hr after removal to prevent air from being pulled into the subdural space.

Fluids and electrolytes: Nothing by mouth (NPO) status for 8-24 hr (or longer if patient is unresponsive). IV fluids are given to maintain normovolemia and balanced electrolyte status. Fluid restrictions are avoided because resulting increased blood viscosity and decreased volume may lead to hypotension, decreased CPP, and increased ischemia. I&O are monitored carefully, and patient usually has an indwelling catheter. Supplementation of electrolytes is done in response to laboratory results. Hypotonic IV solutions, such as 5% dextrose in water (D_5W), are contraindicated because they increase cerebral edema.

Glucose monitoring: Because hyperglycemia is associated with poorer outcomes, glucose is closely monitored and kept under strict control. Intensive insulin therapy may be used during the acute phase when patient is in ICU, with insulin drips and frequent monitoring to keep glucose at less than 110 mg/dL. After stabilization, sliding scale or rainbow coverage to keep glucose at less than 150 mg/dL is usually instituted.

Gastrointestinal (GI) decompression: Initially patient may have a gastric tube for gastric decompression to prevent vomiting and aspiration. With basilar skull fractures, the tube may be inserted through the mouth to avoid passing it via the nose through the fracture area and into the brain.

Nutritional support: Total parenteral nutrition (TPN), intralipids, tube feedings (preferred for gut mucosal integrity), or progressive diet depending on patient's LOC, ability to swallow, and GI tract functioning. If aspiration is considered a risk, a swallowing evaluation should be done before oral intake begins, and a suction machine should be on hand.

Treatment of secondary complications: Cerebral edema, IICP, disseminated intravascular coagulation (DIC), acute respiratory distress syndrome (ARDS), SIADH, cerebral salt-wasting syndrome, diabetes insipidus (DI), infection, seizures, and heterotopic ossification (HO) (development of bone in abnormal places that often occurs after SCI).

Pharmacotherapy: Opioids and other medications that alter mentation are generally avoided, with the possible exception of codeine for pain control.

Antiepileptic drugs (AEDs) (e.g., carbamazepine, phenytoin, fosphenytoin): Prophylaxis for seizures.

Osmotic diuretics (e.g., mannitol) and loop diuretics (e.g., furosemide): Decrease cerebral edema.

Antibiotics and tetanus prophylaxis: Used in the presence of penetrating wounds and basilar fractures.

Antipyretics (e.g., acetaminophen): Reduce fever, so that patient's metabolic needs are not increased.

Analgesics (e.g., acetaminophen, codeine): Decrease pain.

Mild sedatives (e.g., diphenhydramine): Decrease restlessness.

Blood pressure (BP) medications (e.g., dopamine, labetalol): Control hypertension and hypotension so that optimal CBF is maintained and cerebral edema is reduced. Hypotension is especially not well tolerated by these patients. Need for vasopressors such as dopamine and nitroprusside will necessitate transfer to ICU.

Insulin: Controls hyperglycemia. Intensive insulin therapy may be initiated during the acute phase. After stabilization, sliding scale or "rainbow" insulin coverage may be instituted to keep glucose at less than 150 mg/dL.

Phenothiazines (chlorpromazine): Control shivering, which can increase ICP.

Skeletal muscle relaxants (e.g., propofol, atracurium, pancuronium): Decrease the skeletal muscle tension that is seen with abnormal flexion and extension posturing, which can increase ICP. This therapy requires transfer of patient to ICU for intubation and ventilation.

Antianxiety agents (haloperidol, lorazepam, midazolam): Decrease or control agitation. An attempt to identify and relieve cause (e.g., overstimulation, pain) should be made before medicating.

Low-dose heparin, low-molecular-weight heparin (e.g., enoxaparin): Prevents deep vein thrombosis (DVT).

Proton pump inhibitors (e.g., pantoprazole), histamine H_2-receptor blockers (e.g., famotidine), and sucralfate: Reduce gastric acidity and prevent gastric ulcer formation.

Exogenous antidiuretic hormone (ADH) (e.g., vasopressin, desmopressin): Treats DI.

ADH inhibitor (e.g., demeclocycline) and diruetics (e.g., furosemide, bumetanide): Treat syndrome of inappropriate ADH (SIADH). Demeclocycline blocks the action of ADH in the kidney.

Mineralocorticoid that acts at distal renal tubules (e.g., fludrocortisone): Treats cerebral salt-wasting syndrome by inhibiting Na^+ excretion and inducing Na^+ retention.

Bisphosphonate (e.g., etidronate) and nonsteroidal antiinflammatory drugs (NSAID) (e.g., indomethacin): Prevent HO.

Eye drops or ointment: Maintain corneal lubrication.

Stool softeners and laxatives (e.g., docusate sodium, Milk of Magnesia): Prevent constipation and straining at stool, which would increase ICP.

Hypothermia: Hypothalamic dysfunction from swelling or injury may cause hyperthermia. Patient should be kept normothermic (36°-37° C [96.8°-98.6° F]) via antipyretics and cooling measures.

Antithrombus therapy (antiembolism hose, sequential compression devices [SCDs], pneumatic foot pumps): Prevents thrombophlebitis and pulmonary embolism (PE).

Bowel and bladder program: A bowel program is initiated to prevent straining at stool. Patient initially has an indwelling urinary catheter. A bladder training program may be necessary, depending on presence and type of neurologic deficit.

Physical medicine: Physical therapy (PT), occupational therapy (OT), and assistive devices or braces may be prescribed to promote mobility and independence with activities of daily living (ADL), depending on presence and type of neurologic deficit.

Early passive ROM exercises: Prevent contractures and HO.

Speech therapy: Needed to evaluate and aid communication of aphasic or dysarthric patients.

Seizure precautions: Prevent injury in the event of seizure activity, especially for patients with penetrating TBIs.

Cognitive rehabilitation: Promotes highest level of cognitive functioning. Coma stimulation techniques (usually for short periods 2-4×/day) are started on appropriate patients to increase quantity, quality, and duration of responses. Most cognitive recovery occurs in the first 6 mo. Referrals are provided, as appropriate, to cognitive retraining specialist.

Management of SIADH vs. cerebral salt-wasting syndrome: It is critical to distinguish correctly between these two types of hyponatremia (Na$^+$ less than 137 mEq/L) and fluid imbalance because their treatment is so different. SIADH, characterized by inappropriate urinary concentration causing water retention, results in dilutional hyponatremia with increased plasma volume, weight gain, and decreased serum osmolality and is treated with fluid restriction, mild diuresis with furosemide or bumetanide and sometimes demeclocycline (see "Syndrome of Inappropriate Antidiuretic Hormone," p. 409, for more information). Cerebral salt-wasting syndrome, in which the kidneys are unable to conserve Na$^+$, is characterized by true hyponatremia with decreased plasma volume, weight loss, high blood urea nitrogen (BUN) level, decreased serum osmolality, and hypernatriuria and is treated with fluid replacement (IV normal saline), volume expanders, salt tablets, and occasionally fludrocortisone to inhibit Na$^+$ excretion and induce Na$^+$ retention to counteract hyponatremia and volume depletion. If serum Na$^+$ is very low, a hypertonic saline may be used. Ongoing monitoring of serum Na$^+$ and I&O for both are necessary. Usually both syndromes resolve in a week or two.

Management of DI: Characterized by hourly urine output exceeding 200 mL/hr, low urine specific gravity, high serum osmolarity (300 mOsm/kg or more), and hypovolemia. (See p. 404 for more information.)

HO: Abnormal formation of true bone within the extraskeletal soft tissues causing pain, swelling, redness, warmth, and decreased ROM and function and occurring most commonly around the hips. Prevention involves use of etidronate, NSAIDs, ROM exercises, and external beam radiation. Once HO has formed, resection may be necessary. A bone scan will show HO about 7-10 days earlier than an x-ray study.

Surgical procedures

Suturing: Repairs superficial lacerations or dural tears.

Craniotomy, craniectomy: Evacuates hematomas, controls hemorrhage, removes bone fragment or foreign objects, débrides necrotic tissue, elevates depressed fractures, or decompresses the brain.

Trephination (burr holes): Needed to evacuate hematomas or insert intracranial monitoring devices.

Cranioplasty: Repairs traumatic or surgical defects in the skull.

Ventricular puncture, ventriculostomy: Removes excess CSF.

Ventricular shunt: Provides drainage of CSF and reduces ICP. A plastic tube drains the ventricles into the venous or peritoneal spaces through a one-way valve that permits CSF to flow only above a certain pressure gradient.

Endoscopic third ventriculostomy: Provides drainage of CSF in cases of obstructive hydrocephalus. A small hole or holes are made in the third ventricle to enable CSF to flow into the basal cistern for absorption.

Placement of ICP monitoring device: Provides accurate and continual monitoring of patient's ICP. This necessitates transfer of patient to ICU for monitoring.

Repair of CSF leak: Most CSF leaks from dural tears heal themselves in 5-10 days. If they do not, serial LPs or a lumbar subarachnoid drain may be needed to drain CSF, reduce CSF pressure, and promote healing. Radionuclide-labeled materials may be injected into the subarachnoid space and pledgets placed in the nose and ears to find the site of the CSF leak. A blood patch may be used. Surgical repair (e.g., duraplasty) may be required if other methods prove ineffective. Basilar fractures are a common site of CSF leaks and make surgical repair difficult because of location inaccessibility.

With a lumbar drain, patient is on bed rest, with HOB typically elevated up to 15-20 degrees, and is instructed to call for assistance and not to cough, sneeze, or strain. Maintain HOB and collection container securely at prescribed levels. Maintain a sterile occlusive dressing. Possible complications include meningitis or pneumocranium resulting from too rapid drainage of CSF, which causes air to siphon in through the dural tear and creates an intracranial mass effect. If neurologic signs deteriorate, clamp the lumbar drain tubing, place patient flat or in a slight Trendelenburg position, and provide supplemental O_2, which will promote absorption of intracranial air and relieve IICP.

NURSING DIAGNOSES AND INTERVENTIONS

Deficient knowledge related to caretaker's responsibilities for observing patient who is sent home with a concussion

Desired outcomes: Following instruction, caretaker verbalizes knowledge about the observation regimen. Caretaker returns patient to the hospital if neurologic deficits are noted.

Nursing Interventions

- Assess caretaker's facility with language; provide an interpreter or language-appropriate written materials as indicated; and give the following instructions:
- Do not give patient anything stronger than acetaminophen to relieve headache. *Aspirin is usually contraindicated because it can prolong bleeding if it occurs.*
- Assess patient at least q1-2h for first 24 hr as follows: awaken patient; ask patient's name, location, and caretaker's name; monitor for twitching or seizure activity. Return patient to the hospital immediately patient becomes increasingly difficult to awaken; cannot answer questions appropriately; cannot answer at all; becomes confused, restless, or agitated; develops slurred speech; develops twitching or seizures; develops or reports worsening headache or nausea/vomiting; has visual disturbances (e.g., blurred or double vision); develops weakness, numbness, or clumsiness or has difficulty walking; has clear or bloody drainage from nose or ear; or develops a stiff neck. *These may indicate a more severe brain injury.*
- Ensure that patient rests and eats lightly for first day or so after concussion or until feeling well. Over next 2-3 days, patient should avoid alcohol, driving, contact sports, swimming, using power tools, and taking

medication for headache or nausea without calling health care provider. Patient should return to a full schedule slowly.

♦ Inform patient and significant other that some individuals may have post-concussion syndrome, in which they continue to have headaches, dizziness, or lethargy for several weeks or months after a concussion. Patient also may experience sleep disturbance, difficulty concentrating, poor memory, irritability, emotional lability, and difficulty with judgment or abstract thinking. Patient may be very distractible, with hypersensitivity to noise and light. Explain importance of reporting these problems to health care provider, especially if they worsen.

Risk for infection related to inadequate primary defenses secondary to basilar skull fractures, penetrating or open TBIs, or surgical wounds
Desired outcomes: Patient is free of symptoms of infection as evidenced by normothermia; stable or improving LOC; and absence of headache, photophobia, or neck stiffness. Patient verbalizes knowledge about signs and symptoms of infection and importance of reporting them promptly.

Nursing Interventions

♦ Monitor injury site or surgical wounds for persistent erythema, local warmth, pain, hardness, and purulent drainage. Notify health care provider of significant findings. *These may indicate infection is present.*

♦ Be alert to indicators of meningitis or encephalitis such as fever, chills, malaise, back stiffness and pain, nuchal rigidity, photophobia, seizures, ataxia, and sensorimotor deficits. *These can occur after a penetrating, open TBI or cerebral surgical wound.*

♦ When examining scalp lacerations and assessing for foreign bodies or palpable fractures, wear sterile gloves and follow sterile technique. Cleanse area gently, and cover scalp wounds with sterile dressings. *This is to prevent infection.*

♦ Document drainage and its amount, color, and odor. If patient has clear or bloody drainage from nose, throat, or ears, notify health care provider of findings. *This may indicate patient has a dural tear with CSF leakage until proven otherwise.* Note complaints of a salty taste or frequent swallowing. *This may signal CSF dripping down back of the throat.* Bending forward may produce nasal drainage that can be tested for CSF. Inspect dressing and pillowcases for a halo ring (blood encircled by a yellowish stain). *It may indicate CSF drainage.* Clear drainage may be tested with a glucose reagent strip. Drainage may be sent to laboratory to test for chloride (Cl^-). *The presence of glucose and Cl^- (CSF Cl^- is greater than serum Cl^-) in nonsanguineous drainage indicates that the drainage is CSF rather than mucus or saliva.*

♦ If CSF leakage occurs, do not clean ears or nose unless prescribed by health care provider. Place a sterile pad over affected ear or under nose to catch drainage, but do not pack them. Position patient so that fluids can drain. Change dressings when they become damp, and use sterile technique.

♦ Avoid excessive movement. If not contraindicated, place patient on bed rest with HOB in semi-Fowler's position.

♦ With CSF leakage or possible basilar fracture, avoid nasal suction. *This is to prevent introduction of bacteria into the nervous system.* Instruct patient to avoid Valsalva's maneuver, straining with bowel movement, and vigorous coughing. Caution patient not to blow nose, sneeze, or sniff in nasal drainage. *These may may tear the dura and increase CSF flow.*

♦ If patient is intubated, the tube for gastric decompression may be placed orally rather than nasally. If a nasogastric (NG) tube is placed nasally, the health care provider usually performs the intubation. Check tube placement, preferably by x-ray examination, before applying suction. *NG tubes have been known to enter the fracture site and curl up into patient's cranial vault during insertion attempts.* Visually check back of patient's throat for NG tube to help confirm placement.

◆ Individuals with basilar skull fractures generally are placed flat in bed on complete bed rest. *This position helps decrease pressure and amount of CSF draining from a dural tear.*

◆ Patients are given antibiotics and are observed for healing and sealing of the dural tear within 7-10 days. *The antibiotics are to prevent infection.* Teach patient to report any indicators of infection promptly.

Acute pain related to headaches secondary to TBI
Desired outcome: Within 1 hr of intervention, patient's subjective perception of pain decreases, as documented by a pain scale.

Nursing Interventions

◆ Monitor and document duration and character of patient's pain, and rate it on a scale of 0 (no pain) to 10 (worst pain). Monitor for nonverbal indicators of pain such as facial grimacing, muscle tension, guarding, restlessness, increased or decreased motor activity, irritability, anxiety, or sleep disturbance.

◆ Administer analgesics if needed. *Patients with TBIs generally do not have much pain.* Pain is usually relieved by analgesics, such as acetaminophen. Sometimes codeine is prescribed, but as a rule, other narcotics are contraindicated. *That is because they can mask neurologic indicators of IICP and cause respiratory depression.*

◆ For additional nursing interventions, see **Acute pain,** p. 366, in "General Care of Patients with Neurologic Deficits."

Excess fluid volume related to compromised regulatory mechanisms with increased ADH and increased renal resorption secondary to SIADH
Desired outcome: By time of hospital discharge (or within 3 days of injury), patient is normovolemic, as evidenced by stable weight; balanced I&O; urinary output 30 mL/hr or more; urine specific gravity 1.010-1.030; BP within patient's baseline limits; absence of fingerprint edema over the sternum; and orientation to person, place, and time.

Nursing Interventions

◆ Differentiate between SIADH and cerebral salt-wasting syndrome, whose treatments are different (see "Collaborative Management," p. 410, for treatment). *Although both involve hyponatremia, SIADH results in hypervolemia, and cerebral salt-wasting syndrome results in hypovolemia.*

◆ Monitor serum Na^+, I&O, and weight. Expect seizure activity when serum Na^+ level drops below 118 mEq/L. Notify health care provider of significant findings. *This is because serum Na^+ level less than 115 mEq/L may result in loss of reflexes, coma, and death.*

◆ Assess for fingerprint edema over sternum. *This reflects cellular edema. Because fluid is not retained in the interstitium with SIADH, peripheral edema will not necessarily occur.*

◆ Depending on serum Na^+ value, fluids may be restricted to an amount as low as 500-1000 mL/24 hr. Intervene accordingly and as prescribed.

◆ Be aware that free use of salt or salty foods may be prescribed for patient's diet.

◆ For other nursing interventions, see this nursing diagnosis in "Syndrome of Inappropriate Antidiuretic Hormone," p. 410.

Deficient knowledge related to ventricular shunt procedure
Desired outcome: Following explanation, patient verbalizes accurate information about ventricular shunt procedure, including presurgical and postsurgical care.

Nursing Interventions

- Determine patient's understanding of the procedure after health care provider's explanation, including purpose, risks, and anticipated benefits or outcome. Intervene accordingly. Also assess patient's facility with language; provide an interpreter or language-appropriate written materials as indicated.

- Explain that the procedure is performed to enable drainage of CSF when flow is obstructed (e.g., because of presence of a tumor or blood). Shunt types vary but can extend from lateral ventricle of the brain to one of the following: subarachnoid space of the spinal canal, right atrium of the heart, a large vein, or the peritoneal cavity. Patient may have a cranial dressing, as well as a dressing on the neck, chest, or abdomen.

- Explain that it is important to avoid lying on insertion site after the procedure. *This is to prevent putting pressure on shunt mechanism.* The head and neck are kept in alignment. *This is to prevent kinking and compression of the shunt catheter.* Explain that shunt site will be monitored for redness, tenderness, bulging, or fluid collection and that swelling will be assessed along the course of the shunt.

- Most shunts have a shunt valve that is preset to open at a particular pressure to permit CSF flow and does not require "pumping." There also are valves with adjustable programmable opening pressures that are adjusted externally by using a magnet or programming device. Pumping is usually contraindicated for these new shunts, depending on manufacturer recommendations. Some older implants may have a shunt valve that is pumped to control CSF drainage or reflux. These valves may be pumped by compressing them with index or middle finger a certain number of times (e.g., $10 \times q6h$) at prescribed intervals to flush the system of exudate and prevent plugging. Explain that the valve, which is usually located behind or above the ear and is the approximate diameter of a pencil, can be felt to empty and then refill. Malfunction may be noted by either deterioration in neurologic status or failure of the reservoir to refill when pumped.

- Reassure patient and significant other that before hospital discharge, specific instructions will be given about shunt care, recognition of shunt site infection and malfunction, and steps to take should they occur. Kinked tubing and obstructed tubing or valve must be corrected, and movement of the cannula must be prevented. *This can result in inadequate drainage of ventricles. Cannula movement also can result in abdominal viscus perforation or subdural hematoma formation.* Teach signs and symptoms of IICP (i.e., headache; change in LOC such as drowsiness, lethargy, irritability, nausea, personality changes) that should be reported to health care provider. *This may indicate shunt malfunction.* For ventriculoatrial shunts, emboli or endocarditis may occur. For ventriculoperitoneal shunts, ascites may occur.

- For additional nursing interventions, see **Risk for infection,** p. 8, and **Deficient knowledge:** Surgical procedure, p. 1, in "Perioperative Care."

Deficient knowledge related to craniotomy procedure
Desired outcome: Following the explanation, patient verbalizes accurate understanding of the craniotomy procedure, including presurgical and postsurgical care.

Nursing Interventions

- After health care provider's explanation of the procedure, determine patient's level of understanding of purpose, risks, and anticipated benefits or outcome. Intervene accordingly with an interpreter, or reinforce health care provider's explanation as appropriate. Provide and review language-appropriate printed material if available.

- Encourage questions and discuss fears and anxiety. Obtain informed consent. Discuss possibility of cognitive and behavioral changes related to site of surgery. Cognitive and behavioral changes often diminish or disappear in 6 wk to 6 mo.

◆ Explain that a craniotomy is a surgical opening into the skull to remove a hematoma or tumor, repair a ruptured aneurysm, or apply arterial clips or wrap the involved vessel to prevent future rupture. As appropriate, explain that the bone flap may be left open postoperatively to accommodate cerebral edema and prevent compression. When the bone is removed, the procedure is called a craniectomy.

◆ Explain that before surgery, antiseptic shampoos may be given and patient may be started on corticosteroids.

◆ Explain that a baseline neurologic assessment will be done. *This provides a basis for comparison with postoperative neurologic checks.*

◆ During immediate postoperative period, patient is in ICU. Explain the following considerations and interventions that are likely to occur:

- Assessment of VS and neurologic status at least hourly. Patient will be asked to perform a variety of assessment measures, including squeezing tester's hand, moving extremities, extending tongue, and answering questions. Emphasize importance of performing these tasks to the best of patient's ability.

- Changes in body image that can occur because of loss of hair, presence of a head dressing, and potential for and expected duration of facial edema. Suggest use of headpiece, scarf, or wig. *This is for patient concerns regarding change in body image.*

- Presence of SCDs on legs, and possibly an arterial line. *This is for continuous BP monitoring as well as other devices such as ICP monitoring equipment.*

- Possible need for respiratory and airway support, including O_2, intubation, or ventilation. *Typically patients are on a cardiac monitor for 24-48 hr because dysrhythmias are not unusual after posterior fossa surgery or when blood is in CSF.* Respirations will be monitored for irregularity. *That may be a sign of bleeding and brainstem compression.*

- Presence of large head dressing and drains, which will be inspected periodically for bleeding or CSF leakage, which will be reported to health care provider. Stress importance of not pulling or tugging on dressing or drains. Advise that patient should report a sweet or salty taste in mouth. *This may indicate a CSF leak.*

- NPO status for first 24-48 hr. *This is to reduce the risk of vomiting and choking.* Patient may experience a dry throat at this time and will be monitored for swallowing difficulties.

- Periorbital swelling, which usually occurs within 24-48 hr of supratentorial surgery. Explain that relief is obtained with applications of cold or warm compresses around the eyes. Raise HOB, if allowed, with patient lying on nonoperative side. *This may also help reduce edema.*

- Insertion of indwelling urinary catheter. This is to enable accurate measurement of I&O and monitor for problems such as DI.

- Measurement of core temperature (e.g., rectal, tympanic, bladder) at frequent intervals. A rectal probe or bladder catheter temperature probe may be used for continuous monitoring. Oral temperatures are avoided during period cognitive function is decreased.

◆ Teach patient that postsurgical positioning is a key factor during recovery.

- *Supratentorial craniotomy:* Patient maintained with HOB elevated to 30 degrees or as prescribed. Patient will be assisted with turning and usually will be kept off operative site, especially if the lesion was large. Head and neck will be kept in good alignment.

- *Infratentorial craniotomy (for cerebellar or brainstem surgery):* HOB is kept flat or as prescribed. *Sitting may increase risk of venous air embolus with posterior fossa surgery.* Pressure is kept off operative site, especially with a craniectomy; so these patients are kept off their backs for 48 hr. In posterior fossa surgery, the supporting neck muscles are altered.

Logroll patient to alternate sides, keeping head in alignment. A soft cervical collar may be used. *This is to prevent anterior or lateral angulation of the neck.* A small pillow may be used. *This is to provide more comfort for the patient.*

- *For areas of evacuation causing large intracranial space:* Avoid positioning onto operative side immediately after surgery. *This could cause shifting inside the space.*
- *After craniectomy:* Avoid turning onto side from which bone was removed. Label on chart and bed the location of missing bone.
- *Ventricular shunts and chronic subdural heamtomas:* May involve a gradual elevation of HOB to prevent cerebral hemorrhage. For example, HOB may be flat for 24 hr, 15 degrees for next 24 hr, 30 degrees for next 24 hr, 45 degree for next 24 hr, and then 90 degrees.

◆ Explain that bed rest will be enforced immediately after surgery.

◆ For eyelids that do not close or for patient who is less responsive or on sedation, lubricant or saline will be instilled into eyes. If eyes cannot close, an eye shield may be used.

◆ Explain that patient having supratentorial surgery near the area of the pituitary gland or hypothalamus may develop transient DI. (See "Diabetes Insipidus," p. 404, for teaching details.)

◆ Teach patients undergoing infratentorial surgery that they are likely to experience the following:
- Dizziness and hypotension, necessitating a longer period of bed rest.
- Nausea, which should be reported so that antiemetics can be given.
- Swallowing difficulties, extraocular movements, or nystagmus, any of which should be reported promptly. *This may indicate cranial nerve edema.*

◆ Teach patient the following precautions: *These are taken to prevent increased intraabdominal and intrathoracic pressure, which can cause IICP:*
- Exhaling when being turned.
- Not straining at stool.
- Not moving self in bed, but rather letting staff members do all moving.
- Importance of deep breathing, but avoiding coughing and sneezing. If coughing and sneezing are unavoidable, they must be done with an open mouth. *This will minimize pressure buildup.*
- Avoiding hip flexion and lying prone.

◆ For additional precautions against IICP, see **Decreased intracranial adaptive capacity,** p. 363.

◆ Teach patient that precautions are taken for seizures (see **Risk for falls** with risk factors related to oral, musculoskeletal, and airway vulnerability secondary to seizure activity, p. 350).

◆ Teach patient wound care and to report fever; redness; drainage from surgical site, nose, or ears; and increased headache. *These may indicate infection.* Generally, a surgical cap is worn after removal of head dressing. Patient must avoid scratching wound, staples, or sutures and must keep incision dry. When sutures or staples are removed, hair can be shampooed, with care taken not to scrub around incision line. Hair dryers are avoided until hair is regrown. (For more information, see **Risk for infection,** p. 315.)

◆ Explain that nausea; hearing loss; facial weakness or paralysis; diminished or absent blinking; eye dryness; tinnitus; vertigo; headache; and occasionally swallowing, throat, taste, or voice problems may occur. *These may be side effects of acoustic neuroma excision.* Provide prescribed antiemetics, and turn and move patient slowly. *This may decrease the nausea and vertigo.* Speak to patient on unaffected side for best hearing, and place phone and call light on that side of bed. Contralateral routing of signal hearing aids may be tried. *This improves hearing by directing sound from deaf ear to hearing ear via a tiny microphone and transmitter.* Background music or other white noise may mask tinnitus. Awareness of tinnitus eventually should lessen. Balance exercises and walking with assistance will start compensation process by the functioning vestibular system. Watching television or reading may be difficult. *This is because of the vertigo.* Suggest books on tape, listening to the radio, or music as alternatives. Eye dryness may require use of eye drops or ointment. *Impaired eyelid function causes the dryness.*

- For additional nursing interventions, see **Deficient knowledge** related to surgical procedure, p. 1, in "Perioperative Care."

Patient-Family Teaching and Discharge Planning

Patients with TBI can have various degrees of neurologic deficit, ranging from mild to severe. Include verbal and written information about the following:

- Safety measures related to decreased sensation, visual disturbances, motor deficits, and seizure activity.
- Measures that promote communication in the presence of aphasia.
- Wound care and indicators of infection. Instruct patient to avoid scratching sutures and shampoo only after sutures are out. *This is to prevent infection.*
- Indicators of IICP, which include change in LOC, lethargy, headache, nausea, and vomiting and should be reported to health care provider promptly.
- Measures that deal with cognitive or behavioral problems. As appropriate, include home evaluation for safety. Caution significant other that personality can change drastically after TBI. Patient may demonstrate inappropriate social behavior, inappropriate affect, hallucination, delusion, and altered sleep pattern.
- If patient had a concussion, a description of problems that may occur at home and necessitate prompt medical attention (see **Deficient knowledge,** p. 314).
- Referrals to community resources, such as cognitive retraining specialist, head injury rehabilitation centers, visiting nurses association, community support groups, social workers, psychologic therapy, vocational rehabilitation agency, home health agencies, and extended and skilled care facilities. Additional general information can be obtained by accessing the following websites:

  Brain Injury Association, Inc.: www.biausa.org

  Brain Injury Resource Foundation: www.birf.info

  Brain Trauma Foundation www.braintrauma.org

  The Rehabilitation and Research Center at Santa Clara Valley Medical Center (SCVMC): www.tbi-sci.org

❖ ❖ ❖

SECTION FOUR **VASCULAR DISORDERS OF THE NERVOUS SYSTEM**

❖ CEREBRAL ANEURYSM

OVERVIEW/PATHOPHYSIOLOGY

An aneurysm is a localized weakness and dilation of an artery. With cerebral aneurysms, this dilation generally takes one of two forms: *fusiform,* in which the entire circumference of a vessel section is dilated; or *saccular,* in which the side of a vessel is dilated. Saccular aneurysms, which include berry aneurysms, are the most common. Depending on their size and location, unruptured aneurysms can produce neurologic symptoms by compressing brain tissue or cranial nerves. A warning leak may precede a major rupture. Usually, however, the aneurysm causes no symptoms until it ruptures. When this occurs, the hemorrhage usually bleeds into the subarachnoid space, although occasionally it may bleed directly into the intracranial tissue and cause direct neuronal damage. Rupture causes a sudden increase in intracranial pressure (ICP) and a loss of cerebral perfusion pressure (CPP). Brain tissue may be compressed by the expanding mass effect of the bleeding. Cranial nerves and brain tissue are irritated by the presence of blood, and the brain begins to swell. Blood in the subarachnoid space prevents adequate circulation and reabsorption of cerebrospinal fluid (CSF) and thereby increases ICP further. In addition, interruption of blood flow to the areas supplied by the ruptured artery can cause brain ischemia and possibly infarction. Patients may experience permanent neurologic deficits, depending on size and site of the bleed, and development of complications. Prognosis for all types depends on site and size of the ruptured aneurysm, but almost half of affected individuals die immediately.

Common causes of death for individuals who survive the initial rupture include increased ICP (IICP), rebleeding, and vasospasm of the blood vessels. Patients are at greatest risk of rebleeding within the first 24-48 hr after initial rupture. Rebleeding, however, is a significant risk for the first 1-2 wk because of the normal process of clot lysis at the rupture site. Approximately 20% of patients will rebleed within 2 wk. Rebleeding may occur up to 6 mo after initial rupture and is an incentive for early surgery in order to clip or embolize the aneurysm.

Patients also are at risk of experiencing cerebral vasospasm, which decreases cerebral blood flow (CBF) and leads to cerebral ischemia. Cerebral ischemia can increase neurologic deficits and may cause cerebral infarct and death. Vasospasm seems to be directly related to the amount of blood present in the subarachnoid space after rupture. Vasospasm usually starts within 3-4 days after subarachnoid hemorrhage (SAH), peaks in 7-10 days, and usually resolves in about 3 wk.

After rupture, some patients may develop acute or chronic hydrocephalus. The presence of blood in the subarachnoid space appears to damage the arachnoid villi and decrease or prevent CSF reabsorption. This condition increases ICP and leads to possible brain herniation. Other potential complications include seizures, cardiac dysrhythmias, and diabetes insipidus (DI). Syndrome of inappropriate antidiuretic hormone (SIADH) may occur because of pituitary gland or hypothalamus compression or damage, which causes increased secretion of antidiuretic hormone (ADH), leading leads to water retention. Cerebral salt-wasting syndrome can occur because of enhanced release of brain natriuretic peptide that leads to volume depletion.

ASSESSMENT

Signs and symptoms/physical findings: Indicators vary, depending on site and amount of bleeding. Rupture often occurs with exertion, excitement, or sudden rise in BP.

Prodromal (as the aneurysm enlarges but before it ruptures): Transitory symptoms include periodic headaches or episodes of weakness, numbness, tingling on one side, diplopia, blurred vision, ptosis, dizziness, and speech disturbances.

Acute (with leakage and rupture): Sudden and severe headache, nausea and/ or vomiting, loss of consciousness, and neck stiffness are among the most common symptoms.

IICP and herniation: Sudden, severe headache; nausea and vomiting; changes or alteration in level of consciousness (LOC) ranging from confusion, irritability, and restlessness to coma; a falling score on the Glasgow Coma Scale (GCS) (Box 5-3); pupillary dilation and changes in their size and reaction to light; VS changes, such as increasing BP with widening pulse pressure and decreased pulse rate; irregular respiratory pattern.

BOX 5-5	WORLD FEDERATION OF NEUROLOGICAL SURGEONS GRADING SCALE

GRADE	GLASGOW COMA SCALE SCORE	FOCAL NEUROLOGIC DEFICIT
1	15	Absent
2	13–14	Absent
3	13–14	Present
4	7–12	Present or absent
5	<7	Present or absent

From World Federation of Neurological Surgeons (WFNS): *Grading system for subarachnoid hemorrhage scale*. Available at The Internet Stroke Center website: www.strokecenter.org. Accessed May 2009.

Meningeal irritation (caused by blood in the subarachnoid space): Neck stiffness; neck, back, and leg pain; fever; photophobia; seizures; and pain aggravated by neck motion.

Cranial nerve irritation/compression: Blurred vision and other visual disturbances, ptosis, inability to rotate the eyes, difficulty with swallowing or speaking, tinnitus.

Focal symptoms: Sensory loss, motor weakness, or paralysis on one side of the body.

Autonomic disturbance (from increased catecholamines immediately following rupture): ECG changes, flushing, sweating, dilated pupils, hypertension, tachycardia, increased blood sugar, increased temperature, ileus.

Physical assessment: Kernig's and Brudzinski's signs confirm presence of meningeal irritation. (See description in "Bacterial Meningitis," p. 245.)

Grading: Individuals with ruptured aneurysms are often graded according to severity of the bleeding or injury. The World Federation of Neurological Surgeons (WFNS) classification scale is used to grade SAH. This scale uses a grading system based on both the neurologic deficit findings and the GCS score (**BOX 5-5**).

Other scales that may be used for grading include the Hunter and Hess, Fisher, and Carter and Olgilvy. The Hunter and Hess scale, which classifies patients based on symptoms, was the most commonly used scale before the WFNS grading system. The Fisher scale is an index of vasospasm risk based on a computed tomography (CT)-defined hemorrhage and clot pattern. The Carter and Ogilvy grading system stratifies patients based on age, Hunter-Hess grade, Fisher scale, and aneurysm size to predict outcome for surgical management of intracranial aneurysms.

History and risk factors: Aneurysms can be caused by a congenital defect in the arterial wall, degenerative processes (e.g., hypertension, atherosclerosis), vessel trauma, dissection, or infection. People with connective tissue disorders, such as Marfan syndrome, Ehlers-Danlos syndrome, polycystic kidney disease, and coarctation of the aorta, have increased incidence of intracranial aneurysms. Smoking, advanced age, female gender, diabetes, and moderate to heavy alcohol usage also increase the risk. Phenylpropanolamine has been associated with increased risk of hemorrhagic stroke, which includes SAH. The drug is a sympathomimetic central nervous system (CNS) stimulant formerly commonly found in over-the-counter (OTC) cough and cold remedies but is now available only by prescription.

DIAGNOSTIC TESTS

Digital subtraction angiography (DSA): Reveals presence of aneurysm and assesses CBF. This is often considered to be the gold standard for for diagnosis of intracranial aneurysms.

Multidetector computed tomography (MDCT) angiography: Very accurate and fast imaging for decting intracranial aneurysms. This CT angiography study can provide a three-dimensional image and demonstrate relationship of the aneurysm to nearby bony structures. It also allows visualization from any angle.

Cerebral angiography: Used to pinpoint site, structure, and size of aneurysm(s) and presence of vasospasm. This test provides the definitive diagnosis of aneurysm and usually is performed before surgery to exclude presence of vasospasm and review accessibility. Small aneurysms may be missed; vasospasm may "hide" the aneurysm.

CT scan: Reveals presence of aneurysm(s) and site, size, and amount of bleeding from the SAH or intracerebral hemorrhage. The scan also may reveal presence of hydrocephalus and may not identify small aneurysms or those in vasospasm. CT scan may be used 1-2 days after rupture to assess the amount of bleeding to predict risk of vasospasm.

MRI: Reveals presence of even small amounts of blood or small aneurysms that are not visualized with CT scan or angiography. MR angiography is being used in some areas to highlight cerebral vascularity.

Lumbar puncture (LP) and CSF analysis: Reveal presence of bloody CSF, increased CSF pressure, and increased protein. Blood in the CSF indicates that SAH has occurred. This procedure is contraindicated for patients with IICP because of risk of herniation. LP usually is done only when CT scan is negative, nondiagnostic, or unavailable. Usually it is deferred for 6 hr after headache onset to accurately assess for the presence of xanthochromia, a pink or yellow tint in CSF that represents hemoglobin degradation products and indicates that blood has been in the CSF for at least 2 hr. Spectrophotometry can provide laboratory confirmation of xanthochromia.

ECG: About 20% of patients with SAH have myocardial ischemia from the increased circulation of catecholamines. Typical results are nonspecific ST- and T-wave changes, prolonged QRS segments, U waves, and increased QT intervals. ECG changes that reflect myocardial ischemia or infarction are treated in the usual manner. Suspected SAH is a contraindication to thrombolytic and anticoagulant therapy. Low-molecular-weight heparin (e.g., enoxaparin) may be considered after aneurysm clipping.

Skull x-ray examination: Reveals calcification in the wall of a large aneurysm.

CBF studies (e.g., Transcranial Doppler [TCD] sonography, CT xenon inhalation): Monitor for cerebral vasospasms, changes in blood flow states, loss of autoregulation, IICP, and brain death.

Single photon emission computed tomography (SPECT): May be used to identify areas of vasospasm.

COLLABORATIVE MANAGEMENT

Respiratory support: Airway maintenance, intubation, and ventilation as necessary. Monitor oximetry and ABG values and provide O_2 to maintain saturation at 92% or greater. If indicated, O_2 is administered to prevent hypoxia. Preoxygenate before suctioning and limit suctioning to 10 sec. CO_2 retention and the resulting respiratory acidosis can cause vasodilation of the cerebral arteries that leads to cerebral edema, and they are to be avoided. Lowering cerebral CO_2 results in alkalosis, which causes cerebral vasoconstriction and results in decreased CBF and ICP. The vasoconstriction also may cause decreased cerebral O_2 delivery, which could increase injury. Blowing off CO_2 through hyperventilation resulting in $PaCO_2$ less than 35 mm Hg generally is avoided and used only in cases of acute deterioration as a "quick fix" for IICP until other interventions such as mannitol can be instituted or in cases in which IICP is refractory and responds to nothing else. Ideally, CBF measurements, continuous jugular venous oxygen saturation (SjO_2), and brain tissue oxygenation ($PbtO_2$) are considered to monitor for effectiveness (i.e., decreased IICP without decreased cerebral O_2 delivery) if hyperventilation is used as a treatment.

Activity restrictions: Strict bed rest in a quiet, dark room; limitation of visitors; restriction of activities of daily living (ADL). Although active ROM is occasionally permitted, even the alert patient is usually limited to passive ROM. Restraints are avoided because they can result in IICP if the patient struggles against them.

Elevation of head of bed (HOB): Bed elevated to whichever level optimizes CPP or as prescribed. Without monitoring equipment, having the HOB at 30 degrees is considered safe and effective in promoting venous drainage and helping reduce cerebral edema as long as patient is not hypovolemic, which could threaten CPP.

Pharmacotherapy

Antihypertensives (e.g., labetalol, hydralazine): Treat underlying hypertension until aneurysm can be clipped. Desired SBP is usually less than 140 mm Hg, and DBP is less than 100 mm Hg. IV nitroprusside and nitroglycerin are usually avoided, if possible, because of they may cause dilation of cerebral vasculature and increase ICP.

Calcium channel blockers (e.g., nimodipine): Reduce risk of vasospasm.

Laxatives and stool softeners (e.g., docusate sodium, Milk of Magnesia): Prevent straining with bowel movements.

Sedatives/tranquilizers (e.g., phenobarbital): Reduce stress and restlessness and promote rest.

Osmotic diuretics (e.g., mannitol): Reduce severe cerebral edema.

Loop diuretics (e.g., furosemide): Appear to decrease cerebral edema without causing the increase in intracranial blood volume that occurs with mannitol.

Antipyretics (e.g., acetaminophen): Control fever, which increases the metabolic activity of the brain. Aspirin is contraindicated because it prevents platelet adhesion.

Antiepileptic drugs (AEDs) (e.g., carbamazepine, phenytoin, fosphenytoin): Control or prevent seizures.

Analgesics (e.g., acetaminophen, codeine): Manage pain. Aspirin is contraindicated because it prevents platelet adhesion.

Proton pump inhibitors (e.g., pantoprazole), histamine H_2-receptor blockers (e.g., famotidine), and sucralfate: Reduce gastric acidity and prevent gastric ulcer formation.

Low-molecular-weight heparin (e.g., enoxaparin): May be given only after aneurysm clipping or embolization is done and risk of bleeding is past, to help prevent deep vein thrombosis (DVT) while patient is on bed rest; may reduce risk of cerebral vasospasm.

Fluid: Initially fluids are given to keep patient normovolemic. Fluid restriction generally has been abandoned because the resultant increased blood viscosity has been suspected to result in increased risk of vasospasm. Later, after aneurysm clipping, patient may be kept hypervolemic to reduce vasospasm.

Nutrition: Coffee and other stimulants are restricted. Very hot and very cold liquids also may be restricted. A high-fiber diet may be prescribed to prevent constipation. For patients with dysphagia, enteral or parenteral feedings may be necessary. A low-Na^+ (see Box 4-1, for high Na^{++} foods, p. 165), low-cholesterol (see Table 3-1, p. 101) diet is often prescribed to control hypertension and atherosclerosis.

SCDs and antiembolism hose: Help prevent thrombophlebitis and DVT.

Avoiding rectal stimulation: Rectal suppositories, thermometers, enemas, and digital examinations are contraindicated because they can stimulate a type of Valsalva's maneuver in the patient that causes increased intrathoracic pressure and IICP and results in rupture or rebleeding.

Seizure precautions: Prevent patient injury in the event of seizure.

Cardiac monitoring: May be done to assess and treat cardiac dysrhythmias, which are common immediately following SAH.

ICU monitoring: May be necessary, particularly if patient develops cerebral vasospasm or IICP or requires vasopressors.

Surgical management/interventional neuroradiology: Patient's surgical candidacy depends on LOC, extent of neurologic deficit, nature and location of the aneurysm, and presence of vasospasm. Surgical timing for aneurysm repair is based on patient's status and surgeon's preference. Usually surgery is performed within 24-48 hr of the initial bleed to reduce risk of rebleeding. The surgical site is thoroughly irrigated to reduce the amount of blood and blood clots present that could result in vasospasm. Surgery is not performed in the presence of vasospasm. Patients graded 1 or 2 are the best surgical candidates. Computerized electroencephalography (EEG) may be used in the operating room (OR) during the procedure for continuous monitoring of neuronal integrity. Brain activity as recorded on the electroencephalogram (EEG) correlates with CBF and can be used to identify ischemia in the anesthetized patient. Intraoperative angiography, CBF studies, or intraoperative Doppler imaging also may be done to verify adequacy of circulation and security of the clip. Somatosensory evoked potential (SSEP) studies may be performed intraoperatively to monitor for neurologic deficits.

Surgical repair with craniotomy: Isolates the aneurysm and prevents rebleeding; a craniotomy is performed, and the aneurysm is repaired by clipping, ligating, coagulating, wrapping the aneurysm neck with muscle, or encasing the aneurysmal sac in plastic or surgical gauze. Fusiform aneurysms may need a bypass and end-to-end anastomosis of arteries once the fusiform section is dissected and removed. (For information on craniotomy patient care considerations, see "Traumatic Brain Injury," p. 313.)

Endovascular balloon occlusion of aneurysm or parent vessel: A small and extremely flexible catheter is threaded through the femoral artery at the groin and advanced up to the aneurysm or parent vessel. The balloon can be inflated with a liquid that solidifies within 45 min. Balloon occlusion within the aneurysm is ideal, but sometimes the parent vessel (usually the carotid) must be occluded. A test occlusion is done to see whether patient can tolerate parent vessel occlusion. If signs of ischemia occur, the balloon procedure is stopped. A bypass is done, if possible, and balloon occlusion usually is performed a few days later.

Embolization of surgically inaccessible aneurysms: Endovascular techniques are used to place a metal coil (e.g., Guglielmi detachable coil [GDC]) in the area of the aneurysm to cause a thrombus to form that obliterates the aneurysm. An intracranial stent may be used to help hold the coil in place (especially in aneurysms with wide necks) and decrease inflow into the aneurysm in certain instances.

Ventriculostomy: Permits temporary ventricular drainage for acute hydrocephalus.

Daily LPs or lumbar drain: Provide temporary CSF drainage and restore reabsorptive ability of the arachnoid villi by removing blood from the CSF.

Ventricular shunt for ventricular drainage: Enables long-term drainage of CSF in patients who develop chronic hydrocephalus after SAH. (See nursing considerations of ventricular shunt in "Traumatic Brain Injury," p. 314.)

Proton beam: Scleroses inoperable aneurysms. This is a type of external beam radiotherapy.

Management of SIADH vs. cerebral salt-wasting syndrome: Hyponatremia and decreased fluid volume increase risk of vasospasm. It is critical to distinguish correctly between these two types of hyponatremia (Na^+ less than 135 mEq/L) and fluid imbalance because their treatment is so different. SIADH (characterized by inappropriate urinary concentration causing water retention results in a dilutional hyponatremia with increased plasma volume, weight gain, decreased serum osmolality) is treated with fluid restriction, mild diuresis with furosemide or bumetanide and, sometimes, demeclocycline (see "Syndrome of Inappropriate Antidiuretic Hormone," p. 410, for more information).

Cerebral salt-wasting syndrome, in which the kidneys are unable to conserve Na^+ (characterized by a true hyponatremia with decreased plasma volume, weight loss, decreased serum osmolality, hypernatriuria), is treated with fluid replacement (IV normal saline), volume expanders, salt tablets, and occasionally fludrocortisone to inhibit Na^+ excretion and induce Na^+ retention in order to counteract hyponatremia and volume depletion. If serum Na^+ is very low, 3% hypertonic saline may be used. Ongoing monitoring of serum Na^+ and I&O for both syndromes is needed. Usually both resolve in a week or two. Three percent hypertonic saline infusions are used cautiously, and the serum Na^+ level is corrected slowly over several days (no faster than 10 mmol/L/24 hr). Prolonged hyponatremia followed by rapid Na^+ correction may result in central pontine myelinolysis. Fluctuating osmotic forces from the serum Na^+ changes result in cellular edema, which causes compression of fiber tracts and induces demyelination. Characteristic signs and symptoms include spastic tetraplegia, dysphagia, dysarthria, confusion, and horizontal gaze paralysis.

Management of DI: Fluid replacement (usually IV 0.45% or 0.9% NaCl bolus and then 1 mL IV fluid for every 1 mL of urinary output [UO]) and vasopressin or desmopressin, See "Diabetes Insipidus," p. 404, for more information.

Treatments for cerebral vasospasm: There is no completely effective treatment for cerebral vasospasm, but some techniques seem to reduce its incidence or severity. Vasospasm is related to the amount of blood in basal cisterns or cerebral fissures. The presence of lethargy, with or without focal neurologic deficit, is considered diagnostic of vasospasm until proven otherwise. Emergency CT is performed to rule out other pathology such as bleeding or hydrocephalus. The following treatments necessitate ICU monitoring.

Calcium channel blockers (e.g., nimodipine): Reduce vasospasm and promote collateral circulation.

Craniotomy: Done within 48 hr to remove any blood clot that may aggravate vasospasm.

Hypervolemic (e.g., plasma protein fraction, saline, albumin) hypertensive (e.g., dopamine, dobutamine), or hemodilution therapy (HHHT): Usually performed only after aneurysm repair to increase CPP via increased blood volume and arterial pressure to reduce ischemia and resulting neurologic deficits during vasospasm. A volume to attain a dilutional hematocrit (Hct) level of 30%-34% may be given to decrease blood viscosity and improve blood flow. Vasopressors are used to obtain a hypertensive state, usually about a 30% increase in SBP over baseline, in order to achieve an mean arterial pressure (MAP) of 100-110 mm Hg.

Balloon angioplasty: Dilates arteries that are in vasospasm.

Tissue plasminogen activator instillation: Accomplished during aneurysm clipping into the basal cisterns to dissolve any clots to prevent or reduce vasospasm.

TCD: Used on a daily basis to monitor flow velocities in major cerebral arteries so that early vasospasm can be detected and treated.

NURSING DIAGNOSES AND INTERVENTIONS

The priorities of care for these patients revolve around maintenance of adequate cerebral perfusion, prevention of rebleeding, and prevention and treatment of vasospasm. (See "Stroke," p. 328, for a discussion of these issues.) The following nursing diagnoses relate primarily to the patient whose aneurysm is graded 1-3. If the patient's aneurysm is graded 4 or 5, see nursing diagnoses in "Stroke," p. 336, for patient care.

Deficient knowledge related to aneurysms and the potential for rebleeding, rupture, or vasospasm

Desired outcome: Following instruction and on an ongoing basis, patient verbalizes knowledge about the potential for rebleeding and vasospasm, measures to prevent their occurrence, and symptoms to report to the health care staff.

Nursing Interventions

♦ Assess for sensorimotor deficits, such as decreased or absent vision, impaired temperature and pain sensation, unsteady gait, weakness, or paralysis. Document baseline neurologic and physical assessments so that changes in patient status are detected promptly. Teach patient and significant other these indicators, and explain importance of reporting them to staff promptly.

♦ Teach importance of reducing activity level. Strict bed rest may be prescribed. Emphasize necessity of allowing others to help with moving, ADL, and passive ROM. *This is to avoid rebleeding or rupture.* Explain that the number and frequency of visitors will be limited and that individuals whose presence is stressful to patient should not be allowed to visit. The phone may be removed from the room, and television, radio, and reading may be restricted or limited to programs and books that are not overstimulating. The room may be darkened and sedatives and tranquilizers offered. *This is to promote more rest.* Caffeine and other stimulants may be restricted, as well as nicotine. *They can increase risk of vasospasm.* A cool, wet cloth or ice pack may be applied to head/neck. *This also may aid comfort in addition to analgesics.*

♦ Teach patient to:
  • Avoid coughing and sneezing; if they are unavoidable, do so with an open mouth.
  • Breathe deeply at frequent intervals to expand the lungs.
  • Exhale when being turned.
  • Avoid straining with bowel movements.
  • Avoid extreme hip flexion or lying prone.
  • Avoid moving self up in bed. Do not grip, push, or pull on side rails or push feet against mattress or foot of bed. Request help from staff member for all moving and turning. *These measures will prevent a sudden increase in ICP.*

♦ Explain that HOB may be maintained at 30 degrees and patient may be asked to keep head and neck in good alignment. *This is to promote venous return to the heart and reduce cerebral congestion and ICP.*

♦ Explain that patient may be given a high-fiber diet and stool softeners. *This is to promote bowel elimination without straining.*

♦ Describe, as appropriate: AEDs, antihypertensive medications, and a low-Na$^+$, low-cholesterol diet. *These preventive measures are important to reduce risk of complications such as seizures or high BP.*

♦ Teach patient to avoid taking aspirin or aspirin-containing products. *This reduces risk of hemorrhage.*

Risk for disuse syndrome related to prescribed immobilization secondary to risk of aneurysm rupture or rebleeding
Desired outcome: Patient exhibits complete ROM.

Nursing Interventions

♦ To maintain joint mobility, perform passive ROM exercises during period of activity restriction. Even if patient feels well enough to perform assisted or active ROM, these activities are contraindicated because they increase ICP and risk of rupture or rebleeding. Explain rationale for activity limitation.

♦ Maintain joint alignment, and provide support to joints and extremities with pillows, trochanter rolls, sandbags, and other positioning devices.

♦ When patient is no longer on bed rest/activity restrictions, additional strengthening and conditioning exercises may be necessary to counteract effects of prolonged bed rest. Patient may have residual neurologic deficits that necessitate gait training or use of assistive devices to promote mobility. Obtain a physical therapist or occupation therapist referral as appropriate.

For additional nursing interventions, see **Risk for disuse syndrome** in "Prolonged Bed Rest," p. 25.

Self-care deficit (bathing, dressing, toileting) related to imposed activity restrictions secondary to risk of aneurysm rupture or rebleeding
Desired outcome: Care activities are completed for patient during the period of strict bed rest.
◆ Perform care activities, while patient is on bed rest, even if patient does not exhibit signs of neurologic deficit. Explain reason for patient's activity restrictions.
◆ If patient has bathroom privileges, provide a commode as appropriate and assist with transferring as necessary.

Patient-Family Teaching and Discharge Planning

The patient with an aneurysm may have continued deficits when discharged or may be expected to fully recover after surgery. Teaching needs will vary depending on the results of the interventions. Include verbal and written information about the following:
◆ Wound care and indicators of wound infection for patients who have undergone surgery.
◆ Importance of avoiding strenuous physical activity. Check with health care provider regarding activity restrictions and limitations and instruct patient accordingly.
◆ Low-Na^+ (see Box 4-1, for high Na^{++} foods, p. 165), low-cholesterol (see Table 3-1, p. 101) diet if prescribed to control hypertension and atherosclerosis.
◆ Medications, including drug names, rationale, schedule, dosage, precautions, drug/drug and food/drug interactions, and potential side effects.
◆ Signs and symptoms of rupture and rebleeding because patient is at risk for 6 mo after initial bleed.
◆ Care of ventricular shunt, if present. Instructions should include indicators of shunt infection and steps to take in event of shunt infection or malfunction.

Additional Teaching
◆ See teaching and discharge planning section in "Stroke," p. 344, for patients who have residual neurologic deficits.
◆ Referrals to community resources, public health nurse, community support groups, social workers, psychologists, vocational rehabilitation agencies, home health agencies, extended and skilled care facilities, and financial counseling, as needed. Additional general information can be obtained from the following:

Brain Aneurysm Foundation, Inc.: www.bafound.org

The Aneurysm and AVM Foundation: www.taafonline.org

American Stroke Association: www.strokeassociation.org

❖ STROKE

OVERVIEW/PATHOPHYSIOLOGY

A stroke (also known as *cerebrovascular accident* [CVA]) is the sudden disruption of O_2 supply to the nerve cells, generally caused by obstruction or rupture of one or more of the blood vessels that supply the brain. *Ischemic stroke* has three main mechanisms: thrombosis, embolism, and systemic hypoperfusion. Thrombosis or embolism results in a blockage of blood supply to the brain tissue. The resulting ischemia, if prolonged, causes brain tissue necrosis (infarction), cerebral edema, and increased intracranial pressure

(IICP). Most thrombotic strokes are caused by blockage of large vessels as a result of atherosclerosis. Thrombi in small penetrating arteries result in "lacunar" strokes. Most embolic strokes are cardiogenic and the result of emboli produced from valve disease or during atrial fibrillation of the heart. Ischemic stroke caused by systemic hypoperfusion usually is the result of decreased cerebral blood flow (CBF) owing to circulatory failure. Circulatory failure results from too little blood, too-low BP, or failure of the heart to pump blood adequately. Hypoxia from any cause also can produce this syndrome.

A *transient ischemic attack* (TIA), which is a temporary (less than 24 hr) neurologic deficit that resolves completely without permanent damage, occurs when the artery cannot deliver enough blood to meet the O_2 requirement of the brain. However, restoration of blood flow is timely enough to make the ischemia (and deficits) transient, thereby avoiding infarction and permanent damage. TIAs usually are associated with thrombosis but may be caused by any of the ischemic mechanisms just mentioned. TIAs may precede a permanent ischemic stroke by hours, days, months, or years. TIAs are a warning sign, and treatment may prevent a stroke. Most TIAs last an average of 5-10 min, although some can last longer than 1 hr. A *reversible ischemic neurologic deficit* (RIND) lasts longer than 24 hr but otherwise is similar to a TIA.

Hemorrhagic stroke causes neural tissue destruction because of the infiltration and accumulation of blood. Ischemia and infarction may occur distal to the hemorrhage because of interrupted blood supply. Although a cerebral hemorrhage usually results from hypertension or an aneurysm, trauma also can cause hemorrhagic stroke. Bleeding may spread into the brain tissue itself, thus causing an intracerebral hemorrhage, or into the subarachnoid space. Usually there is a large rise in intracranial pressure (ICP) with a hemorrhagic stroke because of cerebral edema and the mass effect of blood. (See "Cerebral Aneurysm," p. 321, for discussion of subarachnoid hemorrhage [SAH].)

A stroke may be classified as a *progressive stroke in evolution,* in which deficits continue to worsen over time, or as a *completed stroke,* in which maximum deficit has been acquired and has persisted for longer than 24 hr. Progressive strokes usually are the result of thrombus formation and often take 1-3 days to become "completed." Embolic strokes typically have sudden onset with maximal deficits. *Stroke syndromes* classically have been described according to the distribution of the vessels (middle cerebral artery, anterior cerebral artery, posterior cerebral artery, vertebral, basilar) that supply particular regions of the brain and will have typical assessment findings. Stroke is the third most common cause of death and the most common cause of neurologic disability. Half the survivors are left permanently disabled or experience another stroke. Improvement may continue for 1-2 yr, but deficits at 6 mo usually are considered permanent.

A *brain attack,* also sometimes called a *code stroke* or *stroke alert,* is a sudden event and medical emergency with the same urgency as for a heart attack. If the stroke is ischemic and the patient qualifies, "time-is-tissue," and the sooner the patient can be treated, the better the outcome. (See "Collaborative Management" section for information on immediate treatment interventions.)

ASSESSMENT

Signs and symptoms/physical findings: Classically, symptoms appear on the side of the body opposite the damaged site. For example, a stroke in the left hemisphere of the brain will produce symptoms in the right arm and leg. However, when the stroke affects the cranial nerves, symptoms of cranial nerve deficit will appear on the same side as the site of injury. Similarly, an obstruction of an anterior cerebral artery can produce bilateral symptoms, as will severe bleeding or multiple emboli. Hemiplegia is fairly common. Initially, patient usually has flaccid paralysis. As spinal cord depression resolves, more normal tone is seen, and hyperactive reflexes occur. Symptoms vary with the size and site of injury and may improve in 2-3 days as the cerebral edema decreases. Changes in mentation, including apathy, irritability, disorientation, memory loss, withdrawal, drowsiness, stupor, or coma; bowel and bladder incontinence; numbness or loss of sensation; weakness or paralysis on part or one side of the body; aphasia; headache; neck stiffness and rigidity; vomiting; seizures; dizziness or syncope; ataxia; and fever may occur. A brainstem infarct leaving the patient completely paralyzed with intact cortical function is called *locked-in syndrome.* With cranial nerve involvement, visual disturbances include diplopia, blindness, and hemianopia. Inequality or fixation of the pupils, nystagmus, tinnitus, and difficulty chewing and swallowing also occur.

Because of the narrow 3-hr window in which it may be possible to reverse the likelihood of permanent neurologic damage, it is critical for the nurse to recognize the signs of a stroke and report them (and to teach patients not to ignore symptoms and to call 911) without delay for the following:

◆ Sudden numbness or weakness of the face, arm, or leg, especially on one side of the body
◆ Sudden confusion, trouble speaking or understanding
◆ Sudden trouble with seeing in one or both eyes
◆ Sudden trouble with walking, dizziness, loss of balance, or coordination
◆ Sudden, severe headache with no known cause

Some stroke resources use the STRO acronym for quick assessment or patient teaching purposes. It stands for *smile, talk, raise arms, (stick) out tongue.* If the patient suddenly cannot do these tasks, then a stroke may be suspected.

A history to determine time of symptom onset is critical inasmuch as this may determine eligibility for treatment. Time of onset is when patient was last known to be "normal," so if patient woke up after sleeping with symptoms, time of onset would be when the patient went to bed "normal" and not when the patient woke up symptomatic.

Papilledema, arteriosclerotic retinal changes, or hemorrhagic retinal areas may be seen on ophthalmic examination. Hyperactive deep tendon reflexes (DTRs), decreased superficial reflexes, and Babinski's sign also may be present. Kernig's or Brudzinski's sign (see "Bacterial Meningitis," p. 245) indicates meningeal irritation.

Other Assessment scales include Glasgow Coma Scale (GCS) and National Institutes of Health Stroke Scale (NIHSS): The GCS (see p. 307) is helpful for quickly assessing level of consciousness (LOC). The NIHSS is a 15-item neurologic evaluation assessment scale. It assesses not only LOC but also deficits and provides a standardized approach to neurologic examinations. An NIHSS total score of 0-1 is normal; 1-4 is a minor stroke; 5-15 is a moderate stroke; 15-20 is a moderately severe stroke; and more than 20 is a severe stroke. The NIHSS score also strongly predicts likelihood of recovery, with higher scores resulting in more disability and poorer outcomes. Use of thrombolytics (e.g., recombinant tissue plasminogen activator [rt-PA]) is considered appropriate for ischemic stroke if the total score is more than 4-6 and there is sustained, nonimproving deficit. The NIHSS is used for assessing effects of thrombolytic therapy and should, at minimum, be done initially as a baseline, 2 hr after treatment, 24 hr after the onset of symptoms, and 7-10 days after symptom onset. (The complete scale with instructions can be obtained at website: http://www.nihstrokescale.org.)

TIA: Typical symptoms include temporary episodes of slurred speech, weakness, numbness or tingling, blindness in one eye, blurred or double vision, dizziness or ataxia, and confusion.

History and risk factors: TIAs; hypertension; atherosclerosis; high serum cholesterol or triglycerides; high homocysteine levels; diabetes mellitus; gout; smoking; obesity; cardiac valve diseases, such as those that may result from rheumatic fever, valve prosthesis, and atrial fibrillation; cardiac surgery; blood dyscrasia; anticoagulant therapy; neck vessel trauma; oral contraceptive use; cocaine or methamphetamine use; family predisposition for arteriovenous malformation (AVM); aneurysm; advanced age; or previous stroke.

BOX 5-6 EVALUATION OF A PATIENT WITH SUSPECTED ACUTE ISCHEMIC STROKE: IMMEDIATE DIAGNOSTIC STUDIES

All Patients
- Brain computed tomography (CT) with noncontrast scan (brain magnetic resonance imaging [MRI] may be considered at qualified centers)
- ECG
- Laboratory values:
  - Serum electrolytes, including blood glucose, BUN, and creatinine
  - Complete blood count (CBC), including differential and platelet count
  - Coagulation: prothrombin time/international normalized ratio (INR) and partial thromboplastin time

Selected Patients
- Hepatic function tests
- Toxicology screen and blood alcohol determination
- Pregnancy test
- Oxygen saturation or arterial blood gas (ABG) tests (if hypoxia is suspected)
- Chest radiography (if lung disease is suspected)
- Lumbar puncture (if subarachnoid hemorrhage is suspected and CT result is negative for blood)
- Electroencephalogram (EEG) (if seizures are suspected)
- Cardiac enzymes if myocardial infarction is suspected

DIAGNOSTIC TESTS

Selection, sequence, and urgency of the following tests are determined by the patient's history and symptoms. For example, a patient whose symptoms have resolved from a TIA will have a different set or sequence of tests compared with the patient who is in coma. Because use of rt-PA is time limited, speed is essential in determining type of stroke (ischemic vs. hemorrhagic) and other contraindications to rt-PA. Obtaining CT scan to determine type of stroke is a top priority along with laboratory tests to assess for contraindications (**BOX 5-6**).

CT scan: Reveals site of infarction, hematoma, and shift of brain structures. CT scan is of particular value in identifying blood released early during hemorrhagic strokes. CT scan is the test of choice for unstable patients. Generally, identifying ischemic areas is difficult until they start to necrose at around 48-72 hr. Xenon-enhanced CT may be done to study CBF. CT angiography may be performed to evaluate blood vessels.

MRI: Reveals site of infarction, hematoma, shift of brain structure, and cerebral edema. MRI diffusion and perfusion weighted studies are of particular value in identifying ischemic strokes early and in differentiating between acute and chronic lesions. Other MR techniques include MR angiography to evaluate vessels and MR spectrography.

Laboratory tests: Certain tests should be done immediately to assess for contraindications if patient is a candidate for thrombolytic therapy. Other tests may done depending on patient's history and comorbidity (e.g., toxicology screen, pregnancy test, blood culture and erythrocyte sedimentation rate (ESR) for endocarditis or vasculitis process, glycosylated hemoglobin [HbA_{1c}] for diabetic patients). Lipid panel, C-reactive protein (CRP), and homocysteine levels also may be obtained.

ECG: Evaluates for atrial fibrillation and myocardial ischemia.

Phonoangiography and Doppler ultrasonography: Identify presence of bruits if the carotid blood vessels are partially occluded. B-mode imaging and duplex scanning also may be done to evaluate the carotid arteries to detect occlusive disease. Dimensional ultrasound improves three-dimensional visualization and includes the potential for quantitative monitoring of plaque volume changes in all three directions (circumference, length, and thickness).

Transcranial Doppler (TCD) ultrasound: Provides information (noninvasively) about pressure and flow in the intracranial arteries.

Swallowing examination/videofluoroscopy: All patients should be screened for dysphagia. Videofluoroscopy identifies problem or pathology, determines most appropriate treatment, and enables teaching of proper swallowing technique. This test is not performed for individuals known to aspirate saliva because it involves swallowing a barium-containing liquid, semisolid, and/or solid.

Positron emission tomography (PET): Provides information on cerebral metabolism and blood flow characteristics. This test is useful in identifying ischemic stroke by showing areas of reduced glucose metabolism.

Single photon emission computed tomography (SPECT): Identifies CBF.

EEG: Shows abnormal nerve impulse transmission and indicates amount of brain wave activity present.

Lumbar puncture (LP) and cerebrospinal fluid (CSF) analysis: Not done routinely, especially in the presence of IICP, but may reveal increase in CSF pressure; clear to bloody CSF, depending on stroke type; and presence of infection or other nonvascular cause for bleeding. Blood in the CSF signals that SAH has occurred.

Cerebral and carotid angiography: If surgery is contemplated, this procedure is done to pinpoint site of rupture or occlusion and identify collateral blood circulation, aneurysms, or AVM.

Digital subtraction angiography (DSA): Visualizes CBF and detects vascular abnormalities, such as stenosis, aneurysm, and hematomas.

Echocardiography (e.g., transthoracic and transesophageal): Evaluates valvular heart structures for thrombus and myocardial walls for mural thrombi that may provide a source of emboli.

Evoked response test: Provides measurement of the brain's ability to process and react to different sensory stimuli. Responses from these sensory stimuli can indicate abnormal areas in the brain.

Electronystagmography: Evaluates patients who have dizziness, vertigo, or balance dysfunction and provides objective assessment of oculomotor and vestibular systems.

COLLABORATIVE MANAGEMENT

Stroke care can be differentiated into these basic types: thrombolytic ischemic stroke care, nonthrombolytic ischemic stroke care (including TIAs), and hemorrhagic stroke care. Care differences center mostly around BP management and use of anticoagulant and antiplatelet agents. For appropriate patients, treatment with rt-PA needs to occur within 3 hr of symptom onset. To achieve this, all people should be educated to recognize warning signs of stroke and immediately call 911. Rapid transport to a hospital, preferably a stroke center, should occur, with the emergency medical technician (EMT) starting the medical history, especially the time of symptom onset, and alerting the hospital before arrival so the stroke team (if available) can be assembled. Upon arrival at the hospital door, the time-to-treatment goal is 60 min and is further broken down into subgoals as shown in **BOX 5-7**:

Intraarterial rt-PA, available at some research centers, may extend the window of opportunity to 6 hr. However, intracerebral bleeding is a major risk factor. Thrombolytic therapy reverses symptoms of stroke by dissolving the clot(s) causing the ischemia before actual cell death occurs. (See "Thrombolytic enzymes" in "Pharmacology" section later.)

Respiratory support: Airway maintenance, intubation, and ventilation as necessary. Monitor oximetry and arterial blood gas (ABG) values and provide O_2 to maintain saturation at 92% or greater. If indicated, O_2 is administered to prevent hypoxia. Preoxygenate before suctioning and limit suctioning to

BOX 5-7   TIME-TO-TREATMENT SUBGOALS
FOR STROKE CARE

TIME	TREATMENT
10 min	Evaluation by physician
15 min	Neurologic expert and "stroke team" (if available) contacted
25 min	Head CT or MRI completed; other data (e.g., laboratory values) collected
45 min	Interpretation of CT or MRI scan completed
	Decision to treat made based upon data, contraindications
60 min	Start of treatment (e.g., rt-PA) in appropriate patients.

CT, Computed tomography; MRI, magnetic resonance imaging; rt-PA, recombinant tissue plasminogen activator.

10 sec. CO_2 retention and the resulting respiratory acidosis can cause vasodilation of the cerebral arteries that lead to cerebral edema, and they are to be avoided. Lowering cerebral CO_2 results in alkalosis, which causes cerebral vasoconstriction and results in decreased CBF and ICP. The vasoconstriction also may cause decreased cerebral O_2 delivery, which could increase injury. Blowing off CO_2 through hyperventilation resulting in $PaCO_2$ less than 35 mm Hg generally is avoided and used only in cases of acute deterioration as a "quick fix" for IICP until other interventions such as mannitol can be instituted or in cases in which IICP is refractory and responds to nothing else. Ideally, CBF measurements, continuous jugular venous oxygen saturation (SjO_2), and brain tissue oxygenation ($PbtO_2$) are considered to monitor for effectiveness (i.e., decreased IICP without decreased cerebral O_2 delivery) if hyperventilation is used as a treatment.

IV fluids: Maintenance of electrolyte balance and normovolemia. IV solutions should be saline rather than glucose. Blood glucose level greater than 150 mg/dL may increase infarct size. Fluid restrictions are avoided because the resulting increased blood viscosity and decreased volume may lead to hypotension, decreasing CPP.

Positioning: Bed rest during acute stage. Activity level is increased as patient's condition improves. The head of bed (HOB) is positioned at whatever level optimizes cerebral perfusion pressure (CPP) or as prescribed. Without monitoring equipment, having HOB at 30 degrees is considered safe and effective in promoting venous drainage and helping reduce cerebral edema as long as patient is not hypovolemic, which could threaten CPP. For patients with hemiplegia, provide firm support for affected arm and avoid pulling on arm, to prevent shoulder subluxation. Elevate hand to prevent shoulder-hand syndrome, characterized by pain, edema, and muscle atrophy.

Diet: Nothing by mouth (NPO) status and possible gastric tube if swallow and gag reflexes are diminished or if patient has decreased LOC. Total parenteral nutrition (TPN) may be needed. A swallowing evaluation should be done before restoring oral intake. A low-Na^+ (see Box 4-1, for high Na^{++} foods, p. 165) and/or low-fat (see Table 3-2, p. 101), low-cholesterol (see Table 3-1, p. 101) diet may be prescribed to minimize other risk factors. Diet may consist of fluids and pureed, soft, or chopped foods or tube feedings, depending on patient's LOC and ability to chew and swallow. A gastrostomy (percutaneous endoscopic gastroscopy [PEG], percutaneous endoscopic jejunoscopy [PEJ]) tube may be required for nutrition, especially in aspiration-prone patients.

Deep vein thrombosis (DVT) prevention: Use of sequential compression devices (SCDs) is recommended for all immobilized patients, although patients receiving thrombolytic therapy should not use these devices for the first 24 hr because of bleeding concerns. Anticoagulants (e.g., enoxaparin) are recommended once risk of bleeding is no longer a consideration.

Pressure ulcer prevention: Meticulous skin care and turning are mandatory. Wheelchair-bound patients need to lift themselves up and shift weight q15-30min and use gel cushions for extra padding. Fingernails are kept clipped to avoid scratches and abrasions. (See p. 722, "Pressure Ulcers," for more details.)

Hyperglycemia prevention: Because hyperglycemia is associated with poorer outcomes, glucose is closely monitored and kept under strict control. Intensive insulin therapy may be used during the acute phase while patient is in intensive care unit (ICU), with insulin drips and frequent monitoring to keep glucose at less than 110-120 mg/dL. After stabilization, sliding scale may used to keep glucose at less than 140-150 mg/dL. A better method to keep blood glucose levels at standard is to determine the total daily dose, divide it equally, and manipulate it based on the last 24-hr glucose profile.

Pharmacotherapy

Thrombolytic enzymes (e.g., rt-PA): Cause lysing of the thrombus or embolus obstructing cerebral arteries in an acute, nonhemorrhagic stroke. These agents are administered by IV infusion and must be given within 3 hr to restore circulation and save brain tissue. Intraarterial thrombolytics also have been used to restore blood flow and may extend treatment window to 6 hr, but intracerebral bleeding is a serious risk factor. Follow standard bleeding precautions accordingly. Ischemic stroke may undergo hemorrhagic transformation after rt-PA administration. High BP may be a factor in hemorrhage, and recommendations are to keep SBP less than 185 mm Hg and DBP less than 110 mm Hg. Intracranial bleeding is considered the cause of neurologic worsening until computed tomography (CT) confirms or refutes hemorrhage.

Anticoagulants: Patients receiving thrombolytics should not be given heparin, warfarin, enoxaparin, or other anticoagulants for 24 hr after rt-PA. Anticoagulants are contraindicated with hemorrhagic stroke while there is still risk of bleeding. Once risk of bleeding is no longer present, low-molecular-weight heparin (e.g., enoxaparin) should be started in nonambulatory patients to prevent DVT formation. Patients with strokes caused by emboli (e.g., with atrial fibrillation, thrombus in heart, or cardiomyopathy) usually are started on long-term warfarin or low-dose low-molecular-weight heparin therapy. Patients with TIAs or ischemic strokes who are not treated with thrombolytics may receive low-molecular-weight heparin (e.g., enoxaparin) or subcutaneous heparin to prevent further thrombosis. Ginkgo biloba and garlic may prolong bleeding times of anticoagulants and should be avoided.

Antihypertensive agents (e.g., labetalol, hydralazine, enalapril): Control very high BP, which may cause cerebral edema and IICP. High SBP may be needed to maintain cerebral perfusion and prevent further ischemia in acute ischemic stroke that is not treated with thrombolytics; therefore, BP may not be substantially lowered initially, or if very high (SBP greater than 220 mm Hg or DBP greater than 120 mm Hg), BP should be lowered slowly. For acute intracerebral hemorrhage, the recommended BP goal is usually SBP less than 180 mm Hg and DBP less than 105 mm Hg. After stabilization, hypertensive patients should be placed on medication (e.g., angiotensin-converting enzyme (ACE) inhibitors, calcium channel blockers, thiazide diuretics) with a goal of obtaining a BP less than 140/90 mm Hg.

Insulin: Usually regular insulin subcutaneously (sliding scale coverage) or intensive insulin therapy (during acute phase) to control hyperglycemia.

Antiplatelet medications (e.g., aspirin, clopidogrel, or aspirin with extended-release dipyridamole): Prevent platelet aggregation that may lead to thrombus formation. Patients with TIAs or those at risk for additional thrombotic strokes may be started on this therapy to prevent future ischemic strokes from thrombosis. It is recommended that most patients with ischemic strokes receive aspirin within 48 hr of stroke. These medications should not be used in the presence of hemorrhagic stroke.

Vasopressors (e.g., dopamine): Treat low BP, which may increase ischemia.

Osmotic diuretics (e.g., mannitol): Prevent or reduce cerebral edema.

Proton pump inhibitors (e.g., pantoprazole), histamine H₂-receptor blockers (e.g., famotidine), and sucralfate: Reduce the risk of GI hemorrhage from gastric ulcer caused by stress.

Antiepileptic drugs (AEDs) (e.g., carbamazepine, phenytoin, fosphenytoin, diazepam): Control and prevent seizures if present.

Sedatives/tranquilizers (e.g., diphenhydramine): Promote rest. These are used cautiously to avoid further impairment of neurologic function.

Analgesics (e.g., acetaminophen): Control headache. If stroke is hemorrhagic, aspirin is avoided because it can increase bleeding.

Stool softeners (e.g., docusate): Prevent straining, which can result in IICP.

Antipyretics (e.g., acetaminophen): Reduce fever, which increases cerebral metabolic needs. During the acute phase, patients may be kept mildly hypothermic with antipyretics and cooling measures (e.g., lowered room temperature, cooling blankets, convection devices) because cooling appears to be neuroprotective.

Hemodilution (e.g., albumin, crystalloid fluids): Promotes hydration via IV fluids and volume expanders to decrease blood viscosity (Hct to 30%-35%) to improve CBF through narrowed arteries.

Statins (lipid-lowering medication, e.g., pravastatin, lovastatin, simvastatin): Reduce risk of future strokes.

Hypervolemic infusions (e.g., plasma protein fraction, whole blood, saline, albumin, hetastarch): Increase CPP via increased blood volume.

Arginine derivaties (e.g., argatroban): Direct thrombin inhibitors that appear to provide safe anticoagulation in acute ischemic stroke.

Treatment of secondary complications: Cerebral edema, IICP, aspiration, pneumonia, DVT, pulmonary embolism (PE), pressure ulcers, syndrome of inappropriate antidiuretic hormone (SIADH), diabetes insipidus (DI), and seizures all may occur. These are treated as necessary.

ROM exercises: Maintain or increase joint function and prevent contractures. Exercises may include passive ROM, active ROM, or active-assistive ROM. Passive ROM is started immediately for all joints.

Physical medicine and rehabilitation program tailored to patient's deficits: Promote early mobilization and help patient maintain mobility and independence with activities of daily living (ADL); may include physical therapy (PT), occupational therapy (OT), and assistive devices or braces. Muscle strengthening exercises, conditioning exercises, swallowing facilitation exercises, and gait training are often prescribed also. Reinforce special mobilization techniques, such as the Bobath Concept or Constraint-Induced Movement Therapy, which focus on restoring bilateral function and incorporating affected side into weight bearing, or Proprioceptive Neuromuscular Facilitation (PNF) stretching, which focuses on using reflex and patterning techniques. In BWSTT, patient's body is supported during therapy (eliminating risk of falls resulting from coordination and balance problems), and legs are supported as well and are moved along a treadmill in a repetitive up-and-down pattern that mimics walking. Patient progressively does more weight bearing, which promotes ambulation and gait recovery. Repeated leg movements can teach the damaged neural pathways to adapt, reorganize, and respond.

Functional electrical stimulation (FES): Improves arm function and reduces shoulder subluxation in the hemiplegic patient.

Speech therapy with swallowing evaluations: Helps aphasic and dysarthric patients. Swallowing evaluations may include modified barium swallows performed with videofluoroscopy, ultrasound, or fiberoptic endoscopy to determine laryngeal/pharyngeal deficits. Aphasia is the partial or complete inability to use or comprehend language and symbols and may occur with dominant (left) hemisphere damage. It is not the result of impaired hearing or intelligence. There are many different types of aphasia. Generally the patient has a combination of types, which vary in severity. *Fluent aphasia* (e.g., Wernicke's, sensory, or receptive aphasia) is characterized by inability to recognize or comprehend spoken words. It is as if a foreign language was being spoken or the patient had word deafness. The patient often is good at responding to nonverbal cues. In *nonfluent aphasia* (e.g., Broca's, motor, or expressive aphasia), the ability to understand and comprehend language is retained, but the patient has difficulty expressing words or naming objects. Gestures, groans, swearing, or nonsense words may be used. A short-term, intense language training program called constraint-induced aphasia therapy (CIAT) includes strategies to constrain nonverbal communication attempts in order to foster stable, long-term improvement in communication skills in stroke survivors.

Bowel and bladder programs: Engaged to prevent constipation and incontinence. The patient initially may have an indwelling catheter but should soon start a bladder program to prevent incontinence or retention.

Carotid endarterectomy: Surgical removal of plaque in the obstructed artery to increase blood supply to the brain. The carotid artery is clamped while the artery is opened, the plaque removed, and the artery sutured or patched. CBF studies and EEG monitoring may be done during the procedure. A shunt is sometimes done while the carotid artery is occluded. This is treatment of choice for patients with TIAs or RINDs or asymptomatic patients with stenosis greater than 70% when a lesion lies at or near the carotid bifurcation. This procedure is not generally performed for patients who have experienced a stroke except to correct a stenosis to the unaffected hemisphere. Patients may be placed in ICU postoperatively if vasoactive BP drugs are needed or if they are neurologically unstable. Hyperperfusion syndrome, with severe unilateral headache, changes in LOC, focal neurologic signs, and possible seizures or intracerebral hemorrhage, is best treated via prevention with strict control of postoperative SBP to 150 mm Hg or less with labetalol, nitroprusside, or nitroglycerin.

Carotid angioplasty and stent: Open up the stenosed carotid vessel. Patients may be placed in ICU postoperatively if vasoactive BP drips are needed or if they are neurologically unstable. Balloon angioplasty and stenting are being performed in some cases to open other stenosed intracranial vessels. Proximal embolic protection devices that deploy occlusion balloons may be used to produce retrograde blood flow to prevent embolization to the brain during stent insertions. After the procedure, aspirin (acetylsalicylic acid [ASA]), clopidogrel, and glycoprotein IIb/IIIa inhibitors (e.g., abciximab) may be prescribed.

Other endovascular procedures to open blockages: Endovascular embolectomy and clot disruption are being done with a number of techniques including lasers, ultrasonography (used to help break down fibrin and dissolve thrombi), microcatheter or microwire clot maceration, intraarterial suction devices, and a variety of clot-retrieval or micro-snare devices, used alone or with intraarterial thrombolysis. Some of these are still in the testing phases.

Burr hole aspiration of hematoma: Performed under stereotaxic CT or ultrasound guidance.

Craniotomy: Performed to evacuate a hematoma, repair a ruptured aneurysm, or apply arterial clips or plastic spray to the involved vessel to prevent further rupture. (See "Traumatic Brain Injury," p. 314, for patient care.)

Social service evaluation: Assists with poststroke discharge needs and assesses for poststroke depression.

Education programs: All patients need stroke education that includes knowledge of stroke warning signs and awareness of need to call 911 for warning signs and of the individual's own risk factors. Education regarding appropriate modifiable risk factors (**BOX 5-8**) should be included.

NURSING DIAGNOSES AND INTERVENTIONS

Unilateral neglect related to disturbed perceptual ability secondary to neurologic insult

BOX 5-8   RISK FACTOR MODIFICATION
FOR ISCHEMIC STROKE PREVENTION

- High blood pressure management with angiotensin-converting enzyme inhibitors, calcium channel blockers, and possibly thiazide diuretic therapy to obtain a goal of blood pressure less than 140/90 mm Hg
- Smoking cessation counseling and nicotine replacement therapies
- Lipid- and cholesterol-lowering therapy with statins
- Antithrombotic and antiplatelet agents
- Weight management
- Regular exercise program
- Diet management (e.g., low fat, low cholesterol, low salt)
- Atrial fibrillation management with anticoagulation (e.g., warfarin)
- Diabetes management with optimal glucose control through diet, oral hypoglycemic agents, or insulin to keep fasting blood sugar at less than 126 mg and maintain hemglobin A_{1c} level between 3% and 6%
- Reduction of alcohol consumption
- Use of supplements that appear to reduce risk factors: B vitamins (e.g., folic acid, B_6, B_{12}) to lower homocysteine levels and omega-3 polyunsaturated fatty acids for their endothelial-protective, antiatherogenic, and antiplatelet aggregation effects

Desired outcome: Following intervention and on an ongoing basis, patient scans the environment and responds to stimuli on affected side.

Nursing Interventions

- Assess patient's ability to recognize objects to right or left of his or her visual midline; perceive body parts as his or her own; perceive pain, touch, and temperature sensations; judge distances; orient self to changes in the environment; differentiate left from right; maintain posture sense; and identify objects by sight, hearing, or touch.
- Assess for neglect of affected side. Neglect of and inattention to stimuli on affected side occur more often with right hemisphere injury. Neglect cannot be totally explained on the basis of loss of physical senses (e.g., both ears are used in hearing, but with auditory neglect, patient may ignore conversation or noises that occur on affected side).
  - *Visual neglect:* Patient does not turn head to see all parts of an object (e.g., may read only half of a page or eat from only one side of plate). When patient exhibits signs of visual neglect, continue to place objects necessary for ADL and call bells on unaffected side and approach patient from that side, gradually increasing stimuli on affected side (e.g., while communicating with patient, physically move across patient's visual boundary and stand on that side to shift patient's attention to neglected side; encourage patient to turn head past the midline and scan entire environment; place patient's food on neglected side, encouraging patient to look to neglected side and name the food before eating; place a bright red tape or ribbon on affected side, and encourage patient to scan and find it). Continuously cue patient to the environment. Initially place patient's unaffected side toward most active part of room, but as compensation occurs, reverse this. As patient begins to compensate, place additional items out of his or her visual field. It is particularly important for patient to scan environment while ambulating. *This is to prevent injury from falls or bumping into things.*
  - *Self-neglect:* Patient does not perceive arm or leg as being a part of the body. For example, when combing or brushing hair, patient attends to only one (unaffected) side of the head. Inadequate self-care and injury may occur. Encourage patient to touch or massage and look at affected

side and make a conscious effort to care for neglected body parts; also, check for proper position. *This is to ensure against contractures and skin breakdown.* Periodically refer to patient's body parts on neglected side. *This is to enhance patient's self-recognition.* Provide affected side with warm washcloth, cold ice chip, rough or soft-surfaced cloth, or similar item. *This is to provide structured tactile stimulation.* When patient is in bed or sitting up in a chair, use side rails or restraints. *This is a safety measure to prevent patient from attempting to get up and falling, which can occur as a result of unawareness of affected side.* Teach patient to use unaffected arm to perform ROM exercises on affected side. Integrate patient's neglected arm into activities. Position arm on bedside table or wheelchair lap board with hand or arm past the midline, where patient can see it. Teach patient to attend to affected side first when performing ADL, consciously look for affected side, monitor its position, and check for exposure to sharp objects and irritants. Instruct patient to take precautions with hot or cold items or when around moving machinery. Provide a mirror so that patient can watch himself or herself shave or brush teeth and hair. If patient needs a lapboard, one that is transparent (e.g., made with plexiglass) will enable patient to view affected leg when sitting. Teach use of arm sling. *This is to support affected arm when out of bed.* Teach teach patient to elevate affected arm when in bed. *This will prevent edema or the arm from hanging or flopping.* Stand on patient's affected side when ambulating with patient.

- *Auditory neglect:* Patient ignores individuals who approach and speak from affected side but communicates with those who approach or speak from unaffected side. Move across auditory boundary while speaking, and continue speaking from patient's neglected side. *This is to stimulate patient's attention to affected side and to to bring patient's attention to that area.*

◆ Arrange environment to maximize performance of ADL by keeping necessary objects, such as call light, on patient's unaffected side. If possible, move bed so that patient's unaffected side faces room's largest section. Approach and speak to patient from unaffected side. Announce yourself if you approach from the affected side. *This is to avoid startling the patient.* Perform activities on unaffected side unless specifically attempting to stimulate neglected side. After attempting to stimulate neglected side, return to patient's unaffected side for activities and communication. Inform significant other about patient's deficit and compensatory interventions.

Impaired physical mobility related to neuromuscular impairment with limited use of the upper and/or lower limbs secondary to stroke
Desired outcome: By at least 24 hr before hospital discharge, patient and significant other demonstrate techniques that promote ambulating and transferring.

Nursing Interventions

◆ Teach methods for turning and moving, by using stronger extremity to move weaker extremity. For example, to move affected leg in bed or when changing from a lying to a sitting position, slide unaffected foot under affected ankle to lift, support, and bring affected leg along in the desired movement.

◆ Encourage patient to make a conscious attempt to look at extremities and check position before moving. Remind patient to make a conscious effort to lift and then extend foot when ambulating.

◆ Instruct patient with impaired sense of balance to compensate by leaning toward stronger side. (The tendency is to lean toward weaker or paralyzed side.) As necessary, remind patient to keep body weight forward over feet when standing. Recommend wearing well-fitting shoes. *This is because slippers tend to slide.*

- Monitor for subluxation of the shoulder (e.g., shoulder pain and tenderness, swelling, decreased ROM, altered appearance of bony prominences). *Shoulder subluxation can occur when weight of the affected arm is unable to be supported by the weakened shoulder muscles, with resulting separation of the shoulder joint.* Never pull on the affected arm. Guide upper extremity movement from the scapula and not from the arm; use a lift sheet to reposition in bed. Ensure that the arm has a firm support surface when patient is sitting. When in bed the patient's shoulder should be positioned slightly forward. *This is to counteract shoulder rotation.* The affected arm should be placed in external rotation when the patient is supine or lying on affected side.
- Encourage repeated shoulder movement, elevation of the arm above cardiac level, and regular fist clenching and reclenching. *This is to prevent shoulder-hand syndrome, a neurovascular condition characterized by pain, edema, and skin and muscle atrophy caused by impairment of the circulatory pumping action of the upper extremity.* Prevent this syndrome with regular, gentle joint ROM exercises and proper arm positioning. Never place arm under the body. When patient is in bed, place arm on abdomen or pillow for support.
- Protect impaired arm with a sling to support arm and shoulder when patient is up. *This is to help maintain anatomic position.* Position patient in correct alignment, and provide a pillow or lapboard for support. Encourage active/passive ROM. *This will improve muscle tone.*
- General principles when transferring include the following:
  - Encourage weight bearing on patient's stronger side. Use a transfer belt to safely support patient during transfers without putting excessive stress on upper extremities. A helper should stand and walk on patient's affected side.
  - Instruct patient to pivot on stronger side and use stronger arm for support.
  - Teach patient that transferring toward unaffected side is generally easiest and safest.
  - Instruct patient to place unaffected side closest to bed or chair to which he or she wishes to transfer.
  - Explain that when transferring, affected leg should be under patient with foot flat on the ground.
  - Position a braced chair or locked wheelchair close to patient's stronger side. If patient requires assistance from staff member, teach patient not to support self by pulling on or placing hands around assistant's neck. Staff members should use their own knees and feet to brace feet and knees of patients who are very weak.
- Obtain physical therapy (PT) and occupational therapy (OT) referrals as appropriate. Reinforce special mobilization techniques per patient's individualized rehabilitation program. These techniques may vary from the general principles mentioned. For example, the Bobath Concept focuses on use of affected side in mobility training so that patient tries to bear weight on affected side and move toward affected side to relearn normal movement patterns and position.

Disturbed sensory perception related to altered sensory reception, transmission, and/or integration secondary to neurologic damage
Desired outcome: Following intervention and on an ongoing basis, patient interacts appropriately with his or her environment and does not exhibit evidence of injury caused by sensory/perceptual deficit.

Nursing Interventions

- Patients who have a dominant (left) hemisphere injury usually have normal awareness of their body and spatial orientation despite possible lack of or decreased pain sensation, position sense, and visual field deficit on right side of body. These patients may need reminders to scan their environment but usually do not exhibit unilateral neglect. They tend to be slow, cautious, and disorganized when approaching an unfamiliar problem and benefit from frequent, accurate, and immediate feedback on their performance. They may respond well to nonverbal encouragement, such as a pat on the back. Give short, simple messages or questions and step-by-step directions. *This is bacause patient is easily distracted and may have poor abstract thinking skills.* Keep conversation on a concrete level (e.g., say "water," not "fluid"; "leg," not "limb"). *This is because of a short attention span and impaired logical reasoning.* Patient may benefit from touching items (e.g., washcloth, comb) while caretaker names them. *This is helpful because patient may have difficulty recognizing items by touch.*

◆ Patients with nondominant (right) hemisphere injury also may have decreased pain sensation, pain sense, and visual field deficit but typically are unconcerned or unaware of or deny deficits or lost abilities. They tend to be impulsive and too quick with movements. Typically, they have impaired judgment about what they can and cannot do and often overestimate their abilities. Encourage these patients to slow down and check each step or task as it is completed. *This is because they are at risk for burns, bruises, cuts, and falls and may need to be restrained from attempting unsafe activities.* They also are more likely to have unilateral neglect than individuals with dominant (left) hemisphere injury (see **Unilateral neglect,** p. 336). These patients generally retain ability to think logically but see specifics rather than the global picture (i.e., can see trees but not the forest). Be careful what you say to the patient or around the patient to others. *This is because it may be taken literally, and that may not be the actual intent of what was said.* Impaired ability to recognize subtle distinctions may occur (e.g., the difference between a fork and spoon may become too subtle to detect).

◆ Patients with apraxia have an inability to carry out previously learned motor tasks, although they may be able to describe them in detail. Have these patients return-demonstrate the task. They may be able to be talked through a task or may be able to talk themselves through a task step by step.

◆ Patients may have visual field deficits in which they can physically see only a portion of the normal visual field. Encourage making a conscious effort to scan the rest of the environment by turning head from side to side. *This is to prevent falls or running into objects.*

◆ Patients with nondominant (right) hemisphere injury also may have the following sensory perceptual alterations:

  • *Impaired ability to recognize, associate, or interpret sounds* (e.g., voice quality, animal noises, musical pieces, types of instruments): Direct patient's attention to a particular sound (e.g., if a cat meows on the television, state that it is the sound a cat makes and point to the cat on the screen).

  • *Visual-spatial misconception:* Patient may have trouble judging distance, size, position, rate of movement, form, and how parts relate to the whole (e.g., patient may underestimate distances and bump into doors or confuse inside and outside of an object, such as an article of clothing). Affected patients may lose their place when reading or adding up numbers and therefore never complete the task. Mark outer aspects of their shoes or tag inside sleeve of a sweater or pair of pants with "L" and "R" designations. *This is to help self-dressing efforts.* These patients will benefit from a structured, consistent environment.

  • *Difficulty recognizing and associating familiar objects:* Affected patients may not recognize dangerous or hazardous objects. *This is because they do not know the purpose of the object.* Assist these individuals with eating. *This is because they may not know purpose of silverware.* Monitor environment for safety hazards, and remove unsafe objects such as scissors from the bedside.

- *Inability to orient self in space:* Affected patients may require a restraint or wheelchair belt for support. They may not know whether they are standing, sitting, or leaning.
- *Misconception of own body and body parts:* Affected patients may not perceive their foot or arm as being a part of their body. Teach them to concentrate on body parts (e.g., by watching feet carefully while walking). Provide a mirror to help them adjust.
- *Impaired ability to recognize objects by means of senses of hearing, vibration, or touch:* Affected patients rely more on visual cues. Keep their environment simple. *This is to reduce sensory overload and enable concentration on visual cues.* Remove distracting stimuli.
- *Trouble recognizing emotional cues:* Patient may not be able to tell from voice, tone, words, or expression when others are happy, sad, or angry.

Impaired verbal communication related to aphasia secondary to cerebrovascular insult
Desired outcome: At least 24 hr before hospital discharge, patient demonstrates improved self-expression and relates decreased frustration with communication.

Nursing Interventions

- ♦ Evaluate nature and severity of patient's aphasia. When doing so, avoid giving nonverbal cues. Assess patient's ability to speak clearly without slurring words, use words appropriately, point or look toward a specific object, follow simple directions, understand yes/no questions, understand complex questions, repeat both simple and complex words, repeat sentences, name objects that are shown, demonstrate or relate purpose or action of objects, fulfill written requests, write requests, and read. When evaluating for aphasia, be aware that patient may be responding to nonverbal cues and may understand less than you think. Use this assessment as the basis for a communication plan.
- ♦ Obtain referral to a speech therapist or pathologist as needed. Provide therapist with a list of words that would enhance patient's independence and/or care. In addition, ask for tips that will help improve communication with patient.
- ♦ Treat patient as an adult. It is not necessary to raise volume of your voice unless patient is hard of hearing. Be respectful.
- ♦ Communicate frequently with the patient. Do not pretend you understand if you do not. Ask patient to repeat by speaking slowly in short phrases. Nonverbal cues, pointing, flash cards of basic needs, pantomine, paper/pen, spelling, or picture board may help communication.General principles for patients who may not recognize or comprehend the spoken word include the following: face patient and establish eye contact, speak slowly and clearly, give patient time to process your communication and answer, keep messages short and simple, stay with one clearly defined subject, avoid questions with multiple choices but rather phrase questions so that they can be answered "yes" or "no," and use same words each time you repeat a statement or question (e.g., pill vs. medication, bathroom vs. toilet). If patient does not understand after repetition, try different words. Use gestures, facial expressions, and pantomime to supplement and reinforce your message. Give short, simple directions, and repeat as needed to ensure understanding. Use concrete terms (e.g., water instead of fluid, leg instead of limb). Keep a record at the bedside of words to be used (e.g., pill rather than medication). *This ensures continuity among staff.* Reduce distractions in the environment, such as television or others' conversations. Try to ensure that patient is well rested. *Fatigue affects ability to communicate.*

- ◆ When helping patient regain use of symbolic language, start with nouns first and progress to more complex statements as indicated, using verbs, pronouns, and adjectives.
- ◆ When patient has difficulty expressing words or naming objects, encourage patient to repeat words after you for practice in verbal expression. Begin with simple words such as "yes" or "no," and progress to others, such as "cup." Progress to more complex statements as indicated. Listen and respond to patient's communication efforts; otherwise patient may give up. Praise accomplishments. Be prepared for labile emotions because these patients become frustrated and emotional when faced with their impaired speech. When improvement is noted, let patient complete your sentence (e.g., "This is a _____"). Keep a list of words patient can say, and add to list as appropriate. Use this list when forming questions patient can answer. Avoid finishing patient's sentences.
- ◆ Avoid labeling patient as belligerent or confused when the problem is aphasia with resultant frustration. *Patients who have lost ability to monitor their verbal output may not produce sensible language but may think they are making sense and not understand why others do not comprehend or respond appropriately to them.* Listen for errors in conversation, and provide feedback.
- ◆ Avoid instructing patient to "wait 5 minutes" because this may not be meaningful. *Patients who have lost ability to recognize number symbols or relationships will have difficulty understanding time concepts or telling time.*
- ◆ Give practice in receiving word images by pointing to an object and clearly stating its name. Watch signals patient gives you.
- ◆ Bring patient back to the subject when drifting occurs by saying, "Let's go back to what we were talking about." *Patients with nondominant (right) hemisphere damage often have no difficulty speaking but they may use excessive detail, give irrelevant information, and go off on a tangent.*
- ◆ Provide a supportive and relaxed environment for patient who is unable to form words or sentences or speak clearly or appropriately. If patient makes an error, do not criticize patient's effort but rather compliment it. Do not react negatively to emotional displays. *This may complicate the patient's frustration even more.* Address and acknowledge patient's frustration over the inability to communicate. Maintain a calm and positive attitude. Ask patient to repeat unclear words, ask for more clues, ask patient to use another word, or have patient point to the object. Observe for nonverbal cues, and anticipate patient's needs. Allow time to listen if patient speaks slowly. To validate patient's message, repeat or rephrase it aloud.
- ◆ Ensure that the call light is available and patient knows how to use it.
- ◆ For additional nursing interventions for patients with dysarthria, see **Impaired verbal communication** in "General Care of Patients with Neurologic Deficits," p. 362. *Dysarthria can complicate aphasia.*

Deficient knowledge related to carotid endarterectomy or carotid angioplasty/stent procedure
Desired outcome: Before surgery, patient verbalizes understanding of the carotid endarterectomy procedure, including the purpose, risks, expected benefits or outcome, and postsurgical care.

Nursing Interventions

- ◆ After health care provider has explained the procedure to the patient, determine patient's level of understanding and facility with language; employ an interpreter or provide language-appropriate written materials, and reinforce or clarify information as needed.

For Patient Undergoing Carotid Endarterectomy

- ◆ Explain that carotid endarterectomy is removal of plaque in the obstructed artery to increase blood supply to the brain.

◆ Describe the following postsurgical assessments:
  • VS and neurologic status at least hourly. Pupils will be monitored with a light, and hands and legs will be tested. *This is to monitor for weakness and equality.* Explain that patient may be asked to swallow, move the tongue, smile, speak, and shrug shoulders. *This is to determine facial drooping, tongue weakness, hoarseness, dysphagia, shoulder weakness, or loss of facial sensation, which are signs of cranial nerve impairment.* Stretching of the cranial nerves during surgery can occur, causing edema, and may leave a temporary deficit. Patient should report any numbness, tingling, or weakness. *This may indicate carotid occlusion.* Superficial temporal and facial pulses will be palpated for strength, quality, and symmetry. *This is to evaluate patency of the external carotid artery.* Patient will be evaluated for gag reflex, tongue deviation, and difficulty with speech.
  • Periodic assessment of the neck for edema, hematoma, bleeding, or tracheal deviation from midline will be performed. Explain that patient should report immediately any respiratory distress, difficulty managing secretions, or sensation of neck tightness. Additional O_2 will most likely be supplied, even without respiratory distress or airway compromise. *This is because manipulation of the carotid sinus may cause temporary loss of normal physiologic response to hypoxia.*
  • Pulse oximetry may be continuously monitored. Report readings less than 92% to health care providers.
  • Frequent BP checks may be performed. *This is because temporary carotid sinus dysfunction may cause BP problems (usually hypertension).* Patient may need vasoactive medications. *They are given to keep SBP within a specified range (usually 100-150 mm Hg) to maintain cerebral perfusion while preventing disruption of graft or sutures.*
◆ HOB must be maintained in prescribed position (flat or elevated), and patient generally is positioned on the side opposite to the operative side.
◆ A closed drainage system with suction may be left in the neck for a day. Ice packs may be prescribed. *This is for the incision, to reduce edema formation and pain.*
◆ Anticoagulant/antiplatelet therapy (e.g., aspirin, warfarin) may be instituted for 3-6 mo after the procedure and may continue longer, depending on patient.
◆ Include home instructions for the following:
  • *Incision care:* Wash gently with soap and water.
  • *Signs of infection:* Incision red, swollen, and painful; drainage, fever greater than 100.5° F (38° C).
  • *Activity restrictions:* No heavy lifting, no driving while neck turning is uncomfortable.
  • *Changes in neurologic status:* Such as alterations in speech, swallowing, vision, and numbness or weakness in arm or leg, especially on opposite side.

For Patients Undergoing Carotid Angioplasty and Stenting
◆ Explain that angioplasty is the opening of a stenosed artery via a slender catheter that is passed through the narrow spot with balloon inflation to open up the obstruction. A stent, which will physically hold the newly unblocked vessel open, also may be placed.
◆ Explain that frequent VS and neurologic checks, including cranial nerves, will be performed. *Cranial nerve problems are less frequent with this procedure because nerves have not been stretched, but they still should be checked.* BP medications will be given. *This is to keep BP within specified parameters.*
◆ Advise patient that because the femoral artery is the usual vessel accessed, groin and distal pulses will be monitored. *This is to assess for bleeding and patency.*
◆ Explain that HOB is usually elevated.

◆ Advise that patients are usually discharged the next day and go home on anticoagulants (e.g., aspirin or ticlopidine).

 Patient-Family Teaching and Discharge Planning

Poststroke care and teaching needs vary depending on the patient's residual limitations or complications. Include verbal and written information about the following:

◆ Symptoms that necessitate prompt attention: sudden weakness, numbness (especially on one side of the body), vision loss or dimming, trouble talking or understanding speech, unexplained dizziness, unsteadiness, or severe headache.
◆ Interventions for safe swallowing and aspiration prevention.
◆ Importance of minimizing or treating the following risk factors: diabetes mellitus, hypertension, high cholesterol, high Na$^+$ intake, obesity, inactivity, smoking, prolonged bed rest, and stressful lifestyle. Also see Box 5-8.
◆ Interventions that increase effective communication in the presence of aphasia or dysarthria. Additional patient information can be obtained by accessing the following:

National Aphasia Association: www.aphasia.org

◆ Referrals to the following as appropriate: public health nurse, psychologic therapy, vocational rehabilitation agency, home health agencies, and extended and skilled care facilities.
◆ For patient information pamphlets, access the following website:
◆ National Institute of Neurological Disorders and Stroke (NINDS) (website): www.ninds.nih.gov
◆ Additional general information, which can be obtained by accessing the following:

American Stroke Association: www.strokeassociation.org

American Stroke Foundation: www.americanstroke.org

National Stroke Association: www.stroke.org

Stroke Information Directory: www.stroke-info.com

Stroke Survivor: www.strokesurvivor.org

The Internet Stroke Center: www.strokecenter.org

❖ ❖ ❖

SECTION FIVE   **SEIZURES AND EPILEPSY**
OVERVIEW/PATHOPHYSIOLOGY

Seizures result from an abnormal, uncontrolled electrical discharge from the neurons of the cerebral cortex in response to a stimulus. If the activity is localized in one portion of the brain, the individual will have a partial seizure, but when it is widespread and diffuse, a generalized seizure occurs. Symptoms vary widely, depending on the involved area of the cerebral cortex. Seizures are generally manifested as an alteration in sensation, behavior, movement, perception, or consciousness lasting from seconds to several minutes. A seizure can be an isolated incident that may not recur once the underlying cause is corrected (e.g., fever, alcohol withdrawal). *Epilepsy* is the term used for recurrent, unprovoked seizures. It is characterized by the occurrence of at least two unprovoked seizures 24 hr apart.

Seizure threshold refers to the amount of stimulation needed to cause neural activity. Although anyone can have a seizure if the stimulus is sufficient, the seizure threshold is lowered in some individuals, and this may result

BOX 5-9   RECOMMENDED CLASSIFICATION
                OF SEIZURES

Generalized Seizures
- Tonic clonic (in any combination)
- Absence
  1. Typical
  2. Atypical
  3. Absence with special features
     - Myoclonic absence
     - Eyelid myoclonia
- Myoclonic
  1. Myoclonic
  2. Myoclonic atonic
  3. Myoclonic tonic
- Clonic
- Tonic
- Atonic
- Epileptic spasms

Focal Seizures
- These can be further described as a function of seizure severity, putative site of origin, elemental sequence of events, or other features.
- Syndromes themselves will no longer be classified as being focal (or localization-related or partial) versus generalized.

From Commission on Classification and Terminology of the International League Against Epilepsy, *Summary of key recommendations from the Commission on Classification and Terminology* (website): www.ilae.org. Accessed May 2009.

in spontaneous seizures. If a trigger stimulus is identified, the individual has what is termed *reflex epilepsy.*

Although a seizure itself generally is not fatal, individuals can be injured by hitting their heads or breaking bones if they lose consciousness and fall to the ground. Seizure activity increases cerebral O_2 consumption by 60% and cerebral blood flow (CBF) by 250%. Instances of prolonged and repeated generalized seizures, *status epilepticus (SE),* can be life-threatening because apnea, hypoxia, acidosis, cerebral edema, dysrhythmias, and cardiovascular collapse can occur.

ASSESSMENT

Signs and symptoms/physical findings: Vary with the type of seizure. It is important to obtain an accurate description of seizure characteristics and duration, as well as any antecedent events, precipitating factors, and postictal phase. The Commission on Classification and Terminology of the International League Against Epilepsy standardized the classification of seizures in 1981. The Commission recommended changes to the old classification system for 2009 (**BOX 5-9**). The following atypes of seizures are the most serious or common:

Generalized tonic-clonic (grand mal): Caused by bilateral electrical activity, usually symmetric from onset, and always involving loss of consciousness. A possible prodromal phase of increased irritability, tension, mood changes, or headache may precede the seizure by hours or days. Patients may experience an aura (a sensory warning, such as a sound, odor, or flash of light) immediately preceding the seizure by seconds or minutes. The seizure usually does not last more than 2-5 min and includes tonic, clonic, and postictal phases. The ictal phase is the seizure itself. The phases are described as follows:

TONIC (RIGID/CONTRACTED MUSCLES WITH EXTENDED LIMBS): Often lasts only 15 sec, usually subsiding in less than 1 min. Symptoms and signs include loss of consciousness, clenched jaws (potential for tongue to be bitten), apnea (may hear a cry as air is forced out of the lungs), and cyanosis. The patient may be incontinent, and pupils may dilate and become nonreactive to light.

CLONIC (RHYTHMIC CONTRACTION AND RELAXATION OF EXTREMITIES AND MUSCLES): May subside in 30 sec but can last 2-4 min. Eyes roll upward, and excessive salivation results in foaming at the mouth. During this phase, the potential is greatest for biting the tongue.

POSTICTAL: The first few minutes after the seizure, the individual may be limp and nonresponsive. Pupils begin to react to light and return to their normal size. After about 5 min, patients may be sleepy, semiconscious, confused, unable to speak clearly, and uncoordinated; have a headache; complain of muscle aches; and have no recollection of the seizure event. This phase usually lasts less than 15 min. Temporary weakness, dysphasia, or hemianopia lasting up to 24 hr after the seizure may be experienced.

Generalized absence (petit mal): Patient has momentary loss of awareness and consciousness with abrupt cessation of voluntary muscle activity. Patient may appear to be daydreaming with a vacant stare and may experience facial, eyelid, or hand twitching. Patient usually does not lose general body muscle tone and so does not fall. The individual resumes previous activity when the seizure ends. There is usually no memory of the seizure, and patients may have difficulty reorienting after the seizure event. This type of seizure can last 1-10 sec, may occur up to 100×/day, and may resolve by puberty. This category is further broken down into typical, atypical, and absence with special features (myoclonic absence or eyelid myoclonia).

Generalized myoclonic: Sudden, very brief contraction or jerking of muscles or muscle groups. Individuals may have a very brief, momentary loss of consciousness with some postictal confusion. This category is further broken down into myoclonic, myoclonic atonic, and myoclonic tonic.

Atonic seizures: Produce a sudden loss of muscle tone. These seizures cause head drops, loss of posture, or sudden collapse. They can result in injuries to the head and face. Protective headgear is sometimes necessary. They are often resistant to drug therapy.

Focal seizures: An irritative focus located in the motor cortex of the frontal lobe causes clonic movement in a particular part of the body, such as the hands or face. These seizures are limited to one hemisphere. The seizure usually lasts several seconds to minutes. There is no loss of consciousness. Other simple, partial seizures include those with somatosensory symptoms (e.g., smells, sounds), autonomic symptoms (e.g., tachycardia, tachypnea, diaphoresis, goose bumps [piloerection], pallor, flushing), or psychic symptoms (e.g., fear, déjà` vu). These seizures can also be described by the seizure activity, the site of origin, or by other features.

SE: State of continuous seizure activity lasting more than 5 min or two or more recurring seizures in which the individual does not completely recover baseline neurologic functioning between seizures. Individuals who suddenly stop taking their antiepileptic drugs (AEDs) are likely to develop this condition. Other common causes are drug withdrawal (e.g., alcohol, sedatives), and fever. *This is a medical emergency,* especially with tonic-clonic seizures, resulting in such potential complications as cerebral anoxia and edema, aspiration, rhabdomyolysis, hyperthermia, and exhaustion. Brain injury may occur in 20-30 min, and irreversible damage may occur in 60 min. Death may ensue. SE can occur in the absence of movement. The patient does not regain consciousness. This nonconvulsive SE may not be life-threatening, but it can cause brain damage and will require continuous electroencephalogram (EEG) monitoring. Expect patients in SE to be transferred to intensive care unit (ICU).

Other classifications: In the 2009 classification system, the term *syndrome* is recommended for epilepsies that have electroclinical characteristics. Other types that are structural-metabolic should be classified by the cause (e.g., stroke). Those with unknown causes should be classified by something such as type or age at onset. Establishing the correct diagnosis of seizure type and, when possible, cause will help with selection of effective AEDs and regimen.

History and risk factors: The seizure threshold is lowered in some individuals. Potential causes for lowered seizure threshold include congenital defects; craniocerebral trauma, particularly that from a penetrating wound; subarachnoid hemorrhage (SAH); stroke; intracranial tumors; infections, such as meningitis or encephalitis; exposure to toxins, such as lead; hypoxia; alcohol or other drug withdrawal; and metabolic and endocrine disorders, such as hypoglycemia, hypocalcemia, uremia, fever, hypoparathyroidism, and excessive hydration. Phenothiazine, tricyclic antidepressants, and alcohol use increase risk of seizure by lowering the seizure threshold. For susceptible individuals, triggers may include emotional tension or stress; physical stimulation, such as loud music, bright, flashing lights, some videos; lack of sleep or food; fatigue; menses or pregnancy; and excessive drug/alcohol use.

DIAGNOSTIC TESTS

Because a variety of problems can precipitate seizures, testing may be extensive. Common tests for initial workup include the following:

Laboratory tests: Rule out metabolic causes, such as hypoglycemia, hyponatremia, or hypocalcemia; kidney and liver problems; toxicology screens; and AED level.

EEG—both sleeping and awake: Reveals abnormal patterns of electrical activity, particularly with such stimuli as flashing lights or hyperventilation. Ambulatory EEGs may record brain activity for 48-72 hr. Generalized tonic-clonic seizures show up as high, fast-voltage spikes in all leads. A normal EEG does not rule out seizures.

MRI: Shows structural lesions causing seizures; also may reveal a space-occupying lesion such as a tumor or hematoma. Fast fluid-attenuated inversion recovery (FLAIR) MRI sequences may be particularly sensitive in finding tumors.

Position emission tomography (PET): Used to check for areas of cerebral glucose hypometabolism that correlate with the irritative seizure-causing focus. This test is useful in partial seizures but is available only in a few centers.

CT scan: Checks for presence of a space-occupying lesion, such as a tumor or hematoma.

Skull x-ray examination: Reveals fractures, tumors, calcifications, or congenital anomalies (pineal shift, ventricular deformity).

Lumbar puncture (LP) and cerebrospinal fluid (CSF) analysis: Ordered if infection such as meningitis is suspected. They also can rule out IICP and determine brain levels of gamma aminobutyric acid (GABA).

Newer diagnostic technologies and combination technologies: Have aided in localizing epileptic activity more precisely. Some of these include the following.

Simultaneous EEG-correlated functional MRI (EEG/fMRI): During this test, *blood O_2 level–dependent* MRI focal changes match up to changes in blood flow.

Subtraction ictal and postictal SPECT co-registered to MRI (SISCOM): Assesses focal changes in cerebral perfusion, which may identify epileptogenic areas.

Magnetic source imaging (MSI): Magnetoencephalography (MEG) information is superimposed on a co-recorded MRI for a noninvasive functional/anatomic imaging technique.

EEG dipole source modeling: Data from EEG and MEG are taken to locate origin of epileptic paroxysm.

Methohexital suppression test: Can distinguish the primary focus in temporal lobe epilepsy with multifocal discharges.

Optical imaging: Noninvasive tool that analyzes seizure activity by measuring dynamic changes in blood flow and O_2 during epileptic activity.

COLLABORATIVE MANAGEMENT

AEDs: Help prevent seizure activity. Monotherapy is usually indicated until either lack of seizure control is evident or toxicity occurs, at which time additional medications are added to the regimen. If patient is seizure free for 2-5 yr, medication tapering over several months and then discontinuation may be attempted under health care provider supervision.

Anticonvulsants (e.g., topiramate, gabapentin, lamotrigine, oxcarbazepine): For general or focal seizures.

Hydantoin derivatives (e.g., oral phenytoin, ethotoin, fosphenytoin): For tonic-clonic, focal seizures.

Valproic acid (oral) and valproate (IV): For absence, tonic-clonic, and mixed seizure types.

Succinimide derivatives (e.g., ethosuximide): For absence seizures.

Barbiturate derivatives (e.g., phenobarbital, primidone): May be used in conjunction with one of the AEDs listed or as monotherapy for tonic-clonic or focal seizures.

Tranquilizers (e.g., clonazepam, diazepam): For myoclonic and atonic seizures. Diazepam gel may be used for rectal administration, particularly for at-home use during seizures.

Treatment of underlying cause: Such as metabolic disorder or infectious process.

Treatment/prevention of osteomalacia (softening of bone): Vitamin D and calcium supplementation with use of certain AEDs such as phenytoin and valproic acid. Weight-bearing exercise and smoking cessation also are promoted. Periodic bone density monitoring is recommended.

Nutrition: A balanced diet spaced evenly throughout the day is recommended to avoid hypoglycemia, which may trigger seizures. Patients are advised to avoid caffeine and alcohol products and to prevent overhydration, which also can precipitate seizure activity. A ketogenic (high-fat, adequate protein, low-carbohydrate) diet appears to reduce seizures in children by producing an acidotic state.

Stress management: Progressive relaxation training, diaphragmatic respiratory training, and biofeedback to reduce seizure frequency and severity.

Counseling or psychotherapy: For patients with poor self-concept or coping difficulties related to the diagnosis.

Herbs/supplements: Supplements such as taurine, selenium, and vitamin D and Asian herbs such as saiko-keishi are being investigated for possible benefit. Some herbs (ginkgo, valerian root, ephedra) may be proconvulsant and should be avoided.

Surgery: Performed to prevent increased or new neurologic deficits. Extensive presurgical testing is done, which may include CT scan and MRI to find structural abnormalities, angiograms to detect vascular abnormalities, 24-hr continuous EEG monitoring, and fMRI. Invasive intracranial EEG monitoring involves electrode placement in epidural, sphenoid, and other brain areas to locate seizure activity, a subdural "grid" applied directly to the cortical surface, and depth electrodes placed in brain tissue to evaluate deep epileptic sources.

Excision or evacuation of tumors or hematomas: Brain tumors or hematomas may be excised or evacuated if they are the source of seizure activity.

Excision of epileptogenic areas: For medically intractable seizures, excision of known epileptogenic areas may be attempted to obtain seizure control. Excision or evacuation may include scar removal (lesionectomy) or cortical resection (e.g., temporal lobectomy for focal seizures) and corpus callostomy (for generalized seizures). Corpus callostomy is considered palliative and is used to partially or completely disconnect the cerebral hemispheres from one another, to limit seizure spread from one hemisphere to the other. Multiple subpial transections consisting of horizontal cuts may be done to prevent spread of the seizure impulse. Surgical procedures require a craniotomy (see "Traumatic Brain Injury," p. 313). Intraoperative mapping by electrocorticography also may be done. Stereotaxic radiosurgery with gamma knife also has been used to ablate epileptogenic areas.

Implanted vagus nerve stimulator (VNS): May have an anticonvulsant effect on partial seizures. Side effects are mostly hoarseness, cough, and sometimes throat discomfort. Educate patient in use of "magnet." When the VNS is deactivated, patient may undergo MRI safely. Patient also should keep external magnet away from credit cards.

Management of SE: *This is a medical emergency.* Anticipate transfer to ICU but do not delay initial interventions.

"ABCs": Assess airway, breathing, and circulation. O_2 therapy, oral airway suctioning, and intubation are implemented as needed to maintain airway and prevent hypoxia. Place patient in left lateral position. Monitor VS, pulse oximetry, heart rhythm, and arterial blood gas (ABG) values. Obtain IV access for fluids and medications.

Assessment of blood glucose (fingerstick) and administration of IV glucose and thiamine: If indicated, to reverse hypoglycemia. If alcohol withdrawal is suspected or a possibility, thiamine should be given before dextrose to protect against an exacerbation of Wernicke's encephalopathy.

Serum laboratory studies: Evaluate for hypoglycemia, electrolyte (e.g., hyponatremia, hypocalcemia, hypomagnesiumia) or metabolic (kidney, liver) imbalances that may be causing seizures. Serum drug screens are performed to assess serum AED level and determine presence of alcohol or other drugs that may be causing the seizures.

Priority administration of IV lorazepam or diazepam within 3-10 min: Initially given as a slow bolus. Sublingual lorazepam, rectal diazepam gel, or nasally administered midazolam may be given if there is no IV access. If the seizure stops, this may be the extent of the interventions if patient is already on AEDs. Monitor for signs of respiratory depression and hypotension.

Priority administration of IV fosphenytoin (loading dose): For patient not already on AEDs or for continuing seizure. Fosphenytoin is the drug of choice for injectable hydantoin. Dosage of fosphenytoin is prescribed in phenytoin equivalents (PEs), may be given by IV or intramuscular (IM) route, and has minimal local tissue irritation. Because hypotension can occur with too-rapid IV administration, infusion rate should not exceed 150 mg PE/min. Continuous ECG, BP, and respiration monitoring should be done when providing IV loading of this agent. Fosphenytoin must be refrigerated and has side effects similar to those of phenytoin with the exception of decreased local tissue irritation. Unique side effects include paresthesia and pruritus. This drug is contraindicated in patients with serious renal disease, renal failure, sinus bradycardia, or atrioventricular (A-V) block. IV phenytoin may be given if fosphenytoin is unavailable. Do not mix phenytoin with other medications and most IV fluids; give it slowly, undiluted, IV push, at no more than 50 mg/min. It should be given only with normal saline IV fluids because it will precipitate in the presence of 5% dextrose in water (D_5W). Monitor for hypotension, apnea, and cardiac dysrhythmias. IV infiltration can cause tissue sloughing.

IV phenobarbital: Prescribed if diazepam and phenytoin are unsuccessful or patient is allergic to other drugs. Monitor for signs of respiratory depression.

IV valproate: Used as a second-line agent.

Intubation and general anesthesia with continuous infusion of propofol, midazolam, barbiturate (e.g., pentobarbital), or neuromuscular blocking agent: For severe cases. Neuromuscular blocking agents may stop movement but will not stop brain activity.

Passive cooling with hypothermia blanket: Used if patient is hyperthermic from seizures or infection.

Continuous EEG monitoring: Evaluates brain activity and response to interventions. When patient is seizure free for 12-24 hr, a slow withdrawal of medication may be attempted.

Glucocorticosteroids (e.g., dexamethasone): Relieve cerebral edema.

Search for underlying cause and its correction, if possible: May include a wide variety of diagnostic tests (see "Diagnostic Tests" section, p. 347).

NURSING DIAGNOSES AND INTERVENTIONS

Risk for falls with risk factors related to oral, musculoskeletal, and airway vulnerability secondary to seizure activity

Desired outcomes: Patient exhibits no signs of oral or musculoskeletal tissue injury or airway compromise after the seizure. Before hospital discharge, patient's significant other verbalizes knowledge of actions necessary during seizure activity.

Nursing Interventions
Seizure Precautions

- Pad side rails with blankets or pillows. Keep side rails up and bed in its lowest position when patient is in bed. Keep bed, wheelchair, or stretcher brakes locked.
- Tape a soft rubber oral airway to the bedside. Remove wooden tongue depressors. *This is because they may splinter.* Keep suction and O_2 equipment readily available. Consider a saline lock for IV access for high-risk patient.
- Use electronic tympanic thermometers for patients at high risk for seizure. *This is to prevent potential breakage of glass thremometers and injury to the patient.*
- Caution patients to lie down and push call button if they experience prodromal or aural warning. Encourage patients to empty mouth of dentures or foreign objects. *This is to prevent choling or aspiration if seizure occurs.*
- Do not allow unsupervised smoking.
- Evaluate need for and provide protective headgear as indicated.

During the Seizure

- Remain with patient and stay calm. Observe for, record, and report type, duration, and characteristics of seizure activity and any postseizure response. This should include, as appropriate, precipitating event, aura, initial location and progression, automatisms, type and duration of movement, changes in level of consciousness (LOC), eye movement (e.g., deviation, nystagmus), pupil size and reaction, bowel and bladder incontinence, head deviation, tongue deviation, or teeth clenching.
- Keep patient in bed if seizure occurs while there, and lower head of bed (HOB) to a flat position. Prevent or break the fall and ease patient to floor if seizure occurs while patient is out of bed. *This will lessen potential injury during fall.*
- If patient's jaws are clenched, do not force an object between the teeth. *This is because this maneuver can break teeth or lacerate oral mucous membranes.* If able to do so safely and without damage to oral tissue, insert an airway device. Tongue depressors should not be used. *This is because because they may splinter.* A rolled washcloth may be used as an alternative. Never put your fingers in patient's mouth.
- Protect patient's head from injury during seizure activity. A towel folded flat or hands may be used. *This will cushion the head and prevent it from striking the ground.* Be sure head position does not occlude airway. Remove objects (e.g., chairs) from environment that patient may strike. Pad floors to protect patient's arms and legs. Remove patient's glasses.
- Do not restrain patient but rather guide patient's movements gently. *This is to prevent further injury.*
- Roll patient into a side-lying position. *This is to promote drainage of secretions and maintain a patent airway.* Use head-tilt/chin-lift maneuver. Provide O_2 and suction as needed.

- Loosen tight clothing, collar, or belt.
- Maintain patient's privacy. Clear nonessential people from the room.
- Administer AEDs as prescribed.

After the Seizure

- Determine whether patient has had SE seizure, in which the seizure is continuous (longer than 5 min), seizure is longer than patient's usual length of time by 1 or 2 min, or patient has two or more seizures without recovering baseline neurologic functioning between seizures. *This condition is life-threatening and can cause cerebral anoxia and edema, aspiration, hyperthermia, and exhaustion.* See "Collaborative Management," p. 348, for treatment.
- Reassure and gently reorient patient. Check neurologic status and VS; ask patient if an aura preceded seizure activity. Record this information and postictal characteristics.
- Provide a quiet, calm environment. *Sounds and stimuli can be confusing to the awakening patient.* Keep talk simple and to a minimum. Speak slowly and with pauses between sentences. Repeating may be necessary. Use room light that is behind, not above, patient. *This is to prevent additional seizures and for patient comfort.* Do not offer food or drink until patient is fully awake. *This is to prevent choking or aspiration.*
- Check patient's tongue for lacerations and body for injuries. Monitor urine for red or cola color. *This may signal rhabdomyolysis or myoglobinuria from muscle damage.* Monitor for weakness or paralysis, dysphasia, or visual disturbances.
- Check finger stick blood glucose value and obtain serum laboratory tests as prescribed.
- Administer AED as prescribed.
- Stay with patient for 15-20 min after the seizure. *Sudden unexplained death in epileptic patients is not understood, but it may be related to central respiratory apnea, which can occur with a seizure.*
- Provide significant other with verbal and written information about the preceding interventions.

Deficient knowledge related to life-threatening environmental factors and preventive measures for seizures

Desired outcomes: Before hospital discharge, patient verbalizes accurate information about measures that may prevent seizures and environmental factors that can be life-threatening in the presence of seizures. Patient exhibits health care measures that reflect this knowledge.

Nursing Interventions

- Assess knowledge of measures that can prevent seizures and environmental hazards that can be life-threatening in the presence of seizure activity. Provide or clarify information as indicated.
- Advise patient to check into state regulations about automobile operation. *Most states require 3 mo to 2 seizure-free yr before an individual can obtain a driver's license.*
- Caution patient to refrain from operating heavy or dangerous equipment, swimming, climbing excessive heights, and possibly even tub bathing until he or she is seizure free for amount of time specified by health care provider. Teach patient to never swim alone, regardless of amount of time he or she has been seizure free. Caution patient to swim only in shallow water and in the company of a strong swimmer. Advise patient that some activities, such as climbing or bicycle riding, require careful risk/benefit evaluation. The patient who decides to ride a bike should wear a helmet and avoid heavy traffic. Contact sports should be avoided. *These are precautions to prevent more serious injuries or death.*

◆ Advise patient to turn temperature of hot water heaters at home down. *This is to prevent scalding if a seizure occurs while patient is in the shower.*

◆ Encourage stress management, progressive relaxation techniques, and diaphragmatic respiratory training. *This is to control emotional stress and hyperventilation, which often trigger seizures.*

◆ Encourage vocational assessment and counseling. *In some occupations, such as bus driver or airline pilot, patient's epilepsy may place others at risk.*

◆ Advise female patients that seizure activity may change (increase or decrease) during menses or pregnancy (especially at 3-4 mo gestation). *Tonic-clonic seizures have caused fetal death. AEDs are associated with birth defects; however, 90% of women have normal pregnancies and healthy children.* Provide birth control information if requested. *Oral contraceptive medication effectiveness may be reduced by many AEDs. Intrauterine devices or other methods may be needed. When seizures in women worsen with hormonal changes, suppressing ovulation with medication may be recommended.*

◆ Advise female patients wanting to get pregnant that they should consult with their health care provider. They should be on folate acid and receive vitamin K during the last 2-4 wk of their pregnancy. *This is to avoid neonatal hemorrhage.*

◆ Teach that use of stimulants (e.g., caffeine) and depressants (e.g., alcohol) should be avoided. *Their use can change the seizure threshold, and withdrawal from stimulants and depressants can increase likelihood of seizures.*

◆ Teach that getting adequate amounts of rest, avoiding physical and emotional stress, and maintaining a nutritious diet are important. *This regimen may help prevent seizure activity.* Meals should be spaced throughout the day. *This is to prevent hypoglycemia.* Advise patient to avoid environments that are likely to have stimuli that trigger seizures. *Stimuli such as flashing lights, video or computer games, poorly adjusted televisions, or loud music appear to trigger seizures.* Patients should monitor for and treat fever early during an illness. *Fever may also trigger seizures.*

◆ Encourage individuals who have seizures that occur without warning to avoid chewing gum or sucking on lozenges. *These may be aspirated during a seizure.*

◆ Encourage patient to wear a MedicAlert bracelet or similar identification or to carry a medical information card.

Deficient knowledge related to purpose, precautions, and side effects of AEDs
Desired outcome: Before hospital discharge, patient verbalizes accurate information about the prescribed AED.

Nursing Interventions

◆ Stress importance of taking prescribed medication regularly and on schedule and not discontinuing medication without health care provider guidance. *Missing a scheduled dose can precipitate a seizure several days later. Abrupt withdrawal of any AED can precipitate seizures. Discontinuing these medications is the most common cause of SE.* Assist patients in finding methods that will help them remember to take their medication and monitor their drug supply to avoid running out. *Drugs may be necessary for duration of patient's life. Medications cannot be taken as needed (prn), and lack of seizures does not mean the drug is unnecessary.* Explain concept of drug half-life and steady blood levels. Patients should consult health care provider before changing from a trade name to a generic medication. *This is because of possible differences in bioavailability.* Explain that drugs are usually withdrawn slowly over 1-2 wk rather than abruptly stopped.

- Encourage patient to keep a drug and seizure chart diary.
- Stress importance of informing health care provider about side effects and keeping appointments for periodic laboratory work. *This determines whether blood levels are therapeutic and assesses for side effects. Many side effects are dose related, and medication can be adjusted based on AED blood levels and symptoms.* Explain signs of AED-related toxicity. Teach patient to report immediately any bruising, bleeding, jaundice, or rash. Vitamin D, vitamin K, and folic acid supplements may be prescribed. *Many AEDs can cause blood dyscrasia or liver damage.*
- Teach patient that grapefruit juice should be avoided. *It can inhibit hepatic metabolism of many AEDs and affect drug levels.* Calcium supplementation should not be taken within 2 hr of AEDs. *It can impact AED absorption.*
- Advise patient to avoid activities that require alertness until central nervous system (CNS) response to the medication has been determined. Splitting the dose or giving main dose at bedtime may help. *This is because AEDs may cause drowsiness.*
- Teach patient to take the drug with food or large amounts of liquid. *Nausea and vomiting are common side effects of most AEDs.* Patients taking valproic acid, topiramate, and zonisamide should not chew the medication. *This is because it may irritate the oral mucous membrane.* Also advise patients taking valproic acid that this drug may produce a false-positive test result for urine ketones, and any visual change should be reported immediately. *It may signal ocular toxicity.*
- Instruct patient to notify health care provider if significant weight gain or weight loss occurs. *This is because it may necessitate a change in dose or scheduling.*
- Teach patient to avoid alcoholic beverages and over-the-counter (OTC) medications containing alcohol. *Long-term alcohol use stimulates the body to metabolize phenytoin more quickly, thus lowering the seizure threshold because of decreased plasma phenytoin levels.* Patients taking phenobarbital or primidone should avoid alcohol. *These drugs potentiate CNS-depressant effects.* Caution patient to avoid OTC medications. *Anticonvulsant agents are potentiated or inhibited by many other drugs, including aspirin and antihistamines, and may affect potency of other medications as well.*
- Other side effects common to AEDs are ataxia, diplopia, nystagmus, and dizziness. Instruct patient to report these symptoms.
- Advise patients taking phenytoin to perform frequent oral hygiene with gum massage and gentle flossing and brush teeth 3-4 ×/day with a soft toothbrush. These patients also should report immediately any measles-like rash. *Phenytoin can cause gingival hypertrophy.*
- Caution patients taking phenytoin that there are two types of this drug. Dilantin Kapseals is absorbed more slowly and is longer acting. It is important not to confuse this extended-release phenytoin with prompt-release phenytoin. Generic phenytoin should not be substituted for Dilantin Kapseals. *Doing so may cause dangerous underdose or overdose.*

Noncompliance with therapy related to denial of the illness or perceived negative consequences of the treatment regimen secondary to social stigma, negative side effects of AEDs, or difficulty with making necessary lifestyle changes

Desired outcome: Before hospital discharge, patient verbalizes knowledge about the disease process and treatment plan, acknowledges consequences of continued nonadhering behavior, explains the experience that caused altering of the prescribed regimen, describes appropriate treatment of side effects or appropriate alternatives, and exhibits health care measures that reflect this knowledge, by following an agreed-on plan of care.

Nursing Interventions

- Assess patient's understanding of the disease process, medical management, and treatment plan. Explain or clarify information as indicated.
- Assess for causes of nonadherence, such as financial constraints, inconvenience, forgetfulness or memory problems, medication side effects, misunderstanding of instructions, or difficulty making significant lifestyle changes or following medication schedule.
- Ensure awareness that stopping medications can be life-threatening. *It may result in SE.* Explain drug half-life and concept of a steady blood level. *Intermittent medication use may be informal experimentation or an effort to gain control.* Explain importance of health care provider guidance if medication is stopped for any reason. Instruct and provide written instructions for patient on how to contact health care provider and importance of follow-up with health care provider and laboratory tests. Explain what to do if a dose is missed and how to refill a prescription if medication is lost or depleted.
- Evaluate patient's perception of vulnerability to the disease process, and be alert to signs of denial of the illness. Evaluate patient's perception of effectiveness or ineffectiveness of treatment. Stress importance of expressing feelings.
- Determine whether a value, cultural conflict, or spiritual conflict is causing nonadherence. Confront myths and stigmas. Provide realistic assessment of risks, and counter misconceptions.
- Discuss methods of dealing with common problems, such as obtaining insurance and job or workplace discrimination.
- Assess patient's support systems. Determine whether presence of a family disruption pattern (whether or not it is caused by patient's illness) is making adherence difficult and "not worth it."
- After the reason for nonadherence is found, intervene accordingly to ensure adherence. If it appears that changing medical treatment plan (e.g., in scheduling medications) may promote adherence, discuss this possibility with health care provider. Provide patient with information about interventions that can minimize drug side effects.
- Encourage involvement with support systems such as local epilepsy centers and national organizations.

Patient-Family Teaching and Discharge Planning

Seizure activity and complications may vary with the type of epilepsy. Instructions should be specific to the patient's diagnosis and needs. Include verbal and written information about the following:

- Reinforcement of knowledge of disease process, pathophysiology, symptoms, and precipitating or aggravating factors.
- Medications, including drug names, purpose, dosage, schedule, precautions, and potential side effects. Also discuss drug/drug, herb/drug, and food/drug interactions and importance of adhering to medication routine.
- Importance of follow-up care and keeping medical appointments. Stress that use of AEDs necessitates periodic monitoring of blood levels to ensure therapeutic medication levels and assessment for side effects. Instruct patient to keep emergency contact numbers for health care provider.
- Seizure first aid. An uncomplicated convulsive seizure in an individual known to have epilepsy is not necessarily a medical emergency. On average, these individuals can continue on about their business after a rest period. An ambulance should be called or medical attention sought if the seizure happens in water; if the individual is injured, pregnant, or diabetic; if the seizure lasts longer than 5 min; if a second seizure starts; if consciousness does not begin to return; or if there is any question that the seizure may have been caused by something other than epilepsy.

- Environmental factors that can be life-threatening in the presence of seizures, measures that may help prevent seizures, and safety interventions during seizures. Review home and personal safety tips. Review state and local laws that apply to individuals with seizure disorders.
- Employment or vocational counseling as needed. Discuss need to avoid overprotection and maintain, as possible, normal work and recreation activities. Review or provide information regarding the Americans with Disabilities Act.
- Risks of using AEDs during pregnancy. Provide birth control information as requested.
- Benefits of joining local support groups.
- Additional general information, which can be obtained by accessing the following websites:

  American Epilepsy Society: www.aesnet.org

  Epilepsy Foundation: www.epilepsyfoundation.org

  International League Against Epilepsy: www.ilae.org

  National Institute of Neurological Disorders and Stroke: NINDS Epilepsy Information Page: www.ninds.nih.gov/disorders/epilepsy/epilepsy.htm

SECTION SIX GENERAL CARE OF PATIENTS WITH NEUROLOGIC DEFICITS

❖ DECREASED LEVEL OF CONSCIOUSNESS AND SENSORIMOTOR DEFICITS

NURSING DIAGNOSES AND INTERVENTIONS

Risk for falls related to weakness, difficulties with balance, or unsteady gait secondary to sensorimotor deficit

Desired outcomes: Patient is free of trauma caused by gait unsteadiness. Before hospital discharge, patient demonstrates proficiency with assistive devices if appropriate.

Nursing Interventions

- Evaluate gait and assess for motor deficits such as weakness, difficulty with balance, tremors, spasticity, or paralysis. *Changes in status should be detected promptly.*
- Assess and document patient's fall risk using a fall risk assessment tool. Identify and communicate patient's fall risk through an armband, identifying wall placard, and/or care plan. In plan of care include appropriate interventions, specific-to-patient lifting/transferring/mobilization aids and techniques, and appropriate amount of assistance needed. *This is to avoid patient and staff injury.* Update as appropriate with changes in patient's status.
- Assist patient as needed when unsteady gait, weakness, or paralysis is noted and instruct patient to ask or call for assistance with ambulation. *This is to avoid falls and further injury.* Frequently check on patients who may forget to call for assistance. Stand on patient's weak side and use a transfer belt. *This is to better assist with balance and support.* Instruct patient to use stronger side for gripping railing when stair climbing or using a cane.
- Orient patient to new surroundings. Keep necessary items (including water, snacks, phone, call light) within easy reach. Assess patient's ability to use

these items. *Patients who are very weak or partially paralyzed may require a tap bell or specially adapted call light.*

◆ Maintain an uncluttered environment with unobstructed walkways. *This will minimize risk of tripping.* Ensure adequate lighting at night (e.g., provide a night light). *This is to help prevent falls in the dark.* In addition, keep side rails up and bed in its lowest position with bed brakes on. Encourage patient to use any needed hearing aids and corrective lenses when ambulating.

◆ For unsteady, weak, or partially paralyzed patient, encourage use of low-heel, nonskid, supportive shoes for walking. Teach use of a wide-based gait. *This provides a broader base of support.* Instruct patient to note foot placement when ambulating or transferring to ensure that foot is flat and in a position of support. Teach, reinforce, and encourage use of an assistive device, such as a cane, walker, or crutches that provides added stability. Teach exercises that strengthen arm and shoulder muscles for using walkers and crutches. Teach safe use of transfer or sliding boards. Teach patients in wheelchairs how and when to lock and unlock wheels. Demonstrate how to secure and support weak or paralyzed arms. *This is to prevent subluxation and injury from falling into wheelchair spokes or wheels.* Patients with poor sitting balance may need a seat or chest belt, H-straps for leg positioning, and a wheelchair with an antitip device. Show how to get on and off elevators. *This is to prevent wheels from catching in gaps between elevator and floor.* Keep wheelchair close to bed. Teach proper use of recliner mechanism or battery precautions on appropriate wheelchairs.

◆ Teach patient to maintain sitting position for a few minutes before assuming standing position for ambulating. *This procedure gives patient time to get feet flat and under patient for balance and minimizes any dizziness that may occur because of rapid position changes.*

◆ Monitor spasticity, antispasmodic medications, and their effect on physical function. *Uncontrolled or severe spasms may cause falls, whereas mild to moderate spasms can be useful in activities of daily living (ADL) and transfers if patient learns to control and trigger them.*

◆ Review with patient and significant other potential safety issues at home, such as loose rugs, hot water temperature, cluttered rooms, lighting, ramps, safety appliances (wall, bath, toilet grab rails; elevated toilet seat; nonslip surface in bathtub or shower), rolling furniture, and activity and rest. *Loose rugs can cause slipping and falling. Temperatures on hot water heaters should be turned down to prevent scalding in the event of a fall in the shower or tub. Furniture in the home may need to be moved to provide clear, safe pathways that avoid sharp corners on furniture, glass cabinets, or large windows patient could fall against. Strategically placed additional lighting also may be needed. Edges of steps in the home may require taping with brightly colored strips to provide sufficient contrast so that edges can be recognized and more safely negotiated. Beds should be modified to prevent rolling. Activity should be balanced with rest periods because fatigue tends to increase unsteadiness and potential for falls. Ramp construction to replace stairs may be needed to prevent falls.*

◆ Seek referral for physical therapy (PT) as appropriate.

Risk for injury related to impaired pain, touch, and temperature sensations secondary to sensory deficit or decreased level of consciousness (LOC)
Desired outcomes: Patient is free of symptoms of injury caused by impaired pain, touch, and temperature sensations. Before hospital discharge, patient and significant other identify factors that increase the potential for injury.

Nursing Interventions

◆ Assess for indicators of sensory deficits, such as decreased or absent vision and impaired temperature and pain sensation. *Changes in status should be detected promptly.*

- Protect patient from exposure to hot food or equipment that can burn the skin. Avoid use of heating pads. Encourage use of sunscreen when outside. Always check temperature of heating devices and bath water before patient is exposed to them. Teach patient and significant other about these precautions. *Burns can result from decreased senstion.*
- Inspect skin twice daily for evidence of irritation. Teach coherent patient to perform self-inspection, and provide mirror for inspecting posterior aspects of the body. Keep skin soft and pliable with emollient lotion.
- Teach patient to inspect placement of limbs with altered sensation. *This is to ensure a safe and supported position and to avoid placing ankles directly on top of each other.* Teach patient to change position q15-30min by lifting self and shifting position side to side and forward to backward. Pad wheelchair seat, preferably with a gel pad. *This will help evenly distribute patient's weight and prevent pressure sores.* Encourage frequent turning while in bed and, if tolerated and not contraindicated, periodic movement into prone position. Have patient lift, not drag, self during transfers. *This is to prevent shearing damage.*
- Give injections in muscles with tone, and avoid injecting more than 1 mL into a flaccid muscle. *This promotes better absorption and less risk of sterile abscess formation.*

Impaired tissue integrity: corneal related to irritation secondary to diminished blink reflex or inability to close the eyes
Desired outcome: Patient's corneas remain clear and intact.

Nursing Interventions

- If patient has a diminished blink reflex (normally, blinking occurs every 5-6 sec), or is stuporous or comatose, assess eyes for irritation or presence of foreign objects. Instill prescribed eyedrops or ointment. *This will provide corneal lubrication.* Instruct coherent patients to make a conscious effort to blink eyes several times each minute. *This is to help prevent corneal irritation.* Indicators of corneal irritation include red, itchy, scratchy, or painful eye; sensation of foreign object in eye; scleral edema; blurred vision; or mucus discharge. Apply eye patches or warm, sterile compresses over closed eyes for relief.
- If the eyes cannot be completely closed, use caution in applying eye shield or taping eyes shut. Consider use of moisture chambers (plastic eye bubbles), protective glasses, soft contacts, or humidifiers. *Semiconscious patients may open eyes underneath and injure their corneas.*
- For chronic eye closure problems, special springs or weights on upper lids may ensure closure. Surgical closure (tarsorrhaphy) also may be necessary.
- Teach patient to avoid exposing eyes to irritants such as talc or baby powder, wind, cold air, smoke, dust, sand, or bright sunlight. Instruct patient not to rub eyes. Patients should be taught to wear glasses. *This is to protect against wind and dust, and tight-fitting goggles should be worn when swimming.*

Imbalanced nutrition: less than body requirements related to inability to ingest food secondary to chewing and swallowing deficits, fatigue, weakness, paresis, paralysis, visual neglect, or decreased LOC
Desired outcome: Patient has adequate nutrition as evidenced by maintenance of or return to baseline body weight by time of hospital discharge.

Nursing Interventions

- Assess alertness, ability to cough and swallow, and gag reflexes before all meals. Keep suction equipment at bedside if indicated.
- Assess for type of diet that can be eaten safely (e.g., soft, semisolid, or chopped foods). A pureed diet may be needed eventually.

◆ Reduce stimuli in the room (e.g., turn off television or radio). Minimize conversation and other disruptions such as phone calls. If patient wears glasses, put them on patient; ensure adequate lighting. *This helps patient focus on eating rather than being distracted.*

◆ Provide analgesics, when needed, before meals. *This may help patient be more comfortable and concentrate on eating.*

◆ Evaluate food preferences and offer small, frequent servings of nutritious food. Encourage significant other to bring in patient's favorite foods if not contraindicated. Plan meals for times when patient is rested; use a warming tray or microwave oven to keep food warm and appetizing until patient is able to eat. Serve cold foods while they are cold.

◆ Provide oral/denture care before feeding. *This is to enhance patient's ability to taste.*

◆ Encourage liquid nutritional supplements. *Try different methods such as making a milkshake, serving over ice, or diluting with carbonated beverages to make them more palatable.*

◆ Cut up foods, unwrap silverware, and otherwise prepare food tray. *This helps the patient with a weak or paralyzed arm to manage the tray with one hand.*

◆ For patient with visual neglect, place food within unaffected visual field. Return during meal to make sure patient has eaten from both sides of the plate. Turn plate around so that any remaining food is in patient's visual field.

◆ Feed or assist very weak or paralyzed patients. If not contraindicated, position patient in a chair or elevate head of bed (HOB) as high as possible. Ensure that patient's head is flexed slightly forward. *This helps to close the airway.* Begin with small amounts of food. Encourage chewing food on unaffected side. Do not hurry patient. Be sure that each bite is completely swallowed before giving another. Encourage patient with hemiplegia to consciously sweep paralyzed side of mouth with the tongue to clear it.

◆ If appropriate, provide assistive devices such as built-up utensil handles, broad-handled spoons, spill-proof cups, rocker knife for cutting, wrist or hand splints with clamps to hold utensils, stabilized plates, sectioned plates, and other devices, and encourage using finger foods. *These promote self-feeding and independence.*

◆ Provide materials for oral hygiene after meals. *This will minimize risk of aspiration of food particles. Good oral hygiene will also help maintain integrity of mucous membranes to minimize risk of stomatitis, which may prevent adequate oral intake.* Provide oral care for patients unable to do so for themselves.

◆ Document your assessment of patient's appetite. Weigh patient regularly (at least weekly). *This is to assess for loss or gain, and if indicated, the need for high-protein or high-calorie supplements.* Obtain dietitian consultation. Patient may need enteral or parenteral nutrition. For additional information, see "Providing Nutritional Support," p. 692.

◆ For weak, debilitated, or partially paralyzed patient, assess support systems, such as family or friends, who can assist patient with meals. Consider referral to an organization that will deliver a daily meal to patient's home.

◆ If appropriate for patient's diagnosis (e.g., multiple sclerosis [MS]), consider referral to a speech pathologist. *This is to teach exercises that enhance ability to swallow.*

◆ For patient with visual problems, assess ability to see food. Identify utensils and foods, and describe their location. Arrange foods in an established pattern to promote independence. For patient with diplopia, consider patching one eye.

◆ For patient with chewing or swallowing difficulties, see nursing interventions in **Impaired swallowing,** p. 367.

Risk for deficient fluid volume related to facial and throat muscle weakness, depressed gag or cough reflex, impaired swallowing, or decreased LOC affecting access to and intake of fluids
Desired outcome: Patient is normovolemic as evidenced by balanced I&O, stable weight, good skin turgor, moist mucous membranes, BP within patient's normal range, heart rate (HR) 100 beats per minute (bpm) or less, normothermia, and urinary output at least 30 mL/hr with a specific gravity 1.030 or less.

Nursing Interventions

- Assess gag reflex, alertness, and ability to cough and swallow before offering fluids. Keep suction equipment at bedside if indicated.
- Monitor I&O to assess for fluid volume imbalance. Involve patient or significant other with keeping fluid intake records. Perform daily weight measurement if patient is at risk. *This will monitor for sudden fluid shifts or imbalances. Patient with neurologic deficit may have great difficulty attaining adequate intake of fluids. A significant I&O imbalance may signal need for enteral or IV therapy to prevent dehydration.*
- Assess for and teach patient and significant other indicators of dehydration, including thirst, poor skin turgor, decreased BP, increased pulse rate, dry skin and mucous membranes, increased body temperature, concentrated urine (specific gravity more than 1.030), and decreased urinary output. *Fever and diarrhea increase fluid loss and increase risk of dehydration.*
- Evaluate fluid preferences (type and temperature). Offer fluids q1-2h. Establish a fluid goal. For nonrestricted patients, encourage a fluid intake of at least 2-3 L/day.
- Feed or assist very weak or paralyzed patients. If not contraindicated, assist patient into high Fowler's position to facilitate oral fluid intake. Instruct patient to flex head slightly forward. *This closes the airway and helps prevent aspiration.* Begin with small amounts of liquid. Instruct patient to sip rather than gulp fluids. Do not hurry patient. In patient at risk for aspiration, use thickened fluids to facilitate patient's ability to swallow the fluid.
- Provide periods of rest. *This prevents fatigue, which can contribute to decreased oral intake.* Provide oral care as needed. *This is to enhance taste perception and prevent stomatitis, which may decrease oral intake.*
- If appropriate, provide assistive devices (e.g., plastic, unbreakable, special-handled, spill-proof cups or straws) to promote independence. Teach patient with hemiparalysis or hemiparesis to tilt head toward unaffected side. *This will facilitate intake.* The individual who is paralyzed (e.g., with spinal cord injury [SCI]) may be able to drink independently via extra-long tubing or a straw connected to a water pitcher.
- For patients with chewing or swallowing difficulties, see nursing interventions under **Impaired swallowing,** p. 367.

Risk for aspiration related to facial and throat muscle weakness, depressed gag or cough reflex, impaired swallowing, or decreased LOC
Desired outcomes: Patient is free of the signs of aspiration as evidenced by respiratory rate (RR) 12-20 breaths/min with normal depth and pattern (eupnea), O_2 saturation greater than 92%, normal color, normal breath sounds, normothermia, and absence of adventitious breath sounds. Following instruction on an ongoing basis, patient or significant other relates measures that prevent aspiration.

Nursing Interventions

- Assess effectiveness of patient's cough and quality, amount, and color of sputum.
- If it is not contraindicated, maintain patient in a side-lying position with HOB elevated. Keep HOB elevated after meals or assist patient into a right

side-lying position. *This is to minimize potential for regurgitation and aspiration.* Provide small, frequent meals. Provide oral hygiene after meals. *This is to prevent aspiration of food particles.*
◆ Assess frequently for presence of obstructive material or secretions in throat or mouth, and suction prn. Turn patient on one side. *This is to facilitate secretion drainage.* Anticipate need for artificial airway if secretions cannot be cleared. Teach significant other the Heimlich maneuver.
◆ For general nursing interventions, see this nursing diagnosis in "Older Adult Care," p. 47.

Self-care deficit related to spasticity, tremors, weakness, paresis, paralysis, or decreasing LOC secondary to sensorimotor deficits
Desired outcome: At least 24 hr before hospital discharge, patient performs care activities independently and demonstrates ability to use adaptive devices for successful completion of ADL. (Totally dependent patient expresses satisfaction with activities that are completed for him or her.)

Nursing Interventions
◆ Assess patient's ability to perform ADL.
◆ As appropriate, demonstrate use of adaptive devices, such as long- or broad-handled combs; long-handled pickup sticks, brushes, and eating utensils; dressing sticks; stocking helpers, Velcro fasteners; elastic waistbands; non-spill cups; and stabilized plates. *These may assist patient in maintaining independent care.* A flexor-hinge splint or universal cuff may aid in brushing teeth and combing hair. Also consider electric toothbrush and electric razor.
◆ Set short-range, realistic goals with patient. *This helps decrease frustration and improves learning.* Acknowledge progress. Encourage continued effort and involvement (e.g., in selection of meals, clothing).
◆ Provide care to totally dependent patient. Assist those who are not totally dependent according to degree of disability. Encourage patient to perform self-care to the maximum ability as defined by patient. Encourage autonomy. Allow sufficient time for task performance; do not hurry patient. Involve significant other with care activities if he or she is comfortable doing so. Ask for patient's input in planning schedules. Supervise activity until patient can safely perform task without help.
◆ Encourage use of electronically controlled wheelchair and other technical advances (e.g., environmental control system). *This will improve mobility of patient and may allow independent operation of electronic devices such as lights, radio, door openers, and window shade openers.*
◆ Provide privacy and a nondistracting environment. Place patient's belongings within reach. Set out items needed to complete self-care tasks in the order they are to be used. Apply any needed adaptive devices such as hand splints.
◆ Encourage patient to wear any prescribed corrective eye lenses or hearing aids.
◆ Provide analgesics to relieve pain. *Pain can hinder self-care activity.*
◆ Provide a rest period before self-care activity, or plan activity for a time when patient is rested. *Fatigue reduces self-care ability.*
◆ Encourage patient or significant other to buy shoes without laces; long-handled shoe horns; front opening garments; wide-legged pants; and clothing that is loose fitting with enlarged arm holes, front fasteners, zipper pulls, elastic waistbands or self-stick (Velcro) closures. Avoid items with small buttons or tight buttonholes. Lay out clothing in the order it will be put on. Advise patient to sit while dressing. A dressing stick may help to pull up pants or retrieve clothing. *This facilitates independent dressing and undressing.*
◆ Place stool in shower if sitting down will enhance self-care with bathing. Bathrooms should have nonslip mats and grab bars. A handheld showerhead and a long-handled bath sponge or a washer mitt with a pocket that holds soap may promote autonomy.

- Provide commode chair, elevated toilet seat, or male or female urinal. *This is to facilitate self-care with elimination.* Teach self-transfer techniques that will enable patient to get to commode or toilet. Keep call light within patient's reach. Instruct patient to call as early as possible so that staff will have time to respond and patient will not have to rush because of urgency. Offer toileting reminders q2h, after meals, and before bedtime.

- Have patient use a long-handled grasper that can hold tissues or washcloth. *Some patients with limited hand or arm mobility may have difficulty with perineal care after elimination and this may help maintain independence.*

- For patient with hemiparesis or hemiparalysis, teach use of stronger or unaffected hand and arm for dressing, eating, bathing, and grooming. Instruct patient to dress weaker side first.

- For patient with visual field deficit, avoid placing items on blind side. Encourage patient to scan environment for needed items by turning head.

- Patient with tremors may find splints, weighted utensils, or wrist weights helpful. Resting head against a high-backed chair may reduce head tremors.

- Obtain referral for occupational therapy (OT). *This is to determine best method for performing activity.*

- Provide consistent caregiver and ADL routine. *Individuals with cognitive defects need simple visual or verbal cues, increased gesture use, demonstration, reminders of next step, and gentle repetition.*

- If indicated, teach patient self-catheterization, or teach technique to caregiver. At-home intermittent catheterization usually is done with clean (not sterile) technique and equipment. The catheter is washed after use in warm, soapy water; rinsed; and placed in a clean plastic sack. Catheter insertion guides are available commercially for female patients with limited upper arm mobility. Crusted catheters are soaked in a solution of half distilled vinegar and half water. Teach patient to monitor and notify health professional of cloudy, foul-smelling, or bloody urine; urine with sediment; chills or fever; pain in lower back or abdomen; or a red or swollen urethral meatus.

- Discuss, as appropriate, changing home environment (e.g., with extended sinks, grab bars, lower closet hooks, wheelchair-accessible shower, modified phones, lowered mirrors, and lever door handles that operate with reduced hand pressure). *This is to improve ADL and independence.*

- Listen and provide opportunities for patient to express self, and communicate that it is normal to have negative feelings about changes in autonomy. Discuss with health care team ways to provide consistent and positive encouragement and strategies that increase independence progressively.

- Assess patient's ability to perform mouth care. Identify performance barriers (e.g., sensorimotor or cognitive deficits). If patient cannot perform mouth care, clean teeth, tongue, and mouth at least twice daily with a soft-bristled toothbrush and nonabrasive toothpaste. If patient is unconscious or at risk for aspiration, turn to a side-lying position. Swab mouth and teeth with sponge-tipped applicator moistened with diluted (half-strength) mouthwash solution, and irrigate mouth with a large syringe. If patient cannot self-manage secretions, use only a small amount of liquid for irrigation each time, and remove secretions with a suction catheter or Yankauer tonsil suction tip. Perform this oral hygiene regimen at least q4h. As appropriate, teach procedure to significant other.

- If patient has decreased LOC or is at risk for aspiration, remove dentures and store them in a water-filled denture cup. *This is to prevent choking or aspiration.*

- For patients with physical disabilities, the following toothbrush adaptations can be made:
  - *For patients with limited hand mobility:* Enlarge toothbrush handle by covering it with a sponge hair roller or aluminum foil (attaching with an elastic band) or by attaching a bicycle handle grip with plaster of Paris.
  - *For patients with limited arm mobility:* Extend toothbrush handle by overlapping another handle or rod over it and taping them together.

Impaired verbal communication related to facial/throat muscle weakness, intubation, or tracheostomy

Desired outcome: Following intervention and on an ongoing basis, patient communicates effectively, either verbally or nonverbally, and relates decreasing frustration with communication.

Nursing Interventions

◆ Assess patient's ability to speak, read, write, and comprehend.

◆ If appropriate, obtain referral to a speech therapist or pathologist. *The therapist can assist patient in strengthening muscles used in speech.* Encourage patient to perform exercises that increase ability to control facial muscles and tongue. These exercises may include holding a sound for 5 sec; singing the scale; reading aloud; and extending tongue and trying to touch chin, nose, or cheek.

◆ Provide a supportive and relaxed environment for patient who is unable to form words or sentences or who is unable to speak clearly or appropriately. Acknowledge frustration over inability to communicate. Explain that patience is needed for both patient and caregiver. Maintain a calm, positive, reassuring attitude. Continue to speak to patient using normal volume unless patient's hearing is impaired. Maintain eye contact to promote focus. Provide enough time for patient to articulate. Ask patient to repeat unclear words. Observe for nonverbal cues; watch patient's lips closely. Do not interrupt or finish sentences. Anticipate needs and phrase questions to allow simple answers, such as "yes" or "no." Provide continuity of care. *These interventions will help to decrease patient's frustration.*

◆ Provide alternative methods of communication if patient is unable to speak (e.g., language board, alphabet cards, picture or letter-number board, flash cards, pad and pencil). Other alternatives are systems that use eye blinks, tongue clicks, or hand squeezes; bell signal taps; or gestures such as hand signals, head nods, pantomime, or pointing. Use communication board for urgent situations. Document method of communication used. *Other staff can use the same effective method.*

◆ If patient's voice is weak and difficult to hear, reduce environmental noise to enhance listener's ability to hear words. Suggest that patient take a deep breath before speaking; provide a voice amplifier if appropriate. Encourage patient to organize thoughts and plan what he or she will say before speaking. Encourage patient to express ideas in short, simple phrases or sentences. Remind patient to speak slowly, exaggerate pronunciation, and use facial expressions. *This will help staff and others understand the patient's speech.*

◆ If patient has swallowing difficulties that result in accumulation of saliva, suction mouth. *This helps to promote clearer speech.*

◆ For patient with muscle rigidity or spasm, massage facial and neck muscles before patient attempts to communicate. *This may relax the muscles and make the speech more clear.*

◆ If patient has a tracheostomy, ensure that a tap bell is within reach. Reassure patient with a temporary tracheostomy that ability to speak will return. For patient with permanent tracheostomy, discuss learning alternate communication systems, such as sign language or esophageal speech. Fenestrated tubes or covering tracheostomy tube opening with a finger will enable speech.

◆ Establish a method of calling for assistance, and ensure that patient knows how to use it. Keep calling device where patient can activate it (e.g., place call bell on nonparalyzed side). Depending on deficit, use a tap bell for weak patient, a pillow pad call light (triggered by arm or head movement), or a sip and puff device (triggered by mouth).

◆ Encourage patient with ability to write to keep a diary or write letters. *This helps to ventilate feelings and to express concerns.* If patient has a weak writing arm, evaluate need for a splint. *This may enable patient to hold a pen or pencil*. Felt-tip markers also are useful. *They require minimal pressure for writing.* Large-barrel pens may be easier for grasping and writing. Patient may be able to type. For patient able to speak, a computer voice recognition program may be used. *This facilitates written and e-mail communication.*

Constipation related to inability to chew and swallow a high-roughage diet, side effects of medications, immobility, and spinal cord involvement
Desired outcome: Within 2-3 days of intervention, patient passes soft, formed stools and regains and maintains his or her normal bowel pattern.

Nursing Interventions

◆ Encourage patient to consume one or two servings of applesauce with added bran, prune juice, or cooked bran cereal each day. If that is not effective, encourage use of natural fiber laxatives such as psyllium (e.g., Metamucil). *A high-roughage diet is ideal for the patient who is immobilized or on prolonged bed rest, but individuals with chewing or swallowing difficulties may be unable to consume such a diet.*
◆ Unless contraindicated, encourage fluid intake to at least 2500 mL/day or more, including liberal amounts of fresh fruit juices.
◆ Start a bowel elimination program including the following elements: setting a regular time of day for attempting a bowel movement, preferably 30 min after eating a meal or drinking a hot beverage; using a commode instead of a bedpan for more natural positioning during elimination; using a medicated suppository 15-30 min before a scheduled attempt; drinking 4 oz of prune juice nightly ; or bearing down by contracting abdominal muscles or applying manual pressure to abdomen. *This is to help increase intraabdominal pressure.* Abdominal and pelvic exercise also may be included in patient's morning and evening routine. Keep a call bell within patient's reach. Assess patient's sitting balance. *This is to ensure safety while on commode.* Patients with SCI with involvement at T8 and above should use extreme caution if use of an enema or suppository is unavoidable. *This is because either can precipitate life-threatening autonomic dysreflexia (AD).* Liberal application of anesthetic jelly into the rectum should precede enema or suppository use. In addition, instruct patient at risk of increased intracranial pressure (IICP) not to bear down with bowel movements. This is because this action can cause increased intraabdominal pressure, which in turn increases intracranial pressure (ICP).
◆ If indicated by patient's diagnosis (e.g., MS), provide instructions for anal digital stimulation to promote reflex bowel evacuation. This intervention is contraindicated for SCI patients with involvement at T8 or above. *This is because it can precipitate life-threatening AD.*
◆ For other nursing interventions, see **Constipation,** p. 29, in "Prolonged Bed Rest."

Decreased intracranial adaptive capacity related to altered blood flow with risk of IICP and herniation secondary to positional factors, increased intrathoracic or intraabdominal pressure, fluid volume excess, hyperthermia, or discomfort secondary to brain injury
Desired outcome: Patient is free of symptoms of IICP and herniation as evidenced by stable or improving Glasgow Coma Scale (GCS) score (Box 5-3); stable or improving sensorimotor functioning; BP within patient's normal range; HR 60-100 bpm; pulse pressure 30-40 mm Hg (difference between SBPs and DBPs); orientation to person, place, and time; normal vision; bilaterally equal and normoreactive pupils; RR 12-20 breaths/min with normal depth and pattern (eupnea); normal gag, corneal, and swallowing reflexes; and absence of headache, nausea, nuchal rigidity, posturing, and seizure activity.

Nursing Interventions

◆ Monitor for and report any indicators of IICP or impending/occurring herniation. *The single most important indicator of early IICP is a change in LOC.*

- *Early indicators of IICP:* Declining GCS score, alterations in LOC ranging from irritability, restlessness, and confusion to lethargy; possible onset of or worsening of headache; beginning pupillary dysfunction (e.g., sluggishness); visual disturbances (e.g., diplopia or blurred vision); onset of or increase in sensorimotor changes or deficits e.g., weakness); onset of or worsening of nausea.

- *Late indicators of IICP:* Generally related to brainstem compression and disruption of cranial nerves and vital centers) such as continued decline in GCS score; continued deterioration in LOC leading to stupor and coma; projectile vomiting; hemiplegia; posturing; widening pulse pressure, decreased HR, and increased SBP; Cheyne-Stokes breathing or other respiratory irregularity; pupillary changes, inequality, dilation, and nonreactivity to light; papilledema; and impaired brainstem reflexes (corneal, gag, swallowing). See "Indicators of IICP" in "Traumatic Brain Injury," p. 309.

- *Brain herniation:* Deep coma, fixed and dilated pupils (first unilateral and then bilateral), posturing progressing to bilateral flaccidity, lost brainstem reflexes, and continuing deterioration in VS and respirations.

◆ If changes occur, prepare for possible transfer of patient to ICU. Insertion of ICP sensors for continuous ICP monitoring, continuous bedside cerebral blood flow (CBF) monitoring (e.g., continuous transcranial Doppler [TCD] sonography), cerebrospinal fluid (CSF) ventricular drainage, vasopressor usage (e.g., dopamine), intubation, mechanical ventilation, propofol sedation, neuromuscular blocking, or barbiturate coma therapy may be necessary. Continuous cardiac monitoring for dysrhythmia also will be done. Intensive insulin therapy may be needed to maintain normal serum glucose values (80-100 mg/dL). A computed tomography (CT) scan may be done, but lumbar puncture (LP) is contraindicated or used with caution in the presence of IICP.

◆ For patients at risk for IICP, preventive measures include ensuring a patent airway, delivering O_2 as prescribed, and limiting suctioning to when it is warranted and for 10 sec at a time. *This is to prevent hypoxia and CO_2 retention, to prevent vasodilation of cerebral arteries.* Monitor arterial blood gas (ABG) or pulse oximetry values. Mechanical hyperventilation, through reduced $PaCO_2$ levels and cerebral vasoconstriction, is important. *This is to reduce ICP, but hyperventilation produces a varied blood flow response and may cause cerebral ischemia.* Hyperventilation (e.g., with Ambu bag or if ventilated to keep $PaCO_2$ to 30-35 mm Hg) is generally used only in cases of acute deterioration until other interventions can be instituted (e.g., mannitol) or in cases in which IICP is refractory and responds to nothing else. CBF measurements and continuous jugular venous oxygen saturation (SjO_2) should be monitored. *This is to check for effectiveness if hyperventilation is used as a treatment.*

◆ Promote venous blood return to the heart to reduce cerebral congestion by maintaining head and neck alignment to avoid hyperextension, flexion, or rotation; ensuring that tracheostomy, endotracheal tube ties, or O_2 tubing does not compress the jugular vein; and avoiding Trendelenburg's position for any reason. Ensure that pillows under patient's head are flat. *This is to keep head is in a neutral rather than flexed position.* HOB should be at whatever level optimizes cerebral perfusion pressure (CPP) or as prescribed. Without monitoring equipment, having the HOB at 30 degrees is considered safe and effective at lowering ICP, as long as patient is not hypovolemic. *This condition could threaten CPP.*

◆ Teach patient to exhale when turning or during activity. Provide passive ROM exercises rather than allow active or assistive exercises. Administer prescribed stool softeners or laxatives to prevent straining at stool; avoid enemas and suppositories because they can cause straining. Instruct patient not to move self in bed because it requires a pushing movement; allow only passive turning; use a pull sheet. Instruct patient to avoid pushing against foot of bed or pulling against side rails. Avoid footboards; use high-top tennis shoes with toe end removed to level of the metatarsal heads instead. Assist patient with sitting up and turning. Instruct patient to avoid coughing and sneezing or, if unavoidable, to do so with an open mouth; provide antitussive for cough as prescribed and antiemetic for vomiting. Instruct patient to avoid hip flexion (increases intraabdominal pressure). Do not place patient in a prone position, and avoid using restraints (straining against them increases ICP). Rather than have patient perform Valsalva's maneuver (*to prevent an air embolism during insertion of a central venous catheter*), health care provider should use a syringe to aspirate air from the catheter lumen. *These interventions are precautions against increased intraabdominal and intrathoracic pressure.*

♦ Administer prescribed isotonic or hypertonic IV fluids. *They are given to maintain normovolemia and balanced electrolyte status.* Fluid restrictions are avoided. *This is because increased blood viscosity and decreased volume may lead to hypotension and thus decrease CPP.* Administer IV fluids only with an infusion control device. *This is to prevent fluid overload.* Keep accurate I&O records. When administering additional IV fluids (e.g., IV drugs), avoid using 5% dextrose in water (D_5W). *This is because its hypotonicity can increase cerebral edema and hyperglycemia that has been associated with inferior neurologic outcomes.*

♦ Help maintain patient's body temperature within normal limits by giving prescribed antipyretics, regulating temperature of the environment, limiting use of blankets, keeping patient's trunk warm to prevent shivering, and administering tepid sponge baths or using hypothermia blanket or convection cooling units to reduce fever. *This is because fever increases metabolic requirements (10% for each 1° C increase) and aggravates hypoxia.* When using a hypothermia blanket, wrap the patient's extremities in blankets or towels. *This prevents shivering, which could increase ICP.* Mild (e.g., 35° C) hypothermia treatment also may be tried.

♦ Administer prescribed osmotic (e.g., mannitol) and loop diuretics (e.g., furosemide). *This is to reduce cerebral edema and reduce blood volume.* Administer BP medications as prescribed. *This is to keep BP within prescribed limits that will promote optimal CBF without increasing cerebral edema. Hypotension is particularly detrimental inasmuch as it directly affects CBF.* Hypertension may be allowed or treated first with drugs such as labetalol. *Vasoactive drugs such as nitroprusside may worsen cerebral edema through vasodilation.* Administer prescribed analgesics promptly and as necessary. *This is because pain can increase ICP.* Barbiturates and opioids usually are contraindicated. *This is because of the potential for masking the signs of IICP and causing respiratory depression.* However, intubated, restless patients are usually sedated.

♦ Administer AEDs as prescribed. *This is to prevent or control seizures, which would increase cerebral metabolism, hypoxia, and CO_2 retention and thereby increase cerebral edema and ICP.*

♦ Monitor bladder drainage tubes for obstruction or kinks. *This is because a distended bladder can increase ICP.*

♦ Provide a quiet and soothing environment. Control noise and other environmental stimuli. Speak softly, use a gentle touch, and avoid jarring the bed. Try to limit painful procedures; avoid tension on tubes (e.g., urinary catheter); and consider limiting pain stimulation testing. Avoid unnecessary touch (e.g., leave BP cuff in place for frequent VS; use automatic recycling BP monitoring devices); and talk softly, explaining procedures before touching. Have patient listen to soft music with erphones. Do not say anything in the presence of the patient that you would not say if he or she were awake. Family discussions should take place outside the room. Limit visitors as necessary. Encourage significant other to speak quietly to patient. *These interventions are to prevent the patient from becoming over-stimulated or emotionally upset, situations that may increase ICP. Relaxation activities may decrease the ICP.*

♦ Individualize care to ensure rest periods and optimal spacing of activities; avoid turning, suctioning, and assessing VS all at one time. *Multiple procedures and nursing care activities can increase ICP.* Plan activities and treatments accordingly so that patient can sleep undisturbed as often as possible. *Rousing patients from sleep has been shown to increase ICP.*

Disturbed sensory perception: visual related to diplopia secondary to neurologic deficit
Desired outcome: Following intervention, patient verbalizes that vision has improved.

Nursing Interventions

♦ Assess for diplopia. If patient has diplopia, provide an eye patch or eye-glasses with one frosted lens. *This is a temporary means of eliminating this condition.* Alternate eye patch q4h.

♦ Orient patient to the environment as needed.

♦ Advise patient of availability of "talking books" (tapes) and large-type reading materials.

♦ Place a sign over patient's bed that indicates patient's visual impairment.

♦ Teach patient that depth perception will be altered and to use visual cues and scanning.

Acute pain related to spasms, headache, and photophobia secondary to neurologic dysfunction
Desired outcomes: Within 1 hr of intervention, patient's subjective perception of discomfort decreases, as documented by a pain scale. Objective indicators, such as grimacing, are absent or diminished.

Nursing Interventions

♦ Assess characteristics (e.g., quality, severity, location, onset, duration, precipitating factors) of patient's pain or spasms. Devise a pain scale with patient, and document discomfort on a scale of 0 (no pain) to 10 (worst pain). Determine patient's acceptable pain level and ways of coping with and relieving pain.

♦ Respond immediately to patient's complaints of pain. Administer analgesics and antispasmodics as prescribed. Consider scheduling doses of analgesia. Document effectiveness of the medication, using pain scale, approximately 30 min after administration. Monitor for untoward effects. Consult health care provider if dose or interval change seems necessary. Teach patient and significant other about importance of timing the pain medication so that it is taken before pain becomes too severe and before major moves. Intrascapular pain may be referred from the stomach, duodenum, or gallbladder; umbilical pain may be from the appendix; and testicular or inner thigh pain may be from the kidneys (e.g., pyelonephritis). *Pain in the patient with SCI often is poorly localized and may be referred.* Evaluate patient for signs of infection or inflammatory process (e.g., tachycardia, restlessness, fever, urinary incontinence that was previously controlled). *Infection/inflammation may also cause pain.*

♦ Teach patient about relationship between anxiety and pain, as well as other factors that enhance pain and spasms (e.g., staying in one position for too long, fatigue, chilling).

♦ Instruct patient and significant other in use of nonpharmacologic pain management techniques such as repositioning; ROM exercises; supporting painful extremity or part; back rubs, acupressure, massage, warm baths, and other tactile distraction; auditory distraction such as listening to soothing music; visual distraction such as television; heat applications such as warm blankets or moist compresses; cold applications such as ice massage; guided imagery; breathing exercises; relaxation tapes and techniques; biofeedback; and a transcutaneous electrical nerve stimulation (TENS) device, as appropriate. See **Health-seeking behaviors:** Relaxation technique effective for stress reduction, p. 106.

♦ Encourage rest periods. Try to provide uninterrupted sleep time at night. *This is to facilitate sleep and relaxation because fatigue tends to exacerbate the pain experience. Pain may result in fatigue, which in turn may cause exaggerated pain and further exhaustion.*

♦ If patient has photophobia, provide a quiet and dark environment. Close the door and curtains, provide sunglasses, and avoid use of artificial lights whenever possible.

♦ If patient's present complaint of pain varies significantly from previous pain or if interventions are ineffective, notify health care provider.

Impaired swallowing related to neuromuscular impairment (e.g., decreased or absent gag reflex, decreased strength or excursion of muscles involved in mastication, perceptual impairment, facial paralysis)
Desired outcome: Before oral foods and fluids are reintroduced, patient exhibits ability to swallow safely without aspirating.

Nursing Interventions

♦ Assess for factors that affect ability to swallow safely, including LOC, gag and cough reflexes, and strength and symmetry of tongue, lip, and facial muscles. Monitor coughing, regurgitation of food and fluid through the nares, drooling, food oozing from the lips, and food trapped in buccal spaces. *These may be signs of impaired swallowing.* Development of a weak, "wet," or hoarse voice during or after eating may be significant. *This may signal potential for impaired swallowing.* Check swallow reflex by first asking patient to swallow own saliva. Place a finger gently on top of larynx. If the larynx elevates with the attempt, a sign that the swallow reflex is intact, next ask patient to swallow 3-5 mL of plain water. *Presence of the cough reflex is essential for patient to relearn swallowing safely.*

♦ Obtain a referral to a speech therapist for patients with a swallowing dysfunction. *The act of swallowing is complex, and interventions vary according to the phase of swallowing that is dysfunctional.* Encourage patient to practice any prescribed exercises (e.g., tongue and jaw ROM, sound phonation such as "gah-gah-gah" to promote elevation of the soft palate); puckering lips; and sticking tongue out to touch nose, chin, and cheeks.

♦ If prescribed, insert a nasogastric (NG) tube for feedings. *Enteral nutrition may be necessary for patient who cannot chew or swallow effectively or safely.* Be aware that an NG tube may desensitize patient and impair reflexive response to food bolus stimulus, thereby hindering ability to relearn to swallow.

♦ Keep suction equipment and a manual resuscitation bag with face mask at patient's bedside. Suction secretions in patient's mouth as necessary.

♦ Ensure that patient is alert and responsive to verbal stimuli before attempting to swallow. *Patients who are drowsy, inattentive, or fatigued have difficulty cooperating are at risk of aspirating.* Provide a rest period before meals or swallowing attempts. *This is to minimize fatigue.* Provide oral hygiene frequently. *This is to enhance taste*

♦ Initial swallowing attempts should be made with plain water. *This is to reduce risk of aspiration.* Progressively add easy-to-swallow food and liquids as patient's ability to swallow improves. Determine which foods and liquids are easiest for patient to swallow. *Semisolid foods of medium* consistency, such as puddings, hot cereals, and casseroles, tend to be easiest to swallow. Thicker liquids, such as nectars, tend to be better tolerated than thin liquids. Commercially available powders (e.g., Thick-It) may be added to liquids. This is to increase their viscosity and make them more easily swallowed. Gravy or sauce added to dry foods often facilitates swallowing. Sticky, mucus-producing foods, such as peanut butter, chocolate, or milk, are often restricted or limited. Avoid nuts, hard candies, or popcorn. These may be aspirated.

◆ To help patient focus on swallowing, reduce stimuli in the room (e.g., turn off television, lower radio volume, minimize conversation, and limit disruptions from phone calls). Caution patient not to talk while eating.

◆ Sit patient in a straight-back chair with feet on the floor. Most patients swallow best when in an upright position. If patient must remain in bed, use high Fowler's position if possible. Support shoulders and neck with pillows. Ensure that head is erect and flexed forward slightly, with chin at the midline and pointing toward chest (i.e., the "chin tuck"). This will minimize risk that food will go into the airway. Stroke anterior side of neck lightly. This may help some patients swallow. Maintain patient in an upright position for at least 30-60 min after eating. This is to prevent regurgitation and aspiration.

◆ Teach patient to break down the act of chewing and swallowing. Encourage concentration and taking adequate time. Talk patient through the following steps:
  • Take small bites or sips (approximately 5 mL each).
  • Place food on tongue.
  • Use tongue to transfer food so that it is directly under teeth on unaffected side of the mouth.
  • Chew food thoroughly.
  • Move food to middle of tongue and hold it there.
  • Flex neck and tuck chin against chest.
  • Hold the breath and think about swallowing.
  • Without breathing, raise tongue to roof of mouth and swallow.
  • Swallow several times if necessary.
  • When mouth is empty, raise chin and clear throat or cough purposefully once or twice.

◆ Start with small amounts of food or liquid. Each bite should not exceed 5 mL (1 tsp). Feed slowly. Ensure that each previous bite has been swallowed. Check mouth for pockets of food. After every few bites of solid food, provide a liquid. This will help clear the mouth. Avoid using a syringe. This is because the force of the fluid, if sprayed, may cause aspiration. Avoid use of drinking straws. Tear a piece out of a Styrofoam cup to make a space for the nose so that patient can drink with neck flexed.

◆ Teach patient who has food pockets in the buccal spaces to periodically sweep mouth with tongue or finger or to clean these areas with a napkin. Apply external pressure to cheek with a finger. This will help remove a trapped food bolus.

◆ Teach patient who has a weak or paralyzed side to place food on side of the face patient can control and to tilt the head toward the stronger side. This will allow gravity to help keep food or liquid on side of the mouth patient can manipulate. Some patients may find that rotating head to weak side is helpful. This will close damaged side of the pharynx and facilitate more effective swallowing.

◆ Patients with loss of oral sensation may be unable to identify foods or fluids of tepid temperature with tongue or oral mucosa. Serve only warm or cool foods to these individuals. This may prevent tissue injury.

◆ Encourage repeated swallowing attempts. This will facilitate movement of food in a patient in a patient with a rigid tongue. Patients with a rigid tongue (e.g., with parkinsonism) have difficulty getting the tongue to move a bolus of food into the pharynx for swallowing. Evaluate patient's swallowing ability at different times of the day. Reschedule mealtimes to times when patient has improved swallowing, or as appropriate, discuss with health care provider the possibility of changing dose schedule of patient's antiparkinsonian medication.

♦ If decreased salivation is contributing to patient's swallowing difficulties, perform one of the following before feeding: swab patient's mouth with a lemon-glycerin sponge; have patient suck on a tart-flavored hard candy, dill pickle, or lemon slice; teach patient to move tongue in a circular motion against inside of cheek; or use artificial saliva. Moisten food with melted butter, broth or other soup, or gravy. Dip dry foods such as toast into coffee or other liquid to soften them. Rinse patient's mouth as needed to remove particles and lubricate mouth. Investigate medications patient is taking for potential side effect of decreased salivation (e.g., antiparkinsonian medications or those with extrapyramidal side effects). *These interventions will help increase salivation.*

♦ Tablets or capsules may be swallowed more easily when added to foods such as puddings or ice cream. Crushed tablets or opened capsules also mix easily into these types of foods. However, check with pharmacist to ensure that crushing a tablet or opening a capsule does not adversely affect its absorption or duration (i.e., slow-release medications should not be crushed). Liquid forms of medications also may be available through the pharmacy.

♦ Teach significant other the Heimlich or abdominal thrust maneuver. *This is a safety measure so that he or she can intervene in the event of choking.*

Risk for imbalanced body temperature related to illness or trauma affecting temperature regulation and inability or decreased ability to perspire, shiver, or vasoconstrict

Desired outcome: Following intervention(s), patient is normothermic, with core temperatures between 36.5° and 37.7° C (97.8° and 100° F).

Nursing Interventions

♦ Monitor rectal, tympanic, or bladder core temperature q4h, or if patient is in spinal shock, q2h.
  - *Observe for signs of hypothermia:* impaired ability to think, disorientation, confusion, drowsiness, apathy, and reduced HR and RR. Monitor for complaints of being too cold, goose bumps (piloerection), and cool skin (in patients with SCI, above level of injury).
  - *Observe for signs of hyperthermia:* flushed face, malaise, rash, respiratory distress, tachycardia, weakness, headache, and irritability. Monitor for complaints of being too warm, sweating, or hot and dry skin (in patients with SCI, above level of injury). *Infection and hypothalamic dysfunction as a result of cerebral insult (trauma, edema) are two common causes of hyperthermia. Rapid development of spinal lesions (e.g., patients in SCI) breaks the connection between the hypothalamus and sympathetic nervous system (SNS) and causes an inability to adapt to environmental temperature. In spinal cord shock, temperatures tend to lower toward the ambient temperature. Inability to vasoconstrict and shiver makes heat conservation difficult; inability to perspire prevents normal cooling.*
  - *Observe for signs of dehydration:* parched mouth, furrowed tongue, dry lips, poor skin turgor, decreased urine output, increased concentration of urine (specific gravity greater than 1.030), and weak, fast pulse.

♦ *For hyperthermia:* Maintain a cool room temperature (20° C [68° F]). Provide a fan or air conditioning to prevent overheating. Remove excess bedding and cover patient with a thin sheet. Give tepid sponge baths. Place cool, wet cloths at patient's head, neck, axilla, and groin. Administer antipyretic agent as prescribed. Use a padded hypothermia blanket (wrap hands and feet in towels or blankets to prevent shivering) or convection cooling device if prescribed. Provide cool drinks. Evaluate for potential infectious cause.

◆ *For hypothermia:* Increase environmental temperature. Protect patient from drafts. Provide warm drinks. Provide extra blankets. Provide warming (hyperthermia) blanket or convection warming device.

◆ Keep feverish patient dry. Change bed linens after diaphoresis. Provide careful skin care when patient is on a hypothermia or hyperthermia blanket. Maintain adequate hydration. Consider insensible water loss from fever. *This may affect total hydration, when measuring I&O.* Unless contraindicated, encourage increased fluid intake in febrile patients. Increase caloric intake. *This is because of increased metabolic needs.* Note whether patient is on steroids. *Steroids may mask fever or infection.*

Deficient knowledge related to neurologic diagnostic tests (electroencephalogram [EEG], PET [positron emission tomography], magnetic resonance imaging [MRI], CT scan, lumbar puncture [LP], myelography, digital subtraction angiography [DSA], cerebral angiography, oculoplethysmography, electromyography (EMG), nerve conduction velocity [NCV], evoked potential [EP] studies, single photon emission CT [SPECT]) related to new treatment experience

Desired outcome: Following explanation and before the procedure, patient verbalizes understanding about the prescribed diagnostic test, including purpose, risks, anticipated benefits, and expectations for the patient before, during, and after the test.

Nursing Interventions

◆ After health care provider has explained diagnostic study, reinforce or clarify information as indicated. Explain who will perform the test, why and where it will be done, and need to report any possible adverse reactions. Describe physical sensations patient may experience and explain cause. Answer questions. Adjust and simplify information to what patient can understand, and repeat several times, as appropriate. Instruct patient regarding any test preparation and give printed, language-appropriate information if available. Obtain signed permit if test is invasive.

◆ Have patient void before the test. This is to prevent discomfort or test interruption.

◆ For tests using contrast media, evaluate for allergies to contrast media. If not contraindicated, fluid intake should be encouraged. *This is to help dilute dye and reduce its nephrotoxicity. Contrast media generally act as osmotic diuretics.* Patients taking metformin generally should hold medication for 6 hr before and 48 hr after procedure (check with health care provider). *This is to reduce risk of lactic acidosis with inadequate renal function.* Oral antihistamine or corticosteroids may be prescribed as a premedication.

◆ If scalp **EEG** is prescribed, explain that this test will indicate amount of brain activity present and may reveal abnormal patterns of electrical activity, particularly with such stimuli as flashing lights or hyperventilation. Explain that an EEG may be performed while patient is either asleep or awake and may sometimes be performed on a continuous basis by telemetry. Cooperation is important. The test may take 40-120 min. Alert EEG staff to medications being taken. In addition, discuss the following as appropriate:

- *Before the test:* antiepileptic drugs (AEDs), sedatives, tranquilizers, and alcohol may be withheld 24-48 hr before test. Patient's hair should be thoroughly washed and dried, but sprays, creams, and oils must be avoided. If a sleep EEG has been prescribed, patient will need to stay awake or limit amount of sleep the night before the test. A normal diet usually is allowed the morning of the test to prevent hypoglycemia, but caffeine-containing foods (e.g., chocolate) and beverages (e.g., coffee, tea, colas) are restricted.

- *During the test:* Small electrode patches are attached to the head. The skin may be lightly abraded. *This is to ensure good contact.* Reassure patient that he or she will not receive any electric shocks. The patient must lie very still during the test and may be asked to watch flashing lights or to hyperventilate. *This is to elicit electrical activity patterns in the brain.*

- *After the test:* Hair washing or acetone swabs will be used. *This is to remove paste used for attaching electrodes.* Medications probably will be reinstated at this time. If needle electrodes were used, avoid washing hair for 24 hr.
- *For ambulatory (telemetry) EEG:* Teach how to keep electrodes in place and how to keep a journal of activity for the 48-72 hr length of the test.
- *For continuous video and EEG recording:* Instruct patient to stay within camera view. *This is so that clinical behavior can be correlated with EEG abnormalities.*

◆ If **PET** is prescribed, explain that this test measures how rapidly tissue consumes or uses a radioisotope and may locate areas of altered cerebral glucose metabolism that correspond to a seizure-causing focus (e.g., increased metabolic activity from rapid nerve firing), areas of ischemia or low metabolism (e.g., Alzheimer's disease), or tumor tissue. In addition, discuss the following as appropriate:

- *Before the test:* The procedure is contraindicated during pregnancy. Alcohol, caffeine, and tobacco may be restricted for 24 hr. *This is to prevent skewing of test results.* Usually food is restricted about 4 hr before the test (water is usually allowed). If patient has diabetes mellitus, the health care provider should give special instructions about a 3-4hr pretest meal and insulin administration. *This is because insulin alters glucose metabolism.* IV and arterial lines will be placed for isotope injection and laboratory blood drawing.
- *During the test:* Explain that the test takes 1-4 hr, and patient is required to be still during that time. Tranquilizers are contraindicated. *This is because they alter glucose metabolism.* The patient is given radioisotope by injection or inhalation. If it will be given by inhalation, a dome-shaped hood will be placed over patient's head. *This is to prevent exhaled tracer from circulating in the room.* Patient may be blindfolded or have ears plugged. *This is to reduce extraneous stimulation.* Patient may be asked to do mental activity such as recitation.
- *After the test:* Encourage fluids if not contraindicated.

◆ If **MRI** has been prescribed, explain that this test may reveal biochemical changes caused by hypoxia or necrosis; by degenerative disease; or by a mass such as a tumor, hemorrhage, tissue shift, or hydrocephalus. This test also may show structural lesions that may be responsible for symptoms such as seizures. *MRI is more useful than CT scanning in evaluating pituitary tumors, acoustic neuromas, posterior fossa tumors, spinal cord tumors and trauma, demyelinating disease, and cerebral atrophy, as well as in situations in which patient is allergic to contrast medium.* In addition, discuss the following as appropriate:

- *Before the test:* Confirm that patient does not have a ferromagnetic implant such as a pacemaker, surgical aneurysm clip, prosthetic heart valve, or umbrella filter for emboli and is not pregnant. Ask about presence of fractures that were treated with metal rods, other implants (cochlear, insulin pumps), or shrapnel or gunshot wounds. *MRI is contraindicated during pregnancy; MRI can deactivate pacemakers, and the strong magnetic field can move ferrous metal aneurysm clips, valves, and umbrella filters within the body, thus putting patient at obvious risk.* The presence of these internal items makes patient ineligible for MRI. Patients with compatible programmable implants (e.g., deep brain stimulator) may need to have them reprogrammed postprocedure. Explain that no exposure to radiation occurs. Claustrophobic patients may need sedation (usually oral) and may be given prism glasses so they can "see out."

Obese patients will need to meet equipment size/weight limitations. "Open" MRI is useful for these types of patients. Patients should void before the test and remove items such as jewelry, hair clips, credit cards, clothing with metal fasteners, and glasses before entering scanner.

- *During the test:* Patient must be able to cope with confined spaces and have ability to lie motionless throughout the 30-90-min test. Confused patients may not be able to cooperate enough even with sedation. A soft, humming sound and "knocking" on-off pulses will be heard. Health care provider may prescribe a sedative. Patient's head, chest, and arms may be restrained. *This is to help the patient lie still.* Patients with metal fillings in teeth or compatible implants may feel a tingling or warmth. Patient may be injected with IV contrast medium, such as gadolinium (Gd), a paramagnetic agent. *This enhances tumor images.* Patient can communicate with radiology staff via a two-way microphone.

- If a **CT scan** has been prescribed, explain that the test may detect masses from tumors, hemorrhage, tissue shift, and hydrocephalus. Serial scans may be performed. *This is to determine the response of a tumor to therapy and to detect a resolution or increase in a hemorrhage.* Xenon-enhanced CT is used to measure CBF. *CT scanning is more useful than MRI in evaluating acute trauma or hemorrhage, supratentorial enhancing tumors, and hydrocephalus, as well as when patient has a pacemaker or internal ferrous metal objects or is uncooperative.* If contrast agents are not used, there are no known complications of CT scans. If a contrast agent is used, discuss the following with patient as indicated:
  - *Before the test:* Allergies to iodine or iodine-containing substances such as shellfish or contrast medium must be reported to health care provider. Food and fluids may be restricted 4 hr before the test. Remove hairpins, wigs and glasses. The test usually lasts 5-30 min. Patient must lie flat and still, the head may be immobilized, and sedation may be prescribed. Explain that the room will be cool. *This is to protect the equipment.*
  - *During the test:* A warm, flushed feeling or burning sensation is normal. Patient also may experience a salty taste with dye injection, nausea, vomiting, or a headache during or after the test. *These sensations are usually the result of administration of the dye.* Patient may be asked to take and hold several deep breaths during scanning.
  - *After the test:* If it is not contraindicated, fluid intake is increased. *This is to ensure elimination of contrast dye via the kidneys.* Patient will be monitored for signs of delayed allergic reaction (e.g., hives, rash, and itching).

- If **LP** has been prescribed, explain that it is performed to remove a sample of CSF for analysis, to determine CSF pressure, or to administer medication. *CSF is evaluated for microorganisms, blood cells, tumor markers, and chemical analysis.* Skin or bone infection at the puncture site is a contraindication. This procedure is performed with great caution in the presence of IICP. *This is because of risk of herniation.* Inability of patient to cooperate, severe degenerative joint disease, and anticoagulant therapy also may preclude use of LP. Also discuss the following as indicated:
  - *Before the test:* Assure patient that the needle will not enter spinal cord. Patient should empty bladder.
  - *During the test:* Patient will be assisted into a side-lying position, with chin tucked into chest and knees drawn up to abdomen (fetal position). *This position curves the spine and widens the intervertebral space for easier insertion of spinal needle.* Patient must lie still during the procedure, and a nurse will assist with maintaining position. An alternate position is sitting flexed over an over-the-bed table with patient's head and arms resting on a pillow. Patient should breathe normally during the test. There may be a short burning sensation when local anesthetic is injected and some local transient pain when the spinal needle is inserted.

Patient will feel pressure as the needle is advanced to the spinal canal. Patient should report any pain or sensations that continue after or differ from these expected discomforts. Patient will be monitored for discomfort, elevated HR, pallor, and clammy skin during the procedure. During the test, the health care provider may ask patient to breathe deeply or may apply jugular pressure.

- *After the test:* Bed rest may not be prescribed if patient has no headache. Generally, however, patient will remain in bed with HOB flat or raised slightly for a prescribed period, usually no more than 4-8 hr; may turn from side to side during this period; and should drink a large amount of fluids unless contraindicated. *These measures will help minimize any postprocedure headache, which is the most common adverse effect of LP.* Patient should report any headache to nurse. *This is so that an ice cap and analgesia, if prescribed, can be administered.* The nurse will check LP site periodically for redness, swelling, and drainage. The nurse also will check VS and neurologic status. Patient should report any neck stiffness, pain, numbness, weakness, or difficulty voiding. For post-LP headache lasting more than 24 hr, IV caffeine may be used, or as a second-line agent, adrenocorticotropic hormone. In the event of a CSF leak or persistent, severe headache lasting several days, the health care provider may place an epidural blood patch.

◆ If **myelography** has been prescribed, explain that it is performed when other diagnostic tests are inconclusive, to delineate or rule out blockage or disruption of the spinal cord. Radiopaque dye is injected into the subarachnoid space of the spine by lumbar or cervical puncture, and the test usually is done in combination with CT. Discuss foregoing LP section with patient. Also discuss the following as indicated:

- *Before the test:* Allergies or sensitivity to iodine, shellfish, and contrast medium; history of medications that could lower the seizure threshold (e.g., phenothiazines, neuroleptics [tricyclics, antidepressants], amphetamines) and AEDs must be reported to radiologist. Foods are withheld for a period, usually 4-8 hr, before the test, but patient should be kept well hydrated. An intestinal preparation may be prescribed.

- *During the test:* Patient may feel transient burning when contrast dye is injected and experience salty taste, headache, or nausea after injection. Patient will need to sit quietly with head up during the 45-60-min procedure. *This enables controlled upward dispersion of the dye.* Patient may feel some discomfort during the procedure.

- *After the test:* VS and peripheral neurologic status should be routinely assessed, and changes from pretest assessments promptly reported to health care provider. Patient should be instructed to report any increased motor or sensory deficit from pretest status, chills, fever, neck stiffness, and redness or swelling at puncture site. Headache occurs in 25%-50% of patients, nausea in 15%-40%, and vomiting in 25%; these adverse effects should be reported. *This is so that comfort measures can be taken.* Nonrestricted persons should drink extra fluids. *This is to replace CSF lost during the test.* The following postmyelogram positions may be used:
  - HOB will be elevated to 30-60 degrees for 8-12 hr. *This is to minimize irritation to cranial nerves and structures.* After 4-6 hr of bed rest, bathroom privileges are permitted, but minimal activity is permitted for 24 hr after the myelogram. Seizures, hallucination, depression, confusion, speech problems, chest pain, and dysrhythmia may occur. *This may happen if water-based contrast reaches the cranial vault.* Phenothiazines and neuroleptics should be held for 24-48 hr after myelograms done using water-based dyes. *This is because they lower the seizure threshold.* Nausea and headache can be treated with appropriate medications. Monitor for back pain, spasms, increased temperature, or difficulty voiding.

- An air contrast myelogram may be done. *This is to avoid side effects of the dyes.* After air is injected, the head must be kept lower than the trunk. *Air gravitating to the cerebrum will cause headache.*

◆ If **DSA** has been prescribed, explain that it is performed to help visualize CBF and detect vascular abnormalities such as stenosis, aneurysm, and hematoma. Patients are expected to lie still for the 30-60-min procedure and hold their breath on command. *Minor movements such as swallowing can distort the results.* Also discuss the following with patient as indicated:
  - *Before the test:* Patient will be assessed for adequate cardiac output to disperse the dye and adequate kidney function to excrete the dye. Allergies to iodine, shellfish, or radiopaque dye must be reported to health care provider. Food and fluids usually are withheld 2-4 hr before the procedure, although clear liquids sometimes are allowed. Patient may feel transient discomfort with needle or catheter insertion, as well as a headache, warm sensation, or metallic taste. *This is the result of dye injection.*
  - *During the test:* Patient must be able to hold breath, remain motionless, and lie flat.
  - *After the test:* Patient will be required to drink large amounts of fluid, if not contraindicated. *This is to promote dye excretion by the kidneys.* Nurses will check venipuncture site for bleeding, redness, and swelling. Patient should be instructed to report itching, rash, hives, or dyspnea. *This may signal delayed dye reaction 2-6 hr after the test.*

◆ If **cerebral angiography** has been prescribed, explain that it enables visualization of cerebral vasculature after injection of a contrast medium and determines site, structure, and size of an aneurysm or arteriovenous malformation (AVM), presence of vasospasm, and site of rupture or obstructed blood flow. It also may show an abnormal perfusion pattern, which suggests presence of a tumor. Severe kidney, liver, or thyroid disease may be contraindications. Also discuss the following with patient as indicated:
  - *Before the test:* Allergies to iodine, shellfish, or radiopaque dyes must be reported to health care provider. Foods and fluids are withheld for 6-10 hr or as prescribed. Local anesthetic is used at puncture site. Patient will feel a warm or burning sensation and have a transient headache or metallic taste sensation. *This is the result of dye administration.* The proposed site may be shaved. If the femoral approach is used, pedal pulses will be checked and their location marked. Document decrease or absence of pedal pulses. If the carotid approach is used, patient's neck circumference will be measured, marked, and recorded. Baseline neurologic status is checked and recorded. *This is for postprocedure comparison so that small changes can be detected early.* Dentures and eyeglasses usually are removed.
  - *During the test:* Patient is expected to lie flat and still for the 60-120-min procedure. Patient's extremities or head may be immobilized with tape or straps.
  - *After the test:* Patient will be on strict bed rest for 6-8 hr, followed by a specified period of bathroom privileges only. VS and pulse quality will be checked frequently (e.g., 15 min × 4; 30 min × 2; 60 min × 4). Patient should notify staff if signs of reaction to the dye occur, including respiratory distress, lightheadedness (hypotension), hives, or itching. Fluids will be encouraged. *This is to eliminate dye and protect against kidney damage.* Puncture site will be checked frequently for bleeding or formation of hematoma. Patient should not be alarmed if bleeding occurs. Manual pressure will be maintained until bleeding stops. A pressure dressing and/or sandbag may then be applied and health care provider notified. Quality of distal pulses and temperature, color, capillary refill, motor function, and sensation in the extremity will be monitored at

frequent intervals and changes reported to health care provider. *Any weakening pulses, pallor, coolness, extremity pain, delayed capillary refill (3 sec or longer), or cyanosis may signal thrombus formation and artery obstruction.* Nerve injury during insertion of needle/catheter is also possible; any paresthesia or weakness should be reported to health care provider. *This is because of proximity to nerves at the puncture site.*

- If the femoral approach was used, patient should keep leg straight for prescribed period (usually 6-8 hr). *This is to minimize risk of bleeding.* Patient will use a bedpan or urinal and eat in a side-lying position during this time.
- A device such as an Angio-Seal or Perclose may be used to attain hemostasis on the femoral artery. If used, patient is usually on bed rest for a period (e.g., 4 hr) but is not required to be flat and still.
- If the brachial approach was used, patient's arm will be immobilized for 6-8 hr or as prescribed. A sign will be posted over patient's bed that cautions against measuring BP or drawing blood in that arm. Patient should report pain or numbness in fingers. *This may indicate nerve compression.*
- If the carotid artery was the puncture site, patient should report any difficulty swallowing or breathing or any weakness or numbness. HOB is usually at 30 degrees. The neck will be checked for increasing circumference (comparing current measurements with preprocedural measurements) or tracheal displacement. *These may signal hematoma formation.* LOC or neurologic status will be monitored. *Changes in LOC or the presence of neurologic deficits may indicate thrombus formation or cerebral emboli from disrupted atherosclerotic plaque causing arterial obstruction.*

◆ If **EMG** and **NCV** studies are prescribed, explain that they are usually are performed together. *This is to diagnose and differentiate between peripheral nerve and muscle disorders.* Also discuss the following with patient as indicated:
- *Before the test:* Bleeding disorders, use of anticoagulants, or extensive skin infection may be contraindications. Fasting is not required, but some stimulants such as coffee, tea, colas, or cigarettes may be restricted for 2-4 hr before the test. Explain that patient cooperation will be necessary during the 20-30-min test.
- *During the test:* Insertion of small needles into muscle will cause some discomfort. The muscle will twitch when electrical stimulus is applied, but that is not painful.
- *After the test:* Needle sites will be monitored. *This is to determine presence of hematomas or inflammation.* Mild analgesia may be used. *This is for any muscle aches.*

◆ If **EP** studies are prescribed, explain that they are used to evaluate integrity of a visual, auditory, or somatosensory nerve pathway by stimulating a sensory organ (e.g., eye, ear) and measuring the time required for the triggered electrical response (the EP) to travel along the pathway and into the brain. A conduction velocity delay indicates damage. Hair is shampooed before the procedure. *This is to remove oil and lotions.* Postprocedure shampooing is also done. *This is to remove electrode paste.* Also discuss the following with patient:
- *Visual evoked response:* Cooperation is needed. Electrodes are placed over occipital region. Prescription glasses should be worn. Patterned (e.g., checkerboard) and flashing lights will provide retinal stimulation. This test is helpful in diagnosing optic neuritis associated with multiple sclerosis (MS).
- *Somatosensory evoked response:* Peripheral nerve responses in upper or lower extremities help evaluate spinal cord function, sensory dysfunction with MS, and nerve root compression.

- *Brainstem auditory evoked responses:* Used to evaluate brainstem function. Auditory stimulation via headphone is provided. A series of clicks will be heard, varying in rate, intensity, and duration. This test does not require patient cooperation. It can help diagnose brainstem lesion in MS, acoustic neuroma, brainstem lesions related to coma, and hearing loss. It also may be used to monitor cranial nerve VIII for surgical injury.

◆ If **SPECT** has been prescribed, explain that this test measures CBF by watching a tracer pass through cerebral circulation. No special preprocedure care or aftercare is needed. Explain the following to the patient:
  - *During the test:* Patient will receive a dose of a salty-tasting solution and an injection with an IV tracer. It is important to lie still during the 60-min scanning. During the test, the table will move, and a large, disk-shaped machine will rotate around patient's head.

◆ After teaching about any of the neurologic diagnostic tests, evaluate patient's level of understanding of the diagnostic test.

SECTION ONE DISORDERS OF THE THYROID GLAND

❖ HYPERTHYROIDISM

OVERVIEW/PATHOPHYSIOLOGY

Hyperthyroidism is a clinical syndrome caused by excessive circulating thyroid hormone. Because thyroid activity affects all body systems, excessive thyroid hormone exaggerates normal body functions and produces a hypermetabolic state.

Lymphocytic ("painless") *thyroiditis* and *postpartum thyroiditis* are autoimmune disorders that result in thyroid inflammation with release of stored thyroid hormone into systemic circulation. Postpartum thyroiditis may ensue several months after delivery and remain active for several months, sometimes followed by hypothyroidism lasting several months.

Subacute (granulomatous) thyroiditis is a viral syndrome resulting in a painful, enlarged, overactive thyroid until the infection is controlled. Hyperthyroid symptoms also result from ingestion of too much thyroid replacement medication.

Graves' disease (diffuse toxic goiter) accounts for approximately 85% of reported cases of hyperthyroidism. It is characterized by spontaneous exacerbations and remissions that appear to be unaffected by therapy. The cause of Graves' disease is unknown, but an immunoglobulin known as *long-acting thyroid stimulator* has been isolated in a majority of patients with this disorder, a finding suggesting that Graves' disease is an autoimmune response.

Thyrotoxic crisis, or *thyroid storm*, is the most severe form of hyperthyroidism. It results from a sudden surge of large amounts of thyroid hormones into the bloodstream that cause an even greater increase in body metabolism. This is a *medical emergency.* Precipitating factors include infection, trauma, and emotional stress, all of which increase demands on body metabolism. Thyrotoxic crisis also can occur following thyroidectomy because of manipulation of the gland during surgery.

ASSESSMENT

Signs and symptoms/physical findings: Tachycardia, palpitations, irregular heart rate (HR), widened pulse pressure, exophthalmos, diplopia, hyperpyrexia, enlargement of the thyroid gland, dependent lower extremity edema, muscle weakness, hyperreflexia, fine tremor, fine hair, thin skin, hypercholesterolemia, impaired glucose tolerance (IGT), stare and/or lid lag, nervousness, irritability, alteration in appetite, weight loss or gain, menstrual irregularities, fatigue, heat intolerance, increased perspiration, frequent defecation or diarrhea, anxiety, tremor, and insomnia. Occasionally male patients may present with gynecomastia.

377

Thyrotoxic crisis (thyroid storm): Acute exacerbation of some or all of the foregoing signs, marked tachycardia, hyperpyrexia, central nervous system (CNS) irritability, and sometimes coma or heart failure.

History and risk factors: Family history of hyperthyroidism and the presence of thyroid nodules or nodular toxic goiters in which one or more thyroid adenomas hyperfunction autonomously are significant risk factors. Amiodarone use has caused thyroid dysfunction in 14%-18% of individuals taking this commonly used antidysrhythmic drug. Patients should have thyroid studies done before the drug is initiated and be monitored subsequently.

DIAGNOSTIC TESTS

Serum thyroid-stimulating hormone (TSH), or thyrotropin: Most commonly used test to detect thyroid dysfunction. It is decreased in the presence of disease.

Serum thyroxine (T_4) or free T_4: Elevated in the presence of disease. It may be more accurate than TSH if patients have been recently treated for hyperthyroidism or if they are receiving high doses of thyroid replacement therapy. T_4 should be monitored along with TSH for the first year of therapy, especially in older adults.

Serum triiodothyronine (T_3) radioimmunoassay (RIA) or free T_3: Elevated in the presence of disease.

Serum thyroid autoantibody assay: Detects TSH receptor antibodies (TRAb) and thyroid-stimulating immunoglobulins (TSIs), which may be present in autoimmune disease.

Doppler ultrasonography: Determines size of the gland and abnormal densities, which can indicate presence of nodules.

Radioactive iodine (^{131}I) uptake and thyroid scan: Clarifies gland size and detects presence of hot or cold nodules.

Radioactive iodine (^{123}I) scintiscan/thyroid scintigraphy: Defines functional characteristics of the gland to help determine cause of hyperthyroidism.

COLLABORATIVE MANAGEMENT

Pharmacotherapy

Antithyroid agents: Propylthiouracil (PTU) and methimazole are the first line therapeutic agents. In milder cases, methimazole is preferred because it is taken once daily, a regimen that increases adherence to therapy. The most severe side effect of these drugs is leukopenia. Patients should discontinue the drug at the first sign of infection and be referred for a complete blood count (CBC). If the blood count is normal, medication is promptly resumed. Rash, another side effect, can be treated easily with antihistamines. For pregnant women, PTU is the drug of choice, because newborn infants have experienced scalp irritation when their mothers took methimazole while pregnant.

Radioactive iodine ablation: Approach used most commonly in the United States to resolve hyperthyroidism permanently. The thyroid is destroyed with radioactive iodine. The process takes 6-18 wk for completion. Severely symptomatic people, those with heart disease, and older adults should receive antithyroid drugs before receiving radioiodine in order to resolve symptoms more quickly. Radioiodine ablation is used for (1) failure to respond to antithyroid drugs, (2) relapse after 1-2 yr of therapy, (3) toxic multinodular goiter, (4) solitary toxic nodules, and (5) noncompliant patients. ^{131}I is the most commonly used agent. Its use usually results in hypothyroidism, which is controlled easily with thyroid hormone replacement therapy. The small amount of radiation present in liquid or capsules does not cause cancer. About 10% of patients treated require a second dose.

β-Adrenergic blocking agents (e.g., atenolol or propranolol): Relieve overactive thyroid symptoms, including tachycardia, anxiety, heat intolerance, and tremor. Once symptoms resolve with other medications or treatments, β-blocking agents may be discontinued.

Mild tranquilizers: Minimize anxiety and promote rest.

Diet: If significant weight loss has occurred, a diet high in calories, protein, carbohydrates, and vitamins is recommended to restore a normal nutritional state.

Thyroidectomy: Surgical removal of the gland may be necessary for patients with extremely enlarged glands that may partially obstruct the trachea or multinodular goiter. Surgery is done infrequently in the United States because most patients receive medical therapy with antithyroid medications or radioactive iodine. The patient is prepared with antithyroid agents until normal thyroid function is achieved (usually 6-8 wk). The most common postoperative complication is hemorrhage at the operative site. Rare but extremely serious complications are hypoparathyroidism, laryngeal nerve injury, and tetany, owing to damage to the parathyroid glands.

NURSING DIAGNOSES AND INTERVENTIONS

Imbalanced nutrition: less than body requirements related to hypermetabolic state and/or inadequate nutrient absorption

Desired outcomes: At least 24 hr before hospital discharge, patient has adequate nutrition as evidenced by stable weight and a positive nitrogen balance. Within 24 hr of the instruction, patient lists types of foods that are necessary to restore a normal nutritional state.

Nursing Interventions

- Provide foods high in calories, protein, carbohydrates, and vitamins. Teach patient about foods that will provide optimal nutrients and encourage between-meal stacks *to maximize intake.*
- Administer vitamin supplements as prescribed, and explain their importance to patient. *Helps replace vitamins lost as a result of the hypermetabolic state.*
- Administer prescribed antidiarrheal medications, which increase absorption of nutrients from the gastrointestinal (GI) tract. *Helps prevent hypermetabolic diarrhea.*
- Weigh patient daily, and report significant losses to health care provider. *Weight loss is common because of hypermetabolism and diarrhea.*

Disturbed sleep pattern related to accelerated metabolism

Desired outcome: Within 48 hr of hospital admission, patient relates attainment of sufficient rest and sleep.

Nursing Interventions

- Adjust care activities to patient's tolerance *to prevent excessive fatigue or activity intolerance.*
- Provide frequent rest periods at least 90 min in duration. If possible, arrange for patient to have bed rest in a quiet, cool room with nonexertional activities such as reading, watching television, working crossword puzzles, or listening to soothing music *to help reduce metabolic rate.*
- Assist with walking up stairs or other exertional activities if needed, *to prevent injury.*
- Administer short-acting sedatives (e.g., lorazepam) as prescribed. After administering these agents, raise side rails and caution patient not to smoke in bed. *Promotes rest.*

Ineffective protection related to risk for thyrotoxic crisis (thyroid storm) secondary to emotional stress, trauma, infection, or surgical manipulation of the gland

Desired outcomes: Patient is free of symptoms of thyroid storm as evidenced by normothermia; BP 90/60 mm Hg or more (or within patient's baseline range); HR 100 beats per minute (bpm) or less; and orientation to person, place, and time. If thyroid storm occurs, it is noted promptly and reported immediately.

Nursing Interventions

◆ Measure and report rectal or core temperature greater than 38.3° C (101° F) *because this often is the first sign of impending thyroid storm.*

◆ Monitor VS hourly for evidence of hypotension and increasing tachycardia and fever in patients in whom thyroid storm is suspected, *to facilitate early detection and treatment.*

◆ Monitor patient for signs of heart failure, which occurs as an effect of thyroid storm: jugular vein distention, crackles (rales), decreased amplitude of peripheral pulses, peripheral edema, and hypotension. Immediately report any significant findings to health care provider, and prepare to transfer patient to the ICU if such findings are noted, *to facilitate early treatment.*

◆ Provide a cool, calm, protected environment to minimize emotional stress. Reassure patient and explain all procedures before performing them. Limit the number of visitors. *Helps reduce metabolic rate.*

◆ Ensure good handwashing and meticulous aseptic technique for dressing changes and invasive procedures. Advise visitors who have contracted or been exposed to a communicable disease to either not enter patient's room or wear a surgical mask, if appropriate. *Reduces the risk for infection, which will further increase metabolic rate.*

◆ Implement emergency treatment if signs of thyroid storm are present:

  • Administer acetaminophen as prescribed *to decrease temperature.* Aspirin is contraindicated because it releases T_4 from protein-binding sites and increases free T_4 levels.

  • Provide cool sponge baths, or apply ice packs to patient's axilla and groin areas. If high temperature continues, obtain prescription for a hypothermia blanket *to decrease fever.*

  • Administer PTU as prescribed *to prevent further synthesis and release of thyroid hormones.*

  • Administer propranolol as prescribed *to block sympathetic nervous system (SNS) effects.*

  • Administer IV fluids as prescribed *to provide adequate hydration and prevent vascular collapse.*

  • Monitor for fluid volume deficit, which may occur because of increased fluid excretion by the kidneys or excessive diaphoresis.

  • Carefully monitor I&O hourly. Decreasing output with normal specific gravity may indicate decreased cardiac output, whereas decreasing output with increased specific gravity can signal dehydration. *Detects fluid overload or inadequate fluid replacement.*

  • Administer sodium iodide as prescribed, 1 hr after administering PTU. If given before PTU, sodium iodide can exacerbate symptoms in susceptible persons.

  • Administer small doses of insulin as prescribed. Hyperglycemia can occur as an effect of thyroid storm because of the hypermetabolic state. *Insulin controls hyperglycemia.*

  • Administer supplemental O_2 as necessary *because O_2 demands are increased as metabolism increases.*

Anxiety related to SNS stimulation
Desired outcomes: Within 24 hr of hospital admission, patient is free of harmful anxiety as evidenced by HR 100 bpm or less, respiratory rate (RR) 12-20 breaths/min with normal depth and pattern (eupnea), and absence of or decrease in irritability and restlessness. Patient and significant others verbalize knowledge about the causes of the patient's behavior.

Nursing Interventions

- Assess for signs of anxiety; administer short-acting sedatives (e.g., alpra-zolam or lorazepam) as prescribed, *to help control nervousness and rest-lessness from SNS stimulation.*
- Provide a quiet, stress-free environment away from loud noises or excessive activity, *to facilitate rest.*
- Limit number of visitors and the amount of time they spend with patient. Advise significant others to avoid discussing stressful topics and refrain from arguing with the patient, *to facilitate rest and decrease anxiety.*
- Administer propranolol as prescribed, *to reduce symptoms of anxiety, tachycardia, and heat intolerance.*
- Reassure patient that anxiety symptoms are related to the disease process and that treatment decreases their severity, *to reduce fear and facilitate coping.*
- Inform significant others that patient's behavior is physiologic and should not be taken personally, *to reduce their anxiety and fears.*

Impaired tissue integrity of the cornea related to dryness that can occur with exophthalmos in persons with Graves' disease
Desired outcome: Within 24 hr of admission, patient's corneas are moist and intact.

Nursing Interventions

- Teach patient to wear dark glasses *to protect the cornea.*
- Administer lubricating eyedrops as prescribed *to supplement lubrication, decrease SNS stimulation, and prevent lid retraction.*
- If appropriate, apply eye shields or tape eyes shut at bedtime *to protect the cornea.*
- Administer thioamides as prescribed *to maintain normal metabolic state and halt progression of exophthalmos.*

Disturbed body image related to exophthalmos or surgical scar
Desired outcome: Within the 24-hr period before hospital discharge, patient verbalizes measures for disguising exophthalmos or surgical scar and exhibits self-acceptance.

Nursing Interventions

- Encourage patient to communicate feelings of frustration *to relieve anxiety and facilitate coping.*
- Advise patient to wear dark glasses *to cover exophthalmos.*
- Suggest patient wear customized jewelry, high-necked clothing such as turtlenecks, or loose-fitting scarves *to cover the scar.*
- Suggest that after incision has healed, patient use makeup colored in his or her skin tone *to decrease visibility of the scar.*
- Caution patient that creams are contraindicated until incision has healed completely, and even then they may not minimize scarring. Increasing vitamin C intake up to 1 g/day may promote healing. Avoiding direct sunlight to the operative site for 6-12 mo *to help prevent hyperpigmentation of the incision.*

Deficient knowledge related to risk for side effects from iodides and thioamides or stopping thioamides abruptly
Desired outcome: Within the 24-hr period before hospital discharge, patient verbalizes knowledge about potential side effects of prescribed medications, signs and symptoms of hypothyroidism and hyperthyroidism, and importance of following the prescribed medical regimen.

Nursing Interventions

- Assess patient's facility with language; engage an interpreter or provide language-appropriate written materials if necessary.
- Explain importance of taking antithyroid medications daily, in divided doses, and at regular intervals as prescribed, *to prevent hypermetabolism and resulting symptoms.*
- Teach indicators of hypothyroidism, which may occur from excessive medication, and signs and symptoms that necessitate medical attention, including cold intolerance, fatigue, lethargy, and peripheral or periorbital edema, *to facilitate early intervention of corrective treatment.*
- Teach side effects of thioamides and symptoms that necessitate medical attention, including appearance of a rash, fever, or pharyngitis, which can occur in the presence of agranulocytosis.
- Alert patients taking iodides to signs of worsening hyperthyroidism, including high body temperature, palpitations, rapid HR, irritability, anxiety, and feelings of restlessness or panic, *to facilitate early intervention if needed.*

Acute pain related to surgical procedure
Desired outcomes: Within 2 hr of surgery, patient's subjective perception of pain decreases, as documented by a pain scale. Objective indicators, such as hesitation before turning or moving the head, are absent or diminished.

Nursing Interventions

- Assess and document patient's pain, including precipitating events. Devise a pain scale with patient, rating pain on a scale of 0 (no pain) to 10 (worst pain).
- Teach patient to clasp hands behind neck when moving *to minimize stress on the incision and help reduce pain.*
- Teach patient to perform gentle neck ROM exercises after health care provider has removed surgical clips and drain, *to help reduce pain.*
- For other interventions, see "Pain," p. 13, in Chapter 1.

Impaired swallowing (or risk for same) related to edema or laryngeal nerve damage resulting from surgical procedure
Desired outcomes: Patient reports swallowing with minimal difficulty, has minimal or absent hoarseness, and is free of symptoms of respiratory dysfunction, as evidenced by RR 12-20 breaths/min with normal depth and pattern (eupnea) and absence of inspiratory stridor. Laryngeal nerve damage, if it occurs, is detected promptly and reported immediately.

Nursing Interventions

- Monitor respiratory status for signs of edema (dyspnea, choking, inspiratory stridor, inability to swallow) and voice for hoarseness. Slight hoarseness is normal after surgery; hoarseness that persists is indicative of laryngeal nerve damage and should be reported to health care provider promptly. If bilateral nerve damage is present, upper airway obstruction can occur.
- Elevate head of bed (HOB) 30-45 degrees. Support patient's head with flat or cervical pillows so that it is in a neutral position with the neck (does not flex or hyperextend) *to minimize edema and incisional stress.*
- Keep tracheostomy set and O_2 equipment at the bedside at all times. Suction upper airway as needed, and use gentle suction to avoid stimulating laryngospasm. *Maintains patent airway.*
- Administer analgesics promptly and as prescribed *to minimize pain and anxiety and enhance patient's ability to swallow.*

Patient-Family Teaching and Discharge Planning

Include verbal and written information about the following:

- Diet high in calories, protein, carbohydrates, and vitamins. Inform patient that as a normal metabolic state is attained, the diet may change.

- Medications, including drug names, purpose, dosage, schedule, precautions, and potential side effects. Also discuss drug/drug, food/drug, and herb/drug interactions.
- Changes that can occur as a result of therapy, including weight gain, normal bowel function, increased strength of skeletal muscles, and return to normal activity levels.
- Importance of continued and frequent medical follow-up; confirm date and time of next appointment.
- Indicators that necessitate medical attention, including fever, rash, or sore throat (side effects of thioamides) and symptoms of hypothyroidism (see p. 383) or worsening hyperthyroidism.
- For patients receiving radioactive iodine, importance of not holding children to the chest for 72 hr following therapy because children are more susceptible to the effects of radiation. There is negligible risk for adults.
- Importance of avoiding physical and emotional stress early in the recuperative stage and maximizing coping mechanisms for dealing with stress.

❖❖ HYPOTHYROIDISM

OVERVIEW/PATHOPHYSIOLOGY

Hypothyroidism occurs from an inadequate amount of circulating thyroid hormone that causes a decrease in metabolic rate that affects all body systems.

Primary hypothyroidism accounts for 90% of cases of hypothyroidism and is caused by pathologic changes in the thyroid itself. The most common cause of the disease in the United States is chronic autoimmune thyroiditis (Hashimoto's disease.) *Secondary hypothyroidism* is caused by dysfunction of the anterior pituitary gland, which results in decreased release of thyroid-stimulating hormone (TSH). *Tertiary hypothyroidism* is caused by a hypothalamic deficiency in the release of thyrotropin-releasing hormone (TRH).

Myxedema, a life-threatening condition, can occur when hypothyroidism is untreated or when a stressor such as infection affects an individual with hypothyroidism. The clinical picture of myxedema coma is that of exaggerated hypothyroidism, with dangerous hypoventilation, hypothermia, hypotension, shock, and possible coma and seizures. Myxedema coma usually develops slowly and has a greater than 50% mortality rate. It requires prompt and aggressive treatment.

ASSESSMENT

Signs and symptoms/physical findings: Early fatigue, weight gain from fluid retention, anorexia, lethargy, cold intolerance, hoarseness, ataxia, memory and mental impairment, decreased concentration, menstrual irregularities or heavy menses, infertility, constipation, depression, muscle cramps, possible presence of goiter, bradycardia, hypothermia, deepened voice, hyperlipidemia, and obesity. Skin may appear yellow and dry, cool, and coarse and hair may be thin, coarse, and brittle. The tongue may be enlarged (macroglossia), and reflexes may be slowed.

Myxedema coma: Hypoventilation, hypoglycemia, hypothermia, hypotension, bradycardia, and shock. Symptoms can progress from mild early in onset to life-threatening.

History and risk factors

Primary hypothyroidism: Dietary iodine deficiency, thyroid gland radioablation for hyperthyroidism management, thyroid atrophy or fibrosis of unknown cause, radiation therapy to the neck, surgical removal of all or part of the gland, drugs that suppress thyroid activity including propylthiouracil (PTU) and iodides, invasion of the thyroid gland by tumor (e.g., lymphoma), drugs including lithium and interferon, or a genetic dysfunction resulting in inability to produce and secrete thyroid hormone.

Secondary hypothyroidism: Pituitary tumors, postpartum necrosis of the pituitary gland, hypophysectomy.

DIAGNOSTIC TESTS

TSH: Most commonly used test to detect thyroid dysfunction. Value will be elevated unless the disease is long standing or severe.

Free T$_4$ index (FTI) and T$_4$ levels: Decreased with hypothyroidism.

Radioactive iodine (^{131}I) scan and uptake: Will be less than 10% in a 24-hr period. In secondary hypothyroidism, uptake increases with administration of exogenous TSH.

Doppler ultrasonography: Used to diagnose gland size and abnormal densities, which may be present if nodules are present.

Thyroid autoantibodies: Presence of thyroperoxidase autoantibodies or antithyroglobulin autoantibodies signals chronic autoimmune thyroiditis.

COLLABORATIVE MANAGEMENT

Oral thyroid hormone: Given early in treatment for primary hypothyroidism. To prevent hyperthyroidism from too much exogenous hormone, patients are started on low doses that are increased gradually, based on serial laboratory tests (TSH and T$_4$) and adjusted until TSH is in a normal range. This therapy is continued for patient's lifetime. For patients with secondary hypothyroidism, thyroid supplements can promote acute symptoms and therefore are contraindicated.

Stool softeners: To minimize constipation owing to decreased gastric secretions and peristalsis.

Diet: High in fiber and protein to help prevent constipation, restriction of Na$^+$ to decrease edema, and reduction in calories to promote weight loss.

Treatment of Myxedema Coma

Intubation and mechanical ventilation: Compensate for decreased ventilatory drive.

IV thyroid supplements: Rapid IV administration of thyroid hormone can precipitate hyperadrenalism. This can be avoided by concomitant administration of IV hydrocortisone.

Treatment of hypotension: Administration of IV isotonic fluids, such as normal saline and lactated Ringer's solution. Hypotonic solutions, such as 5% dextrose in water (D$_5$W), are contraindicated because they can decrease serum Na$^+$ levels further. Because of altered metabolism, these patients respond poorly to vasopressors.

Treatment of hypoglycemia: IV glucose.

Treatment of hyponatremia: Fluids are restricted, or hypertonic (3%) saline is administered, or both.

Treatment of associated illnesses such as infections. Because of alterations in metabolism, patients with hypothyroidism do not tolerate barbiturates and sedatives well, and therefore central nervous system (CNS) depressants are generally contraindicated.

NURSING DIAGNOSES AND INTERVENTIONS

Ineffective breathing pattern (or risk for same) related to upper airway obstruction occurring with enlarged thyroid gland and/or decreased ventilatory drive caused by greatly decreased metabolism

Desired outcome: Patient has an effective breathing pattern as evidenced by respiratory rate (RR) 12-20 breaths/min with normal depth and pattern (eupnea), normal skin color, O$_2$ saturation (Sao$_2$) 95% or more, and absence of adventitious breath sounds. Alternatively, if ineffective breathing pattern occurs, it is detected, reported, and treated promptly.

Nursing Interventions

- Assess rate, depth, and quality of breath sounds, and be alert to presence of adventitious sounds (e.g., from developing pleural effusion) or decreasing or crowing sounds (e.g., from swollen tongue or glottis).
- Monitor for signs of inadequate ventilation, including changes in RR or pattern and circumoral or peripheral cyanosis. Immediately report significant findings to health care provider. *May indicate early myxedema.*
- Measure SaO_2 intermittently or continuously in patients with decreased ventilatory drive *to verify adequacy of oxygenation.*
- Teach patient coughing, deep breathing, and use of incentive spirometer. Suction upper airway prn *to facilitate patent airway.*
- For patient experiencing respiratory distress, be prepared to assist health care provider with intubation or tracheostomy and maintenance of mechanical ventilatory assistance or transfer patient to ICU.

Activity intolerance related to weakness and fatigue secondary to slowed metabolism and decreased cardiac output caused by pericardial effusions, atherosclerosis, and decreased adrenergic stimulation
Desired outcome: During activity patient rates perceived exertion at 3 or less on a 0-10 scale and exhibits cardiac tolerance to activity as evidenced by heart rate (HR) 20 beats per minute (bpm) or less over resting HR, SBP 20 mm Hg or less over or under resting SBP, warm and dry skin, and absence of crackles (rales), murmurs, chest pain, and new dysrhythmias.

Nursing Interventions

- Monitor VS and apical pulse at frequent intervals. Be alert to hypotension, bradycardia, dysrhythmias, complaints of chest pain or discomfort, decreasing urine output, and changes in mentation. Ask patient to rate perceived exertion. Promptly report significant changes to health care provider. *May indicate too little thyroid medication or myxedema.*
- Balance activity with adequate rest *to decrease workload of the heart.*
- Administer IV isotonic solutions as prescribed such as normal saline *to help prevent hypotension.*
- Assist patient with ROM and other in-bed exercises and consult with health care provider about implementation of exercises that require greater cardiac tolerance *to prevent complications of immobility.*

Risk for infection related to compromised immunologic status secondary to alterations in adrenal function
Desired outcome: Patient is free of infection as evidenced by normothermia, absence of adventitious breath sounds, normal urinary pattern and characteristics, and well-healing wounds.

Nursing Interventions

- Assess for early indicators of infection, including fever, erythema, swelling, or discharge from wounds or IV sites; urinary frequency, urgency, or dysuria; cloudy or malodorous urine; presence of adventitious sounds on auscultation of lung fields; and changes in color, consistency, and amount of sputum. Notify health care provider of significant findings *to facilitate early intervention if needed.*
- Provide meticulous care of indwelling catheters *to minimize risk of urinary tract infection (UTI).*
- Use sterile technique when performing dressing changes and invasive procedures *to minimize risk for infection.*
- Provide good skin care *to maintain skin integrity and prevent pressure ulcers.*

◆ Advise visitors who have contracted or been exposed to a communicable disease not to enter patient's room or to wear a surgical mask, if appropriate.

Risk for imbalanced nutrition: more than body requirements related to slowed metabolism

Desired outcomes: Patient does not experience weight gain. Within the 24-hr period before hospital discharge, patient verbalizes understanding of rationale and measures for dietary regimen.

Nursing Interventions

◆ Provide a diet that is high in protein and low in calories. As prescribed, restrict or limit Na^+ and foods high in Na^+ content (see Box 4-1, p. 165). Teach patient about foods to augment and foods to limit or avoid *to decrease edema.*

◆ Provide small, frequent meals of appropriate foods patient particularly enjoys.

◆ Encourage foods that are high in fiber content (e.g., fruits with skins, vegetables, whole grain breads and cereals, nuts) *to improve gastric motility and elimination.*

◆ Administer vitamin supplements as prescribed.

Constipation related to inadequate dietary intake of roughage and fluids, prolonged bed rest, and/or decreased peristalsis secondary to slowed metabolism

Desired outcome: Within 48-72 hr of admission, patient relates attainment of his or her normal pattern of bowel elimination.

Nursing Interventions

◆ Assess current bowel function; document changes.

◆ Monitor for decreasing bowel sounds, presence of distention, and increases in abdominal girth. *These may indicate ileus or obstructive process.*

◆ Encourage patient to maintain a diet with adequate roughage and fluids. Examples of foods high in bulk include fruits with skins, fruit juices, cooked fruits, vegetables, whole grain breads and cereals, and nuts. Ensure that fluid intake in persons without underlying cardiac or renal disease is at least 2-3 L/day *to prevent constipation.*

◆ Administer stool softeners and laxatives as prescribed *to facilitate bowel movement.*

◆ Avoid suppositories and teach patient not to use suppositories, *to stimulate bowel function.* Suppositories are contraindicated because of risk of stimulating the vagus nerve, which would further decrease HR and BP.

◆ Advise patient to increase amount of exercise *to promote bowel regularity.*

Ineffective protection (risk of myxedema coma) related to inadequate response to treatment of hypothyroidism or stressors such as infection

Desired outcomes: Patient is free of symptoms of myxedema coma, as evidenced by HR 60 bpm or greater, BP 90/60 mm Hg or greater (or within patient's normal range), RR 12 breaths/min or more with normal depth and pattern (eupnea), and orientation to person, place, and time. Alternately, if myxedema coma occurs, it is detected, reported, and treated promptly.

Nursing Interventions

◆ Monitor VS at frequent intervals and be alert for bradycardia, hypotension, or decrease in RR. Report SBP less than 90 mm Hg, HR less than 60 bpm, or RR less than 12 breaths/min.

◆ Monitor patient for signs of hypoxia (circumoral or peripheral cyanosis, decrease in level of consciousness [LOC]). Immediately report significant findings to health care providers.

- Avoid external warming measures for patients with hypothyroidism who are hypothermic *because they can produce vasodilation and vascular collapse.*
- Carefully check medication doses and classifications carefully before administration, especially barbiturates and sedatives, which are generally contraindicated *because they may cause excessive sedation, increased ventilatory effort, or decreased LOC.*
- Monitor serum electrolytes and glucose levels. Be especially alert to decreasing Na^+ (less than 137 mEq/L) and glucose (less than 80 mg/dL) *because they may indicate myxedema.*
- Implement emergency care for myxedema coma:
  - Restrict fluids or administer hypertonic saline as prescribed *to correct hyponatremia.*
  - Use infusion control device *to maintain accurate infusion rate of IV fluids.*
  - Administer IV thyroid replacement hormones as prescribed with IV hydrocortisone and IV glucose *to treat hypoglycemia.*
  - Monitor for jugular vein distention, crackles (rales), shortness of breath, peripheral edema, weakening peripheral pulses, and hypotension. Notify health care provider of any significant findings *because they are signs of heart failure.*
  - Prepare to transfer patient to ICU. Keep oral airway and manual resuscitator at the bedside in the event of seizure, coma, or the need for ventilatory assistance.

 Patient-Family Teaching and Discharge Planning

Include verbal and written information about the following:

- Medications, including drug names, purpose, dosage, schedule, precautions, and potential side effects. Also discuss drug/drug, food/drug, and herb/drug interactions. Remind patient that thioamides, iodides, and lithium are contraindicated because they decrease thyroid activity. Be sure patient is aware that thyroid replacement medications are to be taken for life.
- Dietary requirements and restrictions, which may change as hormone replacement therapy takes effect.
- Expected changes that can occur with hormone replacement therapy: increased energy level, weight loss, and decreased peripheral edema. Neuromuscular problems should resolve as well.
- Importance of continued, frequent medical follow-up; confirm date and time of next medical appointment.
- Importance of avoiding physical and emotional stress and ways for patient to maximize coping mechanisms for dealing with stress.
- Signs and symptoms that necessitate medical attention, including fever or other symptoms of upper respiratory, urinary, or oral infections and signs and symptoms of hyperthyroidism, which may result from excessive hormone replacement.
- Inform patient of available resources:

  The American Thyroid Association: www.thyroid.org

  The Thyroid Foundation of America: www.tsh.org

  The Hormone Foundation: www.hormone.org

SECTION TWO # DISORDERS OF THE PARATHYROID GLANDS

The parathyroid glands regulate serum calcium (Ca^{++}) and phosphorus levels via release of parathyroid hormone (PTH). This is accomplished by a negative-feedback mechanism: when serum Ca^{++} levels rise, PTH secretion is suppressed. PTH acts on bone to decrease Ca^{++} binding, and it stimulates the kidneys to increase resorption of Ca^{++}. Parathyroid glands affect serum phosphorus levels in two ways: (1) directly, in that PTH causes increased renal excretion of phosphorus; and (2) indirectly, in that phosphorus and Ca^{++} combine readily to form an insoluble salt, and increased serum phosphorus facilitates this reaction, thus effectively lowering circulating Ca^{++} levels. PTH is also involved in the synthesis of a renal enzyme that catalyzes formation of vitamin D, which, in conjunction with PTH, increases absorption of Ca^{++} from the gastrointestinal (GI) tract.

❖ HYPERPARATHYROIDISM

OVERVIEW/PATHOPHYSIOLOGY

Hyperparathyroidism is a clinical syndrome occurring from excessive secretion of parathyroid hormone (PTH). *Primary hyperparathyroidism* is caused by pathology of one or more of the parathyroid glands. Approximately 80% of these cases are caused by a benign adenoma of one gland, another 10% by multigland involvement, and in rare cases by carcinoma. In this disorder, excessive PTH acts on the skeletal, renal, and gastrointestinal (GI) systems, and the overall effects are increased serum calcium (Ca^{++}) levels and decreased phosphate levels.

Hyperparathyroidism is the second most common cause of hypercalcemia. Incidence of this diagnosis increases dramatically after age 50 yr and is much more prevalent in female patients than in male patients. *Secondary hyperparathyroidism* is usually caused by renal insufficiency with decreased glomerular filtration. Although Ca^{++} and phosphorus are retained because of the lack of renal filtration, the high serum phosphate level depresses Ca^{++} concentration because phosphorus combines with Ca^{++} to form insoluble salts, with resulting hypocalcemia. This hypocalcemia, in turn, stimulates the parathyroid glands to release PTH in an effort to increase serum Ca^{++} levels. Bone resorption occurs because of increased PTH, but absorption of calcium from the GI tract is depressed because of Ca^{++} binding with high-phosphate GI secretions. The overall effects are decreased Ca^{++} levels and increased phosphate levels. *Tertiary hyperparathyroidism* occurs when secondary hyperparathyroidism progresses to a state in which excessive PTH is released independent of serum Ca^{++} levels.

ASSESSMENT

Signs and symptoms/physical findings: Many individuals are asymptomatic. Symptomatic individuals experience nonspecific symptoms such as bone pain, lower extremity weakness, hypotonic muscles, joint hyperextensibility, sensory loss, tongue fasciculations, ataxic gait, fatigue, personality disturbances, emotional lability, constipation, weight loss, renal calculi, nausea, vomiting, anorexia, hardened fingernails, polyuria, hematuria, drowsiness, stupor, and coma. Frequent kidney infections, renal calculi, anemia, arthralgia, pancreatitis, peptic ulcers, and pathologic fractures, and heart disease may occur from Ca^{++} deposits in the tissues.

History and risk factors: Benign adenoma, carcinoma, renal insufficiency.

DIAGNOSTIC TESTS

Serum Ca^{++}: Elevated in primary hyperparathyroidism and low in secondary hyperparathyroidism. This test usually is repeated at least three times to confirm diagnosis. Venous blood is drawn in the morning after patient has been fasting. Because Ca^{++} is bound to protein, test results must be "corrected," based on a simultaneous test for albumin level. Serum Ca^{++} changes by 0.8 mg/dL for each 1 g/dL change in albumin level above or below normal. This represents circulating Ca^{++} available for use by body cells and is considered the "true" Ca^{++} level. To avoid venous stasis, which can produce erroneously high results, care must be taken not to apply the tourniquet too tightly or occlude the vessel for longer than necessary.

Serum PTH: High or inappropriately high for serum Ca^{++} levels.

Plasma phosphorus: Decreased in primary hyperparathyroidism and elevated in secondary hyperparathyroidism.

24-hr urine Ca^{++}: Elevated in primary hyperparathyroidism. This test is often used to rule out other causes of hypercalcemia.

Bone dual-energy x-ray absorptiometry (DEXA) (bone density scan): Will show diminution of bone mass in virtually all patients with hyperparathyroidism, as well as calcification of articular cartilage. X-ray examination of the hands will show subperiosteal resorption of the phalanges.

ECG: May show shortened QT interval, which is reflective of hypercalcemia.

Ultrasound scanning of the parathyroid glands: Used for operative planning when adenoma is suspected.

Radioisotope scan (sestamibi scan): Patient receives radioactive material that is absorbed only by the diseased gland in order to locate the adenoma preoperatively.

COLLABORATIVE MANAGEMENT

For patients without symptoms: Some health care providers may recommend that patient watch and wait to see whether symptoms develop. If patient remains asymptomatic, no further treatment may be necessary.

Surgical Treatment of Hyperparathyroidism

Conventional parathyroidectomy for primary hyperparathyroidism: The most effective form of treatment for patients with symptomatic primary hyperparathyroidism is surgical removal of one or more of the parathyroid glands (parathyroidectomy). The traditional incision is somewhat wider than with thyroidectomy, but the surgery is very similar. Only the affected gland or glands are removed, and, in cases in which all the parathyroid glands are enlarged, $3\frac{1}{2}$ glands are removed. The remaining tissue is enough to provide normal Ca^{++} regulation. In addition to postoperative complications potentially found with thyroidectomy, abnormalities in serum Ca^{++} levels also may be found.

Minimally invasive radioguided parathyroidectomy: A simple 1-inch incision is made, and in many cases the procedure can be done using local anesthesia. The surgeon uses the sestamibi scan as a guide and may use a special probe (similar to a Geiger counter) to locate the tumor for removal. Patients receiving local anesthesia may be able to return home the same day.

Medical Treatment for Hyperparathyroidism

Promotion of Ca^{++} excretion: In the absence of heart failure or renal insufficiency, this is accomplished by forcing fluids orally or giving IV normal saline for patients who are stuporous or nauseated. Volumes up to 1000 mL/hr may be given for short periods.

Increase in salt intake by food or tablet: Because Na^+ competes with Ca^{++} for excretion by the kidneys, increased Na^+ levels will cause the kidneys to excrete more Ca^{++}.

Diet: Limitation of dietary Ca^{++} (e.g., milk, many cheeses, cottage cheese, mustard greens, kale, broccoli) intake to one serving per day.

Hemodialysis in a low-Ca^{++} bath: Sometimes prescribed for severe hypercalcemia to remove Ca^{++} from the plasma.

Pharmacotherapy

Cinacalcet: Initially approved to treat secondary hyperparathyroidism in patients with both renal failure and parathyroid cancer, cinacalcet also performs well in managing primary hyperparathyroidism. Medical treatment for primary hyperparathyroidism is reserved for patients who are poor surgical risks or who have only a mild form of the disease. Ultimate goals of treatment are to provide adequate hydration and reduce serum Ca^{++} levels. Ca^{++} levels greater than 14 mg/dL are life-threatening and necessitate vigorous and immediate treatment if patient is to survive. In secondary hyperparathyroidism, the initial goal is managing the underlying problem, such as renal failure. Unfortunately, even the best management of renal failure does not cure secondary hyperparathyroidism.

Diuretics: Given to prevent volume overload and facilitate diuresis. Loop diuretics (furosemide and bumetanide) are preferred because they increase urinary Ca^{++} excretion. Thiazide diuretics (hydrochlorothiazide, chlorothiazide) are contraindicated because they decrease Ca^{++} excretion.

Oral phosphate supplements: For patients who have not been on recent glucocorticoid (steroid) therapy to help decrease bone resorption of Ca^{++} and bind Ca^{++} in the intestine to limit Ca^{++} absorption. Because these drugs may cause precipitation of insoluble Ca^{++}-phosphate complexes in the soft tissues of the kidneys, lungs, and cardiac conductive system, they are given only to patients with a low serum phosphate level or to those who have normal kidney function. Diarrhea is a common side effect. IV phosphates are avoided except for extreme emergency (Ca^{++} more than 14 mg/dL).

Intramuscular (IM) calcitonin: Decreases bone resorption of Ca^{++} and increases renal clearance. This has limited use, however, because it is short acting and patients commonly become resistant.

IV mithramycin: Inhibits bone resorption and lowers serum and urine Ca^{++} levels. This is the drug of choice for treatment of severe hypercalcemia because it is more effective and works more rapidly than calcitonin. Effects usually are seen within 2 hr. Side effects include bleeding abnormalities, hypocalcemia, and nausea.

IV etidronate: As effective as mithramycin in controlling hypercalcemia but has fewer side effects.

IV etidronate with IV pamidronate: Concomitant use of both medications results in better control of hypercalcemia than using etidronate alone.

Oral steroids: Given for their calciuric effect and to decrease Ca^{++} absorption in the presence of vitamin D intoxication. To avoid immunosuppressive effects of these drugs, they are given in as small a dose as it takes to achieve therapeutic effects. This treatment usually is reserved for hypercalcemia associated with hematologic malignancies.

Treatment for Secondary Hyperparathyroidism

Reduction of dietary phosphorus: Helps prevent formation of insoluble salts, thus increasing available circulating Ca^{++} (e.g., meat, poultry, fish, eggs, cheese, dried beans, and cereals may be limited).

Oral Ca^{++} supplements: Increase serum Ca^{++} levels, which will help prevent further release of PTH.

Aluminum-containing antacids: For patients with chronic renal failure to bind phosphorus in the intestine and prevent resorption.

Oral vitamin D supplements: Given to correct deficiency.

NURSING DIAGNOSES AND INTERVENTIONS

Impaired physical mobility related to neuromuscular weakness and joint pain secondary to increased serum Ca^{++} and altered phosphate levels

Desired outcome: Within 2 days after treatment/interventions, patient demonstrates progression to his or her baseline or optimal level of mobility with decreasing evidence of weakness or joint pain.

Nursing Interventions

- Administer analgesics and antiinflammatory agents as prescribed to minimize discomfort and enhance effectiveness of prescribed or necessary activity. Time exercise activity to coincide with peak effectiveness of the medication.

- ◆ Adjust activity to patient's tolerance and provide rest periods at frequent intervals. Discuss importance of activity with patient, and set realistic short-term and long-term goals in clearly understood terms (e.g., "Ambulate the length of the hall three times, four times a day"). *Conserves energy.*
- ◆ Assist with ambulation as necessary. Provide a walker or cane if appropriate. For patients undergoing IV therapy, provide a stable rolling IV pole *to prevent falls or injury.*
- ◆ Request physical therapy and occupational therapy consultations *to facilitate gradual increase in patient's muscular strength and endurance.*

Risk for deficient fluid volume related to osmotic diuresis, vomiting, or diarrhea caused by oral phosphates
Desired outcome: Patient remains normovolemic as evidenced by balanced I&O, urinary output 30 mL/hr or more, good skin turgor, moist tongue and mucous membrane, brisk capillary refill (less than 2 sec), and BP 90/60 mm Hg or greater or within patient's baseline.

Nursing Interventions

- ◆ Monitor and document I&O. Be alert for signs of dehydration, including decreasing urinary output, dry mucous membranes, poor skin turgor, thirst, furrowed tongue.
- ◆ Monitor serum Ca^{++} levels. Normal range for Ca^{++} is 8.5-10.5 mg/dL. *Decreasing levels signal correction of the fluid volume deficit.*
- ◆ Monitor for hypotension. *Can be caused by oral phosphate supplements.*
- ◆ Encourage oral fluids to 3 L/day unless patient has coexisting renal or cardiac disease, *to prevent dehydration.*
- ◆ Rehydrate with IV fluids (typically normal saline) as prescribed *to prevent dehydration.*
- ◆ Administer prescribed medications (e.g., calcitonin, mithramycin, *to decrease hypercalcemia*; loop diuretics, steroids, *to increase urinary Ca^{++} excretion*).

Risk for trauma (pathologic fractures) related to bone demineralization
Desired outcome: Patient remains free of symptoms of pathologic fractures.

Nursing Interventions

- ◆ Keep bed in its lowest position, keep walkway free of clutter, and assist patient with ambulation and any strenuous activity *to minimize risk of pathologic fractures from falls.*
- ◆ Assess each extremity daily for movement, pain, swelling, or deformity. *These findings may signal pathologic fracture.*
- ◆ Notify health care provider of patient complaints of back or chest pain. *May signal vertebral or rib fracture.*
- ◆ Instruct unstable patient to request help when getting out of bed. Promote use of a cane or walker, and keep call light within patient's reach *to minimize risk for falls.*
- ◆ Pad side rails for patients with severe bone pathology *to help prevent fractures.*
- ◆ Apply chest restraints and/or mitts carefully for patients who are severely confused and may attempt to leave the bed, or arrange for significant other to sit with patient *to minimize risk for injury or falls.*

Risk for constipation related to decreased peristalsis associated with increased serum Ca^{++} level
Desired outcomes: After receiving instructions, patient verbalizes knowledge of measures that promote bowel movement. Within 2-3 days of intervention, patient relates bowel elimination within his or her normal pattern.

Nursing Interventions

◆ Auscultate bowel sounds in each abdominal quadrant for 2-3 min once per shift. Report absence of bowel sounds, *which indicates lack of GI motility.*

◆ Monitor for abdominal pain and distention. *These are physical indicators of constipation.*

◆ Administer stool softeners, suppositories, laxatives, and enemas as prescribed *to facilitate bowel elimination.*

◆ Encourage patient to increase dietary intake of dried fruits, whole grain cereals, nuts, fresh fruits, and vegetables. *Fiber prevents or relieves constipation because it moves through the GI tract unchanged and adds bulk to the stool.*

◆ Teach patient that increasing fluid intake to 3 L/day, if not fluid restricted, *will help promote bowel elimination.*

◆ Encourage as much activity as tolerated. *Activity stimulates peristalsis.*

Ineffective protection related to risk for hypercalcemia, hypocalcemia, tetany, and thyroid storm secondary to surgical procedure or gland manipulation
Desired outcomes: Optimally, patient remains free of symptoms of hypercalcemia, hypocalcemia, tetany, and thyroid storm, as evidenced by respiratory rate (RR) 12-20 breaths/min with normal depth and pattern (eupnea); orientation to person, place, and time; absence of Chvostek's and Trousseau's signs; normal strength and motion in all extremities; heart rate (HR) 60-100 beats per minute (bpm); and normothermia. If hypercalcemia, hypocalcemia, tetany, or thyroid storm occurs, the abnormality is detected and reported promptly.

Nursing Interventions

◆ Monitor for signs of hypercalcemia. Signs include nausea, vomiting, anorexia, abdominal pain, weakness, thirst, dyspnea, and coma. Hypercalcemia can be caused by increased release of PTH secondary to surgical manipulation of the gland.

◆ Monitor for numbness and tingling around the mouth. Also be alert to indicators of tetany: muscle twitching, painful tonic muscle spasms, and grimacing facial spasms. Two tests to assess for tetany are Chvostek's and Trousseau's signs. *Chvostek's sign* is elicited by tapping the face just below the temple where the facial nerve emerges. The sign is positive if twitching occurs along the nose, lip, or side of the face. *Trousseau's sign* is tested by applying BP cuff to the arm, inflating it to slightly higher than SBP, and leaving it inflated for 1-4 min. Carpopedal spasms are indicative of hypocalcemia. Report significant findings to health care provider. *These are early signs of hypocalcemia.*

◆ Keep IV Ca^{++} readily available *for prescribed treatment of hypocalcemia.*

◆ Monitor for signs of thyroid storm, including tachycardia, agitation, and hyperpyrexia. Immediately report presence of these signs to health care provider. Although thyroid storm occurs rarely, it can be caused by a sudden release of excessive amounts of thyroid hormone into the bloodstream from gland manipulation during surgery.

Acute pain or **Chronic pain** related to surgical procedure or to arthralgia caused by bone demineralization
Desired outcomes: Within 1 hr of intervention, patient's subjective perception of pain decreases, as documented by pain scale. Objective indicators, such as grimacing, are absent or diminished.

Nursing Interventions

◆ Monitor for pain, noting and documenting intensity, character, and precipitating factors. Devise a pain scale with patient that rates discomfort from 0 (no pain) to 10 (worst pain).

- Administer analgesics as prescribed, and document their effectiveness.
- Remind patient to notify staff as soon as discomfort occurs so that analgesics can be administered before pain becomes too severe. *Early treatment of pain results in better pain control.*
- Administer analgesics 30-60 min before scheduled activities such as turning or ambulation *to minimize pain during such activities.*
- Teach patient to clasp hands behind neck during postoperative moving *to minimize stress on the incision and thus control pain.*
- Teach gentle ROM exercises for the neck, as well as assisted or active ROM for painful joints *to maintain movement and help minimize pain.*
- Provide comfort measures such as a foam mattress and a foot cradle *to minimize pressure on the extremities.*
- Provide back rubs, especially at bedtime, *to reduce discomfort from prolonged bed rest and promote relaxation.*
- For additional pain interventions, see this nursing diagnosis in "Pain," p. 13.

Deficient knowledge related to risk for side effects from prescribed steroids, phosphate supplements, and mithramycin

Desired outcome: Patient verbalizes knowledge of side effects of prescribed medications and importance of notifying health care provider if these side effects occur.

Nursing Interventions

- Assess patient's facility with language; engage an interpreter or provide language-appropriate written materials if necessary.
- Teach patient about prescribed medications:
  - *Steroids:* Teach importance of monitoring for side effects, including frequent BP checks for hypertension, assessment for mental changes, daily weight measurement for evidence of weight gain, and blood tests for hyperglycemia.
  - *Phosphate supplements*: Explain that diarrhea is a common side effect.
  - *Mithramycin:* Teach that lower extremity petechiae may signal thrombocytopenia; jaundice signals hepatocellular necrosis; and tetany occurs with hypocalcemia. Explain that urinalysis results must be monitored for evidence of proteinuria.
- Explain importance of notifying health care provider promptly if side effects from prescribed medications occur.
- Teach patient that extreme changes in the patient's condition can be life-threatening and must be managed promptly. Patients who cannot reach their health care provider by phone or who cannot get an appointment should proceed to a hospital emergency department for immediate assistance.

Patient-Family Teaching and Discharge Planning

Include verbal and written information about:

- Dietary considerations, including Ca^{++} restriction, increased fluids, and possibly increased Na^+. As appropriate, arrange for a dietary consultation to help patient with meal planning and integration of individual restrictions into family meals.
- Medical follow-up: Emphasize importance and confirm date and time of next appointment.
- Signs and symptoms of hypocalcemia and hypercalcemia (see **Ineffective protection,** p. 392), which necessitate medical attention if they occur.
- Prescribed medications, including drug names, purpose, dosage, schedule, precautions, and potential side effects. Also discuss drug/drug, food/drug, and herb/drug interactions.

◆ Management of incision if surgery was performed, including indications of wound infection (e.g., erythema, local warmth, swelling, discharge, pain, fever) and review of surgeon's instructions regarding wound cleaning and when showering may ensue.

❖ HYPOPARATHYROIDISM

OVERVIEW/PATHOPHYSIOLOGY

Hypoparathyroidism results from the decreased production of parathyroid hormone (PTH). Most commonly this disorder is iatrogenic, caused by damage to or accidental removal of the parathyroid glands during thyroid surgery or radioactive iodine treatment for hyperthyroidism. Damage may be temporary or permanent. If injury occurs in the absence of gland removal, the tissue generally recovers within a period of months and returns to normal functioning. Familial or autoimmune factors also can be significant in the development of hypoparathyroidism because of deficient PTH receptors in target tissues.

ASSESSMENT

Signs and symptoms/physical findings: The primary abnormality with hypoparathyroidism is hypocalcemia; therefore, symptoms can include numbness and tingling around the mouth, fingertips, and sometimes the feet; painful contractions or twitching of skeletal muscles; clonic and tonic spasms; grand mal seizures; laryngeal spasms; carpopedal spasm; nausea; vomiting; dysrhythmias; heart failure; cataracts (from calcium [Ca^{++}] deposits); conjunctivitis; photophobia; cardiorespiratory compromise with bronchial and/or laryngeal spasm, cardiac dysrhythmias, and prolonged QT and ST intervals on ECG. Neuropsychiatric signs of irritability and psychosis also may be present.
History and risk factors: Thyroid radiation or surgery, familial pattern, autoimmune condition.

DIAGNOSTIC TESTS

Serum tests: Levels of ionized Ca^{++} are decreased, phosphate levels are increased, and PTH levels are inappropriately low for the level of serum Ca^{++}.
Skull x-ray examination: May show evidence of increased density and calcification of basal ganglia.
Dual-energy x-ray absorptiometry (DEXA) (bone density scan): May show osteopenia or osteoporosis.

COLLABORATIVE MANAGEMENT

Ca^{++} supplements: Given either by the oral (PO) or IV route, with dosage adjustments based on serum levels of Ca^{++}.
PTH injections: Given to replace lost PTH.
Vitamin D preparations: Facilitates absorption of Ca^{++} from the gastrointestinal (GI) tract.
Sedatives (phenobarbital) and magnesium sulfate: Minimize tetany and seizures.
Aluminum hydroxide gels: Bind phosphorus in the intestines and decreases serum phosphate levels.
Diet: High in Ca^{++} (1 qt milk/day) and low in phosphorus (limit meat, poultry, fish, eggs, cheese, dried beans, and cereals). If hyperphosphatemia persists, it may be necessary to restrict dairy products and egg yolks and provide oral Ca^{++} supplements. Foods high in oxalate, which binds to Ca^{++}, also should be avoided. These include beets, figs, nuts, spinach, black tea, and chocolate.

NURSING DIAGNOSES AND INTERVENTIONS

Activity intolerance related to weakness and fatigue secondary to decreased cardiac contractility

Desired outcome: During activity, patient rates perceived exertion at 3 or less on a 0-10 scale and exhibits cardiac tolerance to activity, as evidenced by heart rate (HR) 20 beats per minute (bpm) or less over resting heart rate HR; SBP 20 mm Hg or less over or under resting SBP; respiratory rate (RR) 12-20 breaths/min with normal depth and pattern (eupnea); normal skin color; warm and dry skin; and absence of crackles (rales), murmurs, chest pain, and new dysrhythmias.

Nursing Interventions

- Monitor for activity intolerance, and ask patient to rate his or her perceived exertion.
- Monitor for heart failure, including increased work of breathing, congested breath sounds, hypotension, tachycardia, pallor, or cyanosis. Report significant findings to health care provider.
- Provide adequate rest periods of at least 90 min in duration *to conserve energy.*
- Administer PO or IV Ca^{++} supplements as prescribed *to replace needed Ca^{++}.*
- Assist patient with ROM and other in-bed exercises *to help prevent complications of inactivity.*

Ineffective protection related to risk for tetany, respiratory distress, and seizures secondary to hypocalcemia
Desired outcome: Patient verbalizes orientation to person, place, and time and is free of symptoms of injury caused by tetany, respiratory distress, and seizures.

Nursing Interventions

- Assess for signs of hypocalcemia: tingling around mouth and in hands, muscle twitching, painful tonic muscle spasms, grimacing facial spasms, and Chvostek's and Trousseau's signs (see p. 392). Report significant findings to health care provider. *These are indicators of tetany.*
- Monitor for respiratory distress, including stridor, wheezing, and dyspnea; report significant findings to health care provider immediately.
- Monitor serum Ca^{++} levels, and note whether levels are increased or decreased. Either extreme will require a change in Ca^{++} therapy. Serum Ca^{++} levels less than 7 mg/dL or more than 14 mg/dL (after being "corrected" with albumin level) are life-threatening. If they occur, notify health care provider immediately *to prevent a life-threatening event.*
- Provide a restful, quiet environment away from loud noises and bright lights *to conserve energy.*
- Administer sedatives and anticonvulsant medications as prescribed *to prevent and/or control seizures.*
- Keep side rails up at all times. Keep an oral airway at the bedside *to minimize the risk for injury and facilitate patent airway.*
- Keep tracheostomy set, O_2 equipment, and IV Ca^{++} at the bedside *for rapid implementation of emergency measures if needed.*

Patient-Family Teaching and Discharge Planning

Include verbal and written information about the following:
- Diet: High in Ca^{++}, low in phosphorus, and low in oxalate. As appropriate, arrange for a dietary consultation so that patient's requirements and restrictions can be integrated into family meal planning.
- Medications, including drug names, purpose, dosage, schedule, precautions, and potential side effects. Also discuss drug/drug, food/drug, and herb/drug interactions.

- Importance of seeking immediate medical attention if signs of worsening hypocalcemia (e.g., tetany) or hypercalcemia (e.g., weakness, fatigue, constipation, polyuria, renal calculi) occur.
- Importance of continued medical follow-up. Confirm date and time of next appointment.

❖ ❖ ❖

SECTION THREE   **DISORDERS OF THE ADRENAL GLANDS**

❖ ADDISON'S DISEASE

OVERVIEW/PATHOPHYSIOLOGY

Addison's disease is a deficiency of adrenocortical hormones following destruction of the adrenal cortex, which can occur suddenly as a result of such stressors as trauma, infection, or surgery but more commonly occurs gradually. As many as 80% of reported cases involve an autoimmune factor, such as polyglandular autoimmune syndrome. *Primary Addison's disease* is a pathologic condition of the adrenal glands themselves, whereas *secondary Addison's disease* is often caused by prior treatment with glucocorticoids or other diseases of the pituitary gland that inhibit pituitary adrenocorticotropic hormone (ACTH) release.

Deficiency of glucocorticoids retards mobilization of tissue protein, inhibits the liver's ability to store glycogen, and thereby causes muscle weakness and hypoglycemia to occur. Wound healing is slowed, and these individuals become particularly susceptible to infection. There is loss of vascular tone in the periphery, as well as decreased vascular response to the catecholamines epinephrine and norepinephrine. Decreased secretion of aldosterone causes Na^+, chloride (Cl^-), and water loss from the kidneys and increased reabsorption of K^+.

Acute adrenal insufficiency, or *addisonian crisis,* is a life-threatening emergency caused by insufficient cortisol and aldosterone. Crisis occurs in patients with acute adrenal insufficiency (Addison's disease) or as an indication of adrenal insufficiency. Crisis usually follows stress (trauma, infection, prolonged fasting), sudden withdrawal of exogenous steroid therapy (the most common cause), bilateral adrenalectomy or removal of an adrenal tumor, sudden destruction of the pituitary gland, or injury to both adrenal glands.

ASSESSMENT

Signs and symptoms/physical findings: Weakness, fatigue, anorexia, nausea, vomiting, abdominal pain, fever, restlessness, emotional instability, and confusion. More acutely ill patients may experience dizziness, postural hypotension, weight loss, arthralgia, amenorrhea, increased skin pigmentation (especially in skin creases, pressure areas, mucous membranes, nipples), small heart size, weakened pulse, sparse axillary hair growth, weight loss, emaciation, and dehydration.

Acute adrenal crisis: Weakness, headache, nausea, vomiting, fever, intractable abdominal pain, cyanosis, and severe hypotension, which can lead to vascular collapse and shock.

History and risk factors: Familial tendency, bilateral adrenalectomy, major trauma or infection, damage to the pituitary gland, or sudden withdrawal of exogenous steroids after long-term use.

DIAGNOSTIC TESTS

Cosyntropin (synthetic adrenocorticotropic hormone 1-24 [ACTH1-24]) stimulation test: Initially a blood sample is drawn to determine baseline level of serum cortisol. Then 0.25 mg cosyntropin is given by IV push, at which time patient may experience nausea and have a sudden urge to urinate, but these side effects resolve quickly. Additional blood samples are drawn 30-60 min later to determine serum cortisol levels. Individuals with adrenal insufficiency demonstrate a slight rise in serum cortisol but not the peak values that would occur in individuals without adrenal insufficiency.

Corticotropin-releasing hormone (CRH) stimulation test: Additional test to determine the cause of adrenal insufficiency when ACTH test is abnormal.

Serum chemistry: K^+ is elevated, Na^+ and Cl^- are decreased, glucose is decreased, and Ca^{++} is elevated.

Plasma ACTH: Markedly increased with primary adrenal disease (more than 200 pg/mL if patient is in, or approaching, crisis); decreased in secondary Addison's disease.

Cultures: When the patient is in addisonian crisis, blood, urine, or sputum cultures may be positive if cause of the crisis is major infection. Meningococcal infections may result in associated Waterhouse-Friderichsen syndrome.

CBC with differential: In crisis there may be associated neutropenia (5000 cells/μL), lymphocytosis (35%-50%), and elevated eosinophils (more than 300 million/L).

Plasma cortisol: Low (less than 5 mcg/dL) on a morning sample can be diagnostic of adrenal insufficiency or crisis, especially when accompanied by elevated plasma ACTH.

Urine Na^+ levels: Increased because of renal Na+ wasting.

CT scan or MRI: May show a decrease in adrenal or pituitary size, which signals glandular destruction from an autoimmune process. Adrenal glands are enlarged in 85% of patients with granulomatous or metastatic disease. Calcification may be seen in tuberculosis (TB), hemorrhage, pheochromocytoma, melanoma, and fungal infection.

Chest x-ray examination: May reveal underlying TB, fungal infection, or cancer in non-addisonian patients.

COLLABORATIVE MANAGEMENT

Pharmacotherapy

Hydrocortisone: For addisonian patients, 15-30 mg is given in twice-daily doses: two-thirds in the morning and one-third at night.

Prednisone: Used if hydrocortisone is ineffective; 5 mg in the morning and 2.5 mg at night.

Fludrocortisone acetate: Because of its Na^+-retention properties, it is used in patients receiving hydrocortisone or prednisone who continue to excrete sodium excessively. If postural hypotension, weakness, or hyperkalemia occurs, dosage is increased; if hypertension, edema, or hypokalemia occurs, dosage is decreased.

Antibiotics or anti-TB therapy: If infection or TB is the cause. Agents are administered after all appropriate specimens for culture have been obtained.

Diet: High in calories, carbohydrates, proteins, and vitamins and provided in small, frequent feedings to enhance nutritional state for these patients, who tend to be anorexic.

For Adrenal Crisis

Intravenous (IV) fluids: Rapid administration of 1-2 L of saline may be provided over 2 hr to correct dehydration or hypovolemic shock.

Pharmacotherapy

Hydrocortisone: 100-300 mg intravenously, in a saline infusion, given rapidly without awaiting serum cortisol level. Initial dosage also may be prescribed for IV push over 1 min. Follow-up IV dosage of 50-100 mg is provided q6h for the first day and then q8h on the second day. When patient is able to resume oral intake, hydrocortisone may be given orally q6h and gradually reduced.

Vasopressors (e.g., norepinephrine, dopamine): Given to maintain adequate systolic blood pressure (SBP) (greater than 90 mm Hg).

Broad-spectrum antibiotics: Administered prophylactically until infecting organisms are identified (bacterial infection often precipitates acute adrenal crisis).

Dextrose 50%: Administered intravenously to rapidly correct hypoglycemic reactions.

Continuous cardiac monitoring: For prompt identification of life-threatening dysrhythmias associated with hypotension and electrolyte imbalances. Patients may have benign ECG changes such as depressed T waves, peaked T waves, and possibly premature ventricular contractions.

Serum chemistry monitoring: Serial monitoring of Na^+, Cl^-, K^+, glucose, CO_2, blood urea nitrogen (BUN), and creatinine to assess patient's return to homeodynamism.

NURSING DIAGNOSES AND INTERVENTIONS

Risk for infection related to compromised immunologic status secondary to decreased adrenal function

Desired outcome: Patient is free of infection as evidenced by normothermia, white blood count (WBC) count $11,000/mm^3$ or less, clear and straw-colored urine, well-healing wounds, negative culture results, and absence of adventitious breath sounds and sore throat.

Nursing Interventions

- Monitor for and report early signs of infection, including fever; leukocytosis; frequency, urgency, dysuria, and cloudy or malodorous urine; persistent erythema, pain, local warmth, swelling, or purulent discharge from wounds or IV site; and complaints of sore throat and pharyngitis. Teach patient these indicators and importance of reporting them to health care provider or staff promptly.
- Culture any drainage as described *to determine presence and type of infectious organism.*
- Monitor temperature q2-4h, and report significant elevation to health care provider.
- Use meticulous sterile technique for all invasive procedures and when changing dressings. Ensure meticulous indwelling catheter care *to help prevent* urinary tract infection (UTI).
- Perform stringent handwashing technique before caring for these patients *to minimize risk for cross contamination and infection.*
- Caution visitors who have contracted or been exposed to a communicable disease to stay out of room or to wear a surgical mask when visiting patient *to minimize risk for infection.*

Ineffective protection related to risk for adrenal crisis

Desired outcomes: Patient is free of symptoms of adrenal crisis, as evidenced by normothermia; BP 90-140/60-100 mm Hg (or within patient's baseline range); heart rate (HR) 60-100 beats per minute (bpm); respiratory rate (RR) 12-20 breaths/min with normal depth and pattern (eupnea); no significant change in mental status; orientation to person, place, and time; and absence of abdominal pain, nausea, vomiting, and headache. If adrenal crisis occurs, it is detected and reported promptly.

Nursing Interventions

- Monitor carefully for headache, nausea, vomiting, fever, abdominal pain, and severe hypotension. Be aware that profound hypotension can lead to vascular collapse and shock. *These are indicators of adrenal crisis.*

◆ Place patient in a quiet room away from loud noises and excessive activity. Caution staff and visitors not to discuss stress-provoking topics with patient. *Stress exacerbates crisis.*

◆ Administer corticosteroids and prophylactic antibiotics as prescribed. These drugs *help prevent adrenal crisis.*

◆ In the presence of adrenal crisis:
  • Administer prescribed vasopressors *to maintain BP.*
  • Administer prescribed hydrocortisone preparations *to replace cortisol.*
  • Administer IV fluids as prescribed *to prevent circulatory collapse.*
  • Monitor VS q15min until stable and then as prescribed. Report significant changes in BP, HR, or RR or pattern to health care provider.
  • Monitor oximetry, report oxygen saturation (SaO_2) 92% or less, and administer O_2 as prescribed.
  • Monitor cardiac rhythm continuously for signs of hypokalemia (increased premature ventricular contractions, depressed T waves) or hyperkalemia (peaked T waves).
  • Monitor capillary glucose levels as required. Report capillary glucose 80 mg/dL or less, and administer glucose replacement as prescribed *to prevent hypoglycemia.*

◆ Monitor for and report signs of Na^+ retention and fluid volume excess (peripheral, pulmonary, and cerebral edema). Be alert to dependent edema, jugular venous distention, edema, crackles (rales), weight gain, severe headache, irritability, mental status changes, and confusion *because they are related to excessive doses of agents used to treat or prevent adrenal crisis.*

◆ Teach symptoms of adrenal crisis to patient and significant other, and stress importance of reporting these symptoms promptly to health care provider or staff member.

Activity intolerance related to generalized weakness and fatigue secondary to decreased cardiac output

Desired outcome: During activity, patient rates perceived exertion at 3 or less on a 0-10 scale and exhibits cardiac tolerance to activity, as evidenced by HR 20 bpm or less over resting HR; SBP 20 mm Hg or less over or under resting SBP; RR 20 breaths/min or less with normal depth and pattern (eupnea); warm and dry skin; and absence of crackles (rales), murmurs, chest pain, and new dysrhythmias.

Nursing Interventions

◆ Monitor VS for tachycardia and tachypnea, hypotension, pallor, and cyanosis. Ask patient to rate perceived exertion. Steroid dosage may need to be increased if positive findings are present, *to minimize symptoms.*

◆ Organize care based on patient's activity tolerance, *to facilitate frequent rest periods.*

◆ Assist patient with ROM and other in-bed exercises, *to prevent complications of immobility.*

Deficient fluid volume related to active loss secondary to diuresis

Desired outcome: Patient becomes normovolemic within 24 hr of hospital admission, as evidenced by balanced I&O, urinary output 30 mL/hr or more, adequate skin turgor, stable weight, and moist tongue and oral mucous membranes.

Nursing Interventions

◆ Monitor I&O and be alert to thirst, poor skin turgor, and furrowed tongue. *These signs indicate fluid volume deficit.*

◆ If deficit is noted, report findings to health care provider and encourage oral fluids *to restore fluid balance.*

- Administer maintenance doses of mineralocorticoid (e.g., fludrocortisone) as prescribed *to promote salt and water retention.*
- Supplement Na⁺ intake as prescribed by adding salt to foods or eating foods relatively high in Na⁺, such as meat, fish, poultry, eggs, and milk. *Corrects hyponatremia.*

 Patient-Family Teaching and Discharge Planning

Include verbal and written information about the following:

- Medications, including drug names, purpose, dosage, schedule, precautions, and potential side effects. Also discuss drug/drug, food/drug, and herb/drug interactions. Ensure that patient understands necessity of lifetime hormone replacement. Emphasize that abrupt withdrawal of steroids can lead to adrenal crisis.
- Diet (e.g., foods to increase, such as those high in Na⁺ [see Box 4-1, p. 165]).
- Instruct patient to seek medical help during periods of emotional or physical stress so that medication dosages can be adjusted accordingly.
- Discuss situations that require immediate medical attention. Include indicators of excessive adrenal hormones (e.g., weight gain, moon face, dependent edema, headache, weakness, irritability), adrenal insufficiency (e.g., progressive fatigue, nausea, vomiting, weakness, postural hypotension), and infections (e.g., upper respiratory infection [URI], wound infection, UTI, oral infection).
- Teach methods for maximizing coping mechanisms to deal with stress, such as diversional activities and relaxation exercises. Explain importance of avoiding physical or emotional stress.
- Discuss the importance of continued medical follow-up. Emphasize need to attend all appointments.
- Discuss the importance of obtaining a MedicAlert bracelet and identification card outlining diagnosis and emergency treatment from:

MedicAlert Foundation: www.medicalert.org

- Provide phone numbers to call if questions or concerns arise about therapy or disease after discharge. Additional general information can be obtained from:

National Adrenal Diseases Foundation: www.medhelp.org/nadf

- Assist patient/significant other with preparation of an emergency kit, including alcohol sponges and syringes with 100 mg of hydrocortisone, to be carried and used for adrenal crisis. Teach technique for intramuscular (IM) administration of medication to patient and significant other.

❖ CUSHING'S DISEASE

OVERVIEW/PATHOPHYSIOLOGY

Cushing's disease (hypercortisolism) is a spectrum of symptoms associated with prolonged elevated plasma concentration of adrenal glucocorticoids (e.g., cortisol). In individuals with normal functioning, the pituitary gland secretes adrenocorticotropic hormone (ACTH), which stimulates the adrenal glands to release adrenal glucocorticoid hormone (cortisol) and mineralocorticoid (aldosterone). This process is regulated by a negative-feedback mechanism in which increasing levels of plasma cortisol suppress ACTH. In pituitary pathologic conditions, the anterior pituitary gland fails to sense the plasma cortisol level, and the results are constant secretion of ACTH and abnormally high levels of glucocorticoid hormones. This situation accounts for approximately 70% of reported cases and is termed *Cushing's disease.* Approximately 90%

of patients with Cushing's disease have a pituitary adenoma. *Cushing's syndrome*, on the other hand, is caused by autonomous adrenal tumors (adenomas or carcinomas) or ACTH-secreting tumors outside the pituitary; or from long-term administration of corticotropin (ACTH) or cortisol (steroids).

ASSESSMENT

Signs and symptoms/physical findings: Actions of excessive *glucocorticoid (cortisol)* secretion include increased protein catabolism; increased production of glucose and glycogen, with resultant hyperglycemia; elevated plasma lipid levels causing atherosclerotic changes in blood vessels, heart, brain, and kidney; decreased bone formation and increased bone resorption resulting in osteoporosis, kyphosis and back pain, especially in the vertebrae; pathologic fractures of long bones; aseptic necrosis, especially of the femoral head; inhibition of the inflammatory response to tissue injury; central obesity with pendulous abdomen and thin legs and arms; moon face (cushingoid facies); fat deposits on the neck and supraclavicular area (buffalo hump); edema; hypertension; thin, transparent skin with multiple ecchymoses; muscle weakness; mental and emotional disturbances (mood lability to psychosis); capillary fragility and easy bruising; renal calculi; thirst and polyuria; changes in menstruation, virilism, and hirsutism in female patients; and impotence in male patients. Actions of excessive *mineralocorticoid (aldosterone)* include Na^+ and water retention, increased renal excretion of K^+, weakness, tingling, muscle spasms, and periods of temporary paralysis.

History and risk factors: Excessive or chronic exogenous steroid ingestion, pituitary tumor.

DIAGNOSTIC TESTS

24-hr urine sample for free cortisol or 17-hydroxycorticosteroid levels: Highly accurate; elevated in the presence of Cushing's disease.

Overnight dexamethasone suppression test: Excludes Cushing's syndrome with 98% certainty. Patient is given a 1-mg tablet of dexamethasone at 11 PM the evening before the test. For patients without Cushing's disease, this dose should suppress plasma cortisol levels at 8 AM the following morning to less than 50% of baseline. False-positive results are possible with concurrent administration of phenytoin, phenobarbital, or primidone.

Serum electrolyte studies: Blood glucose levels drawn after meals are elevated in 80%-90% of patients with Cushing's disease. Serum K^+ levels are decreased.

CT scan or MRI: May show adrenal masses or abnormalities in the sella turcica that indicate pituitary dysfunction or pituitary adenoma.

COLLABORATIVE MANAGEMENT

Transsphenoidal pituitary surgery: Selective resection of pituitary adenoma is the preferred treatment because of low morbidity and few postsurgical complications, although approximately 20% of patients develop diabetes insipidus (DI) because of swelling and trauma to the posterior pituitary where antidiuretic hormone (ADH) is released (See "Diabetes Insipidus," p. 404). CT-guided stereotactic surgery also is an option at some medical centers. After surgery, hydrocortisone replacement therapy is needed for 6-36 mo until normal corticotropic function resumes.

Bilateral adrenalectomy: If selective pituitary resection does not remit symptoms, removal of the adrenal glands may be necessary. Laparoscopic resection is used whenever possible; open resection may be necessary when adrenal neoplasm is suspected.

Adrenocortical inhibitors (e.g., metapyrone, ketoconazole, aminoglutethimide, cyproheptadine): Inhibit production of adrenocortical hormones. Exogenous steroids also may be given in conjunction with adrenocortical inhibitors to prevent hypocortisolism. Adrenocortical inhibitors are used only for short periods, however, because increased ACTH production quickly overcomes their effect.

Irradiation of pituitary gland: Decreases pituitary production of ACTH; used only in patients with a mild form of the disease or in those who are poor surgical candidates.

Diet: Low in calories and carbohydrates to reduce hyperglycemia. Salt is restricted to reduce BP, and foods high in K^+ (see Box 4-2, p. 174) are given to raise serum K^+ levels. If patient has osteoporosis (or to prevent osteoporosis), foods high in vitamin D may be added.

NURSING DIAGNOSES AND INTERVENTIONS

Disturbed body image related to hyperpigmentation, hair loss, and other physical changes associated with increased ACTH production

Desired outcome: Within the 24-hr period before hospital discharge, patient relates attainment of self-acceptance and verbalizes knowledge that symptoms will abate with treatment.

Nursing Interventions

- Spend time with patient when feasible and encourage patient to verbalize feelings and frustrations.
- Reassure patient that symptoms should subside with adequate treatment of the disorder.
- Assist patient with keeping hair well groomed, wearing own gown or pajamas if possible, and performing personal hygiene (e.g., bathing, brushing teeth). Encourage use of cosmetics and toiletries as patient desires *to help improve appearance.*
- See **Disturbed body image,** p. 31, in "Psychosocial Support" for additional information.

Risk for impaired skin integrity related to thinning skin and fragile capillaries secondary to increased cortisol production

Desired outcome: Patient's skin remains intact and nonerythematous.

Nursing Interventions

- Turn immobile patients q2h. Post a turning schedule. Gently massage bony prominences with nonirritating, nonalcoholic lotions *to help prevent pressure ulcers.*
- Place alternating air pressure mattress or other pressure-relief mattress or pad on the bed *to help prevent pressure ulcers.*
- Position foot cradle over the bed to keep bed linen off feet and *to prevent pressure areas on lower extremities.*
- Pad side rails of the bed if patient is confused or disoriented, *to protect skin.*

Ineffective protection related to risk for increased intracranial pressure (IICP), DI, cerebrospinal fluid (CSF) leak, hemorrhage, and infection secondary to transsphenoidal hypophysectomy

Desired outcomes: Optimally, patient demonstrates normal level of mental acuity; verbalizes orientation to person, place, and time; and is free of indicators of injury caused by complications of transsphenoidal hypophysectomy. Immediately after instruction, patient and significant other verbalize understanding of importance of avoiding Valsalva-type maneuvers; describe signs and symptoms of IICP, DI, and infection; and verbalize importance of notifying staff of postnasal drip or excessive swallowing.

Nursing Interventions

- Monitor carefully for change in mental status or level of consciousness (LOC), sluggish or unequal pupils, and changes in respiratory rate (RR) or pattern of respirations. Monitor patient for decreased vision, eye muscle weakness, abnormal extraocular eye movements, double vision, and airway obstruction. Report significant findings to health care provider. Neurologic deterioration may necessitate CT scan. *These are indicators of IICP.*

◆ Measure I&O hourly for 24 hr, and monitor urine specific gravity q1-2h. Report output greater than 200 mL/hr for 2 consecutive hr or a total of 500 mL/hr. Specific gravity less than 1.007 is found with DI. Monitor weight daily for evidence of loss.

◆ Explain signs of DI. DI can occur as a result of the edema caused by manipulating the pituitary stalk and usually is transitory.

◆ Inspect nasal packing at frequent intervals for presence of frank bleeding or CSF leakage. Note the number of times mustache dressing is changed. Expect nasal packing removal in about 3-4 days. Test serous drainage for the presence of CSF using a glucose reagent strip *to detect glucose, which indicates the presence of CSF.*

◆ Monitor patient for complaints of postnasal drip or excessive swallowing, which may signal CSF drainage down the back of the throat. *Immediately report any suspicious drainage.* Because the presence of CSF represents a serious breach in cranial integrity, elevate head of bed (HOB) *to minimize the potential for bacteria entering the brain.*

◆ Elevate HOB 30 degrees *to decrease intracranial pressure (ICP) and swelling.* Dexamethasone may be prescribed to reduce cerebral swelling.

◆ Explain that coughing, sneezing, and other Valsalva-type maneuvers must be avoided *because these actions can stress the operative site and increase ICP, thus causing CSF leakage.*

◆ Teach patient to cough or sneeze with an open mouth if either coughing or sneezing is unavoidable. Remind patient that nose blowing should be avoided until the nasal mucosa is healed (about 1 mo). Advise patient about the importance of mouth breathing and the possibility of having a soft nasal airway.

◆ Obtain prescription for a mild cathartic or stool softener, if indicated, *to prevent straining with bowel movements.*

◆ Do not allow patient to brush teeth. Provide mouthwash (e.g., hydrogen peroxide diluted with water to half strength) and sponge-tipped applicator for oral hygiene. Monitor for erythema or swelling at the suture line. Front teeth should not be brushed until incision has healed (about 10 days). Initially diet will be liquid but will progress quickly to soft food. Advise patient that the sense of smell usually returns in about 2-3 wk and the taste of foods may improve at that time. *These measures prevent disturbance of operative site integrity.*

◆ Apply cold compresses to the eyes if patient has periorbital edema, headache, and tenderness over the sinuses. The transsphenoidal donor site for fat or muscle packing usually is taken from the thigh or abdomen. The donor site is covered with a small dressing. *Cold helps minimize discomfort by decreasing swelling at the site.*

◆ Be alert to and teach the patient to report signs that necessitate medical attention: fever, nuchal rigidity, headache, and photophobia. *These are signs and symptoms of infection.*

 Patient-Family Teaching and Discharge Planning

Include verbal and written information about the following:

◆ Diet, including foods to increase, such as those high in K^+ (see Box 4-2, p. 174), and foods to restrict, including those high in Na^+ (see Box 4-1, p. 165) or carbohydrates. Arrange for a dietary consultation to help patient with meal planning and integration of individual restrictions into family diet. Foods high in calcium (Ca^{++}) and vitamin D may be consumed *for prevention or treatment of osteoporosis.*

- Medications, including drug names, purpose, dosage, schedule, precautions, and potential side effects. Also discuss drug/drug, food/drug, and herb/drug interactions. Advise patient with bilateral adrenalectomy of the necessity for lifetime hormone replacement therapy.
- Importance of continued medical follow-up; confirm date and time of next medical appointment.
- Hormone levels and stress: Because stress stimulates adrenal hormone production, advise patient to seek medical assistance during periods of emotional or physical stress so that medications can be adjusted accordingly. Teach patient to maximize coping mechanisms, such as relaxation exercises or diversional activities.
- Importance of balancing rest and exercise: *Exercise is helpful in preventing or managing osteoporosis.*
- Signs of excessive or deficient adrenal hormone: Inform patient that weight gain, thirst, polyuria, easy bruising, and muscle weakness indicate hormone excess, whereas easy fatigability, weight loss, and abdominal pain indicate hormone deficiency. Any of these indicators necessitates medical attention.
- Infection management: Discuss signs and symptoms of urinary tract infection (UTI), upper respiratory infection (URI), and wound and oral infections and the importance of seeking medical care if they occur.
- Additional information sources: Provide telephone numbers to call and websites that patient can access concerning adrenal disease if questions or concerns arise about therapy or disease after discharge. Additional general information can be obtained by accessing the website:

  The National Adrenal Disease Foundation: www.medhelp.org/nadf

- Importance of obtaining a MedicAlert bracelet and identification card outlining the diagnosis and emergency treatment from:

  MedicAlert Foundation: www.medicalert.org

- The need for an emergency kit stocked with alcohol sponges and syringes filled with 100 mg of hydrocortisone for episodes of acute adrenal insufficiency. Teach patient and significant other technique for intramuscular (IM) administration of medication for emergency treatment.

SECTION FOUR **DISORDERS OF THE PITUITARY GLAND**

❖ DIABETES INSIPIDUS

OVERVIEW/PATHOPHYSIOLOGY

Diabetes insipidus (DI) is a condition that can result from one of several problems. *Central (neurogenic) DI* is caused by a defect in the synthesis of antidiuretic hormone (ADH) by the hypothalamus or release from the posterior pituitary. *Nephrogenic DI* results from a defect in the renal tubular response to ADH that causes impaired renal conservation of water. The primary problem is excessive output of dilute urine. *Neurogenic DI* may be the result of primary DI (i.e., a hypothalamic or pituitary lesion or dominant familial trait), secondary DI (following injury to the hypothalamus or pituitary stalk), or vasopressinase-induced DI, which is seen in the last trimester of pregnancy (caused by a circulating enzyme that destroys vasopressin).

Nephrogenic DI either occurs as a familial X-linked trait or is associated with pyelonephritis, renal amyloidosis, Sjögren's syndrome, sickle cell anemia, myeloma, K^+ depletion, or chronic hypercalcemia. A rare form of DI, termed *psychogenic DI*, is associated with compulsive water drinking. Another form of water consumption–related DI is *dipsogenic DI*, caused by an abnormality in hypothalamic control of the thirst mechanism. This condition is most often idiopathic, but it has been associated with chronic meningitis, granulomatous diseases, multiple sclerosis, and other widely diffuse brain diseases. Patients have severe polydipsia and polyuria. Finally, a lack of vasopressin can develop during pregnancy and can result in *gestagenic DI*. The condition may be treated with vasopressin if severe, but it generally resolves 6-8 wk after delivery.

Except for when it follows infection or trauma, DI onset is usually insidious, with progressively increasing polydipsia and polyuria. DI following trauma or infection has three phases. In the first phase, polydipsia and polyuria immediately follow the injury and last 4-5 days. In the second phase, which lasts about 6 days, the symptoms disappear. In the third phase, the patient experiences continued polydipsia and polyuria. Depending on the degree of injury, the condition can be either temporary or permanent.

The chief danger to patients with DI is dehydration from the inability to take in adequate fluids to balance the excessive output of urine. DI must be differentiated from other syndromes resulting in polyuria. History, physical examination, and simple laboratory procedures assist in diagnosis. Other causes of polyuria include recent lithium or mannitol administration; renal transplantation; renal disease; hyperglycemia; hyperosmolality (early); hypercalcemia; and K^+ depletion, including primary aldosteronism.

ASSESSMENT

Signs and symptoms/physical findings: Polydipsia, polyuria (2-20 L/day) with dilute urine (specific gravity less than 1.007), and dehydration if fluid intake is inadequate. Individuals with cranial injury, disease, or trauma may exhibit impairment of neurologic status, including altered level of consciousness (LOC) and sensory or motor deficits.

History and risk factors: Cranial injury, especially basilar skull fracture; meningitis; primary or metastatic brain tumor; surgery in the pituitary area; cerebral hemorrhage; encephalitis; syphilis; or tuberculosis (TB). Familial incidence rarely is a factor.

DIAGNOSTIC TESTS

Urine osmolality: Decreased (less than 50-200 mOsm/kg) in the presence of disease.

Specific gravity: Decreased (less than 1.007) in the presence of disease.

Serum osmolality: Increased (300 mOsm/kg or more) in the presence of disease.

Vasopressin (desmopressin acetate—i.e., 1-desamino-8-D-arginine vasopressin [DDAVP]) challenge test: After administration of vasopressin subcutaneously or desmopressin by nasal spray (**TABLE 6-1**), urine is collected q15min for 2 hr. Quantity and specific gravity are then measured. Normally, individuals show a concentration of urine but not as pronounced as that of persons with DI; a person with kidney disease has a lesser response to vasopressin. One serious side effect of this test is precipitation of heart failure in susceptible individuals.

Hypertonic saline infusions: A 3% sodium chloride (NaCl) IV solution is infused to assess for subsequent water conservation. Although this test seldom is necessary for diagnosis of DI, it does assist in documentation of changes in the osmotic threshold for ADH release.

Water deprivation (dehydration) test: Although less commonly used today, some health care providers do use this test as a marker.

TABLE 6-1 VASOPRESSIN PREPARATIONS

GENERIC NAME	BRAND NAME	ONSET	DURATION (hr)	USUAL DOSE	ADVANTAGES/ DISADVANTAGES	COMMENTS
Oral						
Desmopressin acetate	DDAVP Desmotabs	Within 1 hr	8	0.2-1.2 mg total daily divided into 3 doses	May be easier or more convenient to use than other preparations	Can be taken with or without food
Nasal						
Vasopressin	Pitressin (20 pressor units/ mL)	Within 1 hr	4-8	5-10 units bid or tid	Action decreased by nasal congestion or discharge or trophy of nasal mucosa	Administer by spray, cotton swab or dropper
Desmopressin acetate	DDAVP (0.1 mg/mL)	Within ½ hr	8-20	0.1-0.4 mL daily in 1-3 doses (10-40 mcg)	See vasopressin above	Administer by spray or nasal tube system; store in refrigerator at 4° C (39.2° F)
Lypressin	Diapid (0.185 mg/mL)	Within ½ hr	3-8	7-14 mcg qid (1 or 2 sprays into each nostril	See vasopressin above	Administer by spray
Subcutaneous						
Vasopressin	Pitressin (20 pressor units/mL)	½-1 hr	2-8	0.25-0.5 mL (5-10 units) q3-4hr prn for increased thirst or increased urine output	May be used as an alternative in patients for whom nasal route is contraindicated	Carbamazepine and chlorpropamide may potentiate antidiuretic effects of all forms of vasopressin
Desmopressin acetate	DDAVP	Within ½ hr	1½-4	0.5-1 mL (2-4 mcg) daily in 2 divided doses		Keep refrigerated at 4° C (39.2° F)
Intramuscular						
Vasopressin	Pitressin (20 pressor units/mL)	½-1 hr	2-8	0.25-0.5 mL (5-10 units) q3-4hr for increased thirst or increased urine output		
Intravenous						
Desmopressin acetate	DDAVP (4 mcg/mL)	Within ½ hr	1½-4	0.5-1 mL (2-4 mcg) daily in 2 divided doses	Generally not for home use	Keep refrigerated at 4° C (39.2° F); dilute in 10-50 mL 0.9% NaCl, and infuse over 15-30 min

bid, Twice daily; *DDAVP,* 1-desamino-8-D-arginine vasopressin; *NaCl,* sodium chloride; *qid,* four times daily; *prn,* as needed [*pro re nata*]; *tid,* three times daily.

Baseline measurements of body weight, serum and urine osmolalities, and urine specific gravity are obtained. Fluids are not permitted, and measurements are repeated hourly. The test is terminated when urine specific gravity exceeds 1.020 and osmolality exceeds 800 mOsm/kg (normal responses), urine specific gravity does not increase for 3 hr (a positive result), or 5% of body weight is lost. The last result is, in itself, an abnormal response, and corresponding urine osmolality will be less than 400 mOsm/kg, which is diagnostic of DI. Because the most serious side effect of this test is severe dehydration, the test should be performed early in the day so that patient can be more closely monitored. Before a firm diagnosis of DI can be made from an abnormal water deprivation test, it is also necessary to demonstrate that the kidneys can respond to vasopressin (see later).

MRI of the brain: Used to identify pituitary lesions that may have caused the DI.

COLLABORATIVE MANAGEMENT

Central, or Neurogenic, DI

Rehydration: Lost water is replaced with IV hypotonic (e.g., 0.45% NaCl) solution. Initial replacement is rapid, necessitating close monitoring of BP, heart rate (HR), and urine output.

Administration of exogenous vasopressin: Replacement therapy for ADH. Several preparations are available (Table 6-1), and it is important to read the package insert carefully to ensure proper administration. Potential side effects include hypertension secondary to vasoconstriction, myocardial infarction (MI) secondary to constriction of coronary vessels, uterine cramps, and increased peristalsis of the gastrointestinal (GI) tract.

Achieving a mild antidiuretic effect: For example, with hydrochlorothiazide, chlorpropamide, carbamazepine, or other medication that increases the action or release of ADH.

Nephrogenic DI

Indomethacin therapy: Short-term treatment is begun with 25 to 50 mg bid/tid. It may be combined with thiazide diuretics, desmopressin, or amiloride.

Therapy with thiazide diuretics (e.g., hydrochlorothiazide, 50-100 mg daily, or chlorthalidone, 50 mg daily): Although it may seem antithetical to treat diuresis with a diuretic, one of the side effects of the thiazide diuretics is blocking of the kidneys' ability to excrete free water, which is the primary problem with DI.

Psychogenic DI

Psychotherapy: Necessary for patients with compulsive water drinking. Thioridazine and lithium should be avoided because they cause polyuria.

Dipsogenic DI

Cannot be effectively treated at this time because DDAVP can eliminate excessive urination but cannot eliminate excessive thirst. Patients must voluntarily reduce fluid intake, and most cannot resist the urge to drink. Patients managed with DDAVP throughout the day develop water intoxication from their uncontrollable thirst/ingestion of fluids. A small dose of DDAVP at bedtime can help reduce the number of times patient voids during the night.

NURSING DIAGNOSES AND INTERVENTIONS

Deficient fluid volume related to active loss secondary to polyuria

Desired outcome: Patient becomes normovolemic within 7 days of onset of symptoms as evidenced by stable weight, balanced I&O, good skin turgor, moist tongue and oral mucous membrane, BP 90-140/60-100 mm Hg (or within patient's normal range), HR 60-100 beats per minute (bpm), urine specific gravity greater than 1.010, and central venous pressure (CVP) 2-6 mm Hg (or 5-12 cm H_2O).

Nursing Interventions

- Monitor I&O, specific gravity, daily weight, and VS closely. Signs of hypovolemia include weight loss, inadequate fluid intake to balance output, thirst, poor skin turgor, decreased specific gravity, furrowed tongue, hypotension, and tachycardia. If available, monitor CVP for evidence of hypotension. *Assesses for hypovolemia.*
- Report the following signs of extreme diuresis to health care provider: (1) urinary output more than 200 mL in each of 2 consecutive hr, (2) urinary output more than 500 mL in any 2-hr period, or (3) urine specific gravity less than 1.002. *Allows for early intervention to minimize the risk for severe dehydration.*
- Provide unrestricted fluids: keep water pitcher full and within easy reach of patient. Explain importance of consuming as much fluid as can be tolerated *to minimize risk for dehydration.*
- Administer vasopressin and antidiuretic agents (or thiazide diuretic for patient with nephrogenic DI) as prescribed *to prevent extreme diuresis.* Ensure that urine output alone is not used to determine whether subsequent doses of desmopressin are required, because of the potential seriousness of side effects.
- Administer IV fluids as prescribed for unconscious patients. Unless otherwise directed, for every mL of urine output, deliver 1 mL of IV fluid *to provide rehydration.*

Ineffective protection related to risk for side effects of vasopressin
Desired outcomes: Optimally, patient demonstrates normal mental acuity; verbalizes orientation to person, place, and time; and is free of signs of injury caused by side effects of vasopressin. As appropriate, patient or significant other demonstrates administration of coronary artery vasodilators by time of hospital discharge.

Nursing Interventions

- Monitor VS and report significant changes, such as SBP elevated more than 20 mm Hg over baseline SBP or HR increased more than 20 bpm over baseline HR. *May indicate side effects of vasopressin.*
- Monitor for changes in mental status or LOC, confusion, weight gain, headache, convulsions, and coma. If these develop, stop the vasopressin, restrict fluids, and notify health care provider. Institute safety measures accordingly, and reorient patient as needed. *These signs indicate water intoxication caused by fluid retention.*
- Keep prescribed coronary artery vasodilators (i.e., nitroglycerin) at the bedside if indicated for use if angina occurs. Teach patient and significant other how to administer these medications. *Manages chest discomfort associated with vasopressin.*

 Patient-Family Teaching and Discharge Planning

Include verbal and written information about the following:
- Importance of medical follow-up; confirm date and time of next visit to health care provider.
- Medications, including drug names, purpose, dosage, schedule, precautions, and potential side effects. Also discuss drug/drug, food/drug, and herb/drug interactions.
- Importance of seeking immediate medical attention if signs of dehydration or water intoxication occur.

- ◆ Recommendations for fluid replacement: guidelines on type and amount of replacement fluids prescribed for patient.
- ◆ Additional information that can be accessed from:

  Diabetes Insipidus Foundation, Inc: www.diabetesinsipidus.org

❖ SYNDROME OF INAPPROPRIATE ANTIDIURETIC HORMONE

OVERVIEW/PATHOPHYSIOLOGY

Syndrome of inappropriate antidiuretic hormone (SIADH) is caused by release of ADH from the pituitary gland without regard to serum osmolality, plasma volume, or BP and results in excessive water retention and hyponatremia. The action of ADH increases reabsorption of water in the last segment of the distal tubules and collecting ducts of the kidney. ADH secretion usually is stimulated by one of three mechanisms: (1) increased serum osmolality, (2) decreased plasma volume, or (3) decreased BP. SIADH requires differential diagnosis to rule out other problems that prompt elevation of vasopressin and resultant hyponatremia because of an appropriate response to hypovolemic or hypotensive stimuli. SIADH is seen in postoperative and oncology patients and in individuals with multiorgan dysfunction syndrome. Sometimes it is present but not diagnosed because of mild or transient symptoms.

In the presence of excessive ADH, water that normally would be excreted is reabsorbed into the circulation, with resulting water retention and eventual water intoxication. The retained water expands extracellular fluid volume and causes serum osmolality and sodium (Na^+) to decrease because of dilutional effects. Decreased serum osmolality causes movement of water into the cells that can result in cerebral edema. Further water retention results in increased glomerular filtration rate and decreased aldosterone secretion, and more Na^+ is filtered out into the urine.

Water intoxication, cerebral edema, and severe hyponatremia cause altered neurologic/mental status, which if untreated, may lead to death.

ASSESSMENT

Signs and symptoms/physical findings: Elevated BP, weight gain without edema (because of loss of Na^+, edema does not accompany the fluid volume excess), decreased urine output with concentrated urine, altered mental status. Signs of water intoxication include altered level of consciousness (LOC), fatigue, headache, diarrhea, anorexia, nausea, vomiting, and seizures.

History and risk factors: Cancers of the lung, pancreas, duodenum, and prostate, which can secrete a biologically active form of ADH. Other common causes include pulmonary disease (e.g., TB, pneumonia, COPD, empyema), acquired immunodeficiency syndrome [AIDS], head trauma, brain tumor, intracerebral hemorrhage, meningitis, and encephalitis. Positive-pressure ventilation, physiologic stress, chronic metabolic illness, and a wide variety of medications (chlorpropamide, acetaminophen, oxytocin, narcotics, general anesthetic, carbamazepine, thiazide diuretics, tricyclic antidepressants, neuroleptics, angiotensin-converting enzyme [ACE] inhibitors, cancer chemotherapy agents) all have been linked to SIADH.

DIAGNOSTIC TESTS

Serum Na^+ level: Decreased to less than 137 mEq/L.
Plasma osmolality: Decreased to less than 275 mOsm/kg.
Urine osmolality: Elevated disproportionately relative to plasma osmolality.
Urine Na^+ level: Increased to more than 200 mEq/L. Urine Na^+ level (e.g., increased) is best evaluated in comparison with serum Na^+ level (e.g., decreased).

Urine specific gravity: More than 1.030.
Plasma ADH level: Elevated.

COLLABORATIVE MANAGEMENT

Fluid restriction: Based on urine output plus insensible losses. Restricting fluids to the amount manageable by the kidneys allows restoration of normal serum Na^+ levels and osmolality without complications from drug therapy.

Isotonic (0.9%) or hypertonic (3%) sodium chloride (NaCl): May be given if patient has severe hyponatremia. Supplemental Na^+ solutions may be administered with IV furosemide or bumetanide or osmotic diuretics, such as mannitol, to promote water excretion.

Lithium or demeclocycline: Inhibits action of ADH on distal renal tubules to promote water excretion.

Treatment of underlying cause: SIADH associated with surgery, trauma, or drugs usually is temporary and self-limiting. In chronic situations, the focus is on treating the underlying cause with surgery (i.e., transsphenoidal hypophysectomy, craniotomy, thoracotomy), radiation therapy, or chemotherapy.

NURSING DIAGNOSES AND INTERVENTIONS

Excess fluid volume related to compromised regulatory mechanisms resulting in increased serum ADH level, excessive renal water reabsorption, and renal Na^+ excretion

Desired outcome: Patient becomes normovolemic (and normonatremic) within 7 days of onset of symptoms or within 7 days following treatment, as evidenced by orientation to person, place, and time; intake that approximates output plus insensible losses; stable weight; central venous pressure (CVP) 2-6 mm Hg; BP 90-140/60-85 mm Hg or within patient's normal range; and heart rate (HR) 60-100 beats per minute (bpm).

Nursing Interventions

◆ Monitor LOC, VS, and I&O at least q4h; measure weight daily. Be alert to decreasing LOC, elevated BP and CVP, urine output less than 30 mL/hr, and weight gain. Promptly report significant findings or changes to health care provider. *These are clinical signs of hypervolemia and hyponatremia.*

◆ Monitor laboratory results: serum Na^+, urine and serum osmolality, and urine specific gravity. Be alert to decreased serum Na^+ and plasma osmolality, urine osmolality elevated disproportionately in relation to plasma osmolality, and increased urine Na^+. Normal values are as follows: urine specific gravity, 1.010-1.020; serum Na^+, 137-147 mEq/L; urine osmolality, 300-1090 mOsm/kg; and serum osmolality, 280-300 mOsm/kg. Report significant findings to health care provider. *Abnormal values are indicators of hyponatremia and water intoxication.*

◆ Maintain fluid restriction as prescribed. Explain necessity of this treatment to patient and significant other. *Do not* keep water or ice chips at the bedside. Ensure precise delivery of IV fluid administered by using a monitoring device *to prevent hypervolemia and water intoxication.*

◆ Elevate head of bed (HOB) 10-20 degrees *to promote venous return and thus reduce ADH release.*

◆ Administer demeclocycline, lithium, furosemide, or bumetanide as prescribed; carefully observe and document patient's response *to determine effectiveness of treatment.*

◆ Administer hypertonic NaCl as prescribed. Rate of administration usually is based on serial serum Na^+ levels. To minimize risk of hypernatremia, make sure that specimens for laboratory tests are drawn on time and results are reported to health care provider promptly. *Manages hyponatremia.*

◆ Institute seizure precautions, including padded side rails, supplemental O_2, and oral airway at the bedside, as well as side rails up at all times when staff member is not present, *to prevent patient injury in the event of seizure related to hyponatremia or brain edema secondary to water intoxication.*

 Patient-Family Teaching and Discharge Planning

Include verbal and written information about the following:

- Importance of fluid restriction for the prescribed period. Assist patient with planning permitted fluid intake (e.g., by saving liquids for social and recreational situations as indicated).
- Safely enriching diet with Na$^+$ and K$^+$ salts, particularly if ongoing diuretic use is prescribed.
- Use of daily weight measurements to assess hydration status.
- Signs of water intoxication and hyponatremia: altered LOC, fatigue, headache, nausea, vomiting, and anorexia, any of which should be reported promptly to health care provider.
- Medications, including drug names, dosage, route, purpose, precautions, and potential side effects. Also discuss drug/drug, food/drug, and herb/drug interactions. Encourage patient to report to health care provider all alternative and complementary health strategies being used.
- Importance of continued medical follow-up; confirm date and time of next medical appointment.
- How to obtain a MedicAlert bracelet and identification card outlining diagnosis and emergency treatment:

MedicAlert Foundation: www.medicalert.org

❖ ❖ ❖

SECTION FIVE DIABETES MELLITUS

❖ GENERAL DISCUSSION

OVERVIEW/PATHOPHYSIOLOGY

Diabetes mellitus (DM) is a disease of chronic hyperglycemia affecting more than 7% (20.8 million) of the total U.S. population, with 14.6 million cases diagnosed and another 6.2 million undiagnosed. It is further estimated that 41 million Americans have prediabetes (AACE DM Practice Guidelines, 2007). Prevalence has increased in a direct relationship with the increasing incidence of obesity (see "Metabolic Syndrome," p. 413). Metabolic, vascular, and neurologic disorders ensue from dysfunctional glucose transport into body cells. Insulin facilitates glucose transport into cells for oxidation and energy production. Food intake, glycogen breakdown, and gluconeogenesis increase the serum glucose level, which stimulates the β islet cells of the pancreas to release needed insulin for transport of glucose from the bloodstream into the cells. At the cellular level, insulin receptors control the rate of transport of glucose into the cells. As glucose leaves the blood, serum levels return to normal (70-110 mg/dL).

Individuals with DM have impaired glucose transport because of decreased or absent insulin secretion and/or ineffective insulin receptors. Carbohydrate, fat, and protein metabolism are abnormal, and patients are unable to store glucose in the liver and muscle as glycogen, store fatty acids and triglycerides in adipose tissue, and transport amino acids into cells normally. DM is classified into the following clinical classes as well as prediabetes:

Type 1 (5%-10%): Complete lack of effective endogenous insulin that causes hyperglycemia and ketosis resulting from β islet cell destruction. This type is precipitated by altered immune responses, genetic factors, and environmental stressors. Certain human leukocyte antigens (HLAs) have been strongly associated with type 1 DM. Affected individuals depend on insulin for survival and prevention of life-threatening diabetic ketoacidosis (DKA).

Type 2 (90%-95%): Metabolic disorder that may range from insulin resistance with moderate insulin deficiency to a severe defect in insulin secretion with insulin resistance that results in severe hyperglycemia without ketosis. Untreated hyperglycemia can result in hyperosmolar hyperglycemic nonketotic syndrome (HHNK). Most individuals with type 2 DM are obese. Insulin resistance is an important contributor to the condition known as *metabolic syndrome.*

Other types: Collectively, these forms of DM were formerly termed *secondary diabetes;* they include:

♦ *Diseases of the exocrine pancreas:* Pancreatitis, cystic fibrosis, hemochromatosis, trauma, infection, pancreatic cancer, and pancreatectomy may result in destruction of β islet cells. All diseases except cancer generally involve extensive pancreatic destruction.

♦ *Drug-induced by insulin antagonists:* Many drugs impair insulin secretion, including phenytoin, steroids (hydrocortisone, dexamethasone), hormones (estrogen), IV pentamidine, nicotinic acid, thyroid hormone, thiazides, interferon-α, and rat poison.

♦ *Endocrine dysfunction/hormonal diseases:* Growth hormone, epinephrine, cortisol, and glucagons antagonize insulin and may be increased when diseases such as acromegaly, Cushing's syndrome, pheochromocytoma, or glucagonoma are present. Presence of excess antagonistic hormones results in reduced insulin action, and in patients with somatostatinoma and aldosteronoma, insulin secretion may be reduced.

♦ *Genetic defects of the β cell:* An autosomal dominant pattern results in severely impaired insulin secretion, most often characterized by hyperglycemia beginning before 25 yr of age; it is also termed maturity-onset diabetes of the young (MODY).

♦ *Genetic defects in insulin action:* A genetic defect manifested as abnormal insulin action is reflected by hyperinsulinemia with mild to severe hyperglycemia. Women with acanthosis nigricans and those with polycystic ovaries may have this type of insulin resistance. Leprechaunism and Rabson-Mendenhall syndrome are two pediatric syndromes in this category.

♦ *Infections:* Infection with one or several different viruses, including rubella virus, coxsackievirus B, cytomegalovirus (CMV), adenovirus, and mumps virus, has resulted in β cell destruction.

♦ *Uncommon immune-mediated diabetes:* Antiinsulin receptor antibodies bind to insulin receptors and can either block or increase binding of insulin, and the result is either hyperglycemia or hypoglycemia. Systemic lupus erythematosus and "stiff-man" syndrome are examples of implicated disorders.

♦ *Other genetic syndromes:* Hyperglycemia has been linked to patients with Down syndrome, Klinefelter syndrome, Turner syndrome, and Wolfram syndrome.

Many of these "secondary" causes have recently become subclassified under type 1 and type 2 DM as possible primary causes of these diseases.

Gestational diabetes mellitus (GDM): Glucose intolerance with hyperglycemia that develops during pregnancy in approximately 4% of pregnant women and results in increased perinatal risk to the child and increased risk (25%) that the mother will develop chronic DM during the next 10-15 yr. This type does not include previously diabetic pregnant women. Deterioration of glucose tolerance is considered "normal" during the third trimester of pregnancy.

Prediabetes with IGT and impaired fasting glucose (IFG): Certain individuals may manifest chronic hyperglycemia without meeting other criteria for DM and are classified as having IGT or IFG, with fasting blood glucose levels 100 mg/dL or more but less than 126 mg/dL or 2-hr oral glucose tolerance test (OGTT) 140 mg/dL or more but less than 200 mg/dL. These persons are at risk for developing DM and cardiovascular disease. IGT was formerly termed *borderline, chemical, latent, subclinical,* or *asymptomatic DM.* At least 20.1 million people in the United States, ages 40 to 74 yr, have prediabetes. Research has shown that some long-term damage to the body, especially heart and circulatory system, already may be occurring during prediabetes. Research also has shown that if blood glucose is controlled when prediabetes is identified, development of type 2 DM can be prevented.

Metabolic syndrome: Also known as *insulin resistance syndrome,* this cluster of conditions occurs together and increases the risk for diabetes, stroke, and heart disease. The presence of a family history of type 2 DM, GDM, hypertension, excess abdominal fat with body mass index (BMI) greater than 25%, hyperlipidemia, elevated cholesterol levels, elevated C-reactive protein levels, and elevated prothrombin levels are risk factors for metabolic syndrome. The Centers for Disease Control and Prevention (Ervin, 2009) has mest estimated that approximately 34% of adults in the United States meet the criteria for metabolic syndrome, which increases with age and BMI. This syndrome is an important contributor to type 2 DM.

ASSESSMENT

Signs and symptoms/physical findings
Hyperglycemia: Fatigue, weakness, weight loss, paresthesias, mild dehydration, polyuria, polydipsia, polyphagia (classic signs of hyperglycemia).

Impending type 1 crisis (DKA): Profound dehydration and hyperglycemia, electrolyte imbalance, metabolic acidosis caused by ketosis, altered mental status, Kussmaul respirations (paroxysmal dyspnea), acetone breath, possible hypovolemic shock (hypotension, weak and rapid pulse), abdominal pain, and possible strokelike symptoms.

Impending type 2 crisis (HHNK): Severe dehydration, hypovolemic shock (hypotension, weak and rapid pulse), severe hyperglycemia, shallow respirations, altered mental status, slight lactic acidosis or normal pH, possible strokelike symptoms.

History and risk factors: Family history of DM; GDM; obesity; metabolic syndrome; Hispanic, Native American, and African American race or ethnicity; altered immune responses; genetic factors; and environmental stressors.

COMPLICATIONS

Potential for acute crisis: DKA and hypoglycemia for type 1; HHNK and hypoglycemia for type 2. All individuals with DM are at higher risk for developing cardiovascular disease, which is preventable in most cases.

Long-term complications: The most important factor in delaying progression to long-term complications is stabilization of blood glucose levels to normal range.

Macroangiopathy: Heart attack and stroke caused by vascular disease affecting the coronary arteries and larger vessels of the brain and lower extremities (peripheral vascular disease). Risk factors are hyperglycemia, hypertension, hypercholesterolemia, smoking, aging, and extended duration of DM.

Microangiopathy: Blindness and renal failure caused by thickening of capillary basement membranes and resulting in retinopathy and nephropathy. Early signs and symptoms include increased leakage of retinal vessels and microalbuminuria.

Neuropathy: Gastroparesis (impaired gastric emptying), lack of sensation (especially in the feet), and neurogenic bladder caused by deterioration of peripheral and autonomic nervous systems that results in impaired or slowed nerve transmission.

Morning hyperglycemia: Blood glucose elevation on awakening. Causes include the following: (1) *insufficient insulin;* the most common cause of hyperglycemia before breakfast is probably inadequate levels of circulating insulin; patient may need a higher dosage, a mixture of insulins, or longer-acting insulin; (2) *dawn phenomenon,* in which glucose remains normal until approximately 3 AM, when the effect of nocturnal growth hormone may elevate glucose in type 1 DM; it may be corrected by changing the time of the evening dose of intermediate-acting insulin injection to bedtime instead of dinnertime; and (3) *Somogyi phenomenon,* in which patient becomes hypoglycemic during the night; compensatory mechanisms to raise glucose levels are activated and result in overcompensation; decreasing the evening dose of intermediate-acting insulin and/or eating a more substantial bedtime snack may correct the problem.

Problems with insulin

Insulin resistance: A problem experienced by most individuals with DM and other diseases at some point in the illness, when the daily insulin requirement to control hyperglycemia and prevent ketosis exceeds 200 units. It is a major contributing factor to metabolic syndrome. It is characterized as one of three anomalies:

- *Prereceptor:* Insulin abnormal or insulin antibodies present
- *Receptor:* Number of insulin receptors decreased or insulin binding to the receptors diminished
- *Postreceptor:* Receptors not appropriately activated by insulin

Local allergic reactions: Soreness, erythema, or induration at the insulin injection site within 2 hr after injection. Reactions are decreasing in frequency with the evolution of more purified insulins. Beef and beef/pork insulins are no longer commercially available in the United States. Pork insulin is used in less than 10% of patients. Use of recombinant human insulin has decreased the number of reactions significantly.

Systemic allergic reactions: With the advent of primarily human insulin and insulin analogs, systemic allergic reactions have become extremely rare. The episode begins with a localized skin reaction, which evolves into generalized urticaria or anaphylaxis. Patients must be desensitized to insulin by progression from minuscule to more normal doses over the course of 1 day, by using a series of subcutaneous injections.

Lipodystrophy: Local disturbance in fat metabolism that results in loss of fat (lipoatrophy) or development of abnormal fatty masses at the injection sites (lipohypertrophy). Lipoatrophy rarely has been seen since the development of U-100 and human source insulins. Rotation of injection sites helps to prevent lipohypertrophy. Individuals experiencing lipohypertrophy should use alternate injection sites until the condition resolves.

DIAGNOSTIC TESTS

Testing for DM should be considered for persons more than 45 yr old, particularly for those who are obese (BMI greater than 25 kg/m^2). If results are normal, testing should be repeated every 3 yr. Younger obese individuals also may warrant testing, particularly if they have a first-degree relative with DM, are physically inactive, are in a high-risk ethnic group (e.g., Latino, Native American, African American, Asian American, or Pacific Islander), are hypertensive (BP greater than 130/80 mm Hg), have a high-density lipoprotein (HDL) cholesterol level less than 35 mg/dL or triglyceride levels greater than 250 mg/dL, have a history of vascular disease or other diseases associated with hyperglycemia, have a history of IFG/IGT, or have polycystic ovary syndrome (PCOS).

The World Health Organization (WHO) and the American Diabetes Association (ADA) define the diagnostic criteria for DM in nonpregnant adults as follows:

Hemoglobin A1c (HbA1c)/glycosylated hemoglobin (glycohemoglobin): Normal range is 4%-7%. Individuals with DM have values greater than 7%. This value is measured to assess control of blood glucose over a preceding 2- to 3-mo period. The larger the percentage of glycosylated hemoglobin, the poorer the blood glucose control. Reducing glycohemoglobin levels to less than 6% may further reduce complications. Kits are now available to monitor this value in the home, and this test is becoming the preferred diagnostic test for monitoring control of blood glucose levels.

Fasting plasma glucose/blood sugar: The preferred diagnostic test; a value greater than 126 mg/dL is indicative of DM. Fasting is defined as no calories consumed or infused for 8 hr before testing.

OGTT: The 2-hr sample during the test is 200 mg/dL or more. The test is poorly reproducible and not performed often in practice. The patient is given a high-glucose solution and undergoes multiple blood sample testings over the following 2 hr.

Casual/random plasma glucose: Measurement is 180 mg/dL or more on at least two occasions. The blood is drawn regardless of food/beverage consumption at any time during the day.

Fasting lipid profile (total, HDL, and low-density lipoprotein [LDL] cholesterol levels; triglyceride level): If total and LDL cholesterol values are elevated, triglyceride value is elevated, or HDL cholesterol level is decreased, the patient is at high risk for developing cardiovascular disease.

Urinalysis for presence of microalbuminuria, ketones, protein, and sediment: If present, may indicate early renal disease caused by hyperglycemia.

Serum creatinine: If elevated, may indicate renal disease secondary to diabetes.

12-lead ECG: If patient has symptoms of cardiovascular disease, an ECG can identify areas of myocardial ischemia, infarction, and active injury.

COLLABORATIVE MANAGEMENT

Control of blood glucose: The American Association of Clinical Endocrinologists (2007) determined that both morbidity and mortality could be reduced for thousands of patients if hyperglycemia was diagnosed at admission and treated throughout hospitalization. Guidelines state that in critically ill patients, blood sugar level should be maintained at 80-110 mg/dL. Non–intensive care patients should be maintained at a premeal level of no more than 110 mg/dL and a maximum level of 180 mg/dL. Benefits of treatment outweigh any potential negative outcomes of low blood sugar.

Point-of-care monitoring of blood glucose: Control of blood glucose is facilitated by a glucose monitoring device, which is designed to provide timely measurement of the glucose level from a small drop of blood. There are many blood glucose meters available. Each meter specifies the type of blood sample needed for testing. Some meters require a much smaller blood sample. Several afford a variety of blood sampling sites, including fingertips, forearms, upper arms, thighs, calves, and hands. This simple technology provides the opportunity for closer monitoring and stabilization of glucose levels, which have been shown to decrease both the incidence and severity of long-term complications. Blood glucose is generally monitored before meals, at bedtime, and possibly during the night (3:00 AM) in order to assess whether a correction dose of short-acting insulin is needed. Self-monitoring by patients has proved extremely useful in reducing complications. The measurement of HbA1c/glycosylated hemoglobin levels is becoming more popular for monitoring adequacy of blood glucose control now that home test kits are available.

Diet: Control of carbohydrates via a Consistent Carbohydrate Diet is the current strategy supported for successful management. The type and amount of carbohydrates consumed must be managed to control the glycemic index (a measure of the effect of carbohydrates on blood glucose). Controlling blood glucose is the key to effective management and prevention of complications. Total grams of carbohydrate consumed should not be reduced to less than 130 g daily because the brain and central nervous system (CNS) are dependent on glucose as an energy source. Carbohydrate intake should be 45%-65% of total calories consumed.

Counting carbohydrates has been practiced increasingly over the past few years. Individuals with type 1 DM require day-to-day consistency in diet and exercise to prevent hypoglycemia. Before a diet is initiated, a medical nutritional therapy team should evaluate patient's lifestyle so that a workable diet for the individual can be recommended. Typically, three daily meals and an evening snack are prescribed. Some fat and protein should be present in all meals and snacks to slow down the elevation of postprandial blood glucose. Adding 10-15 g of fiber will slow the digestion of monosaccharides and disaccharides. For all types of diabetes, refined and simple sugars should be reduced and complex carbohydrates (breads, cereals, pasta, beans) encouraged. Various artificial sweeteners are used in "diet" products. Some contribute calories and must be accounted for in a calorie-restricted diet. Exchange lists may be used for meal planning if this is preferred to carbohydrate counting.

Weight management: A moderate reduction (500-1000 cal/day) of calories results in a gradual but steady loss of weight. Weight loss diets should provide 1000-1200 kcal/day for women and 1200-1600 kcal/day for men, to target a BMI of 25% or less.

Oral hypoglycemic agents: There are many oral medications for the treatment of hyperglycemia, as described in the following paragraphs and in **TABLE 6-2**:

Sulfonylureas (e.g., glyburide, glipizide, glimepiride): Lower blood sugar levels primarily by stimulating production of insulin by the pancreas. To a lesser degree, these agents decrease hepatic glucose production and increase glucose uptake at the cell membrane. All patients taking sulfonylureas can experience hypoglycemia, for example, if a meal is delayed or skipped or activity is increased. Excretion of the medication in patients with impaired renal function may be delayed, also increasing risk of hypoglycemia. Glipizide should be taken 30 min before eating. The other sulfonylureas should be taken with the meal.

Biguanides (e.g., metformin, Glucovance [combination drug consisting of metformin and glyburide]): Metformin lowers blood glucose levels primarily by decreasing hepatic glucose production. It also increases glucose uptake at the cell membrane and increases peripheral glucose use in skeletal muscles. Metformin is often used in combination with sulfonylureas and rarely causes hypoglycemia when used alone. Side effects seen during initial weeks of therapy include nausea, vomiting, diarrhea, and flatulence. Unlike some of the other oral agents, metformin must be given with food and can cause lactic acidosis if given inappropriately.

Metformin should be stopped for severe illness, surgery, dye procedure, or dehydration. Renal function must be assessed before restarting the medication. Serum creatinine should normalize before metformin is reinstituted. Metformin is contraindicated in patients with renal dysfunction (creatinine more than 1.5 mg/dL in male patients and 1.4 mg/dL in female patients), hepatic dysfunction, and alcoholism.

Meglitinide analogs (e.g., glyburide, glipizide, glimepiride, repaglinide, nateglinide: Work by helping the body release insulin in response to rising blood glucose levels as a result of eating. Therefore, these drugs must always be

TABLE 6-2	ORAL HYPOGLYCEMIC AGENTS		
GENERIC NAME (TRADE NAME)	**USUAL DOSE (mg)/ ADMINISTRATION**	**MAXIMUM DOSE (mg)**	**DURATION (hr)**
Sulfonylureas			
Acetohexamide (Dymelor)	250-1500; single or divided	1500	12-24
Chlorpropamide (Diabinese)	100-500; single or divided	750	60
Glipizide (Glucotrol)	5-40; single or divided	40	10-24
Glipizide (Glucotrol XL)	5 – 20 single	20	24
Glimepiride (Amaryl)	1-8; single	8	24
Glyburide (Micronase, Glynase Prestab, DiaBeta)	2.5-20 single or divided	20	12-24
Tolazamide (Tolinase)	100-750; single or divided	1000	12-24
Tolbutamide (Orinase)	500-2000; single or divided	3000	12-24
Biguanides			
Metformin (Glucophage)	1000-2500; divided	2550	7-12
Alpha Glucosidase Inhibitors			
Acarbose (Precose)	50-100; tid with meals	300 daily total	~4
Miglitol (Glyset)	25-100; tid with meals	300 daily total	~4
Meglitinides			
Repaglinide (Prandin)	0.5-2.0; tid before meals	16 daily total	3
Nateglinide (Starlix)	60-120; tid before meals	360 daily total	3
Thiazolidinediones			
Pioglitazone (Actos)	15-30; daily	45 daily total	16-24
Rosiglitazone (Avandia)	4-8; daily	8 daily total	3-4

tid, Three times daily.

taken 15 min before each meal. Repaglinide and nateglinide have a very short half-life and are quickly excreted from the body. Possible side effects of all of these drugs include hypoglycemia (less likely than with sulfonylureas) and cold and flulike symptoms (diarrhea, joint ache, and back pain).

Alpha glucosidase inhibitors (e.g., acarbose, miglitol): Work by slowing digestion of complex carbohydrates that, in turn, reduces glucose absorption. These agents have less effect on fasting blood glucose than on postprandial blood glucose. Patients should take these drugs with the first bite of a meal. Alpha glucosidase inhibitors can be used alone or in combination with other oral agents or insulin. These drugs when given alone do not cause hypoglycemia, but when they are used in combination with insulin or oral agents, hypoglycemia may occur. Alpha glucosidase inhibitors blunt the gastric absorption of glucose. If hypoglycemia occurs after the medication is given, the juice, cola, and candy that are typically used to correct low blood glucose may not be effective. Hypoglycemia should be managed using an alternative such as glucose tabs (dextrose) or 4-6 oz of milk (lactose). These drugs have little interaction with other medications, have a minimal effect on liver and kidney function, and can be safely used in older adults. Diarrhea and flatulence are common initially and subside over time.

Thiazolidinediones or insulin sensitizers (e.g., pioglitazone, rosiglitazone): Improve ability of the cells to use insulin. Insulin resistance is decreased, and the amount of insulin produced does not increase. When used alone, these agents do not cause hypoglycemia. Insulin sensitizers should be taken with a meal. Peak therapeutic effect is attained at 3-12 wk. Increased fluid retention may be noted. Liver function studies must be monitored periodically. These medications are used with caution in patients with hepatic failure and are contraindicated in patients with New York Heart Association (NYHA) class III and class IV heart failure.

Subcutaneous hypoglycemic agents (augment oral hypoglycemic drugs and insulin)

Amylinomimetic compounds (e.g., pramlintide acetate): This analog of the hormone amylin, which is synthesized by β cells of the pancreas, is used for management of type 1 diabetes in patients whose mealtime insulin has not controlled glucose despite repeated adjustments in therapy; or patients with type 2 DM who use mealtime insulin therapy, either with or without a sulfonylurea and/or metformin, and whose blood glucose is not controlled effectively. This drug has been associated with severe hypoglycemia in patients with type 1 DM who take insulin, so it is not viewed as a drug suitable for all patients with DM. Insulin dose adjustments are generally required when this drug is added to an insulin regimen.

Incretin mimetics (e.g., exenatide): Used for added control of blood glucose in patients with type 2 DM who are taking either metformin alone or metformin plus a sulfonylurea and who continue to have hyperglycemia. The drug enhances glucose-dependent insulin secretion by the β cells of the pancreas while suppressing glucagon secretion and slowing gastric emptying.

Insulin and insulin glargine: Examples of short-, intermediate-, and long-acting insulins are shown in **TABLE 6-3**. Glargine is an insulin alternative, and it attains full action within 1 hr of administration and remains at a steady level for 24 hr.

- ◆ *Basal/bolus therapy* is recommended because it promotes tighter control of blood glucose. Basal insulin is either glargine, given once daily at bedtime, or an intermediate-acting insulin generally administered before meals with a prescribed dose of prandial (meal time) insulin. Prandial (bolus) insulin is rapid-acting and includes regular insulin and insulin analogs (insulin aspart, insulin lispro) to mimic the natural action of the pancreas at mealtime. Correction doses are calculated by formula, based on patient's pre-meal blood glucose reading. An NPH/regular mixed insulin [Humulin 70/30] or an NPH/insulin aspart [NovoLog 70/30] or NPH/insulin lispro mixed analog insulin [Humalog 70/30] also may be used to promote better adherence to insulin administration. Basal/bolus therapy precludes use of the longer-acting single-dose insulins, which provide have less adequate control of blood glucose.

- ◆ *Insulin detemir (Levemir)* is another long-acting basal insulin analog that has actions similar to those of glargine (Lantus). The duration of action is up to 24 hr, and the agent is indicated for patients who need long-acting control of hyperglycemia. It should not be diluted or mixed with other insulin preparations. Hypoglycemia is the most common side effect.

Insulin delivery systems

Continuous subcutaneous insulin infusion (CSII)/portable insulin pumps: Devices that deliver a constant basal rate of insulin throughout the day and night with capability of delivering a patient-programmed bolus of insulin at mealtime. A needle or tiny catheter attaches to a pump via long, thin, plastic tubing and remains indwelling in the subcutaneous tissue of the abdomen. Patients program their own pump to deliver the optimal amount of

TABLE 6-3	TYPES OF COMMON INSULIN AND INSULIN ANALOGS				
INSULIN TYPE	**EXAMPLE(S)**	**SUBCUTANEOUS INJECTION ONSET**	**PEAK**	**DURATION**	**MIXTURE/OTHER**
Rapid Acting					
Regular	Humulin R Novolin R Iletin II Pork Regular	30 min	1-2 hr	8-12 hr	NPH, Lente and for IV infusion
Insulin aspart	NovoLog	~15 min	40-50 min	3-5 hr	NPH, Lente and for insulin subcutaneous pumps
Insulin lispro	Humalog	15-30 min	30-90 min	3-5 hr	Human insulin lispro protamine, NPH, Lente
Semilente	Prompt insulin zinc suspension	1-1½ hr	5-10 hr	10-16 hr	Lente
Intermediate Acting					
NPH	Isophane insulin suspension, Humulin N, Novolin N, NPL insulin	1-1½ hr Iletin II Pork (NPH), 1-1½ hr	4-12 hr NPH N Pork 1.3-8.3 hr	20-24 hr	Regular
Human insulin lispro protamine				20-24 hr	Human insulin lispro (Humalog)
Lente	Insulin zinc suspension, Humulin L, Novolin L, Iletin II Pork, Lente L Pork	1-2½ hr	6-16 hr	20-24 hr	Semilente

Continued

TABLE 6-3		TYPES OF COMMON INSULIN AND INSULIN ANALOGS—cont'd				
INSULIN TYPE	EXAMPLE(S)	SUBCUTANEOUS INJECTION ONSET	PEAK	DURATION	MIXTURE/OTHER
Long Acting					
Ultralente	Extended insulin zinc suspension, Humulin U	2-6 hr	7-10 hr	24-36 hr	Regular, Semilente
Insulin detemir	Levemir	30 min	No peak/steady action	24 hr	None
Insulin glargine	Lantus	30 min	No peak/steady	24 hr	None
PZI	Protamine zinc insulin suspension	4-8 hr	14-24 hr	36 hr	Regular
Intermediate/Rapid-Acting Combination					
Premixed insulin	Humalog Mix 75/25 or 50/50	30 min	2-4 hr	20-22 hr	None
Lispro					
Lispro protamine/insulin					
Lispro combinations					
Premixed insulin	NovoLog Mix 70/30	30 min	2-4 hr	20-22 hr	None
Aspart					
Aspart protamine/30% aspart					
Premixed human NPH/ Regular human insulin combinations	Humulin 70/30 or 50/50 Novolin 70/30 or 50/50	30-60 min	2-6 hr	20-24 hr	None

IV, Intravenous.

insulin, based on self-monitoring of blood glucose. Patients should be alert to soreness and erythema at the insertion site, which may indicate abscess or staphylococcal infection. Implantable pumps are commercially available, and clinical trials on a variety of pump technologies and glucose sensors are ongoing. Limiting factors to the use of such pumps are cost and lack of pump glucose monitoring capability.

Injection ports: Subcutaneous access ports inserted into the subcutaneous fat by the patient. These ports may remain in place for up to 3 days. They are constructed similarly to peripheral IV catheters, with introducer needles that are removed when the catheter is appropriately positioned. The device is secured by taping, and patients may use the port for dosage, rather than puncturing the skin.

Jet injectors: Deliver insulin in a fine, pressurized stream through the skin without use of a needle for injection. Absorption, peak, and insulin levels may be altered by the injector, thus necessitating caution for the patient. Typically, onset and peak action occur earlier with these devices. Thorough training must be provided before allowing patients to use these devices independently.

Insulin pens: Small, prefilled insulin cartridges that are inserted into a penlike holder or other housing. After attachment of a specially designed, shorter, and finer disposable needle, the insulin is injected by selecting a dose or depressing a button either once for each 1- to 2-unit increment desired for the dosage (older device) or once for the entire selected dosage (newer device). Although patients must use needles for injection, there is no need for insulin to be drawn up from multidose vials, thus adding to the convenience and accuracy of administration. Patients electing to use these agents should plan on frequent blood glucose testing until use of the new device demonstrates stable glucose control.

Exercise: Exercise is as important as diet and insulin in treating DM. It lowers blood glucose levels, helps maintain normal cholesterol levels, and increases circulation. These effects increase the body's ability to metabolize glucose and help reduce the therapeutic dose of insulin for most patients. The exercise program must be consistent and individualized (especially for individuals with type 1 DM). Patients should be given a complete physical examination and encouraged to incorporate acceptable activities as part of their daily routine. If blood glucose level is greater than 250 mg/dL, exercise acts as a stressor, causing blood glucose to increase rather than decrease. Patients should monitor blood glucose levels with a monitoring device before beginning an exercise program.

Transplantation: Complete or partial pancreatic transplants have been performed, sometimes in conjunction with kidney transplantation. Candidates must thoroughly evaluate risks associated with antirejection medications vs. benefits of pancreatic transplantation. Immune suppression caused by the medications may promote development of opportunistic infections. Transplantation of only β cells is being investigated as an alternative to other methods.

NURSING DIAGNOSES AND INTERVENTIONS

Ineffective peripheral, cardiopulmonary, renal, cerebral, and gastrointestinal tissue perfusion (or risk for same) related to interrupted blood flow secondary to development and progression of macroangiopathy and microangiopathy

Desired outcomes: Optimally, patient has adequate tissue perfusion as evidenced by warmth, sensation, brisk capillary refill time (less than 2 sec), and peripheral pulses greater than 2 on a 0-4 scale in the extremities; BP within his or her optimal range; urinary output 30 mL/hr or more; baseline vision; good appetite; and absence of nausea and vomiting. Patient demonstrates adherence to the therapeutic regimen (essential for promoting optimal tissue perfusion).

Nursing Interventions

◆ Check blood glucose before meals and at bedtime regularly. Urine testing is less reliable and should not be used by patients with reduced renal function. *Promotes optimal blood glucose control.*

◆ Administer basal, prandial, and correction doses of insulin as prescribed *to maximize blood glucose control.*

◆ Check BP q4h, administer antihypertensive medication as prescribed, and alert health care provider of values outside patient's normal range. Hypertension is a common complication of diabetes. *Control of BP is critical in preventing or limiting development of heart disease, stroke, retinopathy, and nephropathy.*

◆ Protect patients with impaired peripheral perfusion from sharp objects or heat (e.g., avoid use of heating pads). *Minimizes the risk of injury when patient has peripheral neuropathy and subsequent loss of sensation.*

◆ Assess capillary refill, temperature, peripheral pulses, and color *to detect venous stasis.*

◆ Teach patient to avoid pressure at back of the knees (e.g., by not crossing legs or "gatching" bed under the knees). Caution patient to avoid garments that constrict circulation to the extremities and lower body. *Minimizes risk for venous stasis.*

◆ Provide a safe environment for patients with diabetic retinopathy. Orient patient to locations of such items as water, tissues, glasses, and call light. *Minimizes risk of falls or other injuries because of diminished eyesight.*

◆ Monitor patients for changes in renal function (e.g., increases in blood urea nitrogen [BUN] [more than 20 mg/dL] and creatinine [more than 1.5 mg/dL] and altered urine output). Approximately half of all persons with type 1 DM develop chronic kidney disease (CKD) and end-stage renal disease. Proteinuria (protein more than 8 mg/dL in a random sample of urine) and microalbuminuria are early indicators of developing CKD. Individuals with DM and with reduced renal function are at significant risk for dehydration and development of acute renal failure (ARF) after exposure to contrast medium. Patients who will receive contrast medium should be well hydrated and possibly receive several doses of oral acetylcysteine (Mucomyst) or an IV bicarbonate infusion to protect the kidneys from contrast-related deterioration. Observe these patients for indicators of ARF. (See "Acute Renal Failure," p. 174, and "Chronic Kidney Disease," p. 181.)

◆ Assess for signs of hypoglycemia (e.g., changes in mentation, apprehension, erratic behavior, trembling, slurred speech, staggering gait, seizure activity). Treat hypoglycemia as prescribed (see discussion in "Collaborative Management," p. 415).

◆ Assist patients when they are getting up suddenly or after prolonged recumbency. Check BP while patient is lying down, sitting, and then standing to document findings. Alert health care provider to significant findings. *Minimizes risk for orthostatic hypotension.*

◆ Administer metoclopramide before meals if prescribed. *Minimizes the risk gastroparesis/impaired gastric emptying with nausea, vomiting, and diarrhea.*

◆ Encourage patient to void q3-4h during the day when neurogenic bladder is present. Intermittent catheterization may be necessary in severe cases. Avoid use of indwelling urinary catheters *because of risk of infection.* (See "Neurogenic Bladder," p. 217.)

Risk for infection related to chronic disease process (e.g., hyperglycemia, neurogenic bladder, poor circulation)

Desired outcome: Patient is asymptomatic for infection as evidenced by normothermia, negative cultures, and WBC count 11,000/mm³ or less. Infection is the most common cause of DKA.

Nursing Interventions

◆ Monitor temperature q4h. Alert health care provider to elevations. *May indicate infection.*
◆ Maintain meticulous sterile technique when changing dressings, performing invasive procedures, or manipulating indwelling catheters *to minimize risk for infection.*
◆ Monitor for indicators of infection:
  • *Upper respiratory infection (URI):* fever, chills, productive cough, crackles, dyspnea, inflamed pharynx, sore throat.
  • *Urinary tract infection (UTI):* burning, urgency, and frequency of urination; cloudy or malodorous urine; fever; chills; tachycardia; diaphoresis; nausea; vomiting; abdominal pain.
  • *Systemic sepsis:* fever, chills, tachycardia, diaphoresis, nausea, vomiting.
  • *Localized infection (IV sites):* erythema, swelling, purulent drainage, warmth.
◆ Consult health care provider about obtaining culture specimens for blood, sputum, and urine during temperature spikes or for wounds that produce purulent drainage *to verify the presence of infection and determine the most appropriate antibiotic therapy.*

Impaired skin integrity (or risk for same) related to altered circulation and sensation secondary to peripheral neuropathy and vascular pathology
Desired outcomes: Patient's lower extremity skin remains intact. Within the 24-hr period before hospital discharge, patient verbalizes and demonstrates knowledge of proper foot care.

Nursing Interventions

◆ Assess integrity of the skin and evaluate proprioceptive sensations, two-point discrimination, and vibration sensation (using a tuning fork on the medial malleolus) *to determine whether patient's sensations are impaired and whether or not patient is able to respond to harmful stimuli.*
◆ Monitor peripheral pulses, comparing quality bilaterally. Be alert to pulse complitudes 2+ or less on a 0-4+ scale *because indicate decreased peripheral circulation.*
◆ Use foot cradle on bed, space boots for ulcerated heels, elbow protectors, and pressure-relief mattress *to prevent pressure points and promote patient comfort.*
◆ Incorporate progressive passive and active exercises into daily routine. Discourage extended rest periods in same position *to alleviate acute discomfort yet prevent hemostasis.*
◆ Teach patient regarding foot care:
  • Wash feet daily with mild soap and warm water; check water temperature with water thermometer or elbow *to prevent burns when decreased sensation is present.*
  • Inspect feet daily for presence of erythema, discoloration, or trauma; use mirrors as necessary for adequate visualization *to detect injury.*
  • Alternate between at least two pairs of properly fitted shoes *to avoid potential for pressure points that can occur by wearing one pair only.*
  • Change socks or stockings daily and wear cotton or wool blends *to prevent infection from moisture or dirt.*
  • Use gentle moisturizers *to soften dry skin,* and avoid areas between toes *to prevent accumulation of lotion, which may harbor bacteria.*

- Cut toenails straight across after softening them during bath. File nails with emery board. *Prevents ingrown toenails.*
- Do not self-treat corns or calluses; visit podiatrist regularly *to prevent injury from corn/callus removal.*
- Attend to any foot injury immediately, and seek medical attention *to avoid any potential complications.*
- Do not go barefoot indoors or outdoors, *to minimize risk for injury.*

Deficient knowledge related to proper insulin administration and dietary precautions for promoting normoglycemia

Desired outcome: Within the 24-hr period before hospital discharge, patient verbalizes and demonstrates knowledge of proper insulin administration, symptoms and treatment of hypoglycemia, and the prescribed dietary regimen.

Nursing Interventions

◆ Assess patient's facility with language; engage an interpreter or provide language-appropriate written materials if necessary.

◆ Teach patient to check the expiration date on the insulin vial and to avoid using it if outdated. Also teach patient proper storage of insulin and the importance of avoiding temperature extremes, *to prevent harm to the medication.*

◆ Teach patient to use the insulin syringe that corresponds with the insulin (e.g., U-100 insulin with U-100 syringes). In the United States, insulin is standardized to U-100 (100 units per mL). Patients must be aware, especially if they travel to other countries, that there are differences in strengths of insulin suspensions, and each strength must be given using the appropriate syringe because U-40 insulin and U-40 syringes are used in some countries.

◆ Explain that intermediate- and long-acting insulins require mixing (contraindicated for intermediate/rapid acting). Demonstrate rolling the insulin vial between the palms to mix contents. Caution patient that vigorous shaking produces air bubbles that can interfere with accurate dose measurement.

◆ Explain that regular prandial insulin (e.g., Novolin or Humalin) should be injected 30 min before eating a meal; newer insulin analogs may be injected immediately before or directly after eating. If patients are unable to finish at least half of a meal, they may be advised to hold their prandial insulin if they are receiving an analog (e.g., NovoLog, Humalog). Because analogs can be given after a meal, dosage is more flexible than with regular human insulins. Explain that either making a change in insulin type or withholding a dose of insulin may be required for the following: when fasting for studies or surgery, when not eating because of nausea/vomiting, or when hypoglycemic. Remind patient that stress from illness or infection can increase insulin requirements (or necessitate insulin therapy for one whose DM is normally controlled with oral hypoglycemics) and that increased exercise will necessitate additional food intake *to prevent hypoglycemia when no change is made in insulin dose.* Adjustments are always individually based and require clarification with patient's health care provider *to ensure accuracy of insulin dosage and schedule.*

◆ Provide a chart that depicts injection site rotations. Explain that injection sites should be at least 1 inch apart *to minimize the risk for lipodystrophy.*

◆ Explain importance of inserting the needle perpendicular to the skin rather than at an angle. Very thin persons may need to use a 45-degree angle. *Ensures deep subcutaneous administration of insulin.*

- Ensure patient understands and demonstrates the technique and *timing for home monitoring of blood glucose using* a commercial kit, which provides ongoing data reflecting the degree of control and may identify necessary changes in diet and medication before severe metabolic changes occur. *Allows for patient's self-control and psychologic security.*
- Caution patient about importance of following a diet that is controlled in carbohydrates, low in fat, and high in fiber. Stress that diet is the sole method of control for many individuals with type 2 DM. Adequate nutrition, consistent carbohydrates, and controlled calories are essential *to maintain normoglycemia and effectively control blood fats, especially cholesterol and triglycerides.*
- Teach patient how to count carbohydrates. The "magic number" used for counting carbohydrates is 15, because 15 g of carbohydrate = one serving of carbohydrate. Many carbohydrate-controlled diets allow four servings of carbohydrates per meal. Complex carbohydrates raise blood glucose levels more gradually than do simple carbohydrates and are preferred. *Complex carbohydrates they have a lower glycemic index than simple carbohydrates.*
- For patients who experience low blood glucose at night, discuss commercially available long-acting carbohydrate sources *to minimize nighttime hypoglycemia.*

Patient-Family Teaching and Discharge Planning

Include verbal and written information about the following:
- Importance of carrying a diabetic identification card, wearing a MedicAlert bracelet or necklace, and having the identification card outline the diagnosis and emergency treatment. Contact the MedicAlert Foundation for more information:

MedicAlert Foundation: www.medicalert.org

- Recognizing warning signs of both hyperglycemia and hypoglycemia, treatment, and factors that contribute to both conditions.
- Emphasize importance of disclosing all alternative and complementary health practices being used *because some may affect blood glucose or possibly lead to adverse drug reactions.*
- Remind patient that stress from illness or infection can increase insulin requirements (or necessitate insulin therapy for one whose DM is normally controlled with oral hypoglycemics) and that increased exercise will necessitate additional food intake *to prevent hypoglycemia* when no change is made in insulin dosage under normoglycemic conditions. Blood glucose at a level greater than 250 mg/dL at the beginning of exercise will make the exercise a stressor that elevates rather than decreases the glucose level.
- Drugs that potentiate **hyperglycemia:** estrogens, corticosteroids, thyroid preparations, diuretics, phenytoin, glucagon, and drugs containing sugar (e.g., cough syrup).
- Drugs that potentiate **hypoglycemia:** salicylates, sulfonamides, tetracyclines, methyldopa, anabolic steroids, acetaminophen, monoamine oxidase (MAO) inhibitors, ethanol, haloperidol, and marijuana. Propranolol and other β-adrenergic blocking agents may mask the signs of and inhibit recovery from hypoglycemia. Patients using combinations of newer agents (i.e., alpha glucosidase inhibitors, meglitinides, thiazolidinediones) must be particularly careful to follow directions regarding taking drugs before meals (or with meals), along with other specifics for each drug, *to avoid causing hypoglycemia.*

- Home monitoring of blood glucose using commercial kits and possibly daily urine testing for glucose and ketones, which provide ongoing data reflecting degree of control and may identify necessary changes in diet and medication before severe metabolic changes occur. In addition, kits for monitoring glycohemoglobin (HbA1c) are available for home use and may assist patients in determining overall effectiveness of their diabetes management regimen.
- Importance of daily exercise, maintenance of normal body weight, and yearly medical evaluation. Stress that each exercise program must be individualized (especially for persons with type 1 DM) and implemented consistently. Patient should have a complete physical examination and then be encouraged to incorporate acceptable exercise activities into his or her daily routine.
- Review of diet that is consistent in carbohydrates, low in fat, and high in fiber as an effective means of controlling blood fats, especially cholesterol and triglycerides. Patients who gained weight before developing type 2 DM are sometimes able to normalize their blood glucose by losing weight and maintaining ideal body weight.
- Mixing insulins properly by drawing up the regular first, followed by the intermediate- or long-acting insulin. Insulin analogs (Humalog, NovoLog) and glargine (Lantus) should not be mixed with other insulin preparations.
- Use of syringe magnifiers that can be used by patients with poor visual acuity. Other products that permit safe and accurate filling of syringes are also available.
- Rotating injection sites and injecting insulin at room temperature. Provide a chart showing possible injection sites, and describe the system for site rotation. Complications related to insulin injections, including lipodystrophy, insulin resistance, and allergic reactions, should be discussed thoroughly.
- Importance of daily meticulous skin, wound, and foot care.
- Necessity of annual eye examination for early detection and treatment of retinopathy.
- Scheduling dental checkups at least every 6 mo to help prevent periodontal disease, a major problem for individuals with DM. The mouth often is the primary site of origination for low-grade infections.
- Medications, including purpose, dosage, schedule, precautions, interactions, and potential side effects for all medications used. Also discuss drug/drug, food/drug, and herb/drug interactions.
- Identifying available resources for ongoing assistance and information, including nurses, dietitian, patient's health care provider, and other individuals with DM in patient care unit. Other resources include the local chapter of the ADA and the local library for free access to current materials on diabetes. The following is a list of resources available to patients:

American Diabetes Association: www.diabetes.org

Canadian Diabetes Association: www.diabetes.ca

Juvenile Diabetes Research Foundation International (JDRF): www.jdrf.org

Joslin Diabetes Center: www.joslin.org

National Diabetes Information Clearinghouse (NDIC): www.niddk.nih.gov/health/diabetes/ndic.htm

American Heart Association, National Center: www.americanheart.org

Can-Am-Care (diabetes care store brand availability guide): www.canamcare.com

❖ DIABETIC KETOACIDOSIS

OVERVIEW/PATHOPHYSIOLOGY

Diabetic ketoacidosis (DKA) is a life-threatening condition caused by extreme lack of effective insulin and resulting in major hyperglycemia and acidosis from abnormal carbohydrate, fat, and protein metabolism, occuring in persons with diabetes mellitus (DM). The intracellular environment is unable to receive necessary glucose for oxidation and energy production without insulin to facilitate transport of glucose from the bloodstream across the cell membrane. Impairment of glucose uptake results in hyperglycemia, while the intracellular environment continues to lack necessary nutrients. Glucagon secretion increases and causes available body stores of food substances to be broken down in an attempt to provide cell nourishment. Impaired amino acid transport, protein synthesis, and protein degradation facilitate protein catabolism, with a resultant increase in serum amino acids, whereas fat breakdown results in elevated free fatty acids (FFA) and glycerol. The liver converts the newly available amino acids, fatty acids, and glycerol into glucose (gluconeogenesis) in an attempt to provide nourishment for the cells, but instead the hyperglycemia worsens because of the lack of insulin to transport glucose into the cells. The liver also produces ketone bodies from available FFA, and ketone bodies cause mild to severe acidosis. As ketone bodies increase in the extracellular fluid, the hydrogen ions within the ketones are exchanged with K^+ ions from within the cells. Thus intracellular K^+ is released into the extracellular fluid and then to circulating fluid, where it is excreted by the kidneys into the urine. Hyperglycemia acts as an osmotic diuretic, by causing severe fluid and electrolyte losses that lead to hypovolemic shock if untreated. Individuals with severe DKA may lose nearly 500 mEq of Na^+, chloride (Cl^-), and K^+, along with approximately 7 L of water in 24 hr.

ASSESSMENT

Sign and symptoms/physical findings: See **TABLE 6-4**.
History and risk factors: Too little insulin, illness, lack of compliance with dietary restrictions.

DIAGNOSTIC TESTS

See Table 6-4.

COLLABORATIVE MANAGEMENT

The goals of treatment are to lower the high blood glucose level by giving insulin and to replace fluids lost through polyuria and vomiting.
Fluid replacement: Usually, normal saline or 0.45% saline is administered until plasma glucose falls to 200-300 mg/dL. After that, dextrose-containing solutions usually are given to prevent rebound hypoglycemia. Initially, IV fluids are administered rapidly (i.e., 2000 mL infused during the first 2 hr of treatment and 150-250 mL/hr thereafter until BP stabilizes).
Rapid-acting insulin: Usually given by continuous IV infusion for rapid action and because poor tissue perfusion caused by dehydration sometimes makes the subcutaneous route less effective. Initial dose may vary from 10 to 25 units, or about 0.3 unit/kg. Patient is maintained on 5-10 unit/hr, or 0.1 unit/kg/hr as a continuous infusion administered through a separate IV tubing and controlled with an infusion control device. Dosage is adjusted based on serial glucose levels and resolution of ketosis. Insulin drip should be adjusted using a formula that considers the patient's sensitivity to insulin. When formulas are used, the sensitivity number is reflected as a variable multiplier that increases with higher levels of insulin resistance. Insulin analogs (e.g., NovoLog, Humalog) may be used in place of regular insulin to lower blood glucose levels.

TABLE 6-4   COMPARISONS OF DIABETIC KETOACIDOSIS, HYPEROSMOLAR HYPERGLYCEMIC NONKETOTIC SYNDROME, AND HYPOGLYCEMIA

	DKA	HHNK	HYPOGLYCEMIA
Type of Diabetes **Signs, Symptoms/** **Physical** **Assessment**	Usually type 1 Symptoms are a result mainly of hyperglycemia, intracellular hypoglycemia, hypotension or impending hypovolemic shock, and fluid-electrolyte imbalance with possible acid-base imbalance	Usually type 2 Same as DKA	Symptoms result from intracellular hypoglycemia and hypotension/impending "insulin" shock (vasogenic)
Neurologic	Altered LOC (confusion, lethargy, irritability, coma); strokelike symptoms (unilateral/bilateral weakness, paralysis, numbness, paresthesia); fatigue	Same as DKA; also possible seizures and tremors	Tremors, trembling, shaking, confusion, apprehension, erratic behavior; may be same as DKA
Respiratory	Deep, rapid Kussmaul respirations	Shallow, rapid (tachypneic) breathing	Usually rapid (tachypneic) breathing
Cardiovascular	Tachycardia, hypotension, ECG changes	Same as DKA	Same as DKA, possibly with diaphoresis
Metabolic/GI/ **Endocrine**	Polyuria, polyphagia, polydipsia, fruity "acetone" breath, abdominal pain, weight loss, fatigue, generalized weakness, nausea, vomiting	Polyuria, polyphagia, polydipsia, fatigue, generalized weakness, nausea, vomiting	Hunger, nausea, eructation
Integumentary	Dry, flushed skin; poor turgor; dry mucous membranes	Same as DKA	Cool, clammy, pale skin
VS monitoring	BP low (more than 20% below normal); HR more than 100 bpm; CVP less than 2 mm Hg (less than 5 cm H_2O); temperature normal	BP low (more than 20% below normal); HR more than 100 bpm; CVP less than 2 mm Hg (less than 5 cm H_2O); temperature possibly elevated	BP normal to low; HR more than 100 bpm; CVP usually unchanged
Diagnostic Tests/ **Laboratory Values**	Values reflect dehydration/metabolic acidosis (ketosis) secondary to hyperglycemia, abnormal lipolysis, and osmotic diuresis; fluid loss 6.5 L or more	Values reflect dehydration secondary to hyperglycemia, osmotic diuresis, and possible lactic acidosis from hypoperfusion; fluid loss 9 L or more	Values reflect hypoglycemia, possibly with vasodilation owing to insulin shock

Hgb/Hct	Elevated	Same as DKA	Unchanged to slightly decreased
Serum BUN/ Creatinine	Elevated	Same as DKA	Normal
Serum Electrolytes	Initially elevated, then decreased	Same as DKA	Usually unchanged
Serum Glucose	250-800 mg/dL (+ ketones)	400-1800 mg/dL (– ketones)	15-50 mg/dL
ABGs	pH 6.8-7.3; HCO_3^- 12-20 mEq/L; CO_2 15-25 mEq/L	pH 7.3-7.5; HCO_3^- 20-26 mEq/L; CO_2 30-40 mEq/L	pH 7.3-7.5; HCO_3^- 20-26 mEq/L; CO_2 30-40 mEq/L
Serum Osmolality	300-350 mOsm/L	More than 350 mOsm/L	Less than 280 mOsm/L
Urine Glucose/ Acetone	Positive/positive	Positive/negative	Negative/negative
Onset	Hours to days	More than 1 day	Minutes to hours
History/Risk Factors for Development of Crisis	Undiagnosed DM, infections, acute pancreatitis, uremia, insulin resistance *Medications:* digitalis intoxication; omission/reduction of insulin dosage; failure to increase insulin to compensate for stress of infections, injury, emotional problems, or surgery	Undiagnosed DM; infections, especially gram negative; acromegaly; Cushing's syndrome; thyrotoxicosis, acute pancreatitis, hyperalimentation pancreatic carcinoma; cranial; trauma/subdural hematoma; uremia, hemodialysis, peritoneal dialysis; burns, heat stroke; pneumonia, MI, stroke *Medications:* loop and thiazide diuretics (i.e., hydrochlorothiazide, chlorthalidone, furosemide); diazoxide; glucocorticoids (i.e., hydrocortisone, dexamethasone); propranolol (Inderal); phenytoin (Dilantin); sodium bicarbonate	Excessive dose of insulin; excessive dose of sulfonylureas/oral hypoglycemic agents; skipping meals; too much exercise with controlled blood glucose without extra food intake *Medications:* insulin, sulfonylureas (Tables 6-2 and 6-3)
Mortality	10% or less	10%-25%	Less than 0.1%

ABGs, Arterial blood gases; *BP,* blood pressure; *BUN,* blood urea nitrogen; *CVP,* central venous pressure; *DKA,* diabetic ketoacidosis; *DM,* diabetes mellitus; *ECG,* electrocardiogram; *GI,* gastrointestinal; *Hct,* hematocrit; *Hgb,* hemoglobin; *HHNK,* hyperosmolar hyperglycemic nonketotic syndrome; *HR,* heart rate; *LOC,* level of consciousness; *MI,* myocardial infarction; *VS,* vital signs.

Restoration of electrolyte balance: Na^+ and Cl^- are replaced with IV normal saline. K^+ must be monitored and corrected carefully. Before treatment there is a risk of hyperkalemia from excess transport of intracellular K^+ to extracellular spaces. After initiation of treatment, K^+ returns to the intracellular compartment through accelerated transport into cells via insulin and following correction of acidosis, and therefore the patient is at risk for becoming hypokalemic. Use of phosphorus replacement is controversial, but if phosphorus levels remain low, potassium phosphate solutions can be used to assist with K^+ and phosphate replacement.

IV bicarbonate: For pH less than 7.10. Its use is limited because acidosis will be corrected by hydration, BP stabilization, and insulin therapy. Excessive use of sodium bicarbonate can produce alkalosis, hyperosmolality, and respiratory depression.

Insertion of gastric tube: Prevents aspiration of gastric contents, particularly in comatose patients.

Treatment of underlying cause: For example, infection is treated with appropriate antibiotics, and medications are evaluated along with diet and patient's habits.

Treatment/prevention of complications: For example, arterial thrombosis, stroke, renal failure, acute respiratory distress syndrome (ARDS), multiple organ failure, heart failure, cerebral edema, malignant dysrhythmias, and death from irreversible hypovolemic shock.

NURSING DIAGNOSES AND INTERVENTIONS

Deficient fluid volume related to failure of regulatory mechanisms or decreased circulating volume secondary to hyperglycemia with osmotic diuresis

Desired outcome: Patient becomes normovolemic within 10 hr of treatment, as evidenced by BP 90/60 mm Hg or more (or within patient's normal range), heart rate (HR) 60-100 beats per minute (bpm), central venous pressure (CVP) 2-6 mm Hg (5-12 cm H_2O), good skin turgor, moist and pink mucous membranes, specific gravity less than 1.020, balanced I&O, and urinary output 30 mL/hr or more.

Nursing Interventions

- Monitor VS q15min until stable for 1 hr. Notify health care provider promptly of the following: HR greater than 120 bpm, BP less than 90/60 or decreased 20 mm Hg or more from baseline, and CVP less than 2 mm Hg (or less than 5 cm H_2O). *These indicate hypovolemia related to osmotic diuresis or vomiting.*

- Monitor for poor skin turgor, dry mucous membranes, sunken and soft eyeballs, tachycardia, and orthostatic hypotension. *These are physical indicators of dehydration.*

- Weigh patient daily, measure I&O accurately, and monitor urinary specific gravity. Report urine specific gravity of more than 1.020 in the presence of other indicators of dehydration or urine output less than 30 mL/hr for 2 consecutive hr. *Decreasing urinary output may signal diminishing intravascular fluid volume or impending renal failure.*

- Administer IV fluids as prescribed. Be alert to indicators of fluid overload, which can occur with rapid infusion of fluids: jugular vein distention, dyspnea, crackles (rales), CVP greater than 6 mm Hg (greater than 12 cm H_2O). *Ensures adequate rehydration.*

- Administer insulin as prescribed *to correct or stabilize existing hyperglycemia.*

- Before initiating treatment, be aware that insulin, when added to IV solutions, may be absorbed by the container and plastic tubing. Flush the tubing with at least 30 mL of the insulin-containing IV solution *to ensure that maximum adsorption of the insulin by the container and tubing has occurred before patient use.*

- Monitor laboratory results for abnormalities. Serum K^+ should decline until it reaches normal levels and may drop below normal. Promptly report to health care provider serum K^+ levels less than 3.5 mEq/L. Observe for clinical manifestations of the electrolyte, glucose, and acid-base imbalances associated with DKA as follows:
  - *Hyperkalemia:* Lethargy, nausea, hyperactive bowel sounds with diarrhea, numbness or tingling in extremities, muscle weakness.
  - *Hypokalemia:* Muscle weakness, hypotension, anorexia, drowsiness, hypoactive bowel sounds.
  - *Hyponatremia:* Headache, malaise, muscle weakness, abdominal cramps, nausea, seizures, coma.
  - *Hypophosphatemia:* Muscle weakness, progressive encephalopathy possibly leading to coma.
  - *Hypomagnesemia:* Anorexia, nausea, vomiting, lethargy, weakness, personality changes, tetany, tremor or muscle fasciculations, seizures, confusion progressing to coma.
  - *Hypochloremia:* Hypertonicity of muscles, tetany, depressed respirations.
  - *Hypoglycemia:* Headache, impaired mentation, agitation, dizziness, nausea, pallor, tremors, tachycardia, diaphoresis.
  - *Metabolic acidosis:* Lassitude, nausea, vomiting, Kussmaul respirations, lethargy progressing to coma.

Risk for infection related to inadequate secondary defenses (suppressed inflammatory response) secondary to protein depletion
Desired outcome: Patient is free of infection as evidenced by normothermia, HR 100 bpm or less, BP within patient's normal range, WBC count 11,000/mm^3 or less, and negative culture results.

Nursing Interventions

- Monitor patient for evidence of infection. Monitor laboratory results for increased WBC count, and culture purulent drainage as prescribed. *Detects presence of infection.*
- Use meticulous handwashing when caring for patient. Rotate peripheral IV sites q48-72h, depending on agency policy. Discontinue central lines as soon as feasible, and when lines are in place, handle carefully. Schedule dressing changes according to agency policy, and inspect site(s) for signs of local infection, including erythema, swelling, or purulent drainage. Document the presence of any of these indicators, and notify health care provider. *Minimizes the risk for infection and facilitates early intervention when signs of infection are noted.*
- Provide good skin care. Use pressure-relief mattress on the bed or air circulation beds, *to help prevent skin breakdown.*
- Use meticulous sterile technique when caring for or inserting indwelling urinary catheters. Limit use of indwelling urethral catheters to those patients who are unable to void in a bedpan or when continuous assessment of urine output is essential, *to minimize risk of bacterial entry and subsequent urinary tract infection (UTI).*
- Encourage hourly use of incentive spirometry while patient is awake, along with deep-breathing and coughing exercises, *to help prevent pulmonary infection.*

Risk for injury with risk factors related to altered cerebral function secondary to dehydration or cerebral edema associated with DKA
Desired outcome: Patient verbalizes orientation to person, place, and time and does not demonstrate significant change in mental status; normal breath sounds are auscultated over patient's airway; and patient's oral cavity and musculoskeletal system remain intact and free of injury.

Nursing Interventions

♦ Monitor patient's mental status; orientation; level of consciousness (LOC); and respiratory status, especially airway patency, at frequent intervals. Keep an appropriate-size oral airway, manual resuscitator and mask, and supplemental O_2 at the bedside *to facilitate resuscitation if needed.*

♦ Maintain bed in lowest position, keep side rails up at all times, and use soft restraints as necessary. *Reduces likelihood of injury or falls.*

♦ Insert gastric tube in comatose patients, as prescribed. Attach gastric tube to low, intermittent suction, and assess patency q4h *to decrease likelihood of aspiration.*

♦ Elevate head of bed (HOB) to 45 degrees *to minimize risk of aspiration.*

Ineffective peripheral tissue perfusion (or risk for same) related to interrupted venous or arterial flow secondary to increased blood viscosity, increased platelet aggregation and adhesiveness, and patient immobility
Desired outcomes: Optimally, patient has adequate peripheral perfusion, as evidenced by peripheral pulses greater than 2+ on a 0-4+ scale; warm skin; brisk capillary refill (refill time less than 2 sec); and absence of swelling, bluish discoloration, erythema, and discomfort in calves and thighs. Alternatively, if signs of altered peripheral tissue perfusion occur, they are detected and reported promptly.

Nursing Interventions

♦ Monitor hematocrit (Hct) results. Normal values are 40%-54% (in males) and 37%-47% (in females). A return to normal values within 24-48 hr *indicates proper fluid replacement.*

♦ Assess for a falling blood urea nitrogen (BUN) value. Normal BUN is 6-20 mg/dL. *Indicates improved tissue perfusion and renal function.*

♦ Assess peripheral pulses q2-4h. Report immediately any decrease in amplitude or absence of pulse(s) to health care provider *because these signs may indicate compromised peripheral perfusion.*

♦ Be alert to erythema, pain, tenderness, warmth, and swelling over area of thrombus and bluish discoloration, paleness, coolness, and dilation of superficial veins in distal extremities, especially lower extremities. Arterial thrombosis may produce pain, paresthesia (especially loss of sensation of light touch and two-point discrimination), cyanosis with delayed capillary refill, mottling, and coolness of the extremity. Report significant findings to health care provider immediately. *These are indicators of deep vein thrombosis (DVT).*

♦ Encourage active exercises to all extremities q2h, calf pumping, and ankle circles q1h in patients susceptible to DVT, *to increase blood flow to the tissues.*

♦ Encourage fluid intake to more than 2500 mL/day unless contraindicated, *to decrease the potential for hemoconcentration.*

♦ Apply antiembolic hose, elastic (Ace) wraps, pneumatic alternating pressure stockings, or pneumatic foot pumps as prescribed, *to aid in the prevention of thrombosis.*

Deficient knowledge related to cause, prevention, and treatment of DKA
Desired outcome: Within the 24-hr period before hospital discharge, patient verbalizes understanding of the cause, prevention, and treatment of DKA.

Nursing Interventions

♦ Assess patient's facility with language; engage an interpreter or provide language-appropriate written materials if necessary.

- Determine patient's knowledge about DKA and its treatment. As needed, explain disease process of DKA and the common early symptoms of worsening hyperglycemia, including polyuria, polydipsia, polyphagia, dry and flushed skin, and increased irritability (Table 6-4).
- Assess patient's ability to engage in self-management of blood glucose monitoring and control. Explore whether patient psychologically accepts the disease as a significant health challenge.
- Stress importance of maintaining a consistent controlled-carbohydrate diet, exercise, and insulin regimen for optimal control of serum glucose levels and prevention of adverse physical effects of DM, such as peripheral neuropathies and increased atherosclerosis.
- Explain importance of blood glucose monitoring during episodes of stress, injury, and illness. Testing urine ketones may be advised. Blood glucose greater than 250 mg/dL and appearance of large amounts of urine ketones should be reported to health care provider *so that insulin dose can be increased.* Caution that DKA necessitates professional medical management and cannot be self-treated.
- Discuss "sick day management" with patient, including *not* stopping insulin or skipping doses, increasing frequency of blood glucose testing to monitor more closely for hyperglycemia, and testing urine for ketones if ill or vomiting.
- Review testing and insulin administration procedure as indicated. Teach patient that insulin or insulin analog must be taken 1-4 ×/day as prescribed and that lifetime insulin therapy is necessary *to achieve control of blood glucose.*
- Remind patient of importance of maintaining adequate oral fluid intake during illness despite anorexia or nausea.
- Teach importance of receiving prompt treatment if indicators of hypoglycemia (dizziness, impaired mentation, irritability, pallor, and tremors) or hyperglycemia (polyuria, polydipsia, polyphagia or increasingly dry and flushed skin) occur.
- Explain importance of dietary changes as prescribed by health care provider (see "Diabetes Mellitus," p. 411).
- Explain causes for adjustments in insulin dose: (1) increased or decreased food or carbohydrate intake; and (2) any physical (e.g., exercise) or emotional stress (see "Diabetes Mellitus," p. 411).
- Remind patient that alternative and complementary health strategies may alter blood glucose levels and prompt a need for adjustment of medications. All methods used should be reported to health care provider.
- Explain that persons with diabetes are susceptible to infection. Preventive measures, such as good hygiene, meticulous daily foot care, and avoiding persons with infections are necessary *to prevent infection.* In addition, teach patient and significant other to be alert to wounds or cuts that do not heal, burning or pain with urination, and a productive cough.
- Instruct patient to implement the following therapy when ill for any reason:
  - Do not alter insulin (Novolin, Humulin), insulin analog (Humalog, NovoLog), or oral diabetes or hyperglycemia medication dosage unless health care provider has prescribed a supplemental regimen.
  - Perform blood glucose monitoring and urine ketone checks q3h, and promptly report glucose greater than 250 mg/dL and positive ketones to health care provider.
  - Implement small, frequent meals of soft, easily digestible, nourishing foods if regular meals are not tolerated.
  - Maintain adequate hydration, particularly if diarrhea, vomiting, or fever is persistent.

- Use a balance of regular sodas or juices and water *to ensure adequate calories yet prevent hyperosmolality caused by sugars in the beverages.*
- Report any of the foregoing conditions to the health care provider *to gain further insight into treatment modalities and to prevent dehydration.*
- Provide website address of the American Diabetes Association (ADA) for information on acquiring pamphlets and magazines related to the disease, its complications, and appropriate treatment:

  American Diabetes Association: www.diabetes.org

 Patient-Family Teaching and Discharge Planning

See **Deficient knowledge:** related of cause, prevention, and treatment of DKA, in this section.

❖ HYPEROSMOLAR HYPERGLYCEMIC NONKETOTIC SYNDROME

OVERVIEW/PATHOPHYSIOLOGY

Hyperosmolar hyperglycemic nonketotic syndrome (HHNK), also known as hyperosmolar coma, nonketotic hyperosmolar coma, hyperosmolar nonketotic syndrome, hyperosmolar hyperglycemic nonketotic coma, and nonketotic hyperglycemic hyperosmolar coma, is a life-threatening emergency resulting from a lack of effective insulin, or severe insulin resistance, that causes extreme hyperglycemia. Affected patients often are older adults, with undiagnosed or inadequately treated type 2 diabetes mellitus (DM). Often HHNK is precipitated by a stressor, such as trauma, injury, or infection, that increases insulin demand.

It is believed that enough insulin to prevent acidosis resulting from lipolysis and formation of ketone bodies is effective at the cellular level. Without adequate insulin to facilitate transport into cells, or with severe insulin resistance, glucose molecules accumulate in the bloodstream and cause serum hyperosmolality with resultant osmotic diuresis and simultaneous loss of electrolytes, most notably K^+, Na^+, and phosphate. Patients may lose up to 25% of their total body water. Fluids are pulled from individual body cells by increasing serum hyperosmolality and extracellular fluid loss, with consequent intracellular dehydration and body cell shrinkage. Neurologic deficits (i.e., slowed mentation, confusion, seizures, strokelike symptoms, coma) can occur as a result. Loss of extracellular fluid stimulates aldosterone release, which facilitates Na^+ retention and prevents further loss of K^+. However, aldosterone cannot halt severe dehydration. As extracellular volume decreases, blood viscosity increases, causing slowing of blood flow. Thromboemboli are common because of increased blood viscosity, enhanced platelet aggregation and adhesiveness, and possibly patient immobility. Cardiac workload is increased and may lead to myocardial infarction (MI). Renal blood flow is decreased, potentially resulting in renal impairment or failure. Stroke may result from thromboemboli or decreased cerebral perfusion. These severe complications, in addition to the initial precipitating disorder, contribute to a mortality of 10%-25%.

Unlike in diabetic ketoacidosis (DKA), in which acidosis produces severe symptoms requiring fairly prompt hospitalization, symptoms of HHNK develop more slowly and often are nonspecific. The cardinal symptoms of polyuria and polydipsia are noted first but may be ignored by older persons or their families. Neurologic deficits may be mistaken for senility. The similarity of these symptoms to those of other disease processes common to this age group may delay differential diagnosis and treatment and thus allow progression of pathophysiologic processes with resultant hypovolemic shock and multiple organ failure.

ASSESSMENT

Signs and symptoms/physical findings: Patients with HHNK usually are older than 50 yr of age and may have preexisting cardiac or pulmonary disorders. Assessment results often cannot be evaluated based on accepted normal values. Evaluate results based on what is normal or optimal for the individual patient. Central venous pressure (CVP), heart rate (HR), and BP should be evaluated in terms of deviations from patient's baseline and concurrent clinical status. See Table 6-4.

History and risk factors: Most commonly associated with type 2 DM, acute or chronic illness, or infection.

DIAGNOSTIC TESTS

Serum glucose: 400-1800 mg/dL.

Serum chemistry: Serum values change as osmotic diuresis progresses. At late stages, patient may reflect the following electrolyte values/losses:

◆ Na^+: 125-160 mEq/L. Although patient has lost large quantities of Na^+, osmotic diuresis causes abnormally high blood concentration. The Na^+ value may appear high despite probable Na+ deficits.
◆ K^+: less than 3.5 mEq/L.
◆ $Chloride$ (Cl^-): less than 95 mEq/L.
◆ $Phosphorus:$ less than 1.7 mEq/L.
◆ $Magnesium:$ less than 1.5 mEq/L.

Serum osmolality: Will be greater than 350 mOsm/L. A quick bedside calculation of serum osmolality can be obtained by using the following formula:

$$2(Na^+ + K^+) + BUN(mg/dL)/2.8 + Glucose(mg/dL)/18 = mOsm/L$$
$$For\ example: Na^+ = 140; K^+ = 4.5; BUN = 20; glucose = 120$$
$$2(140 + 4.5) + 20/2.8 + 120/18 = 2(144.5) + 7 + 6.7$$
$$289 + 7 + 6.7 = 302.7\ mOsm/L$$

◆ See Table 6-4 for a discussion of other diagnostic tests.

COLLABORATIVE MANAGEMENT

Fluid replacement: Usually 0.9% normal saline (NS) or 0.45% saline is administered at 200-300 mL/hr until the plasma glucose is 200-300 mg/dL. For the first 2 hr of fluid infusion, more than 1000 mL/hr may be initiated to correct the hypovolemia and hypotension; 6-20 L may be given in the first 24 hr. Dextrose solutions (e.g., 5% dextrose in half-normal saline [$D_5\frac{1}{2}NS$] or D_5NS) are administered when blood glucose reaches 200-300 mg/dL. CVP measurements, coupled with thorough cardiovascular and pulmonary physical assessments, can be used to guide therapy and assess tolerance to the rapid fluid infusion.

Rapid-acting insulin: Initial dose of 10-25 units (0.3 unit/kg) followed by continuous infusion of 5-10 units/hr (0.1 unit/kg/hr) of regular insulin until blood glucose level is lowered to 200-250 mg/dL, at which time the infusion should be decreased to 2-3 units/hr. Subcutaneous administration is less predictable if patient is hypotensive because tissue perfusion is decreased throughout the body, sometimes profoundly to the skin. Dosage is adjusted based on serial glucose levels and resolution of ketosis. Insulin drip adjustments are made using a formula that considers patient's sensitivity to insulin. When formulas are used, the sensitivity number is reflected as a variable multiplier, which increases with higher levels of insulin resistance. If the insulin is ineffective in reducing blood glucose, insulin resistance is considered as a cause. Insulin analogs (e.g., lispro [Humalog]) also may be used to lower blood glucose levels.

Restoration of electrolyte balance: Na^+ and Cl^- are replaced with IV normal saline, and K^+ is replaced with 10-40 mEq of potassium chloride (KCl) or potassium phosphate if patient also needs phosphorus replacement. All electrolytes are replaced carefully because fluids and electrolytes will be shifting between fluid compartments as fluids are replaced and insulin is administered.

Supportive care: Protective measures are instituted for those who are neurologically impaired or in a coma. These measures include seizure precautions, endotracheal intubation, placement of indwelling urinary catheter, insertion of a gastric tube, and use of a pressure-relieving mattress or specialty bed and possibly restraints for patients who are confused or agitated.

Prevention of complications of HHNK: Measures to prevent arterial thrombosis, stroke, renal failure, heart failure, multiple organ failure, cerebral edema, malignant dysrhythmias, and gram-negative sepsis (from infection that may have caused the problem to ensue).

NURSING DIAGNOSES AND INTERVENTIONS

Deficient knowledge related to causes, prevention, and treatment of HHNK
Desired outcome: Within the 24-hr period before hospital discharge, patient and significant other verbalize understanding of causes, prevention, and treatment of HHNK.

Nursing Interventions

- Assess patient's facility with language; engage an interpreter or provide language-appropriate written materials if necessary.
- Determine patient's understanding of HHNK and its treatment. As needed, explain the disease process of DM and HHNK and common early symptoms of worsening diabetes, including polyuria, polydipsia, polyphagia, dry and flushed skin, and increased irritability. Enable patient to verbalize fears and feelings about the diagnosis. *Ensures patient understanding and allows opportunity to correct any misconceptions.*
- Teach importance of testing urine acetone and blood glucose levels as prescribed before meals and at bedtime. Explain that blood glucose greater than 200 mg/dL should be reported to health care provider *so that insulin dose can be increased.*
- Stress importance of dietary changes as prescribed by health care provider. Typically, the person with type 2 DM is obese and is on a reduced-calorie diet with fixed amounts of carbohydrate, fat, and protein. Explain that fats should be polyunsaturated and proteins chosen from low-fat sources *to help minimize risk for HHNK.*
- Teach importance of eating three meals per day at regularly scheduled times and a bedtime snack. Explain that increased or decreased food intake will necessitate adjustment in insulin dosage. Provide referral to a dietitian as needed *to minimize risk for HHNK.*
- Reinforce the importance of taking oral hypoglycemic agents as prescribed. In addition, explain that exogenous insulin or insulin analogs may be required during periods of physical and emotional stress and that blood glucose levels should be monitored closely during these times *to prevent HHNK and its complications.*

- Explain to patients with type 2 DM that regular exercise, especially aerobic exercise such as walking or swimming, maintains blood glucose levels. *Aerobic exercise is most effective in lowering blood glucose levels.*
- Caution patient always to monitor blood glucose level before exercise. A level greater than 250 mg/dL is indicative of abnormal metabolism. *In this case, exercise would be a stressor, resulting in further elevation of blood glucose.*
- Explain need for measures to prevent infection, such as good hygiene and meticulous daily foot care. Stress importance of avoiding exposure to communicable diseases. In addition, teach patient and significant other to be alert to wounds or cuts that do not heal, burning or pain with urination, and cough that is productive of sputum.
- Provide booklets or pamphlets from the American Diabetes Association (ADA) or pharmaceutical companies about diabetes and appropriate treatment.

 Patient-Family Teaching and Discharge Planning

See **Deficient knowledge** related to causes, prevention, and treatment of HHNK, in this section.

❖ HYPOGLYCEMIA

OVERVIEW/PATHOPHYSIOLOGY

Hypoglycemia is a lowering of blood glucose caused by an excessive dose of insulin or oral hypoglycemic agents, skipping meals, or too much exercise without a concomitant increase in food intake. Unlike diabetic ketoacidosis (DKA) and hyperosmolar hyperglycemic nonketotic syndrome (HHNK), hypoglycemia can have a sudden onset, and its course is precipitous if it is left untreated. Typically, hypoglycemia occurs during the time of peak action of the insulin/hypoglycemic agent, particularly at night when patient is asleep and has not eaten an adequate bedtime snack.

ASSESSMENT

Signs and symptoms/physical findings: The patient usually becomes symptomatic when blood glucose is less than 50 mg/dL or a relatively significant drop in blood glucose occurs (e.g., when an older person's blood glucose drops to 90 mg/dL from 180-200 mg/dL). See Table 6-4.

History and risk factors: Type 1 or type 2 diabetes mellitus (DM), excessive dose of insulin or oral hypoglycemic agents, skipping meals, or too much exercise without a concomitant increase in food intake. Alcohol consumption also can cause hypoglycemia because it depletes glycogen stores and increases insulin levels.

COLLABORATIVE MANAGEMENT

Administration of rapid-acting sugar: 10-15 g of a fast-acting sugar (e.g., 4 oz fruit juice or nondiet soda, 2-3 tsp honey or table sugar, 5-10 Lifesavers or other small hard candies, or 2-4 commercially manufactured glucose tablets) is given by mouth. If symptoms persist for more than 15 min, treatment is repeated. After resolution of the event, patient should continue to consume a protein/complex carbohydrate snack, such as cheese or peanut butter on crackers/whole grain bread, or milk with crackers/bread.

Glucagon: For patients unable to swallow, 1 mg glucagon is injected subcutaneously or by the intramuscular (IM) route. Glucagon stimulates the liver to break down stored glycogen into glucose and usually results in patient's regaining consciousness in 15-30 min, at which time patient should be given a fast-acting sugar followed by the snack just described. Patients and their significant others are instructed in glucagon administration as a part of their diabetes education. Glucagon is used rarely in the hospital setting.

50% Dextrose: Hospitalized patients may receive an IV injection of 10-30 mL of 50% dextrose (D_{50}), which usually revives the unconscious individual in less than 10 min. Dosage of D_{50} is individualized to the level of the blood glucose. Patients may experience hyperglycemia and headache after D_{50}, particularly if they are given 50 mL. These individuals may benefit from a protein or complex carbohydrate snack once consciousness is regained unless blood glucose has been elevated to more than 200 mg/dL. If patient has frequent episodes of hypoglycemia, an alteration in dietary composition or insulin administration should be evaluated.

Differentiate from alcohol stupor: Mentation changes caused by severe hypoglycemia can be indistinguishable from those caused by alcoholic stupor. If hypoglycemic symptoms are misdiagnosed as alcoholic stupor and an individual with hypoglycemic is left to "sleep it off," death can ensue.

NURSING DIAGNOSES AND INTERVENTIONS

Ineffective protection related to risk for brain damage or death secondary to hypoglycemia

Desired outcome: Within 10-30 min of intervention, patient is alert with no significant change from usual mental status and verbalizes orientation to person, place, and time.

Nursing Interventions

- Treat hypoglycemia as an emergency situation. *Hypoglycemia requires immediate intervention because, if severe, it can lead to brain damage and death.* When the cause of coma in a person with DM is unknown, immediately draw a blood sample for evaluation of glucose and prepare to administer IV D_{50}, *to quickly reverse the hypoglycemic state.*
- Administer a fast-acting carbohydrate (see "Collaborative Management," earlier). Notify health care provider if patient is incoherent, unresponsive, or incapable of taking carbohydrates by mouth. If any of these indicators occur, access an IV site and prepare to administer prescribed 10-30 mL D_{50} by IV push, *to restore consciousness within 10 min.*
- Continue to monitor blood glucose levels q15-30 min, *to identify recurrence of hypoglycemia.*
- Once patient is alert, ask about most recent food intake. Any situations preventing food intake, such as nausea, vomiting, dislike of hospital food related to cultural preferences, or fasting for a scheduled test, should be identified so that they can be addressed immediately, *to prevent recurrence of hypoglycemia.*
- If food intake has been adequate, consult health care provider about a reduction in daily dose of antihyperglycemic medication, *to prevent future hypoglycemic episodes.*
- Consider use of a commercially available long-acting carbohydrate at bedtime to help prevent nocturnal hypoglycemia. Sometimes hypoglycemia leads to rebound hyperglycemia (Somogyi phenomenon). If hypoglycemia goes undetected, the rebound hyperglycemia may be inappropriately treated with increased insulin. Suspect the Somogyi phenomenon if wide fluctuations in blood glucose occur over several hours. Notify health care

provider if these changes are observed, *to prevent nocturnal or rebound hypoglycemia.*

Ineffective protection related to neurosensory alterations with risk of seizures secondary to hypoglycemia
Desired outcomes: Within 4 hr of the event, patient verbalizes orientation to person, place, and time and is free of signs of trauma caused by seizures or altered level of consciousness (LOC). Alternatively, if patient experiences a seizure, it is detected, reported, and treated promptly.

Nursing Interventions

- Monitor LOC at frequent intervals. Anticipate seizure potential in the presence of severe hypoglycemia, and have airway, protective padding, and suction equipment at bedside. Keep all side rails raised, *to prevent injury if seizures occur.*
- Notify health care provider of any seizure activity; do not leave patient unattended if a seizure occurs, *to prevent injury.*
- Place call light within patient's reach, and have patient demonstrate its proper use every shift. Patient's inability to use call light properly necessitates assessments at least q30min. If necessary, consider moving patient to a room next to nurses' station, *to provide for close monitoring.*
- Keep all potentially harmful objects, such as knives, forks, and hot beverages, out of patient's reach, *to prevent injury.*
- Obtain a prescription for soft restraints if necessary. Explain these safety precautions to patient and significant other. *Prevents patient from wandering and causing self-injury.*
- See "Seizures and Epilepsy," p. 344.

Deficient knowledge related to disease process, diagnostic testing, indicators of hypoglycemia, and therapeutic regimen
Desired outcome: Within the 24-hr period before hospital discharge, patient verbalizes knowledge about DM, including testing and management, indicators of hypoglycemia, and therapeutic regimen.

Nursing Interventions

- Assess patient's facility with language; engage an interpreter or provide language-appropriate written materials if necessary.
- Assess patient's knowledge about DM, including diagnostic testing and management. Provide information or clarify as appropriate, *to verify patient understanding and correct misconceptions.*
- Review indicators and immediate interventions for hypoglycemia with patient, *to help minimize the risk for recurrence of hypoglycemia.*
- Evaluate current diet for adequate nutritional requirements, caloric content, and patient satisfaction. Assist patient in making acceptable and realistic changes. Consider patient's activity level and need for changes to achieve normoglycemia. Refer patient and significant other to dietitian as needed, *to help prevent hypoglycemia.*
- Review with patient the onset, peak action, and duration of hypoglycemic medication. Advise patient to avoid drugs that contribute to hypoglycemia (salicylates, sulfonamides, methyldopa, anabolic steroids, acetaminophen, ethanol, haloperidol, marijuana).
- Stress importance of testing blood glucose at the time symptoms of hypoglycemia occur.
- Explain that injection of insulin into a site that is about to be exercised heavily (e.g., a jogger's thigh) will result in quicker insulin absorption and possible hypoglycemia.

◆ Inform patient that a change in the type of medication may require a change in dose. Caution about the need to follow prescription directions precisely to prevent hypoglycemia.

 Patient-Family Teaching and Discharge Planning

See **Deficient knowledge** related to disease process, diagnostic testing, indicators of hypoglycemia, and therapeutic regimen, in this section. See also "General Discussion," p. 411, for general care of patients with DM.

Gastrointestinal Disorders

SECTION ONE ## DISORDERS OF THE MOUTH AND ESOPHAGUS

❖ STOMATITIS

OVERVIEW/PATHOPHYSIOLOGY

Inflammatory and infectious diseases of the mouth are commonly overlooked in the debilitated hospitalized patient. *Stomatitis* (inflammation of the mouth and mucous membrane) is the term generally applied to a variety of mouth disorders characterized by mucosal cell destruction and disruption of the mucosal lining.

ASSESSMENT

Signs and symptoms/physical findings: Oral pain; sensitivity to hot, spicy foods; foul taste; oral bleeding or drainage; fever; xerostomia (dry mouth); burning sensation in the lips; difficulty chewing or swallowing; poorly fitting dentures.

The oral mucosa appears swollen, red, and ulcerated; the lymph glands may be swollen; and the breath is often foul smelling. The lips may have cracks, fissures, blisters, ulcers, and lesions; the tongue may appear dry and cracked and contain masses, lesions, or exudate.

History and risk factors: Typically occurs secondary to systemic disease and infection; nutritional and fluid deficiencies; poorly fitting dentures; neglect of oral hygiene; side effects of drugs; or exposure to oral irritants such as alcohol, smoking, or smokeless tobacco. Patients with leukemia or neoplastic disease of the head and neck are at increased risk for stomatitis. It is one of the major side effects of radiation therapy and cancer chemotherapy, and it occurs in more than 30% of this population. It also is commonly seen in patients older than 65 yr of age, patients in the ICU, and individuals with human immunodeficiency virus (HIV) infection.

DIAGNOSTIC TESTS

In most incidences, diagnosis of the causative factor is made by history and physical examination. However, the following tests may be used in selected patients.

Culture: May be taken of the lesion or drainage to identify the offending organism. The most common organism is *Candida albicans,* followed by herpes simplex virus 1.

Platelet count: Done if any bleeding is present.

COLLABORATIVE MANAGEMENT

Treatment varies, depending on the type of impairment and its cause.

Identification and attempt to control or remove causative factor(s): If appropriate (e.g., if poor nutrition is the cause of stomatitis, the goal is to improve nutrition and follow through with other treatments that may be necessary, such as antibiotics).

Oral hygiene/mouth irrigations: Teeth should be brushed with a fluoride-containing dentifrice and a soft-bristle toothbrush. The tongue also should be lightly brushed and the mouth rinsed with sterile normal saline solution after brushing. Mouthwashes may be used to loosen debris, but use of commercial mouthwashes, especially those containing alcohol, should be avoided. The accepted mouthwash, in particular for immunosuppressed patients with stomatitis, is sodium bicarbonate with normal saline. A typical solution is made with 15 mL of sodium bicarbonate and 500 mL of normal saline. Oral hygiene should be repeated 4-5×/day or even more frequently, depending on degree of oral mucosal impairment.

Pharmacotherapy

Local/systemic analgesics and local anesthetics (e.g., lidocaine [Xylocaine] jelly): For relief of pain.

Topical/systemic steroids: Reduce inflammation and promote healing in severe conditions.

Antibiotic, antifungal, and antiviral agents: Used to combat infection.

Vitamins: Correct deficiencies (e.g., vitamin C to strengthen connective tissue in the gums; niacin and riboflavin to promote efficient cellular growth).

Dietary management: Typically, a diet high in protein to promote wound healing, high in calories for protein sparing, and high in vitamins to correct the specific deficiency. Usually, hot and spicy foods are restricted, and consistency of the food ranges from liquid to regular, as tolerated. Fluids are encouraged. Severe cases necessitating hospitalization also may require treatment with nutritional support, that is, enteral feeding or total parenteral nutrition (TPN) if unable to insert feeding tube.

Cauterization of ulcerations: If required.

Dental restoration and repair: If needed.

Adequate rest: For optimal tissue repair.

NURSING DIAGNOSES AND INTERVENTIONS

Impaired oral mucous membrane (stomatitis) related to ineffective oral hygiene, dehydration, irritants, or pathologic condition

Desired outcomes: Patient demonstrates oral hygiene interventions and complies with the therapeutic regimen within 12-24 hr of instruction. Patient's oral mucosal condition improves, as evidenced by intact mucous membrane, moist and intact tongue and lips, and absence of pain and lesions.

Nursing Interventions

- Inspect mouth 3 ×/day for inflammation, lesions, and bleeding. Report significant findings to health care provider.
- Administer analgesics; corticosteroids; anesthetics, and mouthwashes (described in the next list item) as prescribed. Avoid commercial mouthwashes. *This is because they are high in alcohol.* For mild stomatitis, provide mouth care after every meal and before bedtime. For moderate stomatitis, provide mouth care q4h; for severe stomatitis, provide mouth care q2h and twice at night or even hourly if indicated.
- Prepare a solution containing 15 mL of sodium bicarbonate and 500 mL of normal saline. Instruct patient to rinse mouth with the solution (as often as indicated by assessments described earlier). *This is to provide local relief and promote healing.* Warm saline solution may be used. *This provides some heat and aids in cleansing mucous membranes.* Avoid solutions containing hydrogen peroxide.

- Instruct patient to brush teeth after meals and at bedtime, with a soft-bristle toothbrush and nonabrasive toothpaste. Patients with severe stomatitis who have dentures should remove them until the oral mucosa has healed. Dietary alterations may be necessary (e.g., changing to a full liquid or pureed diet). *This will reduce the irritation.* A dietary or nutritional consultation may be helpful.
- Use disposable foam swabs to stimulate gums and clean the oral cavity. Avoid use of lemon and glycerin swabs. *This is because glycerin is hydrophilic and will cause excessive drying of oral membranes.* If platelet levels are at least as high as 50,000/mm^3, encourage gentle flossing of teeth twice daily, using unwaxed floss.
- Advise patient to use lip emollients, such as lanolin or any nonpetroleum surgical lubricant. *This will keep the lips lubricated and avoid drying and cracking.*
- Advise patient to avoid irritants, including alcohol; tobacco products; and foods that are hot, spicy, and rough in texture.
- Offer ice or flavored ice pops. *This is to help anesthetize the mouth.*

Deficient knowledge related to disease process, treatment, and factors that potentiate oral bleeding
Desired outcome: Within the 24-hr period before hospital discharge, patient verbalizes knowledge about the cause, preventive measures, and treatment of stomatitis and factors that potentiate oral bleeding.

Nursing Interventions

- Assess patient's facility with language; engage an interpreter or provide language-appropriate written materials if necessary.
- Describe causes of patient's stomatitis, and remind patient that the best treatment is prevention.
- Explain importance of meticulous, frequent oral hygiene and periodic dental examinations.
- Advise patient to avoid substances such as alcohol; tobacco; hot, spicy, and rough foods. *This is because they can be irritating to the mouth lesions.*
- Teach importance of discontinuing flossing when platelet count drops below 50,000/mm^3, or as suggested by health care provider, and discontinuing brushing when count drops below 30,000/mm^3, or per health care provider's instructions, to avoid possible bleeding. Instead, instruct patient to perform oral hygiene using mouth irrigation technique described in **Impaired oral mucous membrane**, immediately preceding.

Imbalanced nutrition: less than body requirements related to inability to ingest food secondary to discomfort with chewing and swallowing
Desired outcome: At least 24 hr before hospital discharge, patient exhibits adequate progress toward optimal nutrition, as evidenced by stable weight, serum protein 6-8 g/dL, serum albumin 3.5-5.5 g/dL, and a balanced or positive N state.

Nursing Interventions

- Assess patient's ability to chew and swallow.
- Monitor I&O. Unless contraindicated, ensure patient has optimal hydration (at least 2-3 L/day) and a diet that is high in protein, calories, and essential vitamins and minerals. Drinks high in calories and protein are especially helpful. Consider adding Polycose to beverages and powdered milk or protein powder to food preparations. Alert health care provider if need for IV or nasogastric (NG) tube feedings becomes apparent.
- Provide any special equipment such as straws, nipples, or syringes. *This is to facilitate ingestion.*

- Encourage intake of soft foods (e.g., cooked cereals, soups, gelatin, ice cream). *This is to reduce mouth pain.*
- Encourage mouth care after every meal or more frequently. *This is to minimize risk of infection caused by nonintact oral mucosa.*

Patient-Family Teaching and Discharge Planning

When providing patient-family teaching, include verbal and written information about the following:

- Essentials of diet, medications, and oral hygiene; adaptations that may be required at home; and importance of monitoring for changes in level of consciousness (LOC), which will necessitate precautions to prevent aspiration during oral hygiene.
- Importance of notifying health care provider if any of the following recurs or worsens: oral pain, fever, drainage, continuous bleeding, inability to eat or drink, progressive weight loss.
- Necessity for follow-up care; reconfirm date and time of next medical appointment.
- Importance of visiting dentist at least twice per year.

❖ HIATAL HERNIA, GASTROESOPHAGEAL REFLUX DISEASE, AND BARRETT'S ESOPHAGUS

OVERVIEW/PATHOPHYSIOLOGY

Hiatal hernia is a herniation of the esophagogastric junction and a portion of the stomach into the chest through the esophageal hiatus of the diaphragm. Hernias are classified as acquired or congenital. Acquired hernias include sliding, paraesophageal, and mixed as the most common classifications. In a sliding hernia, intraabdominal pressure increases, enabling a portion of the lower esophagus and stomach to rise up into the chest. In paraesophageal hernias, the esophagogastric junction remains in place and the stomach fundus or greater curvature squeezes into the chest through the esophageal hiatus. Complications of hiatal hernia include aspiration of reflux contents; ulceration; hemorrhage; stricture; gastritis; and in severe cases, strangulation of the herniated tissue. The most common type of hiatal hernia is the sliding hernia, which accounts for most of adult hiatal hernias. The incidence of hiatal hernia increases with age.

Diagnosis of diaphragmatic hernia is often suspected on the basis of reflux symptoms. However, gastroesophageal reflux disease (GERD) is not caused by any one abnormality. The multiple factors that determine whether GERD is present include (1) efficacy of the antireflux mechanism, (2) volume of gastric contents (in the stomach), (3) potency of refluxed material, (4) efficiency of esophageal clearance, and (5) resistance of the esophageal tissue to injury and the ability for tissue repair. By definition, however, the patient must have several episodes of reflux for reflux disease to be present. Barrett's esophagus is a condition caused by chronic gastric reflux that injures the esophageal squamous epithelium. Abnormal columnar epithelium replaces the injured squamous epithelium. Seen predominantly. The incidence of Barrett's esophagus is increasing. It is predominantly seen in white males. Complications include esophagitis, strictures, and ulcers. Although not all patients develop esophageal adenocarcinoma, GERD and Barrett's esophagus are the most important risk factors.

ASSESSMENT

Signs and symptoms/physical findings: Many individuals are asymptomatic unless esophageal reflux is present. Reflux often occurs 1-4 hr after eating and while sleeping or reclining, with stress, and with increased intraabdominal pressure. Heartburn (often worse with recumbency), belching, regurgitation, vomiting, retrosternal or substernal chest pain (dull, full, heavy), hiccups, mild or occult bleeding in vomitus or stools, and mild anemia also may occur. Dysphagia can occur and is associated with advanced disease and greater potential for complications. The older adult often presents with symptoms of pneumonitis caused by aspiration of reflux contents into the pulmonary system. Peptic stricture of the esophagus is a serious sequela of aggressive reflux esophagitis. Barrett's esophagus can cause additional signs and symptoms, including chronic cough and hoarseness. Some patients have few symptoms, possibly from desensitized esophageal tissue.

Physical assessment: Auscultation of peristaltic sounds in the chest, presence of palpitations, abdominal distention. These findings are not diagnostic, nor are they usually helpful in making the diagnosis.

History and risk factors: History and causative factors for acquired hernias include degenerative changes (aging), trauma, kyphoscoliosis (a curvature of the spine), increased intraabdominal pressure, and surgery. Increased intraabdominal pressure can occur with coughing, straining, bending, vomiting, obesity, pregnancy, trauma, constricting clothing, ascites, and severe physical exertion. GERD is the result of incompetence of the lower esophageal sphincter (LES) that allows regurgitation of acidic gastric contents into the esophagus. Chronic gastric reflux is found in patients with Barrett's esophagus. Male gender and older age are also risk factors for esophageal problems.

DIAGNOSTIC TESTS

For most patients with reflux, obtaining a complete history is sufficient for starting therapy without the necessity of comprehensive diagnostic tests.

Barium swallow: The most specific diagnostic test for revealing hernias and gastroesophageal and diaphragmatic abnormalities. With fluoroscopy, a hiatal hernia appears as a barium-containing outpouching at the lower end of the esophagus. It may be necessary for the patient to be in Trendelenburg's position for the hernia to appear on x-ray film. Although gastric barium moves into the esophagus with reflux, the degree of esophagitis is not easily demonstrated radiographically. Scintigraphic techniques using a technetium-99m–labeled solid meal have been used to quantify the degree of esophageal reflux.

Chest x-ray examination: Reveals large hernias that look like air bubbles in the chest; infiltrates will be seen in lower lobes of the lungs if aspiration has occurred.

Upper endoscopy and biopsy: Used as initial evaluation when symptoms persist, are refractory to treatment, or worsen. These methods aid in differentiating between hiatal hernia and gastroesophageal lesion, exclude the possibility of neoplasm, and assess type and severity of esophagitis. They are the primary diagnostic tools for Barrett's esophagus. Patients diagnosed with Barrett's esophagus should be screened with esophagogastroduodenoscopy (EGD) and biopsy from yearly to every 5 yr.

Esophageal motility studies: Identify primary and secondary motor dysfunction before surgical repair of the hernia is performed. Included are manometry, which graphically records resting pressures and peristaltic wave pressures, and pH probe, which shows a low (acidic) value in the presence of gastroesophageal reflux.

Gastric analysis: Assesses bleeding, which can occur if ulceration is present.

CBC: May reveal anemic condition if bleeding ulcers are present.

Stool occult blood test: Positive if bleeding has occurred.

ECG: Rules out cardiac origin of pain.

COLLABORATIVE MANAGEMENT

Conservative medical management, which is successful in most cases, is preferred over surgical intervention. The goal is to prevent or reduce gastric reflux caused by increased intraabdominal pressure and increased gastric acid production.

Dietary management: Small, frequent meals; bland foods; weight reduction for obese individuals; food restriction 2-3 hr before reclining; refraining from fatty foods, acidic foods, chocolate, and alcohol. Meals low in fat and high in protein increase LES tone and decrease reflux. Restricting intake of irritants such as caffeine, nicotine, and nonsteroidal antiinflammatory drugs (NSAIDs) is important. Restricting tight clothing around the waist may also help. The cornerstone for many patients with reflux is a change in lifestyle.

Elevation of head of bed (HOB): Using 4- to 6-inch blocks to prevent postural reflux at night, depending on reflux severity.

Pharmacotherapy

Proton pump inhibitors (PPIs) (e.g., omeprazole, lansoprazole, pantoprazole, esomeprazole, rabeprazole): Provide significant remission of symptoms in many patients and are prescribed most often for their healing properties.

Histamine H₂-receptor blockers (e.g., cimetidine, ranitidine, famotidine, nizatidine): Work by suppressing acid secretion in the stomach. Over-the-counter (OTC) use should not continue for more than 1-2 wk before consultation with a medical professional.

Antacids: Do not add to the effectiveness of the H_2-receptor blockers but may be useful when side effects of the H_2-receptor blockers preclude their use. Antacids should not be taken at the same time as PPIs and H_2-receptor blockers because antacids interfere with the effectiveness of these drugs.

Prokinetic agents (e.g., metoclopramide): Augment peristalsis of the esophagus and stomach and increase LES pressure.

Antiemetics, cough suppressants, and stool softeners: Prevent increased intraabdominal pressure from vomiting, coughing, and straining with bowel movements.

Surgery: Indicated in some patients to restore gastroesophageal integrity and prevent reflux if symptoms do not resolve and complications (obstruction, bleeding, aspiration) occur. The most common procedure is a fundoplication, in which a portion of the upper stomach is wrapped around the distal esophagus and sutured to itself to prevent reflux from recurring. Typically, an abdominal rather than a thoracic approach is used. Laparoscopic approaches may also be used.

Postsurgical management: Includes chest physiotherapy to prevent respiratory complications; IV fluids and electrolytes until bowel sounds are present; a gradual increase in diet as tolerated after the return of peristalsis; and, in some cases, gastric tubes for decompression and feeding.

NURSING DIAGNOSES AND INTERVENTIONS

Deficient knowledge related to disease process and treatment for hiatal hernia, GERD, or Barrett's esophagus

Desired outcome: Within the 24-hr period before hospital discharge, patient verbalizes knowledge about the cause and therapeutic regimen for hiatal hernia, reflux disease, or Barrett's esophagus.

Nursing Interventions

◆ Assess patient's facility with language; engage an interpreter or provide language-appropriate written materials if necessary.

◆ Assess patient's knowledge about the disorder, its treatment, and methods used to prevent symptoms and their complications. Provide instructions as appropriate. *The main treatment for these disorders is lifestyle change, so patient needs to understand the methods for making those changes.*

◆ Explain the following methods of dietary management: eating a low-fat, high-protein diet; eating small, frequent meals; eating slowly; chewing well to avoid reflux; avoiding extremely hot or cold foods; limiting stimulants of gastric acid, such as alcohol, caffeine, chocolate, fatty or spicy foods, peppermint, citrus fruit/juices, and nicotine; and losing weight if appropriate. *These interventions will help reduce symptoms of the disease and may prevent surgery.*

♦ Advise patient to drink water after eating. *This is to cleanse the esophagus of residual food, which can irritate esophageal lining.*

♦ Advise patient to avoid smoking. *It may increase aerophagia, acid exposure, and belching.*

♦ Explain the following alterations in body positions and activities: avoiding supine position for 2-3 hr after eating; sleeping on right side with HOB elevated on 4- to 6-inch blocks to promote gastric emptying; for 2-3 hr after eating, avoiding bending, coughing, lifting heavy objects, straining with bowel movements, strenuous exercise, and clothing that is too tight around waist.

♦ Stress importance of following prescribed pharmacologic regimen: PPIs, H$_2$-receptor blockers, antacids, sucralfate, or prokinetic agents. *It is important to continue with the prescribed medications even if symptoms no longer are persistent.*

♦ Explain chronic nature of these conditions, including follow-up, support, education, and adherence to pharmacologic therapy. *This is because the disease management is a life-long process.*

Acute pain, nausea, or feeling of fullness related to gastroesophageal reflux and increased intraabdominal pressure

Desired outcomes: Patient's subjective perception of discomfort decreases within 1 hr of intervention, as documented by pain scale. Nonverbal indicators, such as grimacing, are absent or diminished.

Nursing Interventions

♦ Assess and document amount and character of discomfort. Devise a pain scale with patient, rating discomfort from 0 (no pain) to 10 (worst pain). Administer medications as prescribed and then document their effectiveness using pain scale.

♦ Encourage patient to follow dietary and activity restrictions.

♦ If prescribed, insert nasogastric (NG) tube and connect it to suction. *This is to reduce pressure on diaphragm and relieve vomiting.*

♦ Raise HOB or have patient turn from side to side. *Position change may reduce pain.*

♦ For additional information, see "Pain," p. 13, in Chapter 1.

For Patients with a Fundoplication

Ineffective breathing pattern related to guarding secondary to pain of thoracic incision or chest tube insertion

Desired outcome: Patient's respiratory rate (RR) is 12-20 breaths/min with normal depth and pattern (eupnea) within 1 hr after pain-relieving intervention.

Nursing Interventions

♦ If a thoracic rather than abdominal approach was used, chest tubes may be present. Assess insertion site and suction apparatus for integrity, patency, function, and character of drainage. Tape all chest tube insertion sites.

♦ Be alert for dyspnea, cyanosis, sharp chest pain. *These are indicators of a pneumothorax.* (See "Pneumothorax/Hemothorax," p. 75, for care of the patient with a chest tube.)

♦ Encourage and assist patient with coughing, deep breathing, incentive spirometry, and turning q2-4h, and note the quality of breath sounds, cough, and sputum.

♦ Teach patient how to splint incision with hands, a folded blanket, or pillow. *This is to facilitate coughing and deep breathing.*

- Medicate patient about $1/2$ hr before major moves such as ambulation and turning. *This is to enhance compliance with postoperative routine.* If patient-controlled analgesia (PCA) is available, advise its use accordingly. Be aware that opioid analgesics will depress respirations.
- Reassure patient that sutures and tubes will remain intact with coughing and deep breathing.

Patient-Family Teaching and Discharge Planning

When providing patient-family teaching, include verbal and written information about the following:

- Importance of dietary management and activity (see **Deficient knowledge**, p. 446).
- Medications, including drug names, dosage, schedule, purpose, precautions, and potential side effects. Also discuss drug/drug, herb/drug, and food/drug interactions.
- Indicators that signal recurrence of hernia or reflux (which happens only rarely after surgery): dysphagia, hematemesis, increased pain.
- Importance of follow-up care; reconfirm date and time of next medical appointment.
- Care of incision, including dressing changes. Ensure that patient verbalizes indicators of infection (e.g., increasing pain, local warmth, fever, purulent drainage, swelling, foul odor).
- Procedure for enteral feedings and care of tubes if appropriate. Initiate a visiting nurse referral for follow-up as needed.
- Community resources for weight reduction and smoking cessation. Refer patient to a smoking cessation program as appropriate. Additional resources, including free brochures, can be found at:

Agency for Health Care Policy and Research (AHCPR): www.ahrq.gov or www.ahrq.gov/consumer. Select the links listed under "Quit Smoking."

National Cancer Institute: www.nci.nih.gov. A link to the stop smoking website is available or can be accessed directly at www.smokefree.gov.

SECTION TWO DISORDERS OF THE STOMACH AND INTESTINES

❖ PEPTIC ULCERS

OVERVIEW/PATHOPHYSIOLOGY

Peptic ulcers are erosions of the upper gastrointestinal (GI) tract mucosa that may extend through the muscularis mucosa and into the muscularis propria. They may occur anywhere the mucosa is exposed to the erosive action of gastric acid and pepsin. Commonly, ulcers are gastric or duodenal, but the esophagus, surgically created stomas, and other areas of the upper GI tract may be affected. Autodigestion of mucosal tissue and ulceration are associated with increased acidity of the stomach juices or increased sensitivity of the mucosal surfaces to erosion. Erosions can penetrate deeply into the mucosal layers and become a chronic problem, or they can be more superficial and manifest as an acute problem resulting from severe physiologic or psychologic trauma, infection, or shock (stress ulceration of the stomach or duodenum). Both duodenal and gastric ulcers can occur in association with a high-stress lifestyle, smoking, or use of irritating drugs, as well as being secondary to other diseases. Ulceration may occur as a part of Zollinger-Ellison syndrome, in which gastrinomas (gastrin-secreting tumors) of the pancreas or other organs develop. Gastric acid hypersecretion and ulceration subsequently occur. However, the most common causes of peptic ulcer disease are use of nonsteroidal antiinflammatory drugs (NSAIDs) and infection with *Helicobacter pylori (H. pylori).*

H. pylori, a gram-negative, spiral-shaped bacterium with four to six flagella on one pole, was first isolated from gastric biopsy material in 1983. *H. pylori* can reside below the mucosa of the stomach because it produces the enzyme *urease,* which hydrolyses urea to ammonia and carbon dioxide and provides a buffering alkaline halo. Infection can go undetected for years because there may be no symptoms until gastric or duodenal ulceration or gastritis occurs. Transmission of *H. pylori* has been determined to be by fecal-oral and oral-oral routes of transmission. A high duodenal acid load is one of the characteristics of duodenal ulcer disease inasmuch as it reduces concentration of bile acids that normally inhibit growth of *H. pylori.* Gastric ulcers tend to occur on the lesser curvature of the stomach. Ulcers in both locations are characterized by slow healing leading to metaplasia. In turn, greater colonization with *H. pylori* causes slow healing and results in a vicious cycle.

Serious and disabling complications, such as hemorrhage, GI obstruction, perforation, peritonitis, or intractable ulcer pain, are common. With treatment, ulcer healing usually occurs within 4-6 wk (gastric ulcers can take as long as 12-16 wk to heal), but there is potential for recurrence at the same or another site.

ASSESSMENT

Signs and symptoms/physical findings: Burning, gnawing, dull pain typically with onset 1-3 hr after eating. Discomfort occurs more often between meals and at night. With duodenal ulcer, eating usually alleviates discomfort; with gastric ulcer, pain often worsens after meals. Older persons have less sensory perception in the stomach and may not experience pain as a symptom. In addition, 40% of patients with active ulcers deny abdominal pain. However, on examination there may be findings of ulceration, gastritis, and other conditions. Even so, pain symptoms warrant further investigation.

Hematemesis, melena, dizziness, and syncope are associated with an actively bleeding ulcer. Sudden, severe epigastric pain, often radiating to the right shoulder, suggests perforation of an ulcer. Pain described as piercing through to the back suggests penetration of the ulcer into adjacent posterior structures in the abdomen.

Typically there is tenderness over the involved area of the abdomen. With perforation, there will be severe pain (see "Peritonitis," p. 461, for more information) and rebound tenderness. With penetration, the pain is usually altered by changes in back position (extension or flexion).

History and risk factors: NSAID use; chronic or acute stress; smoking; use of irritating agents such as caffeine, alcohol, corticosteroids, salicylates, reserpine, indomethacin, or phenylbutazone; disorders of the endocrine glands, pancreas, or liver; and hypersecretory conditions, such as Zollinger-Ellison syndrome.

DIAGNOSTIC TESTS

Barium swallow: Uses contrast agent (e.g., barium) to detect abnormalities. Patient should maintain nothing by mouth (NPO) status and not smoke for at least 8 hr before the test. Postprocedure care involves administration of prescribed laxatives and enemas to facilitate passage of the barium and prevent constipation and fecal impaction.

Endoscopy: Allows visualization of the stomach (gastroscopy), duodenum (duodenoscopy), both stomach and duodenum (gastroduodenoscopy), or the esophagus, stomach, and duodenum (EGD) via passage of a lighted, flexible fiberoptic tube. Patient is NPO for 8-12 hr before the procedure, and written consent is required. Before the test, a sedative is administered to relax the patient, and an opioid analgesic may be given to prevent pain. Local anesthetic may be sprayed into the posterior pharynx to ease passage of the tube. A biopsy may be performed as part of the endoscopy procedure. Biopsied tissue may be sent for histologic examination and for culture and sensitivity to identify *H. pylori* infection. Postprocedure care involves maintaining NPO status for $\frac{1}{2}$-1 hr; ensuring return of the gag reflex before allowing the patient to eat (if local anesthetic was used); administering throat lozenges or analgesics as prescribed; and monitoring for complications, such as bleeding or perforation (e.g., hematemesis, pain, dyspnea, tachycardia, hypotension).

Stool for occult blood: Positive if bleeding is present.

Other laboratory tests: CBC reveals a decrease in hemoglobin (Hgb), hematocrit (Hct), and RBCs when acute or chronic blood loss accompanies ulceration. Serum antigen identifies exposure to *H. pylori* infection. However, antibody test results remain positive many months after successful therapy and are not reliable for assessing therapy effectiveness. A breath test is available to identify *H. pylori* infection by detecting carbon dioxide and ammonia as byproducts of the action of the bacterium's urease in the patient's expired air. Histologic identification of the microorganism and culture are other direct tests for *H. pylori*. Direct testing and stool antigen assay require discontinuation of all drugs that suppress *H. pylori* for 2 wk before testing.

COLLABORATIVE MANAGEMENT

Conservative management is preferred over surgical intervention, with the therapy aimed at decreasing hyperacidity, healing the ulcer, relieving symptoms, and preventing complications.

Lifestyle alterations: Smoking cessation, decreased consumption of alcohol, avoidance of irritating drugs, and stress reduction therapies.

Activity as tolerated with adequate rest: So that tissue repair can occur. The patient who is anemic from bleeding ulcers requires activity limitations and more assistance with activities of daily living (ADL) because of fatigue.

Dietary management: Well-balanced diet with avoidance of foods that are not tolerated. Three meals per day are recommended, with elimination of bedtime snacks. Consumption of caffeine and alcohol should be reduced or eliminated. For acute episodes of upper GI hemorrhage, the patient is NPO and is given IV fluid and electrolyte replacement, with foods and fluids introduced orally after bleeding subsides.

Pharmacotherapy

Histamine H_2-receptor blockers (e.g., cimetidine, ranitidine, nizatidine, famotidine): Administered by the oral (PO) or IV route to suppress secretion of gastric acid and facilitate ulcer healing. These drugs also can be used prophylactically for limited periods, especially in patients susceptible to stress ulceration. Because antacids can reduce their absorption, these medications should be administered with meals at least 1 hr apart from antacids.

Sucralfate: An antiulcer agent that coats the ulcer with a protective barrier so that healing can occur. However, it is now considered outmoded as primary therapy for ulcer disease.

Antacids: Administered orally or through nasogastric (NG) tube to provide symptomatic relief; not used as primary therapy.

Proton pump inhibitors (PPIs) (e.g., omeprazole, lansoprazole, pantoprazole, rabeprazole, esomeprazole): Deactivate the enzyme system that pumps hydrogen ions (H^+) from the parietal cells, thus inhibiting gastric acid secretion; used for short-term treatment of active duodenal and gastric ulcers and for long-term treatment of hypersecretory conditions.

Misoprostol: Synthetic prostaglandin E_1 analog that enhances the normal mucosal protective mechanisms of the body and decreases acid secretion. The drug is used in the healing and prevention of NSAID-induced ulcers but is not a first-line agent. Caution must be used when giving this drug to women of childbearing years who could be pregnant because the drug can cause abortion.

Eradication therapy for H. pylori: Indicated for patients in whom *H. pylori* is cultured. Eradication may be obtained with any one of the following regimens: (1) a PPI, clarithromycin 500 mg twice daily, and either amoxicillin or metronidazole for 2 wk; (2) ranitidine, bismuth citrate, clarithromycin 500 mg twice daily, and amoxicillin, metronidazole, or tetracycline for 2 wk; or (3) a PPI, bismuth, metronidazole, and tetracycline for 1-2 wk. Giving PPIs with antimicrobials increases the intragastric pH needed for antimicrobials to be effective.

NSAID ulcer treatment: NSAIDs should be discontinued to enable the ulcer to heal. If patient is also infected with *H. pylori,* therapy for that cause is instituted. For patients with rheumatoid arthritis, prednisone may be used until the ulcer is healed.

NG tube with gastric lavage: For acute, severe GI bleeding, to clear blood from the stomach before endoscopy and to prevent accumulation of clotted blood. For this procedure, the patient should be in semi-Fowler's position or higher. A large-bore NG tube or an Ewald tube is inserted. Gastric contents are aspirated, followed by instillation of 100-250 mL of room-temperature normal saline or tap water, as prescribed, and reaspiration. The process is repeated until returns are clear or light pink and clot free. IV vasopressin may be administered to diminish uncontrolled bleeding before surgery.

Surgical interventions: Indicated for hemorrhage, intractable ulcers, GI obstruction, and perforation. Common surgical procedures include the following, singly or in combination.

Pyloroplasty: Remodeling of the pyloric valve between the stomach and duodenum. This may involve enlargement to relieve obstruction and facilitate gastric emptying or tightening to reduce duodenal reflux into the stomach.

Vagotomy: Severing of the vagus nerve branches to inhibit gastric acid secretion. This may be done at the following three levels:

TRUNCAL VAGOTOMY: Severs vagus nerves at the gastroesophageal junction, thereby reducing gastric acid production and gastric mobility. Use of this procedure has declined recently, but it may be performed in older persons and high-risk patients.

SELECTIVE VAGOTOMY: Severs branches of the vagus nerve that innervate the distal two-thirds of the stomach, thereby reducing gastric acid production but maintaining antral function and thus having little impact on gastric motility.

PARIETAL CELL, OR SUPERSELECTIVE, VAGOTOMY: Severs only branches of the vagus nerve that innervate the parietal cells responsible for gastric acid production.

Subtotal gastrectomy: Removal of distal part of the stomach with anastomosis to the duodenum in a gastroduodenostomy (Billroth I for gastric ulcer and gastric outlet obstruction) or removal of part of the stomach and the duodenum with anastomosis to the jejunum in a gastrojejunostomy (Billroth II for duodenal ulcer). Vagotomy may accompany subtotal gastrectomy.

Postsurgical care: Involves temporary GI decompression with NG tube; analgesics for pain; IV fluid and electrolyte replacement; symptomatic relief of dumping syndrome (rapid gastric emptying characterized by abdominal fullness, weakness, diaphoresis, fatigue, tachycardia, palpitations, dizziness) with a low-carbohydrate, high-fat, high-protein diet, small meals without liquids, and supine position after meals; treatment of pernicious anemia (decreased production of intrinsic factor secondary to removal of that part of the stomach that contains the parietal cells) with vitamin B_{12} injections; and treatment with iron supplements for iron-deficiency anemia (which might occur secondary to loss of blood or iron-absorbing surface in the GI tract). Prevention of hypoventilation (and subsequent atelectasis) and hypoxemia with deep-breathing exercises is especially important in patients who have had abdominal surgery (see "Atelectasis," p. 57).

NURSING DIAGNOSES AND INTERVENTIONS

Ineffective protection related to risk for bleeding, obstruction, and perforation secondary to ulcerative process

Desired outcome: Patient is free of signs and symptoms of bleeding, obstruction, perforation, and peritonitis, as evidenced by negative results for occult blood testing, passage of stool and flatus, soft and nondistended abdomen, good appetite, and normothermia.

Nursing Interventions

- Assess for hematemesis and melena, and check any NG aspirate, emesis, and stools for occult blood. *These are indicators of bleeding.* Report positive findings.
- Monitor results of CBC and coagulation studies. Be alert for hematocrit (Hct) less than 40% (male) or less than 37% (female) and hemoglobin (Hgb) less than 14 g/dL (male) or less than 12 g/dL (female); partial thromboplastin time (PTT) greater than 70 sec or prothrombin time (PT) greater than 12.5 sec.
- If indicated, insert gastric tube. *This is to evacuate blood from stomach.* Monitor for bleeding, and perform gastric lavage as prescribed. Do not use gastric tubes in patients who have or are suspected of having esophageal varices. *This is because the procedure may increase bleeding from the varices.*
- If patient is actively bleeding or if Hct is low, administer O_2. Monitor O_2 saturation (SaO_2) via oximetry. *This is to evaluate systemic oxygenation status.* Report SaO_2 less than 92%.
- Monitor and note abdominal pain, abnormal (increased peristalsis, "rushes," or "tinkles") or absent bowel sounds, distention, anorexia, nausea, vomiting, and inability to pass stool or flatus. *These are indicators of obstruction.* (See "Intestinal Obstructive Processes," p. 457, for more information.)
- Be alert to sudden or severe abdominal pain, distention and abdominal rigidity, fever, nausea, and vomiting. *These are indicators of perforation and peritonitis.* Notify health care provider immediately of significant findings. (See "Peritonitis," p. 461, for more information.)
- Teach signs and symptoms of GI complications and importance of reporting them promptly to staff or health care provider if they occur.

Impaired tissue integrity related to exposure to chemical irritants (gastric acid, pepsin)

Desired outcomes: Patient verbalizes knowledge of necessary lifestyle alterations within the 24-hr period before hospital discharge and demonstrates compliance with medical recommendations for peptic ulcer throughout the hospital stay. Gastric and duodenal mucosal tissues heal and remain intact as evidenced by reduced or absent pain and absence of bleeding.

Nursing Interventions

- Advise patient to avoid foods and drugs such as coffee, caffeine, alcohol, aspirin, and NSAIDs. *These are associated with pain and increased acid secretion.*
- Administer *H. pylori* eradication therapy as prescribed for *H. pylori*–associated ulceration.
- Administer acid suppression therapy as prescribed for acute episodes of ulceration.
- Stress importance of taking medications at prescribed intervals and not just for symptomatic relief of pain. *It is important to continue with the prescribed medications even if symptoms no longer are persistent.*

♦ Refer patient to community resources and support groups for assistance in smoking or alcohol cessation. *Smoking and alcohol can exacerbate disease symptoms.*

Patient-Family Teaching and Discharge Planning

When providing patient-family teaching, include verbal and written information about the following:

♦ Importance of following prescribed diet to facilitate ulcer healing, prevent exacerbation or recurrence, or control postsurgical dumping syndrome. If appropriate, arrange consultation with dietitian.
♦ Medications, including drug names, rationale, dosage, schedule, precautions, and potential side effects. Also discuss drug/drug, food/drug, and herb/drug interactions.
♦ Signs and symptoms of exacerbation and recurrence, as well as potential complications.
♦ Care of incision line and dressing change technique, as necessary.
♦ Signs of wound infection, including persistent redness, swelling, purulent drainage, local warmth, fever, and foul odor.
♦ Role of lifestyle alterations in preventing exacerbation or recurrence of ulcer, including smoking cessation, stress reduction, decreasing or eliminating consumption of alcohol, and avoidance of irritating foods and drugs. Note that histamine H_2-receptor blockers are more effective in individuals who are nonsmokers.
♦ Referral to health care specialist for assistance with stress reduction as necessary.
♦ Referrals to local community support groups (e.g., Alcoholics Anonymous [AA]). Additional resources include:

American Gastroenterological Association: www.gastro.org

Alcoholics Anonymous: www.aa.org

❖ MALABSORPTION/MALDIGESTION

OVERVIEW/PATHOPHYSIOLOGY

Malabsorption or maldigestion refers to a condition in which a specific nutrient or variety of nutrients is inadequately digested or absorbed from the gastrointestinal (GI) tract. Although there is a slight distinction between the two terms, *malabsorption* is used more commonly. Causes of malabsorption are varied and can include the following.

Postsurgical malabsorption: Seen in individuals after subtotal gastrectomy with gastrojejunostomy and gastric bypass surgery because of rapid gastric emptying and decreased intestinal transit time. There is also delayed mixing of biliary and pancreatic secretions with food as a result of altered anatomy.

Inadequate presence of digestive substances in the GI tract: Examples are lactase enzyme deficiency, which is characterized by an inability to digest and absorb lactose, a disaccharide found in milk and dairy products; bile deficiency secondary to liver and gallbladder disease and biliary tract obstruction, which is characterized by the inability to digest and absorb fats and fat-soluble vitamins; and pancreatic secretion deficiency secondary to pancreatic insufficiency or obstruction to the flow of pancreatic secretions, as seen with pancreatic disorders or cystic fibrosis.

Inadequate absorptive space in the GI tract: This occurs secondary to GI surgery (especially ileal resection) or trauma and is characterized by general nutrient malabsorption (short bowel syndrome).

Mucosal lesions that impair absorption: Mucosal changes occur secondary to intestinal invasion of microorganisms endemic to tropical islands (tropical sprue) or ingestion of gluten in the diet (celiac disease, nontropical sprue, gluten-induced enteropathy). Grains with gluten include rye, barley, oats, and wheat. With Whipple's disease, which is a rare disorder, small bowel lipo-dystrophy occurs, resulting in impaired absorption.

Inflammatory conditions of the GI tract: For example, ulcerative colitis (UC) (see p. 476) and Crohn's disease (CD) (see p. 484) involve significant diarrhea with malabsorption and deficiencies of various nutrients. Inflammation and mucosal ulceration secondary to chemotherapy also can impair digestion and absorption.

Use of drugs that alter intestinal fluids or mucosa: Includes antacids, mineral oil, broad-spectrum antibiotics, hypocholesterolemic agents, antiinflammatory agents, oral hypoglycemics, and oral KCl, all of which can affect absorption of specific nutrients.

Overgrowth of microbes in the GI tract: Overgrowth is secondary to diverticula (outpouchings) of the small intestine, inadequate gastric acid secretion (e.g., secondary to total or partial gastrectomy or aggressive antisecretory therapy), immunologic defects, gastroenteritis, blind loop syndrome, and intestinal obstruction.

Excessive use of enemas or cathartics: Nutrients pass too rapidly through the intestinal tract to be absorbed. Complications can include specific or generalized malnutrition, fluid and electrolyte imbalances, and acid-base imbalances.

ASSESSMENT

Signs and symptoms/physical findings: Vary depending on specific nutrients that are not absorbed. Patient may have unexplained weight loss with muscle atrophy, despite normal or increased appetite; diarrhea; steatorrhea (greasy, pale, foul-smelling stools); bloating; excessive flatus; abdominal cramping; and indicators of specific nutrient deficiencies (e.g., anemia with iron or vitamin B_{12} deficiency; tetany and paresthesias with calcium (Ca^{++}) deficiency; bleeding or easy bruising with vitamin K deficiency).

History and risk factors: GI surgery; excessive use of enemas or cathartics; diseases that cause diarrhea; immunologic defects; diverticulosis; liver, pancreatic, or gallbladder disease; inflammatory/infectious disorders of the intestinal tract; medications that increase GI motility and cause diarrhea; chemotherapy.

DIAGNOSTIC TESTS

Quantitative stool fat test (72-hr fecal fat): The gold standard test for fat malabsorption. A high-fat diet is ingested for 2 days and then continued for 3 more days, during which time the 72-hr collection is obtained. Normal fat excretion is less than 7 g/day. A false-negative result occurs if inadequate fat is ingested, and a false-positive result occurs if a mineral oil laxative or suppository is given before stool collection.

Qualitative stool fat test (Sudan stain): Test requires intake of 100 g fat per day. High sensitivity and specificity is present when fat malabsorption exceeds 10 g/day.

Stool culture: Diagnoses pathogens or bacterial overgrowth.

Schilling's test: Analysis of a 24-hr urine specimen collected after intramuscular (IM) injection of nonradioactive vitamin B_{12} followed by ingestion of radioactive vitamin B_{12} will reveal below-normal levels of B_{12}. Further testing, during which intrinsic factor is administered, will facilitate diagnosis of pernicious anemia from malabsorption or renal disease.

D-Xylose tolerance test: Shows inadequate presence of xylose (an easily absorbed monosaccharide) in a 5-hr collection of urine after oral administration. This test is used to distinguish small intestine mucosal malabsorption from pancreatic insufficiency.

Serum tests: Show depressed levels of carotene, Ca^{++}, magnesium, and other electrolytes and minerals, depending on specific malabsorption problem. In addition, serum albumin, total iron-binding capacity, and transferrin may be decreased because of protein depletion.

Hydrogen breath test: For bacterial overgrowth, which causes increased excretion of hydrogen in the breath.

Barium swallow: Facilitates diagnosis of the specific cause of malabsorption (e.g., diverticula of the small intestine). (For a description, see "Peptic Ulcers," p. 448.) Small bowel follow-through is accomplished by serial x-ray examinations as the barium progresses through the small intestines.

CT scan of the abdomen: Facilitates diagnosis, especially for pancreatic involvement. Patients are on nothing-by-mouth (NPO) status 3-4 hr before the procedure. If contrast will be used, patients should be assessed in advance for allergy to iodine. Patients may be required to hold several deep breaths during scanning. Oral or IV fluids should be adequate to ensure elimination of the dye via the kidneys after the procedure.

Endoscopy with or without biopsy: Visualization of the small (duodeno-scopy) or large (colonoscopy) bowel through a lighted, flexible tube (endoscope) that is inserted through the mouth (duodenoscopy) or anus (colo-noscopy). The patient is on NPO status before the procedure. Written consent is required. Sedation is prescribed to relax the patient; atropine may be administered to decrease GI secretions; and glucagon may be administered to facilitate passage of the tube through the pylorus. Tissue samples may be taken for examination, including culture and cytologic evaluation. Hemorrhage and perforation are potential complications, and VS should be monitored closely for 4-8 hr after the procedure.

Endoscopic retrograde cholangiopancreatography (ERCP): Involves passage of an endoscope into the duodenum to the ampulla of Vater (distal end of the pancreatic and common bile duct drainage system) for visualization. A contrast medium is injected through the scope into the pancreatic ducts or biliary ducts (common bile duct, cystic duct, hepatic ducts), and x-ray images are taken. This test is diagnostic for pancreatic disease and common bile duct pathology (stricture, obstruction, choledocholithiasis). Patient is on NPO status for 8-12 hr before the test and must be assessed for allergies to iodine (and/or to shellfish) before undergoing the test. Written consent is required. Oral or IV fluid should be adequate to ensure elimination of dye via the kidneys after the procedure. A rare but potentially fatal complication of ERCP is acute pancreatitis; monitor for increasing abdominal pain, tachycardia, hypotension, abdominal distention, nausea, and vomiting.

Secretin stimulation test: Gold standard test for pancreatic insufficiency. A collecting tube is passed into the duodenum of the patient who is on NPO status. IV secretin and/or cholecystokinin are given, and the duodenal secretions are collected and analyzed for bicarbonate and trypsin levels, which are decreased with pancreatic insufficiency. Written consent is required.

COLLABORATIVE MANAGEMENT

Management varies, depending on specific cause of malabsorption and nutrient deficiencies that are exhibited.

Activity as tolerated: Patient may be fatigued and require limited activity as a consequence of diarrhea, malnutrition, and associated anemia.

Dietary management: A low-residue diet may be useful for controlling diarrhea. For lactase deficiency, a low-lactose diet (avoidance of milk and milk products) is prescribed, and for nontropical sprue, a gluten-free diet is prescribed (**BOX 7-1**). Until specific problems (e.g., liver or gallbladder disorders) are corrected, dietary intake of fats is avoided. Any specific nutrient deficiencies are corrected. For the seriously malnourished patient, parenteral nutrition may be necessary.

BOX 7-1	GUIDELINES FOR LOW-RESIDUE, HIGH-RESIDUE, AND GLUTEN-FREE DIETS

Low-Residue Diet
- *Encouraged:* Enriched/refined breads and cereals; rice and pasta dishes
- *To be avoided:* Fruits, vegetables, whole-wheat products (cereals and breads)

High-Residue Diet
- *Encouraged:* Fruits, vegetables, large amounts of fluid, whole-grain breads and cereals
- *To be avoided:* Highly refined cereals and pasta (e.g., white rice, white bread, white spaghetti or noodles, ice cream)

Gluten-Free Diet
- *Encouraged (if allowed):* Rice, corn, eggs, potatoes; breads made from rice flour, cornmeal, soybean flour, gluten-free wheat starch, and potato starch; cereals made from corn or rice (grits, cornmeal mush, cooked cream of rice, puffed rice, rice flakes); pasta made from rice or corn flour; homemade ice cream; tapioca pudding
- *To be avoided if they contain wheat, barley, rye, or oats:* Cereals and bakery goods, coffee substitutes, sauces, commercially prepared luncheon meats, gravies, noodles, macaroni, spaghetti, flour tortillas, crackers, cakes, cookies, pastries, puddings, commercial ice cream, alcoholic beverages

IV fluids and electrolytes: As necessary to rehydrate and correct electrolyte imbalances.

Pharmacotherapy

Mineral, vitamin, and electrolyte supplements: Correct specific deficiencies. Vitamin D levels and serum and urinary Ca^{++} levels should be monitored to prevent vitamin D toxicity.

Antibiotics: For treatment of bacterial overgrowth or pathogenic infection (e.g., *Clostridium difficile*). Use of specific drugs is based on culture results when possible.

Antihyperlipidemic agents (e.g., cholestyramine): May be given to control diarrhea when it is associated with ileal resection.

Surgical intervention: May be necessary to correct specific disorders that precipitate malabsorption, such as biliary tract obstruction or stricture of the sphincter of Oddi.

NURSING DIAGNOSES AND INTERVENTIONS

Diarrhea (with bloating, excessive flatus, and abdominal cramping) related to malabsorption in the bowel

Desired outcome: Patient is free of discomfort from diarrhea and other symptoms of malabsorption at least 24 hr before hospital discharge, as evidenced by passage of normal stools (soft, semiformed) and absence of excessive flatus and cramping.

Nursing Interventions

◆ Assess and document presence of GI discomfort and symptoms, including onset and duration of symptoms and precipitating and palliative factors. Instruct patient to avoid foods associated with symptoms.

◆ Teach importance of dietary compliance in treatment for some malabsorptive disorders. *Dietary restriction, such as a low-lactose diet with lactase intolerance or a gluten-free diet with nontropical sprue, may be necessary to prevent symptoms.* Have patient plan a 3-day menu that includes and excludes foods from lists in Box 7-1 as appropriate.

◆ If an infectious source of diarrhea is suspected (e.g., *C. difficile),* collect a stool specimen for culture and sensitivity.

Risk for deficient fluid volume related to excessive loss with diarrhea
Desired outcome: Patient is normovolemic, as evidenced by good skin turgor, moist mucous membranes, urinary output at least 30 mL/hr, heart rate (HR) 100 beats per minute (bpm) or less, absence of orthostatic SBP changes, and absence of thirst.

Nursing Interventions

◆ Assess for weight loss, tachycardia, hypotension, poor skin turgor, dry skin and mucous membranes, thirst, and decreased urinary output. *These indicate fluid volume deficit.* Consult health care provider for hypotension or urinary output less than 30 mL/hr for 2 consecutive hr.
◆ Ensure precise maintenance and documentation of fluid I&O records and daily weights.
◆ Administer IV fluids and parenteral nutrients as prescribed.
◆ As appropriate, encourage intake of water and/or noncaffeinated clear liquids.
◆ Encourage prescribed dietary compliance. *This is for relief of symptomatic diarrhea.*
◆ Administer medications, and teach patient self-administration of medications as prescribed. *This is to help control diarrhea or treat underlying condition.* For assessment of nutrient deficiencies, see "Providing Nutritional Support," p. 692.

Patient-Family Teaching and Discharge Planning

When providing patient-family teaching, include verbal and written information about the following:
◆ Use of medications, including drug names, purpose, dosage, schedule, precautions, and potential side effects. Also discuss drug/drug, food/drug, and herb/drug interactions.
◆ Prescribed dietary replacement of deficiency nutrients and dietary management of symptoms, if appropriate.
◆ Need to ensure adequate oral fluid intake during episodes of diarrhea to avoid dehydration.
◆ Problems that necessitate medical attention: nutrient deficiencies, fluid volume deficit, and acid-base imbalances.
◆ Phone numbers to call if questions or concerns arise about therapy or disease after discharge. Additional resources include:

National Institute of Diabetes and Digestive and Kidney Diseases: www.niddk.nih. gov

Gluten Intolerance Group (GIG) of North America: www.gluten.net

American Dietetic Association: www.eatright.org

World Gastroenterology Association: www.worldgastroenterology.org

❖ INTESTINAL OBSTRUCTIVE PROCESSES

OVERVIEW/PATHOPHYSIOLOGY

Obstruction of the gastrointestinal (GI) tract is a condition in which normal peristaltic transport of GI contents does not take place. Therefore, digestion and absorption of foods and fluids and elimination of wastes are impaired or totally blocked. Furthermore, GI fluids become hypertonic and thus precipitate osmotic fluid loss from the body into the GI lumen. Subsequently, nutritional status and fluid and electrolyte status are compromised, and distention occurs. Increased pressure in the GI tract also can result in perforation and peritonitis or necrosis of the GI mucosa. The three most common causes of intestinal obstruction are adhesions, hernias, and neoplasms. Adhesions cause most cases of small bowel obstruction (SBO), then hernias, and lastly, neoplasms. Obstruction also can occur anywhere along the GI tract, but most commonly at the pyloric area of the stomach or in the small bowel because of adhesions in the ileum. Obstruction can occur as a result of the inflammation and edema that accompany GI disease (peptic ulcers, diverticulitis, colitis, gastroenteritis, trauma); adynamic (paralytic) ileus secondary to peritoneal insult, such as surgery or peritonitis; diminished GI motility because of hypokalemia, intestinal pseudoobstruction, uremia, diabetes mellitus (DM), or use of opioids, diuretics, or anticholinergic drugs; volvulus; or incarcerated hernia. When obstruction is prolonged or infarction or perforation of intestinal tissue occurs, sepsis is likely.

ASSESSMENT

Signs and symptoms/physical findings: Severe, crampy pain; vomiting; back pain; restlessness; hiccoughs; belching; and inability to pass stool or flatus (accompanied by a feeling of fullness). Symptoms vary, depending on the type and site of obstruction. In SBO, pain may be severe and episodic with vomiting (possibly projectile), late abdominal distention, and little to no stool or pencil-like stool. In large bowel obstruction, pain may be moderate but continuous with vomiting occurring late, extreme abdominal distention, and little to no stool. In paralytic ileus, pain and vomiting are usually absent or mild, abdominal distention is present, and there may be little or no stool passed.

Abdominal distention, abdominal tenderness, high-pitched ("tinkles") and intermittent bowel sounds may be noted above the point of obstruction. Bowel sounds are absent or diminished with paralytic ileus. Patients may have decreased urinary output, poor skin turgor, and dry skin and mucous membranes associated with intravascular volume depletion. Bleeding may be noted on rectal examination if strangulation is present along with severe pain, vomiting, and a rigid, tender, distended abdomen. Bleeding may also indicate the presence of a tumor.

History and risk factors: Abdominal hernia, recent or past abdominal surgery, GI inflammation or perforation secondary to various disease processes, DM, chronic renal failure, or use of opioids, diuretics, or anticholinergics.

DIAGNOSTIC TESTS

CBC count: WBCs usually are elevated secondary to inflammation. Marked leukocytosis is usually present with intestinal strangulation. Hematocrit (Hct) and hemoglobin (Hgb) may be elevated because of hemoconcentration.

X-ray examination of abdomen: Reveals distention of bowel loops with air and fluid proximal to the obstruction. The presence of free air under the diaphragm suggests intestinal perforation.

Serial x-ray examinations: Along with physical examinations, determine whether obstruction is resolving.

Contrast studies: Used to determine presence and location of obstruction in patients with atypical clinical signs. Barium or meglumine diatrizoate (Gastrografin) is commonly used as the contrast agent. Barium enema (to exclude colon obstruction) should precede barium swallow. Barium will not advance past the site of obstruction. For more information, see "Peptic Ulcers," p. 448.

Aspiration of fecal matter from nasogastric (NG) or intestinal tube: Fecal matter, identified by its characteristic foul odor, is an indication of obstruction.

Endoscopy (sigmoidoscopy, colonoscopy): Identifies tumor, stricture, inflammation, or other sources of colonic obstruction.

TABLE 7-1	GASTRIC/INTESTINAL TUBES USED IN OBSTRUCTIVE PROCESSES	
TUBE	**OBSTRUCTIVE PROCESS**	**PURPOSE**
Gastric tube*	Pyloric obstruction, small bowel obstruction, paralytic ileus	Decompresses GI tract of retained fluids, alleviates abdominal distention, relieves edema in intestinal wall, prevents vomiting, promotes comfort
Intestinal tube*† (e.g., single-lumen Cantor or Harris tube or double-lumen Miller-Abbott tube)	Small or large bowel obstruction, paralytic ileus	Same as for gastric tube; presence of tube may promote return of peristalsis in paralytic ileus; tube may relieve edema sufficiently to relieve obstruction, thereby avoiding need for surgery

*In some cases, gastric and intestinal tubes are used together.
†Long intestinal tubes are indicated primarily when obstruction is partial.
GI, Gastrointestinal.

COLLABORATIVE MANAGEMENT

The specific cause of obstruction must be identified quickly so that appropriate treatment can be instituted and complications prevented. In the interim, management is supportive and aimed at maintaining nutritional and fluid and electrolyte balance and promoting comfort.

Activity as tolerated: With paralytic ileus, patient is encouraged to ambulate to promote return of peristalsis. With other forms of obstruction, activity may be limited because of pain or complications.

Dietary management: Patient is on nothing-by-mouth (NPO) status until obstruction is resolved (or bowel sounds return in paralytic ileus).

IV fluid and electrolyte support: Lactated Ringer's or isotonic saline solutions (or isotonic dextrose/saline combinations) are commonly prescribed. Volume of IV fluid required often depends on the amount of gastric or intestinal tube drainage (replacement fluids often prescribed mL for mL). K^+ is added to IV fluids to correct or prevent hypokalemia. Total parenteral nutrition (TPN) may be indicated to meet nutritional needs if obstruction or recovery is prolonged.

GI decompression: Accomplished via gastric or intestinal tube connected to low, intermittent suction (**TABLE 7-1**).

Urinary catheterization: Allows close monitoring of urinary output.

Pharmacotherapy

Antibiotics: Prevent or treat infection.

Analgesics: For pain relief. Opioid analgesics are not administrated until surgical evaluation has been completed because they can mask symptoms and interfere with diagnosis. Opioids, such as morphine, can decrease intestinal motility and increase nausea and vomiting.

Antiemetic agents (e.g., hydroxyzine, ondansetron, granisetron, prochlorperazine, promethazine): For relief of nausea and vomiting.

GI stimulants (e.g., metoclopramide, dexpanthenol): Used perioperatively to minimize paralytic ileus. They are given cautiously because stimulant action may cause perforation in ischemic bowel. Metoclopramide is used in management of diabetic gastric stasis.

Surgical intervention: Indicated for complete bowel obstruction that does not resolve. In some cases, inflammatory processes subside, and obstruction resolves without surgery. Paralytic ileus generally resolves in 2-3 days without any treatment. In most other cases, surgery is indicated to identify and relieve obstruction source. Exploratory laparotomy is performed when diagnosis is uncertain. When diagnosis is known, the indicated surgery is performed (e.g., pyloroplasty for pyloric obstruction or bowel resection with or without colostomy for removal of tumor or adhesions). When carcinomatosis is present, nonsurgical management may be indicated.

NURSING DIAGNOSES AND INTERVENTIONS

Acute pain (with nausea, and distention) related to obstructive process or malfunction of gastric or intestinal drainage tube
Desired outcomes: Patient's subjective perception of discomfort decreases within 8 hr of admission and is absent by hospital discharge, as documented by a pain scale. Nonverbal indicators, such as grimacing, are absent or diminished.

Nursing Interventions

◆ Assess and document degree of discomfort at least q4h. Investigate pain characteristics such as severity, character, location, duration, precipitating/alleviating factors, and nonverbal indicators. Devise a pain scale with patient, rating discomfort from 0 (no discomfort) to 10 (worst discomfort).
◆ Be alert to vomiting and distention, depending on type of obstructive process.
◆ Teach nonpharmacologic methods of pain relief: distraction, back rubs, conversation, relaxation therapy.
◆ Administer prescribed analgesics and antiemetic agents as indicated. Instruct patient to request analgesia before pain becomes severe. Assess and document degree of relief obtained using pain scale. Be aware that opioid analgesics contribute to intestinal hypomotility.
◆ Maintain patency and proper functioning of gastric or intestinal tube.
  • Maintain connection to low, intermittent suction or as prescribed.
  • Irrigate tube with 30 mL of normal saline as needed (prn) or as prescribed.
  • Secure gastric tube with tape or other adhesive. *This keeps it properly positioned in stomach.*
  • Avoid occlusion of vent side of sump suction tubes. *This is because it may result in vacuum occlusion of the tube and excessive suction and injury to gastric mucosa.*
◆ Keep head of bed (HOB) elevated 30-45 degrees as permitted. *This is to promote comfort and facilitate ventilation.* A slightly Trendelenburg, right side-lying position may be helpful. *This is to reduce gas pains in patients with paralytic ileus.*
◆ Encourage turning in bed and activity as permitted. *This will promote peristalsis.*
◆ Provide oral care at frequent intervals. *Frequent brushing of teeth and rinsing of mouth will alleviate dryness.* Provide lubricant for lips.
◆ Provide mouth rinses at frequent intervals. Apply water-soluble lubricant to naris. Apply viscous lidocaine solution to naris or back of throat. *These interventions are to alleviate nose and pharyngeal discomfort from tube.*

Risk for deficient fluid volume related to excessive loss secondary to obstructive process and subsequent vomiting or gastric decompression of large volumes of GI fluids and decreased intake secondary to fluid restrictions
Desired outcome: Patient is normovolemic, as evidenced by good skin turgor, moist mucous membranes, urinary output at least 30 mL/hr, urinary specific gravity 1.010-1.025, stable weight, heart rate (HR) less than 100 beats per minute (bpm), absence of orthostatic SBP changes, and absence of thirst.

Nursing Interventions

♦ Ensure precise measurement and documentation of fluid I&O. Weigh patient daily.

♦ Take special note of amount and character of GI aspirate. Check GI aspirate for electrolyte loss or pH as prescribed.

♦ Administer appropriate IV fluids at prescribed rate. Replace volume of GI fluids aspirated by suction if prescribed.

♦ Take careful note of character and amount of GI aspirate. Check GI aspirate for electrolyte loss (collect specimen for laboratory analysis) or pH as prescribed.

♦ For other interventions, see **Risk for deficient fluid volume,** p. 5, in "Perioperative Care."

 Patient-Family Teaching and Discharge Planning

When providing patient-family teaching, include verbal and written information about the following:

♦ Specific disease process that precipitated obstruction and methods to prevent recurrence, such as compliance with prescribed therapies.

♦ Symptoms of recurring obstruction to report to health care provider.

♦ Medications, including drug names, purpose, dosage, schedule, precautions, and potential side effects. Also discuss drug/drug, food/drug, and herb/drug interactions.

❖ PERITONITIS

OVERVIEW/PATHOPHYSIOLOGY

Peritonitis is the inflammatory response of the peritoneum to offending chemical and bacterial agents invading the peritoneal cavity. The inflammatory process can be local or generalized and may be classified as primary, secondary, or tertiary, depending on pathogenesis of the inflammation. Primary peritonitis (e.g., spontaneous bacterial peritonitis) occurs without a recognizable cause. Secondary peritonitis is caused by abdominal injury or rupture of abdominal organs. Common precipitating events or factors include abdominal trauma, postoperative leakage of gastrointestinal (GI) contents or blood into the peritoneal cavity, intestinal ischemia, ruptured or inflamed abdominal organs, poor sterile technique (e.g., with peritoneal dialysis), and direct contamination of the bloodstream. Tertiary peritonitis is a persistent abdominal sepsis without a focus of infection, and it may follow treatment for a previous episode of peritonitis. The peritoneum responds to invasive agents by attempting to localize the infection with a shift of the omentum to wall off the inflamed area. Inflammation of the peritoneum results in tissue edema, development of fibrinous exudate, and hypermotility of the tract. As the disease progresses, paralytic ileus occurs, and intestinal fluid, which then cannot be reabsorbed, leaks into the peritoneal cavity. As a result of the fluid shift, cardiac output and tissue perfusion are reduced, leading to impaired cardiac and renal function. If infection or inflammation continues, respiratory failure and shock can ensue. Peritonitis often is progressive and can be fatal. It is the most common cause of death following abdominal surgery, and risk of death is dictated by the patient's overall health, including nutritional and immune status and organ function.

ASSESSMENT

Signs and symptoms/physical findings

Early findings: Acute abdominal pain with movement, anorexia, nausea, vomiting, chills, fever, rigor, malaise, weakness, hiccoughs, diaphoresis, absence of bowel sounds, and abdominal distention and rigidity ("boardlike abdomen").

Later findings: May include manifestations of dehydration (e.g., thirst, dry mucous membranes, oliguria, concentrated urine, poor skin turgor). There may be tachycardia, hypotension, and shallow and rapid respirations caused by abdominal distention and discomfort. Often the patient assumes a supine position with knees flexed or a side-lying position with knees drawn up toward the chest. Palpation usually elicits signs of peritoneal irritation as shown by distention, abdominal rigidity with general or localized tenderness, guarding, and rebound or cough tenderness. However, as many as one-fourth of these patients will have minimal or no indications of peritoneal irritation. Auscultation findings include hyperactive bowel sounds during the gradual development of peritonitis and absence of bowel sounds or infrequent high-pitched sounds ("tinkling" or "squeaky") during later stages if paralytic ileus occurs. Mild ascites may be present, as demonstrated by shifting areas of dullness on percussion.

History and risk factors: Abdominal surgery, peptic ulcer disease, cholecystitis, acute necrotizing pancreatitis, GI disorders, acute salpingitis, ruptured appendix or diverticulum, trauma, peritoneal dialysis.

DIAGNOSTIC TESTS

Serum tests: May reveal presence of leukocytosis, usually with a shift to the left (may be the only sign of tertiary peritonitis); hemoconcentration; elevated BUN; and electrolyte imbalance, particularly hypokalemia. Hypoalbuminemia and prolonged prothrombin time (PT), in combination with leukocytosis, are especially characteristic.

ABG values: May reveal hypoxemia (PaO_2 less than 80 mm Hg) or acidosis (pH less than 7.40).

Urinalysis: Often performed to rule out genitourinary involvement (e.g., pyelonephritis).

Paracentesis for peritoneal aspiration with culture and sensitivity: May be performed to determine presence of blood, bacteria, bile, pus, and amylase content and identify causative organism. Gram stain of ascitic fluid is positive in only about 25% of these patients. Ascitic fluid with a WBC count greater than 500/mm^3 with more than 25% polymorphonuclear leukocytes is especially characteristic. Blood–ascitic fluid albumin gradient greater than 1.1 g/dL, reduced pH of ascitic fluid (less than 7.31), and serum lactic acid elevation greater than 33 mg/dL aid in confirmation of the diagnosis.

Abdominal x-ray examination: Determines presence of distended loops of bowel and abnormal levels of fluid and gas, which usually collect in the large and small bowel in the presence of a perforation or obstruction. "Free air" under the diaphragm also may be visualized and indicates a perforated viscus.

Chest x-ray examination: Abdominal distention may elevate the diaphragm. Pain from peritonitis may limit respiratory excursion and lead to associated infiltrates in the lower lobes. In later stages, changes in serum osmolality allow for pleural effusions to occur.

Contrast x-ray examination: May be used to identify specific intestinal pathologic conditions. Water-soluble contrast (e.g., meglumine diatrizoate) may be used to evaluate suspected upper GI perforation.

CT scan and ultrasound: May be used to evaluate abdominal pain and more clearly delineate nondistinct areas found by plain abdominal x-ray examination. Magnetic resonance imaging (MRI) has not been an effective adjunct in abdominal surveys because of motion artifacts.

Radionuclide scans: Such as gallium, hepatoiminodiacetic acid (HIDA), and liver-spleen scans, may be used to identify intraabdominal abscess.

COLLABORATIVE MANAGEMENT

Bed rest: With patient in semi-Fowler's or high Fowler's position to promote fluid shift to the lower abdomen, which will reduce pressure on the diaphragm and enable deeper and easier respirations. Raising the knees will lower stress on the abdominal wall.

Nasogastric (NG) or intestinal tube: Inserted to reduce or prevent GI distention, nausea, and vomiting (Table 7-1).

IV fluids, electrolyte therapy, and parenteral feedings: Correct fluid, electrolyte, and nutritional disorders. Daily measurements of serum electrolytes and calculations of fluid volume are performed to determine necessary types of fluid and electrolyte replacement. A urinary catheter is inserted to facilitate careful I&O measurement. Crystalloids, colloids (albumin, human plasma protein fraction [Plasmanate]), blood, and blood products may be administered to correct hypovolemia, hypoproteinemia, and anemia. Patient is on nothing-by-mouth (NPO) status during the acute phase, and oral fluids are not resumed until patient has passed flatus and the gastric tube has been removed. Total parenteral nutrition (TPN) usually is initiated in early stages to promote nutrition and protein replacement.

Cardiovascular monitoring: A central venous pressure (CVP) catheter may be inserted in critically ill patients. CVP values should be maintained at 2-6 mm Hg (5-12 cm H_2O). A pulmonary artery (i.e., Swan-Ganz) catheter may be inserted if patient is unstable or develops hypovolemic shock.

Pharmacotherapy

Antibiotics (e.g., cephalosporins [cefotaxime, cefepime], aminoglycosides [gentamicin], ampicillin, floxacin, metronidazole): Combination broad-spectrum antibiotic therapy is promptly initiated to cover gram-negative bacilli and anaerobic bacteria. Single-drug therapy also may be effective with drugs such as imipenem and cilastatin sodium. Antibiotics are commonly administered by the IV route or may be directly instilled into the peritoneal cavity via surgically placed catheters. (Antifungal agents may be required for fungal infections.)

Analgesics and sedatives: Relieve severe pain and discomfort once diagnosis has been confirmed. Because potent analgesics can mask diagnostic symptoms, opioids should not be administered until surgical evaluation has been completed.

O_2 therapy: Often prescribed to support increased metabolic needs or treat hypoxia.

Surgical intervention: Required to repair perforations; may be needed to remove the source of infection, drain the abscess or accumulated fluids, and prevent recurrent infection. Intervention can include removal of an organ, such as the appendix or gallbladder. Drains usually are inserted to enable continued removal of purulent drainage and excessive fluids. Intestinal decompression may be employed to decrease massive abdominal distention. Intraoperative and postoperative irrigation, with or without antibiotic solutions, may be indicated if bowel contents have grossly contaminated the peritoneal cavity. Fluoroscopically guided drainage catheters may be inserted for tertiary peritonitis if collection is attainable.

Peritoneal lavage: May be used if patient does not respond to the interventions just mentioned or is a surgical risk. Rapid dialysis exchanges may be performed along with antibiotic lavages.

NURSING DIAGNOSES AND INTERVENTIONS

Acute pain, nausea, and abdominal distention related to inflammatory process, fever, and tissue damage

Desired outcomes: Patient's subjective perception of pain decreases within 1 hr of intervention, as documented by a pain scale. Nonverbal indicators, such as grimacing and abdominal guarding, are absent or diminished.

Nursing Interventions

♦ Assess and document character and severity of discomfort q1-2h. Devise a pain scale with patient, rating discomfort on a scale of 0 (no pain) to 10 (worst pain).

- After diagnosis has been made, administer opioids, other analgesics, and sedatives as prescribed. *This is to promote comfort and rest.* Encourage patient to request analgesic before pain becomes severe. Document relief obtained, using the pain scale.
- Keep patient on bed rest. *This is to minimize pain, which can be aggravated by activity.*
- Instruct patient in methods to splint abdomen. *This helps to reduce pain on movement, coughing, and deep breathing.*
- Provide a restful and quiet environment.
- Keep patient in a position of comfort, usually semi-Fowler's position with knees bent.
- Explain all procedures. *This is to help minimize anxiety, which can exacerbate discomfort.*
- Offer mouth care and lip moisturizers at frequent intervals. *This is to help relieve discomfort/nausea from continuous or intermittent suction, dehydration, and NPO status.*
- Administer antiemetics (e.g., hydroxyzine, ondansetron, prochlorperazine, promethazine) as prescribed. Instruct patient to request medication *before* nausea becomes severe. *This is to combat nausea and vomiting as soon as possible and to promote comfort.*
- See "Stomatitis," p. 442, for mouth care interventions.

Impaired gas exchange related to alveolar hypoventilation and decreased depth of respirations secondary to guarding with abdominal pain or distention
Desired outcomes: Patient has an effective breathing pattern, as evidenced by PaO$_2$ at least 80 mm Hg; O$_2$ saturation (SaO$_2$) greater than 92%; BP at least 90/60 mm Hg (or within patient's baseline range); heart rate (HR) 100 beats per minute (bpm) or less; and orientation to person, place, and time. Eupnea occurs within 1 hr after pain-relieving intervention.

Nursing Interventions

- Monitor arterial blood gas (ABG) analysis and oximetry results, and be alert to indicators of hypoxemia, including PaO$_2$ less than 80 mm Hg and low O$_2$ saturation (92% or less), and to the following clinical signs: hypotension, tachycardia, tachypnea, restlessness, confusion or altered mental status, central nervous system (CNS) depression, and possibly cyanosis.
- Auscultate lung fields. *This is to assess ventilation and detect pulmonary complications.*
- Keep patient in semi-Fowler's or high Fowler's position. *This is to aid respiratory effort; encourage deep breathing to enhance oxygenation and coughing to clear pulmonary secretions.* Instruct patient in splinting abdomen. *This is to reduce pain during the respiratory hygiene routine.*
- Administer O$_2$ as prescribed.

Ineffective protection related to risk for worsening/recurring peritonitis or development of septic shock secondary to inflammatory process
Desired outcome: Patient is free of symptoms of worsening/recurring peritonitis or septic shock, as evidenced by normothermia, BP at least 90/60 mm Hg (or within patient's normal range), HR 100 bpm or less, absence of chills, presence of eupnea, urinary output at least 30 mL/hr, CVP 2-6 mm Hg (5-12 cm H$_2$O), decreasing abdominal girth measurements, and minimal tenderness to palpation.

Nursing Interventions

- Assess abdomen q1-2h during acute phase and q4h once patient is stabilized. Measure abdominal girth; use a permanent marker to identify placement of tape measure to ensure consistent measurement by caregivers. *This is to monitor for increasing distention.* Auscultate bowel sounds. *This is to assess motility.* Bowel sounds initially may be frequent but later are absent.

Lightly palpate abdomen for evidence of increasing rigidity or tenderness, which indicates disease progression. If patient experiences increased pain on removal of your hand, rebound tenderness is present. Notify health care provider of significant findings.

◆ If prescribed, insert gastric tube and connect it to suction. *This is to prevent or decrease distention.*

◆ Monitor VS at least q2h and more frequently if patient's condition is unstable. Assess for increased temperature, hypotension, tachycardia, shallow and rapid respirations, urine output less than 30 mL/hr, and CVP less than 2 mm Hg (less than 5 cm H_2O). *These may indicate septic shock.* In the early (warm) stage of shock, skin usually is warm, pink, and dry secondary to peripheral venous pooling, and BP and CVP begin to drop. In the late (cold) stage of shock, extremities become pale and cool. *This is because of decreasing tissue perfusion.*

◆ Administer antibiotics as prescribed; ensure close adherence to schedules. *This maintains bactericidal serum levels.* Collect peak and trough antibiotic determinations as prescribed.

◆ Monitor CBC for presence of leukocytosis. *This signals infection.* Monitor hemoconcentration (increased hematocrit [Hct] and hemoglobin [Hgb]). *This may indicate decreased plasma volume. With peritonitis, WBC count usually is greater than 20,000/mm³.* Notify health care provider of significant findings.

◆ Maintain sterile technique with dressing changes and all invasive procedures.

◆ Teach signs and symptoms of recurring peritonitis and importance of reporting them promptly if they occur: fever, chills, abdominal pain, vomiting, and abdominal distention.

Imbalanced nutrition: less than body requirements related to vomiting and intestinal suctioning
Desired outcome: By at least 24 hr before hospital discharge, patient demonstrates optimal progress toward adequate nutritional status, as evidenced by stable weight, balanced or positive N state, serum protein 6-8 g/dL, and serum albumin 3.5-5.5 g/dL.

Nursing Interventions

◆ Keep patient on NPO status as prescribed during acute phase. If patient has an ileus, an NG tube will be inserted to decompress the abdomen. Reintroduce oral fluids gradually once motility has returned, as evidenced by presence of bowel sounds, decreased distention, and passage of flatus.

◆ Support patient with peripheral parenteral nutrition (PPN) or TPN, as prescribed, depending on duration of acute phase (usually by day 5).

◆ Administer replacement fluids, electrolytes, and vitamins as prescribed.

◆ Instruct patient in rationale for tube placement and NPO status; underlying pathologic condition (as appropriate); need for close monitoring of fluid I&O; and, eventually, diet advancement.

Patient-Family Teaching and Discharge Planning

When providing patient-family teaching, include verbal and written information about the following:

◆ Medications, including drug names, dosage, schedule, purpose, precautions, and potential side effects. Also discuss drug/drug, food/drug, and herb/drug interactions.

◆ Activity alterations as prescribed by health care provider, such as avoiding heavy lifting (more than 10 lb), resting after periods of fatigue, getting maximum amounts of rest, and gradually increasing activities to tolerance.

◆ Notifying health care provider of the following indicators of recurrence: fever, chills, abdominal pain, vomiting, abdominal distention.

◆ If patient has undergone surgery, indicators of wound infection: fever, pain, chills, incisional swelling, persistent erythema, purulent drainage.
◆ Importance of follow-up medical care; confirm date and time of next medical appointment.

❖❖ APPENDICITIS

OVERVIEW/PATHOPHYSIOLOGY

Appendicitis is the most commonly occurring inflammatory lesion of the bowel and one of the most common reasons for abdominal surgery. Appendicitis occurs most often in adolescents and young adults, especially males. The appendix is a blind, narrow tube that extends from the inferior portion of the cecum and does not serve any known useful function. Appendicitis is usually caused by obstruction of the appendiceal lumen by a fecalith (hardened bit of fecal material), inflammation, a foreign body, or a neoplasm. Obstruction prevents drainage of secretions that are produced by epithelial cells in the lumen and thereby increases intraluminal pressure and compresses mucosal blood vessels. This tension eventually impairs local blood flow and can lead to necrosis and perforation. Inflammation and infection result from normal bacteria invading the devitalized wall. Mild cases of appendicitis can heal spontaneously, but severe inflammation can lead to a ruptured appendix, which can cause local or generalized peritonitis.

ASSESSMENT

Signs and symptoms/physical findings: Vary because of differences in anatomy, size, and age. Physical assessment is performed in four steps— (1) inspection, (2) auscultation, (3) percussion, and (4) palpation—in that order, to delay stimulating the abdomen by palpation and percussion, which can affect bowel sounds.

Early stage: Onset of abdominal pain usually occurs in either the epigastric or the umbilical area, and the pain may be vague and diffuse or associated with mild cramping. Abdominal discomfort is accompanied by fever and nausea. Vomiting is not always present.

Intermediate (acute) stage: Over a period of a few hours, pain shifts from the midabdomen or epigastrium to the right lower quadrant (RLQ) at McBurney's point (approximately 2 inches from the anterior superior iliac spine on a line drawn from the umbilicus) and is aggravated by walking, coughing, and movement. Pain may be accompanied by a sensation of constipation (gas-stoppage sensation). Anorexia, malaise, occasionally diarrhea, and diminished peristalsis also can occur.

Patient experiences pain in the RLQ elicited by *light* palpation of the abdomen; presence of rebound tenderness; RLQ guarding, rigidity, and muscle spasms; tachycardia; low-grade fever; absent or diminished bowel sounds; and pain elicited with rectal examination. A palpable, tender mass may be felt in the peritoneal pouch if the appendix lies within the pelvis.

Acute appendicitis with perforation: Increasing, generalized pain; recurrence of vomiting. Patient usually exhibits temperature increases to more than 38.5° C (101.4° F) and generalized abdominal rigidity. Typically, patient remains rigid with flexed knees. Presence of abscess can result in a tender, palpable mass. The abdomen may be distended.

History and risk factors: Occurs at any age but is most common in children and tends to occur on its own, with no particular causes related to lifestyle or genetics.

DIAGNOSTIC TESTS

WBC with differential: Reveals presence of leukocytosis and an increase in neutrophils. A shift to the left with more than 75% neutrophils is a consistent finding in later stages of appendicitis.

Urinalysis: Rules out genitourinary conditions mimicking appendicitis; may reveal microscopic hematuria and pyuria. Analysis results usually are normal.

Abdominal x-ray examination: May reveal presence of a fecalith. About half of these patients may have x-ray findings of localized air-fluid levels, increased soft tissue density in the RLQ, and indications of localized ileus. If perforation has occurred, the presence of free air is noted. Barium enemas do not aid in diagnosis.

IV pyelogram (IVP): May be performed to rule out ureteral stone or pyelitis.

Abdominal ultrasound: May be done to rule out appendicitis or conditions that mimic it, such as Crohn's disease (CD), diverticulitis, or gastroenteritis.

Abdominal CT scan: Has high accuracy rate overall and is often used instead of or in addition to abdominal x-ray examination.

COLLABORATIVE MANAGEMENT

Preoperative Care

Bed rest: For observation.

Nothing-by-mouth (NPO) status: Parenteral fluids begun if surgery is imminent.

Pharmacotherapy

Opioids: For pain but usually not given until diagnosis is made so symptoms are not masked.

Antibiotics: Prevent systemic infection.

Tranquilizing agents: For sedation.

Gastric tube: Inserted for gastric suction and lavage, if needed.

Surgery

Appendectomy: Performed as soon as diagnosis is confirmed and fluid imbalance and systemic reactions have been controlled. The appendix is removed through an incision made over McBurney's point or through a right paramedian incision. In the presence of abscess, rupture, or peritonitis, an incisional drain is inserted.

Laparoscopic appendectomy incidental to gynecologic procedures (e.g., endometriosis involving the appendix) or for acute or chronic appendicitis (in the absence of rupture or signs of peritonitis) is as effective as open laparotomy. Advantages to this technique over traditional surgery include earlier ambulation and hospital discharge, decreased risk of wound infection, improved cosmesis, and less pain.

Postoperative Care

Activities: Ambulation on day of surgery. Patient may be hospitalized for 1-2 days and frequently recovers in extended recovery units with discharge on postoperative day 1 or 2 if no complications have developed. Normal activities are resumed 2-3 wk after surgery.

Diet: Advances from clear liquids to soft solids; parenteral fluids are continued if required.

Pharmacotherapy

Antibiotics: May be used prophylactically or in the presence of infection.

Mild laxatives: Given if necessary, but enemas continue to be contraindicated during first few postoperative weeks until adequate healing has occurred and bowel function has been restored.

Analgesics: For postoperative pain.

NURSING DIAGNOSES AND INTERVENTIONS

Risk for infection related to inadequate primary defenses (danger of rupture, peritonitis, abscess formation) secondary to inflammatory process

Desired outcomes: Patient is free of infection as evidenced by normothermia, heart rate (HR) 100 beats per minute (bpm) or less, BP at least 90/60 mm Hg, respiratory rate (RR) 12-20 breaths/min with normal depth and pattern of respirations (eupnea), absence of chills, soft and nondistended abdomen, and bowel sounds 5-34/min in each abdominal quadrant. Following instruction, patient verbalizes rationale for not administering enemas or laxatives preoperatively and enemas postoperatively and demonstrates compliance with the therapeutic regimen.

Nursing Interventions

- Assess and document quality, location, and duration of pain. Be alert to pain that becomes accentuated and generalized or to presence of recurrent vomiting, and note whether patient assumes side-lying or supine position with flexed knees. *Any of these signs can signal worsening appendicitis, which can lead to rupture.* Be alert to pain that worsens and then disappears. *This is a signal that rupture may have occurred.*
- Monitor for ambulation with a limp or pain with hip extension. *Retrocecal abscess may irritate the psoas muscle as it traverses the area of posterior RLQ of the abdomen and result in pain with hip extension.*
- Monitor VS for elevated temperature, increased pulse rate, hypotension, and shallow/rapid respirations; assess abdomen for presence of rigidity, distention, and decreased or absent bowel sounds. *These can occur with rupture.* Report significant findings to health care provider.
- Caution patient about the danger of preoperative self-treatment with enemas and laxatives. *This is because they increase peristalsis, which increases risk of perforation.* If constipation occurs postoperatively, health care provider may prescribe laxatives/stool softeners at bedtime after the third day. Remind patient that enemas should be avoided until approved by health care provider (usually several weeks after surgery). Teach anti-constipation diet with added roughage and fluid intake.
- Teach postoperative incisional care, as well as care of drains if patient is to be discharged with them.
- Provide instructions for prescribed antibiotics if patient is to be discharged with them.
- See "Peritonitis," p. 461, for more information.

Acute pain (with nausea) related to inflammatory process
Desired outcomes: Within 1-2 hr of pain-relieving intervention, patient's subjective perception of pain decreases, as documented by pain scale. Objective indicators, such as grimacing, are absent or diminished.

Nursing Interventions

- Assess and document quality, location, and duration of pain. Devise a pain scale with patient, rating discomfort from 0 (no pain) to 10 (worst pain). Be aware of characteristics of discomfort during the following stages of appendicitis.
  - *Early stage:* Abdominal pain (either epigastric or umbilical) that may be vague and diffuse, nausea and vomiting, fever, and sensitivity over appendix area.
  - *Intermediate (acute) stage:* Pain that shifts from epigastrium to RLQ at McBurney's point (approximately 2 inches from anterior superior iliac spine on a line drawn from umbilicus) and is aggravated by walking or coughing. The pain may be accompanied by a sensation of constipation (gas-stoppage sensation). Anorexia, malaise, occasional diarrhea, and diminished peristalsis also can occur.
  - *Acute appendicitis with perforation:* Increasing, generalized pain; recurrence of vomiting; increasing abdominal rigidity.
- Medicate with antiemetics, sedatives, and analgesics as prescribed; evaluate and document patient's response, using the pain scale. Encourage patient to request medication before symptoms become severe.

- Keep patient on NPO status before surgery; after surgery, nausea and vomiting usually disappear. If prescribed, insert gastric tube. *This is for decompression.*
- Teach technique for slow, diaphragmatic breathing. *This is to reduce stress and help relax tense muscles.*
- Help position patient for optimal comfort. *Many patients find comfort in a side-lying position with knees bent, whereas others find relief when supine with pillows under knees.* Avoid pressure on popliteal area.

 Patient-Family Teaching and Discharge Planning

When providing patient-family teaching, include verbal and written information about the following:

- Medications, including drug names, dosage, purpose, schedule, precautions, and potential side effects. Also discuss drug/drug, food/drug, and herb/drug interactions
- Care of incision, including dressing changes and bathing restrictions if appropriate.
- Indicators of infection: fever, chills, incisional pain, redness, swelling, and purulent drainage.
- Postsurgical activity precautions: avoid lifting heavy objects (more than 10 lb) for the first 6 wk or as directed, be alert to and rest after symptoms of fatigue, get maximum rest, gradually increase activities to tolerance.
- Importance of avoiding enemas for the first few postoperative weeks. Caution patient about need to check with health care provider before using an enema.

❖ ❖ ❖

SECTION THREE **INTESTINAL INFLAMMATORY PROCESSES**

❖ DIVERTICULOSIS AND DIVERTICULITIS

OVERVIEW/PATHOPHYSIOLOGY

Diverticulosis is characterized by acquired small pouches or sacs (diverticula) in the colon formed by herniation of mucosal and submucosal linings through the muscular layers of the intestine. Although diverticula can be found anywhere in the colon, they are most often found in the sigmoid colon because it is the narrowest part of the colon; harbors the firmest stool; and, as a result, must generate higher intraluminal pressures than in the rest of the colon. It is theorized that diverticula develop secondary to a low-residue (low-fiber) diet and increased intracolonic pressure, such as that created with straining to have a bowel movement. Diverticular disease is common in Western countries but uncommon in countries, such as Asia, where high-fiber diets are the norm. Prevalence of colonic diverticula increases with age, from about 5% at 40 yr of age, to 30% at 60 yr of age, to 65% by 85 yr of age. Men and women are equally affected.

Diverticulitis is a complication of diverticulosis. It is an inflammatory process that is theorized to begin with a single diverticulum, followed by trapping of in the sigmoid colon, to be caused by the irritating presence of trapped and fecal material within the diverticulum, resulting in irritation of the bowel wall. When the obstructing fecal plug *(fecalith)* remains and bacteria proliferate, inflammation can spread from the thin wall at the apex of the diverticulum to peridiverticular tissue. This inflammatory process creates edema that may compromise blood flow to the diverticulum, with resulting tissue ischemia. If unrelieved, tissue ischemia eventually may allow perforation of the diverticulum. The resulting infection can be localized (diverticular abscess) or more extensive (peritonitis) and life-threatening. Intestinal obstruction or an internal fistula from the inflamed segment of the colon to surrounding hollow organs also can develop.

ASSESSMENT

Signs and symptoms/physical findings: Presence of tender, palpable mass, usually in the left lower quadrant (LLQ); rebound tenderness secondary to infection or abscess formation; abdominal distention; hypoactive or hyperactive bowel sounds; and, possibly, absence of stool on rectal examination. Often the patient assumes a side-lying position with knees flexed to relieve pain. Tachycardia, hypotension, and shallow respirations can be present if there is severe abdominal discomfort. With massive hemorrhage, the presenting symptom may be hypovolemic shock.

Diverticulosis: Lower gastrointestinal (GI) bleeding that may be minute or may manifest as massive hemorrhage (hematochezia) that can be life-threatening. Such hemorrhage is usually self-limiting. Other findings include symptoms of irritable bowel syndrome, such as steady or crampy abdominal pain in the LLQ associated with alternating constipation or diarrhea and increased flatulence. Up to 80% of patients may be asymptomatic.

Diverticulitis: See the indicators for diverticulosis. Pain may be mild to severe, crampy or aching, or described as similar to that of appendicitis, only occurring in the LLQ. Cecal diverticulitis presents with findings similar to those in appendicitis. Passing flatus or stool may reduce pain. In addition, fever, nausea, vomiting, and obstipation can be present if obstruction or peritonitis occurs. Fistulas to the bladder, vagina, or skin and gas or stool elimination from the involved site also may be present.

History and risk factors: Low-fiber diet, high intake of red meat, chronic dehydration, colonic spasms, constipation, increasing age, and conditions that cause weakness in colon wall (e.g., Marfan syndrome).

DIAGNOSTIC TESTS
Diverticulosis

Barium enema: Determines presence and number of diverticula.
CBC: Determines whether anemia is present.
Rigid sigmoidoscopy or colonoscopy: Reveals presence of diverticula, thickening of bowel wall, diverticular openings, and stricture (decrease in intraluminal size from scarring following repeated attacks). If multiple diverticula or strictures are found at the beginning of the procedure, the procedure may be aborted because of potential for perforation. The patient then may undergo barium enema or computed tomography (CT) colography. Sigmoidoscopy and colonoscopy are contraindicated during acute attacks.

Diverticulitis

Abdominal x-ray examination: Determines presence of abnormal gas and fluid levels, which collect in the intestine above the affected area of the colon and indicate the presence and degree of bowel obstruction or ileus, and reveals presence of free air in the peritoneal cavity that signals noncontainment of diverticular perforation. These films also may show the presence of air in the urinary bladder if a colovesical fistula is present.
CBC with differential: Usually reveals leukocytosis with a shift to the left and increased neutrophils, indicating presence of infection. Critical value: WBCs greater than 30,000/mm^3.
Blood culture: May reveal presence of bacteremia in severely ill patients.
Urinalysis: Rules out bladder involvement; may show RBCs and WBCs in the presence of colovesical fistula.

Barium enema: Supports diagnosis of diverticulitis by demonstrating the presence of barium outside the lumen of the colon or outside a diverticulum, fistula or fistulas leading from the colon, intramural abscess, or pericolic mass. This examination should be deferred during the acute phase of illness if perforation is suspected. Water-soluble agents can be used if risk of perforation is great or fistula formation is suspected.

CT scan: Demonstrates diverticula, changes in the colon wall that indicate diverticulitis (effacement of pericolonic fat), and related abscesses and fistulas. Oral or IV contrast may be used to enhance imaging. Because this examination is noninvasive, it can be used in acutely ill or septic individuals for whom barium enema studies can be hazardous. CT scan also can be combined with percutaneous drainage of localized abscesses in selected patients.

GI bleeding scan (technetium-99m–sulfur colloid, technetium-99m–labeled RBCs) and mesenteric angiography: Identifies active bleeding sites during lower GI hemorrhage.

MRI and ultrasound: May aid in clarifying abnormal findings.

COLLABORATIVE MANAGEMENT
Diverticulosis

The goal of medical therapy for uncomplicated disease is to relieve symptoms and prevent or postpone complications, with the focus on increasing dietary fiber and providing medication therapy.

High-residue high-fiber diet: Including fruits and vegetables and use of wheat bran in the form of 100% bran cereal or 2 tbsp/day (10-25 g/day) of unprocessed bran, to increase moisture content of the stool and thus soften stool to promote elimination and reduce intracolonic pressure (Box 7-1). Fluid intake also should be encouraged (2500-3000 mL/day).

Pharmacotherapy

Bulk laxatives (e.g., psyllium [Metamucil] 1-2 tsp orally twice daily): Can replace bran in the diet.

Diverticulitis

The goal of medical therapy is to rest the bowel, resolve infection and inflammation, and prevent or decrease severity of complications. More than 70% of patients improve with medical therapy.

For outpatients: For outpatients (mild symptoms and no peritoneal signs), the following treatment plan is indicated.

Clear liquid diet with no or low-fiber intake: Promotes bowel rest. Diet may be advanced when symptoms improve, usually in 2 to 3 days.

Pharmacotherapy

Oral antibiotics (e.g., amoxicillin plus clavulanate potassium, metronidazole plus either ciprofloxacin or trimethoprim-sulfamethoxazole): Treat infection. Broad-spectrum antibiotics with anaerobic activity should be continued for 7 to 10 days or until patient is afebrile for 3 to 5 days.

For *hospitalized patients* with diverticulitis: Patients may need hospitalization if high fever, leukocytosis, or peritoneal signs are present. For these patients, the following treatment plan is Indicated.

Bed rest and NPO status: Promote physical, emotional, and bowel rest.

Gastric suction: Relieves nausea, vomiting, or abdominal distention if present.

Parenteral replacement of fluids, electrolytes, and blood products: As indicated by laboratory test results to maintain intravascular volumes, electrolyte and acid-base balance, urinary output, and caloric intake.

Pharmacotherapy

Parenteral antibiotics (e.g., an aminoglycoside plus metronidazole or a second- or third-generation cephalosporin): Limit secondary infection. Broad-spectrum antibiotics with both aerobic and anaerobic activity should be continued for 7 to 10 days.

Analgesics (e.g., meperidine): Relieve pain. Meperidine produces analgesia and decreases GI motility and spasm. Use of morphine and other opiates is contraindicated because they increase intraluminal pressure in the sigmoid colon and thus potentially increase risk of perforation.

Percutaneous drainage of abscesses: Localized abdominal abscess can be drained with a percutaneous catheter placed by an interventional radiologist. If ineffective, colonic resection may be required.

Emergency diverting colostomy: In severely unstable patients (e.g., those with advanced peritonitis), a transverse colostomy for stool diversion can be created using local anesthesia. This procedure creates a "double-barreled" colostomy; the proximal barrel empties stool from the GI tract, whereas the distal barrel (or mucous fistula) allows rest of the distal diseased colon. After patient stabilizes, more definitive surgery may be performed. Hartmann's procedure involves removal of the inflamed bowel, creation of a temporary colostomy, and temporary closure of the distal colon. After 3-6 mo, the patient returns for takedown of the temporary colostomy and reanastomosis to the distal colon. Referral to wound, ostomy, and continence (WOC)/enterostomal therapy (ET) nurse should be initiated as soon as surgery with resulting ostomy is anticipated or immediately postoperatively.

NURSING DIAGNOSES AND INTERVENTIONS

Ineffective health maintenance (for patients with diverticulosis) related to need for increased dietary fiber and fluid intake

Desired outcome: Before hospital or outpatient clinic discharge, patient verbalizes understanding of recommendations and rationale for increased dietary fiber and fluid intake.

Nursing Interventions

- Teach patient that the National Research Council advises increasing fiber intake by consuming five or more servings of fresh fruits and vegetables and six or more servings of legumes, whole-grain breads, and cereals per day. The American Dietetic Association recommends 20-35 g of fiber daily.
- Teach patient that inadequate fluid intake in the presence of a high-bulk diet may lead to constipation. Emphasize importance of maintaining a fluid intake of 2500-3000 mL/day to provide adequate fluids.

 Patient-Family Teaching and Discharge Planning

When providing patient-family teaching, include verbal and written information about the following:

- Medications, including drug names, rationale, dosage, schedule, precautions, and potential side effects. Also discuss drug/drug, herb/drug, and food/drug interactions.
- Signs and symptoms that necessitate medical attention, including fever; nausea or vomiting; cloudy or malodorous urine; diarrhea or constipation; change in stoma color from the normal bright and shiny red; peristomal skin irritation; and incisional pain, increased local skin temperature, drainage, swelling, or redness.
- Importance of a normal diet that includes all food groups (meat, eggs, and fish; fruits and vegetables; milk and cheese; cereal and breads) and drinking adequate fluids (at least 2500-3000 mL/day). Also teach patient to add fiber to diet in the form of uncooked fruits and vegetables, and whole-grain cereals with addition of bran in the form of 100% bran cereal or 2 tbsp/day of coarse, unprocessed bran, which can be taken with milk or juice or sprinkled over cereal. Because bran initially may cause abdominal distention and excessive flatus, instruct patient to begin with 1 tbsp/day and increase gradually over a period of 6 to 8 wk. Caution patient to avoid nuts and berries and foods with seeds.

- Gradual resumption of activities of daily living (ADL), excluding heavy lifting (more than 10 lb), pushing, or pulling for 6 wk to prevent development of incisional herniation.
- Care of incision, dressing changes, and permission to take baths or showers once sutures and drains are removed. (Some surgeons may allow showers with sutures still in place.)
- Care of stoma and peristomal skin, if applicable; use of ostomy skin barriers, pouches, and accessory equipment; and method for obtaining supplies.
- Importance of follow-up care with health care provider; confirm date and time of next appointment.
- Referral to community resources, including WOC/ET nurse, local ostomy organization, and home health care agency. Additional resources include:

National Institutes of Health: www.nlm.nih.gov/medlineplus/tutorials/colostomy/ htm/index.htm

United Ostomy Association of America: www.uoaa.org

❖ POLYPS/FAMILIAL ADENOMATOUS POLYPOSIS

OVERVIEW/PATHOPHYSIOLOGY

Polypoid colon tumors may be single or multiple, sessile or pedunculated. The adenomatous polyp is the most common clinical. The histologic type significance of these polyps derives from their tendency to become malignant. Familial adenomatous polyposis (FAP) is characterized by, but distinct from, frequent colon polyp formation. FAP is also known as familial polyposis coli and adenomatous polyposis coli. In this disorder, the glandular epithelia of the colon and rectum undergo excessive proliferation throughout the mucous membranes, leading to formation of sessile or pedunculated polyps. These are soft and red or purplish red, vary in size from a few millimeters to several centimeters, and range in number from a few to several thousand. They can be found anywhere along the entire length of the colon, but the rectum is almost always involved. Every individual with untreated familial polyposis will develop cancer because at some point in time one or more of these polyps will undergo malignant degeneration. This is a hereditary disease passed from generation to generation as an autosomal dominant trait, and it appears most often during late childhood through the early 30s. The hallmark is development of more than 100 adenomatous polyps in the colon.

ASSESSMENT

Signs and symptoms/physical findings

Polyps: Generally no symptoms but may have blood in stool.

FAP: Mild, early symptoms, such as diarrhea or melena, although many patients remain asymptomatic for years. Once malignant degeneration has begun, these symptoms become more pronounced, and there can be intermittent or constant colicky pain. Tenesmus and a frequent urge to defecate also may be features. If blood loss is significant, anemia, weight loss, loss of appetite, and fatigue can occur. In the presence of a well-developed malignant growth, a mass can be palpated on abdominal examination. Digital rectal examination may detect the presence of polyps.

History and risk factors

Polyps: Polyp development is related to chronic constipation or other colon problems and low-fiber diet.

FAP: Family history of FAP, mild colicky abdominal discomfort with or without diarrhea, the presence of blood in stools.

DIAGNOSTIC TESTS

Genetic testing: Confirms diagnosis of FAP and determines which at-risk individuals should undergo colon evaluation and appropriate regular colon screenings by proctosigmoidoscopy or colonoscopy.

Proctosigmoidoscopy or colonoscopy: Visualizes polyposis.

Biopsy: Confirms diagnosis. Histopathologic criteria for malignant potential are polyp size, histologic type, and degree of dysplasia.

X-ray examination with barium enema and air contrast: Determines disease extent.

CBC: Detects presence of anemia.

COLLABORATIVE MANAGEMENT

Because colorectal cancer is inevitable, appearing approximately 10-15 yr after onset of polyposis if the colon is not removed, surgical resection is the treatment of choice for FAP. Once the diagnosis has been made, it is not advisable to delay surgery. (Polyps generally develop by a mean age of 15 yr, and adenomatous polyps develop by the age of 35 yr. Colorectal cancer will develop by age 50 yr if colectomy is not performed.)

Proctocolectomy: Surgical cure via removal of colon and rectum with continent (Kock) ileostomy, conventional (Brooke) ileostomy, or ileoanal reservoir (ileal pouch anal anastomosis [IPAA]) for fecal diversion (see "Fecal Diversions," p. 491). Referral to a wound, ostomy, and continence (WOC)/enterostomal therapy (ET) nurse should be initiated as soon as surgery is anticipated.

Colectomy with preservation of rectum and ileorectal anastomosis: After this procedure, follow-up proctoscopies are necessary at frequent intervals to assess the rectum for further evidence of disease or malignant changes and fulguration of polyps.

Radiation or chemotherapy: May be indicated as adjuvant therapy or for advanced malignant disease.

Nonsteroidal antiinflammatory drugs (NSAIDs) and selective cyclooxygenase-2 inhibitors (COX-2 selective agents): These agents have demonstrated effectiveness in polyp suppression and promotion of adenoma regression. Effective polyp control may delay need for eventual proctectomy and possibly reduce cancer risk. Although it may be premature to recommend these agents for primary treatment of unoperated FAP, they may be useful for patients who have had colectomy with ileorectal anastomosis, in order to decrease the number and size of polyps in the rectal stump.

NURSING DIAGNOSES AND INTERVENTIONS

Ineffective health maintenance related to need for increased dietary fiber and fluid intake

Desired outcome: Before hospital discharge, patient verbalizes understanding of recommendations and rationale for increased dietary fiber and fluid intake and sources of dietary insoluble fiber.

Nursing Interventions

◆ Instruct patients that the National Research Council advises increasing fiber intake by consuming five or more servings of fresh fruits and vegetables and six or more servings of legumes, whole-grain breads, and cereals per day. The American Dietetic Association recommends 20-35 g of fiber daily.

◆ Explain that increased insoluble fiber is important. *This is because it seems to reduce exposure of the bowel mucosa to potential carcinogens by reducing intestinal transit time and diluting carcinogens in bulky stools.*

◆ Teach sources of insoluble dietary fiber (e.g., wheat bran; navy, kidney, pinto, and lima beans; skins of fruits and vegetables; raspberries and strawberries; sesame and poppy seeds). *This is so patient can understand how many foods contain fiber and that choices are available.*

◆ Emphasize importance of maintaining a fluid intake of 2500-3000 mL/day to provide adequate fluids. *This is because inadequate fluid intake in the presence of a high-bulk diet may lead to constipation.*

Health-seeking behaviors related to recommendations for follow-up diagnostic care after colon resection or polypectomy for malignant polyps
Desired outcome: Before hospital discharge, patient and/or significant other verbalize accurate information about recommendations for follow-up diagnostic care.

Nursing Interventions

For patients who have had colorectal cancer resection

◆ Teach that colonoscopy is recommended 6-12 mo after surgery, followed by yearly colonoscopy for 2 consecutive yr; if results of the aforementioned are negative, colonoscopy or air contrast barium enema (ACBaE) plus proctosigmoidoscopy is performed every 3 yr thereafter.
◆ Explain that fecal occult blood testing is performed every year.
◆ Remind patient that serum carcinoembryonic antigen (CEA) levels are measured at regular intervals (three times at 6-mo intervals, then annually for 5 yr).

For postpolypectomy patients with malignant polyps

◆ Teach that a colonoscopy is performed within 6 mo of polypectomy; if results of this second examination are negative, colonoscopy is performed every 2 yr. However, if the second examination result is positive, colonoscopy is performed at yearly intervals until negative, and then colonoscopy is performed at 2-yr intervals.
◆ Explain that fecal occult blood testing is performed between colonoscopies.

Patient-Family Teaching and Discharge Planning

When providing patient-family teaching, include verbal and written information about the following:

◆ Importance of informing all close family members that because familial polyposis is inherited, periodic examinations of rectum and colon are essential. Genetic testing may be considered.
◆ Medications, including drug names, rationale, dosage, schedule, precautions, and potential side effects. Also discuss drug/drug, herb/drug, and food/drug interactions.
◆ Signs and symptoms that necessitate medical attention, including fever, nausea and vomiting, diarrhea, or constipation.
◆ If an intestinal stoma is present, importance of reporting change in stoma color from the normal bright and shiny red; presence of peristomal skin irritation; and incisional pain, local increased temperature, drainage, swelling, or redness.
◆ Importance of a normal diet that includes all food groups (meat, eggs, and fish; fruits and vegetables; milk, yogurt, and cheese; and cereals and breads) with recommendations for increasing dietary fiber intake and fluids (at least 2500-3000 mL/day).
◆ Enteral or parenteral feeding instructions if patient is to supplement diet or is on NPO status.
◆ Gradual resumption of activities of daily living (ADL), excluding heavy lifting (more than 10 lb), pushing, or pulling for 6 wk to prevent incisional herniation.
◆ Care of incision and perianal wounds, including dressing changes, and bathing once sutures and drains are removed. Sitz baths may be recommended for perianal wound.

- If stoma is present, care of stoma and peristomal skin; use of ostomy skin barriers, pouches, and accessory equipment; and method for obtaining supplies.
- Importance of follow-up care with health care provider (or WOC/ET nurse if appropriate); confirm date and time of next appointment.
- Recommendations for follow-up diagnostic care after colon resection or polypectomy.
- Referral to community resources, including home health care agency, and, if appropriate, WOC/ET nurse. Additional resources include:

United Ostomy Association of America: www.uoaa.org

❖ ULCERATIVE COLITIS

OVERVIEW/PATHOPHYSIOLOGY

Ulcerative colitis (UC) is a nonspecific, chronic inflammatory disease of the mucosa and submucosa of the colon. Generally the disease begins in the rectum and sigmoid colon, but it can extend proximally and uninterrupted as far as the cecum. In many cases, the rectum (proctitis) or rectosigmoid colon (proctosigmoiditis) is affected; but the disease may extend to the splenic flexure (left-sided or distal colitis); in some cases, the disease extends proximally to involve the entire colon (pancolitis). A few centimeters of distal ileum may also be affected. This is sometimes referred to as *backwash ileitis,* and it occurs in only a small number of patients with UC involving the entire colon. In a majority of patients, extent of colonic involvement is maintained from onset through the disease course, with the patient experiencing flare-ups and remissions. UC initially affects the mucosal layer. Eventually, small mucosal layer abscesses form that ultimately penetrate the submucosa and spread horizontally, allowing sloughing of the mucosa, thus creating ulcerative lesions. The muscular layer (muscularis) generally is not affected, but the serosal layer may show congested and dilated blood vessels.

The cause of UC is unknown, but theories posit an interaction of external agents, host responses, and genetic immunologic factors creating the pathogenic responses. In a genetically susceptible subject, an outside agent or substance, such as a bacterium, virus, or other antigen, interacts with the body's immune system to trigger the disease or may cause damage to the intestinal wall, thereby initiating or accelerating the disease process. The resulting inflammatory response continues unregulated by the immune system. As a result, inflammation continues to damage the intestinal wall, resulting in symptoms of UC.

UC can occur at any age, but it is generally diagnosed in the third decade of life, with a second peak in the fifth and sixth decades. There is no difference in gender distribution; however, men are more likely than women to be diagnosed in the fifth and sixth decades of life. Incidence is higher in the white population and in Ashkenazi Jews than in nonwhite populations and in people of non-Jewish descent. UC is more prevalent in urban areas and developed countries with temperate climates than in rural areas and more southern countries. It is more common in nonsmokers and former smokers, a finding suggesting that smoking has a protective effect and may decrease the severity of symptoms. Appendectomy before age 20 yr may reduce risk (**TABLE 7-2**).

ASSESSMENT

Signs and symptoms/physical findings: Bloody diarrhea (the cardinal symptom). The clinical picture can vary from acute episodes with frequent discharge of watery stools mixed with blood, pus, and mucus, accompanied by fever, abdominal pain, rectal urgency, and tenesmus, to loose or frequent stools, to formed stools coated with a little blood. However, nearly two-thirds of patients have crampy abdominal pain and varying degrees of fever,

TABLE 7-2	COMPARISON OF FEATURES OF ULCERATIVE COLITIS AND CROHN'S DISEASE	
FEATURE	**ULCERATIVE COLITIS**	**CROHN'S DISEASE**
Incidence		
Age at onset	Any age, but 10-14 yr is most common	Any age, but 10-30 yr is most common
Family history	Less common	More common
Gender	Equal in men and women	Equal in men and women
Cancer risk	Increased	Increased
Pathophysiology		
Location of lesions	Colon and rectum	All of GI tract from mouth to anus
Inflammation/ulceration	Mucosal layer involved	Entire intestinal wall involved
Granulomas	Rare	Common
Thickened mesentery	Rare	Common
Fistulas and abscesses	Rare	Common
Strictures/obstruction	Rare	Common
Small bowel involvement	None	May occur
Clinical Manifestations		
Abdominal pain	Occasional	Common
Diarrhea	Common	Common
Bloody stools	Common	May occur
Abdominal mass	Rare	Common
Small intestine malabsorption	Rare	Common
Steatorrhea	Rare	Common
Potential for malignancy	Common	Common
Proctoscopy results	Involvement of rectum	Involvement of rectum may occur
Clinical course	Remissions/exacerbations	Remissions/exacerbations

GI, Gastrointestinal.
Modified from McCance KL, Huether SE: *Pathophysiology: the biologic basis for disease in adults and children,* ed 5, St Louis, Mosby, 2006.

vomiting, anorexia, weight loss, and dehydration. Remissions and exacerbations are common. Extracolonic manifestations also can occur, including polyarthritis, skin lesions (erythema nodosum, pyoderma gangrenosum), liver impairment, and ophthalmic complications (iritis, uveitis). Extracolonic manifestations may precede overt bowel disease, and their clinical activity may be related or unrelated to the clinical activity of the bowel disease.

With mild disease, there is no significant abdominal tenderness; left lower quadrant (LLQ) cramps are commonly relieved by defecation. With moderate disease, abdominal pain and tenderness may be present; mild fever (temperature 99°-100° F [37° C–38° C]), anemia (hematocrit [Hct] 30%-40%), and hypoalbuminemia (3.0-3.5 g/dL) may be present. With severe disease, abdominal pain and tenderness are characteristic, especially in the LLQ; distention and a tender, spastic anus also may be features; fever (temperature greater than 100° F [38° C]), severe anemia (Hct less than 30%), and impaired nutrition with hypoalbuminemia (less than 3.0 g/dL) and weight loss are present. On rectal examination, the mucosa may feel gritty, and the examining gloved finger may be covered with blood, mucus, or pus (Table 7-2).

History and risk factors: Duration of active disease more than 10 yr, pancolitis, and family history of colonic cancer, white race, and nonsmoker. The most firmly established risk factor for developing inflammatory bowel disease (IBD) is a positive family history. There is a 10-fold increase in risk of IBD in first-degree relatives of patients with UC. Individuals with UC develop colonic adenocarcinomas at 10 × the rate of the general population.

DIAGNOSTIC TESTS

Stool examination: Reveals presence of frank or occult blood. Stool cultures and smears rule out bacterial and parasitic disorders. Collect specimens before barium enema is performed.

Sigmoidoscopy: Reveals red, granular, hyperemic, and extremely friable mucosa; strips of inflamed mucosa undermined by surrounding ulcerations, which form pseudopolyps; and thick exudate composed of blood, pus, and mucus. Enemas should not be given before the examination because they can produce hyperemia and edema and may cause exacerbation of the disease. A limited prep may be given to facilitate visualization during exam.

Colonoscopy: Helps determine extent of the disease and differentiates UC from Crohn's disease (CD) through both endoscopic appearance and histologic examination of biopsy tissues. Serial colonoscopy is also performed to monitor patients with chronic UC at risk for colon carcinoma. This test may be contraindicated in patients with acute disease because of risk of perforation or hemorrhage.

Rectal biopsy: Aids in differentiating UC from carcinoma and other inflammatory processes.

Barium enema: Reveals mucosal irregularity from fine serrations to ragged ulcerations, narrowing and shortening of the colon, presence of pseudopolyps, loss of haustral markings, and presence of spasms and irritability. Double-contrast technique may facilitate detection of superficial mucosal lesions. With a double-contrast technique, barium is instilled into the colon as with a conventional barium enema, but most of the barium is then withdrawn, and the colon is inflated with air, a maneuver that causes a thin coating of barium to line the intestinal wall. The double-contrast technique has become the standard method for evaluating patients for colitis. Because they produce hyperemia and edema, which may cause exacerbation of the disease, irritant cathartics and enemas should not be given before the examination.

Abdominal plain x-ray (flat plate) examinations: An important tool for screening severely ill patients when colonoscopy and barium enema are contraindicated. An abdominal flat plate examination may reveal fecal residue, appearance of mucosal margins, widening or thickening of visible haustra, and colonic wall diameter. In patients with suspected ileus, obstruction, or perforation, the flat plate film reveals abnormal gas and fluid levels or presence of free air in the peritoneal cavity.

CT scan: Used to identify suspected complications of UC (i.e., toxic megacolon, pneumatosis coli).

Serum antibody testing: Several serum antibodies are being evaluated for aiding in the development of noninvasive diagnostic techniques for UC. Some of these tests have been found to be useful in differentiating UC from CD.

Radionuclide imaging: Used to identify extent of disease activity, especially when colonoscopy and barium enema are contraindicated. Injections of indium-111–labeled autologous leukocytes are used to identify areas of active inflammation.

Blood tests: Anemia, with hypochromic microcytic red blood indices in severe disease, usually is present because of blood loss, iron deficiency, and bone marrow depression. WBC count may be normal to markedly elevated in severe disease. Sedimentation rate usually is increased according to illness severity. Hypoalbuminemia and negative N state occur in moderately severe to severe disease and result from decreased protein intake, decreased albumin synthesis in the debilitated condition, and increased metabolic needs. Electrolyte imbalance is common; hypokalemia is often present because of colonic losses (diarrhea) and renal losses in patients taking high doses of corticosteroids. Bicarbonate may be decreased because of colonic losses and may signal metabolic acidosis.

COLLABORATIVE MANAGEMENT

Medical therapy is symptomatic. The goals are to terminate the acute attack, induce remission, maintain remission, maintain quality of life, and prevent complications related to both disease and therapy.

Parenteral replacement of fluids, electrolytes, and blood products: Maintains acutely ill patient, as indicated by laboratory test results.

Physical and emotional rest: Including bed rest and limitation of visitors.

Pharmacotherapy

Sedatives and tranquilizers: Promote rest and reduce anxiety.

Hydrophilic colloids (e.g., kaolin and pectin mixture) and anticholinergic and antidiarrheal preparations (e.g., tinctures of belladonna and opium, diphenoxylate hydrochloride, loperamide, codeine phosphate): Relieve cramping and diarrhea. Opiates and anticholinergics should be administered with extreme caution because they contribute to development of toxic megacolon.

Antiinflammatory agents (e.g., corticosteroids): Reduce mucosal inflammation. Dosage and routes of administration vary with disease severity and extent. In patients with mild disease limited to the rectum and sigmoid colon, rectal instillation of steroids (enema or suppository) may induce or maintain remission. In patients with more extensive (pancolonic) or more active disease, oral corticosteroid therapy with prednisone or prednisolone usually is initiated. In severely ill patients, IV corticosteroids are given. Once clinical remission is achieved, IV and oral corticosteroids are tapered until discontinuation because these medications have not been shown to prolong remission or prevent future exacerbations.

Aminosalicylates (e.g., sulfasalazine): Help maintain remissions. Sulfasalazine is effective in the treatment of mild to moderate attacks of UC and appears to decrease frequency of subsequent relapses. Sulfasalazine is considered inferior to corticosteroids in the treatment of severe attacks of disease; once remission has been attained by use of corticosteroid therapy, sulfasalazine appears to be superior to systemic corticosteroids in maintenance of remission.

When administered orally, sulfasalazine is broken down by colonic bacteria into its two constituents: 5-aminosalicylic acid (5-ASA), which is considered the active therapeutic component; and sulfapyridine, which is the carrier and responsible for side effects experienced by more than one-third of individuals receiving this drug. To avoid side effects of sulfapyridine, several agents have been developed using a variety of delivery mechanisms that allow release of the active agent in the colon or ileum. These agents include the 5-ASA derivatives: mesalamine (in enteric-coated and time-release forms), olsalazine, and balsalazide. These three agents are useful alternatives for patients unable to tolerate sulfapyridine; however, these agents have their own side effects.

Topical therapy with 5-ASA given by retention enemas for patients with proctosigmoiditis (involvement to 40 cm) and as suppositories for patients with proctitis has provided encouraging results. If relapses occur after cessation of interim topical therapy, maintenance therapy may be accomplished with 5-ASA enemas once a day or suppositories twice a day. Although the therapeutic benefit of 5-ASA enemas is the same as that achieved with hydrocortisone enemas, 5-ASA therapy is preferred because of systemic side effects from corticosteroids. A combination of mesalamine enema and oral mesalamine can be more effective than the oral form alone.

Immunosuppressive (immunomodulatory) therapy: Reduces inflammation in patients not responding to steroids and sulfasalazine and in patients unwilling or unable to undergo colectomy, or as an alternative to steroid dependency.

Immunosuppressive therapy has been used to maintain remission in patients with frequent relapses. Therapy for 3-6 mo may be required to achieve therapeutic response, and patients need to be closely monitored for hematologic toxicity.

Antibiotics: Limit secondary infection. Antibiotics are not indicated in the management of mild to moderate disease because infectious agents generally are not thought to be responsible for UC.

Nutritional management: Varies with patient's condition. In severely ill patients, total parenteral nutrition (TPN) along with nothing-by-mouth (NPO) status is prescribed to replace nutritional deficits while allowing complete bowel rest and improving patient's nutritional status before surgery. For less severely ill patients, a low-residue elemental diet provides good nutrition with low fecal volume to allow bowel rest. A bland, high-protein, high-calorie, low-residue diet with vitamin and mineral supplements and exclusion of raw fruits and vegetables provides good nutrition and decreases diarrhea. Milk and gluten products are restricted, to reduce cramping and diarrhea in patients with lactose and gluten intolerance (Box 7-1).

Biologic agents (e.g., infliximab): To control inflammation, heal mucous membranes, and eliminate the use of corticosteroids in patients with moderately to severely active colitis who have had poor response to therapy.

Probiotics: Restore balance to the intestinal environment by use of beneficial bacteria, with resulting reduction in inflammation. Health benefits appear to be strain-specific; *Lactobacillus acidophilus, Saccharomyces boulardii,* and VSL #3 (a proprietary blend of eight strains of bacteria) are most promising. Probiotics are available in capsule, powder, tablet, and liquid forms, as well as in live-culture yogurt (live-culture soy yogurt if patient is lactose-intolerant). Other than for "pouchitis," probiotics are effective in the colon only.

Fish oils: Decrease inflammation. Omega-3 fatty acids found in fish oil appear to benefit patients with active UC, but they do not appear effective in maintaining remission. They must be taken in large amounts.

Referral to mental health practitioner: As indicated for supportive psychotherapy for patient who has difficulty dealing with any type of chronic or disabling illness.

Surgical interventions: Indicated only when the disease is intractable to medical management or when patient develops a disabling complication. Total proctocolectomy cures UC and results in construction of a permanent fecal diversion, such as a Brooke ileostomy, continent (Kock pouch) ileostomy, or ileoanal reservoir, now more commonly referred to as ileal pouch anal anastomosis (IPAA). See "Fecal Diversions," p. 491, for additional details. Referral to a WOC/ET nurse should be initiated as soon as surgery is anticipated.

Postoperative management: Includes routine chest physiotherapy to prevent respiratory complications, IV fluid and electrolyte replacement or TPN as the patient's condition warrants, nasogastric (NG) tube for decompression until bowel sounds are present and patient is eliminating flatus or stool, gradual resumption of diet as tolerated following NG tube removal and return of bowel function, aseptic incisional care to prevent infection, and fecal diversion care and teaching. (Some surgeons are no longer inserting NG tubes and begin feeding patients soon after recovery from anesthesia.)

Referral to a wound, ostomy, and continence (WOC)/enterostomal therapy (ET) nurse: If referral was not initiated preoperatively.

NURSING DIAGNOSES AND INTERVENTIONS

Deficient fluid volume related to active loss secondary to diarrhea and GI bleeding/hemorrhage

Desired outcome: Patient is normovolemic within 24 hr of admission, as evidenced by balanced I&O, urine output 30 mL/hr or more, urine specific gravity less than 1.030, good skin turgor, moist mucous membranes, stable weight, BP 90/60 mm Hg or more (or within patient's normal range), and respiratory rate (RR) 12-20 breaths/min.

Nursing Interventions

♦ Monitor I&O and urine specific gravity; weigh patient daily; and monitor laboratory values. *This is to evaluate fluid, electrolyte, and hematologic status.* (Optimal values: serum K^+ 3.5 mEq/L or greater, Hct 40%-54% [male] and 37%-47% [female], Hgb 14-18 g/dL [male] and 12-16 g/dL [female], and BBC count of 4.5-6.0 million/mm^3 [male] and 4.0-5.5 million/mm^3 [female]. Critical values: K^+ less than 2.5 or greater than 6.5 mEq/L, Hct less than 15% or greater than 60%, and hemoglobin (Hgb) less than 5.0 g/dL or greater than 20 g/dL.)

♦ Monitor frequency and consistency of stool. For frequent bowel movements, keep a stool count; measure liquid stools. Assess and record presence of blood, mucus, fat, and undigested food.

♦ Monitor for thirst, poor skin turgor (may not be a reliable indicator of hydration in the older adult), dryness of mucous membranes, fever, and concentrated (specific gravity greater than 1.030) and decreased urinary output. *These are indicators of dehydration.*

♦ Monitor for hypotension, increased heart rate (HR) and RR, pallor, diaphoresis, and restlessness. Assess stool for quality (e.g., is it grossly bloody and liquid?) and quantity (e.g., is it mostly blood or mostly stool?). *These are signs of hemorrhage.* Report significant findings to health care provider.

♦ Maintain parenteral replacement of fluids, electrolytes, and vitamins as prescribed.

♦ Administer blood products and iron as prescribed. *This is to correct existing anemia and losses caused by hemorrhage.*

♦ Provide bland, high-protein, high-calorie, low-residue diet, as prescribed when patient is taking food orally. Determine incidence of cramping, diarrhea, and flatulence. *This assesses tolerance to diet.*

Ineffective protection related to risk of perforation secondary to deeply inflamed colonic mucosa
Desired outcome: Patient is free of signs of perforation, as evidenced by normothermia; HR 60-100 beats per minute (bpm); RR 12-20 breaths/min with normal depth and pattern of respirations (eupnea); normal bowel sounds; absence of abdominal distention, tympany, or rebound tenderness; negative culture results; no mental status changes, and orientation to person, place, and time.

Nursing Interventions

♦ Monitor for fever, chills, increased RR and HR, diaphoresis, and increased abdominal discomfort. *These findings can occur with perforation of the colon and potentially result in localized abscess or generalized fecal peritonitis and septicemia.* Assess patients on corticosteroid therapy carefully. *Systemic therapy with corticosteroids and antibiotics can mask the development of this complication.* Monitor patient's WBC count. *Patients with severe UC can have markedly elevated WBC counts: greater than 20,000/mm^3 and occasionally as high as 50,000/mm^3.* (Critical values: WBC counts less than 2500 or greater than 30,000/mm^3).

♦ Report any evidence of sudden abdominal distention associated with preceding symptoms. *They can signal toxic megacolon.* Note in particular patients with hypokalemia, barium enema examinations, and those on opiates and anticholinergics. *These factors can contribute to development of toxic megacolon.*

♦ If surgery is indicated, prepare patient and explain need for interventions. *Surgery to prevent perforation is indicated in patients with fulminant disease or toxic megacolon whose condition worsens or does not improve in 48-72 hr.*

♦ If patient has a sudden temperature elevation, culture blood and specimens from other sites as prescribed. Monitor culture reports, and notify health care provider promptly of any positive cultures.

- Administer antibiotics as prescribed and in a timely fashion.
- Evaluate mental status, orientation, and level of consciousness (LOC) q2-4h.

Acute pain (and nausea, and abdominal cramping) related to intestinal inflammatory process
Desired outcomes: Within 4 hr of intervention, patient's subjective perception of discomfort decreases as documented by pain scale. Objective indicators, such as grimacing, are absent or diminished.

Nursing Interventions

- Monitor and document characteristics of discomfort, and assess whether it is associated with ingestion of certain foods or medications or with emotional stress. Devise a pain scale with patient, rating discomfort from 0 (no pain) to 10 (worst pain). Eliminate foods that cause cramping and discomfort.
- As prescribed, maintain patient on NPO status or TPN. *This is to provide bowel rest.*
- Provide nasal and oral care at frequent intervals. *This is to lessen discomfort from NPO status or an NG tube.*
- Keep patient's environment quiet. Facilitate coordination of health care providers. *This is to provide rest periods between care activities.* Allow 90 min for undisturbed rest.
- Administer sedatives and tranquilizers as prescribed. *This is to promote rest and reduce anxiety.*
- Administer hydrophilic colloids, anticholinergics, and antidiarrheal medications as prescribed. *These help to relieve cramping and diarrhea.* Instruct the patient to request medication before discomfort becomes severe.
- Reassess patient and document degree of relief obtained, rated according to the pain scale.
- Observe for intensification of symptoms. *This can indicate the presence of complications.* Notify health care provider of significant findings.

Diarrhea related to inflammatory process of the intestines
Desired outcome: Patient's stools become normal in consistency, and frequency is lessened within 3 days of admission.

Nursing Interventions

- Monitor and record amount, frequency, and character of stools. When possible, measure liquid stools.
- Provide covered bedpan, commode, or bathroom that is easily accessible and ready to use at all times.
- Empty bedpan and commode immediately after use. *This is to control odor and decrease patient's anxiety and self-consciousness.*
- Administer hydrophilic colloids, anticholinergics, and antidiarrheal medications as prescribed. *This is to decrease fluidity and number of stools.*
- Administer topical corticosteroid preparations and antibiotics via retention enema, as prescribed. *This is to relieve local inflammation.* If patient has difficulty retaining the enema for the prescribed amount of time, consult health care provider about use of corticosteroid foam. *It is easier to retain and administer.*
- Monitor serum electrolytes, particularly K^+, for abnormalities. Alert health care provider to K^+ less than 3.5 mEq/L. *This can cause numbness, nausea, vomiting, palpitations, fainting confusion, or more serious symptoms.* (Critical value: serum K^+ less than 2.5 mEq/L.)

Risk for impaired skin integrity (perineal/perianal) related to persistent diarrhea

Desired outcome: Patient's perineal/perianal skin remains intact with no erythema.

Nursing Interventions

♦ Provide materials or assist patient with cleansing and drying perineal area after each bowel movement. Use a nonirritating cleansing agent.

♦ Apply protective skin care products (skin preparations, gels, or barrier films). *This is to prevent irritation from frequent liquid stools.*

♦ Administer hydrophilic colloids, anticholinergics, and antidiarrheal medications as prescribed. *This is to decrease fluidity and number of stools.*

 Patient-Family Teaching and Discharge Planning

When providing patient-family teaching, include verbal and written information about the following:

♦ Medications, including drug names, rationale, dosage, schedule, route of administration, precautions, and potential side effects. Also discuss drug/drug, herb/drug, and food/drug interactions. Caution patients receiving high-dose steroid therapy about abrupt discontinuation of steroids, to prevent precipitation of adrenal crisis. Withdrawal symptoms include weakness, lethargy, restlessness, anorexia, nausea, and muscle tenderness. Instruct patient to notify health care provider if these symptoms occur.

♦ Signs and symptoms that necessitate medical attention, including fever, nausea and vomiting, diarrhea or constipation, and any significant change in appearance and frequency of stools. Any of these findings can signal exacerbation of the disease.

♦ Dietary management to promote nutritional and fluid needs and prevent abdominal cramping, discomfort, and diarrhea.

♦ Importance of perineal care after bowel movements.

♦ Enteral or parenteral feeding instructions if patient is to supplement diet or is on NPO status.

♦ Importance of follow-up medical care, particularly for patients with long-standing disease, because many of them develop colonic adenocarcinoma.

♦ Referral to a mental health specialist if recommended by health care provider.

♦ Referral to community resources. Additional information can be found at:

Crohn's & Colitis Foundation of America, Inc.: www.ccfa.org

National Institutes of Health: www.nlm.nih.gov/medlineplus/ulcerativecolitis.html

Additional Teaching, if Patient Has a Fecal Diversion

♦ Care of incision, dressing changes, and permission to take baths or showers once sutures and drains are removed.

♦ Care of stoma, peristomal/perianal skin, or perineal wound; use of ostomy equipment; and method for obtaining supplies. Sitz baths may be indicated for perineal wound.

♦ Medications that are contraindicated (e.g., laxatives) or that may not be well tolerated or absorbed (e.g., antibiotics, enteric-coated tablets, long-acting tablets).

♦ Gradual resumption of activities of daily living (ADL), excluding heavy lifting (more than 10 lb), pushing, or pulling for 6-8 wk to prevent incisional herniation.

♦ Importance of reporting signs and symptoms that require medical attention, such as change in stoma color from the normal bright and shiny red; peristomal or perianal skin irritation; diarrhea; incisional pain, local increased temperature, drainage, swelling, or redness; signs and symptoms of fluid and electrolyte imbalance; and signs and symptoms of mechanical or functional obstruction.

◆ Referral to community resources, including home health care agency, WOC/ET nurse, and the local ostomy association. Additional information can be found at:

National Institutes of Health: www.nlm.nih.gov/medlineplus/ostomy.html

United Ostomy Association of America: www.uoaa.org

❖ CROHN'S DISEASE

OVERVIEW/PATHOPHYSIOLOGY

Crohn's disease (CD), also known as *regional enteritis, granulomatous colitis,* or *transmural colitis,* is a chronic inflammatory disease that can involve any part of the gastrointestinal (GI) tract from the mouth to the anus. Usually the disease occurs segmentally and demonstrates discontinuous areas of disease with segments of healthy bowel in between. In 45%-50% of cases, the end of the ileum and cecum/ascending colon are involved (ileocolitis); in 35% of cases, the terminal ileum is affected (ileitis); and in 20% of cases, the colon alone is affected (Crohn's colitis). Small numbers of patients have involvement of the jejunum, duodenum, stomach, esophagus, and mouth; in these cases, the ileum, colon, or both are also involved. Approximately 30%-35% of patients have perianal fistulas, fissures, or abscesses. The disease affects all layers of the bowel: the mucosa, submucosa, circular and longitudinal muscles, and serosa, thus predisposing to intestinal strictures and fistulas. A family history of this disease or ulcerative colitis (UC) occurs in 15%-20% of affected patients.

The cause of CD is unknown, but theories include infection, immunologic factors, environmental factors, and genetic predisposition. In a genetically susceptible subject, an outside agent or substance, such as a bacterium, virus, or other antigen, interacts with the body's immune system to trigger the disease or may cause damage to the intestinal wall that initiates or accelerates the disease process. The resulting inflammatory response continues unregulated by the immune system. As a result, inflammation continues to damage the intestinal wall and causes the symptoms of CD. The disease is generally diagnosed between the ages of 15 and 35 yr, but it also can occur in young children and in people 70 yr of age or older. Prevalence is slightly higher in women than in men. CD is seen more frequently in the white population and in Ashkenazi Jews than in nonwhite populations and in people of non-Jewish descent. It is more prevalent in urban areas and developed countries with temperate climates than in rural areas and more southern countries. However, increasing incidence is in Japan and South America (Table 7-2).

ASSESSMENT

Signs and symptoms/physical findings: Clinical presentation varies as a direct reflection of the location of the inflammatory process and its extent, severity, and relationship to contiguous structures. Sometimes onset is abrupt, and the patient can appear to have appendicitis, UC, intestinal obstruction, or fever of obscure origin. Acute manifestations include right lower quadrant (RLQ) pain, tenderness, spasm, flatulence, nausea, fever, and diarrhea. A more typical picture is insidious onset with more persistent but less severe symptoms, such as vague abdominal pain, unexplained anemia, and fever. Diarrhea—liquid, soft, or mushy stools—is the most common symptom. The presence of gross blood is rare. Abdominal pain is a common symptom, and it may be colicky or crampy, initiated by meals, centered in the lower abdomen, and relieved by defecation because of chronic partial obstruction of the small intestine, colon, or both. As the disease progresses, anorexia, malnutrition, weight loss, anemia, lassitude, malaise, and fever can occur in addition to fluid, electrolyte, and metabolic disturbances. See Table 7-2 for a comparison of UC and CD.

In early stages, examination is often normal but may demonstrate mild tenderness in the abdomen over the affected bowel. In more advanced disease, a palpable mass may be present, especially in the RLQ with terminal ileum involvement. Persistent rectal fissure, large ulcers, perirectal abscess, or rectal fistula is the first indication of disease in 15%-25% of patients with small bowel involvement and in 50%-75% of patients with colonic involvement. Rectovaginal, abdominal, and enterovesical fistulas also may develop. Extraintestinal manifestations characteristic of UC do occur, but less commonly (10%-20%).

History and risk factors: There is a 20-fold increase in risk of IBD in first-degree relatives of individuals with CD. Cigarette smoking has been shown to increase the risk of developing CD and is associated with resistance to medical therapy and recurrence of disease after surgery.

DIAGNOSTIC TESTS

Stool examination: Usually reveals occult blood; frank blood may be noted in stools of patients with colonic involvement or with ulcerations and fistulas of the rectum. A few patients have the presenting symptom of bloody diarrhea. Stool cultures and smears rule out bacterial and parasitic disorders. Specimens are also examined for fecal fat.

Sigmoidoscopy: Evaluates possible colonic involvement and obtains rectal biopsy. The finding of granulomas on mucosal biopsy argues strongly for the diagnosis of CD. However, because granulomas are more numerous in the submucosa, suction biopsy of the rectum provides deeper, larger, and less traumatized specimens for a better diagnostic yield than does mucosal biopsy obtained through an endoscope.

Colonoscopy: May help differentiate CD from UC. Characteristic patchy inflammation (skip lesion) rules out UC. However, colonoscopy usually does not add useful diagnostic information in the presence of positive findings from sigmoidoscopy or radiologic examination. When diagnosis is unclear and there is a question of malignancy, colonoscopy provides the means of directly visualizing mucosal changes and obtaining biopsies, brushings, and washings for cytologic examination. Colonoscopy also may assist in planning for surgery by documenting the extent of colonic disease. Because of risk of perforation, this procedure may be contraindicated in patients with acute phases of Crohn's colitis or when deep ulcerations or fistulas are known to be present.

Endoscopic ultrasonography: Aids in diagnosis of perirectal fistula and abscesses and in detecting transmural depth of inflammation in the bowel or esophagus, by using an endoscopically placed ultrasound probe.

Small bowel enteroscopy: Permits visualization of the upper GI tract to identify areas of inflammation and bleeding to the level of the midjejunum.

Wireless capsule: Permits visualization of the small intestine to identify abnormalities. The patient swallows a large capsule that contains a small disposable camera; images are transmitted to a receiver on the patient's waist. Use is contraindicated if strictures exist, because strictures can prevent the capsule from progressing through the intestine; surgical removal of the capsule may be required.

Barium enema and upper GI series with small bowel follow-through: Contribute to diagnosis of CD. Involvement of only the terminal ileum or segmental involvement of the colon or small intestine almost always indicates CD. Thickened bowel wall with stricture (string sign) separated by segments of normal bowel, cobblestone appearance, and presence of fistulas and skip lesions are common findings. A double-contrast barium enema technique may increase sensitivity in detecting early or subtle changes. Barium enema may be contraindicated in patients with acute phases of Crohn's colitis because of risk of perforation. Upper GI barium series is contraindicated in patients in whom intestinal obstruction is suspected.

CT scan: Complements information gathered via endoscopy and conventional radiography. In advanced disease, CT scanning clearly delineates extraluminal complications (e.g., abscess, phlegmon [a diffuse inflammatory process with exudate], bowel wall thickening, mesenteric inflammation). CT has been used also to percutaneously drain fistulas (colovesicular, enterovesicular, colovaginal, enterocolonic) and to evaluate perirectal disease, enterocutaneous fistula, and sinus tracts.

Serum antibody testing: In difficult to diagnose cases, may be helpful in differentiating CD from UC.

Radionuclide imaging: IV indium-111–labeled or technetium-99–labeled leukocytes migrate to areas of active inflammation and are then identified by scans performed after 4 and 24 hr. This procedure aids in differentiating CD from UC and in evaluating abscess and fistula formation.

Blood tests: Nonspecific for diagnosis of CD but help determine whether the inflammatory process is active and evaluate patient's overall condition. Anemia may be present and may be microcytic because of iron deficiency from chronic blood loss and bone marrow depression secondary to chronic inflammatory process or megaloblastic because of folic acid or vitamin B_{12} deficiency (usually seen only in patients with extensive ileitis causing malabsorption). Increased WBC count and sedimentation rate reflect disease activity and inflammation. Hypoalbuminemia corresponds with disease activity and results from decreased protein intake, extensive malabsorption, and significant enteric loss of protein. Hypokalemia is seen in patients with chronic diarrhea; hypophosphatemia and hypocalcemia are seen in patients with significant malabsorption. Findings on liver function studies may be abnormal as a consequence of pericholangitis.

Urinalysis and urine culture: May reveal urinary tract infection secondary to enterovesicular fistula.

Tests for malabsorption: Because patients with active, extensive disease (especially when it involves the small intestine) may develop malabsorption and malnutrition, the following tests are clinically significant: D-xylose tolerance test (for upper jejunal involvement); Schilling's test (for ileal involvement); serum albumin, carotene, calcium (Ca^{++}), and phosphorus levels; and fecal fat (steatorrhea). (See also "Malabsorption/Maldigestion," p. 453.)

COLLABORATIVE MANAGEMENT

Initial treatment is nonoperative, individualized, and based on symptomatic relief. Medical treatment is most likely to be successful early in the course of disease, before permanent structural changes have occurred.

Parenteral replacement of fluids, electrolytes, and blood products: Maintenance therapy for acute exacerbation as indicated by laboratory test results.

Physical and emotional rest: Complete bed rest and assistance with activities of daily living (ADL) during acute phases.

Pharmacotherapy

Sedatives and tranquilizers: Promote rest and reduce anxiety.

Antidiarrheal medications: Decrease diarrhea and cramping. Codeine or loperamide often reduces diarrhea with a concomitant decrease in abdominal cramping. Anticholinergics are not recommended because they may mask obstructive symptoms and precipitate toxic megacolon. For these reasons, antidiarrheal medications should be administered with caution. If patient does not respond appropriately to standard antidiarrheal medications and mild sedation, the presence of obstruction, bowel perforation, or abscess formation is suspected.

Aminosalicylates (e.g., sulfasalazines): Treat acute exacerbations of colonic and ileocolonic disease. Sulfasalazine appears to be more effective in patients with mild to moderate disease limited to the colon than in those with disease limited to the small bowel. Sulfasalazine has not been shown to prevent recurrence of CD, but patients who respond tend to benefit from long-term therapy and tend to relapse when the agent is discontinued. Because sulfasalazine impairs folate absorption, patients receive folic acid supplements during treatment.

5-Aminosalicylic acid (5-ASA) preparations (e.g., oral: mesalamine, olsalazine; topical: mesalamine): Used for maintenance therapy. These agents appear to be effective in preventing recurrence in patients who have recently undergone surgical resection.

Corticosteroids (may be oral, topical or parenteral): Reduce active inflammatory response, decrease edema in moderate to severe forms, and control exacerbations. Prednisone is effective in diminishing activity of the disease process but is more beneficial in patients with small bowel involvement than it is in those with disease limited to the colon. As active disease subsides, prednisone is tapered with the goal of eliminating the drug. However, many patients with CD become steroid dependent, meaning they are symptomatic with low-dose therapy (5-15 mg/day) or with total discontinuation of the drug. In some cases of chronic disease, continuous corticosteroid therapy may be necessary. Budesonide is a nonsystemic steroidal agent that reduces side effects seen with traditional steroids. It is approved for treatment of mild to moderate, active CD involving the ileum and cecum/ascending colon. It is used for flares but not commonly used for maintenance therapy. Topical therapy with hydrocortisone has controlled inflammation via retention enemas for patients with proctosigmoiditis (involvement to 40 cm), and suppositories have been used for patients with Crohn's proctitis.

Immunosuppressive immunomodulatory agents (e.g., azathioprine, 6-mercaptopurine [6-MP], cyclosporine, methotrexate): Allow dosage reduction or withdrawal of corticosteroids in steroid-dependent patients, for maintenance therapy with a lower relapse rate, and to aid in healing and reduce drainage of perianal fistulas. IV cyclosporine has been used to treat refractory CD and treatment-resistant fistulas. Oral cyclosporine has not proved effective for maintenance therapy because relapse occurs when dosage is reduced or stopped. Because of frequency and severity of toxicity and side effects, short-term IV administration has proved to be the best method for cyclosporine. Parenteral (intramuscular [IM], subcutaneous) methotrexate provides both immunosuppressive and antiinflammatory effects and allows for reduction or cessation of steroid therapy in some patients with chronically active CD.

Biologic agents (e.g., infliximab): Block tumor necrosis factor-α (TNF-α), a protein that escalates inflammation. One of these agents, infliximab, is approved for treatment and maintenance of remission in moderate to severe, active disease that is unresponsive to conventional therapy and for treatment and maintenance of remission in fistulizing disease. It is administered by the IV route. Infusion reactions have been reported, and a skin test for tuberculosis (TB) should be performed before therapy is initiated. Smoking may reduce response to infliximab.

Antibiotics (e.g., metronidazole, ciprofloxacin): Control suppurative complications (e.g., bacterial overgrowth) and perianal fistulas in patients with mild to moderate colonic or ileocolonic CD. In patients who are allergic, intolerant, or unresponsive to sulfasalazine, metronidazole appears to be effective in colonic disease and in promoting healing of perianal disease. Long-term use of metronidazole is limited because of potential for peripheral neuropathy and other side effects. Patients with bacterial overgrowth in the small intestine may be treated with broad-spectrum antibiotics. Ciprofloxacin may be useful in treating patients who are intolerant or unresponsive to metronidazole therapy.

Nutritional management: A major adjunct to standard medical therapy. During acute exacerbations, total parenteral nutrition (TPN) and nothing-by mouth (NPO) status can be used to replace nutritional deficits and allow complete bowel rest. Elemental diets that are free of bulk and residue, low in fat, and digested in the upper jejunum provide good nutrition with low fecal volume, to allow bowel rest in selected patients. Use of elemental diets is being investigated for effectiveness as primary therapy, as an alternative to steroids and bowel rest, in treating patients with acute CD. Bland diets low in residue, roughage, and fat but high in protein, calories, carbohydrates, and vitamins provide good nutrition and reduce excessive stimulation of the bowel. A diet free of milk, milk products, gas-forming foods, alcohol, and iced beverages reduces cramping and diarrhea. When remission occurs, a less restricted diet can be tailored to the individual patient, with exclusion of foods known to precipitate symptoms. Personal exclusion diets have been associated with a decrease in the number of relapses, but further research is needed to substantiate these findings. Patients with involvement of the small intestine often require supplementation of vitamins and minerals, especially Ca^{++}, iron, folate, and magnesium, secondary to malabsorption or to compensate for foods excluded from the diet. Patients with extensive ileal disease or resection often require vitamin B_{12} replacement, and if bile salt deficiency exists, cholestyramine and medium-chain triglycerides (MCTs) may be needed to control diarrhea and reduce fat malabsorption and steatorrhea. Vitamin D deficiency is common in these patients and may require supplementation with cholecalciferol. (See also "Providing Nutritional Support," p. 688, and "Malabsorption/Maldigestion," p. 453.)

Probiotics: Restore balance to the intestinal environment by use of beneficial bacteria, with resulting reduction in inflammation. Health benefits appear to be strain-specific; *Lactobacillus acidophilus, Saccharomyces boulardii,* and VSL #3 (a proprietary blend of eight strains of bacteria) are most promising. Probiotics are available in capsule, powder, tablet, and liquid forms, as well as in live-culture yogurt (live-culture soy yogurt if lactose intolerant).

Referral to mental health practitioner for supportive psychotherapy: If indicated, because of the chronic and progressive nature of CD.

Surgical management: Because surgery is not a cure for CD, it is reserved for complications rather than used as a primary form of therapy. Common indications for surgery include bowel obstruction, internal and enterocutaneous fistulas, intraabdominal abscesses, perianal disease, failure of medical therapy, complications of therapy, and cancer secondary to long-standing CD. Conservative resection of the affected bowel segments with restoration of bowel continuity, with preservation of as much of the intestine as possible, is the preferred surgical approach. If small bowel strictures are present, strictureplasty is a surgical technique that widens the strictured area without removing any of the small intestine. Laparoscopic surgery is now in use for selected patients. If fecal diversion using an ostomy is required, the type of diversion used will depend on the location and amount of intestinal segment(s) to be resected. (For details, see "Fecal Diversions," p. 491.) After surgery, disease may recur at the site of anastomosis. Use of 5-ASA agents and immunomodulators may reduce these recurrences.

Referral to a wound, ostomy, and continence (WOC)/enterostomal therapy (ET) nurse: Should be initiated as soon as surgery resulting in an ostomy is anticipated or immediately postoperatively.

NURSING DIAGNOSES AND INTERVENTIONS

Deficient fluid volume related to active loss secondary to diarrhea or presence of GI fistula

Desired outcomes: Patient is normovolemic within 24 hr of admission, as evidenced by balanced I&O, urinary output 30 mL/hr or more, specific gravity 1.010-1.030, BP 90/60 mm Hg or higher (or within patient's normal range), respiratory rate (RR) 12-20 breaths/min, stable weight, good skin turgor, and moist mucous membranes. Patient reports that diarrhea is controlled.

Nursing Interventions

◆ Monitor I&O and urinary specific gravity, weigh patient daily, and monitor laboratory values. *This is to evaluate fluid and electrolyte status.* (Optimal values: serum K^+ 3.5-5.0 mEq/L, serum Na^+ 137-147 mEq/L, and serum chloride [Cl$^-$] 95-108 mEq/L. Critical values: K$^+$ less than 2.5 or more than 6.5 mEq/L, Na$^+$ less than 120 or more than 160 mEq/L, Cl$^-$ less than 80 or more than115 mEq/L.)

♦ Monitor frequency and consistency of stools. Keep a stool count, and measure volume of liquid stools. Assess and record presence of blood, mucus, fat, or undigested food.

♦ Monitor for thirst, poor skin turgor, dryness of mucous membranes, fever, and concentrated (specific gravity greater than 1.030) and decreased urinary output. *These are indicators of dehydration.*

♦ Maintain patient on parenteral replacement of fluids, electrolytes, and vitamins as prescribed. *This is to promote anabolism and healing.*

♦ When patient is taking food orally, provide bland, high-protein, high-calorie, low-fat, low-residue diet, as prescribed. Determine incidence of cramping, diarrhea, and flatulence. *This is to assess for tolerance to diet.* Modify diet plan accordingly.

Risk for infection/ineffective protection related to risk for complications caused by intestinal inflammatory disorder
Desired outcome: Patient is free from indicators of infection and intraabdominal injury, as evidenced by normothermia; heart rate (HR) 60-100 beats per minute (bpm); RR 12-20 breaths/min; normal bowel sounds; absence of abdominal distention, rigidity, or localized pain and tenderness; absence of nausea and vomiting; negative culture results; no significant change in mental status; and orientation to person, place, and time.

Nursing Interventions

♦ Monitor for abdominal distention, abdominal rigidity, and increased episodes of nausea and vomiting. *These are indicators of intestinal obstruction.* Carefully check patients on opiates or antidiarrheal medications. *Contributing factors to development of intestinal obstruction include use of opiates and prolonged use of antidiarrheal medication.*

♦ Monitor for fever, increased RR and HR, chills, diaphoresis, and increased abdominal discomfort. *These may occur with intestinal perforation, abscess or fistula formation, or generalized fecal peritonitis and septicemia.* Assess patients, in particular, who are on corticosteroids or antibiotics. *Systemic therapy with corticosteroids and antibiotics can mask development of preceding complications.*

♦ Evaluate mental status, orientation, and level of consciousness (LOC) q2-4h.

♦ Obtain cultures of blood, urine, fistulas, or other possible sources of infection, as prescribed, if patient has a sudden temperature elevation. Monitor culture reports, and notify health care provider promptly of any positive results. *Abscesses or fistulas to abdominal wall, bladder, or vagina are common in CD, as well as abscesses or fistulas to other loops of small bowel and colon.*

♦ If draining fistulas or abscesses are present, change dressings and pouching system or irrigate tubes or drains as prescribed. Note color, character, and odor of all drainage. Report presence of foul-smelling or abnormal drainage or loss of tube/drain patency. Refer to a WOC/ET nurse for fistula management as needed.

♦ Administer antibiotics as prescribed and on prescribed schedule to maintain therapeutic serum level.

♦ Use good handwashing technique before and after caring for patient and by disposing of dressings and drainage using proper infection control techniques (see "Infection Prevention and Control," p. 743). *This is to prevent transmission of potentially infectious organisms.*

Acute pain, nausea, and abdominal cramping related to intestinal inflammatory process

Desired outcomes: Patient's subjective perception of discomfort decreases within 4 hr of intervention, as documented by pain scale. Objective indicators, such as grimacing, are absent or diminished.

Nursing Interventions

◆ Monitor and document characteristics of discomfort, and assess whether it is associated with ingestion of certain foods or with emotional stress. Devise a pain scale with patient, rating discomfort from 0 (no discomfort) to 10 (worst discomfort). Eliminate foods that cause cramping and discomfort.

◆ As prescribed, keep patient on NPO status and provide parenteral nutrition. *This is to allow bowel rest.*

◆ Administer antidiarrheal medications and analgesics as prescribed. *This is to reduce abdominal discomfort.* Instruct patient to request analgesic before pain becomes severe.

◆ Provide nasal and oral care at frequent intervals. *This is to reduce abdominal discomfort.*

◆ Administer antiemetic medications before meals. *This is to enhance appetite when nausea is a problem.*

◆ Using pain scale, reassess patient and document relief obtained. For additional information, see "Pain," p. 13, in Chapter 1.

Diarrhea related to intestinal inflammatory process
Desired outcome: Patient reports a reduction in frequency of stools and a return to more normal stool consistency within 3 days of hospital admission.

Nursing Interventions

◆ If patient is experiencing frequent and urgent passage of loose stools, provide covered bedpan or commode or be sure bathroom is easily accessible and ready to use at all times.

◆ Empty bedpan or commode promptly. *This is to control odor and decrease patient's anxiety and self-consciousness.*

◆ Administer antidiarrheal medication as prescribed. *This is to decrease fluidity and number of stools.*

◆ If bile salt deficiency is contributing to diarrhea (because of ileal disease or resection), administer cholestyramine as prescribed. *This is to control diarrhea.*

◆ Eliminate or decrease fat content in the diet. *This is because it can increase diarrhea in individuals with malabsorption syndromes.* Also, restrict foods and beverages such as raw vegetables and fruits; whole-grain cereals; condiments; gas-forming foods; alcohol; iced and carbonated beverages; and, in lactose-intolerant patients, milk and milk products. *These foods can precipitate diarrhea and cramping.*

Activity intolerance related to generalized weakness secondary to intestinal inflammatory process
Desired outcome: Patient adheres to prescribed rest regimen and sets appropriate goals for self-care as the condition improves (optimally within 3-7 days of admission).

Nursing Interventions

◆ Keep patient's environment quiet. *This is to facilitate rest.*

◆ Assist patient with ADL and plan nursing care to provide maximum rest periods. *This is because adequate rest is necessary to sustain remission.* Facilitate coordination of health care providers. *This is to allow rest periods between care activities.* Allow 90 min for undisturbed rest.

◆ As prescribed, administer sedatives and tranquilizers. *This is to promote rest and reduce anxiety.*

♦ As patient's physical condition improves, encourage self-care to greatest extent possible and assist patient with setting realistic, attainable goals.
♦ For additional information, see **Risk for activity intolerance,** p. 23, in "Prolonged Bed Rest."

 Patient-Family Teaching and Discharge Planning

When providing patient-family teaching, include verbal and written information about the following:

♦ Medications, including drug names, rationale, dosage, schedule, route of administration, precautions, and potential side effects. Also discuss drug/drug, herb/drug, and food/drug interactions.
♦ Signs and symptoms that necessitate medical attention, including fever, nausea and vomiting, abdominal discomfort, any significant change in appearance and frequency of stools, or passage of stool through the vagina or stool mixed with urine, any of which can signal recurrence or complications of CD.
♦ Importance of dietary management to promote nutritional and fluid maintenance and prevent abdominal cramping, discomfort, and diarrhea.
♦ Importance of perineal/perianal skin care after bowel movements.
♦ Importance of balancing activities with rest periods, even during remission, because adequate rest is necessary to sustain remission.
♦ Importance of follow-up medical care, including supportive psychotherapy, because of the chronic and progressive nature of CD.
♦ Referral to community resources. Additional information can be found at:

Crohn's & Colitis Foundation of America, Inc.: www.ccfa.org

United Ostomy Association of America: www.uoaa.org

Additional Teaching, if Patient Has a Fecal Diversion

♦ Care of incision, dressing changes, and bathing.
♦ Care of stoma and peristomal skin, use of ostomy equipment, and method for obtaining supplies.
♦ Gradual resumption of ADL, excluding heavy lifting (more than 10 lb), pushing, or pulling for 6-8 wk to prevent incisional herniation.
♦ Referral to community resources, including home health care agency, WOC/ET nurse, and local ostomy association.
♦ Importance of reporting signs and symptoms that require medical attention, such as change in stoma color from the normal bright and shiny red; lesions of stomal mucosa that may indicate recurrence of disease; peristomal skin irritation; diarrhea or constipation, fever, chills, abdominal pain, distention, nausea, and vomiting; and incisional pain, local increased temperature, drainage, swelling, or redness.

❖ FECAL DIVERSIONS

For a discussion of Diverticulitis, see p. 469; "Polyps/Familial Adenomatous Polyposis," p. 473; "Ulcerative Colitis," p. 476; and "Crohn's Disease," p. 484.

SURGICAL INTERVENTIONS

It is sometimes necessary to interrupt continuity of the bowel because of intestinal disease or its complications. A fecal diversion may be necessary to divert stool around a diseased portion of the bowel or, more commonly, out of the body. A fecal diversion can be located anywhere along the bowel, depending on location of the diseased or injured portion, and it can be permanent or temporary. The most common sites for fecal diversion are the colon and ileum. The more distal the colostomy, the more formed the fecal matter will be.

Colostomy: Created surgically by bringing a portion of the colon to the surface of the abdomen. An opening in the exteriorized colon permits elimination of flatus and stool through the stoma. Any part of the colon may be diverted into a colostomy.

Transverse colostomy: Most commonly created stoma to divert feces on a temporary basis. Surgical indications include relief of bowel obstruction before definitive surgery for tumors, inflammation, or diverticulitis and colon perforation secondary to trauma. Stool can be liquid to pastelike or soft and unformed, and bowel elimination is unpredictable. A temporary colostomy may be double barreled, with a proximal stoma through which stool is eliminated and a distal stoma, called a *mucous fistula,* adjacent to the proximal stoma. More commonly, a loop colostomy is created with a supporting rod placed beneath it until the exteriorized loop of colon heals to the skin.

Descending or sigmoid colostomy: Usually a permanent fecal diversion. Rectal cancer is the most common cause for surgical intervention. Stool is usually formed, and some individuals may have stool elimination at predictable times. In a permanent colostomy, the severed end of the colon is brought to the abdominal skin surface. The diseased or injured portion of the colon and/or rectum is resected and removed. To create the stoma, the colon above the skin surface is rolled back on itself to expose the mucosal surface of the intestine. The end of the cuff is sutured to the subcutaneous tissues with absorbable sutures to hold it in place as it heals.

Temporary colostomy: Typically created when there is significant inflammation in the diseased portion of the bowel (e.g., perforated diverticulum or ulcerative colitis [UC]). When a temporary colostomy is created, the severed end of the colon is brought through the abdominal wall as for a permanent colostomy. The diseased or injured portion of the colon is resected and removed. The remaining rectum or rectosigmoid is oversewn, left in the peritoneal cavity, and is referred to as *Hartmann's pouch.* After the inflammatory process has resolved (e.g., 3-6 mo), the colostomy is taken down and reattached to the bowel of Hartmann's pouch, thus reconstructing continuity of the bowel and normal bowel elimination.

Cecostomy or ascending colostomy: Not a common procedure. A temporary diverting colostomy is used to bypass an unresectable tumor. The stool from an ascending colostomy is soft, unformed, pastelike, semiliquid, or liquid, and bowel elimination is unpredictable. Surgical procedure is similar to that with transverse colostomies.

Ileostomy

Conventional (Brooke) ileostomy: Created by bringing a distal portion of the resected ileum through the abdominal wall. A permanent ileostomy is created by the same procedure discussed with a permanent colostomy. Surgical indications include UC, Crohn's disease (CD), and familial adenomatous polyposis (FAP) requiring excision of the entire colon and rectum. For any ileostomy, the output is usually liquid and is eliminated continually. The more proximal the ileostomy, the more active are digestive enzymes within the stool and the greater their potential for irritation to exposed skin around the stoma. A collection pouch is worn over the stoma on the abdomen to collect gas and fecal discharge.

Temporary ileostomy: Usually a loop stoma with or without a supporting rod in place beneath the loop of the ileum until the exteriorized loop of ileum heals to the skin. The purpose is to divert the fecal stream away from a more distal anastomotic site or fistula repair until healing has occurred.

Continent (Kock pouch) ileostomy: An intraabdominal pouch constructed from approximately 30 cm of distal ileum. Intussusception of a 10-cm portion of ileum is performed to form an outlet nipple valve from the pouch to the skin of the abdomen, where a stoma is constructed flush with the skin. The intraabdominal pouch is continent for gas and fecal discharge and is emptied approximately 4×/day by inserting a catheter through the stoma. No external pouch is needed, and an adhesive bandage (Band-Aid) or small dressing is worn over the stoma to collect mucus. Surgical indications include UC and FAP requiring removal of the colon and rectum. CD is generally a contraindication to this procedure because the disease can recur in the pouch, necessitating its removal. A long-term complication of Kock pouch is pouchitis, with symptoms and signs as discussed. See under IPAA in the next paragraph, with the exception that tenesmus is not a symptom for a patient with a Kock pouch.

Ileal pouch and anastomosis (IPAA) or restorative proctocolectomy: A two-stage surgical procedure developed to preserve fecal continence and prevent the need for a permanent ileostomy. During the first stage after total colectomy and removal of the rectal mucosa, an ileal reservoir or pouch is constructed and lowered into position in the pelvis just above the rectal cuff. Then the ileal outlet from the pouch is brought down through the cuff of the rectal muscle and anastomosed to the anal canal. The anal sphincter is preserved, and the resulting ileal pouch provides a storage place for feces. A temporary diverting ileostomy is required for 2-3 mo to allow healing of the anastomosis. The second stage occurs when the diverting ileostomy is taken down and fecal continuity is restored. Initially, the patient experiences fecal incontinence and 10 or more bowel movements per day. After 3-6 mo, the patient experiences decreased urgency and frequency with 4-8 bowel movements per day. This procedure is an option for patients requiring colectomy for UC or FAP. Its use is controversial in patients with CD. It is contraindicated with incontinence problems. *Pouchitis* is a long-term complication of IPAA. Its cause is unknown, but the condition may result from stasis of bacteria in the ileal pouch. Symptoms and signs include increased stool frequency, cramping, tenesmus, and bleeding. Pouchitis is effectively treated with metronidazole or ciprofloxacin. Probiotics also may be effective in preventing and maintaining remission in patients with recurrent pouchitis.

NURSING DIAGNOSES AND INTERVENTIONS

Risk for impaired peristomal skin integrity related to risk factors from exposure to effluent or sensitivity to appliance material, *and*

Impaired tissue integrity (stomal) (or risk for same) related to improperly fitted appliance resulting in impaired circulation

Desired outcome: Patient's stomal and peristomal skin and tissue remain nonerythemic and intact.

Nursing Interventions

After colostomy or conventional ileostomy (permanent or temporary)

- Apply a pectin, gelatin, methylcellulose-based, or synthetic solid-form skin barrier around the stoma. *This is to protect peristomal skin from irritation caused by contact with stool.*

- Cut an opening in skin barrier the exact circumference of stoma or as recommended by manufacturer. Remove release paper and apply sticky surface directly to peristomal skin. For some pouching systems, the skin barrier may be a separate barrier to be used with an adhesive-backed pouch, part of a two-piece system, or an integral part of a one-piece pouch system. Pectin-based paste also may be used. *This is to "caulk" around the barrier and compensate for irregular surfaces on peristomal skin. A pectin-based paste may prevent undermining of barrier with stool and protect skin immediately adjacent to stoma.*

- Remove skin barrier and inspect skin q3-4 days. Monitor peristomal skin for changes (e.g., erythema, erosion, serous drainage, bleeding, induration). *These may signal presence of infection, irritation, or sensitivity to materials placed on skin.* Carefully document abnormal findings, and report them to health care provider. Discontinue use of irritating materials, and substitute other materials. Patch test patient's abdominal skin. *This is to determine sensitivity to suspected materials.*

◆ Recalibrate skin barrier opening to size of stoma with each change. *Stomas become less edematous over a period of weeks after surgery, necessitating changes in size of skin barrier opening.* The skin barrier opening should be the exact circumference of the stoma. *This is to prevent contact of stool with skin.* Commercial templates are available to aid in estimating size of the opening needed for the skin barrier.

◆ Apply a two-piece pouch system or a pouch with access cap. *This is so that stoma can be inspected for viability q12-24h in the immediate postoperative period.* A mature stoma is red, with overlying mucus. A nonmature stoma is red and moist where the mucous membrane is exposed but can be a darker, mottled, grayish red with a transparent or translucent film of serosa elsewhere.

◆ Cleanse skin with warm water when removing skin barrier and pouch for routine care. Dry peristomal skin completely. *This helps the skin retain its normal integrity and barrier function and helps pouch materials adhere well.*

◆ Empty pouch when it is one-third to one-half full of stool or gas. *This is to maintain a secure pouch seal.*

After continent ileostomy (kock pouch)

◆ Avoid stress on ileostomy catheter and its securing suture. As prescribed, maintain catheter on low, continuous suction or gravity drainage. The catheter is inserted through the stoma into the continent ileostomy pouch during surgery. *This is to prevent stress on nipple valve and maintain pouch decompression so that suture lines are allowed to heal without stress or tension.*

◆ Monitor site for erythema, induration, drainage, or erosion around the stoma.

◆ Check catheter q2h for patency, and irrigate with sterile saline (30 mL). *This is to prevent obstruction.* Notify health care provider if solution cannot be instilled, if there are no returns from catheter, or if leakage of irrigating solution or pouch contents appears around catheter.

◆ Change 4 × 4 dressing around stoma q2h or as often as it becomes wet. *This is to prevent peristomal skin irritation.* Drainage will be serosanguineous at first and mixed with mucus. Report presence of frank bleeding to health care provider.

◆ Assess stoma for viability with each dressing change. It should be red and moist and shiny with mucus. *A stoma that is pale, dark purple to black, or dull in appearance may indicate circulatory impairment.*

After IPAA

◆ Perform routine care for diverting ileostomy (see earlier discussion).

◆ Maintain perineal/perianal skin integrity by gently cleansing the area with water and cotton balls or soft tissues. *After first stage of the operation, patient may have incontinence of mucus.* Use absorbent pad at night. *This is to absorb oozing mucus.* Avoid using soap. *This can cause itching or irritation.*

◆ After second stage of the operation (when ileostomy is taken down), expect patient to experience frequency and urgency of defecation.

◆ Wash perineal/perianal area with warm water or commercial perineal/perianal cleansing solution, and use squeeze bottle, cotton balls, or soft tissues. Do not use toilet paper. *It can cause irritation.* If desired, dry the area with a hair dryer on a cool setting.

◆ Provide sitz baths. *This is to promote comfort and help clean perineal/perianal area.*

◆ Apply protective skin sealants or ointments. Skin sealants containing alcohol should not be used on irritated or eroded skin. *This is because the high alcohol content can cause a painful burning sensation.*

Bowel incontinence related to disruption of normal function with fecal diversion

Desired outcomes: Within 2-4 days after surgery, patient has bowel sounds and eliminates gas and stool via the fecal diversion. Within 3 days after teaching has been initiated, patient verbalizes understanding of measures that will maintain normal elimination pattern and demonstrates care techniques specific to the fecal diversion.

Nursing Interventions

After colostomy and conventional ileostomy (permanent and temporary)

◆ Empty stool from bottom opening of pouch and assess quality and quantity of stool, and document return of normal bowel function. Record volume of liquid stool and its color and consistency.

◆ If colostomy is not eliminating stool after 3-4 days and bowel sounds have returned, gently insert a gloved, lubricated finger into the stoma. *This is to determine presence of stricture at skin or fascial levels and note presence of any stool within reach of examining finger.* Health care provider may prescribe colostomy irrigation. *This is to stimulate elimination of gas and stool.* (For procedure, see **Deficient knowledge** related to colostomy irrigation procedure, p. 496.)

After continent ileostomy (kock pouch)

◆ Monitor I&O, and record amount, color, and consistency of output.

◆ Expect aspiration of bright red blood or serosanguineous liquid drainage from Kock pouch during early postoperative period.

◆ As gastrointestinal (GI) function returns after 3-4 days, expect drainage to change in color from blood-tinged to greenish brown liquid. When ileal output appears, suction (if used) is discontinued, and pouch catheter is placed to facilitate gravity drainage.

◆ As patient's diet progresses from clear liquids to solid food, ileal output thickens. Check and irrigate catheter q2h and as needed. *This is to maintain patency.* If patient reports abdominal fullness in an area of pouch along with decreased fecal output, check catheter placement and patency.

◆ When patient is alert and taking food by mouth, teach catheter irrigation procedure, which should be performed q2h; demonstrate how to empty pouch contents through the catheter into the toilet.

◆ Before hospital discharge, teach patient how to remove and reinsert catheter.

After IPAA

◆ Monitor I&O, and observe quantity, quality, and consistency of output from diverting ileostomy and reservoir. Monitor patient for temperature elevation accompanied by perianal pain and discharge of purulent, bloody mucus from drains and anal orifice. *These signal infection.* Report significant findings to health care provider.

◆ If drains are present, irrigate them as prescribed. *This is done to maintain patency, decrease stress on suture lines, and decrease incidence of infection.*

◆ After first stage of the operation, patient may experience oozing of mucus. Advise patient to wear small pad to avoid soiling outer garments.

◆ After second stage of the operation (when ileostomy is taken down), expect incontinence and 15-20 bowel movements per day with urgency when patient is on a clear-liquid diet. Assist with perianal care, and apply protective skin care products. The catheter can be placed in the reservoir and connected to a gravity drainage bag overnight. *This is done if nocturnal incontinence is especially troublesome.*

◆ Expect the number of bowel movements to decrease to 6-12/day and consistency to thicken when patient is eating solid foods.

◆ Administer hydrophilic colloids and antidiarrheal medications as prescribed. *This is to decrease fluidity and frequency of stools.*

◆ Provide diet consultation. *This is done so that patient can avoid foods that cause liquid stools (spinach, raw fruits, highly seasoned foods, green beans, broccoli, prune and grape juices, alcohol) and increase intake of foods that result in thick stools (cheese, ripe bananas, applesauce, creamy peanut butter, gelatin, pasta).*

◆ Reassure patient that frequency and urgency are temporary and that as the reservoir expands and absorbs fluid, bowel movements should become thicker and less frequent.

Disturbed body image related to presence of fecal diversion
Desired outcome: Within 5-7 days after surgery, patient demonstrates actions that reflect beginning acceptance of the fecal diversion and incorporates changes into self-concept as evidenced by acknowledging body changes, viewing the stoma, and participating in the care of the fecal diversion.

Nursing Interventions

◆ Expect the following fears, which may be expressed by patients experiencing a fecal diversion: physical, social, and work activities will be curtailed significantly; rejection, isolation, and feelings of uncleanliness will occur; everyone will know about the altered pattern of fecal elimination; and loss of voluntary control may occur. *Many patients view incontinence as a return to infancy, and this is very distressing.*

◆ Encourage patient to discuss feelings and fears; clarify any misconceptions. Involve family members in discussions. *They too may have anxieties and misconceptions.*

◆ Provide a calm and quiet environment for patient and significant other to discuss the surgery. Initiate an open, honest discussion. Monitor carefully for and listen closely to expressed or nonverbalized needs. *Each patient will react differently to the surgical procedure.*

◆ Encourage acceptance of fecal diversion by having patient participate in care. Assure patient that education offers a means of control.

◆ Assure patient that physical, social, and work activities will not be affected by the presence of a fecal diversion.

◆ Expect patient to have fears about sexual acceptance, although these fears usually are not expressed overtly. Concerns center on change in body image; fears about odor and worries that the ostomy appliance will interfere with sexual intercourse; conception, pregnancy, and discomfort from perianal wound and scar in women; and impotence and failure to ejaculate in men, especially after more radical dissection of the pelvis in patient with cancer. Arrange for a consultation with someone who can speak openly and honestly about these problems.

◆ Consult patient's health care provider about a visit by another person with an ostomy. *Patients gain reassurance and build positive attitudes by seeing a healthy, active person who has undergone the same type of surgery.*

Deficient knowledge related to colostomy irrigation procedure
Desired outcome: Within 3 days after initiation of teaching, patient demonstrates proficiency with the procedure for colostomy irrigation.

Nursing Interventions

◆ Teach prescribed colostomy irrigation to patient with permanent descending or sigmoid colostomy. Colostomy irrigation is performed daily or every other day so that wearing a pouch becomes unnecessary. An appropriate candidate is a patient who has one or two formed stools each day at predictable times (same as normal stool elimination pattern before illness). In addition, the patient must be able to manipulate the equipment, remember the technique, and be willing to spend approximately 1 hr/day performing the procedure. It may take 4-6 wk for the patient to have stool elimination regulated with irrigation.

Instruct patient about the following steps:

♦ Position the irrigating sleeve over the colostomy, and center the stoma in the opening. Secure the sleeve in place with an adhesive disk on the sleeve or with a sleeve belt.

♦ Fill the enema/irrigation container with 500-1000 mL (1-2 pints) warm water. With patient in a sitting position on the toilet or on a chair facing the toilet, position the sleeve so that it empties into the toilet. Hang the enema/ irrigation container so that the bottom surface is at patient's shoulder level.

♦ Open the slide or roller clamp and flush the tubing with the water to remove air from the tubing; reclamp the tubing.

♦ Gently dilate the stoma with a gloved finger lubricated with water-soluble lubricant. *This enables patient to identify the direction of the intestinal lumen.* Lubricate the cone and catheter, and slowly insert them into the stoma. If a cone and catheter are used, insert the catheter no more than 3 inches. Hold the cone gently, but firmly, in place against the stoma. *This is to prevent backflow of irrigant.*

♦ Allow water to slowly enter the stoma from the container through the tubing; it should take 15 min for fluid to enter the colon. If cramping occurs while water is flowing, stop the flow and leave the cone in place until cramping passes; then the flow of water may be resumed. If cramping does not resolve, the colon is probably ready to evacuate and should be allowed to do so.

♦ After water has entered the colon, advise patient to hold the cone in place for a few seconds and then gently remove it. The sleeve should be left in place for 30-40 min. *This is to allow water and stool to be eliminated.*

♦ When elimination is complete, remove the irrigation sleeve and cleanse and dry the peristomal area.

♦ Apply a small dressing or security pouch over the colostomy between irrigations.

📝 Patient-Family Teaching and Discharge Planning

When providing patient-family teaching, include verbal and written information about the following:

♦ Medications, including drug names, rationale, dosage, schedule, route of administration, precautions, and potential side effects. Also discuss drug/ drug, herb/drug, and food/drug interactions.

♦ Importance of dietary management to promote nutritional and fluid maintenance.

♦ Care of incision, dressing changes, and permission to take baths or showers once sutures and drains are removed.

♦ Care of the stoma, care of peristomal and perianal skin, use of ostomy equipment, and method for obtaining supplies.

♦ Gradual resumption of activities of daily living (ADL), excluding heavy lifting (more than 10 lb), pushing, or pulling for 6-8 wk to prevent development of incisional herniation.

♦ Importance of follow-up care with a health care provider and wound, ostomy, and continence (WOC)/enterostomal therapy (ET) nurse; confirm date and time of next appointment.

♦ Importance of reporting signs and symptoms that require medical attention, such as change in stoma color from normal bright and shiny red; peristomal or perianal skin irritation; any significant changes in appearance, frequency, and consistency of stools; fever, chills, abdominal pain, or distention; and incisional pain, increased local warmth, drainage, swelling, or redness; and signs and symptoms of pouchitis, including diarrhea, cramping, tenesmus, and bleeding.

◆ Referral to community resources including home health care agency, WOC/ET nurse, and local ostomy association. Additional resources include the following:

International Ostomy Association: www.ostomyinternational.org

United Ostomy Association of America: www.uoaa.org

❖ ❖ ❖

SECTION FOUR **ABDOMINAL TRAUMA**

OVERVIEW/PATHOPHYSIOLOGY

Abdominal trauma accounts for several million emergency department visits in the United States annually. Abdominal trauma may cause serious injury to major organs. It is essential to understand the mechanism of the injury (blunt, penetrating, or combination) and abdominal organs affected to avoid complications in the recovery period. Astute serial assessments in the posttraumatic period may prevent serious consequences and avoid life-threatening situations. Abdominal injuries often are associated with multisystem trauma. See also discussions under "Pneumothorax/Hemothorax," p. 75; "Spinal Cord Injury," p. 287; and "Traumatic Brain Injury," p. 314.

Common injuries to abdominal organs may be predicted with knowledge of the injury mechanism and location (**TABLE 7-3**). Thoracic and musculoskeletal trauma, especially below the fourth rib, may be associated with abdominal trauma. Solid organs (liver, kidneys, spleen) tend to fracture and bleed with trauma; hollow organs (stomach, intestines) may collapse or rupture, releasing caustic substances into the peritoneum. Injury also may result from movement of organs within the body, particularly at the transition between rigidly fixed and mobile organs. Injury to the urinary bladder is not common but may be associated with pelvic fractures. Rectal and vaginal exams are necessary to assess for bleeding.

Blunt trauma may be caused by falls, assaults, motor vehicle collisions, or sports injuries. These blunt injuries involve direct transmission of energy to solid or hollow organs and most commonly affect the spleen and liver. Splenic injury should be suspected in the presence of left lower rib fractures. Rupture may not be immediately obvious, thus reinforcing the need for ongoing assessments. Pain radiating to the left shoulder (Kehr's sign) may indicate blood beneath the diaphragm from splenic bleeding. Pain radiating to the right shoulder may indicate injury to the liver. Other organs that may be affected by blunt trauma include the kidneys and, occasionally, the pancreas and small and large intestines. Bleeding is the most common complication, resulting in increased morbidity and mortality. Abdominal vessels are injured in about 10% of patients with blunt abdominal trauma, and these injuries can quickly lead to shock and death if they are not recognized. Signs of blood loss may be nonspecific. Young, healthy patients can lose 50% of blood volume and appear stable.

Penetrating trauma may be caused by gunshot, stabbing, or impalement. If the lower esophagus and stomach are injured by penetration, complications from release of irritating gastric fluids into the peritoneum and free air below the diaphragm may be present. Penetrating injuries may occur to the liver, small intestine, and mesentery. The external appearance of the wound may not accurately reflect internal damage.

TABLE 7-3	SIGNS AND SYMPTOMS OF INJURY TO SPECIFIC ORGANS
ORGAN	**SIGNS AND SYMPTOMS**
Spleen	Signs and symptoms of peritoneal irritation (Box 7-2)
	Signs and symptoms of hemorrhage
	Left-sided rib fractures
	Left upper quadrant abdominal pain
	Kehr's sign (pain referred to left shoulder)
Liver	Signs and symptoms of peritoneal irritation (Box 7-2)
	Signs and symptoms of hemorrhage
	Elevated diaphragm on right side
	Right-sided rib fractures
Pancreas	Epigastric pain
	Grey Turner's sign (flank ecchymosis)
	Elevated amylase/lipase
Esophagus/stomach/small intestine	Signs and symptoms of peritoneal irritation (Box 7-2)
	Signs and symptoms of shock
	Absent bowel sounds
	Frank blood in nasogastric aspirate
	Increased pain with inspiration or sudden motion
Colon/rectum	Signs and symptoms of peritoneal irritation (Box 7-2)
	Blood in stools
	Pain with rectal examination
Major vessels	Signs and symptoms of peritoneal irritation (Box 7-2)

ASSESSMENT

Signs and symptoms/physical findings: As with all trauma patients, immediate life-threatening problems are identified, and treatment is begun before the more detailed secondary and focused assessments. *It is extremely important that recently injured patients be evaluated for peritoneal signs (**BOX 7-2**) by the same professional at hourly intervals. Notify health care provider immediately if patient develops peritoneal signs, evidence of shock, gastric or rectal bleeding, or gross hematuria.*

VS and hemodynamic measurements: VS should be assessed frequently to detect changes early. Gradual or sudden changes may be the heralding signs of hemorrhage following trauma, with tachycardia, impaired capillary refill, and hypotension being key indicators of bleeding or shock. Ventilatory excursion may be diminished because of pain, thoracic injury, or limited diaphragmatic movement caused by abdominal distention.

Pain: Mild tenderness to severe abdominal pain may be present, with pain either localized to the site of injury or diffuse. Blood or fluid collection within the peritoneum causes irritation and pain, with consequent involuntary guarding, distention, rigidity, and rebound tenderness.

Gastrointestinal (GI) symptoms: Nausea and vomiting may be present following blunt or penetrating trauma secondary to bleeding or obstruction. Absence of signs and symptoms, especially in patients who have sustained head or spinal cord injury, does not exclude the presence of major abdominal injury.

Inspection: Abrasions and ecchymoses are suggestive of underlying injury. For example, ecchymosis over the left upper quadrant (LUQ) suggests possible splenic injury. Ecchymotic areas around the umbilicus or flanks are suggestive of retroperitoneal bleeding. Erythema and ecchymosis across the lower abdomen suggest intestinal or bladder injury, caused by lap belts. Ecchymoses may take hours to days to develop, depending on rate of blood loss. Abdominal distention may signal bleeding, free air, or inflammation.

BOX 7-2	SIGNS AND SYMPTOMS SUGGESTIVE OF PERITONEAL IRRITATION

- Generalized abdominal pain or tenderness
- Guarding of abdomen
- Abdominal wall rigidity
- Rebound tenderness
- Abdominal pain with movement or coughing
- Abdominal distention
- Decreased or absent bowel sounds

Auscultation: Auscultate before percussion and palpation to avoid stimulating the bowel and confounding assessment findings. Bowel sounds may be decreased or absent in patients with abdominal organ injury, intraperitoneal bleeding, or recent surgery. However, the presence of bowel sounds does not exclude significant abdominal injury. Bowel sounds in the chest could indicate a ruptured diaphragm with small bowel herniation into the thorax. Bowel sounds should be auscultated frequently, especially in the first 24-48 hr after injury. Absence of bowel sounds is suggestive of ileus or other complications, such as bleeding, peritonitis, or bowel infarction. Presence of an abdominal bruit (turbulent blood flow through vessels) could indicate arterial injury.

Percussion and palpation: Percuss and palpate painful areas last. If patient's pain is severe, do not percuss or palpate, inasmuch as more advanced studies are indicated for evaluation. Percussion may reveal unusually large areas of dullness over ruptured blood-filled organs (e.g., a fixed area of dullness in the LUQ suggests a ruptured spleen). Tympany suggests the presence of gas. Tenderness or pain to palpation suggests abdominal injury. Blood or fluid in the abdomen can result in signs and symptoms of peritoneal irritation (Box 7-2).

DIAGNOSTIC TESTS

Blood studies

WBC count: Leukocytosis is expected immediately after injury. Splenic injuries in particular result in rapid development of a moderate to high WBC count. A later increase in WBCs or a shift to the left reflects an increase in the number of neutrophils, which signals inflammatory response and possible intraabdominal infection. In patients with abdominal trauma, ruptured abdominal viscera must be considered as a potential source of infection.

Platelet count: Mild thrombocytosis is seen immediately after traumatic injury. After massive hemorrhage, thrombocytopenia may be noted. Platelet transfusion usually is not required unless spontaneous bleeding is present.

Glucose: Initially elevated because of catecholamine release and insulin resistance associated with major trauma. Glucose metabolism is abnormal after major hepatic resection, and patients should be monitored to prevent hypoglycemic episodes.

Amylase: Elevated serum levels are associated with pancreatic or upper small bowel injury, but values may be normal even with severe injury to these organs.

Liver function tests: Elevations reflect hepatic injury.

ABG values: May reveal respiratory compromise or metabolic acidosis.

Other blood testing: A type and crossmatch may be done if blood replacement is anticipated. A flow sheet for serial laboratory values will help pinpoint changes that may otherwise go unnoticed.

X-ray examination: Initially, flat and upright chest x-ray films will exclude chest injuries (commonly associated with abdominal trauma) and establish a baseline. Subsequent chest x-ray examinations aid in detecting complications, such as atelectasis and pneumonia. In addition, chest and pelvic x-ray examinations may reveal fractures, missiles, foreign bodies, free intraperitoneal air, hematoma, or hemorrhage. Plain abdominal films are not useful in blunt trauma because they cannot define blood in the peritoneum.

Ultrasound: A rapid, noninvasive assessment tool for detecting intraabdominal hemorrhage. The Focused Assessment Sonogram for Trauma (FAST) has a sensitivity, specificity, and accuracy rate of more than 90% in detecting 100 mL or more of intraabdominal blood or fluid. It cannot image the retroperitoneum, nor can it determine the etiology of the bleeding. A single negative FAST result cannot absolutely exclude intraabdominal bleeding.

CT scan: Can reveal organ-specific blunt abdominal injury and quantify the amount of blood in the abdomen. It images the ureters and can detect extravasation of urine. Disadvantages are the expense and time required to perform the exam. Patients with positive CT scan require diagnostic laparotomy. A patient in unstable condition should be accompanied by a nurse during the CT scan.

Diagnostic peritoneal lavage (DPL): Involves insertion of a peritoneal dialysis catheter into the peritoneum to check for intraabdominal bleeding. This procedure is much less commonly performed since FAST and CT scan have become available. It may be indicated for confirmed or suspected blunt abdominal trauma for the following patients: (1) those in whom signs and symptoms of abdominal injury are obscured by intoxication, head or spinal cord trauma, opioids, or unconsciousness; and (2) any patient with equivocal assessment findings. DPL is unnecessary for patients who have obvious intraabdominal bleeding or other indications for immediate laparotomy (see "Surgical Considerations," p. 502).

Laparotomy: Enables complete evaluation of the abdomen and retroperitoneum. It is mandatory in all patients with hypotension, penetration of the abdominal wall, peritonitis, and air in the abdomen and in most patients with organ-specific injury noted on CT scan.

Occult blood: Gastric contents, urine, and stool are tested for occult blood because bleeding can occur as a result of direct injury and later complications.

Angiography: Angiography is performed rarely, but it may be needed with blunt trauma to evaluate injury to spleen, liver, pancreas, duodenum, and retroperitoneal vessels when other diagnostic findings are equivocal. Because of the large amount of contrast material used during this procedure, ensure adequate hydration and monitor urine output closely for 24-48 hr, especially in older patients or patients with preexisting cardiovascular or renal disease. Decreased urinary output and increased blood urea nitrogen (BUN) and serum creatinine may indicate contrast-associated acute tubular necrosis.

COLLABORATIVE MANAGEMENT

O_2 therapy: Individuals sustaining abdominal trauma are likely to be tachypneic, with the potential for poor ventilatory effort. Supplemental O_2 is delivered until patient's ABG or oximetry values while breathing room air are acceptable.

Fluid management: Massive blood loss is commonly associated with abdominal injuries. Restoration and maintenance of adequate volume are essential. Initially, Ringer's lactate or similar balanced salt solution is given. Packed RBCs are given to replace blood loss, especially with hemoglobin (Hgb) less than 9.0. Patients with abdominal trauma must have two large-bore IV lines inserted peripherally or centrally. Anticipate aggressive fluid replacement.

Gastric intubation: Gastric decompression prevents accumulation of gas or fluid in the stomach and reduces the chance of aspiration. Aspirated contents can be checked for blood to aid in diagnosis of lower esophageal, gastric, or duodenal injury. The tube usually remains in place until bowel function returns, as detected by positive bowel sounds, passage of flatus, and decreased gastric output via the tube.

Urinary drainage: An indwelling catheter is inserted to obtain a specimen for urinalysis and for a urine pregnancy test (female patients of childbearing age), to monitor urine output, and to guide fluid replacement. An indwelling catheter is not inserted if urinary tract injury is suspected.

Pharmacotherapy

Antibiotics: Abdominal trauma is associated with a high incidence of intraabdominal abscess, sepsis, and wound infection. Individuals with suspected intestinal injury are given parenteral, broad-spectrum antibiotics prophylactically for several days. If infection is present, antibiotics may be continued for several weeks.

Analgesics: May be delivered intermittently by the nurse. IV analgesics are recommended for management of pain, usually via patient-controlled pumps. As pain severity lessens, alternative analgesics such as nonsteroidal antiinflammatory drugs (NSAIDs) may be prescribed if not contraindicated by patient history or gastric bleeding.

Tetanus prophylaxis: Tetanus immune globulin (IG) and tetanus toxoid are considered, based on Centers for Disease Control and Prevention recommendations (available at www.cdc.gov).

Proton pump inhibitors (PPIs) or histamine H_2-receptor blockers: May be indicated to prevent ulcers. If the patient was taking these drugs before the trauma, signs and symptoms of peritonitis may be delayed.

Nutrition: Patients with abdominal trauma have complex nutritional needs because of the hypermetabolic state associated with major trauma and traumatic or surgical disruption of normal GI function. Often infection and sepsis contribute to negative N state and increased metabolic needs. Prompt initiation of enteric feedings and administration of supplemental calories, proteins, vitamins, and minerals are essential for healing. Parenteral feedings are given if the patient cannot have oral feedings.

Surgical considerations for penetrating abdominal injuries: Mandatory surgical exploration vs. observation and selective surgery, especially with stab wounds, remains controversial. Patients without obvious injury or peritoneal signs generally are observed for positive peritoneal signs and stability of VS. Indications for laparotomy include one or more of the following: (1) penetrating injury suspected of invading the peritoneum, (2) positive peritoneal signs (Box 7-2), (3) shock, (4) GI hemorrhage, (5) free air in the peritoneal cavity as seen on x-ray film, (6) evisceration, (7) massive hematuria, or (8) positive DPL or CT scan results.

Surgical considerations for nonpenetrating abdominal injuries: Physical examination alone will lead to an unacceptable rate of missed injuries. Therefore, additional diagnostic tests such as DPL, ultrasound, or CT scan are necessary to evaluate need for surgery in selected abdominal trauma patients. This is particularly true for patients who are intoxicated or unconscious or who have sustained head or spinal cord trauma. Immediate laparotomy for blunt abdominal trauma is indicated under the following circumstances: (1) clear signs of peritoneal irritation (Box 7-2); (2) free air in the peritoneum; (3) hypotension caused by suspected abdominal injury or persistent and unexplained hypotension; (4) positive DPL; (5) GI aspirate or rectal smear positive for blood; or (6) other positive diagnostic tests, such as CT scan, FAST, or arteriogram. Carefully evaluated stable patients with blunt abdominal trauma may be admitted to the critical care unit for observation. These patients should be evaluated in the same manner as that just described for patients with penetrating abdominal injuries. It is important to note that damage to retroperitoneal organs, such as the pancreas and duodenum, may not result in significant signs and symptoms for 6-12 hr or longer. Relatively slow bleeding from abdominal viscera may not be clinically apparent for 12 hr or longer after the initial injury. In addition, nurses should be aware that such complications as bowel obstruction may develop days or weeks after the traumatic event. The need for vigilant assessment in caring for these patients cannot be overemphasized.

NURSING DIAGNOSES AND INTERVENTIONS

Ineffective breathing pattern related to pain from injury or surgical incision, chemical irritation of blood or bile on pleural tissue, and diaphragmatic elevation caused by abdominal distention

Desired outcome: Within 24 hr of admission or surgery, patient is eupneic with respiratory rate (RR) 12-20 breaths/min and clear breath sounds.

Nursing Interventions

- Note quality of breath sounds, RR, presence/absence of cough, and sputum characteristics.
- Monitor oximetry readings q2-4h, and report O_2 saturation (Sao_2) less than 92%.
- Administer supplemental O_2 as prescribed. Monitor and document effectiveness.
- Encourage and assist patient with coughing, deep breathing, incentive spirometry, and turning q2-4h.
- Administer analgesics at dose and frequency. *This relieves pain and associated impaired chest excursion.*
- Instruct patient how to splint abdomen. *This is to reduce pain on movement, coughing, and deep breathing.*
- For additional interventions, see **Ineffective breathing pattern,** p. 5, in "Perioperative Care."

Deficient fluid volume related to active loss secondary to bleeding/hemorrhage

Desired outcomes: Within 4 hr of admission or on definitive repair (e.g., surgery), patient is normovolemic, as evidenced by SBP 90 mm Hg or higher (or within patient's baseline range), heart rate (HR) 60-100 beats per minute (bpm), central venous pressure (CVP) 2-6 mm Hg (5-12 cm H_2O), urinary output at least 30 mL/hr, warm extremities, brisk capillary refill (2 sec or less), distal pulses at least 2+ on a 0-4+ scale, and absence of orthostasis.

Nursing Interventions

- In recently injured patients, monitor BP hourly or more frequently in the presence of obvious bleeding or unstable VS. Be alert to increasing DBP and decreasing SBP. *Even a small but sudden decrease in SBP signals need to notify health care provider, especially with a trauma patient in whom the extent of injury is unknown. Most trauma patients are young, and excellent neurovascular compensation results in a near-normal BP until there is large intravascular volume depletion.* In stable postoperative patients, perform routine VS assessment.
- Be alert to decreasing BP, tachycardia, tachypnea, confusion, lethargy, come, delayed capillary refill, cool, pale skin, low CVP, and low urinary output. *These are clinical indicators of fluid volume deficit.* Report them immediately.
- Monitor HR and cardiovascular status hourly until patient's condition is stable. Note and report sudden increases or decreases in HR, especially if associated with indicators of fluid volume deficit, as noted earlier.
- In patient with evidence of volume depletion or active blood loss, administer prescribed fluids rapidly through one or more large-caliber (18-gauge or larger) IV catheters. Evaluate patency of IV catheters frequently during rapid volume resuscitation. Monitor patient closely. *This is to avoid fluid volume overload and complications such as heart failure (see p. 107) and pulmonary edema (see p. 110).* Large volumes of fluid require warming. *This is to prevent hypothermia.*
- Measure CVP q1-4h if indicated. Be alert to low or decreasing values. Report sudden decreases in CVP.

♦ Measure urinary output hourly (or when patient voids). Be alert to decreasing urinary output and to infrequent voidings. *Low urine output usually reflects inadequate intravascular volume in abdominal trauma patients.*

♦ Estimate ongoing blood loss. Measure all bloody drainage from drainage tubes or catheters, and note drainage color (e.g., coffee grounds, burgundy, bright red). Monitor for, and measure when possible, bloody stools. Note frequency of dressing changes resulting from saturation with blood. *This is to estimate amount of blood lost via wound site.* Note and report significant increases in amount of drainage, especially if it is bloody.

Acute pain related to irritation caused by intraperitoneal blood or secretions, actual trauma or surgical incision, and manipulation of organs during surgery

Desired outcomes: Within 4 hr of admission, patient's subjective perception of pain decreases, as documented by pain scale. Nonverbal indicators, such as grimacing, are absent or diminished. Patient's pain is controlled without sedation.

Nursing Interventions

♦ Evaluate for the presence of preoperative and postoperative pain. *Preoperative pain is anticipated and is a vital diagnostic aid. The location and character of postoperative pain also can be important. Incisional and some visceral pain can be anticipated, but intense or prolonged pain, especially when accompanied by other peritoneal signs, can signal bleeding, bowel infarction, infection, or other complications.* Devise a pain scale with patient, rating discomfort from 0 (no pain) to 10 (worst pain). Recognize that autonomic nervous system response to pain can complicate assessment of abdominal injury and hypovolemia. For details, see "Pain," p. 13, in Chapter 1.

♦ Administer analgesics as prescribed and indicated. *An alert patient should not suffer severe pain while awaiting surgical evaluation.* Administer postoperatively prescribed analgesics on a continual or regular schedule promptly with additional analgesia as needed, or provide patient-controlled analgesia (PCA) as prescribed and document effectiveness. *Analgesics are helpful in relieving pain and in aiding the recovery process by promoting greater ventilatory excursion.* Encourage patient to request analgesic before pain becomes severe.

♦ Recognize that opioid analgesics can decrease GI motility and may delay return to normal bowel function.

♦ Be aware that intoxication often is involved in traumatic events; therefore, victims may be drug or alcohol users with a higher-than-average tolerance for opioids. *They may need adjusted dosages.* Observe for signs of intoxication and/or withdrawal. *They may suffer symptoms of alcohol withdrawal (tremors, weakness, tachycardia, elevated BP, delusions, agitation, hallucinations) or narcotic withdrawal (lacrimation, rhinorrhea, anxiety, tremors, muscle twitching, mydriasis, nausea, abdominal cramps, vomiting) that need recognition and treatment.*

♦ Supplement analgesics with nonpharmacologic maneuvers (e.g., positioning, back rubs, distraction). This is to aid in pain reduction. Provide these instructions to patient and family members.

Risk for infection related to inadequate primary defenses secondary to disruption of the GI tract (particularly of the terminal ileum and colon) and traumatically inflicted open wound, multiple indwelling catheters and drainage tubes, and compromised immune state caused by blood loss and metabolic response to trauma

Desired outcome: Patient is free of infection, as evidenced by temperature less than 37.7° C (100° F); HR 100 bpm or less; no significant changes in mental status; orientation to person, place, and time; and absence of unusual

TABLE 7-4	CHARACTERISTICS OF GASTROINTESTINAL DRAINAGE
SOURCE	**COMPOSITION AND USUAL CHARACTER**
Mouth and oropharynx	Saliva; thin, clear, watery; pH 7.0
Stomach	Hydrochloric acid, gastrin, pepsin, mucus; thin, brownish to greenish; acidic
Pancreas	Enzymes and bicarbonate; thin, watery, yellowish brown; alkaline; usually abundant after surgery
Biliary tract	Bile, including bile salts and electrolytes; bright yellow to brownish green
Duodenum	Digestive enzymes, mucus, products of digestion; thin, bright yellow to light brown, may be greenish; alkaline
Jejunum	Enzymes, mucus, products of digestion; brown, watery with particles
Ileum	Enzymes, mucus, digestive products, greater amounts of bacteria; brown, liquid feculent
Colon	Digestive products, mucus, large amounts of bacteria; brown to dark brown, semiformed to firm stool
Postoperative (GI surgery)	Initial drainage expected to contain fresh blood; later drainage mixed with old blood and then approaches normal composition
Infection present	Drainage cloudy, may be thicker than usual; strong odor; unusual drain site often erythematous and warm

GI, Gastrointestinal.

erythema, edema, tenderness, warmth, or drainage at surgical incisions or wound sites.

Nursing Interventions

♦ Monitor VS, and note temperature increases and associated increases in HR and RR. *These may indicate infection present.* Notify health care provider of sudden temperature elevations.
♦ Evaluate mental status, orientation, and level of consciousness (LOC) q8h. Note mental status changes, confusion, or deterioration from baseline LOC.
♦ Ensure patency of all surgically placed tubes or drains. Irrigate or attach to low-pressure suction as prescribed. Maintain continuity of closed drainage systems; use sterile technique when emptying drainage and recharging suction containers. Promptly report loss of tube patency.
♦ Evaluate incisions and wound sites for unusual erythema, warmth, tenderness, edema, delayed healing, and purulent or unusual drainage. *This is to watch for evidence of infection.*
♦ Note amount, color, character, and odor of all drainage. Report presence of foul-smelling or abnormal drainage (**TABLE 7-4** describes normal or expected drainage).
♦ Administer antibiotics in a timely fashion. Reschedule parenteral antibiotics if a dose is delayed more than 1 hr. *Failure to administer antibiotics on schedule may result in inadequate blood levels and treatment failure.* Check blood levels as indicated (e.g., with vancomycin and gentamicin).
♦ As prescribed, administer pneumococcal vaccine to patients with total splenectomy. *This is to minimize risk of postsplenectomy sepsis.*
♦ Administer tetanus IG and tetanus toxoid as prescribed.
♦ Change dressings, one at a time, using sterile technique. *This is to prevent cross-contamination from wounds.*
♦ Use drains, closed drainage systems, or drainage bags to remove and collect GI secretions. *This is to avoid contamination of surgical incision site.*

♦ If patient has or develops evisceration, do not reinsert tissue or organs. Place a sterile, saline-soaked gauze over evisceration, and cover with a sterile towel until the evisceration can be evaluated by the surgeon. Keep patient on bed rest with bed in semi-Fowler's position with knees bent. Maintain nothing-by-mouth (NPO) status for patient, and anticipate need for emergency surgery.

Ineffective gastrointestinal tissue perfusion (or risk for same) related to interrupted blood flow to abdominal viscera secondary to vascular disruption or occlusion or related to moderate to severe hypovolemia caused by hemorrhage

Desired outcomes: Patient has adequate GI tissue perfusion, as evidenced by normoactive bowel sounds; soft, nondistended abdomen; and return of bowel elimination. Gastric secretions, drainage, and excretions are negative for occult blood.

Nursing Interventions

♦ Auscultate for bowel sounds hourly in recently injured patients and q8h during recovery phase. Report prolonged or sudden absence of bowel sounds. *This is because these signs may signal bowel ischemia or infarction.* Anticipate absent or diminished bowel sounds for up to 72 hr after surgery.
♦ Evaluate patient for peritoneal signs (Box 7-2), which may occur acutely secondary to injury or may not develop until days or weeks later if complications caused by slow bleeding or other mechanisms occur.
♦ Ensure adequate intravascular volume (see discussion in **Deficient fluid volume,** p. 503).
♦ Evaluate laboratory data (e.g., serial hematocrit [Hct] and elevated liver enzymes) or organ ischemia. *This is to check for evidence of bleeding or organ ischemia.*
♦ Document amount and character of GI secretions, drainage, and excretions. Note changes suggestive of bleeding (presence of frank or occult blood), infection (e.g., increased or purulent drainage), or obstruction (e.g., failure to eliminate flatus or stool within 72 hr after surgery).

Risk for impaired skin integrity related to risk of exposure to irritating GI drainage *and*
Impaired tissue integrity (or risk for same) related to direct trauma and surgery, catabolic post-traumatic state, and altered circulation
Desired outcome: Patient exhibits wound healing, and skin remains nonerythemic and intact.

Nursing Interventions

♦ Promptly change all dressings that become soiled with drainage or blood.
♦ Protect skin surrounding tubes, drains, or fistulas, and keep the areas clean and free from drainage. *Gastric and intestinal secretions and drainage are irritating and can lead to skin excoriation.* If necessary, apply ointments, skin barriers, or drainage bags. Apply reusable dressing supports such as Montgomery straps or tubular mesh gauze. *This is to prevent excessive injury to surrounding skin.* Consult the enterostomal therapy (ET) nurse for complex or involved cases.
♦ Inspect wounds, fistulas, and drain sites. *This is to observe for signs of irritation, infection, and ischemia.*
♦ Identify infected and devitalized tissue. Aid in the removal of this tissue by irrigation, wound packing, or preparing patient for surgical débridement.
♦ Ensure adequate protein and calorie intake. *This can promote tissue healing* (see **Imbalanced nutrition: less than body requirements,** immediately following).
♦ For more information, see "Managing Wound Care," p. 716.

Imbalanced nutrition: less than body requirements related to decreased intake secondary to disruption of GI tract integrity (traumatic or surgical) and increased need secondary to hypermetabolic posttrauma state

Desired outcome: By at least 24 hr before hospital discharge, patient has adequate nutrition as evidenced by maintenance of baseline body weight and positive or balanced N state.

Nursing Interventions

- Collaborate with health care provider, dietitian, and pharmacist about nutrition plan. *This is to estimate patient's metabolic needs based on type of injury, activity level, and nutritional status before injury.*
- Consider patient's specific injuries when planning nutrition (e.g., expect patients with hepatic or pancreatic injury to have difficulty with blood sugar regulation; patients with trauma to upper GI tract may be fed enterally, but feeding tube must be placed distal to the injury; disruption of GI tract may require feeding gastrostomy or jejunostomy; patients with major hepatic trauma may have difficulty with protein tolerance).
- Ensure patency of gastric or intestinal tubes. *This is to maintain decompression and encourage healing and return of bowel function.* Use caution and consult surgeon before irrigating nasogastric (NG) or other tubes that have been placed in or near recently sutured organs.
- Confirm placement of feeding tube before each tube feeding. After initial insertion, check x-ray film for position of feeding tube. *Insufflation with air and aspiration of stomach contents do not always confirm placement of small-bore feeding tubes.* Mark to determine tube migration, secure tubing in place, and reassess q4h and before each feeding. Assess aspirate for pH less than 5 for gastric tube placement. *Acid blockade drugs may alter pH.*
- Do not start enteral feeding until bowel function returns (i.e., bowel sounds are present, and patient experiences hunger).
- Consider administration of prescribed nonnarcotic analgesics (e.g., ketorolac). *Opioid analgesics decrease GI motility and may contribute to nausea, vomiting, abdominal distention, and ileus.*
- For more information, see "Providing Nutritional Support," p. 692.

Posttrauma syndrome related to life-threatening accident or event resulting in trauma

Desired outcomes: By at least 24 hr before hospital discharge, patient verbalizes aspects of the psychosocial impact of the event and does not exhibit signs of severe stress reaction, such as display of inconsistent affect, suicidal or homicidal behavior, or extreme agitation or depression. Patient cooperates with treatment plan.

Nursing Interventions

- Evaluate mental status at regular intervals. Be alert to display of affect inconsistent with statements or behavior, suicidal or homicidal statements or actions, extreme agitation or depression, and failure to cooperate with instructions related to care. *These are indicators of severe stress reaction.* Many victims of major abdominal trauma sustain life-threatening injury. Patient is often aware of the situation and fears death. Even after the physical condition stabilizes, patient may have a prolonged or severe reaction triggered by recollection of the trauma.
- Consult specialists such as psychiatrist, psychologist, psychiatric nurse practitioner, or pastoral counselor if patient displays signs of severe stress reaction described previously.
- Observe for severe pain, alcohol intoxication or withdrawal, electrolyte imbalance, metabolic encephalopathy, impaired cerebral perfusion. *These are organic causes that may contribute to posttraumatic response.*

♦ For other interventions, see nursing diagnosis in "Psychosocial Support," p. 31.

 Patient-Family Teaching and Discharge Planning

Anticipate extended physical and emotional rehabilitation for patient and significant other. When providing patient-family teaching, include verbal and written information about the following:

♦ Self-management: Assessment of patient's ability to manage own care should be completed before hospital discharge. Identification of support persons to assist with care should be initiated early.

♦ Probable need for emotional care, even for patients who have not required extensive physical rehabilitation. Provide referrals to support groups for trauma patients and family members.

♦ Availability of rehabilitation programs, extended care facilities, and home health agencies for patients unable to accomplish self-care on hospital discharge.

♦ Availability of rehabilitation programs for substance abuse, as indicated. Immediately after the traumatic event, patient and family members are very impressionable, thus making this period an ideal time for the substance abuser to begin to resolve the problem.

♦ Medications, including drug names, purpose, dosage, schedule, precautions, and potential side effects. Also discuss drug/drug, herb/drug, and food/drug interactions. Encourage patients taking antibiotics to take medications for prescribed length of time, even though they may be asymptomatic. If patient received tetanus immunization, ensure that he or she receives a wallet-size card documenting the immunization.

♦ Wound and catheter care: Have patient or caregiver describe and demonstrate proper technique before hospital discharge.

♦ Activity: Restrictions and recommendations should be reviewed thoroughly with patient and caregivers. An at-home assessment may be necessary if activity is severely limited or adaptations are necessary. Consider referral to OT or PT.

♦ Diet/nutrition: Review diet recommendations with patient/family. If enteral or parenteral feeding is necessary, have patient or caregiver describe and demonstrate correct technique before hospital discharge. Home health care services may be warranted for support and evaluation.

♦ Importance of seeking medical attention if indicators of infection or bowel obstruction occur (e.g., fever, severe or unusual abdominal pain, nausea and vomiting, unusual drainage from wounds or incisions, a change in bowel habits).

♦ Injury prevention: Following traumatic injury, patient and family members are especially likely to respond to injury prevention education. Provide instructions on proper seatbelt applications (across pelvic girdle rather than across soft tissue of lower abdomen), safety for infants and children, and other factors suitable for individuals involved.

❖ ❖ ❖

SECTION FIVE **HEPATIC AND BILIARY DISORDERS**

❖❖ **HEPATITIS**

OVERVIEW/PATHOPHYSIOLOGY

Viral hepatitis may be caused by one of five viruses that are capable of infecting the liver: hepatitis A virus (HAV), hepatitis B virus (HBV), hepatitis C virus (HCV), hepatitis D or delta virus (HDV), or hepatitis E virus (HEV). A sixth virus, hepatitis G virus (HGV), has been isolated in a few cases of hepatitis caused by other viruses of the five common strains. It is not known what the role of HGV is in liver disease, nor are clinical manifestations, natural history, or pathogenesis known. However, HGV has been found in a small percentage of blood donors, sometimes along with other hepatotropic viruses and sometimes alone. It also has been found in IV drug users, hemodialysis patients, and patients with hemophilia. Although symptoms are similar among all the hepatitis virus infections, immunologic and epidemiologic characteristics are different (**TABLE 7-5**). When hepatocytes are damaged, necrosis and autolysis can occur that in turn lead to abnormal liver functioning. Generally these changes are completely reversible after the acute phase. In some cases, however, massive necrosis can lead to acute liver failure and death.

Chronic hepatitis is inflammation of the liver for more than 6 mo. The term is used to describe a spectrum of inflammatory liver diseases ranging from mild chronic persistent hepatitis to severe chronic active hepatitis. Forms of chronic hepatitis are associated with infection with HBV, HCV, and HDV; viral infections such as cytomegalovirus (CMV); excessive alcohol consumption; inflammatory bowel disease (IBD); and autoimmunity (chronic active lupoid hepatitis). *Alcoholic hepatitis* occurs as a result of tissue necrosis caused by alcohol abuse; it is nonviral and noninfectious. Generally it is a precursor to cirrhosis (see p. 515), but it may occur simultaneously with cirrhosis.

Jaundice is discoloration of body tissues from increased serum levels of bilirubin (total serum bilirubin more than 2.5 mg/dL). Jaundice may be seen in any patient with impaired hepatic function and occurs as bilirubin begins to be excreted through the skin. There is also increased excretion of urobilinogen and bilirubin by the kidneys that results in darker, almost brownish, urine. Jaundice is classified as follows.

Prehepatic (hemolytic): Caused by increased production of bilirubin following erythrocyte destruction. Prehepatic jaundice is implicated when the indirect (unconjugated) serum bilirubin is more than 0.8 mg/dL.

Hepatic (hepatocellular): Caused by dysfunction of the liver cells (hepatocytes) that reduces their ability to remove bilirubin from the blood and form it into bile. Hepatic jaundice is also implicated with indirect serum bilirubin and is associated with hepatitis.

Posthepatic (obstructive): Caused by an obstruction of the flow of bile out of the liver and resulting in backed-up bile through the hepatocytes to the blood. Posthepatic jaundice is implicated when direct serum bilirubin is more than 0.3 mg/dL.

ASSESSMENT

Signs and symptoms/physical findings: Nausea, vomiting, malaise, anorexia, muscle or joint aches, fatigue, irritability, slight to moderate temperature increases, epigastric discomfort, dark urine, clay-colored stools, pruritus, aversion to smoking.

Acute hepatic failure: Nausea, vomiting, and abdominal pain tend to be more severe. Jaundice is likely to appear earlier and deepen more rapidly. Mental status changes (possibly progressing to encephalopathy), coma, seizures, ascites, sharp rise in temperature, significant leukocytosis, "coffee grounds" emesis, gastrointestinal (GI) hemorrhage, purpura, shock, oliguria, and azotemia all may be present. Jaundice is present; palpation of lymph nodes and abdomen may reveal lymphadenopathy, hepatomegaly, and splenomegaly. Liver size usually is small in acute hepatic failure.

History and risk factors: Clotting disorders, multiple blood transfusions, excessive alcohol ingestion, parenteral drug use, exposure to hepatotoxic chemicals or medications, travel to developing countries.

TABLE 7-5	TYPES AND CHARACTERISTICS OF VIRAL HEPATITIS				
CHARACTERISTIC	HEPATITIS A VIRUS (HAV) INFECTION	HEPATITIS B VIRUS (HBV) INFECTION	HEPATITIS C VIRUS (HCV) INFECTION	HEPATITIS D VIRUS (HDV) INFECTION	HEPATITIS E VIRUS (HEV) INFECTION
Mode(s) of Transmission	Fecal-oral; food-borne most common; parenteral transmission rare; most infectious 2 wk before symptoms appear	Contact with blood or serum; perinatal transmission; sexual contact; often transmitted by chronic carriers; most infectious before symptoms appear and for 4-6 mo after acute infection	Contact with blood or serum; perinatal transmission rare unless mother is HIV infected; often transmitted by chronic carriers; most infectious 1-2 wk before symptoms appear	Similar to HBV; can cause infection only if individual already has HBV; blood infectious throughout HDV infection	Fecal-oral; food-borne; water-borne
Population most affected	Children; individuals living in or traveling to areas with poor sanitation	Injecting drug users; health care and public safety workers exposed to blood; patients and staff of institutions for the developmentally disabled; homosexual men; men and women with multiple heterosexual partners; young children of infected mothers; recipients of certain blood products; hemodialysis patients	Injecting drug users; individuals who received blood products before 1991; potential risk to health care and safety workers exposed to blood	Injecting drug users; patients with hemophilia; recipients of multiple blood transfusions; infects only individuals who are already HBV positive	Individuals living in or traveling to countries where sanitation is poor
Incubation	2-6 wk	6 wk-6 mo	15-150 days	30-150 days	1-2 mo
Serum marker(s) of acute infection	Anti-HAV; IgM	HBsAg, anti-HBc IgM	HCV RNA (anti-HCV)	Anti-HDV IgM	Anti-HEV IgM

Measures to reduce exposure	Handwashing; good personal hygiene; sanitation; appropriate infection control measures (Appendix 1)	Handwashing; good personal hygiene; appropriate infection control measures; autoclaving all nondisposable items; careful handling of needles/sharps; not reusing needles; discarding needles/sharps in special containers	Same as for HBV	Same as for HBV	Same as for HAV
Prophylaxis	Sanitation measures; immunization; immunoglobulin within 1-2 wk of exposure	Screening donated blood; protective devices for health care or safety workers; immunization; use of condoms; HBIG for known exposure to HBsAg-contaminated material	Screening donated blood; protective devices for health care or safety workers; no vaccine available	Immunization against HBV	Effectiveness of immunoglobulin not known
Other information	Symptoms usually mild; rarely causes fulminant hepatic failure; epidemics can occur	HBsAg persists in carrier state; chronic hepatitis may develop; fulminant hepatic failure may occur; this is the most complex hepatitis virus	Carrier state and chronic hepatitis may develop; fulminant hepatic failure may occur	Increased risk of serious complications including fulminant hepatic failure and death; carrier state and chronic hepatitis may develop	Sporadic cases as well as outbreaks have occurred (not in the United States), mostly in countries where sanitation is a problem; does not produce chronic hepatitis, cirrhosis, or a chronic carrier state

HBcAg, Hepatitis B core antigen; *HBIG*, hepatitis B immunoglobulin; *HBsAg*, hepatitis B surface antigen; *HIV*, human immunodeficiency virus; *IgG*, immunoglobulin G; *IgM*, immunoglobulin M; *RNA*, ribonucleic acid.

DIAGNOSTIC TESTS

Hematologic tests

Immunoglobulins (IG): See Table 7-5 for serum markers for acute infection for each of the five viruses. Chronic infection markers are recognized for HBV, HCV, and HDV. They are HBV surface antigen (HBsAG) and anti-HBc immunoglobulin G (IgG) for hepatitis B; anti-HCV (enzyme-linked immunosorbent assay [ELISA]) RIBA for hepatitis C; and anti-HDV IgG for hepatitis D.

Serum enzymes: Aspartate aminotransferase (AST) and alanine aminotransferase (ALT) are initially elevated and then drop. γ-Glutamyl transpeptidase (GGT) is elevated early in liver disease and persists as long as cellular damage continues.

Total bilirubin: Is elevated.

PT: Is prolonged.

Differential WBC count: Reveals leukocytosis, monocytosis, and atypical lymphocytes.

Urine tests: Reveal elevation of urobilinogen, mild proteinuria, and mild bilirubinuria.

Liver biopsy: Performed percutaneously or via laparoscopy to collect a specimen for histologic examination to confirm differential diagnosis.

COLLABORATIVE MANAGEMENT

Monitoring of activity level: Bed rest may be indicated when symptoms are severe, with a gradual return to normal activity as symptoms subside.

Diet: In general, dietary management consists of giving palatable meals as tolerated without overfeeding. If oral intake is substantially decreased, parenteral or enteral nutrition may be initiated. Na^+ restrictions may be indicated in the presence of fluid retention. Protein is moderately restricted or eliminated, depending on the degree of mental status changes (i.e., encephalopathy). If no mental status changes are noted, normal amounts of high biologic value protein are indicated to facilitate tissue healing. All alcoholic beverages are strictly forbidden. Vitamins usually are given, and folic acid may be indicated in alcoholic hepatitis.

Management of pruritus: Alkaline soaps are restricted; emollients and lipid creams (e.g., Eucerin) are prescribed. Antihistamines and tranquilizers, if used, are administered with caution and in low doses because they are metabolized by the liver. See **BOX 7-3** for a list of hepatotoxic drugs.

Pharmacotherapy

Parenteral vitamin K: For patients with prolonged PT. Patients with severe hepatic failure may not respond to vitamin K and therefore may require transfusions of fresh frozen plasma.

Antihistamines (e.g., diphenhydramine): For symptomatic relief of pruritus. However, they may cause excessive sedation.

Antiemetics (e.g., hydroxyzine, ondansetron): For patients with nausea. Avoid phenothiazines, such as prochlorperazine (Compazine), because they cause excessive sedation.

IG: Given routinely to all close personal contacts of patients with HAV infection.

Hepatitis B IG (HBIG): Recommended for individuals exposed to HBsAg-contaminated material.

HAV vaccine: Recommended for people with potential for exposure to HAV.

HBV vaccines: Developed for prevention of hepatitis, they reduce the incidence of HBV infection by approximately 92%. Immunization is recommended for all health care workers and others with risk of exposure to blood and body secretions. Vaccination against HBV is now recommended for all newborns and children.

BOX 7-3	DRUGS THAT CAN CAUSE HEPATOTOXICITY

Prescription Drugs
- Allopurinol
- Amiodarone
- Androgenic steroids
- Carbamazepine
- Carmustine (BCNU)
- Chlorpromazine (CPZ)
- Cyclosporine
- Dantrolene
- Diazepam
- Erythromycin
- Glucocorticoids
- Haloperidol
- Halothane (and related anesthetics)
- Isoniazid (INH)
- Ketoconazole
- MAO inhibitors
- Mercaptopurine (6-MP)
- Methotrexate (MTX)
- Methyldopa
- Mitomycin
- Oral contraceptives
- Oxacillin
- Phenindione
- Phenylbutazone
- Phenytoin sodium
- Rifampin
- Sulfonamides

Nonprescription Drugs
- Acetaminophen
- Alcohol
- Aspirin and other salicylates
- Other NSAIDs
- Vitamin A

BCNU, Bischloroethy/nitrosourea; *MAO,* monoamine oxidase; *NSAIDs,* nonsteroidal antiinflammatory drugs.

Corticosteroids: May be used, particularly for patients with alcoholic hepatitis, to control symptoms and reduce abnormal liver function.

Recombinant interferon: An antiviral agent that inhibits viral replication. Combination therapy using pegylated interferon-α and ribavirin (an antiviral agent) has been proved effective in treatment of chronic hepatitis, although not in HAV or HBV infection.

Restriction of hepatotoxic drugs: See Box 7-3.

NURSING DIAGNOSES AND INTERVENTIONS

Fatigue related to decreased metabolic energy production secondary to liver dysfunction, which causes faulty absorption, metabolism, and storage of nutrients

Desired outcome: By at least 24 hr before hospital discharge, patient relates decreasing fatigue and increasing energy.

Nursing Interventions

- Determine food preferences. Encourage significant other to bring in desirable foods if permitted.
- Encourage small, frequent feedings, and provide emotional support during meals. Consult dietitian regarding increased intake of carbohydrates or other high-energy food sources within prescribed dietary limitations. Record intake.
- Obtain prescription for vitamin and mineral supplements if appropriate.
- Provide rest periods of at least 90 min before and after activities and treatments. Avoid activity immediately after meals. *This is to decrease fatigue and encourage compliance with activities and treatments.*
- Keep frequently used objects within easy reach.
- Decrease environmental stimuli; provide back massage and relaxation tapes. *This is to promote rest and sleep.*

- Administer acid suppression therapy, antiemetics, antidiarrheal medications, and cathartics as prescribed. *This is to minimize gastric distress and promote absorption of nutrients.*

Deficient knowledge related to causes of hepatitis and modes of transmission
Desired outcome: Within the 24-hr period before hospital discharge, patient verbalizes knowledge about the causes of hepatitis and measures that help prevent transmission.

Nursing Interventions

- Assess patient's knowledge about disease process, and educate as necessary. (Do not make moral judgments about alcohol/drug use or sexual behavior.)
- Teach patient and significant other to wear gloves and use good handwashing technique if contact with body fluids such as urine, blood, wound exudate, feces is possible. *This is to avoid transmission or recurrence of disease.*
- If appropriate, advise patients with HAV infection that crowded living conditions with poor sanitation should be avoided. *This is to prevent recurrence.*
- Remind patients with HBV and HCV infection that they should modify sexual behavior as directed by health care provider. Explain that blood donation is no longer possible.
- Advise patients with HBV infection that their sexual partners should receive HBV vaccine.
- Refer patient to drug treatment programs as necessary.

Risk for impaired skin integrity related to pruritus secondary to hepatic dysfunction
Desired outcome: Patient's skin remains intact.

Nursing Interventions

- Use tepid water or emollient baths, avoid alkaline soap, and apply emollient lotions at frequent intervals. *This is to keep the skin moist.*
- Encourage patient not to scratch skin and to keep nails short and smooth. Suggest use of knuckles if patient must scratch. Wrap or place gloves on patient's hands (especially comatose patients).
- Treat any skin lesion promptly and change soiled linen as soon as possible. *This is to prevent infection.*
- Administer antihistamines as prescribed; observe closely for excessive sedation.
- Encourage patient to wear loose, soft clothing; provide soft linens (cotton is best).
- Keep environment cool.

Ineffective protection related to increased risk of bleeding secondary to decreased vitamin K absorption, thrombocytopenia
Desired outcome: Patient is free of bleeding as evidenced by negative tests for occult blood in the feces and urine, absence of ecchymotic areas, and absence of bleeding at the gums and injection sites.

Nursing Interventions

- Monitor PT levels daily for increases; optimal range is 10.5-13.5 sec.
- Monitor platelet count daily for thrombocytopenia; optimal range is 150,000-400,000/mm^3.
- Monitor hematocrit (Hct) and hemoglobin (Hgb) daily for decreases. *They may indicate occult bleeding.* Optimal ranges are Hct 40%-54%

(male) and 37%-47% (female), Hgb 14-18 g/dL (male) and 12-16 g/dL (female).

♦ Handle patient gently (e.g., when turning or transferring). *This is to prevent bruising.*
♦ Minimize intramuscular (IM) injections. Rotate sites, and use small-gauge needles. Apply moderate pressure after an injection, but do not massage site. Administer medications orally or by the IV route when possible.
♦ Observe for ecchymotic areas. Inspect gums, and test urine and feces. *This is to observe for bleeding.*
♦ Teach patient to use electric razor and soft-bristle toothbrush. *This is to prevent cuts and bleeding.*
♦ Administer vitamin K as prescribed.

 Patient-Family Teaching and Discharge Planning

When providing patient-family teaching, include verbal and written information about the following:

♦ Importance of rest and getting adequate nutrition. When appropriate, provide a list of high biologic value protein food sources or protein foods to avoid and sample menus to demonstrate how these foods may be incorporated into or excluded from the diet. Instruct patient to eat frequent, small meals; to eat slowly; and to chew all food thoroughly. Teach patient to rest for 30-60 min after meals. Initiate dietitian consult as needed for diet instruction.
♦ Importance of avoiding hepatotoxic agents, including over-the-counter (OTC) drugs (Box 7-3).
♦ Prescribed medications (e.g., multivitamins), including drug names, purpose, dosage, schedule, potential side effects, and precautions. Also discuss drug/drug, food/drug, and herb/drug interactions.
♦ Importance of informing health care providers, dentists, and other health care workers of hepatitis diagnosis.
♦ Potential complications, including delayed healing, skin injury, and bleeding tendencies.
♦ Importance of avoiding alcohol during recovery, and referral to alcohol/drug treatment programs as appropriate. Additional resources include the following:

CDC Division of Hepatitis Resources: www.cdc.gov/hepatitis/Resources/index. htm

Hepatitis Foundation International: www.hepfi.org

❖ CIRRHOSIS

OVERVIEW/PATHOPHYSIOLOGY

Cirrhosis is a chronic, serious disease in which normal configuration of the liver is changed, resulting in cell death. When new cells are formed, the resulting scarring causes disruption of blood and lymph flow. Although pathologic changes do not occur for many years, structural changes gradually lead to total liver dysfunction. Manifestations of cirrhosis are related to hepatocellular necrosis and portal hypertension. Complications caused by cellular failure are similar to those of acute hepatitis and include inability to metabolize bilirubin and resultant jaundice; difficulty producing serum proteins, including albumin and certain clotting factors; hyperdynamic circulation and decreased vasomotor tone; pulmonary changes (ventilation/perfusion mismatch) and sometimes cyanosis; changes in N metabolism (e.g., inability to convert ammonia to urea); and difficulty metabolizing some hormones (especially the sex hormones). Complications related to portal hypertension include development of ascites, bleeding esophageal and gastric varices, portal-systemic collateral vessels, encephalopathy, and splenomegaly.

Alcoholic (Laënnec's) cirrhosis: Associated with long-term alcohol abuse; accounts for 50% of all cirrhosis cases. Changes in liver structure caused by cirrhosis are irreversible, but compensation of liver function can be achieved if the liver is protected from further damage by alcohol cessation and proper nutrition. The histologic definition of this form of cirrhosis is micronodular cirrhosis.

Postnecrotic cirrhosis: Associated with a history of viral hepatitis (hepatitis B virus [HBV] or hepatitis C virus [HCV]) or hepatic damage from drugs or toxins and is the leading type of cirrhosis in the Western world, Asia, and Africa. This type appears to predispose the patient to the development of a hepatoma. The histologic definition of this form of cirrhosis is macronodular cirrhosis.

Biliary cirrhosis: Associated with chronic retention of bile and inflammation of bile ducts; accounts for 15% of all cirrhosis cases. The histologic definition of this form of cirrhosis is mixed nodular cirrhosis; it may be further classified as follows.

Primary biliary cirrhosis (PBC) (nonsuppurative destructive cholangitis): An inflammatory disease of intrahepatic bile ducts, this slowly progressive disease has other findings, including steatorrhea, xanthomatous (yellow tumors) neuropathy, osteoporosis, and portal hypertension. Hypercholesterolemia, hyperlipidemia, and hepatomegaly are found in approximately 85% of patients with PBC.

Secondary biliary cirrhosis: Results from chronic obstruction to bile flow, usually from an obstruction outside the liver, such as calculi, neoplasms, or biliary atresia.

ASSESSMENT

Signs and symptoms/physical findings: Many patients with cirrhosis have no symptoms. Others exhibit symptoms in varying degrees, depending on the degree of impaired hepatocellular function. Symptoms and signs may include weakness, fatigability, weight loss, pruritus, fever, anorexia, nausea, occasional vomiting, abdominal pain, diarrhea, menstrual abnormalities, sterility, impotence, loss of libido, hematemesis. Urine may be dark (brownish) because of the presence of urobilinogen, and stools may be pale and clay-colored because of the absence of bilirubin. Jaundice, hepatomegaly, ascites, peripheral edema, pleural effusion, and fetor hepaticus (a musty, sweetish odor on the breath) may be present. There may be slight changes in personality and behavior, which can progress to coma (a result of hepatic encephalopathy); spider angiomas, testicular atrophy, gynecomastia, pectoral and axillary alopecia (a result of hormonal changes); splenomegaly; hemorrhoids (a result of portal hypertension complications); spider nevi; purpuric lesions; and palmar erythema. Asterixis (i.e., jerking movements of the hands and wrists when the wrists are dorsiflexed with the fingers extended) may be present in advanced cirrhosis.

History and risk factors: Excessive alcohol ingestion; hepatitis B, C, or D infection; exposure to hepatotoxic drugs (Box 7-3) or chemicals; biliary or metabolic disease; poor nutrition.

DIAGNOSTIC TESTS

Blood studies/biochemical tests

Hematologic: RBCs are decreased in hypersplenism and decreased with hemorrhage. WBCs are decreased with hypersplenism and increased with infection. Platelet counts are less than normal.

Bilirubin levels: Elevated because of failure in hepatocyte metabolism and obstruction in some instances. Very high or persistently elevated levels are considered a poor prognostic sign.

Alkaline phosphatase levels: Normal to mildly elevated in most cases; in PBC levels are elevated 2-3 × normal.

AST and ALT levels: Usually elevated to more than 300 units with acute failure and normal or mildly elevated with chronic failure. ALT is more specific for hepatocellular damage.

Albumin levels: Reduced, especially with ascites. Persistently low levels suggest a poor prognosis. This test is not a perfect indicator of liver function because it is affected by poor nutrition and fluid status.

International normalized ratio (INR): Elevated with severe hepatocellular dysfunction because the liver synthesizes clotting factors, particularly vitamin K–dependent factors.

Electrolytes

NA^+ *LEVELS:* Normal to low. Na^+ is retained but is associated with water retention, which results in normal serum Na^+ levels or even dilutional hyponatremia. Often severe hyponatremia is present in the terminal stage and is associated with tense ascites and hepatorenal syndrome.

K^+ *LEVELS:* Slightly reduced unless patient has renal insufficiency, which would result in hyperkalemia. Chronic hypokalemic acidosis is common in patients with chronic alcoholic liver disease.

Glucose levels: Hypoglycemia possible because of impaired gluconeogenesis and glycogen depletion in patients with severe or terminal liver disease.

BUN levels: May be slightly decreased because of failure of Krebs cycle enzymes in the liver or elevated because of bleeding or renal insufficiency.

Ammonia levels: Elevation expected because of inability of the failing liver to convert ammonia to urea and shunting of intestinal blood via collateral vessels. Gastrointestinal (GI) hemorrhage or an increase in intestinal protein from dietary intake increases ammonia levels. Keep patient on nothing-by-mouth (NPO) status except for water for 8 hr before drawing the ammonia level. Notify laboratory of all antibiotics taken by patient because they may lower the ammonia level.

Coagulation: Prothrombin time (PT) is prolonged and, in severe liver disease, unresponsive to vitamin K therapy. Coagulation abnormalities usually involve factor V but also may involve factors II, VII, IX, and X.

Urine tests: Urine bilirubin is increased; urobilinogen is normal or increased; and proteinuria may be present.

Liver biopsy: Obtains a specimen of liver for microscopic analysis and diagnosis of cirrhosis, hepatitis, or other liver disease. After local anesthetic is administered and patient's skin is prepared, a large needle is inserted into the eighth or ninth intercostal space in the midaxillary line. It is critical that patient hold his or her breath at the end of expiration to elevate the liver maximally. Patient movement or failure to sustain expiration can result in puncture through the lung rather than the liver. Type and crossmatching sometimes are performed before the procedure in anticipation of hemorrhagic complications. Percutaneous liver biopsy is contraindicated in patients with markedly prolonged PT or very low platelet counts because of the risk of hemorrhage. In these patients, a transvenous biopsy via the jugular or hepatic vein may be attempted instead (see **BOX 7-4** for care of patients undergoing liver biopsy). Open liver biopsy, or minilaparotomy, also may be done for liver biopsy.

Barium swallow: Used in nonemergency situations (i.e., for patients without active bleeding) to verify the presence of gastroesophageal varices. Patient should be on NPO status from midnight until completion of the test. Because of the constipating effects of barium, enemas should be given on patient's return from the procedure.

Radiologic studies: Ultrasound differentiates hemolytic and hepatocellular jaundice from obstructive jaundice and shows hepatomegaly and intrahepatic tumors. Computed tomography (CT) scan of the liver/spleen is performed to evaluate size and location of tumors and nodules and to rule out gallbladder

BOX 7-4	NURSING CARE OF THE PATIENT UNDERGOING LIVER BIOPSY

Prebiopsy
- Explain procedure to patient and significant other.

Intrabiopsy
- Assist patient with remaining motionless.
- Coach patient in sustaining exhalation during puncture (or manually ventilate intubated patient to prevent lung inflation during puncture) to prevent pneumothorax.

Postbiopsy
- Auscultate breath sounds immediately after procedure and at 1- to 2-hr intervals for 6-8 hr after procedure to detect pneumothorax or hemothorax (unlikely but serious complications). Diminished sounds on the right side and tachypnea suggest pneumothorax or hemothorax.
- Position patient on the right side for several hours after biopsy, to tamponade (stop blood flow) puncture site.
- Enforce bed rest for 8-12 hr after biopsy to minimize risk of hemorrhage from puncture site.
- Administer analgesics as prescribed. Avoid NSAIDs, which may affect clotting, and hepatotoxins (Box 7-3).
- Monitor patient for indicators of peritonitis or intraperitoneal bleeding, which can occur as a result of puncture of blood vessels or major bile duct: severe abdominal pain, abdominal distention and rigidity, rebound tenderness, nausea, vomiting, tachycardia, tachypnea, pallor, decreased blood pressure, and rising temperature.

NSAIDs, Nonsteroidal antiinflammatory drugs.

disease. Percutaneous transhepatic cholangiography reveals extent of obstruction via contrast dye. Endoscopic retrograde cholangiopancreatography (ERCP) is a fiberoptic technique used to show obstructions of the common bile and pancreatic ducts as potential causes of jaundice. Liver scans enable visualization of the spleen and liver via injection of radioisotopes. After injection of the dye, patient may experience nausea, vomiting, and transient elevated temperature.

Angiographic studies: Establish portal vein patency and visualize portosystemic collateral vessels to determine cause of and effective treatment for variceal bleeding. Portal venous anatomy must be established before such operations as portal systemic shunt or hepatic transplantation. In patients with previously constructed surgical shunts, loss of patency may be confirmed as a factor leading to the present bleeding episode. See **BOX 7-5** for nursing implications with angiographic studies.

- The most common procedure is portal venography by indirect angiography. The femoral artery is catheterized, and contrast material is injected into the splenic artery. Contrast material flows through the spleen into the splenic and portal veins.
- Hepatic vein wedge pressure is measured by introducing a balloon catheter into the femoral vein and threading it into a hepatic vein branch.
- Direct access to the portal vein may be achieved through transhepatic portography. During this procedure, varices may be obliterated by injection of thrombin or Gelfoam into veins that supply the varices. Transhepatic portography involves a direct puncture through the liver and has many of the same risks as liver biopsy. Patients returning from this procedure should be positioned on their right side and monitored closely.

Esophagoscopy: Visualizes the esophagus and stomach directly via a fiberoptic esophagoscope. Varices in the esophagus and upper portion of the

BOX 7-5 NURSING CARE OF THE PATIENT
UNDERGOING ANGIOGRAPHIC STUDIES

Preprocedure
- Explain procedure to patient and significant other.
- Maintain NPO status for 8 hr before procedure.
- Verify patency of IV catheter.
- Note allergies to seafood, iodine, and contrast material.
- Administer sedatives as prescribed. Be aware that dosage usually is reduced if cirrhosis or hepatitis is diagnosed.

Intraprocedure
- Assist radiology personnel with positioning and draping patient.
- Monitor VS q15min or more often for evidence of anaphylaxis or hemorrhagic shock.

Postprocedure
- Check VS q15min initially and q1-2h once patient's condition has stabilized.
- Maintain patient in supine position.
- Keep pressure dressing and sandbag over puncture site for 6-8 hr.
- Evaluate distal pulses and perfusion in affected extremity q1-2h for 8 hr. Arterial thrombosis and large hematomas that compromise femoral blood flow may develop as a result of manipulation of the artery and clotting abnormalities associated with liver disease.
- Promote adequate hydration via PO intake or IV fluids as indicated.
- Monitor urine output q1-2h, and report volume less than 30 mL/hr.

IV, Intravenous; *NPO,* nothing by mouth; *PO,* by mouth; *VS,* vital signs.

stomach are identified, and attempts are made to identify the exact source of bleeding. Variceal bleeding may be treated by sclerotherapy, electrocautery, laser, vasoconstrictive agents, or other methods during the endoscopic procedure (see "Collaborative Management," following). See **BOX 7-6** for nursing implications with esophagoscopy.

Peritoneoscopy or laparoscopy: Visualizes the liver and allows for biopsy.

Electroencephalogram (EEG): Traces the electrical impulses of the brain to detect or confirm encephalopathy. Changes on the EEG occur very early, usually before behavioral or biochemical alterations.

Psychometric testing (e.g., Reitan number connection [trail-making] test): Evaluates for hepatic encephalopathy. Patient's speed and accuracy at connecting a series of numbered circles are evaluated at intervals. A daily handwriting test is an easy check of intellectual deterioration or improvement.

COLLABORATIVE MANAGEMENT

Treatment of underlying causes: For example, exposure to hepatotoxins, use of alcohol, biliary obstruction.

Pharmacotherapy: Opioids and sedatives, which are metabolized by the liver, are contraindicated. Small doses of benzodiazepines with a short half-life, such as oxazepam, may be administered if absolutely necessary. See Box 7-3 for a list of hepatotoxic drugs.

Ursodeoxycholic acid (UDCA) (e.g., ursodiol): Occurs naturally in the bile, where its role is controlling serum cholesterol concentration. As a drug, it is used as a surgical alternative for dissolving gallstones made of cholesterol. Treatment lasts several months.

Diuretics: Reduce edema. K^+-sparing diuretics (e.g., spironolactone) often are used if there is no response to salt restriction. If indicated, teach patient to avoid excessive ingestion of K^+-rich foods or salt substitutes. Weight loss in ascitic patients should not exceed 1-1.5 lb/day (0.5-0.7 kg/day).

BOX 7-6	NURSING CARE OF THE PATIENT UNDERGOING ESOPHAGOSCOPY

Preprocedure
- Explain procedure to patient and significant other.
- Maintain NPO status for 8 hr before procedure.
- Clear stomach of blood and gastric contents immediately before endoscope is passed.
- Verify patency of two large-bore IV catheters, which are used for rapid administration of fluids and medications.
- Administer sedatives as prescribed. Be aware that dosage usually is reduced if cirrhosis or hepatitis is diagnosed.

Intraprocedure
- Maintain patient in side-lying position to reduce likelihood of aspiration.
- Have pharyngeal and tracheal suction readily available.
- Monitor LOC, VS, and oxygenation status during procedure.

Postprocedure
- Maintain side-lying position until patient is fully alert.
- Note evidence of change in rate of hemorrhage.
- Be alert for immediate complications, such as aspiration pneumonia (evidenced by difficulty breathing, diminished breath sounds, coarse crackles, rhonchi) and perforation (rare—evidenced by severe retrosternal pain and bleeding).

IV, Intravenous; *LOC,* level of consciousness; *NPO,* nothing by mouth; *VS,* vital signs.

Neomycin or metronidazole: Controls intestinal flora that aggravate encephalopathy.

Lactulose: Neutralizes intraluminal ammonia in the intestine in an attempt to control encephalopathy.

Propranolol: Reduces portal vein BP to aid in controlling bleeding esophageal or gastric varices.

Vasopressin: Used with acute variceal bleeding to vasoconstrict mesenteric blood vessels and reduce portal blood flow. Nitroglycerin also is commonly administered to counteract the potential for myocardial ischemia or other serious cardiovascular side effects.

Hematinics (e.g., ferrous sulfate): Control anemia. They are used to replace iron after abnormal blood loss.

Blood coagulants: Control bleeding.

Laxatives and stool softeners: Prevent straining and rupture of varices.

Antihistamines (e.g., diphenhydramine) or cholestyramine: For pruritus.

Topical anesthetics: For hemorrhoids.

Supplemental vitamins and minerals: Such as folic acid for macrocytic anemia and vitamin K for prolonged PT.

Dietary management: With fluid retention and ascites, Na^+ and fluids are restricted. Usually half the calories are supplied as carbohydrates. Protein is restricted in hepatic coma or precoma because the action of intestinal bacteria on protein increases blood ammonia levels; increased ammonia levels cause or worsen the coma state. Parenteral or enteral nutrition is administered in the presence of bleeding or coma.

Bed rest: In the presence of fever, infection.

Treatment of complications

GI hemorrhage: Upper GI hemorrhage is common in patients with chronic liver disease and can result from esophageal varices, portal hypertensive gastropathy, duodenal or gastric ulcers, or Mallory-Weiss tear (mucosal laceration at the juncture of the distal esophagus and proximal stomach). Early diagnosis is essential to enable appropriate intervention.

ESOPHAGEAL VARICES: The therapeutic goal is to reduce portal hypertension and blood flow.

♦ Pharmacotherapy includes β-blockers, vasopressin, and somatostatin.
♦ Gastroesophageal balloon tamponade (using Minnesota, Linton, or Seng-staken-Blakemore tubes) applies direct pressure on acutely bleeding varices until definitive therapy is possible. Complications can include airway obstruction, pulmonary aspiration, gastroesophageal mucosal pressure necrosis, and esophageal rupture.
♦ Endoscopic therapies include variceal sclerosis, using sodium morrhuate or sodium tetradecyl sulfate, electrocautery, laser cautery, topical vasoconstrictive agents, or variceal band ligation. Complications include pain, fever, dysphagia, ulcerations, bleeding, perforation, pulmonary problems, and bacteremia.
♦ Portosystemic shunt procedures are used to divert portal blood flow away from the liver. Transjugular intrahepatic portosystemic shunting (TIPS) (preferred for refractory ascites) is a nonoperative procedure that achieves portal decompression by transvenous placement of a stent between the hepatic and portal veins. Surgical shunts, such as portacaval or distal splenorenal shunts, may be performed if medical therapies are unsuccessful. Operative mortality is much higher for emergent vs. elective procedures. Postsurgical complications include disseminated intravascular coagulation (DIC), bacterial infections, heart failure, and variceal bleeding.

PORTAL HYPERTENSIVE GASTROPATHY: Results in bleeding from the gastric mucosa from severe portal hypertension. Treatment focuses on reducing portal vein BP with propranolol or a portosystemic shunt.

Ascites: Dietary management may include Na^+ and fluid restrictions. Diuretics, usually aldosterone antagonists, are often given to minimize fluid collection. If indicated, surgical management includes a peritoneovenous (LeVeen or Denver) shunt, which provides a route for reinfusion of ascitic fluid into the venous system. Monitor for these potential complications: cardiac or renal overload (see "Heart Failure," p. 107; "Pulmonary Hypertension," p. 118), shunt occlusion, DIC (see p. 562), hemorrhage, infection, and extravasation of ascitic fluid from incisions. Large-volume paracentesis may be indicated in patients with massive ascites when it is refractory to diuretics and severe respiratory distress is present. IV albumin may be infused to replete intravascular volume but cost-benefit effectiveness is not proved.

Hepatic encephalopathy (hepatic coma): Ammonia is the most easily identified toxin. Dietary management includes restriction of protein from the diet to decrease blood ammonia levels, giving sweetened fruit juices to provide the necessary carbohydrates for energy, and administering parenteral/enteral nutrition if the patient is comatose. Pharmacologic management includes neomycin to inhibit intestinal bacteria and magnesium sulfate or enemas to cleanse the intestines after GI bleeding. Lactulose is administered to neutralize ammonia and aid in evacuating stool to improve mentation. The following drugs are contraindicated: barbiturates and opioids (because of the inability of the liver to detoxify them), K^+-depleting diuretics (aldosterone antagonists are the first-line choice because edema is related to inadequate detoxification of aldosterone), and ammonia-containing medications or food, which would cause or worsen hepatic coma.

Spontaneous bacterial peritonitis: Occurs in cirrhotic patients with ascites. Abdominal pain, worsening ascites, fever, and progressive encephalopathy suggest peritonitis. Mortality is high. See "Peritonitis," p. 461, for treatment.

Irreversible end-stage liver disease: Individuals with irreversible liver failure caused by chronic active hepatitis, PBC, sclerosing cholangitis, alcoholic cirrhosis, metabolic liver disease, acute fulminant hepatic necrosis, and other conditions may be considered for liver transplantation. Severe liver failure is manifested by serum bilirubin more than 10 mg/dL, albumin less than 2.5 g/dL, and PT more than 5 sec beyond the control. Patient must be refractory to all medical and other surgical treatments and have no absolute contraindications to transplantation (e.g., active substance abuse, metastatic disease). Patients are referred to specialized medical centers where they receive extensive preoperative evaluation and preparation.

NURSING DIAGNOSES AND INTERVENTIONS

Imbalanced nutrition: less than body requirements related to anorexia, nausea, or malabsorption

Desired outcome: By at least 24 hr before hospital discharge, patient demonstrates progress toward adequate nutritional status, as evidenced by stable weight, balanced or positive N state, serum protein 6-8 g/dL, and serum albumin 3.5-5.5 g/dL.

Nursing Interventions

- Explain dietary restrictions; remember that Na^+ and fluids are restricted (see Box 4-2, p. 174, for a list of foods high in Na^+). Encourage patient to eat foods that are permitted within dietary restrictions. If the ammonia level rises (normal levels are whole blood 70-200 mcg/dL and plasma 56-150 mcg/dL), protein and foods high in ammonia also will be restricted.
- Monitor I&O; weigh patient daily.
- Encourage small, frequent meals and have nourishing foods available to patient at night. Encourage significant other to bring desirable foods as permitted. *This is to ensure adequate nutrition.*
- Administer vitamin and mineral supplements as prescribed.
- Administer acid suppression agents, antiemetics, and cathartics, as prescribed. *This is to decrease gastric distress.*
- Implement prescribed measures to relieve/mobilize ascites and decrease pressure on intraabdominal structures.
- Promote bed rest. *This helps reduce metabolic demands on the liver.*
- Provide soft diet if patient has esophageal varices that are not bleeding. Patients with bleeding esophageal varices are on NPO status.
- Discuss need for feeding supplements and enteral or parenteral nutrition (see "Providing Nutritional Support," p. 692) with health care provider if appropriate.

Impaired gas exchange related to alveolar hypoventilation secondary to shallow breathing occurring with ascites or pleural effusion, altered O_2-carrying capacity of the blood secondary to erythrocytopenia, and possible ventilation/perfusion mismatching

Desired outcome: Within 24 hr of admission, patient has adequate gas exchange, as evidenced by $Paco_2$ 45 mm Hg or less, Pao_2 less than 80 mm Hg, O_2 saturation (Sao_2) greater than 92%, and respiratory rate (RR) 12-20 breaths/min with normal depth and pattern of respirations (eupnea).

Nursing Interventions

- During complaints of dyspnea or orthopnea, assist patient into semi-Fowler's or high Fowler's position. *This is to promote gas exchange.*
- Administer O_2 as prescribed.
- Monitor arterial blood gas (ABG) values and pulse oximetry; notify health care provider of Pao_2 less than 80 mm Hg or Sao_2 92% or less.
- Encourage patient to change positions and deep breathe at frequent intervals. *This helps promote gas exchange.* If secretions are present, ensure that patient coughs frequently.
- Notify health care provider of spiking temperatures, chills, diaphoresis, and adventitious breath sounds. *These are indicators of respiratory infection.*
- Position patient in a side-lying position during episodes of vomiting. *This is to prevent aspiration.*

♦ Obtain baseline abdominal girth measurement, and measure girth either daily or every shift. Measure around same circumferential area each time; mark site with indelible ink. Report significant findings to health care provider.

Ineffective protection related to increased risk of esophageal bleeding secondary to portal hypertension and altered clotting factors
Desired outcomes: Patient is free of esophageal bleeding, as evidenced by BP at least 90/60 mm Hg; heart rate (HR) 100 beats per minute (bpm) or less; warm extremities; distal pulse magnitude greater than 2+ on a 0-4+ scale; brisk capillary refill (refill time less than 2 sec); and orientation to person, place, and time.

Nursing Interventions

♦ Monitor VS q4h (or more frequently if values are outside of patient's baseline values). Be alert to hypotension and increased HR, as well as cool extremities, delayed capillary refill, decreased amplitude of distal pulses, mental status changes, and decreasing level of consciousness (LOC). *These are physical indicators of hypovolemia and hemorrhage.*
♦ Teach patient to avoid swallowing rough or spicy foods, hot foods, hot liquids, alcohol. *These are chemically or mechanically irritating and therefore injurious to the esophagus.*
♦ Instruct patient to avoid coughing, sneezing, lifting, or vomiting. *These are actions that increase intraabdominothoracic pressure.*
♦ Administer stool softeners as prescribed. *This helps prevent straining with defecation.*
♦ Inspect stools for presence of blood. *This would signal bleeding within the GI tract.* Perform stool occult blood test as indicated.
♦ Monitor PT for abnormality (normal range is 10.5-13.5 sec), and assess for altered VS, irritability, air hunger, pallor, weakness, melena, and hematemesis. *These signs may indicate bleeding.*
♦ As appropriate, encourage intake of foods rich in vitamin K (e.g., spinach, cabbage, liver). *This is to help decrease PT.*
♦ As often as possible, avoid invasive procedures such as giving injections and taking rectal temperatures.
♦ Monitor patient undergoing injection sclerotherapy for increased HR, decreased BP, pallor, weakness, and air hunger. *These are signs of perforation.* If they occur, notify health care provider immediately, keep patient on NPO status, and prepare for gastric suction. Administer antibiotics as prescribed to prevent infection.

Disturbed sensory perception related to increased risk of neurosensory changes secondary to hepatic coma occurring with cerebral accumulation of ammonia or GI bleeding
Desired outcome: Patient verbalizes orientation to person, place, and time; exhibits intact signature; and is free of symptoms of injury caused by neurosensory changes.

Nursing Interventions

♦ Perform a baseline assessment of patient's personality characteristics, LOC, and orientation. Enlist aid of significant other to help determine slight changes in personality or behavior.
♦ Have patient demonstrate signature daily. Be alert to generalized muscle twitching and asterixis (flapping tremor induced by dorsiflexion of wrist and extension of fingers). *These signs may indicate increasing ammonia levels.*
♦ Remind patient to avoid protein and foods high in ammonia, such as gelatin, onions, and strong cheeses. *The diseased liver cannot convert*

ammonia to urea, and buildup of ammonia adds to progression of hepatic encephalopathy.

◆ Monitor for melena or hematemesis. *These are indicators of GI bleeding. GI bleeding can precipitate hepatic coma.* Report bleeding promptly to health care provider, and obtain prescription for cleansing enemas if indicated.

◆ Protect patient against injury (e.g., keep side rails up and bed in its lowest position, and assist patient with ambulation when need is determined). *Injury can occur when patient is in a confused state.*

◆ Use caution when administering sedatives, antihistamines, and other agents affecting the central nervous system (CNS). Avoid opiate analgesics and phenothiazines.

Excess fluid volume related to compromised regulatory mechanism with sequestration of fluids secondary to portal hypertension and hepatocellular failure

Desired outcome: By at least 24 hr before hospital discharge, patient is normovolemic, as evidenced by stable or decreasing abdominal girth, RR 12-20 breaths/min with normal depth and pattern (eupnea), HR 100 bpm or less, edema severity 1+ or less on a 0-4+ scale, and absence of crackles (rales).

Nursing Interventions

◆ Obtain baseline abdominal girth measurement. Place patient in supine position and mark abdomen with indelible ink. *This is to ensure serial measurements from same circumferential site.* Measure girth daily or every shift as appropriate.

◆ Monitor weight and I&O. Output should be equal to or exceed intake. Weight loss should not exceed 0.23 kg/day ($\frac{1}{2}$ lb/day). Assess degree of edema, from 1+ (barely detectable) to 4+ (deep, persistent pitting), and document accordingly.

◆ Be alert to dyspnea, basilar crackles that do not clear with coughing, orthopnea, and tachypnea. *These are clinical indicators of pulmonary edema.*

◆ Give frequent mouth care, and provide ice chips. *This is to help minimize thirst.*

◆ Monitor serum Na^+ and K^+ values and report abnormalities to health care provider. Optimal values are serum Na^+ 137-147 mEq/L and serum K^+ 3.5-5.0 mEq/L. Restrict Na^+ and replace K^+ as prescribed.

◆ Remind patient to avoid food and nonfood items that contain Na^+, such as antacids and baking soda.

◆ Elevate extremities. *This is to decrease peripheral edema.* Apply antiembolism hose (AEH) support stockings, sequential compression devices, or pneumatic foot compression devices as prescribed.

◆ Monitor for hemorrhage accordingly (see **Ineffective protection,** p. 565). *Rapid increases in intravascular volume can precipitate variceal hemorrhage in susceptible patients.*

◆ Teach patient to inhale against resistance, by using a blow bottle to facilitate flow of ascitic fluid through the shunt (if a LeVeen peritoneovenous or Denver shunt is in place). *Inhaling against resistance raises intraperitoneal pressure sufficiently to enable ascitic fluid to flow through the shunt.* In addition, provide instructions about the following: importance of lifestyle changes such as low-Na^+ diet, abstinence from alcohol, practicing breathing exercises, obtaining daily weight and abdominal girth measurements, and monitoring I&O and edema.

Patient-Family Teaching and Discharge Planning

When providing patient-family teaching, include verbal and written information about the following:

- Medications, including drug names, purpose, dosage, schedule, precautions, and potential side effects. Also discuss drug/drug, food/drug, and herb/drug interactions.
- Dietary restrictions, in particular that of Na^+ (see Box 4-2, p. 174), protein, and ammonia.
- Potential need for lifestyle changes, including avoiding alcoholic beverages. Stress that alcohol cessation is a major factor in survival of this disease. Include appropriate referrals (e.g., to Alcoholics Anonymous, Al-Anon, and Alateen). As appropriate, provide referrals to community nursing support agencies.
- Awareness of hepatotoxic agents (Box 7-3), especially over-the-counter (OTC) drugs, including acetaminophen and aspirin.
- Importance of breathing exercises when ascites is present.
- Indicators of variceal bleeding/hemorrhage (i.e., vomiting blood, change in LOC) and need to inform health care provider if they occur.
- Phone numbers to call if questions or concerns arise about therapy or disease after discharge.

Additional information can be found at:

American Liver Foundation: www.liverfoundation.org

National Institute of Diabetes and Digestive and Kidney Diseases: www.niddk.nih. gov

National Library of Medicine/National Institutes of Health: www.nlm.nih.gov/ medlineplus/liverdiseases.html

- For patients awaiting transplantation, provide the following information as appropriate:

The United Network for Organ Sharing: www.unos.org

❖ CHOLELITHIASIS, CHOLECYSTITIS, AND CHOLANGITIS

OVERVIEW/PATHOPHYSIOLOGY

Gallstones may be found anywhere in the biliary system. They may cause pain and other symptoms or remain asymptomatic for years. *Cholelithiasis* is characterized by the presence of stones in the gallbladder. *Choledocholithiasis* is the term used to describe gallstones that have migrated to the common bile duct. Gallstones are classified as cholesterol or pigment stones. Cholesterol stones are more common in the United States and represent approximately 80% of cases. Black-pigment stones result from an increase of calcium (Ca^{++}) and unconjugated bilirubin and are associated with cirrhosis and chronic hemolysis. Brown-pigment stones are the predominant type found in native Asians and may be associated with bacterial infection of the bile. Precipitating factors for stone formation include disturbances in metabolism, biliary stasis, obstruction, hypertriglyceridemia, and infection. Gallstones are especially prevalent among women who are multiparous, are taking estrogen therapy, or use oral contraceptives. Other risk factors include obesity, dietary intake of fats, sedentary lifestyle, and familial tendencies. The incidence increases with age; about one of every three persons who reach 75 yr of age has gallstones. Cholelithiasis is commonly seen in disease states such as diabetes mellitus (DM), regional enteritis, and certain blood dyscrasias. Usually cholelithiasis is asymptomatic until a stone becomes lodged in the cystic tract. If the obstruction is unrelieved, biliary colic (intermittent painful episodes) and cholecystitis can ensue.

Cholecystitis is most commonly associated with cystic duct obstructions caused by impacted gallstones; however, it may also result from stasis, bacterial infection, or ischemia of the gallbladder. Cholecystitis involves acute inflammation of the gallbladder and is associated with pain, tenderness, and fever. With obstruction, structural changes such as swelling and thickening of the gallbladder walls can occur. If the edema is prolonged, the walls become scarred and fibrosed, and the constant pressure of bile can lead to mucosal irritation. As a complication of the impaired circulation and edema, pressure ischemia and necrosis can develop, resulting in gangrene or perforation. With chronic cholecystitis, stones almost always are present, and the gallbladder walls are thickened and fibrosed.

Cholangitis is the most serious complication of gallstones and is more difficult to diagnose than either cholelithiasis or cholecystitis. It is caused by an impacted stone in the common bowel duct, and it results in bile stasis, bacteremia, and septicemia if left untreated. Cholangitis is most likely to occur when an already infected bile duct becomes obstructed. Mortality rate is high if the condition is not recognized and treated early.

ASSESSMENT

Signs and symptoms/physical findings

Cholelithiasis: History of intolerance to fats and occasional discomfort after eating. As the stone moves through the duct or becomes lodged, a sudden onset of mild, aching pain occurs in the midepigastrium after eating (especially after a high-fat meal) and increases in intensity during a colic attack, potentially radiating to the right upper quadrant (RUQ) and right subscapular region. Nausea, vomiting, tachycardia, mild fever, and diaphoresis also can occur. Many individuals with gallstones are entirely asymptomatic. Palpation of the RUQ reveals a tender abdomen during a colic attack. Otherwise, between attacks, the examination is usually normal.

Cholecystitis: History of intolerance to fats and discomfort after eating, including regurgitation, flatulence, belching, epigastric heaviness, indigestion, heartburn, chronic upper abdominal pain, and nausea. Amber-colored urine, clay-colored stools, pruritus, jaundice, steatorrhea, fever, and bleeding tendencies can be present if there is bile obstruction. Symptoms may be vague. An acute attack may last 7-10 days, but it usually resolves in several hours. Palpation elicits tenderness localized behind the inferior margin of the liver. With progressive symptoms, a tender, globular mass may be palpated behind the lower border of the liver. Rebound tenderness and guarding also may be present. With the patient taking a deep breath, palpation over the RUQ elicits Murphy's sign (pain and inability to inspire when the examiner's hand comes in contact with the gallbladder).

Cholangitis: Fever is present in nearly all patients with bacterial cholangitis. Jaundice, chills, mild and transient pain, mental confusion, and lethargy are part of the presenting symptoms. Leukocytosis and elevated bilirubin are present in most cases. RUQ tenderness is present in most cases. Peritoneal signs are not common and occur in only a few patients. Hypotension and mental confusion are present in patients with severe cases.

History and risk factors: Excessive body weight, increasing age, diet, and being female. The five Fs of cholelithiasis are (1) female, (2) fair complexion, (3) fat or obese, (4) fertile or has had children, (5) 40 (forty) yr of age or older.

DIAGNOSTIC TESTS

Ultrasonography: The preferred test for confirming the presence of gallstones, as well as their number, color, and size. Ultrasound examination of the gallbladder and biliary tract may be used to determine gallstone location and detect tumors.

Radiologic studies: For example, oral cholangiogram, IV cholangiogram, nuclear scans, and percutaneous transhepatic cholangiogram may be performed to determine patency of biliary or cystic ducts and help rule out other conditions that mimic gallstone disease. Chest, abdominal, upper gastrointestinal (GI), and barium enema x-ray examinations often are used to rule out pulmonary or other GI disorders.

Hepatoiminodiacetic acid (HIDA) scan: Radioisotopic scan that is highly sensitive for diagnosis of acute cholecystitis. HIDA is injected by the IV route, absorbed in the liver, and then excreted in the biliary system. An obstructing stone in the cystic duct prevents HIDA from filling the gallbladder.

Oral cholecystogram: Measures gallbladder function and demonstrates number and size of gallstones. This test requires ingestion of iodine-based tablets (e.g., Telepaque) at night, with x-ray films taken the following morning. Failure to visualize the gallbladder indicates a nonfunctioning gallbladder, usually because of complete obstruction of the cystic duct or chronic irritation of the gallbladder wall. Diarrhea may be caused by the iodine tablets and sometimes results in nonvisualization of the gallbladder. Ultrasound often takes the place of this test.

CT scan: Detects dilated bile ducts and the presence of gallbladder cysts, tumors, abscesses, perforated gallbladder, and other complications of gallbladder disease.

Endoscopic retrograde cholangiopancreatography (ERCP): Used for visualization and evaluation of the biliary tree or pancreatic duct. This is the gold standard for diagnosing choledocholithiasis.

ECG: Rules out cardiac disease.

CBC with differential: Assesses for presence of infection or blood loss.

Blood studies

PT: Assesses for prolonged clotting time secondary to faulty vitamin K absorption.

Serum liver enzyme test: Usually normal in cholecystitis but often abnormal in the presence of prolonged cholecystitis or common duct stones.

Bilirubin tests (serum and urine) and urobilinogen tests (urine and fecal): Used to differentiate among hemolytic disorders, hepatocellular disease, and obstructive disease. Usually bilirubin in the plasma and urine are increased with biliary disease.

COLLABORATIVE MANAGEMENT

Pharmacologic therapy

Analgesics (e.g., Nonsteroidal antiinflammatory drugs [NSAIDs] or opioid analgesics): May be indicated, depending on pain severity. For postoperative patients, epidural, continuous IV, and patient-controlled infusions of opioid analgesics are used with increasing frequency and superior efficacy (see Chapter 1, "Pain," p. 13, for more information).

Acid suppression therapy: Neutralizes gastric hyperacidity and reduces associated pain.

Antibiotics: For infection.

Antiemetics (e.g., hydroxyzine, ondansetron, prochlorperazine, promethazine): For nausea and vomiting.

Bile sequestrant therapy (e.g., cholestyramine, colestipol): Binds with bile salts in the intestine to facilitate their excretion and may be given to provide relief from pruritus caused by prolonged obstructive jaundice.

Gallstone-solubilizing agents (e.g., ursodeoxycholic acid [UDCA], ursodiol]): May be used in patients with a working gallbladder and relatively small, uncalcified (cholesterol) stones to reduce stone size and eventually dissolve them. Indicated for patients in whom open or laparoscopic cholecystectomy is contraindicated and in cases of uncomplicated gallstone disease. Treatment duration ranges from months to years with variable results and considerable expense. Patients should be advised of the many potential drug interactions, serious side effects, and need for careful follow-up treatment.

Chemical dissolution of cholesterol gallstones with a solvent (e.g., monoctanoin): May be used in patients with a functioning gallbladder and an unobstructed biliary tract. The solvent is infused via a T-tube or endoscopically placed catheter. Oral solubilizing agents are administered after chemical dissolution to prevent recurrence of stones.

Dietary management: Varies according to patient's condition. During an acute attack, nothing-by-mouth (NPO) status with IV fluids may be instituted. With severe nausea and vomiting, a gastric tube is inserted and attached to low, intermittent suction. Diet advances to patient's tolerance, and small, frequent feedings of a low-fat diet are recommended for both acute and chronic conditions.

ERCP: The common bile duct may be cannulated, and if a stone is present, an endoscopic sphincterotomy (a technique that cuts the opening of the bile duct) can be performed with stone extraction via a snare or balloon catheter.

Nonoperative biliary stone removal: One method of stone extraction, which is performed using fluoroscopy in the radiology department. The stone is removed with a basket that is inserted via a catheter or T-tube through a surgically created sinus tract into the common duct. If this technique is unsuccessful, forceps are used to manipulate the stone. A cholangiogram is done before and after the procedure. If the x-ray findings are normal after the procedure, the T-tube is removed; if stones are still present, a new T-tube or catheter is inserted, and the patient returns the following day for the same procedure. This technique may be ideal for an individual who is not a good surgical candidate.

Lithotripsy: Gallstones, like kidney stones, can be fragmented by exposure to extracorporeal shock waves. The stones are broken up into small granules that can be passed through the intestine or dissolved with ursodiol. Patients are carefully selected and evaluated before therapy. During the approximately 1-hr procedure the patient is mildly sedated and may feel some RUQ tenderness immediately after the procedure. Common stone recurrence and follow-up drug therapy make this an expensive option.

Surgical interventions: Usually required for relief of long-term symptoms of cholelithiasis and for acute cholecystitis. Surgery is the best treatment choice for patients with frequent or severe episodes of biliary pain, cholecystitis, DM, or suspected gallbladder cancer. The type of surgery depends on severity and length of illness, site of obstruction, and patient's condition. The following procedures may be performed.

Laparoscopic cholecystectomy (removal of the gallbladder): The standard modality for gallstone treatment. Three to four small incisions are made in the abdominal wall. A laparoscope and specialized, long-handled instruments are used to resect the gallbladder with electrocautery or laser cautery. Although laparoscopic cholecystectomy is more costly, surgical complications are fewer and postoperative recovery is more rapid (hospital stay less than 24 hr) than with conventional cholecystectomy.

Cholecystectomy: If laparoscopic cholecystectomy is unsuccessful (or contraindicated), an open cholecystectomy is done via a right subcostal incision. The gallbladder is excised, and the cystic duct, vein, and artery are ligated. A closed drainage system may be needed for drainage of blood, serum, and bile from the gallbladder bed. The drain is brought out through a separate stab wound away from the incision. An intraoperative cholangiogram is done if stones are suspected in the common bile duct; that is, a small catheter is threaded through the amputated cystic duct, and radiopaque dye is injected. If stones are identified, a common duct exploration (CDE) is done to remove the stones, by using either gallbladder scoops or embolectomy catheters. Because of edema after the CDE, a T-tube may be inserted to drain bile until the edema resolves and patency of the common bile duct returns.

Cholecystotomy: Opening and draining the gallbladder in grossly septic or unstable patients. This is a palliative surgery and is generally followed by more definitive cholecystectomy once the patient is stable.

Choledochotomy: Opening the common bile duct to remove stones.
Choledochoduodenostomy or choledochojejunostomy: Anastomosis of the common bile duct to the duodenum or jejunum; done for neoplasms involving the duodenum or common bile duct.

NURSING DIAGNOSES AND INTERVENTIONS

Acute pain (nausea, spasms, and itching) related to obstructive or inflammatory process
Desired outcomes: Patient's subjective perception of discomfort decreases within 1 hr of intervention, as documented by pain scale. Nonverbal indicators, such as grimacing, are absent or diminished.

Nursing Interventions

- Monitor patient for pain or other discomfort. Devise a pain scale with patient, rating discomfort on a scale of 0 (no pain) to 10 (worst pain).
- Put patient in a low-Fowler's position. *This will minimize pressure in the RUQ.*
- Teach patient to avoid fatty and rough or fibrous foods. *This is to prevent nausea and spasms.*
- Administer bile salt binding agent (e.g., cholestyramine) as prescribed. Provide cool Alpha Keri baths and cold water or ice for topical application and use soft linens on the bed. *This is to reduce itching.*
- For additional interventions, see "Pain," p. 13, in Chapter 1.

Ineffective protection related to recurrence of biliary obstruction
Desired outcomes: Patient is free of symptoms of postsurgical perforation, as evidenced by diminishing dark brown drainage of less than 1000 mL/day and the presence of a soft and nondistended abdomen. Patient is free of symptoms of recurring biliary obstruction, as evidenced by normal skin color, brown-colored stools, and straw-colored urine.

Nursing Interventions

- Monitor color of the skin, sclera, urine, and stool. *If obstruction recurs and bile is forced back into the bloodstream, jaundice will be present, urine will be amber, and stools will be clay colored (clay color is normal if bile is drained via a T-tube). Brown color should return to stools once bile begins to drain normally into the duodenum.*
- Note and record color, amount, odor, and consistency of drainage from T-tube or wound drain q2h on day of surgery and at least every shift thereafter. Initially drainage will be dark brown with small amounts of blood and can amount to 500-1000 mL/day. Report greater amounts of blood or drainage to health care provider. Amount should subside gradually as swelling diminishes in common duct and drainage into duodenum normalizes.
- Ensure that drainage collection devices are positioned lower than level of the common bile duct. *This is to prevent reflux of drainage when patient is ambulating.*
- Be alert to abdominal distention, rigidity, and complaints of diaphragmatic irritation along with cessation or significant decrease in amount of drainage. If these occur, notify health care provider immediately and anticipate tube replacement with a 14Fr catheter.

Patient-Family Teaching and Discharge Planning

When providing patient-family teaching, include verbal and written information about the following:

- Notifying health care provider if the following indicators of recurrent biliary obstruction occur: dark urine, pruritus, jaundice, clay-colored stools. Inform patient that loose stools may occur for several months as the body adjusts to the continuous flow of bile.
- Medications, including drug names, dosage, schedule, purpose, precautions, and potential side effects. Also discuss drug/drug, food/drug, and herb/drug interactions.
- Care of dressings and tubes if patient is discharged with them, and monitoring of incision and drain sites for signs of infection (e.g., fever, persistent redness, pain, purulent discharge, swelling, increased local warmth).
- Importance of maintaining a diet low in fat and eating frequent, small meals for medically managed patients.
- Importance of follow-up appointments with health care provider; reconfirm time and date of next appointment.
- Avoiding alcoholic beverages during first 2 mo postoperatively, to minimize risk of pancreatic involvement.
- Necessity for postsurgical activity precautions: avoid lifting heavy objects (more than 10 lb) for first 4-6 wk or as directed, rest after periods of fatigue, get maximum amounts of rest, and gradually increase activities to tolerance. Postsurgical patients may experience fatty food intolerance (e.g., flatulence, cramps, diarrhea) for several months postoperatively until the body acclimates to loss of the gallbladder.
- Additional information can be found at:

  National Institute of Diabetes and Digestive and Kidney Diseases: www.niddk.nih. gov

❖ ❖ ❖

SECTION SIX **PANCREATITIS**

OVERVIEW/PATHOPHYSIOLOGY

Pancreatitis, which can be acute or chronic, is an inflammation of the pancreas with varying degrees of edema, hemorrhage, and necrosis. The damage can lead to fibrosis, stricture, and calcifications. Acute pancreatitis occurs when pancreatic ductal flow becomes obstructed and digestive enzymes escape from the pancreatic duct into surrounding tissue. Self-destruction of the pancreas produces edema, hemorrhage, and necrosis of pancreatic and surrounding tissue. Biochemical abnormalities and disruption of cardiopulmonary, renal, metabolic, and gastrointestinal (GI) function are likely. Pancreatitis has been associated with gallstones, alcoholism, surgical manipulation, abdominal trauma, abdominal vascular disease, heavy metal poisoning, infectious agents (viral, bacterial, mycoplasma, parasitic), and some allergic reactions. Pancreatitis also is associated with familial hyperlipidemia and can be induced by endoscopic retrograde cholangiopancreatography (ERCP). Most cases of acute pancreatitis are mild, require a short hospitalization, and leave no long-term adverse effects. Severe acute pancreatitis (SAP), involving multiple organ failure, occurs in approximately 25% of cases but accounts for 98% of deaths associated with acute pancreatitis. Complications of acute pancreatitis include pancreatic abscess, hemorrhage, pancreatic pseudocyst, fistula formation, and transient hypoglycemia. Acute, life-threatening complications include renal failure, hemorrhagic pancreatitis, septicemia, acute respiratory distress syndrome (ARDS), shock, and disseminated intravascular coagulation (DIC).

Chronic pancreatitis is characterized by varying degrees of pancreatic insufficiency, which results in decreased production of enzymes and bicarbonate and malabsorption of fats and proteins. The digestion of fat is affected most severely. As a result, high fat content in the bowel stimulates water and electrolyte secretion, which produces diarrhea. The action of bacteria on fecal fat produces flatus, fatty stools (steatorrhea), and abdominal cramps. Often diabetes mellitus (DM) occurs as a result of chronic pancreatitis because of damage to the insulin-producing β cells and resultant deficient insulin production. Chronic pancreatitis is associated with complications of DM, chronic pain, maldigestion, pseudocysts, and bleeding.

ASSESSMENT

Signs and symptoms/physical findings

Acute pancreatitis: Symptoms vary according to severity of the attack. Sudden onset of constant, severe epigastric pain often occurs after a large meal or alcohol intake. Pain frequently radiates to the back or left shoulder and is relieved somewhat by a sitting position with the spine flexed. It is caused by biliary tree obstruction, enzymes irritating pancreatic and surrounding tissue, and the resulting edema. Nausea and vomiting, sometimes with persistent retching, usually occur and are caused by bowel hypermotility or ileus. Pain may be increased after vomiting because of increased pressure on the ducts that leads to further obstructions of secretions and tissue damage. Fever is usually present as well as hypotension and tachycardia. Jaundice suggests biliary tree obstruction. Extreme malaise, restlessness, respiratory distress, and diminished urinary output may be present. Hypovolemic shock may be present with hemorrhagic events, or distributive shock may occur secondary to systemic inflammatory response syndrome. Other symptoms that may occur include diminished or absent bowel sounds, suggesting the presence of ileus; mild to moderate ascites; generalized abdominal tenderness; tachypnea, crackles (rales) at lung bases related to atelectasis, and interstitial fluid accumulation; diminished ventilatory excursion related to splinting and guarding with pain; low-grade fever (temperatures of 37.7°-38.8° C [100°-102° F]) or pronounced fever with abscess or sepsis. Agitation, confusion, and altered mental status may result from electrolyte/metabolic abnormalities or acute alcohol withdrawal. Gray-blue discoloration of the flank (Grey Turner's sign) or blue-red discoloration around the umbilicus (Cullen's sign) sometimes is present with pancreatic hemorrhage.

Chronic pancreatitis: Constant, dull epigastric pain; steatorrhea resulting from malabsorption of fats and protein; severe weight loss; and onset of symptoms of DM: polydipsia, polyuria, polyphagia. In addition, chemical addiction is often seen because of the chronic pain.

History and risk factors: Biliary tract disease; chronic excessive alcohol consumption; physical trauma to the abdomen (especially in young people); peptic ulcer disease; viral infection; ERCP; cystic fibrosis; neoplasms; shock; and use of certain medications, such as estrogen-containing oral contraceptives, glucocorticoids, sulfonamides, chlorothiazides, and azathioprine.

DIAGNOSTIC TESTS

Blood studies

Amylase: When significantly elevated (more than 500 units/dL), rules out acute abdomen conditions, such as cholecystitis, appendicitis, bowel infarction/obstruction, and perforated peptic ulcer, and confirms the presence of pancreatitis. These levels return to normal 48-72 hr after onset of acute symptoms, even though clinical indicators may continue. Sensitivity is limited in patients with alcoholic pancreatitis and hypertriglyceridemia.

Lipase: Has higher specificity and sensitivity than serum amylase. It rises more slowly than serum amylase and persists longer. Both lipase and amylase levels reflect the degree of necrosis of pancreatic tissue. Higher cost and the few additional benefits of this test limit its use.

Glucose: Hyperglycemia occurs because of interference with β cell function. It is transient with acute pancreatitis but common with chronic pancreatitis, during which DM is likely to develop.

Serum K⁺: Hyperkalemia occurs in the presence of tissue damage, metabolic acidosis, and renal failure in severe cases.

Serum calcium (Ca⁺⁺) and magnesium: May be lower than normal. On electro cardiogram (ECG), hypocalcemia is evidenced by prolonged QT segment with a normal T wave.

CBC: Elevated WBC count caused by inflammatory process. Polymorpho-nuclear bodies may increase if bacterial peritonitis is present secondary to duodenal rupture. Hct may be elevated or decreased.

BUN/serum creatinine: Evaluate renal function.

Urinalysis: May show presence of glycosuria, which can signal the onset of DM. Elevated urine amylase levels are useful diagnostically when serum levels have dropped off. An elevated specific gravity reflects the presence of dehydration.

Abdominal x-ray examination: May show dilation of the small or large bowel and presence of pancreatic calcification in chronic pancreatitis.

MRI or CT scan: May reveal an enlarged and edematous pancreatic head, or abscess, pseudocyst, or calcification.

Magnetic resonance cholangiopancreatography (MR-CP): May be used to visualize pancreatic and common bile ducts if ERCP is not feasible.

ERCP: A combined endoscopic-radiographic tool that is used to study the degree of pancreatic disease via assessment of biliary-pancreatic ductal systems. It allows direct visualization of the ampulla of Vater, diagnoses biliary stones and duct stenosis, and distinguishes cancer of the pancreas from pancreatic calculi. ERCP is not performed until the acute episode has subsided.

Secretin stimulation test: Diagnoses chronic pancreatitis.

COLLABORATIVE MANAGEMENT

Medical goals are to reduce stimuli for pancreatic secretions to permit healing, provide supportive therapy/treatments during acute exacerbation, and prevent and treat complications.

For Acute Pancreatitis

Fluid and electrolyte replacement/monitoring: Maintains adequate circulating blood volume (e.g., parenteral solutions and blood volume expanders, such as albumin and plasma protein fraction). Close monitoring of urinary output is accomplished to assess for renal complications.

NPO status and nasogastric (NG) suction: Initiated early in the course of illness to decrease stimulus for pancreatic secretions and reduce stress in the GI tract. After acute pain and ileus have resolved, the patient is given clear liquids, and diet is advanced as tolerated.

Nutritional support: Enteral feedings are being used with increasing frequency but should be infused past the ligament of Treitz to avoid pancreatic stimulation. Parenteral nutrition typically is instituted when distal enteral feedings are unobtainable or unsuccessful within 5-7 days. Strict glycemic control needs to be maintained during parenteral nutritional support.

Bed rest: Reduces metabolic demands on the body.

Ruling out underlying factors (e.g., hyperparathyroidism, hyperlipoproteinemia): These factors can contribute to the development of pancreatitis.

Pharmacotherapy

Analgesics (e.g., meperidine, morphine, pentazocine): For pain. Both morphine and meperidine may cause spasms at the sphincter of Oddi, although meperidine may be less likely to do so. However, large doses and prolonged use of meperidine can lead to seizures. Response varies with the individual.

TABLE 7-6	HISTAMINE H$_2$-RECEPTOR BLOCKERS		
GENERIC NAME	**TRADE NAME**	**USUAL DOSAGE**	**COMMENTS**
Cimetidine	Tagamet Tagamet HB	800-1200 mg/day*	Reduces hepatic blood flow; inhibits metabolism of some drugs in the liver
Ranitidine	Zantac Zantac 150 or 300 Zantac EFFERdose	150-300 mg/day*	5-12× more potent than cimetidine; fewer drug interactions than with cimetidine
Famotidine	Pepcid Mylanta AR	40-120 mg/day*	30-100× more potent than cimetidine
Nizatidine	Axid Axid AR	150-300 mg/day†	

*Oral, intramuscular, or intravenous (IV) administration or continuous IV infusion titrated to gastric pH value.
†Available in oral form only.

Broad-spectrum antibiotics: For infection or abscess if present or suspected. Definitive agreement regarding significant reduction in mortality rates using antibiotics for severe acute pancreatitis (SAP) is not available, although studies are in progress.

Steroids: Reduce inflammation in certain types of pancreatitis when infection is not a problem.

Histamine H$_2$-receptor blockers: Reduce gastric acid secretion, which stimulates pancreatic enzymes (**TABLE 7-6**).

Antiemetics (e.g., hydroxyzine, ondansetron, prochlorperazine, promethazine): For nausea and vomiting.

Antacids: Neutralize gastric acid and reduce associated pain.

Other pharmacotherapies: Atropine (to reduce sphincter of Oddi spasm), glucagon, somatostatin, aprotinin, and indomethacin.

Peritoneal lavage: Removes toxic factors present in peritoneal exudate and can result in immediate clinical improvement. The procedure is similar to peritoneal dialysis. A soft lavage catheter is positioned in the peritoneum, and continual lavage is instituted for 2-7 days, depending on the patient's clinical course. Because it is invasive, it is not routinely used.

Surgery: In general, nonsurgical management of acute pancreatitis is preferred. Surgical interventions may not improve the patient's condition, and the risk of respiratory and other complications is great. Because symptoms of acute pancreatitis are easily confused with those of other acute abdominal emergencies that require urgent surgery, exploratory laparotomy is necessary for some patients. For unstable patients with SAP, prompt surgical débridement sometimes is necessary to limit vessel erosion and bleeding or to remove necrotic, infected tissue. Surgery in these patients carries a high mortality rate, and complications are numerous.

For Chronic Pancreatitis

For exacerbations: See treatment for acute pancreatitis.

Alcohol rehabilitation: If alcoholism is the cause of pancreatitis.

Long-term pain management: With lowest effective dose of analgesic. Acetaminophen is used for initial pain control, but pain may require oral opioids using the lowest effective dose. Referral to a pain management team is recommended for these patients. Nerve blocks that interfere with transmission of pain sensations along visceral nerve fibers are effective in the relief of pancreatic pain. Bilateral splanchnic nerve or left celiac ganglion blocks may be performed.

Oral enzyme supplements (e.g., pancreatin, pancrelipase): Used to treat maldigestion.

Histamine H₂-receptor blockers: Used as with acute pancreatitis.

Diet: High in carbohydrates and protein and low in fat; avoidance of spicy foods, caffeine, and nicotine.

Insulin therapy: May be required to ensure adequate carbohydrate metabolism if endocrine function is impaired. Laboratory values of fasting blood sugar and bedside monitoring of blood glucose will reveal abnormalities in blood glucose levels and direct the appropriate insulin therapy (see "Diabetes Mellitus," p. 411, for more information).

Surgical interventions: Indicated when pancreatitis is caused by an obstructive process, such as gallstone formation or cancer. When gallstones are the cause of the pancreatitis, surgical removal of the stone(s) and usually the gallbladder is performed (see "Cholelithiasis, Cholecystitis, and Cholangitis," p. 525). The surgery is performed when the acute symptoms of pancreatitis have abated. A common duct exploration (CDE) may be done at the time of surgery to retrieve all stones.

NURSING DIAGNOSES AND INTERVENTIONS

Deficient fluid volume related to active loss secondary to NG suctioning, vomiting, diaphoresis, or pooling of fluids in the abdomen and retroperitoneum

Desired outcome: Patient is normovolemic within 8 hr of admission, as evidenced by heart rate (HR) 60-100 beats per minute (bpm), central venous pressure (CVP) 2-6 mm Hg (5-12 cm H₂O), brisk capillary refill (refill time less than 2 sec), peripheral pulse amplitude greater than 2+ on a 0-4+ scale, urinary output at least 30 mL/hr, and stable weight and abdominal girth measurements.

Nursing Interventions

- Monitor VS q2-4h, and be alert to falling BP and increasing HR. *These can occur with moderate to severe fluid loss.*
- Measure I&O and CVP, if available, q2-4h. Be alert to and report I&O imbalances. *This is because fluid loss requires immediate replacement to prevent shock and acute renal failure. CVP less than 2 mm Hg can occur with volume-related hypotension.* Measure orthostatic VS initially and q8h. Be alert to decreasing BP and increasing HR on standing. *These suggest the need for crystalloid and/or colloid volume expansion.* Weigh patient daily, and note trends. Correlate weights with I&O ratios.
- Administer plasma volume expanders as prescribed. Monitor closely for fluid overload and pulmonary edema.
- Administer electrolytes (K⁺, Ca⁺⁺) as prescribed. *This is to prevent cardiac dysrhythmias and tetany.*
- Be alert for presence of Chvostek's sign (facial muscle spasm) and Trousseau's sign (carpopedal spasm), muscle twitching, tetany, or irritability. *These can occur with electrolyte loss and may be indicators of hypocalcemia.*
- Monitor values of the following for irregularities: hematocrit (Hct), hemoglobin (Hgb), Ca⁺⁺, glucose, blood urea nitrogen (BUN), serum creatinine, and K⁺. Normal values are as follows: Hct 40%-54% (male) and 37%-47% (female); Hgb 14-18 g/dL (male) and 12-16 g/dL (female); Ca⁺⁺ 8.5-10.5 mg/dL (4.3-5.3 mEq/L); glucose less than 145 mg/dL (2 hr postprandial) and 65-110 mg/dL (fasting); BUN 6-20 mg/dL; and K⁺ 3.5-5.0 mEq/L.

Acute pain related to inflammatory process of the pancreas

Desired outcomes: Within 6 hr of intervention, patient's subjective perception of discomfort decreases, and pain is controlled within 24 hr, as documented by pain scale. Nonverbal indicators, such as splinting of abdominal muscles, are absent or diminished.

Nursing Interventions

◆ Assess for and document degree and character of patient's discomfort. Devise a pain scale with patient, rating discomfort on a scale of 0 (no pain) to 10 (worst pain).

◆ Assess patient's previous responses to pain and previously effective pain relief measures. Consider possible cultural and spiritual influences.

◆ Ensure that patient maintains limited activity or bed rest. *This is to minimize pancreatic secretions and pain and to maximize needed rest.*

◆ Maintain nothing-by-mouth (NPO) status. *This is to minimize stimulation of pancreatic secretions.* Monitor NG tube function, and maintain patency.

◆ Administer analgesics, histamine H_2-receptor blockers (Table 7-6), antiemetics, and other medications as prescribed; be alert to patient's response to medications, and use pain scale. Instruct patient to request analgesic before pain becomes severe. Optimally, analgesics are administered via patient-controlled pumps. Transdermal analgesic or small, frequent doses of IV opiates usually are more effective than intramuscular (IM) injections. Avoid IM injections in individuals with clotting or bleeding complications. Note bowel pattern. *Opioid analgesics decrease intestinal motility and delay return to normal bowel function.*

◆ Assist patient in attaining a position of comfort. Suggest a sitting or supine position with knees flexed. *This often helps to relax abdominal muscles.*

◆ Emphasize nonpharmacologic pain interventions (e.g., relaxation techniques, distraction, guided imagery, massage). *These interventions are especially important for patients who develop chronic pancreatitis and are prone to chemical dependence.* (See **Health-seeking behaviors:** Relaxation technique effective for stress reduction, p. 106.)

◆ Prepare significant other for personality changes and behavioral alterations associated with extreme pain and opioid analgesic. *This is because pancreatitis can be very painful. Family members sometimes misinterpret patient's lethargic condition or unpleasant disposition and may even blame themselves.* Reassure family members that these are normal responses.

◆ Monitor patient's respiratory pattern, pulse oximetry, and level of consciousness (LOC) closely. *This is because both respiration and LOC may be depressed by the large amount of opioids usually required to control pain. Continuous pulse oximetry identifies decreasing O_2 saturation (SaO_2) associated with hypoventilation (report SaO_2 less than 92%).*

◆ Consider referral to a pain management team.

◆ For additional pain interventions, see "Pain," p. 13, in Chapter 1.

Impaired gas exchange (or risk for same) related to ventilation/perfusion mismatching secondary to atelectasis or accumulating pulmonary fluid
Desired outcome: Patient has adequate gas exchange, as evidenced by RR 12-20 breaths/min with normal depth and pattern (eupnea); O_2 saturation greater than 92%; no significant changes in mental status; orientation to person, place, and time; and breath sounds that are clear and audible throughout the lung fields.

Nursing Interventions

◆ Monitor and document respiratory rate (RR) q2-4h as indicated by patient's condition. Note pattern, degree of excursion, and whether patient uses accessory muscles of respiration. Report significant deviations from baseline to health care provider.

◆ Auscultate both lung fields q4-8h. Note presence of abnormal (crackles [rales], rhonchi, wheezes) or diminished breath sounds.

◆ Monitor sputum production. *This is to note secretions indicating respiratory tract infection or pulmonary edema.*

◆ Be alert to changes in mental status, restlessness, agitation, and alterations in mentation. *These may be early signs of hypoxia.*

◆ Monitor pulse oximetry q8h or as indicated (report Sao_2 92% or less). Monitor arterial blood gas (ABG) results as available (report Pao_2 less than 80 mm Hg).

◆ Administer O_2 as prescribed. Monitor O_2 delivery system at regular intervals.

◆ Maintain body position that optimizes ventilation and oxygenation. Elevate head of bed (HOB) 30 degrees or higher, depending on patient comfort. If pleural effusion or other defect is present on one side, position patient with unaffected lung dependent to maximize ventilation/perfusion relationship.

◆ Avoid overaggressive fluid resuscitation.

◆ Explain to patient and significant other that pancreatitis results in decreased production of surfactant and pain limits adequate respiratory excursion, thus increasing the potential for hypostatic pneumonia.

◆ Teach use of hyperinflation device (e.g., incentive spirometer). *The emphasis of this therapy is on inhalation to expand the lungs maximally.* Ensure that patient inhales slowly and deeply 2× normal tidal volume and holds the breath at least 5 sec at end of inspiration. A regimen of 10 breaths/hr is recommended. *This is to maintain adequate alveolar inflation. Deep breathing expands alveoli and aids in mobilizing secretions to the airways, whereas coughing further mobilizes and clears secretions.*

◆ When appropriate, teach methods of splinting wounds or upper abdomen. *This is to enable coughing.*

◆ Instruct patients who cannot cough effectively in cascade cough. *This is a succession of more short and forceful exhalations that may be beneficial even if patient cannot cough effectively.*

◆ Encourage activity as prescribed. *This is to help mobilize secretions and promote effective airway clearance.*

Risk for infection related to risk of tissue destruction with resulting necrosis secondary to release of pancreatic enzymes

Desired outcome: Patient remains free of infection, as evidenced by body temperature less than 37.7° C (less than 100° F); negative culture results; HR 60-100 bpm; RR 12-20 breaths/min; BP within patient's normal range; and orientation to person, place, and time.

Nursing Interventions

◆ Check patient's temperature q4h. *Hypothermia may precede hyperthermia in some individuals.*

◆ If there is a sudden elevation in temperature, obtain specimens for culture of blood, sputum, urine, wound, drains, and other sites as indicated. Monitor culture reports, and report findings promptly to health care provider.

◆ Evaluate patient's mental status, orientation, and LOC q4-8h.

◆ Monitor BP, HR, and RR q4h. Be alert to increases in HR and RR. *These are associated with temperature elevations.*

◆ Administer parenteral antibiotics in a timely fashion. *This is to maintain bactericidal serum levels.* Reschedule antibiotics if a dose is delayed for more than 1 hr. *Failure to administer antibiotics on schedule can result in inadequate blood levels and treatment failure.*

◆ Observe all secretions and drainage. *This is to check for changes in appearance or odor that may signal infection.*

◆ Use good handwashing technique before and after caring for patient and dispose of dressings and drainage carefully. *This is to prevent transmission of potentially infectious agents.*

Imbalanced nutrition: less than body requirements related to anorexia, dietary restrictions, and digestive dysfunction

Desired outcomes: Patient maintains baseline body weight and exhibits a positive or balanced N state on N studies by 24 hr before hospital discharge.

Nursing Interventions

♦ Initiate parenteral nutrition, and adjust insulin amounts according to capillary blood glucose levels, as prescribed.

♦ Provide oral hygiene at frequent intervals. *This is to enhance appetite and minimize nausea.*

♦ Monitor capillary blood sugar levels for presence of hyperglycemia, and be alert to dysphagia, polydipsia, and polyuria. *These can occur with a hyperglycemic state.* These indicators reflect need for health care provider evaluation and intervention to ensure proper metabolism of carbohydrates.

♦ When the gastric tube is removed, provide diet as prescribed (e.g., small, high-carbohydrate, low-fat meals at frequent intervals [6/day] with protein added according to patient's tolerance). Instruct patient to avoid coffee, tea, alcohol, and nicotine or other gastric irritants. *These stimulants increase pancreatic enzyme secretion.*

♦ Weigh patient daily to assess gain or loss. *Progressive weight loss may signal need to change diet or provide enzyme replacement therapy.*

♦ Note amount and degree of steatorrhea (foamy, foul-smelling stools high in fat content). *This may indicate fat intolerance.* As prescribed, administer pancreatic enzyme supplements, which are given before introducing fat into the diet.

♦ If prescribed, administer other dietary supplements. *This is to support nutrition and caloric intake.* These may include products that consist of medium-chain triglycerides (MCTs), such as Isocal or MCT oil. *These supplements do not require pancreatic enzymes for absorption.*

♦ Avoid administering pancreatin with hot foods or drinks. *The heat will deactivate enzyme activity.*

♦ Provide meals in small feedings throughout the day. *This is to help alleviate bloating, nausea, and cramps.*

 Patient-Family Teaching and Discharge Planning

When providing patient-family teaching, include verbal and written information about the following:

♦ Cause for current episode of pancreatitis, if known, so that recurrence may be avoided.

♦ Alcohol consumption, which can cause or exacerbate chronic pancreatitis.

♦ Diet: frequent, small meals that are high in carbohydrates and protein. Food should be bland until gradual return to normal diet is prescribed. Remind patient to avoid enzyme stimulants, such as coffee, tea, nicotine, and alcohol.

♦ Medications, including drug names, purpose, dosage, schedule, precautions, and potential side effects. Also discuss drug/drug, food/drug, and herb/drug interactions.

♦ Signs and symptoms of DM, including fatigue, weight loss, polydipsia, polyuria, and polyphagia.

♦ Necessity of medical follow-up; confirm time and date of next medical appointment.

♦ Potential for recurrence of steatorrhea, as evidenced by foamy, foul-smelling stools that are high in fat content, because steatorrhea can indicate recurrence of disease process or ineffectiveness of drug therapy. This should be reported to health care provider.

◆ Weighing daily at home; importance of reporting weight loss to health care provider.

◆ If surgery was performed, the indicators of wound infection: redness, swelling, discharge, fever, pain, or increased local warmth.

◆ Availability of chemical dependency programs to prevent/treat drug dependence, which is a common occurrence with chronic pancreatitis; or to treat alcoholism.

◆ Additional resources can be found at:

Alcoholics Anonymous: www.aa.org

Narcotics Anonymous: www.na.org

The National Pancreas Foundation: www.pancreasfoundation.com

National Institute of Diabetes and Digestive and Kidney Diseases: www.niddk.nih. gov

Hematologic Disorders

SECTION ONE **DISORDERS OF THE RED BLOOD CELLS**

Anemia is a common hematopoietic disorder defined as reduced RBC volume (hematocrit [Hct]) or reduced concentration of hemoglobin (Hgb). Consideration of the patient's intravascular volume (i.e., hydration status) is essential for proper interpretation of Hct and Hgb values. The general effects of anemia are the result of a deficiency in the O_2-carrying mechanism, although some effects are related to varied pathogenetic factors.

Anemias can be classified in two ways: (1) those involving diminished production or accelerated loss of RBCs (etiology) or (2) those involving cell size (morphology). For details, see **TABLES 8-1** and **8-2**. Three common types of anemias are discussed in this section: anemia of chronic disease, hemolytic and sickle cell anemia, and hypoplastic (aplastic) anemia.

❖ ANEMIA OF CHRONIC DISEASE

OVERVIEW/PATHOPHYSIOLOGY

Erythropoietin (EPO) is a naturally occurring protein hormone produced and released by the kidneys (90%) and liver (10%). The kidneys are stimulated to release EPO in response to low blood oxygenation. EPO then stimulates stem cells in the bone marrow to develop and produce RBCs. Individuals with decreased renal function (e.g., chronic kidney disease [CKD]) often become anemic because their kidneys cannot produce EPO. In other chronic conditions, bone marrow fails to compensate for decreased RBC survival adequately by increasing RBC production. In these cases, EPO rarely is an important cause of underproduction of RBCs except in renal failure. However, the development of recombinant human EPO (epoetin alfa) has provided dramatic benefits for patients with CKD, patients receiving chemotherapy for cancer, and patients undergoing treatment for human immunodeficiency virus (HIV) infection.

ASSESSMENT

Signs and symptoms/physical findings

Acute indicators: Fatigue, decreased ability to concentrate, cold sensitivity, tachycardia, tachypnea, pale mucous membranes, vertigo, menstrual irregularities, and loss of libido.

Chronic indicators: Patient may be asymptomatic or have brittle hair and nails. In the presence of severe and chronic disease, exertional dyspnea, pale

TABLE 8-1	ETIOLOGIC (PATHOPHYSIOLOGIC) CLASSIFICATIONS OF ANEMIA	
TYPE	**CAUSE**	**DISEASES**
Decreased or defective production of erythrocytes	Altered hemoglobin synthesis	Iron deficiency
		Thalassemia
		Anemia of chronic inflammation or disease
	Altered DNA synthesis from deficient nutrients	Pernicious anemia (decreased vitamin B$_{12}$, folate)
	Stem cell dysfunction	Aplastic anemia, myeloproliferative leukemia or dysplasia
	Bone marrow infiltration	Carcinoma, lymphoma, multiple myeloma
	Autoimmune disease or idiopathic	Pure red cell aplasia
Increased erythrocyte destruction	Blood loss	Acute (hemorrhage, trauma)
		Chronic (gastrointestinal bleeding, menorrhagia)
	Hemolysis (intrinsic)	Hereditary spherocytosis, sickle cell trait or disease, pyruvate kinase deficiency, glucose-6-phosphate dehydrogenase (G6PD) deficiency
	Hemolysis (extrinsic)	Warm or cold antibody disease, infection (malarial, clostridial), erythrocyte trauma (hemolytic uremic syndrome, TTP, mechanical cardiac valve, paravalvular leak), splenic sequestration, burns

TTP, Thrombotic thrombocytopenic purpura.

mucous membranes, vertigo, dysphagia, stomatitis, and tongue inflammation may be present.

History and risk factors: CKD, dialysis therapy, cancer within the bone marrow (e.g., leukemia), cancer chemotherapy, or therapy for HIV infection.

DIAGNOSTIC TESTS

Blood count: Usually RBCs and Hgb are decreased. Hct is low because the percentage of RBCs in the total blood volume is decreased.

Ferritin: Normal or increased. However, if it is less than 30 mcg/L, there is a coexisting iron deficiency.

Peripheral blood smear to examine RBC indices: Normocytic and normochromic erythrocytes (normal or slightly low mean corpuscular volume [MCV]).

Total iron-binding capacity: Decreased.

Reticulocyte count: Normal to slightly elevated.

Serum iron levels: Decreased.

TABLE 8-2   MORPHOLOGIC CLASSIFICATIONS OF ANEMIA

TYPE OF ANEMIA*	NAME OF DISORDER AND CLINICAL CONDITION	UNDERLYING CAUSE OF DISORDER	LABORATORY FINDINGS		
			LOW	NORMAL	HIGH
Macrocytic-normochromic—large, abnormally shaped erythrocytes but normal hemoglobin concentrations	*Pernicious anemia*—lack of vitamin B_{12}; abnormal DNA and RNA synthesis in the erythroblast; premature cell death	Congenital or acquired deficiency in IF needed for absorption of dietary vitamin B_{12}; acquired can result from chronic gastritis, gastrectomy, myelodysplasia, use of antiretroviral drugs	Hgb, Hct, reticulocytes, serum B_{12}	Total iron-binding capacity, folate, free erythrocyte protoporphyrin	MCV, plasma iron, ferritin, bilirubin (slight) transferrin (slight)
	Folate-deficiency anemia—lack of folate for erythropoiesis; premature cell death	Dietary folate deficiency, medications	Hgb, Hct, reticulocytes, folate	Total iron-binding capacity, serum B_{12} free erythrocyte protoporphyrin	MCV, plasma iron, ferritin, bilirubin (slight), transferrin (slight)
Microcytic-hypochromic anemia—small, abnormally shaped erythrocytes and reduced hemoglobin concentration	*Iron-deficiency anemia*—lack of folate for erythropoiesis; premature cell death	Chronic blood loss; dietary iron deficiency, disruption of iron metabolism	Hgb, Hct, MCV, plasma iron, ferritin, transferrin	Reticulocytes (or slightly high), serum B_{12}, folate, bilirubin	Total iron-binding capacity, free erythrocyte protoporphyrin
	Sideroblastic anemia—dysfunctional iron uptake by erythrocytes and heme synthesis	Congenital dysfunction of iron metabolism of erythroblasts; acquired dysfunction of iron metabolism from drugs or toxins	Hgb, Hct, MCV	Reticulocytes (or slightly high), total iron-binding capacity, serum B_{12}, folate, free erythrocyte protoporphyrin (or high)	Plasma iron, bilirubin
	Thalassemia—impaired synthesis of alpha or beta chain of hemoglobin A	Congenital defect of globin molecule synthesis	MCV, Hct (mild)	Platelets, RBC (or increased)	Reticulocytes (or normal), WBCs

Continued

TABLE 8-2　MORPHOLOGIC CLASSIFICATIONS OF ANEMIA—cont'd

TYPE OF ANEMIA*	NAME OF DISORDER AND CLINICAL CONDITION	UNDERLYING CAUSE OF DISORDER	LABORATORY FINDINGS		
			LOW	NORMAL	HIGH
Normocytic-normochromic anemia—destruction or depletion of erythrocytes	Aplastic anemia—insufficient erythropoiesis	Depressed stem cell differentiation leading to bone marrow failure	Hgb (or normal), Hct (or WNL), reticulocytes	MCV (or slightly high), total iron-binding capacity, ferritin, serum B_{12}, folate, bilirubin, transferrin	Plasma iron, free erythrocyte protoporphyrin
	Posthemorrhagic anemia—blood loss	Acute or chronic hemorrhage that stimulates increased erythropoiesis, depleting iron losses	Hgb (or normal), Hct (or normal), MCV (may be slight)	Plasma iron, MCV (or slightly high), total iron-binding capacity, ferritin, serum B_{12}, folate, bilirubin, free erythrocyte protoporphyrin, transferrin	Reticulocytes
	Hemolytic anemia—destruction of erythrocytes in circulation	Any condition that increases fragility of erythrocytes	Hgb, Hct	MCV (or high), plasma iron (or high), total iron-binding capacity, ferritin, serum B_{12}, folate, free erythrocyte protoporphyrin, transferrin	Reticulocytes, bilirubin (slight), LDH
	Sickle cell anemia—abnormal hemoglobin synthesis and cell shape, increasing cell damage and destruction	Congenital dysfunction of hemoglobin synthesis	Serum erythropoietin, haptoglobin	MCV	WBCs, nucleated red cells, reticulocytes, bilirubin, platelet
	Anemia of chronic disease—abnormally increased demand for new erythrocytes because of the disease and/or treatment	Chronic infection, inflammation, malignancy, liver disease, chronic renal failure	Hgb, Hct, plasma iron (may be slight), total iron-binding capacity, transferrin (may be slight)	Reticulocytes, MCV (may be low), ferritin, serum B_{12}, folate, bilirubin, free erythrocyte protoporphyrin (or slightly high)	Possibly ferritin

*Macrocytic, Higher MCV; microcytic, lower MCV; hyperchromic, higher MCHC; hypochromic, lower MCHC.
_____ ____. ___ ____, _____, ____, _____; LDH, lactate dehydrase; MCV, mean corpuscular volume; RBC, red blood cell; WBC, white blood cell; WNL, within normal limits.

COLLABORATIVE MANAGEMENT

The goal of collaborative management is correction of the underlying cause (e.g., kidney transplantation, treatment of leukemia).

EPO replacement: Recombinant EPO (epoetin alfa), 50 to 150 units/kg by the IV route 3 ×/wk, or 600 units/kg subcutaneously 1 ×/wk or darbepoetin alfa 200 mcg every 2 wk. Although side effects are few, deep vein thrombosis (DVT) may occur. Patients with renal insufficiency must be observed for hypertension and iron deficiency.

Iron replacement: Replenishes Hgb and depleted iron if needed.

Packed RBCs: Replenishes RBCs when Hgb is dangerously low.

NURSING DIAGNOSES AND INTERVENTIONS

Activity intolerance related to anemia

Desired outcome: After treatment, Hgb and Hct levels are within medical goals, and patient perceives exertion at 3 or less on a 0-10 scale and tolerates activity, as evidenced by respiratory rate (RR) 12-20 breaths/min, presence of eupnea, heart rate (HR) 100 beats per minute (bpm) or less, and absence of dizziness and headaches.

Nursing Interventions

- Assess patient for dyspnea on exertion, dizziness, palpations, headaches, and verbalization of increased exertion level. Ask patient to rate perceived exertion, *to correctly interpret patient's breathing difficulty.*
- Monitor oximetry as indicated. Report O_2 saturation 92% or less. Administer oxygen as prescribed, and encourage deep breathing *to augment oxygen delivery to the tissues.*
- Assess patient for ambulatory ability and implement appropriate strategies *to minimize risk for falls and/or injury.*
- Facilitate coordination of care allowing time for at least 90 min of rest as needed between care activities, *to provide periods of undisturbed rest.*
- Encourage gradually increasing activities to patient's tolerance. Set mutually agreed on goals with patient (e.g., "Let's plan this morning's activity goals. Do you think you could walk up and down the hall once, or twice?" or appropriate amount, depending on patient's tolerance). *Allows time for patient's condition to improve.*
- Reassure patient that symptoms usually are relieved and tolerance for activity increases with therapy. *May reduce anxiety, which depletes energy.*
- Administer blood components (usually packed RBCs) as prescribed. Double-check type and crossmatching and patient identifiers with a colleague, and monitor for and report signs of transfusion reaction. *Replenishes needed RBCs.*

 Patient-Family Teaching and Discharge Planning

Include verbal and written information about the following:

- Importance of a well-balanced diet, especially iron intake, if appropriate, which is found in foods such as red meat, dark green vegetables, legumes, and certain fruits (apricots, figs, raisins). Refer to clinical dietitian as prescribed.
- Special instructions for taking iron, if appropriate, depending on type prescribed. Therapy may need to be continued for 4-6 mo to replace iron stores adequately.
- Necessity for EPO replacement therapy to be continued for duration of the underlying condition.
- When self-administering EPO, importance of *not* shaking medication vial before taking it. *Shaking the vial may denature glycoprotein in the solution and render it biologically inactive.* Any discolored solution or solution with particulate matter should not be used.

- Other medications, including drug names, dosage, purpose, schedule, precautions, and potential side effects. Also discuss drug/drug, herb/drug, and food/drug interactions.
- Risks and benefits of RBC transfusion (as explained by health care provider) and necessity for signed consent for the transfusion.

❖ HEMOLYTIC AND SICKLE CELL ANEMIA

OVERVIEW/PATHOPHYSIOLOGY

Hemolytic anemia is characterized by abnormal or premature destruction of RBCs. Hemolysis can occur because of intrinsic or extrinsic factors (Table 8-1), for example, from a foreign antigen (e.g., from a transfusion reaction) or an autoimmune reaction in which the hemolytic agent is intrinsic to the patient's body. Other possible causes include exposure to radiation and ingestion of certain medications (e.g., sulfisoxazole, phenytoin, methyldopa). Acquired hemolytic anemia is usually the result of an abnormal immune response that causes premature destruction of RBCs.

Hemolytic crisis: Individuals with chronic hemolytic anemia may do relatively well for a time, but many factors can precipitate a hemolytic crisis or acute hemolysis (i.e., an individual with mild hemolytic anemia can become severely anemic with an acute infectious process or with any other physiologic or emotional stressor, including surgery, trauma, or emotional upset). Widespread hemolysis causes an acute decrease in O_2-carrying capacity of the blood that results in decreased O_2 delivery to the tissues. Organ congestion from the hemolyzed blood cells occurs, and it precipitates organ dysfunction and a shock state. Although medical therapy has improved the general prognosis of these patients, there is still an overall decrease in life expectancy.

Sickle cell anemia is a genetic disorder of hemoglobin (Hgb) synthesis characterized by the presence of 50% or more sickle Hgb (HbS). It results in abnormal, crescent-shaped, rigid, and elongated erythrocytes. Because of their abnormal shape and rigidity, these "sickled" RBCs interfere with circulation because they are not pliable like normal cells. Because they cannot get through the microcirculation smoothly, they are destroyed in the process (hemolysis). Vasoocclusive phenomena and hemolysis are the clinical hallmarks of sickle cell disease. *Sickle cell anemia* can affect almost every body system through decreased O_2 delivery, decreased circulation caused by occlusion of the vessels by RBCs, and the inflammatory process leading to infection. *Sickle cell disease* occurs when the gene is inherited from both parents (homozygous). A carrier state for *sickle cell trait* exists when it is inherited from only one parent (heterozygous).

Acute chest syndrome (ACS): ACS is the leading cause of death in adolescents and adults with sickle cell disease. Infection is believed to be the etiologic disorder in most cases, but ACS also can occur because of thrombosis, infarction, fat embolism, and atelectasis.

ASSESSMENT

Signs and symptoms/physical findings

Chronic indicators: Pallor (e.g., conjunctival), fatigue, dyspnea on exertion, and intermittent dizziness, all of which depend on anemia severity; distorted skeletal growth, and increased potential for hematogenic osteomyelitis in children and adolescents; and jaundice, arthritis, cholelithiasis, retinopathy, renal failure, skin ulcers, and chronic organ damage (heart, liver, lungs) from chronic hemolytic anemia.

Acute indicators (hemolytic crisis): Fever; headache; visual blurring or temporary blindness; severe abdominal pain; vomiting; splenomegaly; hepatomegaly; back, lower leg, and joint pain; priapism; palpitations; shortness of breath (because of pulmonary sequestration, anemia, infection); aplastic crisis (resulting from transient marrow suppression by viruses); chills; lymphadenopathy; decreased urinary output; and stroke. Peripheral nerve damage can result in paralysis or paresthesias. Occasionally a low-grade fever may occur 1-2 days after a crisis event. Attacks last a few hours to a few days and resolve spontaneously.

ACS: Chest pain, fever, cough.

History and risk factors: Family history, African-American race, and less commonly, hereditary descendants of Greece and southern Italy.

DIAGNOSTIC TESTS

Sickle cell test (Sickledex): Screens for sickle cell anemia or its trait.

Hgb electrophoresis: Discriminates among Hgb AS, sickle cell trait, and Hgb SS, sickle cell anemia.

Cold agglutinin titer: Markedly elevated (greater than 1:1000). This test measures antibodies that are able to clump RBCs at cold temperatures.

Hgb and Hct: Decreased because of RBC destruction.

Serum tests

Lactate dehydrogenase (LDH): Elevated because of release of this enzyme when RBCs are destroyed.

Bilirubin: Elevated because the liver cannot process the excess that occurs from rapid RBC destruction.

Urine and fecal urobilinogen: Levels increased. These are more sensitive indicators of RBC destruction than serum bilirubin levels.

Bone marrow aspiration: Reveals erythroid hyperplasia, especially with chronic hemolytic anemia.

Reticulocyte count: Elevated because of the rapid destruction of RBCs.

Serum haptoglobin: Decreased because the Hgb released from hemolyzed RBCs is bound to haptoglobin.

Chorionic biopsy: Determines presence of sickle cell disease in the first 6-8 wk of pregnancy.

COLLABORATIVE MANAGEMENT

The goals of treatment for sickle cell anemia are relieving symptoms and preventing crisis and complications.

Elimination or discontinuation of causative factor: If possible (e.g., chemical, drug, incompatible blood).

Volume replacement: Adequate hydration is important to prevent complications from decreased organ perfusion secondary to hemolysis or sickle cell vascular congestion.

O$_2$ therapy: Routine pulse oximetry determines need for oxygen therapy for patients who are hypoxemic (e.g., O$_2$ saturation 92% or less).

Supportive therapy for shock state: For example, antibiotics, vasopressors.

Transfusion: For circulatory failure or severe anemic anoxia if it occurs. Especially at risk are older persons and those with limited cardiopulmonary reserves. A conservative approach is taken and the patient's Hgb is usually not raised greater than 10 g/dL because of increased viscosity with higher levels, development of alloantibodies, and iron overload.

Iron chelation: Agents such as deferoxamine mesylate may be used to bind iron so that chronically transfused patients (i.e., those with sickle cell disease or thalassemia) have a reduced risk of iron overload, which can lead to end-organ damage to the liver and heart.

Erythrocytapheresis (RBC exchange or partial exchange): A procedure that removes abnormal RBCs and infuses healthy RBCs with or without normal saline to correct the anemia. It is used for younger patients with a history of stroke or for individuals with pulmonary or cardiac disease.

Corticosteroids: Help stabilize cell membranes and decrease the inflammatory response.

Folic acid: Helps prevent hemolytic crisis by increasing RBC production in individuals with chronic hemolytic anemias.

Hydroxyurea: Decreases painful sickling episodes by stimulating the production of fetal Hgb.

Rituximab: Monoclonal antibody given by the IV route weekly for 4 wk as an antibody suppressant.

Danazol: Androgen with unknown mechanism of action.

IV immune globulin: Causes binding of antibodies so that they are less likely to cause hemolysis.

Immunosuppressive agents (e.g., cyclophosphamide, azathioprine, or cyclosporine): Suppress the antibodies causing RBC lysis.

Influenza and pneumococcal vaccinations: Prevent infection that may trigger crisis.

Splenectomy: Provides symptomatic relief, depending on anemia cause. It also may be done prophylactically to reduce the potential for rupture and massive blood loss. The spleen is the site of RBC destruction.

Stem cell transplant from human leukocyte antigen (HLA)–matched donor following high-dose chemotherapy: Can be curative in young patients with sickle cell disease. This treatment potentially ablates the genetic disorder and restores normal hematopoiesis. However, it can have acute and delayed risks of morbidity and mortality.

Pain management: Aggressive use of opioids and other analgesics in acute crisis; meperidine is contraindicated because of increased side effects, including seizures, in high doses.

NURSING DIAGNOSES AND INTERVENTIONS

Acute pain or Chronic pain related to joint hemolysis secondary to hemolytic crisis or sickle cell disease

Desired outcomes: Within 1 hr of intervention, patient's subjective perception of discomfort decreases, as documented by pain scale. Objective indicators, such as grimacing, are absent or diminished. Lifestyle behaviors are not compromised because of discomfort.

Nursing Interventions

- Monitor for pain by having patient rate discomfort on a scale of 0 (no pain) to 10 (worst pain) *to determine patient's perception of pain/discomfort.*
- Instruct patient to request analgesic before pain becomes too intense. Pain is easier to control if treated before it becomes severe.
- Administer analgesia as prescribed *to relieve and/or control pain.*
- Reassure patient that acute pain will subside when acute hemolytic episode is over. If chronic pain persists, ensure that a plan for pain management upon discharge is addressed by health care provider.
- Assist with positioning as needed *to promote comfort.*
- Apply moist heat packs to painful joints, but use cautiously for patients with decreased peripheral sensations. *Increases circulation and decreases pain.*
- Apply elastic stockings or wraps, if prescribed, *to protect skin, support joints, and promote circulation.*

Ineffective peripheral and cardiopulmonary tissue perfusion related to inflammatory process and occlusion of blood vessels with RBCs

Desired outcome: Following treatment, patient has adequate peripheral and cardiopulmonary perfusion, as evidenced by SBP 10 mm Hg or less lower than baseline SBP, peripheral pulses 2+ or more on a 0-4+ scale, heart rate

(HR) 100 beats per minute (bpm) or less, respiratory rate (RR) 12-20 breaths/ min with normal depth and pattern (eupnea), and normal skin color.

Nursing Interventions

◆ Assess SBP at frequent intervals, and report significant drops (more than 10 mm Hg from baseline readings).
◆ Assess peripheral pulses. Be alert to pulses 2+ or less on a 0-4+ scale. *Indicates degree of peripheral perfusion.*
◆ Monitor for decreased BP, increased HR, decreased pulse amplitude, dyspnea, and decreased urine output. *Indicate cardiac depression.*
◆ Assess for and report increased RR, dyspnea, shortness of breath, cyanosis, and pallor; pulse oximetry; O_2 saturation 92%, or less, *which could signal ACS.*
◆ *Monitor lips, tongue, oral* mucosa, and nail beds. These areas are especially important to monitor in dark-skinned individuals because pallor is difficult to assess. *Indicates hypoxia or respiratory dysfunction.*
◆ Administer oxygen as prescribed, *to counter hypoxemia if present.*
◆ Assist with ROM exercises and positioning. *Be aware that exercise should be avoided if any early signs of hemolytic crisis appear because exercise can aggravate hemolysis.* In the absence of crisis, *exercise enhances tissue perfusion and maintains and increases joint mobility.*
◆ Report significant findings to patient's health care provider.

Risk for impaired skin integrity or **Impaired tissue integrity** related to altered circulation (occlusion of the vessels), resulting in impaired oxygen transport to tissues and skin
Desired outcome: Patient's skin and tissue remain nonerythematous and intact.

Nursing Interventions

◆ Assess patient's skin, especially over bony prominences and extremities. Document changes in integrity, such as erythema, increased warmth, and blisters.
◆ Keep extremities warm *to promote circulation.*
◆ Encourage moderate exercises or ROM every hour while awake. Avoid any activity or exercise if signs and symptoms of hemolytic crisis are present. *Promotes circulation.*
◆ Caution patient about importance of avoiding trauma or injury to skin and tissues.
◆ Apply dry, sterile dressings or transparent or hydrocolloidal dressing materials such as Duoderm, Comfeel, Op-Site, or Tegaderm to areas of tissue breakdown. Use a bed cradle if indicated to keep linens and blankets off patient's tissue and skin. Use sterile technique *to help prevent infection.*

Patient-Family Teaching and Discharge Planning

Include verbal and written information about the following:
◆ Rationale of treatment plan and importance of medical follow-up.
◆ Importance of ensuring that fluid intake is adequate to promote organ and tissue perfusion and avoiding high altitudes for individuals who are hypoxemic.
◆ Phone numbers and contact person for local and/or national support groups available for sickle cell anemia, such as:

Sickle Cell Disease Association of America: http://SickleCellDisease.org

◆ Indicators of hemolytic crisis, including jaundice, dyspnea, shortness of breath, joint or abdominal pain, decreasing BP, and increased HR; and factors that precipitate hemolytic crisis, such as emotional stress, physical stress, infection, trauma, chemicals, and toxic drug reactions (e.g., to penicillin, methyldopa, sulfonamides, quinine).

◆ Importance of maintaining a calm environment. Teach stress reduction techniques, such as meditation and relaxation exercises.

◆ Importance of hygiene and avoiding infectious processes, such as upper respiratory infections, and getting appropriate immunizations and prompt medical attention if infection occurs.

◆ Necessity to avoid intake of iron and citrus with meals (citrus increases absorption of iron) to help minimize abnormal RBC proliferation.

◆ Medications, including drug names, purpose, schedule, dosage, precautions, and potential side effects. Discuss drug/drug, herb/drug, and food/drug interactions. Over-the-counter (OTC) drugs must be avoided unless approved by primary health care provider, along with alcohol and smoking. Corticosteriods increase the risk for gastrointestinal (GI) hemorrhage, delayed wound healing, and increased appetite. Review need to take medication with food, immediately take missed doses, and avoid precipitously discontinuing medication.

◆ Risks and benefits of RBC transfusion (as explained by health care provider) and necessity for patient to sign consent for the transfusion.

◆ Birth control options and referrals for genetic counseling and any needed psychosocial support for living with a chronic illness.

◆ Importance of obtaining a MedicAlert bracelet and identification card outlining diagnosis and emergency treatment:

MedicAlert Foundation: www.medicalert.org

❖ APLASTIC ANEMIA

OVERVIEW/PATHOPHYSIOLOGY

Aplastic anemia results from inability of erythrocyte-producing organs, specifically bone marrow stem cells, to produce erythrocytes. Causes of aplastic anemia are varied but can include use of antineoplastic or antimicrobial agents, infectious process, systemic lupus erythematosus (SLE), pregnancy, hepatitis, and radiation. Approximately half of patients with aplastic anemia have had exposure to drugs or chemical agents (benzene, insecticides), whereas the remaining half have had immunologic disorders. For no identified etiology, the cause is believed to be a T-cell–mediated autoimmune disorder attacking the patient's own bone marrow. Aplastic anemia most often involves pancytopenia—depressed production of all three bone marrow elements: erythrocytes, platelets, and granulocytes (especially neutrophils) without abnormal cellular morphologies. Usually the onset is insidious, but it can evolve quickly in some cases. Prognosis usually is poor.

ASSESSMENT

Signs and symptoms/physical findings
Chronic indicators: Weakness, fatigue, pallor, dysphagia, and extremity numbness and tingling.
Acute indicators: Fever and infection (because of decreased neutrophils), bleeding (because of thrombocytopenia), dizziness, dyspnea on exertion, progressive weakness, and oral ulcerations.
History and risk factors: Exposure to chemical toxins or radiation; use of medications, such as chloramphenicol or phenytoin; viral infections, such as hepatitis C; antineoplastic therapy.

DIAGNOSTIC TESTS

Complete blood count (CBC) with differential: Decreased hemoglobin (Hgb), WBCs, RBCs, and platelets; however, RBCs usually appear to be normal morphologically.
Platelet count: Low.

Bone marrow aspiration and biopsy: Usually reveal hypocellular or hypoplastic tissue with a fatty and fibrous appearance.

Reticulocyte count: This test, a determinant of bone marrow function and RBC production, shows a marked decrease because of inability of the bone marrow to respond.

Peripheral blood smear: May show nucleated RBCs.

Cultures: If infection is suspected.

COLLABORATIVE MANAGEMENT

The goals of collaborative management are determination of anemia cause and removal or treatment of causative agent, if possible.

Transfusion with packed RBCs: See **TABLE 8-3**. Because of the potential for antibody formation, patients considered candidates for bone marrow transplantation (BMT) should be given leukocyte-poor, irradiated, and cytomegalovirus (CMV)–negative blood products (if patient is CMV negative).

Transfusion with concentrated platelets: Maintains platelet count at greater than 10,000/mm^3 or per health care provider threshold. Hemorrhage occurrence is less common when platelet count is above this level (Table 8-3), but because frequent platelet transfusions can result in platelet antibody formation, conservative use may be warranted.

Treatment with antithymocyte globulin (ATG) and cyclosporine: Suppresses autoimmune response. It is used as standard therapy in adults older than 50 yr of age and before allogeneic stem cell transplant or BMT in patients less than 50 yr of age. Response may take 4-12 wk.

Corticosteroids: Given to prevent complications of serum sickness from ATG.

Allogeneic hematopoietic stem cell transplantation (HSCT) or BMT: Standard treatment for patients less than 50 yr old who do not respond to ATG. Bone marrow is aspirated from a donor's pelvic bones or apheresed from the donor's peripheral blood and then filtered and infused into the patient. Optimally, donated marrow is antigen compatible (using human leukocyte antigen [HLA] tissue typing) and from an identical twin or sibling. However, only about one-third of potential bone marrow transplant recipients have an HLA-matched sibling donor. Use of unrelated donors is possible through the National Marrow Donor Program.

Antibiotic therapy: If infection is present.

Androgen therapy (e.g., oxymetholone): Enhances production of erythropoietin (EPO). It may be used as maintenance therapy in conjunction with ATG and corticosteroids.

O$_2$ therapy: If anemia is severe.

NURSING DIAGNOSES AND INTERVENTIONS

Risk for infection related to neutropenia

Desired outcomes: Optimally, patient is free of infection, as evidenced by normothermia; full, but not bounding, heart rate (HR) of 100 beats per minute (bpm) or less; respiratory rate (RR) 12-20 breaths/min with normal depth and pattern (eupnea); and stable BP.

Nursing Interventions

- Thoroughly assess for infection: low-grade fever, shortness of breath (versus adventitious breath sounds), slight chills, slight change in mentation, or BP changes. Signs of infection may be subtle because lack of neutrophils reduces the febrile and inflammatory response.

- Monitor for and report any signs of local infection, such as sore throat or erythematous or draining wounds. With decreased or absent neutrophils, pus may not form; therefore, it is important to look for other signs of infection.

- Report any signs of systemic infection (e.g., temperature higher than 100.4° F [38° C]) or subtle signs of septic shock promptly, *to facilitate early treatment.*

TABLE 8-3	COMMONLY USED BLOOD PRODUCTS*†		
PRODUCT	**APPROXIMATE VOLUME**	**INDICATIONS**	**PRECAUTIONS/COMMENTS**
Whole blood	500-510 mL (450 mL of whole blood; 50-60 mL of anticoagulants)	Symptomatic anemia; acute, severe blood loss; hypovolemic shock; increases both RBC mass and plasma; whole blood transfusion is used rarely today except for autologous transfusion; patient with hematologic disorders is not usually considered an autologous donor; specific blood components are given in lieu of whole blood	Must be ABO identical and Rh compatible
Packed RBCs	250 mL	Symptomatic anemia; to increase RBC mass and O₂-carrying capacity of blood	*Do not* mix with dextrose solutions; always prime tubing with normal saline Use tubing with microaggregate filter Observe for dyspnea, orthopnea, cyanosis, and anxiety as signs of circulatory overload; monitor vital signs Administer as rapidly as indicated but not to exceed 4 hr Must be ABO identical and Rh compatible Leukocyte-depleted RBCs may be used to reduce risk of antibody formation and nonhemolytic reactions Irradiated RBCs may be used to prevent graft-versus-host disease in patients who are immunocompromised Packed RBCs have less volume than whole blood, thus reducing risk of fluid overload
Fresh frozen plasma	250 mL	Treatment of choice for combined coagulation factor deficiencies and factor II, V, and XI deficiencies; alternate treatment for factor VII, VIII, IX, and X deficiencies when concentrates are not available	Always prime with normal saline; use tubing with microaggregate filter; administer over 1.5-2 hr Must be ABO identical Supplies clotting factors

Continued

Random-donor platelet concentrate	50 mL	Treatment of choice for thrombocytopenia resulting from leukemia, aplastic anemia, and chemotherapy treatment, and diseases that increase destruction or loss; usually contraindicated in TTP and HIT	Usual dose is 10-15 mg/kg of body weight Transfuse within 24 hr of thawing Do not use if patient needs volume expansion Keep rate of infusion at less than 4 hr Usual dose is 0.1 unit/kg of body weight to increase platelet count to 25,000/mm^3
			Administer as rapidly as tolerated ABO compatibility is preferable Effectiveness is decreased by fever, sepsis, and splenomegaly Febrile reactions are common; premedication with diphenhydramine and acetaminophen recommended as prophylaxis Always prime with normal saline; use tubing with microaggregate filter; special filters are available for removing leukocytes and thus decreasing risk of alloimmunization to HLA Platelets must be infused within 4 hr of initiation and ideally within 30 to 60 min
Platelet concentrate by platelet pheresis (single-donor platelets)	200 mL, but may vary	Treatment for thrombocytopenic patients who are refractory to random-donor platelets	Involves removing donor's venous blood, removing platelets by differential centrifuge, and returning blood to donor Approximately 3-4 L of whole blood is processed to obtain a therapeutic dose of platelets May use special donors who are HLA-matched to patient Always prime with normal saline; use tubing with microaggregate filter
Cryoprecipitate (factor VIII)	10-25 mL	For acute bleeding in hemophilia (factor VIII deficiency) and fibrinogen deficiency (factor XIII deficiency); occasionally used to control bleeding in anemic patients	Made from fresh frozen plasma Infuse immediately on thawing, 1-2 mL/min in 8-12 hr to achieve desired effect

TABLE 8-3   COMMONLY USED BLOOD PRODUCTS*† —cont'd

PRODUCT	APPROXIMATE VOLUME	INDICATIONS	PRECAUTIONS/COMMENTS
AHG (factor VIII) concentrates	20 mL	Alternate treatment for hemophilia A	Allergic and febrile reactions occur frequently Administer by syringe or component drip set Can store at refrigerator temperature, making it convenient for persons with hemophilia during travel Can precipitate clotting
Factor II, VII, IX, X concentrate	20 mL	Treatment of choice for acute bleeding with hemophilia B and factor IX deficiencies	Allergic and febrile reactions occur occasionally Contraindicated in liver disease
Albumin‡	50 or 250 mL	Hypovolemic shock, hypoalbuminemia, protein replacement for burn injury patients	Osmotically equal to 5× its volume of plasma Used as a volume expander in conjunction with crystalloids; also used in hypoalbuminemic states Expensive
Plasma protein fraction‡	250 mL (83% albumin with some α and β globulins)	Volume expansion	Certain lots reported to result in hypotension, possibly related to vasoactive amines used in preparation Not a common treatment
Granulocyte transfusion (collected from a single donor)	200 mL, but may vary	Neutropenia related to treatment, myeloproliferative disorder, or aplastic anemia with impending infection and septic shock	Febrile and allergic symptoms are frequent; must be ABO compatible and should be irradiated

AHG, Antihemophilic globulin; *HIT*, heparin-induced thrombocytopenia; *HLA*, human leukocyte antigen; *TTP*, thrombotic thrombocytopenic purpura; *RBC*, red blood cell.
*DNA recombinant technology may decrease complications from factor concentrates.
†When administering blood products, it is important to recognize that most blood products have risk associated with delivery. Risks include transmission of human immunodeficiency virus, hepatitis B and hepatitis C viruses, cytomegalovirus, and human T-cell leukemia/lymphoma virus (HTLV-I).
‡These products carry no risk of disease transmission.

- Obtain blood culture, as ordered, before implementation of antibiotic therapy, *to facilitate identification of pathogenic organisms.*
- Administer antibiotics stat as prescribed, *to minimize injury from infection.*
- Perform meticulous handwashing before patient contact and maintain sterile technique with procedures such as central line dressing changes. **Handwashing is the most important factor in reducing the risk of infection!** *Helps minimizes the risk for infection.*
- Strive to ensure that all health care providers and visitors are free from infection and have not had exposure to infectious diseases. Restrict number of visitors, *to reduce infection via communicable disease.*
- Implement "protective isolation" or "neutropenic precautions" for these patients, following agency policy. Protective isolation is sometimes instituted if neutrophil count is less than 500/mm³, *to help minimize the risk for infection.*
- Discuss potential for allogeneic BMT or HSCT with patient, if appropriate.
- Ensure that patient performs oral care at frequent intervals to prevent oral lesions. Patient should use a soft bristle toothbrush at least 4 ×/day; if bleeding or irritation occurs, a sponge-type swab and/or nonalcoholic rinse or normal saline may be used. *Prevents bleeding and infection from oral lesions.*
- Provide and encourage adequate hygiene, especially handwashing. Avoid giving medications or taking temperature rectally. Perianal hygiene is important, *to prevent rectal abscess.*
- Avoid invasive procedures, if possible, *to minimize risk of introducing pathogens.*
- Encourage ambulation, deep breathing, turning, and coughing, to avoid pneumonia and skin breakdown. *Prevents problems of immobility.*
- Arrange for patient to have a private room when possible, *to permit optimal environmental control and protection.*
- For patient who is severely immunocompromised because of allogeneic HSCT, ensure that he or she is cared for in an appropriate environment, such as a high efficiency particulate air (HEPA)–filtered room, *to minimize risk of exposure to Aspergillus and other fungal spores.* See "Infection Prevention and Control," p. 743, for more information.

Deficient knowledge related to risk for bleeding (caused by low platelet count) and measures that can help prevent it
Desired outcome: Patient has minimal bleeding resulting from staff's, patient's, and family's interventions.

Nursing Interventions

- Assess patient's facility with language; engage an interpreter or provide language-appropriate written materials as indicated.
- Assess patient for occult and subtle signs of bleeding, such as hematuria, hemoptysis, hematemesis, hematochezia or melena, petechiae, hematomas, change in mental status, and acute abdominal pain.
- Monitor platelet count daily and coagulation studies at least weekly or as indicated, *to detect dangerously low levels and monitor treatment effectiveness.*
- Ensure that there is a current type and crossmatch in the blood bank in the event acute bleeding occurs. *Provides supportive RBCs if needed.*
- When possible, avoid venipuncture. If performed, apply pressure on site for 5-10 min or until bleeding stops. Post "bleeding precautions" sign to notify other health care workers.
- Teach patient and significant others about the potential for bleeding and importance of monitoring for hematuria, melena, frank bleeding from the mouth, epistaxis, coughing up blood (hemoptysis), excessive vaginal bleeding (menometrorrhagia), headache, or vision changes and notifying staff promptly if they occur.

- Prevent or promptly control retching, vomiting, coughing, and straining with bowel movements. *These actions can trigger bleeding.*
- Explain importance of maintaining regularity with bowel movements, *to prevent straining and potential bleeding.*
- Monitor intake of fluid (should be greater than 2.5 L/day) and dietary fiber; administer stool softeners as indicated, *to prevent straining and potential bleeding.*
- Teach patient to use an electric razor and soft-bristle toothbrush and avoid blowing nose forcefully (dab instead), bending down (head lower than the heart), potentially traumatic procedures (e.g., enemas, rectal temperatures), and high-risk recreational lifestyle, *to reduce the potential for bleeding.*
- Caution patient to avoid using aspirin, aspirin products, or nonsteroidal antiinflammatory drugs (NSAIDs), which decrease platelet aggregation and *increase the potential for bleeding.*
- Discourage smoking and excessive alcohol consumption, *to minimize risk for bleeding.*
- Explain that concentrated platelets usually are transfused to keep platelet count greater than 10,000/mm^3, but this will vary depending on health care provider's concern regarding patient's development of platelet antibodies and becoming refractory to platelet transfusions. *Helps prevent hemorrhage when platelet count is maintained above this level* (Table 8-3).

Ineffective protection related to neurosensory and musculoskeletal alterations secondary to tissue hypoxia occurring with decreased production of erythrocytes
Desired outcome: Patient verbalizes orientation to person, place, and time and is free of symptoms of injury caused by neurosensory alterations.

Nursing Interventions

- Perform neurologic checks, including orientation, mental status assessments, pupillary reaction to light, level of consciousness (LOC), and motor response to evaluate cerebral perfusion. If signs of decreasing cerebral perfusion occur, establish precautionary measures (e.g., bed in lowest position) to protect patient from injury and falls. Pad side rails if indicated and initiate a fall prevention plan; use restraints only after all other measures have failed *to prevent injury and/or bleeding.*
- Request one-on-one supervision by family or staff member if patient becomes confused or restless.
- Assess sensorimotor status. Be alert to paresthesias, decreased muscle strength, and altered gait. *Helps evaluate nervous system oxygenation.*
- Prevent injury from heat or cold applications. *Patients with paresthesias cannot sense heat or cold.*
- Do not allow patient to ambulate unassisted if muscle or gait alterations are present. Carefully assess patient's reliability in adhering with assisted ambulation, *to minimize risk for injury.*
- As indicated, monitor oximetry; report O$_2$ saturation 92% or less. Administer oxygen as prescribed, *to prevent hypoxia.*
- Teach and encourage deep breathing. Cue patient q1-2h while awake. *Augments oxygen delivery to the tissues.*
- Report indicators of a worsening condition promptly to patient's health care provider.

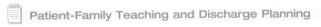 Patient-Family Teaching and Discharge Planning

Include verbal and written information about the following:

- Medications, including drug names, purpose, dosage, schedule, precautions, and potential side effects. Also discuss drug/drug, herb/drug, and food/drug interactions.

- Indicators of systemic infection, including fever, malaise, and fatigue, as well as signs and symptoms of upper respiratory infection, urinary tract infection, and wound infection.
- Importance of avoiding exposure to individuals known to have acute infections; preventing trauma, abrasions, and breakdown of skin; and maintaining good nutritional intake to enhance resistance to infections.
- Signs of bleeding/hemorrhage that necessitate medical attention: melena, hematuria, epistaxis, hemoptysis (coughing up blood), excessive vaginal bleeding (menometrorrhagia), ecchymosis, and bleeding gums.
- Measures to prevent hemorrhage, such as using electric razor and soft-bristle toothbrush and avoiding activities that can traumatize tissues.
- Importance of reporting general symptoms of anemia, including fatigue, weakness, paresthesias, palpitations, or exertional dyspnea. Discuss fall and injury prevention plan.
- Importance of avoiding aspirin, aspirin products, or NSAIDs in the presence of a bleeding disorder.
- Risks and benefits of blood product transfusion explained by health care provider and necessity of patient's signed consent to the transfusion.
- Phone numbers to call if questions or concerns arise about therapy or disease after discharge. In addition, some cities have local support groups for patients who may require HSCT or BMT. Information for these patients can be obtained by contacting:

National Bone Marrow Transplant Link: http://www.nbmtlink.org

❖ POLYCYTHEMIA

OVERVIEW/PATHOPHYSIOLOGY

Polycythemia is a chronic disorder characterized by excessive production of RBCs, platelets, and myelocytes. As production of these elements increases, blood volume, blood viscosity, and hemoglobin (Hgb) concentration increase and cause an excessive workload for the heart and congestion of some organs (e.g., liver, kidney).

Secondary polycythemia results from an abnormal increase in erythropoietin (EPO) production (e.g., because of hypoxia that occurs with chronic lung disease or prolonged living in altitudes greater than 10,000 ft) or from renal tumors. *Polycythemia vera* is a primary disorder of unknown cause resulting in increased RBC mass, leukocytosis, and slight thrombocytosis. Because of increased viscosity and decreased microcirculation, mortality is high if the condition is left untreated. In addition, there is potential for this disorder to evolve into other hematopoietic disorders, such as acute leukemia.

ASSESSMENT

Signs and symptoms/physical findings: Fatigue, muscle pain, headache, dizziness, paresthesias, visual disturbances, dyspnea, thrombophlebitis, joint pain, painful pruritus, night sweats, chest pain, and a feeling of "fullness," especially in the head; hypertension, engorgement of retinal blood veins, crackles (rales), weight loss, cyanosis, changes in mentation or mood (delirium, psychotic depression, mania), ruddy complexion (especially palmar aspects of hands and plantar surfaces of feet), splenomegaly, hepatomegaly, gastrointestinal (GI) disturbances (ulcers, GI bleeding).

History and risk factors: Family history, male gender, Jewish descent, middle to older age, chronic lung disease, high altitudes, renal tumors.

DIAGNOSTIC TESTS

CBC: Increased RBC mass (8-12 million/mm^3), Hgb (18-25 g/dL), hematocrit (Hct) (more than 54% in men and 49% in women), and leukocytes; and overproduction of thrombocytes.

Platelet count: Elevated as a result of increased production.

Bone marrow aspiration: Reveals RBC proliferation.

Uric acid levels: May be increased because of increased nucleoprotein, an end product of RBC breakdown.

EPO levels: Elevated in secondary polycythemia and decreased in polycythemia vera.

O_2 saturation: Normal (greater than 92%).

COLLABORATIVE MANAGEMENT

The goal of collaborative management is reduction Hct levels by reducing RBC production.

Phlebotomy: Blood withdrawn from the vein to decrease blood volume (and decrease Hct to 45%). Usually 500 mL is removed every 2-4 days until Hct is 42%-47%. For the older adult, 250-300 mL is removed.

Myelosuppressive therapy: Chemotherapy agents are given to inhibit bone marrow function, for example, hydroxyurea (preferred), busulfan, and/or radioactive phosphorus (especially for older persons and those refractory to other agents). Myeloablative chemotherapy followed by hematopoietic stem cell transplant from a human leukocyte antigen (HLA)-matched donor to reconstitute patient's bone marrow may be used in younger patients who do not respond to other therapies.

Radioactive phosphorus: Reduces the number of RBCs.

Histamine antagonists: Provide symptomatic relief of pruritus.

Recombinant interferon-α: Increases immune recognition of abnormal cells in myeloid metaplasia and splenomegaly.

Low-dose aspirin: Alleviates microvascular symptoms; often used with interferon-α and phlebotomy.

Anagrelide: Reduces platelet formation from megakaryocytes; may be used with interferon-α in younger patients or with hydroxyurea in older patients.

NURSING DIAGNOSES AND INTERVENTIONS

Acute pain related to headache, angina, pruritus, and abdominal and joint discomfort secondary to altered circulation because of blood hyperviscosity

Desired outcomes: Within 1 hr of intervention, patient's subjective perception of discomfort decreases, as documented by pain scale. Objective indicators, such as grimacing, are absent or diminished. Lifestyle behaviors are not compromised because of discomfort.

Nursing Interventions

- Assess for presence of headache, angina, abdominal pain, and joint pain. Devise a pain scale with patient, rating discomfort from 0 (no pain) to 10 (worst pain).
- In the presence of joint or skin discomfort, rest the joint and elevate the extremity; apply cool compresses or ice. In the presence of pruritus, skin may become painful and swollen, exacerbated by heat or exposure to water. *Helps eases discomfort.*
- Administer analgesics as prescribed. Topical antihistamines or lotions generally are not helpful. Avoid analgesics containing aspirin or other nonsteroidal antiinflammatory drugs (NSAIDs). *Prevents exacerbation of bleeding associated with thrombocytosis (high number of ineffective platelets).*
- Instruct patient to request analgesic before pain becomes too intense. *Pain is easier to control if treated before it becomes severe.*
- Encourage use of nonpharmacologic measures such as relaxation and distraction, *to help control pain.*
- Monitor for calf pain and tenderness. *Indicates peripheral thrombosis.*
- Report significant findings to patient's health care provider.

Ineffective renal, peripheral, and cerebral tissue perfusion related to blood hyperviscosity

Desired outcome: Following treatment, patient has adequate renal, peripheral, and cerebral perfusion, as evidenced by urinary output 30 mL/hr or more; peripheral pulses 2+ or more on a scale of 0-4+; distal extremity warmth; adequate (baseline) muscle strength; no mental status changes; and orientation to person, place, and time.

Nursing Interventions

- Assess peripheral pulses. Be alert to pulse 2+ or less on a scale of 0-4+ and coolness in distal extremities. *Determines peripheral perfusion.*
- Monitor I&O; report urine output less than 30 mL/hr in the presence of adequate intake. *Signals congestion and decreased perfusion.*
- Monitor for muscle weakness and decreased sensation and level of consciousness (LOC). If these indicators are present, protect patient by assisting with ambulation or initiating other fall prevention measures, depending on degree of deficit. *Indicates impending neurologic damage.*
- Provide prescribed IV hydration and encourage fluid intake in the absence of signs of cardiac and renal failure, *to decrease blood viscosity.*
- Encourage patient to change position q1h when in bed or to exercise and ambulate to tolerance *to enhance circulation.*
- Instruct patient to avoid tight clothing, *to prevent restriction of preipheral circulation.*
- Administer myelosuppressive agents, as prescribed, *to inhibit proliferation of RBCs.*
- If patient smokes, encourage enrollment in a smoking cessation program because *smoking significantly increases potential of a thromboembolic event.*
- Report significant findings to patient's health care provider.

Imbalanced nutrition: less than body requirements related to anorexia secondary to feelings of fullness occurring with organ system congestion

Desired outcome: By at least 24 hr before hospital discharge, patient exhibits adequate nutrition, as evidenced by maintenance of or return to baseline body weight or a 1- to 2-lb weight gain.

Nursing Interventions

- Weigh patient daily, *to identify trend.*
- Monitor fluid volume intake; encourage intake, if necessary, *to prevent dehydration.*
- Serve small, frequent meals, documenting intake. *Encourages intake.*
- Request that family bring patient's favorite foods if unavailable in hospital. *Encourages intake.*
- Advise patient to avoid spicy foods and to eat mild foods *because they are better tolerated.*
- Teach patient to avoid intake of iron and citrus with meals (citrus increases absorption of iron), *to help minimize abnormal RBC proliferation and iron overload.*
- As indicated, obtain dietary consultation, *to facilitate weight maintenance or weight gain.*
- Teach patient or significant other how to record and maintain fluid and food intake diary, *to evaluate adequacy of food/fluid intake.*

Ineffective cerebral and cardiopulmonary tissue perfusion (or risk for same) related to hypovolemia secondary to phlebotomy

Desired outcome: Patient has adequate cerebral and cardiopulmonary perfusion, as evidenced by no mental status changes; orientation to person, place, and time; heart rate (HR) 100 beats per minute (bpm) or less; BP 90/60 mm Hg or greater (or within patient's baseline range); absence of chest pain; and respiratory rate (RR) 20 breaths/min or less.

Nursing Interventions

◆ Assess for tachycardia, hypotension, chest pain, or dizziness during procedure; notify patient's health care provider of significant findings. *Indicates decreased perfusion.*

◆ During phlebotomy procedure, keep patient recumbent, *to prevent dizziness or hypotension.*

◆ After the procedure, assist patient with sitting position for 5-10 min before ambulation, *to prevent orthostatic hypotension.*

◆ Teach patients, especially those who are older and chronically ill, about potential for orthostatic hypotension and need for caution when standing for at least 2-3 days after phlebotomy, *to prevent falls.*

 Patient-Family Teaching and Discharge Planning

Include verbal and written information about the following:

◆ Need for continued medical follow-up, including potential for phlebotomy.

◆ Medications, including drug names, purpose, dosage, schedule, precautions, and potential side effects. Also discuss drug/drug, herb/drug, and food/drug interactions.

◆ Importance of augmenting fluid intake (e.g., greater than 2.5 L/day) to decrease blood viscosity and avoiding smoking; provide smoking cessation information as appropriate.

◆ Signs and symptoms that necessitate medical attention: angina, muscle weakness, numbness and tingling of extremities, decreased tolerance to activity, mental status changes, joint pain, and bleeding.

◆ Nutrition: importance of maintaining balanced diet to increase resistance to infection and limiting dietary or supplemental intake of iron to help minimize abnormal RBC proliferation and iron overload.

❖ ❖ ❖

SECTION TWO # DISORDERS OF COAGULATION

Adequate coagulation requires proper formation and function of clotting factors and platelets working together to form a clot. Hemostasis occurs in four major phases: (1) vascular (blood vessel injury and exposure of the subendothelium), (2) formation of a platelet plug, (3) development of a fibrin clot on the platelet plug, and (4) ultimate lysis of the clot.

Platelets form the primary hemostatic plug and provide the surface upon which fibrin formation occurs. At the time of vascular injury, platelets migrate to the site and adhere to collagen fibrils in the vascular subendothelium and subsequently to each other to form a temporary plug to stop the bleeding. They also help activate the clotting factors.

Formation of a visible fibrin clot on the platelet plug is the conclusion of a complex series of reactions involving different clotting factors in the blood that are identified by Roman numerals I through XIII. All are plasma proteins except factor III (thromboplastin, a lipoprotein released from injured tissue) and factor IV (calcium ion, an electrolyte). When vessel injury occurs, these factors interact with the platelet plug to form the end product, a clot. The clots that are formed are eventually dissolved by the fibrinolytic system.

❖ THROMBOCYTOPENIA

OVERVIEW/PATHOPHYSIOLOGY

Thrombocytopenia is a common coagulation disorder that results from a decreased number of platelets. It can be congenital or acquired, and it is classified according to cause. Causes include *deficient production of thrombocytes*, as occurs with bone marrow disease (e.g., leukemia, aplastic anemia) or *accelerated platelet destruction* occurring from loss or increased use, as in hemolytic anemia, disseminated intravascular coagulation (DIC), or damage by prosthetic heart valves, as well as hypersplenism and hypothermia. Potential triggers include an autoimmune disorder, severe vascular injury, and spleen malfunction. In addition, thrombocytopenia can occur as a side effect of certain medications, such as heparin. Regardless of cause or trigger, the disorder affects coagulation and hemostasis. With chemical-induced thrombocytopenia, prognosis is good after withdrawal of the offending drug. Prognosis for other types depends on the form of thrombocytopenia and the individual's baseline health status and response to treatment. Thrombocytopenia may be the first sign of systemic lupus erythematosus (SLE) or infection.

Thrombotic thrombocytopenic purpura (TTP) is an acute, often fatal disorder caused by deficiency of a plasma enzyme that normally inactivates the von Willebrand clotting factor (vWF) when it is not needed. vWF is the most important protein that mediates platelet adhesion to damaged endothelial surfaces. *Idiopathic thrombocytopenic purpura (ITP)* is believed to be an immune disorder specifically involving antiplatelet immunoglobulin G (IgG), which destroys platelets. The acute form is most often seen in children (2-6 yr of age) and may be related to a previous viral infection. The chronic form is seen more often in adults (18-50 yr of age) and is of unknown origin.

Heparin-induced thrombocytopenia (HIT) is a disorder in which heparin triggers an antibody response; the heparin-antibody complexes bind to platelet surfaces, causing activated platelets to aggregate. This process leads to further thrombosis and, because of increased utilization, thrombocytopenia. Because the platelets are activated (although low in number), HIT is uniquely associated with both arterial and venous thrombosis rather than bleeding.

ASSESSMENT

Signs and symptoms/physical findings

Chronic indicators: Long history of mild bleeding or hemorrhagic episodes from the mouth, nose, gastrointestinal (GI) tract, or genitourinary (GU) tract. Increased bruising (ecchymosis) and petechiae also have been noted.

Acute indicators: Fever, splenomegaly, acute and severe bleeding episodes, weakness, lethargy, malaise, hemorrhage into mucous membranes, gum bleeding, and GU or GI bleeding. Prolonged bleeding can lead to a shock state with tachycardia, shortness of breath, and decreased level of consciousness (LOC). Optic fundal hemorrhage decreases vision and often precedes potentially fatal intracranial hemorrhage. With TTP and HIT, the individual may exhibit signs associated with platelet thrombus formation, such as skin necrosis, and ischemic organ failure (decreased renal function, or neurologic changes).

History and risk factors: Recent infection, myeloproliferative disease, or aplastic anemia; recent vaccination; binge alcohol consumption; positive family history of thrombocytopenia; or use of chlorothiazide, digitalis, quinidine, rifampin, sulfisoxazole, chloramphenicol, phenytoin, or heparin.

DIAGNOSTIC TESTS

Platelet count: Can vary from only slightly decreased to nearly absent. A count less than 100,000/mm^3 is significantly decreased; a count less than 20,000/mm^3 results in a serious risk of hemorrhage.

Peripheral blood smear: May reveal megathrombocytes (large platelets), which are present during premature destruction of platelets, as well as reticulocytosis and fragmented RBCs.

LDH: May be elevated.

Bilirubin: Increased.

CBC: Low hemoglobin (Hgb) and hematocrit (Hct) levels because of blood loss; WBC count usually within normal range.

Coagulation studies

Bleeding time: Increased because of decreased platelets.

Partial thromboplastin time (PTT): May be increased or normal.

Prothrombin time (PT): May be increased or normal.

International normalized ratio (INR): Increased.

International sensitivity index (ISI): Increased.

Bone marrow aspiration: Reveals increased number of megakaryocytes (platelet precursors) in the presence of ITP and HIT but may be decreased in other causes of thrombocytopenia.

Antibody screen: May be positive because of the presence of IgG platelet antibodies or positive HIT antibody tests.

COLLABORATIVE MANAGEMENT

The goal of collaborative management of throbocytopenia is treatment of underlying cause or removal of precipitating agent.

Platelet transfusion: Used if platelet destruction or deficient formation is the primary cause of the disorder (Table 8-3) or risk of increased microthrombi and organ ischemia is not of primary concern. It provides only temporary relief because the half-life of platelets is only 3-4 days and may be even shorter with ITP (i.e., minutes to hours). Platelet transfusions should be avoided in patients with TTP or active HIT except in life-threatening or organ-threatening hemorrhage. If used, human leukocyte antigen (HLA)-matched or crossmatched platelets may improve clinical response.

Corticosteroids: Enhance vascular integrity or diminish platelet destruction.

Intravenous immunoglobulin G (IV IgG): Increases platelet count by impeding the antibody production that destroys platelets.

Recombinant interleukin 11: Stimulates megakaryocyte differentiation and platelet production in patients with cancer who have thrombocytopenia, but clinical benefit over use of platelets is controversial.

IV anti-D immune globulin: Increases platelet count by impeding production of antibodies that destroy platelets.

Splenectomy: Removal of the organ responsible for platelet destruction. This is considered viable treatment unless patient has acute bleeding, severe deficiency of platelets, or a cardiac disorder that contraindicates surgery.

Inoculation: In anticipation of splenectomy, vaccination for pneumococcal, meningococcal, and *Haemophilus influenzae* infection should be done.

Plasma exchange via apheresis: Removes the antibody or immune complex; used for short-term therapy and is often a lifesaving and emergency treatment for TTP.

ε-Aminocaproic acid: Inhibits fibrinolysis (clot breakdown), which may be helpful in controlling bleeding resulting from severe thrombocytopenia.

Alternative anticoagulants: For example, lepirudin and argatroban, which may be used to prevent new thromboses.

NURSING DIAGNOSES AND INTERVENTIONS

Ineffective protection related to increased risk of bleeding secondary to decreased platelet count

Desired outcome: Patient is free of the signs of bleeding, as evidenced by secretions and excretions negative for blood, BP 90/60 mm Hg or greater or within patient's baseline range, heart rate (HR) 100 beats per minute (bpm) or less, respiratory rate (RR) 12-20 breaths/min with normal depth and pattern (eupnea), and absence of bruising or active bleeding.

Nursing Interventions

♦ Monitor VS and assess for hematuria, melena, epistaxis, hematemesis, hemoptysis, menometrorrhagia, bleeding gums, petechiae, or severe ecchymosis. Teach patient to be alert to and report these indicators promptly, as well as any headache or changes in vision. *Indicates dangerously low platelet count.*

♦ Monitor platelet count daily and coagulation studies at least weekly or as prescribed and inform health care provider of significant findings. *Detects trends so that corrective measures can be taken if needed.*

♦ Ensure that there is a current type and crossmatch in the blood bank in the event acute bleeding occurs and supportive RBC transfusions are needed *to counter acute bleeding.*

♦ Prevent or promptly control retching, vomiting, coughing, and straining with bowel movements. *These trigger bleeding.*

♦ When possible, avoid venipuncture. If performed, apply pressure on site for 5-10 min or until bleeding stops, *to minimize risk for bleeding.*

♦ Avoid giving intramuscular (IM) injections. If injections are necessary, use subcutaneous route with a small-gauge needle, *to minimize risk for bleeding.*

♦ Advise patient to avoid straining at stool and coughing, which increase intracranial pressure and can result in intracranial hemorrhage. Obtain prescription for stool softeners, if indicated, *to prevent constipation.*

♦ Administer corticosteroids as prescribed, *to help minimize platelet destruction.*

♦ Teach patient to use electric razor and soft-bristle toothbrush, *to minimize risk for bleeding.*

♦ Teach patient that alcohol consumption, smoking, and use of aspirin or other nonsteroidal antiinflammatory drugs (NSAIDs) increases the risk for bleeding, *to minimize the risk for bleeding.*

♦ Administer premedications and platelets as prescribed. Double-check type with a colleague, and monitor for and report chills, back pain, dyspnea, hives, and wheezing. *Indicate transfusion reaction.*

♦ Assure that patient was informed by health care provider about risks and benefits of platelet transfusion before patient signs consent to the transfusion. *Ensures informed consent.*

Ineffective cerebral, peripheral, and renal tissue perfusion (or risk for same) related to interrupted blood flow secondary to presence of thrombotic component, which results in sensitization and clumping of platelets in the blood vessels

Desired outcome: Patient's cerebral, peripheral, and renal perfusions are adequate, as evidenced by no mental status changes; orientation to person, place, and time; normoreactive pupillary responses; absence of headaches, dizziness, and visual disturbances; peripheral pulses greater than 2+ on a 0-4+ scale; and urine output 30 mL/hr or more.

Nursing Interventions

♦ Assess for changes in mental status, level of consciousness (LOC), and pupillary response.

♦ Monitor for headaches, dizziness, or visual disturbances. *Indicates decreased tissue perfusion.*

♦ Palpate peripheral pulses on all extremities. Be alert to pulses 2+ or less on a 0-4+ scale. Assess distal extremities for color, warmth, and character of pulses, *to compare right/left perfusion.*

♦ Assess urine output. Urine output 30 mL/hr or more for 2 consecutive hr. *Indicates adequate renal perfusion.*

♦ Use a bed cradle, *to decrease pressure on tissues of lower extremities.*

♦ Monitor I&O. Patient should be well hydrated (2-3 L/day), *to increase perfusion of the small vessels.*

♦ Choose chairs with or provide padding on seats, *to prevent occluding popliteal vessels.*

Acute pain related to joint discomfort secondary to hemorrhagic episodes or blood extravasation into the tissues

Desired outcomes: Within 1 hr of intervention, patient's subjective perception of discomfort decreases, as documented by pain scale. Objective indicators, such as grimacing, are absent or diminished.

Nursing Interventions

- Monitor patient for presence of fatigue, malaise, and joint pain. Devise a pain scale with patient, rating discomfort on a scale of 0 (no pain) to 10 (worst pain).
- Maintain a calm, restful environment, *to help control pain/discomfort.*
- Facilitate coordination of care providers to provide rest periods as needed between care activities. *Allows time for periods of undisturbed rest.*
- Elevate legs, support legs with pillows, and avoid gatching bed at the knee, *to minimize joint discomfort in lower extremities.*
- Place socks on patient's feet for warmth and *to increase comfort.*
- Administer analgesics as prescribed. Reassess pain and document relief obtained, using the pain scale. *Reduces and controls pain.*
- Avoid intake of aspirin and other NSAIDs because their antiplatelet actions increase the risk for bleeding.
- Instruct patient to request analgesic before pain becomes severe. Pain is easier to control if treated before it becomes severe.

Patient-Family Teaching and Discharge Planning

Include verbal and written information about the following:

- Importance of preventing trauma, which can cause bleeding.
- Seeking medical attention for any signs of bleeding, clotting, hematuria, melena, hematemesis, hemoptysis, menometrorrhagia, oozing from mucous membranes, or petechiae.
- Signs and symptoms of common infections, such as upper respiratory, urinary tract, and wound infections.
- The importance of regular medical follow-up for laboratory studies.
- If prescribed, side effects of steroids, including weight gain, headache, capillary fragility, hypertension, moon facies, thinning of arms and legs, mood changes, acne, buffalo hump, edema formation, risk of gastrointestinal (GI) hemorrhage, delayed wound healing, and increased appetite. Review need to take medication with food, immediately take missed doses, and not precipitously discontinue medication.
- Other medications, including drug names, dosage, purpose, schedule, precautions, and potential side effects. Also discuss drug/drug, herb/drug, and food/drug interactions.
- Importance of obtaining a MedicAlert bracelet and identification card outlining diagnosis and emergency treatment from:

    MedicAlert Foundation: www.medicalert.org

❖ DISSEMINATED INTRAVASCULAR COAGULATION

OVERVIEW/PATHOPHYSIOLOGY

Disseminated intravascular coagulation (DIC) is an acute coagulation disorder characterized by paradoxic clotting and hemorrhage. The sequence usually progresses from massive clot formation, depletion of clotting factors, and activation of diffuse fibrinolysis to hemorrhage (**FIGURE 8-1**). DIC occurs secondary to widespread coagulation factors in the bloodstream caused by an acute condition or reaction (see risk factors, later). Although clotting and

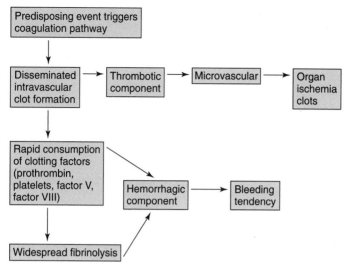

FIGURE 8-1 ◆ Overview of DIC syndrome.

bleeding occur simultaneously, organ failure related to thromboses of vital organs (e.g., renal, pulmonary) is usually the primary life-threatening concern. Prompt assessment of the disorder can result in a good prognosis. Usually, affected patients are transferred to the ICU for careful monitoring and aggressive therapy. DIC may be classified as *low-grade* (compensated or chronic) or *fulminant* (acute).

ASSESSMENT

Signs and symptoms/physical findings: Bleeding of abrupt onset, oozing from venipuncture sites or mucosal surfaces; bleeding from surgical sites; and presence of hematuria, blood in stool (melena or hematochezia), spontaneous ecchymosis (bruising), petechiae, purpura fulminans, pallor, or mottled skin; vaginal bleeding (menometrorrhagia), nose bleed (epistaxis), mucous membrane bleeding or oozing; joint pain and swelling; decreased urine output (hypoperfusion); signs of gastrointestinal (GI) bleeding, such as guarding; distention (increasing abdominal girth measurements); hyperactive, hypoactive, or absent bowel sounds; and a rigid, boardlike abdomen. With significant hemorrhage, patients may exhibit SBP less than 90 mm Hg and DBP less than 60 mm Hg; HR greater than 100 bpm; peripheral pulse amplitude 2+ or less on a 0-4+ scale; respiratory rate (RR) greater than 22 breaths/min; shortness of breath; urinary output less than 30 mL/hr; secretions and excretions positive for blood; cool, pale, clammy skin; lack of orientation to person, place, and time; changes in mental status; or headache (intracranial hemorrhage).

History and risk factors: Extensive surgery, burns, shock, infections, sepsis, neoplastic diseases, or abruptio placentae; extensive destruction of blood vessel walls caused by eclampsia, anoxia, or heat stroke; or damage to blood cells caused by hemolysis, sickle cell disease, or transfusion reactions; trauma; hepatic disease; hypovolemic shock; severe hemolytic reaction; or hypoxia (**BOX 8-1**).

DIAGNOSTIC TESTS

Serum fibrinogen: Low because of abnormal consumption of clotting factors in the formation of fibrin clots.
Platelet count: Less than 250,000/mm³.

| BOX 8-1 | CLINICAL CONDITIONS THAT CAN PRECIPITATE DISSEMINATED INTRAVASCULAR COAGULATION |

Obstetric
- Abruptio placentae
- Toxemia
- Amniotic fluid embolism
- Septic abortion
- Retained dead fetus

Tissue Damage
- Surgery
- Trauma
- Burns
- Prolonged extracorporeal circulation
- Transplant rejection
- Heat stroke

Hemolytic Processes
- Transfusion reaction
- Acute hemolysis secondary to infection or immunologic disorder

Miscellaneous
- Fat or pulmonary embolism
- Snakebite
- Neoplastic disorders (leukemias, solid tumors, or metastatic disease and their related treatments)
- Acute anoxia

GI Disorders
- Cirrhosis
- Hepatic necrosis
- Pancreatitis
- Peritoneovenous shunts
- Necrotizing enterocolitis

Infections
- Viral
- Bacterial
- Rickettsial
- Protozoal

Vascular Disorders
- Shock
- Aneurysm
- Giant hemangioma

GI, Gastrointestinal.

Fibrin split products (FSPs), also known as fibrin degradation products (FDPs): Increased, indicating widespread dissolution of clots. Fibrinolysis produces FSPs as an end product.

D-dimers: They are increased in DIC as byproducts of fibrinolysis. When coupled with increased FDPs, they are considered diagnostic of DIC.

PT: Normal, low, or possibly increased because of depletion of clotting factors.

PTT: Normal, low, or possibly high because of depletion of clotting factors.

Peripheral blood smear: Shows fragmented RBCs (i.e., histiocytes).

COLLABORATIVE MANAGEMENT

The goals of collaborative management of DIC are the identification and treatment of underlying disorder.

Hemodynamic and cardiovascular support: Fluid management, oxygen supplementation, and invasive monitoring.

Anticoagulant therapy: Although this therapy is controversial, heparin may be administered to interfere with the coagulation process and activation of the fibrinolytic system in an attempt to prevent clot formation within organs. Heparin dose is regulated and determined by PTT. Warfarin may be used in compensated DIC.

Replacement of platelets and clotting factors: Platelets may be replaced if they are less than $50,000/mm^3$, by administering *fresh frozen plasma* and *cryoprecipitate* to maintain fibrinogen level greater than 100 mg/dL. However, this is done conservatively because clotting factor replacement can cause further vascular clotting in essential organs.

ε-**Aminocaproic acid:** Only given when severe hemorrhage is the underlying casues because this drug inhibits fibrinolysis and causes further clotting.

Antithrombin III: May be used in patients with low antithrombin levels. It inhibits procoagulants and the fibrinolytic process and is especially helpful in patients with sepsis. It also has antiinflammatory effects.

NURSING DIAGNOSES AND INTERVENTIONS

Ineffective cardiopulmonary, peripheral, renal, and cerebral tissue perfusion related to coagulation/fibrinolysis processes

Desired outcome: Following treatment, patient has adequate cardiopulmonary, peripheral, renal, and cerebral perfusion, as evidenced by BP 90/60 mm Hg or greater and heart rate (HR) 100 beats per minute (bpm) or less (or within patient's baseline range); peripheral pulse 2+ or greater on a 0-4+ scale; urinary output 30 mL/hr or more; equal and normoreactive pupils; normal/baseline motor function; orientation to person, place, and time; and no mental status changes.

Nursing Interventions

- Assess for coagulation and bleeding, *to facilitate early treatment.*
- Monitor VS. Be alert to and report decreased BP, increased HR, or decreased of peripheral pulses. *Signals progression to digital ischemia and gangrene.*
- Perform neurologic checks, including orientation, mental status assessments, pupillary reaction to light, level of consciousness (LOC), and motor response to evaluate cerebral perfusion, and protect patient from injury by implementing fall precautions as appropriate. *Signs of impaired cerebral perfusion.*
- Monitor I&O; report output less than 30 mL/hr in the presence of adequate intake. *Indicates renal vessel thrombosis.*
- Monitor for hemorrhage from surgical wounds, GI and genitourinary (GU) tracts, and mucous membranes. *Can occur after fibrinolysis.*
- Monitor oxygen saturation via pulse oximetry q4h or as indicated; report oxygen saturation 92% or less, *to detect decreased perfusion.*
- Monitor laboratory work for values suggestive of DIC (see "Diagnostic Tests," earlier) and report significant findings to patient's health care provider.
- Prepare for emergency blood product transfusion, medical support, and transfer to ICU if condition worsens.

Ineffective protection related to increased risk of bleeding secondary to hemorrhagic component of DIC

Desired outcome: Patient is free of signs of bleeding, as evidenced by SBP 90 mm Hg or greater; HR 100 bpm or less (or within patient's normal range); RR 12-20 breaths/min with normal depth and pattern (eupnea); urinary output of 30 mL/hr or more; secretions and excretions negative for blood; stable abdominal girth measurements; orientation to person, place, and time; and no changes in mental status.

Nursing Interventions

- Monitor VS and LOC at frequent intervals; report significant changes. Be alert to hypotension, tachycardia, dyspnea, disorientation, and changes in mental status, which can signal hemorrhage. *Indicate bleeding and hypoperfusion.*
- Inflate BP cuff only as high as needed to obtain BP reading. Frequent BP readings may cause bleeding under the cuff. Rotate arm use *to reduce repeated trauma.*
- Monitor for abdominal pain, abdominal distention, changes in bowel sounds, and a boardlike abdomen. *Indicates GI bleeding.*

◆ Assess puncture sites regularly for oozing or bleeding. When possible, treat bleeding sites with ice, pressure, rest, and elevation. Some health care providers promote use of thrombin-soaked gauze, such as Gelfoam or topical thrombin powder, *to reduce external bleeding or oozing.*

◆ Be alert for joint pain, headache, visual changes. *Indicates bleeding and possible retinal hemorrhage.*

◆ Monitor coagulation and other hematologic laboratory values *to detect trends.*

◆ Prevent or promptly control symptoms, such as retching, vomiting, coughing, and straining with bowel movements *because they can trigger bleeding.*

◆ Use a reagent-screening agent to check stool, urine, emesis, and nasogastric drainage, *to detect blood.*

◆ Avoid giving intramuscular (IM) injections, and minimize venipunctures as appropriate; post "bleeding precautions" to notify all health care providers that venipuncture sites may require additional manual pressure *to prevent or stop bleeding.*

◆ Administer blood products (packed RBCs, platelets, fresh frozen plasma [Table 8-3]) and IV fluids as prescribed *to replace losses.*

◆ Teach patient to use electric shaver and soft-bristle toothbrush and avoid forceful nose blowing (dab instead), bending down (head lower than the heart), and potentially traumatic procedures (e.g., enemas, rectal temperatures), *to minimize risk for bleeding.*

◆ Report significant findings to patient's health care provider. Prepare for emergency blood product transfusion, medical support, and transfer to ICU if condition worsens.

Risk for impaired skin integrity or **Impaired tissue integrity** related to altered circulation secondary to hemorrhage and thrombosis

Desired outcome: Patient's skin and tissue remain nonerythemic and intact.

Nursing Interventions

◆ Assess patient's skin, and note erythema that does not clear after removal of pressure or changes in color, temperature, and sensation. *Indicates decreased perfusion that can lead to tissue damage.*

◆ Eliminate or minimize pressure points by ensuring that patient turns q2h and by using sheepskin on elbows and heels and enhanced pressure-distribution mattress padding. Do not pull on extremities when turning patient, *to prevent injury.*

◆ As prescribed, encourage active ROM of all extremities q2h, *to reduce pressure and enhance circulation.*

◆ Keep patient's extremities warm, *to prevent tissue hypoxia.*

◆ Use alternatives to tape to hold dressings in place, such as gauze wraps or net gauze, *to prevent tearing skin.*

◆ If patient has areas of breakdown, see "Managing Wound Care," p. 716.

Patient-Family Teaching and Discharge Planning

See patient's primary diagnosis.

Musculoskeletal Disorders

ARTHRITIC DISORDERS

Arthritic disorders are among the most common disorders causing pain and disability in individuals over the age of 15 yr in the United States. *Arthritis* is simply defined as inflammation of a joint. Arthritis is an often predominant manifestation of more than 100 diffuse joint and connective tissue diseases, including osteoarthritis (OA), fibromyalgia, gouty arthritis, rheumatoid arthritis (RA), Reiter's syndrome, ankylosing spondylitis, systemic lupus erythematosus, and psoriatic arthritis. OA and RA, which are often seen in hospitalized patients, are discussed in this section (**TABLE 9-1**).

❖ OSTEOARTHRITIS

OVERVIEW/PATHOPHYSIOLOGY

Osteoarthritis (OA) is the most prevalent articular disease in adults 65 yr of age and older. OA has been known by many names, including degenerative joint disease (DJD), degenerative arthritis, and hypertrophic arthritis. It is no longer regarded as a wear-and-tear condition that occurs as a normal result of aging. In fact, joint changes that result from arthritis can be distinguished readily from age-related changes in articular cartilage of an asymptomatic older adult. In OA, chondrocytes within the joint fail to synthesize good-quality matrix in terms of both resistance and elasticity; resulting defective the bony cartilage is more prone to deterioration. OA is recognized as a process in which all joint structures produce new tissue in response to joint injury or cartilage destruction. This chronic, progressive disease is characterized by gradual loss of articular cartilage combined with thickening of the subchondral bone and formation of bony outgrowths (osteophytes) at the joint margins. Affected individuals experience increasing pain, deformity, and loss of function. Prevalence of OA varies among different populations, but it is a universal human problem that actually may begin by 20-30 yr of age. A majority of people are affected by 40 yr of age, but few experience symptoms until after 50 to 60 yr of age. Before 50 yr of age, men are affected more often than women. After 50 yr of age, however, incidence of OA is twice as great in women as in men.

OA may be classified as either idiopathic or secondary. *Idiopathic OA* occurs in individuals with no history of joint injury or disease or of systemic illness that could contribute to the development of arthritis. *Secondary OA* occurs from wear and tear, joint injury, or disease.

OA is characterized by *site specificity,* with certain synovial joints showing higher disease prevalence. These include the weight-bearing joints (hips, knees); cervical and lumbar spine; distal interphalangeal (DIP), proximal

TABLE 9-1	DIFFERENTIAL DIAGNOSIS OF OSTEOARTHRITIS AND RHEUMATOID ARTHRITIS	

FEATURE	OSTEOARTHRITIS	RHEUMATOID ARTHRITIS
Age at onset	4th-5th decade	2nd-5th decade
Gender ratio	3:1 female	2:1 female
Disease course	Variable, progressive	Remissions and exacerbations
Symptoms	Localized	Systemic
Commonly affected joints	Weight-bearing joints (knees, hips), spine, MCP, DIP, PIP	Small joints (PIP, DIP, MTP)
Joint involvement	Asymmetric	Symmetric
Joint effusions	Uncommon	Common
Synovial fluid	Usually normal	Decreased viscosity; WBCs 3000-25,000/mm³
Nodules	Heberden's and Bouchard's nodes	Rheumatoid nodules over bony prominences, extensor surfaces, juxtaarticular regions
Pain	Follows activity, improves with rest	Pain at rest, nocturnal pain
Duration of stiffness	Minutes; after prolonged rest (articular gelling)	Hours; most severe after rest
Weakness	Usually localized, mild to moderate	Often pronounced
Fatigue	Not typical	Often severe, especially in the afternoon
X-ray examination	Osteophytes, subchondral cysts, sclerosis; asymmetric narrowing of joint space	Osteoporosis related to steroid use; erosions, narrowed joint space; subluxation in advancing disease
Rheumatoid factor assay results	Negative	Positive in approximately 80% of patients

DIP, Distal interphalangeal; *MCP,* metacarpophalangeal; *MTP,* metatarsophalangeal; *PIP,* proximal interphalangeal; *WBCs,* white blood cells.

interphalangeal (PIP), and metacarpophalangeal (MCP) joints in the hands; and metatarsophalangeal (MTP) joints in the feet (bunion deformity, or hallux valgus). The hips are most often affected in men and the hands in women, especially after menopause.

ASSESSMENT

Signs and symptoms/physical findings

Early disease: Joint pain and stiffness, "aching" asymmetric pain that increases with joint use, such as climbing stairs, standing, and walking; pain subsides with rest.

Progressive disease: Night pain; pain at rest; increased pain during cool, damp, and rainy weather; joint stiffness to pain with initial movement; early morning stiffness lasting less than 30 min; stiffness after periods of rest or inactivity (articular gelling or gel phenomenon) resolving within several minutes; squeaking, creaking, or grating of joints with movement (crepitus); bony enlargement of affected joints that are tender when palpated; reduced ROM; locking of joints during movement accompanied by mild effusion and soft tissue swelling; crepitation during passive movement; deformities including Heberden's nodes on DIP joints and Bouchard's nodes on PIP joints of the hands; joint malalignment, typically a varus deformity resulting from cartilage loss in the medial compartment of knee; leg length discrepancy in advanced hip OA; muscular atrophy secondary to joint splinting for pain relief.

History and risk factors: Aging may be one influence on the deterioration of cartilage in arthritic joints, but additional evidence suggests existence of an autosomal recessive trait for gene defects that causes premature cartilage destruction. Prevalence of OA in postmenopausal women also suggests involvement of one or more hormonal factors in initiation of the disease. Secondary OA occurs from any condition or event that directly damages or overloads articular cartilage or causes joint instability that can result in arthritic changes. *Secondary OA* typically occurs in younger individuals as a manifestation of congenital processes (e.g., Legg-Calvé-Perthes disease), trauma, repetitive occupational stress, joint hemorrhage, or infection.

DIAGNOSTIC TESTS

OA almost always can be diagnosed by history and physical examination.

Laboratory tests: Rule out other arthropathic conditions (e.g., rheumatoid arthritis [RA], septic arthritis) and establish baselines before starting therapy.

CBC: Suggested for patients who will be taking nonsteroidal antiinflammatory drugs (NSAIDs) for arthritis symptom management, with additional CBCs prescribed periodically to screen for anemia caused by occult gastrointestinal (GI) bleeding.

Renal and liver function tests: For older adults starting aspirin or NSAID therapy, with further testing done every 6 mo to monitor for occasional side effects such as electrolyte imbalance, hepatitis, or renal insufficiency.

Rheumatoid factor (RF) assay and erythrocyte sedimentation rate (ESR): Neither test excludes a diagnosis of OA in the older patient. About 20% of healthy older adults are in fact RF-seropositive, and ESR tends to rise with age. ESR evaluation is useful to rule out chronic conditions such as polymyalgia rheumatica.

Synovial fluid analysis: Reliable method for differentiating OA from other arthritic disorders.

X-ray examination: Radiographic findings do not always correlate with severity of patient's clinical symptoms. With disease progression, x-ray examination reveals joint space narrowing, osteophytes at joint margins, subchondral cysts, and altered shape of bone ends that suggests bone remodeling.

MRI: Much more sensitive than x-ray examination in marking progression of joint destruction.

COLLABORATIVE MANAGEMENT

Exercise: Identified by American College of Rheumatology as a critical part of OA management to improve strength, endurance, and flexibility and ability to walk or perform daily tasks. Inactivity may increase arthritis problems. Low-impact exercise, walking, swimming, and water aerobics are often well tolerated by people with arthritis. In addition, quadriceps-strengthening exercises improve joint stability for people with knee OA.

Joint protection: Principles include need for a balance of rest and activity. An affected joint should be rested and weight bearing restricted during periods of acute inflammation. Splints or braces should be used to maintain the joint in a functional position if necessary. Joint immobilization should not exceed 1 wk to prevent additional stiffness from prolonged rest. Modification of occupational and recreational activity also may be needed to protect the joint from stress, and use of assistive devices may be beneficial.

Weight reduction: Obesity is clearly associated with increased incidence of OA. Nutritional counseling will benefit obese patients who need to lose weight in order to control arthritis symptoms and slow disease progression.

Heat and cold applications: Thermal therapy may lessen pain and stiffness. Ice can be helpful during episodes of acute inflammation, whereas heat therapy may be beneficial for stiffness. Heat therapy is delivered via numerous modalities, including hot packs, ultrasound, whirlpool, paraffin wax, and massage.

Topical analgesics: For pain relief. Capsaicin cream in particular has shown significant reduction of knee pain when used along with regular arthritis medications. Necessity for several applications daily often leads to poor adherence to treatment. Topical analgesics should not be used in combination with heat treatments because of risk of burns.

Corticosteroids: Systemic therapy is not indicated in OA because of its side effects, but intraarticular injections of glucocorticoids are often used to treat inflamed joints. Injections should be separated by 3-4 mo because of risk of damage to intraarticular structures by residual corticosteroid crystals.

Viscosupplementation: Hyaluronic acid has been administered via intraarticular injections for treatment of knee OA because of its potential to supplement joint lubrication by synovial fluid. Clinical studies have shown mixed results.

Biologic agents

Glucosamine sulfate and chondroitin sulfate: Neither supplement is directly incorporated into the extracellular matrix; the rapid action of these supplements suggests an antiinflammatory effect, with relief for mild to moderate pain similar to that achieved with NSAIDs. These supplements should be taken with regular medications for 6-8 wk; if symptoms do not improve, these products probably will not work for affected persons.

S-adenosyl-L-methionine (SAMe): The dietary supplement SAMe is believed to play a role in cell growth and repair and also may provide arthritis pain relief.

Pharmacotherapy: Medications are aimed at pain management only because no drug can reverse the effects of OA.

Acetaminophen: Recommended by the American College of Rheumatology as the initial treatment for OA pain, with doses up to 1000 mg 4 ×/day. If acetaminophen proves ineffective, low-dose over-the-counter (OTC) ibuprofen or nonacetylated salicylates are recommended for patients with normal renal function and no prior history of GI problems.

NSAIDs: Ibuprofen, naproxen, diclofenac, and meloxicam are indicated if pain persists or worsens. NSAIDs may increase patient's risk for gastric ulceration or renal impairment because of inhibition of cyclooxygenase-1 (COX-1), which reduces prostaglandin levels in the stomach and kidneys. Traditional NSAIDs can be taken with a proton pump inhibitor to minimize GI effects.

Celecoxib: For severe or continued pain. Celecoxib (Celebrex) with cyclooxygenase-2 (COX-2) selectivity has shown less GI toxicity.

Salicylates (e.g., aspirin): These drugs are still preferred by many patients and doctors for pain management. An opioid analgesic can be safely added to acetaminophen or NSAID therapy if pain is unremitting.

Complementary and alternative treatment: Many therapies have become popular with patients seeking relief of arthritis symptoms. Although some modalities such as wearing copper or magnetic bracelets are harmless and possibly worthless, other treatments such as bee venom injections may lead to severe toxicities. A few therapies such as acupuncture have shown modest beneficial effects in arthritis pain management. Movement therapies (e.g., tai chi, yoga) provide a low-impact form of exercise. Some herbal supplements (e.g., ginger) have been shown to reduce the pain and inflammation of arthritis, but the person with arthritis should be encouraged to discuss use of herbal products with the health care provider.

Surgical interventions: Initial treatment may be through procedures that preserve natural tissues, including debridement, cartilage transplantation, osteotomy, and arthrodesis (fusion). Joint arthroplasty traditionally has been reserved for older patients, but if disease progression indicates, the procedure may be performed on a younger adult with the expectation that revision will be needed in the future.

NURSING DIAGNOSES AND INTERVENTIONS

Chronic pain or Acute pain related to arthritic joint changes and associated therapy
Desired outcomes: Within 1-2 hr of intervention, patient's subjective perception of pain decreases as documented by a pain intensity scale. Patient demonstrates ability to perform activities of daily living (ADL) with minimal discomfort.

Nursing Interventions

◆ Assist patient in use of a pain intensity rating scale with 0 (no pain) to 10 (worst pain imaginable). *This is to evaluate pain and analgesic relief.*
◆ Administer simple analgesics, NSAIDs, and opioid analgesics as prescribed and reassess their effectiveness in approximately 1 hr using pain intensity rating scale. Document preintervention and postintervention pain scores. *Determines medication effectiveness.*
◆ Teach patient about use of epidural or patient-controlled analgesia (PCA) as needed.
◆ Advise patient to coordinate time of peak effectiveness of analgesic or NSAID with periods of exercise or other use of arthritic joints. *This is to minimize pain.*
◆ Teach patient to use nonpharmacologic methods of pain management, including guided imagery, relaxation, massage, distraction, biofeedback, heat or cold therapy, and music therapy. *This helps to minimize pain.*
◆ Supplement other pain management strategies with traditional nursing interventions such as back rubs, repositioning, and encouraging patient to discuss impact of chronic disease.
◆ Encourage patient to use principles of joint protection, which include a balance of rest and activity. *This facilitates movement while minimizing pain.*

Deficient knowledge related to risk for interaction between NSAIDs and herbal products
Desired outcome: Within 1-2 hr of instruction, patient verbalizes understanding of potential interactions between NSAIDs and herbal products that potentiate bleeding.

Nursing Interventions

◆ Assess patient's use of language; engage an interpreter or provide language-appropriate written materials if necessary.
◆ Determine patient's use of NSAIDs and herbal products that potentiate bleeding (e.g., ginkgo, ginger, turmeric, chamomile, kelp, horse chestnut, garlic, dong quai).
◆ Teach risks associated with NSAIDs, which may be potentiated by concomitant use of herbal products. *This prevents interactions that can increase risk for bleeding.*
◆ Teach patient to monitor for black or tarry stools, hematuria, and coughing up or vomiting blood. *These indicate occult bleeding.*
◆ Advise patient to discuss with health care provider use of herbal products while taking NSAIDs for arthritis symptom management. *Helps prevent harmful interactions.*

Impaired physical mobility related to musculoskeletal impairment or walking with assistive device
Desired outcomes: Within 1 wk of instruction, patient demonstrates adequate upper body strength for use of an assistive device. Patient demonstrates appropriate use of assistive device on flat and uneven surfaces.

Nursing Interventions

- Ensure patient has necessary strength of upper extremities for using prescribed assistive device before beginning gait training. *Facilitates successful adaptation to device.*
- Teach armchair push-ups. *Helps patient attain and maintain triceps muscle strength necessary for use of assistive device.*
- Ensure that assistive device is appropriately sized to patient (i.e., height of walker, crutches, or cane allows patient to have approximately 15 degrees of elbow flexion when ambulating). Crutch tops should rest 1-1.5 inches (width of two fingers) below axillae. *Prevents upper extremity paresthesia caused by pressure on brachial plexus.*
- Describe and demonstrate use of prescribed assistive device, and supervise return demonstration. *Ensures patient's ability to ambulate safely with the device.*
- Begin ambulation in small increments on a flat surface and progress to all surfaces patient is expected to encounter; ensure that patient can safely get into and out of a motor vehicle. *This helps prevent falls.*

Ineffective sexuality patterns related to pain, decreased joint function, or body image changes that interfere with sexual performance
Desired outcome: Within 1 wk of intervention, patient describes increased physical and psychologic comfort during sexual intimacy.

Nursing Interventions

- Discuss possible problems with sexual performance related to decreased joint function or pain. *Enhances patient's knowledge and understanding.*
- Encourage patient to verbalize feelings related to body image changes that may impact interest in sexual intimacy. *This helps decrease anxiety.*
- Instruct patient about disease process and alternative positions. *Facilitates comfort during sexual intercourse.*
- Encourage patient to use relaxation strategies (e.g., warm bath). *Helps to alleviate pain and stiffness before sexual intercourse.*
- Encourage use of analgesics before sexual intercourse. *Enables easier movement.*
- Discuss the importance of caressing and holding in a relationship if intercourse is difficult. *Facilitates and preserves intimacy.*

Patient-Family Teaching and Discharge Planning

Include verbal and written information about the following:

- Medications and supplements, including names, dosage, purpose, schedule, precautions, and potential side effects. Also discuss drug/drug, herb/drug, and food/drug interactions.
- Importance of laboratory follow-up (e.g., blood or urine testing) for needed monitoring while patient is taking selected medications.
- Importance of joint protection, with balance of rest and activity.
- Use, care, and replacement of orthotics and assistive devices.
- If surgery was performed, any precautions related to procedure, wound care, and signs of infection (i.e., persistent redness or pain, swelling or localized warmth, fever, purulent drainage) or other complications of surgery.
- Importance of follow-up care, date of next appointment, and a telephone number to call if questions arise.
- Referral to community resources, including local arthritis support activities and the Arthritis Foundation (website): www.arthritis.org
- Additional information on arthritis may be available through the following:

  National Institute of Arthritis and Musculoskeletal and Skin Diseases (NIAMS): www.nih.gov/niams/health%20info

❖ RHEUMATOID ARTHRITIS

OVERVIEW/PATHOPHYSIOLOGY

Rheumatoid arthritis (RA) is a chronic systemic disease associated with severe morbidity and functional decline caused by inflammation of connective tissue, primarily in the synovial joints. The mortality rate for people with RA is double that of the general population, particularly if the disease is not well controlled. Individuals with RA are at increased risk for heart attack and stroke. Although no single known cause for RA exists, theory suggests that RA occurs in a susceptible host who initially experiences an immune response to an antigen. Because complex genetic factors appear to be involved, the antigen is probably not the same in all patients. Autoimmunity has been suggested as a cause because of the association of RA with the occurrence of rheumatoid factor (RF), the antibody against an abnormal immunoglobulin G (IgG).

The immune response appears to center on synovial tissue, where disease changes are first seen. Synovitis develops when immune complexes are deposited onto the synovial membrane or superficial articular cartilage. As hypertrophied synovium invades surrounding tissues, highly vascularized fibrous exudate *(pannus)* forms to cover the entire articular cartilage. Pannus also scars and shortens adjacent tendons and ligaments to create the laxity, subluxation, and contractures characteristic of RA.

ASSESSMENT

Signs and symptoms/physical findings: Fatigue; anorexia; weight loss; generalized stiffness that becomes localized as time progresses; morning joint stiffness lasting 1-4 hr; joint pain and swelling, especially in hands and wrists, although knees, ankles, and MTP joints also may be affected; increasing difficulty with mobility and performance of activities of daily living (ADL); spindle-shaped fingers with swan-neck and boutonniere deformities from flexion contractures that occur with disease progression; ulnar deviation with a "zigzag" wrist deformity; metatarsal head subluxation and hallux valgus (bunion) in the feet that leads to walking disability and pain; symmetric (bilateral) joints that are swollen, red, warm, and tender with decreased ROM; subcutaneous nodules over bony prominences, extensor surfaces, or juxtaarticular areas; hoarseness if nodules have invaded the vocal cords; and guarded movement and gait abnormalities resulting from joint changes.

History and risk factors: Women are affected two to three times more often than men. Genetic studies have confirmed a familial tendency. Unlike in osteoarthritis (OA), no environmental factors have been identified as disease precipitators.

DIAGNOSTIC TESTS

Diagnosis of RA is based primarily on physical findings and patient history. Radiographic studies are not usually needed to make a diagnosis. Laboratory results are helpful in confirming diagnosis and monitoring disease progression.

RF: Positive in about 85% of patients. Higher titers appear to be correlated with severe and unremitting disease. However, the RF titer has little prognostic value, and serial titers have no usefulness in following disease process.

Antinuclear antibodies: Elevated titers seen in 5%-20% of patients.

Erythrocyte sedimentation rate (ESR), C-reactive protein (CRP): Elevation is a general indicator of active inflammation.

Synovial fluid analysis: Fluid is opaque with cloudy yellow appearance, with elevated WBC count and polymorphonuclear leukocytes in the presence of RA. Glucose level will be lower than serum glucose.

X-ray examination of affected joints: Radiographs may be inconclusive in early disease, but baseline films, especially of the hands, aid in monitoring disease progression. Presence of erosions also helps determine prognosis. In advanced disease, loss of articular cartilage leads to narrowed joint space.

Subluxation and joint malalignment can be identified on x-ray film and reflect changes noted on physical examination. Osteopenia or osteoporosis may be evident in the patient with RA who has been treated with corticosteroids.

Bone scan: Detects early synovial changes.

Arthroscopy: Reveals pale, hypertrophic synovium with destruction of cartilage and formation of fibrous scar tissue.

COLLABORATIVE MANAGEMENT

Pharmacotherapy: Pharmacotherapy remains the cornerstone of an interdisciplinary approach to care.

Disease-modifying antirheumatic drugs (DMARDs): These drugs have been shown to control active synovitis and prevent joint erosions and damage. The early use of DMARDs is critical because these drugs do not heal erosions or reverse other effects of established RA. Methotrexate is most commonly prescribed by rheumatologists in the United States. Gold has been a standard therapy since the 1940s. Other DMARDs include leflunomide, sulfasalazine, penicillamine, cyclosporine, and cyclophosphamide.

Tumor necrosis factor inhibitors: These agents interfere with cell surface antigens of modulating cytokines to manage RA symptoms in patients with moderate to severe disease who have not responded to DMARDs. Adalimumab, etanercept, and infliximab block a cytokine known as tumor necrosis factor-α (TNF-α), whereas anakinra blocks interleukin-1 (IL-1). TNF inhibitors are frequently given with a DMARD. Adalimumab, etanercept, and anakinra are given by subcutaneous injection, a route that may be problematic for self-administration by patients with RA who have muscle weakness and deformities of advanced disease. Infliximab is administered by IV infusion over 2 hr in a physician's office, clinic, or hospital.

NSAIDs (ibuprofen, naproxen, diclofenac, meloxicam, celecoxib): These drugs provide largely equal analgesic and antiinflammatory effects in the treatment of RA. They do not affect disease progression, and their use in alleviating RA symptoms may in fact delay initiation of DMARD therapy or referral to a rheumatologist. Patients who have had myocardial infarction (MI), transient ischemic attack (TIA), or stroke and who require antiplatelet therapy can safely use the cyclooxygenase-2 (COX-2) inhibitor celecoxib (Celebrex) because it has no effect on bleeding time or platelet aggregation.

Corticosteroids: Injection of corticosteroids directly into affected joints can temporarily relieve the pain and inflammation of RA exacerbations. Long-term use of oral corticosteroids, however, has been associated with development of avascular necrosis (AVN) or osteoporosis. Low-dose prednisone (less than 10 mg) may be useful in selected patients to minimize disease activity until the prescribed DMARD becomes therapeutic, but it should not be a mainstay of treatment.

Antimalarials (hydroxychloroquine, chloroquine): Mechanism of action is unknown, but it is thought to alter innate immunity. These drugs are used most commonly for patients with mild or nonerosive disease and are given in combination with methotrexate and sulfasalazine.

Joint protection: Inflammation appears to resolve more quickly in a splinted joint.

Therapeutic exercise: ROM, stretching, strengthening, and conditioning exercises preserve function, increase muscle strength, and improve overall endurance. Low-resistance endurance exercises such as bicycling, swimming, golf, and dancing are also appropriate for overall fitness. Performance of progressive muscle contraction and relaxation, however, tends to exacerbate the pain of RA.

Heat and cold therapy: Thermotherapy is an important adjunct to exercise. Heat treatments can be delivered superficially (hot packs, paraffin baths) or deeply (ultrasound). Cold applications may provide greater relief during acute episodes of pain exacerbation.

Assistive devices: Sock donners, long-handled reachers and brushes, raised toilet seats, and other devices may help minimize stress on joints. Clothing can be adapted to encourage independence in dressing (e.g., zipper pulls, Velcro closures).

Nutritional therapy: Research has shown several positive connections between food or nutritional supplements (e.g., omega-3 fatty acids) and some types of arthritis, including RA. However, there are also many claims that special diets, foods, or supplements can cause harm in arthritis. Some specific diets that are known to have harmful side effects include those that rely on large doses of alfalfa, copper salts, or zinc or the so-called immune power diet or the low-calorie/low-fat/low-protein diet. Patients who are taking methotrexate may experience folic acid deficiency that requires supplementation.

Alternative therapies: See discussion in "Osteoarthritis," p. 567.

Surgical interventions: Arthroscopy may be performed to diagnose joint disease or to treat RA by allowing removal of loose bodies or abrasion of cartilage. Synovectomy prevents pannus formation through removal of inflamed synovium; it may be appropriate when one or two joints are affected more severely than others. Carpal tunnel release, tarsal tunnel release, ganglionectomy, tendon repair, and removal of Baker's cysts may correct concurrent connective tissue defects associated with RA. Osteotomy corrects bony malalignment resulting from medial or lateral joint erosion, whereas arthrodesis allows for a stable, painless joint through fusion of surfaces in severely affected joints with extremely weak periarticular tissues and muscle atrophy. Implant arthroplasty is performed to replace eroded joints with Silastic implants that correct deformity and allow greater ROM. Total joint arthroplasty improves joint function by replacing eroded surfaces with prostheses.

NURSING DIAGNOSES AND INTERVENTIONS

Fatigue related to state of discomfort, effects of prolonged mobility, and psychoemotional demands of chronic illness

Desired outcome: Within 24 hr of instruction and interventions, patient verbalizes a reduction in fatigue.

Nursing Interventions

- Investigate patient's sleep pattern and suggest strategies (e.g., warm bath at bedtime). *Helps facilitate rest.*
- Assist patient to evaluate food preparation methods that may contribute to fatigue and suggest changes (e.g., set table for next day's breakfast before going to bed at night, use convenience foods whenever possible). *These activities help minimize fatigue.*
- Assess patient's ability to manage pain and encourage use of interventions. *Maximizes quality of rest periods.*
- Encourage patient to pace activities and allow adequate rest periods during the day. *Reduces fatigue.*
- Assess patient's stress or psychoemotional distress. Suggest coping strategies or refer patient to appropriate clinical specialist in psychiatric nursing. *Helps minimize stress.*
- Discuss rationale for a stepped approach to exercise that increases endurance and strength without fatiguing patient. Encourage patient to set realistic exercise goals and share them with associated health care providers.
- Instruct patient in use of assistive devices *to minimize fatigue.*
- Assist patient to evaluate time that fatigue occurs, its relationship with necessary activities, and activities that relieve or aggravate symptoms.

Disturbed body image related to development of joint deformities

Desired outcome: Within 1 mo of intervention, patient verbalizes positive adjustment to body image changes.

Nursing Interventions

◆ Provide anticipatory counseling about possible joint deformities/body image changes following initial diagnosis, including ways for patient to prepare for reaction of others.

◆ Routinely assess patient for negative body image, as indicated by refusal to discuss or participate in care, withdrawal from social contacts, and avoidance of intimate relationships. *This facilitates identification of negative body image so that corrective actions can be implemented.*

◆ Assess patient for negative feelings about body image linked specifically to use of assistive devices/mobility aids.

◆ Ask patient to complete the Baird Body Image Assessment Tool or other self-assessment survey. *Helps determine subjective response to physical changes.*

◆ Use survey results (Baird Body Image Assessment) along with patient statements *to help patient consider meaning and impact of any physical changes.*

◆ Demonstrate positive regard for patient and acceptance of any physical changes associated with chronic illness. *Helps patient accept physical changes.*

Dressing/grooming self-care deficit related to pain and limitations in joint ROM

Desired outcome: Within 1 wk of instruction, patient verbalizes/exhibits increased independence in dressing/grooming.

Nursing Interventions

◆ Determine impact of pain and limitations in joint ROM on dressing/grooming activities.

◆ Assess pain and ROM in joints used in dressing/grooming (e.g., small joints in hands; elbows, shoulders, knees). *This determines the need for intervention.*

◆ Teach patient to coordinate time of peak effectiveness of prescribed analgesics and antiinflammatory drugs with periods of joint use. *This helps minimize pain while dressing/grooming.*

◆ Teach patient to perform exercises during joint use for dressing/grooming. *This increases joint flexibility and decreases pain.*

◆ Refer patient to occupational therapist to evaluate need for dressing/grooming aids (e.g., buttoner, Velcro clothing closures, elastic shoe laces).

Patient-Family Teaching and Discharge Planning

Provide verbal and written information about the following:

◆ Treatment regimen, including physical therapy (PT) and exercises, systemic rest/principles of joint protection, and thermotherapy.

◆ Medications and supplements, including names, dosage, schedule, precautions, and potential side effects. Also discuss drug/drug, herb/drug, and food/drug interactions.

◆ Potential complications of disease and therapy, as well as need to recognize and seek medical attention promptly if they occur.

◆ Potential concurrent pathologic conditions, such as pericarditis and ocular lesions, and need to report them promptly to health care provider.

◆ Use, care, and replacement of splints, orthotics, and assistive devices.

◆ Use of adjunctive aids as appropriate, including long-handled reacher, long-handled shoehorn, elastic shoelaces, Velcro fasteners, crutches, walker, and cane.

◆ Referral to visiting/public health or home health nurse as necessary for ongoing care after discharge.

◆ Importance of laboratory follow-up (e.g., blood or urine testing) when taking selected medications and the importance of keeping follow-up appointments. Include date of next appointment and telephone number to call if questions arise.

◆ Referral to community resources, including local arthritis support activities:

Arthritis Foundation: www.arthritis.org

American Academy of Pediatrics: www.aap.org

National Institute of Arthritis and Musculoskeletal and Skin Diseases (NIAMS): www.nih.gov/niams/health%20info

❖ ❖ ❖

SECTION TWO MUSCULAR AND CONNECTIVE TISSUE DISORDERS

❖ LIGAMENTOUS INJURIES

OVERVIEW/PATHOPHYSIOLOGY

Injury occurs when the ligament is stressed in a direction other than the one in which it accepts the stress, or when stress exceeds inherent structural strength. Ligament tears usually result from direct trauma or transmission of force to a joint (e.g., injury to shoulder ligaments resulting from twisting the distal arm). Tears can be longitudinal, transverse, tangential, complete, or partial and can involve avulsion fractures at the ligament origin or insertion. Severity of ankle sprains is described as *grade 1* (first degree, least severe) to *grade 3* (third degree, most severe). Grading is based on edema/hemorrhage, pain, ROM, decreased ligament strength, and joint stability.

ASSESSMENT

Signs and symptoms/physical findings: Description of feeling a tear or hearing a "pop" when the injury occurred, localized ecchymosis, edema, tenderness, weakness or joint instability, pain, joint effusion, and limited ROM or inability to use the joint for ambulation or activities of daily living (ADL).

History and risk factors: Trauma, injury.

DIAGNOSTIC TESTS

Diagnosis is based primarily on patient's complaints, mechanism of injury, and physical assessment.

X-ray examination: Rules out additional skeletal injury. Stressing the weakened joint during x-ray examination may reveal an enlarged joint space.

Arthroscopy: Rules out concurrent intraarticular pathology or trauma.

Talar tilt test: Determines mediolateral joint instability.

Anterior drawer test: Determines anterior joint instability.

COLLABORATIVE MANAGEMENT

Uncomplicated injuries: The acronym RICE (rest, ice, elevation, compression) describes standard treatment for ligamentous injuries. *Rest* involves splinting, casting, or bracing and/or avoiding active use of the affected joint. Plaster or fiberglass previously prepared splints and air or gel splints may be used. Use of *ice* (cryotherapy) is well established as a means of controlling inflammation from trauma. *Compression* via elastic wraps prevents swelling and supports joints. *Elevation* decreases further edema formation while aiding resolution of existing edema. In addition, nonsteroidal antiinflammatory drugs (NSAIDs) may be used for analgesic and antiinflammatory effects.

Surgical repair: For injuries resulting in grossly unstable joints, surgery allows removal of a nonviable ligament or suture repair of the stretched ligament with the use of strong, absorbable suture material. Following avulsion injury (ligament torn from bone) without fracture, the ligament may be reattached to its insertion site by using bone staples or passing a suture through holes drilled into the affected bony area. Additional procedures may involve use of prosthetic devices to stent, temporarily replace, or augment ligament repairs.

ROM and muscle-strengthening exercises: Treatment may begin after an appropriate period of joint immobilization (several days to 3 wk).

NURSING DIAGNOSES AND INTERVENTIONS

Deficient knowledge related to therapies and exercise for involved extremity

Desired outcome: Within 30 min of instruction, patient verbalizes understanding of suggested treatments and returns demonstration of prescribed exercises.

Nursing Interventions

- Assess patient's facility with language; engage an interpreter or provide language-appropriate written materials if necessary.
- Teach pathophysiology of injury and concomitant inflammatory response. Provide instructions concerning need for a graded muscle-strengthening and joint ROM exercise regimen. *This enables return of normal joint function.*
- Teach use of RICE interventions for 3-5 days, depending on severity of injury. Encourage use of ice for first 48-72 hr to prevent excessive edema; advise patient to cover ice with at least two layers of terry cloth. *Protects skin from injury.*
- Avoid ice application for patients with suspected compartment syndrome or those with peripheral vascular disease, decreased local sensation, coagulation disorders, or a similar pathologic condition. *Minimizes the potential for thermal injury.*
- Explain each prescribed exercise in detail, including rationale. An effective method is to teach an appropriate exercise, demonstrate it, and then have patient return the demonstration. *This helps ensure patient's understanding of exercise.*
- Provide written instructions that describe the exercises, and list frequency and number of repetitions for each one. Include a phone number in case patient has questions after hospital discharge.

Risk for peripheral neurovascular dysfunction related to use of compressive dressing to decrease swelling after ligamentous injury

Desired outcomes: Patient has adequate peripheral neurovascular function in the involved limb, as evidenced by normal muscle tone, brisk (less than 2 sec) capillary refill (or capillary refill consistent with the contralateral extremity), minimal edema or tautness, and absence of paresthesia. Patient verbalizes understanding of the importance of reporting symptoms indicative of impaired neurovascular function.

Nursing Interventions

- Monitor temperature (circulation), movement, and sensation in affected extremity when elastic wrap or brace is prescribed following ligamentous injury. *Determines neurovascular status.*
- Apply ice and elevate affected extremity when appropriate. *When acute compartment syndrome is suspected, ice and elevation are contraindicated. These may further compromise vascular supply.*
- Teach patient symptoms that should be immediately reported, including any changes in temperature, sensation, or ability to move affected extremity. *These are symptoms of neurovascular compromise.*

♦ Contact health care provider promptly if change in neurovascular condition is noted, and adjust dressing. *Adjusting dressing relieves pressure over affected extremity.*

 Patient-Family Teaching and Discharge Planning

Include verbal and written information about the following:
♦ Prescribed therapies, including RICE interventions, exercise, and external supports.
♦ Potential complications that require immediate medical intervention, including subluxation/dislocation and neurovascular deficit.
♦ For ADL and ambulation, a demonstration of independence in use of assistive devices before hospital discharge.
♦ Medications and supplements, including names, rationale, dosage, schedule, precautions, and side effects. Also discuss drug/drug, herb/drug, and food/drug interactions.
♦ Importance of follow-up care, date of next appointment, and a telephone number to call if questions arise.

❖ ANTERIOR CRUCIATE LIGAMENT TEARS

OVERVIEW/PATHOPHYSIOLOGY

The anterior cruciate ligament (ACL) prevents excessive forward motion and internal rotation of the tibia. Injury to this ligament can result in strain, microtears, partial tears, complete tears, or avulsion of tibial or femoral attachments. Untreated ACL tears result in gross instability, which eventually can cause osteoarthritis (OA).

ASSESSMENT

Signs and symptoms/physical findings: Joint effusion, restricted ROM and joint instability, pain, and sensation of the knee giving way.
History and risk factors: Stresses that result in tears including forceful contraction of the quadriceps muscles combined with restricted extension, "clipping" injuries incurred in football, forced pivoting on the knee, or excessive forward motion of the tibia, which can occur when stopping quickly while running or skiing.

DIAGNOSTIC TESTS

Radiographic studies: Physical examination findings may strongly suggest ACL injury. If appropriate, radiographic studies may be performed to confirm or rule out ligamentous damage. Anteroposterior (AP), lateral, and patellar views of the knee and intercondylar notch views with and without stress on the joint may be obtained to determine the presence of abnormal joint contours.
Lachman's test: Results are positive if the ACL is torn. Patient's knee is partially flexed at 15-20 degrees, and the foot is planted flat on the examining table. The examiner then pulls the patient's tibia forward while holding the femur stable. Excessive forward movement of the tibia is evidenced by a convex curve of the patellar tendon, which is indicative of an ACL tear.
Drawer test: Performed with the patient's knee flexed at 60-90 degrees and the foot planted flat on the table. The tibia is pulled forward as the femur is stabilized. Excessive forward movement (6 mm or more) indicates a tear. The test is then repeated with the foot externally rotated 15 degrees to assess concurrent injury of medial joint structures (meniscus or periarticular ligaments). Finally, the test is repeated with the foot internally rotated 30 degrees to assess concurrent lateral joint injury.

Pivot shift maneuver (jerk test): Provides evidence of anterolateral instability of the knee. The tibia is internally rotated with one hand while the other hand is used to apply valgus stress on the knee. The knee is then flexed 20-30 degrees. The result is positive when the tibia subluxates anteriorly as evidenced by a palpable "clunk" on the lateral aspect of the knee.

MRI: Enables identification of ACL tears and other soft tissues not visible on x-ray film.

Arthroscopy: Enables direct visualization of the ACL injury to determine extent of damage and to assess need for surgery.

COLLABORATIVE MANAGEMENT

The type of therapy is determined by type of injury, length of time since original injury, concurrent joint pathology, and patient's age and functional goals.

RICE: Rest, ice, compression and elevation. See "Ligamentous injuries," p. 577.

Bracing: Provides primary support for an incompletely torn ACL or supplements other ligaments and menisci associated with the affected joint. Functional braces provide support and immobilization following reconstruction and allow controlled ROM in rehabilitation. Several types of commercial braces are available to provide AP, lateral, and rotational stability to the joint.

Physical therapy (PT): Concurrent PT strengthens periarticular structures and muscles.

Surgery: ACL surgery should be considered for all persons who wish to return to sports or activities that require lateral pivoting of the knee or for those who experience recurrent instability.

Primary ACL repair: Involves direct suturing of the torn ligament during arthrotomy or arthroscopy. Suture is heavy and nonabsorbable and is used in repairing incomplete tears that are less than 6 wk old.

ACL reconstruction: Involves use of either anatomic graft (autograft or allograft) or synthetic graft replacements. Autografts are commonly taken from the patellar tendon, although the semitendinosus tendon or hamstring tendon also may be used. Allograft (cadaver) patellar tendon also has been used for repair but is not generally the first choice. Use of a continuous passive movement (CPM) machine often immediately follows ACL reconstruction, and extensive PT follows to help with ROM and strengthening. A protective brace is often recommended for athletic activities after rehabilitation. Most reconstructive procedures are performed by arthroscopy, which permits dramatically less joint trauma, early hospital discharge or even outpatient surgery, and excellent long-term results.

NURSING DIAGNOSES AND INTERVENTIONS

Acute pain related to surgical repair and rehabilitation therapy

Desired outcomes: Within 1-2 hr of intervention, patient's subjective perception of pain decreases as documented by pain intensity rating scale. Patient demonstrates ability to perform activities of daily living (ADL) with minimal complaints of discomfort.

Nursing Interventions

- Assist patient in use of pain intensity rating scale based on 0 (no pain) to 10 (worst pain imaginable). *This allows for accurate evaluation of pain and analgesic relief.*
- Administer simple analgesics, nonsteroidal antiinflammatory drugs (NSAIDs), and opioid analgesics as prescribed, and reassess their effectiveness in approximately 1 hr using pain intensity rating scale. *Helps determine pain control effectiveness.*

◆ If intraarticular anesthetic or opioid was administered intraoperatively, advise patient that lack of pain in the immediate postoperative period does not mean that it is allowable to move the joint excessively.

◆ Instruct hospitalized surgical patient in use of patient-controlled analgesia (PCA) or epidural analgesia if prescribed. *This helps to minimize pain.*

◆ Monitor effectiveness of patient's pain management (PCA or epidural) while observing for excessive sedation, respiratory depression, and decreased level of consciousness.

◆ Closely observe for hemorrhage at the surgical site. *NSAIDs increase the potential for excessive bleeding.*

◆ Avoid administration of NSAIDs during epidural analgesia. *This reduces the risk of bleeding into the epidural space, bleeding that may create pressure on spinal nerves.*

◆ Advise patient to coordinate time of peak effectiveness of analgesics with periods of exercise or ambulation. *Minimizes pain and facilitates ambulation/exercise.*

◆ Teach patient to use nonpharmacologic methods of pain management, including guided imagery, relaxation, massage, distraction, biofeedback, heat or cold therapy, and music therapy. *These methods help minimize pain.*

◆ Supplement other pain management strategies with traditional nursing interventions such as back rubs and repositioning. *These help minimize pain.*

Deficient knowledge related to CPM and other prescribed exercises for involved extremity
Desired outcome: Within 30 min of instruction, patient verbalizes understanding of CPM machine use and returns a demonstration of prescribed exercises.

Nursing Interventions

◆ Assess patient's facility with language; engage an interpreter or provide language-appropriate written materials if necessary.

◆ Provide instructions for muscle-strengthening and joint ROM exercise regimen. An effective method is to teach appropriate exercise, demonstrate it, and then have patient return the demonstration. Provide written instructions that describe the exercises and list the frequency and number of repetitions for each one. *Facilitates return of normal joint function.*

◆ Teach use of CPM machine for rehabilitation and restoration of joint ROM. For patient with prescribed postdischarge CPM, ensure understanding of need to use CPM machine for appropriate amount of time each day. *Decreases risk for misuse or potential injury.*

Patient-Family Teaching and Discharge Planning

Include verbal and written information about the following:

◆ Use of any external support devices (elastic wraps, knee immobilizer, orthosis), including care of the device, care of skin beneath the device, and monitoring for areas of skin irritation or neurovascular deficit.

◆ Prescribed exercise regimen, including how exercise is performed, number of repetitions, frequency of exercise, and rationale for exercise performance.

◆ Use of CPM for rehabilitation and joint ROM, including need to use CPM machine for appropriate amount of time each day.

◆ Ambulation with assistive device, including patient's demonstration of independence on level and uneven ground.

◆ Medications and supplements, including names, rationale, dosage, schedule, precautions, and side effects. Also discuss drug/drug, herb/drug, and food/drug interactions.

- Indications of wound infection that require medical attention, including erythema, edema, joint effusion, purulent discharge, local warmth, pain, and fever.
- Importance of follow-up care, date of next appointment, and a telephone number to call if questions arise.

❖ DISLOCATION/SUBLUXATION

OVERVIEW/PATHOPHYSIOLOGY

A *dislocation* occurs when contact between opposing joint surfaces is completely interrupted. A *subluxation* is an incomplete dislocation in which joint surfaces are partially in contact. Some subluxations are associated with pronounced connective tissue disease, such as the ulnar deviation of phalanges and metacarpals seen with severe rheumatoid arthritis (RA). Complications include recurrent dislocation, joint contracture, neurovascular injury, and eventual traumatic arthritis.

ASSESSMENT

Signs and symptoms/physical findings: Vary with the joint involved, but include significant pain and loss of normal joint mobility; changes in normal joint contour and length of the affected extremity are likely. Although any joint can dislocate, some joints are more susceptible than others.

History and risk factors: Most dislocations and subluxations are the result of trauma and can involve permanent periarticular damage, including fractures.

DIAGNOSTIC TESTS

X-ray examination: Anteroposterior (AP) and lateral views, oblique view, or other special approach. Because muscle spasm commonly forces dislocated bones back into normal alignment, it may be necessary to stress the joint to permit visualization of the injury (stress film).

CT scans or MRI: may be needed to aid in diagnosis.

Bone scans: May reveal nondisplaced avulsion fractures, areas of recent excessive stress, or bony insertions of joint ligaments following dislocation.

Arthrocentesis: Aspirated fluid may show blood from trauma or excessive fluid from joint effusion. Free fat globules in joint aspirate signal a fracture involving joint surfaces.

Arthroscopy: May be used to rule out injury to joint surfaces or intraarticular structures.

COLLABORATIVE MANAGEMENT

Interventions vary with the degree of subluxation or dislocation and the joint involved. Shoulder dislocation is the most common dislocation treated in emergency departments, whereas traumatically dislocated knee is much less common. Prompt diagnosis is critical, and assessment must include any associated neurovascular injury. Many patients are discharged from the hospital with instructions to use temporary immobilization of the affected part, thermotherapy, elevation, and analgesics/nonsteroidal antiinflammatory drugs (NSAIDs).

Immediate reduction: Preferred to decrease likelihood of inflammation and muscle spasm. If immediate reduction is not possible, patient may require NSAIDs and muscle relaxants before a later attempt may be made at joint reduction. A splint, harness, or padding may be needed for up to 8 wk after acute dislocation until pain is adequately decreased and muscular function provides sufficient support.

Manual reduction: Many joints can be manually reduced by using local or general anesthesia. Occasionally open reduction and internal fixation (ORIF) with screws, pins, or wires may be needed to maintain reduction.

Exercise regimen: After satisfactory joint stability has been achieved, patient may begin an exercise regimen to improve muscle strength and joint ROM. Strengthening muscles surrounding the joint will help prevent future dislocation. For persons involved in strenuous sports or heavy work, the affected joint may be protected by elastic bandage or tape wraps, pads, or support stockings. Long-term problems may be prevented by allowing adequate time for an injured joint to rest and heal before resumption of full activity.

NURSING DIAGNOSES AND INTERVENTIONS

SEE "Osteoarthritis," p. 571, for **Pain** related to arthritic joint changes and associated therapy, "Rheumatoid Arthritis," p. 576, for **Dressing/grooming self-care deficit** related to pain and limitations in joint range of motion, and "Ligamentous Injuries," p. 578, for **Deficient knowledge** related to therapies and exercise for involved extremity.

 Patient-Family Teaching and Discharge Planning

Include verbal and written information about the following:
- Therapy for home use, including thermotherapy, elevation, and exercises.
- Use and care of immobilization devices.
- Assessment of neurovascular status at least 4 × daily, including need to report symptoms such as numbness and tingling or coolness in extremity to health care provider immediately.
- Medications and supplements, including names, rationale, dosage, schedule, precautions, and potential side effects. Also discuss drug/drug, herb/drug, and food/drug interactions.
- Importance of follow-up care, date of next appointment, and telephone number to call if questions arise.

❖ ACUTE COMPARTMENT SYNDROME

OVERVIEW/PATHOPHYSIOLOGY

Acute compartment syndrome results from interruption in local blood flow to muscles within an anatomic myofascial compartment. This progressive disorder is associated with changes in compartmental tissue pressures from internal sources (e.g., edema, hemorrhage), external sources (e.g., tight casts/dressings, circumferential eschar formation), or alteration in local blood flow because of venostasis or venospasm. Edema within a myofascial compartment eventually can cause ischemia that damages the capillary endothelium and leads to leakage of fluid into the interstitial space, thus contributing to a self-perpetuating cycle. Similarly, impaired venous return from a compartment can lead to distention and to distention that can eventually disrupt fluid dynamics of the capillary bed. Volkmann's ischemic contracture of the forearm and "march gangrene" (anterior tibial compartment syndrome) are possible sequelae of this process. In addition, arterial injury may result from direct trauma or the presence of fracture fragments; the resultant reflex vasospasm has been implicated as a potential cause of acute compartment syndrome. Systemic hypotension also increases risk of compartment syndrome by further aggravating effects of decreased local blood flow.

Because muscle requires large amounts of blood to meet its needs, tissue necrosis may occur rapidly if blood supply is inadequate. Irreversible ischemia can contribute to development of a functionally useless, disfigured limb distal to the injury. Complications of acute compartment syndrome include infection; renal failure from excessive release of myoglobin (myoglobinuria); hyperkalemia resulting from K^+ loss from injured muscle cells; and metabolic acidosis caused by release of accumulated lactic acid from injured muscle, contracture, and amputation.

ASSESSMENT

Signs and symptoms/physical findings: The hallmark early finding is pain greater than normally expected for the injury or need for increasing amounts of opioid analgesic. Pain increases when pressure is applied over the involved compartment or from passive movement as a result of a stretch of muscles within the compartment. Other physical indicators include paresthesia ("pins and needles") and decreased sensation to light touch or pinprick (including two-point discrimination); edema is occasionally visible and muscles are stiff on palpation ("doughy" muscle); extremity may become pale and cool distal to extremity if pressure is not relieved; slowed capillary refill and impaired venous return are possible indicators of impaired distal circulation; weakness in affected muscle groups may precede pseudoparalysis, which is caused by patient's avoidance of movements that stress the involved compartment. Pulselessness and true paralysis are late findings.

History and risk factors: Any cast or dressing that adversely affects tissue circulation can result in an iatrogenic compartment syndrome that is seen most commonly following trauma or surgery involving the elbow, wrist, knee, or ankle. Fractures of the humerus, radius, ulna, tibia, and/or fibula also may precede development of compartment syndrome.

DIAGNOSTIC TESTS

Although laboratory findings are not unique to this condition, untreated acute compartment syndrome can lead to muscle necrosis with evidence of myoglobin in the urine and high serum creatine kinase levels. However, these findings indicate that muscle damage has already occurred and may be related to other injuries.

Compartment pressure measurement: Can be used to confirm suspected diagnosis of acute compartment syndrome. Measurement can be accomplished with a variety of devices, but handheld instruments such as the transducer-tipped catheter are now generally available in patient care areas. Normal tissue pressure is between 0 and 8 mm Hg; sustained pressure greater than 30 mm Hg is considered significantly elevated. Permanent muscle damage can begin after 4-12 hr of ischemia. Nerves appear to be more sensitive than muscle to the effects of increased pressure, and damage can occur after approximately 8 hr of pressure elevation.

Arteriogram and venogram: Rule out vasospasm, thrombus, embolus, or arterial trauma. Arterial trauma can specifically lead to acute compartment syndrome, especially in patient with a supracondylar humeral fracture. Angiography is not useful in identifying compartment syndrome. Pulse oximetry also has not been proved reliable in identifying vascular compromise in distal extremities.

Doppler ultrasound: May be used to assess peripheral circulation.

EMG and nerve conduction tests: May be done to rule out intrinsic muscle or nerve pathology.

MRI: May show muscle ischemia.

COLLABORATIVE MANAGEMENT

Conservative measures: A fractured limb is elevated to promote venous return, and ice is applied to cause vasoconstriction in the area of injury. If acute compartment syndrome is suspected, however, ice and elevation are contraindicated because they may contribute to decreased vascular supply. The affected limb should be kept at heart level. Adequate hydration also will help preserve mean arterial BP. Larger than normal doses of opioids with other analgesics such as aspirin or acetaminophen may be needed for pain control.

When swelling places patient at risk for acute compartment syndrome, the constricting device (e.g., cast, splint, circumferential dressing) must be loosened down to skin level. To allow uninhibited swelling after cast application, bivalving (splitting both sides) may be performed. Adequate immobilization should then be maintained by wrapping a dressing carefully around the split cast.

Fasciotomy: May be necessary if conservative measures fail to control progressive symptoms. Fasciotomy involves surgical incision of the fascia for the entire length of the involved compartment to decompress tissues and remove any restriction to swelling. In the lower leg, all compartments are incised (i.e., anterior, lateral, and superficial and deep posterior compartments).

Surgical repair of a lacerated artery: Performed if arterial injury is the cause of compartment syndrome. If vasospasm is the suspected cause, some surgeons will expose the involved artery and apply topical papaverine to control the problem; if this is unsuccessful, resection of the involved artery with reanastomosis may be necessary.

NURSING DIAGNOSES AND INTERVENTIONS

For Patients at Risk for Acute Compartment Syndrome

Risk for peripheral neurovascular dysfunction related to interruption of capillary blood flow secondary to increased pressure within the myofascial compartment

Desired outcomes: Patient has adequate peripheral neurovascular function in the involved extremity, as evidenced by normal muscle tone, brisk (less than 2 sec) capillary refill time (or capillary refill consistent with the contralateral extremity), normal tissue pressures (8 mm Hg or less), minimal edema or tautness, and absence of paresthesia. Patient verbalizes understanding of importance of reporting symptoms indicative of impaired neurovascular function.

Nursing Interventions

◆ Monitor neurovascular condition at regular intervals by checking temperature (circulation), movement, and sensation in affected extremity. *Detects neurovascular compromise.* Apply ice and elevate affected extremity when appropriate. When acute compartment syndrome is suspected, ice and elevation are contraindicated *because they may further compromise vascular supply.*

◆ Assess to determine whether passive stretching of digits and pressure over limb compartments increase pain. *Likely indicates compartment syndrome.*

◆ Teach symptoms of neurovascular compromise that should be immediately reported, including any changes in temperature, sensation, or ability to move affected extremity.

◆ Monitor tissue pressures as prescribed if an intracompartmental pressure device is available. Alert health care provider to pressures greater than 8 mm Hg. *Sustained high pressures may signal developing compartment syndrome.*

◆ In response to changes in neurovascular condition, contact health care provider promptly and adjust dressing. *Relieves pressure over affected extremity.*

For Patient Experiencing Acute Compartment Syndrome

Acute pain related to tissue ischemia secondary to compartment swelling
Desired outcomes: Within 8 hr of intervention, patient's subjective perception of pain decreases as documented by pain intensity rating scale. Patient verbalizes understanding of the need to report uncontrolled or increasing pain.

Nursing Interventions

◆ Assist in use of pain intensity rating scale of 0 (no pain) to 10 (worst pain imaginable) *to evaluate pain and analgesic relief.*

◆ Administer simple analgesics, nonsteroidal antiinflammatory drugs (NSAIDs), and opioid analgesics as prescribed, and reassess their effectiveness in approximately 1 hr using pain intensity rating scale. Document preintervention and postintervention pain scores. *Determines analgesia effectiveness.*

◆ Adjust medication regimen to patient's needs; document effectiveness of analgesia.

◆ Prevent pressure on involved compartment and neurovascular structures. *Pressure on affected area increases pain.*

◆ Assess for unrelenting pain in a patient with a fasciotomy and report immediately. *Signals incomplete fasciotomy.*

◆ Assess for pain that increases several days after a fasciotomy. *Signals compartmental infection.*

◆ Continue to monitor temperature (circulation), movement, and sensation in affected extremity *to evaluate neurovascular function.*

 Patient-Family Teaching and Discharge Planning

Include verbal and written information about the following:

◆ Development of acute compartment syndrome, appropriate use of elevation and ice, and loosening of restrictive dressings.

◆ Monitoring for vascular changes in patient who has undergone vascular surgery (exploration or resection). Teach patient to be alert to color changes (pallor, cyanosis, duskiness), coolness, diminished pulses, and increasing time for capillary refill.

◆ Monitoring for signs and symptoms of wound infection, including redness/warmth and/or purulent drainage from wound.

◆ Seeking medical attention promptly if signs and symptoms of neurovascular dysfunction or wound infection develop.

◆ Follow-up care, date of next appointment, and telephone number to call if questions arise.

❖ ❖ ❖

SECTION THREE   **SKELETAL DISORDERS**

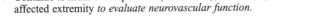

❖ **OSTEOMYELITIS**

OVERVIEW/PATHOPHYSIOLOGY

Osteomyelitis is a severe pyogenic infection of bone and surrounding tissue. Bone infection is accompanied by occlusion of blood vessels that in turn causes bone necrosis and local spread of infection. Although osteomyelitis often remains localized, it can spread through the bone marrow, cortex, and periosteum. There are two types of *acute osteomyelitis: direct or contiguous inoculation osteomyelitis* results from direct or continuous inoculation of microorganisms into bone via open fractures, penetrating wounds, diagnostic bone marrow aspiration, or surgery such as total joint arthroplasty; *hematogenic osteomyelitis* occurs through vascular seeding following bacteremia or septic arthritis, or by infection from contiguous soft tissues (especially from ischemic, diabetic, or neurotrophic ulcers). Recurrent urinary tract infections also may be linked to development of osteomyelitis. Acute hematogenic osteomyelitis most commonly results from infection by *Staphylococcus aureus* (60%), but it also can be caused by *Escherichia coli, Pseudomonas* species, *Klebsiella, Enterobacter, Proteus, Salmonella, Streptococcus* (groups

A, B, and G), and *Haemophilus influenzae.* In addition, infection can be caused by viruses or fungi. As many as 25% of cases of osteomyelitis involve multiple infectious agents. *Chronic osteomyelitis* can result from delayed diagnosis or ineffective treatment and is characterized by persistent multiple draining sinus tracts. It is often polymicrobial.

ASSESSMENT

Signs and symptoms/physical findings: Osteomyelitis often manifests with a slow, insidious progression of symptoms.

Acute osteomyelitis: Localized erythema, warmth, and pain are typical. Fever and malaise are possible, but adults do not always appear acutely ill with other systemic signs. However, fever and malaise suggest osteomyelitis in a person with localized bone pain. Pseudoparalysis is often found in children who refuse to move an adjacent joint because of pain. Vertebral osteomyelitis produces localized back pain with paravertebral muscle spasm that is unresponsive to conservative treatment.

Chronic osteomyelitis: Bone infection persists intermittently for years as a result of delayed or inadequate treatment of the acute condition. It typically flares up after minor trauma or lowered systemic resistance. Edema and erythema over the involved bone, weakness, irritability, and generalized signs of sepsis can occur. Sometimes the only symptom is persistent purulent drainage from an old pocket or sinus tract. With development of implant arthroplasty osteomyelitis, symptoms involve septic loosening (demonstrated radiographically) and pain 3-5 mo postoperatively.

History and risk factors: Patients at risk for osteomyelitis include older adults and those who are undernourished, have diabetes mellitus (DM), or COPD. Susceptibility also increases in individuals with recurrent urinary tract infections, sickle cell disease, acquired immunodeficiency syndrome (AIDS), immunosuppression, or chronic joint disease, as well as those with lifestyles that include alcholism, long-term steroid use, or IV drug use. In addition, the present of an orthopedic device, recent orthopedic surgery, or an open fracture increases the individual's risk for osteomyelitis.

DIAGNOSTIC TESTS

Laboratory studies: The WBC count may be normal, especially in adults, but the erythrocyte sedimentation rate (ESR) and C-reactive protein (CRP) levels usually are elevated in the presence of osteomyelitis. Recognition of these laboratory changes facilitates initiation of antibiotic treatment while awaiting other results such as those of blood culture or joint aspirate analysis.

Bone biopsy: Provides infectious material for accurate culture and sensitivity studies. This study is limited to large bones because of risk of fracture in small bones. Bone biopsy is considered positive when there is evidence of necrosis, acute or chronic inflammatory cells (including polymorphonuclear leukocytes), and aggregates of lymphocytes and/or plasma cells.

Cultures of blood or sequestrum (a piece of necrotic bone separated from surrounding bone as a result of infection): Anaerobic and aerobic cultures can identify causative organism via Gram stain or culture and sensitivity. Culture of sinus drainage is unreliable for diagnosing underlying osteomyelitis.

X-ray examination: May reveal subtle areas of radiolucency (osteonecrosis) and new bone formation. After 3-4 wk, x-ray films show bone destruction, soft tissue swelling, periosteal elevation, loss of vertebral body height or narrowing of the adjacent infected intervertebral disk space, and destruction of end plates above and below the disk.

MRI: Used increasingly for definitive diagnosis of osteomyelitis. MRI is able to distinguish between bone and soft tissue infection and can detect osteomyelitis earlier than computed tomography (CT) scans and x-ray examinations.

Bone scans: Can detect lesions 24-72 hr after onset of infection; may reveal areas of increased vascularity ("hot spots") that can indicate osteomyelitis. Bone scans show abnormalities earlier than x-ray films but cannot distinguish among infections, tumors, and fractures.

COLLABORATIVE MANAGEMENT

Antibiotic therapy (e.g., cefazolin, vancomycin, ticarcillin, fluoroquinolones): When agent-specific antibiosis is possible after blood or wound culture, high doses of IV antibiotics may be given frequently for 4-8 wk, followed by 4-8 wk of oral antibiotic therapy. When the infective agent is not specifically identified, broad-spectrum antibiotic IV therapy may be required for a longer period as determined by patient's response. Topical antibiotics also can be infused into the wound via drains and are continued until three successive negative cultures are obtained. As an alternative or adjunct, antibiotic-impregnated polymethylmethacrylate (PMMA) beads may be packed into affected sites; their primary benefit is the provision of high local concentrations of antibiotic while systemic antibiotic levels remain low. After several weeks of treatment, the wound is reopened, the beads are removed, and bone graft is packed in the deficit. Intramedullary or intraarticular antibiotic solutions also may be used. Serial bone scans and ESR testing can be prescribed to evaluate effectiveness of antibiotic therapy.

Immobilization of affected extremity with splint, cast, or traction device: Relieves pain and decreases potential for pathologic fracture.

Surgical decompression of infected bone: May be followed by primary closure when a small area is involved. When large areas are affected, myocutaneous flaps may be needed to cover denuded bone. Sometimes the area is left open to drain with healing by secondary intention or with secondary closure.

Amputation: Rarely performed but may be required for extremities in which persistent infection severely limits function.

Hyperbaric O$_2$: Sometimes effective in treating refractory osteomyelitis associated with adjacent pressure necrosis.

NURSING DIAGNOSES AND INTERVENTIONS

Risk for infection related to disease chronicity

Desired outcomes: At the time of hospital discharge, patient is free of symptoms of infection, as evidenced by normal body temperature and WBC count 11,000/mm^3 or less. Within 24 hr of instruction, patient verbalizes understanding of the potential chronicity of osteomyelitis and importance of strict adherence to prescribed antibiotic therapy.

Nursing Interventions

- Teach patient about the disease and potential for chronic infection. Stress importance of adherence to prescribed antibiotic therapy.
- Monitor for fever, increasing pain, and laboratory data indicative of infection (e.g., increased ESR).
- Assess exposed wounds for warmth/erythema, increasing or purulent drainage, increasing wound size, edema, and localized tenderness. *These may indicate continued infection.*
- After primary closure or wound grafting, continue to assess operative area. *This is to observe for symptoms of infection.*
- Assess for neurovascular dysfunction. *This can signal infection or pressure from inflamed tissues.*
- Assess for fever, oral monilial growth (e.g., black or furry tongue, complaint of sore mouth or tongue), nausea, and diarrhea. *These symptoms may signal superimposed infections, especially fungal.* If a venous access device (VAD) is used for antibiotic administration, monitor infusion site closely. *This is to observe for irritation that does not respond to usual treatments*

with topical antibiotics. As indicated, obtain cultures of suspicious inflammation.

Deficient knowledge related to maintenance of Groshong catheter, peripherally inserted central catheter (PICC), or other VAD for long-term intermittent antibiotic therapy

Desired outcome: By at least 24 hr before hospital discharge, patient demonstrates care of the catheter and verbalizes understanding of signs of infection and air embolus.

Nursing Interventions

◆ Assess patient's facility with language; engage an interpreter or provide language-appropriate written materials if necessary.

◆ Teach patient how to care for the VAD and monitor entry site for signs and symptoms of inflammation or infection. *This is important if antibiotic therapy is to be continued at home.*

◆ Demonstrate dressing change using sterile technique and following hospital protocol for the procedure. Have patient or significant other return demonstration before hospital discharge. If appropriate, arrange for a visit by a home health nurse to assist in care of the VAD.

◆ If appropriate, caution patient about the importance of keeping tubing clamped unless aspirating or injecting solutions into the catheter. *Some IV catheters do not require clamping (e.g., Groshong catheters).* Teach patient and significant other to be alert for signs and symptoms of air embolism: labored breathing, cyanosis, cough, chest pain, syncope. If an air embolus is suspected, explain that patient should be rolled immediately to the left side and placed in Trendelenburg position while catheter is reclamped; medical assistance should be obtained as quickly as possible.

◆ Teach patient the importance of preventing inadvertent puncture or breakage of the tubing, as well as the need to check for kinks or cracks daily. Explain the necessity of taping all tube junctures, *to prevent accidental separation,* and of positioning clamp over tape tabs, *to minimize stress on tubing.*

Impaired physical mobility related to musculoskeletal pain and immobilization devices

Desired outcomes: By at least 24 hr before hospital discharge, patient maintains appropriate body alignment with external fixation devices in place or demonstrates setup and use of home traction device. Patient verbalizes understanding of use of analgesics and adjunctive methods to decrease pain when performing prescribed exercises or activity.

Nursing Interventions

◆ Teach proper body alignment, most commonly with joints in neutral position. If an orthotic device is used to maintain position, teach application of the device and assessment of areas of excess pressure beneath the device. *This is to prevent the risk of tissue necrosis.* Teach exercises and ROM to do when the device is removed.

◆ Teach patient and significant other active and/or passive ROM of adjacent joints q8h as appropriate.

◆ When appropriate, teach patient and significant other setup and maintenance of home traction, including signs and symptoms of complications (e.g., pressure necrosis, impaired neurovascular function).

◆ Instruct patient and significant other in the care of an extremity in an external fixator, including identification of problems associated with the fixator, performance of prescribed exercises, assessment of neurovascular status of the limb, and assessment of pin sites for signs of infection.

◆ Instruct patient and significant other in the care of a casted extremity, including cast care, assessment of neurovascular status of the distal extremity, assessment of evidence of pressure necrosis beneath cast, performance of prescribed exercises, and prevention of skin maceration and disuse osteoporosis.

◆ Instruct patient and significant other in the use of analgesics and nonpharmacologic pain management methods.

 Patient-Family Teaching and Discharge Planning

When providing patient-family teaching, give instructions related to the particular device (e.g., external fixator, cast) patient has and the specific care needed. Include verbal and written information about the following:

◆ Necessary patient care after hospital discharge (e.g., analgesia, dressing changes, warm soaks, ROM exercises, activity limitations, use of ambulatory aids). Involve significant other in care during hospitalization to familiarize him or her with care activities after discharge.

◆ When parenteral antibiotic therapy is to be given at home via a long-term VAD, method of administering medications and care of device used.

◆ Medications and supplements, including names, rationale, dosage, schedule, precautions, and potential side effects. Also discuss drug/drug, herb/drug, and food/drug interactions.

◆ Signs and symptoms of potential complications and adverse effects of medications.

◆ Involving a home health nurse as appropriate to ensure adequate follow-up after hospital discharge.

◆ Importance of follow-up care, date of next appointment, and telephone number to call if questions arise.

❖ FRACTURES

OVERVIEW/PATHOPHYSIOLOGY

A fracture is a break in continuity of a bone. It occurs when stress is placed on the bone that exceeds its biologic loading capacity. Most commonly, the stress is the result of trauma. Pathologic fractures can occur when the bone's decreased loading capacity cannot tolerate even normal stress, as with osteoporosis. See **TABLE 9-2** for examples of fracture classification.

Severe complications of fractures can occur. Chronic fracture can result from *delayed union,* which is failure of bone fragments to unite within the normally accepted time frame for that bone's healing. *Nonunion* is demonstrated by nonalignment and lost function secondary to loss of bony rigidity. *Pseudoarthrosis* is a state in which the fracture fails to heal and a false joint develops at the fracture site. *Avascular necrosis (AVN)* occurs when the fracture interrupts blood supply to a segment of bone, which eventually dies. *Myositis ossificans* involves heterotopic bone formation (abnormal, out of the normal area) and occurs most commonly in the arms, thighs, and hips. *Complex regional pain syndrome* (or *reflex sympathetic dystrophy*) is an incompletely understood process that results in chronic pain out of proportion to the injury, with reduced function, joint stiffness, and trophic changes in soft tissue and skin following a traumatic event such as a fracture. Other fracture complications include altered sensation, limb length discrepancy, and chronic lymphatic or venous stasis.

ASSESSMENT

Signs and symptoms/physical findings: Include loss of normal bony or limb contours, edema, ecchymosis, limb shortening, decreased ROM of adjacent joints, and false motion (occurs outside a joint). Patient may describe crepitus, but this should not be elicited by health care provider because of risk of injury to surrounding soft tissues. Complicated or complex fractures can present with

TABLE 9-2	TYPES OF FRACTURES
TYPE	**DESCRIPTION**
Complete Fractures	
Closed fracture	Fracture with skin covering bone intact
Open fracture	Fracture with communicating wound between bone and skin
Comminuted fracture	Fracture with multiple bone fragments
Linear fracture	Fracture line parallel to long axis of bone
Oblique fracture	Fracture line at 45-degree angle to long axis of bone
Spiral fracture	Fracture line encircling bone
Transverse fracture	Fracture line perpendicular to long axis of bone
Impacted fracture	Fracture fragments are pushed into each other
Pathologic fracture	Fracture occurs at a point in the bone weakened by disease
Avulsion fracture	Fragment of bone connected to a ligament or tendon breaks off from main bone
Compression fracture	Fracture wedged or squeezed together on one side of bone
Displaced fracture	Fracture with one, both, or all fragments out of normal alignment
Extracapsular fracture	Fracture close to the joint but remaining outside the joint
Intracapsular fracture	Fragment extending into or within the joint capsule
Incomplete Fractures	
Greenstick fracture	Fracture with break on one cortex of bone with splintering of inner bone surface
Torus fracture	Fracture with buckling of cortex
Bowing fracture	Fracture with bending of the bone
Stress fracture	Microfracture
Transchondral fracture	Fracture with separation of cartilaginous joint surface from main bone shaft

Modified from McCance KL, Huether SE: *Pathophysiology: the biologic basis for disease in adults and children,* ed 5, St Louis, 2006, Mosby.

signs and symptoms of perforated internal organs, neurovascular dysfunction, joint effusion, or excessive joint laxity. Open fractures involve a break in the skin and a wound in the area of suspected fracture, or bone may be exposed in the wound (**TABLE 9-3**).

Acute indicators: Fractures cause insidious and progressive pain or sudden onset of severe pain usually associated with trauma or physical stress, such as jogging, strenuous exercise, or a fall. In the event of pathologic fracture, patient typically describes signs and symptoms associated with the underlying pathology (see "Benign Neoplasms," p. 595).

DIAGNOSTIC TESTS

Most fractures are identified easily with standard anteroposterior (AP) and lateral x-ray examination. Occasionally special radiographic views are needed, such as the mortise view with bimalleolar ankle fractures (showing joint spaces in the fibula, tibia, and talus) or x-ray examination through the open mouth to identify fractures of the odontoid process. Magnetic resonance imaging (MRI) may be useful in evaluating complicated fractures, but its ability to identify different bone densities is limited. Intraarticular fractures may be diagnosed with arthroscopy. Bone scans, computed tomography (CT) scans, tomograms, stereoscopic films, and arthrograms also can be used.

TABLE 9-3	GUSTILO-ANDERSON CLASSIFICATION OF OPEN FRACTURES	
TYPE	**WOUND DESCRIPTION**	**OTHER CRITERIA**
I	Less than 1 cm long (so-called puncture wounds)	
II	1-10 cm long	
IIIA	More than 10 cm long, coverage available	Segmental fractures, farm injuries, or any injury occurring in a highly contaminated environment High-velocity gunshot injuries
IIIB	10 cm long, requiring soft tissue coverage procedure	Periosteal stripping
IIIC		With vascular injury requiring repair

Modified from Canale S, Beaty J: *Campbell's operative orthopaedics*, ed 11, St Louis, 2007, Mosby.

COLLABORATIVE MANAGEMENT

Any patient with a suspected fracture should be treated as though a fracture is present until it is ruled out. Interventions should include immobilization of the affected area and careful monitoring of neurovascular function distal to the injury. Any restrictions to swelling (e.g., from rings, wristwatches, or bracelets) should be removed before they can contribute to neurovascular dysfunction. Once a fracture is diagnosed, treatment varies with fracture complexity and patient's age, concurrent health problems, and functional goals. The general treatment goal is to provide bone immobilization until healing occurs; the length of time varies with the type of fracture.

Bed rest: May be all that is required to maintain reduction for simple, uncomplicated fractures in the posterior elements of vertebrae or the pelvis.

Reduction: Enables restoration of fracture fragments to their normal anatomic alignment. *Closed reduction* is accomplished by applying manual traction to the area of injury to attain realignment of minimally displaced fracture fragments. Patient may need to receive general, regional, or local anesthesia for this procedure, which can be quite painful. *Open reduction* involves visualization and realignment of fracture fragments through a surgical incision. Internal fixation is then performed using plates, screws, rods, or pins to maintain fragment position.

Immobilization devices such as casts, collars, splints, or slings/swathes: Used to keep realigned fracture fragments in their normal anatomic position while bone healing occurs. Splints often serve as an initial treatment because they can be applied and removed more quickly than casts, but splints also may be the definitive treatment depending on the injury. Casts generally offer more effective immobilization than splints. Fiberglass and thermoplastic casts, which are lighter, more durable, and faster drying than Plaster of Paris casts, are typically used. In addition, prefabricated immobilizers are commercially available; some of them also offer a means of applying cold to an injury.

External fixation: Consists of skeletal pins (similar to Kirschner wires or Steinmann pins) that penetrate fracture fragments and are attached to universal joints. These joints are in turn attached to rods, which provide stabilization and form a frame around the fractured limb for immobilization. The external fixator is left in place until sufficient soft tissue repair or bony callus formation allows either application of a cast or complete removal of any form of immobilization. Sometimes the external fixation rods are removed and the skeletal pins are left in place, to be incorporated into the cast for further limb immobilization until the fracture has healed. An external fixator can be used to treat massive open comminuted fractures with extensive soft tissue injury or neurovascular injury in which there is increased risk of infection. External fixation is also the treatment of choice for infected nonunion, segmental bone loss, limb-lengthening procedures, joint fusion (arthrodesis), and multiple trauma with injuries involving other body systems.

Traction: Has somewhat limited application in adult patients because of surgical advances in fracture repair. If surgery must be delayed until a patient is medically stable following femoral fracture, skin traction via Buck's boot may be prescribed. The actual fracture repair is now more likely to be accomplished through open reduction with internal fixation (ORIF). Skeletal traction applied means of tongs or halo vest may be used for cervical fractures, but a wide variety of collars and orthotics are more commonly used to provide support for some simple fractures; a collar also may be used to maintain stability of more complex fractures following traction or ORIF. Skeletal traction is most often used for patients with multiple traumas who are not immediate candidates for ORIF. Treatment for upper extremity fractures is more likely to be accomplished with a sling and swathe or with external fixation than with traction. Pelvic fractures are also commonly treated with ORIF or external fixation.

Progressive ROM and muscle-strengthening exercises: Prescribed after the designated period of immobilization to help patient regain joint function.

Continuous passive movement (CPM): Accomplished by using a machine that places a joint through repeated extension and flexion. It may be used as an adjunctive therapy for certain extremity fractures or after total joint arthroplasty.

Electrical bone stimulation: Has proved to be effective in situations in which fracture healing has been delayed. Devices may be incorporated into an overlying cast or completely implanted in the area of the fracture.

NURSING DIAGNOSES AND INTERVENTIONS

Dressing, bathing self-care deficit related to physical limitations secondary to cast, immobilizer, or orthotic devices

Desired outcome: Within 48 hr of initiation of immobilization, patient demonstrates independence with activities of daily living (ADL).

Nursing Interventions

◆ For patients with insufficient strength to manipulate immobilized extremities to enable independence in self-care, incorporate a structured exercise regimen. *This will increase strength and endurance.* Direct the regimen toward development of those muscle groups needed for specific activity deficit.

◆ Use assistive devices liberally. These may include a sock donner, long-handled reacher, enlarged handles on eating utensils, and elevated toilet seat. *This is to maximize independence in self-care.*

◆ As appropriate, use adaptive clothing (e.g., garments with Velcro fasteners). *This will help to accommodate cast or external fixator.*

◆ Refer to physical therapy or occupational therapy for patient instruction on use of self-care aids.

◆ Refer to care management/social services department of hospital for assistance with funding for purchasing assistive equipment or arranging home help.

◆ Ensure that patient receives appropriate treatment as prescribed for pain. *This is because pain management is an essential element for enhancing self-care.*

◆ When needed, teach significant other how to assist patient with self-care activities.

Risk for impaired skin integrity and/or **Impaired tissue integrity** related to irritation and pressure secondary to presence of an immobilization device (e.g., cast, splint)

Desired outcomes: Within 8 hr of immobilization device application, patient verbalizes knowledge about indicators of pressure necrosis. Patient relates absence of discomfort under immobilization device and exhibits intact skin when the device is removed.

Nursing Interventions

◆ When assisting with application of cast or other immobilization device, ensure that adequate padding is put on bony prominences of affected extremity.

◆ While a cast is drying, handle it only with the palms of the hands. *This is to avoid pressure points caused by finger indentations.* Ensure that all cast surfaces are alternately exposed to air. *This will facilitate drying.*

◆ Petal edges of plaster casts with tape or moleskin. *This is to prevent cast crumbs from falling into cast and causing pressure areas.* Pad surfaces of other immobilization devices. *This is to avoid excessive pressure on underlying skin.*

◆ Instruct patient never to insert anything between immobilization device and skin (e.g., coat hanger or stick). *This is to prevent skin irritation or lesions that might not heal under the cast.* In presence of severe itching, advise patient to notify health care provider, who may prescribe a medication to relieve itching.

◆ Teach indicators of pressure necrosis under immobilization device such as pain, burning sensation, foul odor from opening, or drainage on the device.

Deficient knowledge related to function of external fixation, performance of pin care, and signs and symptoms of pin site infection

Desired outcomes: By at least 24 hr before hospital discharge, patient verbalizes knowledge of rationale for the external fixator and indicators of pin site infection. Patient also demonstrates performance of pin care.

Nursing Interventions

◆ Assess patient's facility with language; engage an interpreter or provide language-appropriate written materials if necessary.

◆ Teach rationale for use of fixator with type of fracture or injury, and emphasize benefits to patient.

◆ Instruct patient and significant other in pin care as prescribed by health care provider. If prescribed, teach patient and significant other how to apply antibacterial ointments and small dressings to pin sites.

◆ Instruct patient and significant other to *avoid* using external fixator as a handle or support for moving extremity. *Repeated use of external fixator in this manner may lead to loosening of skeletal pins.* Teach patient and significant other to support extremity with pillows, two hands, slings, and other devices as necessary. *This will prevent stress on skeletal pins.*

◆ Teach patient to monitor pin sites for persistent redness, swelling, drainage, increasing pain, and local warmth. Monitoring should also include pain, local warmth, and increasing temperature (greater than 101° F [38.3° C]). *These signs are indicators of infection.* Instruct patient to report significant findings immediately to health care provider.

◆ If orthotics are added to the external fixator, ensure that patient and significant other are aware of purpose of the orthotic, know how to check for areas of excessive pressure, and know schedule for adjunctive/ROM exercises. *These exercises may be added to prevent wrist drop, footdrop, or similar joint contractures,*

◆ Advise patient of need for maintaining adequate fracture immobilization and for follow-up care. *This is to ensure that device is functioning properly.*

Constipation related to decreased mobility and use of opioid analgesics
Desired outcomes: Within 8 hr of immobilization device application, patient verbalizes understanding of strategies to maintain normal bowel elimination. Patient maintains bowel elimination in his or her normal pattern.

Nursing Interventions

- Teach current influences on bowel elimination (e.g., decreased mobility, use of opioid analgesics, prescription for regular diet).
- Encourage choice of diet items that will facilitate normal bowel elimination (e.g., high-fiber foods).
- If not contraindicated, encourage patient to drink adequate fluids. *This helps ensure to ensure soft stool.*
- If patient desires, request prescription for stool softener and/or bulk-forming laxative. *This is to maintain normal bowel elimination.* Reassess bowel elimination for response to medication.
- Encourage mobility to the extent of prescribed activity parameters.

 Patient-Family Teaching and Discharge Planning

When providing patient-family teaching, focus on information based on the type of fracture and device the patient will have when discharged. Include verbal and written information about the following:

- Medications and supplements, including names, dosage, purpose, schedule, precautions, and potential side effects. Also discuss drug/drug, herb/drug, and food/drug interactions.
- Use of nonpharmacologic methods of pain management.
- Appropriate use of elevation and thermotherapy.
- Importance of performing prescribed exercises.
- Rationale for therapy (i.e., casting, external fixation, internal fixation).
- Precautions of therapy, as follows:
  - *Casts:* Caring for cast, monitoring neurovascular function of distal extremity and for evidence of pressure necrosis beneath cast, preventing skin maceration, preventing disuse osteoporosis.
  - *Internal fixation devices:* Caring for wound, noting signs of wound infection and monitoring for delayed infection, following appropriate weight-bearing prescription for lower extremity fracture.
  - *External fixator:* Demonstrating pin care, monitoring pin sites for signs of infection, knowing when to notify health care provider of problems with fixator, using prescribed orthotics, monitoring neurovascular function of distal extremity.
- Use of assistive devices/ambulatory aids. Ensure that patient can perform return demonstration and is independent with devices/aids before hospital discharge.
- Materials necessary for wound care at home, with names of agencies that can provide additional supplies.
- Importance of follow-up care, date of next appointment, and telephone number to call if questions arise.
- For all patients who receive allograft bone for bone graft and who have questions about these grafts, resources for information include the following organizations:

  American Red Cross: http://www.redcross.org

  AlloSource: www.allosource.org

❖ BENIGN NEOPLASMS

OVERVIEW/PATHOPHYSIOLOGY

The exact incidence of benign bone tumors is unknown because many cause no pain and therefore escape patient's notice. These tumors are often found incidentally when patient undergoes x-ray examination to evaluate another condition. Among the most common benign bone tumors are osteochondromas, chondromas, osteoid osteomas, and giant cell tumors. *Osteochondromas* are cartilage-capped bony protuberances that can occur on any bone but tend to occur near the ends of long bones such as the femur or humerus. Individuals less than 20 yr of age are most commonly affected. *Chondromas* may occur at any age but tend to develop in adults. They are located in the marrow cavity of a bone. Because they are usually positive on bone scan, they raise the concern of malignancy. If imaging is questionable or the lesion is painful, biopsy is probably needed. *Osteoid osteomas* tend to occur in the long bones of young adults. Pain, usually worse at night, is typically relieved by low-dose aspirin. *Giant cell tumors* are also solitary lesions characterized by osteoclast-like giant cells and stromal cells that originate within the epiphysis of adults. They are most commonly found around the proximal humerus, distal radius, sacrum, or knee in the area of the fused epiphyseal growth plate in individuals 30-40 yr of age. Giant cell tumors may erode the parent bone and produce soft tissue extensions. They are usually treated by curettage but are known for their tendency to recur, which can complicate surgical management.

ASSESSMENT

Signs and symptoms/physical findings

Osteochondromas: Somewhat easily noted because of their outward growth near joints. Patient complains of mechanical irritation of surrounding musculotendinous structures and may note pain with specific movements of the involved area.

Chondromas: Usually asymptomatic and detected when an x-ray film is taken for another reason.

Osteoid osteomas: Physical examination may reveal atrophy of regional muscles.

Giant cell tumors: Cause pain before a mass becomes palpable.

History and risk factors: Strong familial tendency with some osteochondromas and genetic links (autosomal dominant) in several others.

DIAGNOSTIC TESTS

X-ray examination (anteroposterior [AP] and lateral views): Most commonly used for preliminary diagnosis; also useful for interval monitoring.

CT and bone scans: Commonly performed to clarify extent of the tumor.

Angiograms and tomograms: Performed as needed.

MRI: May be useful in determining precise areas for surgical resection.

SURGICAL INTERVENTION

If tumors are locally aggressive and cause weakness, fracture, destruction, or bone pain, surgical intervention will become necessary. Resection can require allografting, prosthetic replacement, or use of methylmethacrylate to replace resected bone. When removal is possible, curettage (scraping) of the bone is usually done.

NURSING DIAGNOSES AND INTERVENTIONS

Acute pain related to surgical repair and rehabilitation therapy

Desired outcomes: Within 1-2 hr of intervention, patient's subjective perception of pain decreases as documented by pain intensity rating scale. Patient demonstrates ability to perform activities of daily living (ADL) with minimal complaints of discomfort.

Nursing Interventions

◆ Assist patient in use of pain intensity rating scale of 0 (no pain) to 10 (worst pain imaginable). *This is to evaluate pain and effectiveness of analgesics.*

- ◆ Administer simple analgesics, nonsteroidal antiinflammatory drugs (NSAIDs), and opioid analgesics as prescribed, and reassess their effectiveness in approximately 1 hr using pain intensity rating scale.
- ◆ If appropriate, instruct hospitalized surgical patient in use of patient-controlled analgesia (PCA) or epidural analgesia. Verify with another nurse that PCA or epidural pump contains prescribed medication and concentration with prescribed settings for patient dosing, continuous infusion, and/ or clinician bolus.
- ◆ If PCA or epidural analgesia is used, monitor effectiveness of patient's pain management while observing for excessive sedation, respiratory depression, and decreased level of consciousness. *These symptoms may indicate need for reversal agent.* Ensure that appropriate reversal agent is readily available; most commonly naloxone is used for opioid-induced side effects, and ephedrine is given for hypotensive crisis associated with epidural administration of anesthetics such as bupivacaine.
- ◆ Because of potential for excessive bleeding following NSAID administration, closely observe for hemorrhage at surgical site. NSAIDs should not be prescribed during administration of epidural analgesia. *This is because of risk of bleeding into the epidural space that may create pressure on spinal nerves.*
- ◆ Advise patient to coordinate time of peak effectiveness of analgesics with periods of exercise or ambulation.
- ◆ Teach patient to use nonpharmacologic methods of pain management, including guided imagery, relaxation, massage, distraction, biofeedback, heat or cold therapy, and music therapy.
- ◆ Supplement other pain management strategies with traditional nursing interventions such as back rubs, repositioning, and encouraging patient to verbalize feelings regarding impact of the injury.

Impaired physical mobility related to musculoskeletal pain and immobilization devices

Desired outcomes: By at least 24 hr before hospital discharge, patient maintains appropriate body alignment with external fixation devices in place or demonstrates setup and use of home traction device. Patient verbalizes understanding of use of analgesics and adjunctive methods to decrease pain when performing prescribed exercises or activity.

Nursing Interventions

- ◆ Teach proper body alignment, most commonly with joints in neutral position. If an orthotic device is used to maintain position, teach application of the device and assessment of areas of excess pressure beneath the device. *This is to prevent the risk of tissue necrosis.* Teach exercises and ROM to do when the device is removed.
- ◆ Teach patient and significant other active and/or passive ROM of adjacent joints q8h as appropriate.
- ◆ Instruct patient and significant other in use of analgesics and nonpharmacologic pain management methods.

Patient-Family Teaching and Discharge Planning

When providing patient-family teaching, focus on information based on the type of surgery (e.g., resection with allograft, curettage, prosthetic replacement) and device the patient will have when discharged. Include verbal and written information about the following:

- ◆ Description of disease process and recommended treatment.
- ◆ Medications and supplements, including names, dosage, purpose, schedule, precautions, and potential side effects. Also discuss drug/drug, herb/drug, and food/drug interactions.

◆ Use of nonpharmacologic methods of pain management.
◆ Any precautions related to procedure, wound care and signs of infection (i.e., persistent redness or pain, swelling or localized warmth, fever, purulent drainage), or other complications of surgery.
◆ For patients with casts and orthotics, care of extremity and immobilization device.
◆ Importance of follow-up care, date of next appointment, and telephone number to call if questions arise.
◆ For patients who receive allograft bone for bone graft and who have questions about these grafts, resources for information include the following organizations:

American Red Cross: http://www.redcross.org

AlloSource: www.allosource.org

❖ OSTEOPOROSIS

OVERVIEW/PATHOPHYSIOLOGY

Osteoporosis ("porous bone") is the most common metabolic bone disease. It is characterized by reduction in both bone mass and bone strength, while bone size remains constant. These changes make bone more brittle and susceptible to fractures. Osteoporosis affects 10 million people in the United States, whereas 18 million more have low bone mass. Osteoporosis is responsible for up to 1.5 million fractures annually.

One in three women and one in six men have the disease; women are four times more likely than men to develop osteoporosis. Because of its prevalence and effects, instruction on osteoporosis prevention should be a routine part of health teaching for children, adolescents, and adults.

The World Health Organization (WHO) has defined the diagnostic categories for osteoporosis, and the National Institutes of Health has defined two major types of osteoporosis (**BOX 9-1**).

Signs and symptoms/physical findings: Because of the insidious onset of osteoporosis, most individuals are not diagnosed until they experience an acute fracture or receive radiographic evidence from x-ray examinations obtained for other conditions (e.g., chest x-ray examination to confirm pneumonia). Vertebral compression fractures can develop gradually, with resulting back discomfort and loss of height. Severe chronic flexion of the vertebral spine (kyphosis or "dowager's hump") may inhibit function of multiple organ systems (e.g., gastrointestinal [GI], respiratory). With severe spinal deformities, patient often describes difficulty in obtaining clothes that fit well.

History and risk factors: Summarized in **BOX 9-2**.

DIAGNOSTIC TESTS

Laboratory tests: Cannot accurately determine bone density or fracture risk, but serum and urinary markers of bone remodeling can help in determining disease cause. For example, urinary calcium may be elevated even if serum calcium is normal. Biochemical markers of bone resorption (e.g., osteocalcin) may be useful for both initial assessment and for monitoring treatment effectiveness for confirmed disease.

Standard anteroposterior (AP) and lateral x-ray examinations of the spine: Provide a diagnosis for osteoporotic fractures or kyphosis. These studies have limited use in diagnosing disease before a fracture, however, because changes are not evident on plain films until at least 30% of bone mineral density (BMD) has been lost.

Bone mineral density (BMD) tests: Can measure amount of bone in specific areas of the skeleton to predict risk of fracture. Dual energy x-ray absorptiometry (DEXA) is the gold standard modality for measuring bone density by

BOX 9-1   CLASSIFICATIONS OF OSTEOPOROSIS

Bone Mineral Density

The WHO uses the following four diagnostic categories using BMD to define the category:

- Normal: BMD not more than 1 SD below the young adult mean; T score higher than −1
- Osteopenia: BMD between 1 and 2.5 SD below the young adult mean; T score between −1 and −2.5
- Osteoporosis: BMD 2.5 SD or more below the young adult mean; T score at or below −2.5
- Severe osteoporosis: BMD of 2.5 SD or more below the young adult mean with one or more fragility fractures

Primary versus Secondary

Osteoporosis is also classified as primary or secondary:

- Primary: the most common type and is divided by age groups:
  - Idiopathic: found in young adults not related to other diseases
  - Juvenile: found in boys and girls before puberty
  - Postmenopausal: found in women after menopause
  - Senile: found in elderly individuals
- Secondary: found when osteoporosis is related to another disease or drugs; contributing factors include congenital conditions, diet, drugs, endocrine disease, and other diseases such as rheumatoid arthritis or leukemia

BMD, Bone mineral density; *SD,* standard deviation; *WHO,* World Health Organization.
Modified from Classification of Osteoporosis, MerckMedicus Modules, Merck and Company 2001-2009, accessed at http://www.merckmedicus.com/pp/us/hcp/diseasemodules/osteoporosis/default.jsp February 2010; National Institutes of Health. Osteoporosis Prevention, Diagnosis, and Therapy. NIH Consensus Statement 2000. accessed at http://consensus.nih.gov/2000/2000osteoporosis111html.htm, February 2010.

testing bone mass in the spine, hip, and wrist. This method is precise and economical; short procedure times mean minimal radiation exposure. Quantitative computed tomography (QCT) measures bone density at sites throughout the body but is most often used in the spine. It is accurate but costly and delivers a considerable amount of radiation. In the heel, quantitative ultrasound (QUS) compares favorably with density measurements obtained by DEXA. It is also an easy, low-cost, radiation-free diagnostic aid.

Bone biopsy: Useful in differential diagnosis of metabolic bone diseases such as osteoporosis and osteomalacia. It also can be useful for diagnosis in individuals with early onset of osteoporosis (age less than 50 yr) or those with severe demineralization.

COLLABORATIVE MANAGEMENT

Appropriate nutrition and supplements: The foundation of osteoporosis prevention and treatment. Consistent calcium intake alone cannot prevent or cure osteoporosis, but it is an important part of an overall prevention or treatment program.

Premenopausal women (older than 18 yr) need 1000 mg of calcium daily. After menopause, requirements rise to 1200 mg daily. Adolescents (13-18 yr) need 1300 mg of calcium daily to maintain bone health. Oral calcium supplements (as calcium carbonate) may help perimenopausal women who have inadequate dietary intake and may compensate for inadequate intestinal absorption of calcium in postmenopausal women. Vitamin D is needed for adequate intestinal absorption and usage of calcium. Research is showing that vitamin D may be as important as calcium in preventing or reversing

BOX 9-2   RISK FACTORS FOR OSTEOPOROSIS

Genetic
- Family history of osteoporosis
- White race
- Age over 50 yr
- Female sex

Anthropometric
- Small structure
- Fair/pale skinned
- Thin build

Hormonal and Metabolic
- Early menopause
- Late menarche
- Nulliparity
- Obesity
- Hypogonadism
- Gaucher disease
- Cushing syndrome
- Weight below normal
- Acidosis

Dietary
- Low intake of calcium and vitamin D
- Low endogenous magnesium
- Excessive protein/inadequate protein intake
- Excessive sodium intake
- High caffeine intake
- Anorexia
- Malabsorption

Lifestyle
- Sedentary habits
- Smoking
- Excessive alcohol consumption

Concurrent
- Hyperparathyroidism

Illness and Trauma
- Renal insufficiency, hypercalciuria
- Rheumatoid arthritis
- Spinal cord injury
- Systemic lupus erythematosus

Liver Disease
- Bone marrow disease (multiple myeloma, thalassemia)

Drugs
- Corticosteroids
- Phenytoin (Dilantin)
- Gonadotropin-releasing hormone agonists
- Loop diuretics
- Methotrexate
- Thyroid replacements
- Heparin
- Cyclosporine
- Depomedroxyprogesterone acetate

Modified from McCance KL, Huether SE: *Pathophysiology: the biologic basis for disease in adults and children*, ed 5, St Louis, 2006, Mosby.

osteoporosis. Dietary sources include dairy products and vitamin-enriched cereals.

Supplements can be taken when necessary, but excessive intake is discouraged because of risk of toxicity. Recommended amounts of vitamin D include 400-800 units; supplementation is typically needed only during periods of low sunlight exposure and should not exceed 800 units without health care provider's prescription. Excessive and unsupervised calcium supplementation can lead to hypercalcemia, hypercalciuria, and kidney stones as potential side effects.

Weight-bearing exercise: Contributes to bone density and prevents bone loss. Individuals who have established osteoporosis should avoid vigorous unsupervised exercise. In particular, their exercise regimen should avoid spinal flexion through activities such as toe touches and sit-ups. Rotational exercises such as golf and bowling may lead to vertebral injury by creating excessive compressive forces.

Pharmacotherapy

Hormone replacement therapy: Historically, estrogen therapy has been prescribed to stabilize postmenopausal bone loss. It is now generally recommended that hormone replacement therapy not be routinely prescribed for postmenopausal women. Instead, women are encouraged to talk to their health care providers about their personal risks and benefits from any therapy.

Benefits should be weighed against any risk of heart disease, stroke, and breast cancer, and health care providers should identify other prevention and treatment options when appropriate.

Calcitonin: Exerts a powerful inhibitory effect on osteoclasts to prevent bone resorption. It also has been used prophylactically in patients with low BMD but no other symptoms of osteoporosis. Calcitonin can be administered subcutaneously, intramuscularly, or via intranasal spray. It should be taken in conjunction with a high-calcium diet or with calcium supplementation and adequate amounts of vitamin D.

Bisphosphonates (e.g., alendronate, ibandronate, risedronate): Act to reduce further loss of bone density. They are nonhormonal oral preparations for prevention of osteoporosis or treatment of postmenopausal disease. The highly selective inhibition of osteoclast activity is greater than that of calcitonin and is accomplished without disturbing normal bone formation. Concomitant use of biphosphonates and estrogen is not recommended currently because of lack of clinical data to determine interaction of these drugs.

Selective estrogen receptor modulators (SERMs) (e.g., raloxifene): Maximize the effect of estrogen on bone and minimize negative effects on the breast and endometrium. Studies have documented increased BMD in the spine and femoral neck, as well as a reduction in risk of vertebral fractures.

Synthetic human parathyroid hormone (PTH) (e.g., teriparatide): Used for treatment of osteoporosis in postmenopausal women at high risk for fracture; it is also approved to increase bone mass in men with primary or hypogonadal osteoporosis. Daily injections stimulate new bone formation and lead to increased BMD.

Topical progesterone cream: Promoted for treatment of menopausal symptoms; has been shown to provide significant relief from vasomotor symptoms such as hot flashes. However, research is still needed to determine any impact it may have on bone density.

NURSING DIAGNOSES AND INTERVENTIONS

Health-seeking behaviors related to prevention of osteoporosis, its treatment, and importance of adequate dietary calcium intake/supplementation

Desired outcome: Within 48 hr of instruction, patient verbalizes knowledge of the disease process, possible treatments, and importance of adequate calcium intake.

Nursing Interventions

- Ensure that patient understands the silent nature of osteoporosis and realizes that treatment may be less effective if not initiated until symptoms arise.
- Ensure that health care provider has recommended or approves use of calcium supplements for patient. Excessive calcium intake can lead to nephrolithiasis in susceptible individuals.
- Teach patient that the most effective form is calcium carbonate, which delivers approximately 40% calcium. *Calcium supplements come in numerous forms, and some are more effective than others.* Bone meal and dolomite should be avoided. *This is because they may contain high amounts of lead or other toxic substances.*
- Teach patient to recognize amount of elemental calcium available in supplements. Remind patient of need for sunlight, 15 min/day. *This is to enable vitamin D activation.* Have patient talk with health care provider about supplementation, if needed.
- Teach patient not to take calcium and iron supplements at the same time. *This is because iron absorption will be impaired.* Patient's medication profile should be evaluated to advise appropriate timing of supplements. *This is because calcium also may reduce absorption of some other*

medications. Teach patient to take calcium 2 hr before or after meals. *Foods such as red meats, spinach, bran, or whole-grain products and colas may inhibit calcium absorption.* Calcium should be taken at bedtime. *This is because it is best absorbed at night.*

◆ Caution patient to avoid taking more than 500-600 mg of calcium at one time and to spread doses over entire day. Remind patient to drink a full glass of water with each supplement. *This is to minimize risk of developing renal calculi.*

Risk for injury related to decreased bone density secondary to osteoporosis

Desired outcome: Within 24 hr of instruction, patient describes strategies to decrease risk for fall or fracture.

Nursing Interventions

◆ Identify factors that can contribute to falls (e.g., confusion/dementia, cardiovascular disorders, decreased mobility, generalized weakness, abnormal elimination needs, impaired vision or hearing, use of medications that affect BP or balance) via a fall risk assessment tool. Refer to health care provider for additional evaluation of any identified deficits as necessary.

◆ Instruct patient and family about need to reduce/eliminate environmental hazards. *They may increase risk for falls in the home.*

◆ Encourage patient to avoid unnecessarily limiting activity because of fear of falling. *Inactivity can place individual at greater risk for fractures.*

◆ Instruct patient to avoid lifting objects heavier than 5-10 pounds. *This is because of risk of compression fractures.* Patients interested in holding young grandchildren should be encouraged to have child crawl, climb, or be placed in lap.

◆ Teach exercise regimen that improves balance. *This is to decrease risk of falls.* Aerobic walking and strength training via upper and lower body exercises have been shown to improve standing balance.

◆ Encourage adequate calcium and vitamin D intake. *This will minimize risk of fracture if a fall occurs.*

Imbalanced nutrition: less than body requirements related to insufficient intake of calcium and vitamin D

Desired outcomes: Within 24 hr of instruction, patient demonstrates adequate intake of calcium and vitamin D. Patient plans a 3-day menu that provides sufficient intake of both.

Nursing Interventions

◆ Teach recommended daily intake for calcium.

◆ Verify patient's ability to select foods high in calcium, including cheese and milk. If patient is unable to tolerate dairy products, explore other food choices that can ensure adequate calcium intake (e.g., broccoli, sardines).

◆ Provide sample menus that include adequate daily amounts of calcium and vitamin D. Guide patient in developing a 3-day menu that includes appropriate intake of foods containing calcium and vitamin D.

◆ Teach necessity for appropriate exposure to sunlight. *This is to prevent vitamin D deficiency.* If patient has limited exposure to sunlight (e.g., resident of a long-term care facility), discuss supplementation. *This is to ensure adequate calcium absorption.*

Patient-Family Teaching and Discharge Planning

◆ When providing patient-family teaching, include verbal and written information about the following:

- Description of disease process and recommended treatment.
- Medications and supplements, including names, dosage, purpose, schedule, precautions, and potential side effects. Also discuss drug/drug, herb/drug, and food/drug interactions.
- Dietary regimen to ensure adequate intake of calcium.
- Prescribed exercise regimen, including need to avoid movements that twist or compress the spine (e.g., sit-ups).
- Importance of establishing fall prevention measures in the home (e.g., placing handrail in tub or shower, installing night-lights, avoiding use of throw rugs). Arrange for home visit from a nurse or physical therapist as necessary.
- Importance of reporting to health care provider any indicators of pathologic fracture (e.g., deformity, pain, edema, ecchymosis, limb shortening, false motion, decreased ROM, or crepitus) or indicators of vertebral fractures (e.g., paresthesias, weakness, paralysis, or loss of bowel or bladder function) that may signal spinal cord or nerve compression.
- Importance of follow-up care, date of next appointment, and telephone number to call if questions arise.
- Referral to community resources, including local osteoporosis support activities. Resources for information include the following organizations:

National Osteoporosis Foundation: www.nof.org

National Institute of Arthritis and Musculoskeletal and Skin Diseases (NIAMS): www.niams.nih.gov

❖ ❖ ❖

SECTION FOUR **MUSCULOSKELETAL SURGICAL PROCEDURES**

 AMPUTATION

OVERVIEW/PATHOPHYSIOLOGY

Amputation is the removal of part or all of a limb through bone. Lower extremity amputation may be the treatment of choice for complications of diabetes mellitus (DM) such as peripheral vascular disease (PVD) and for osteomyelitis or severe trauma. PVD accounts for most of the lower extremity amputations. Rarely, amputation may be necessary because of congenital limb deficiencies in infants and children. Amputation also may be needed because of metabolic disorders (e.g., Paget's disease) or massive muscle necrosis that results from an acute embolic or thrombotic event. Patient also may have a tumor of bone or soft tissue, but amputation in this case is much less common than in the past because of the advent of sophisticated limb salvage procedures. Although most lower extremity amputations are performed because of disease, most upper extremity amputations are the result of trauma. Amputation and prosthesis use may offer patient improved functional ability.

ASSESSMENT

Signs and symptoms/physical findings: Findings before the amputation are as follows:

Chronic disease: Complaints of extremity pain in a definable muscle group (usually calf muscles) precipitated by exercise and promptly relieved by rest. This pain is distinguished from that of diabetic neuropathy, which is distributed along dermatomes rather than confined to a specific muscle group; neuropathy is also constant and unrelated to exercise. The affected limb is often dark red (rubor) when it is dependent; atrophy of skin and subcutaneous tissue may be apparent.

Trauma: A mangled extremity is common with high-energy injuries. Patient may have multiple injuries, and surgical priority must be given to those injuries that may be life-threatening. Trauma may result in complete amputation, near or partial amputation, or segmental amputation of an extremity.

DIAGNOSTIC TESTS

Ankle-arm index (ankle-brachial index [ABI]): The most widely used non-invasive test for evaluating PVD. BP is measured at the ankle and in the arm while patient is at rest. Measurements are then repeated at both sites after patient has walked 5 min on a treadmill. ABI is calculated by dividing the highest BP at the ankle by the highest recorded pressure in either arm. ABI results are used to predict severity of the vascular disease (**BOX 9-3**). Decreased ABI with exercise is a sensitive indicator that significant PVD is present.

Doppler ultrasound: Evaluates blood flow to the extremities. It can reliably distinguish exercise-related effects from severe ischemia.

Transcutaneous O_2 pressure: Measured after O_2 sensors are applied to the skin. By determining O_2 tension (desired value is 30-50 mm Hg), the surgeon can map out areas of lesser perfusion in the affected extremity. This test offers the most accurate assessment of blood supply and the best prediction of residual limb healing potential.

Angiography: Confirms circulatory impairment to determine appropriate level for amputation. This invasive study involves radiographic imaging after injection of a radiopaque substance into a blood vessel.

Single photon emission computed tomography (SPECT): Uses a radioactive isotope (xenon-133) injected intradermally at the midpoint of the intended incision for amputation. Skin clearance of this agent reflects skin blood flow as a measure of the appropriate level of amputation.

COLLABORATIVE MANAGEMENT

Amputation: An open (guillotine) amputation is performed when patient has a severe infection that requires immediate treatment. To prevent retraction, traction may be applied to the skin flaps and the wound left open; wound closure is performed at a later time. Skin grafting may be needed to obtain closure if the wound has no skin flaps. Patients who are candidates for this procedure also may have other debilitating illnesses that preclude the longer anesthesia time needed for a closed procedure. Closed amputation is more commonly performed for treatment of vascular disease than for trauma or infection. Skin flaps are prepared and closed over the surgical site at the time of the primary procedure.

BOX 9-3	ANKLE-BRACHIAL INDEX RESULTS
ABI VALUE	**INTERPRETATION**
1.0-1.3	Normal range
0.08-0.99	Some arterial disease/mild blockage
0.5-0.79	Moderate arterial disease/moderate blockage
Less than 0.5	Severe arterial disease/severe blockage

ABI, Ankle-brachial index.

Selection of the level of amputation depends on the degree of pain, infection, or necrosis. In addition, sufficient residual limb must remain to enable fitting with a functional prosthesis. Blood supply at the level of amputation must be adequate to achieve skin healing. Individuals with lower extremity amputations expend more energy in ambulation than people without amputations. Ambulation with a below-knee amputation (BKA) requires 40% more energy; 60% more energy is expended with an above-knee amputation (AKA).

Postoperative care: Focuses on pain management with attention to phantom limb sensation, promotion of residual limb healing, prevention of complications such as contracture or infection, and assistance with attaining optimal mobility through a prescribed rehabilitation program.

Pharmacotherapy

ANALGESICS: For postoperative pain. Use of patient-controlled analgesia (PCA) in the immediate postoperative period facilitates early ambulation that helps in preventing flexion contractures. Epidural medication for PCA may provide better postoperative pain control.

ANTIBIOTICS: To prevent infection in surgical area.

TRICYCLIC ANTIDEPRESSANTS (e.g., AMITRIPTYLINE, DOXEPIN): Used to elevate mood and alleviate insomnia.

β-BLOCKERS (e.g., PROPRANOLOL): May be used to control a constant dull ache.

ANTICONVULSANTS (e.g., PHENYTOIN, CARBAMAZEPINE): May be used to treat stabbing pain.

Prosthestic consultation: Prosthetic technology has advanced in recent years. Proper fitting and teaching how to apply and use the device are very important. Patient should be referred to a prosthetist for evaluation.

Physical therapy (PT): To assist patient in the use of supportive devices and exercises to maintain strength and flexibility.

Psychologic assessment: Should be done along with supporting patient in psychosocial recovery following amputation. Whether amputation is the result of trauma, chronic illness, or cancer, patient is likely to experience a period of grieving. Disbelief and anger often mark patient's initial response. Patient may believe that attainment of independence and future goals is unlikely. Insomnia and somatic complaints are common. Later, as patient begins to adjust to the amputation, sadness and tears are often observed. Patient typically retains a stereotyped image of disability and unattractiveness following amputation. Sometimes these emotions are suppressed during rehabilitation and reemerge as time passes.

NURSING DIAGNOSES AND INTERVENTIONS

Risk for disuse syndrome related to severe pain and immobility secondary to amputation

Desired outcomes: Within 24 hr of instruction, patient verbalizes understanding of the prescribed exercise regimen and performs exercises independently. Patient is free of symptoms of contracture as evidenced by complete range of motion (ROM) of joints and maintenance of muscle mass.

Nursing Interventions

- Manage patient's pain. This helps to encourage optimal movement.
- Elevate affected extremity for first 24 hr postoperatively. Assist in performance of ROM exercises. *This preserves the mobility of proximal joints.* Elevation and ROM exercises are indicated only if prescribed by health care provider. *A residual limb with deficient vascular supply must not be elevated.*
- On the second postoperative day, ensure that patient keeps residual limb flat when at res. *This is to decrease risk for flexion contracture.* Other

strategies to prevent contracture include assisting patient to lie prone for 1-hr periods 4 ×/day and teaching patient to perform prescribed exercises that increase strength of muscle extensors. Prescribed exercises may include the following:

- *AKA:* Have patient attempt to straighten hip from a flexed position against resistance or perform gluteal-setting exercises.
- *BKA:* Have patient attempt to straighten knee against resistance or perform quadriceps exercises. Patient also should perform exercises for AKA.

Deficient knowledge related to care of the residual limb and prosthesis; signs and symptoms of skin irritation or pressure necrosis

Desired outcomes: Within 24 hr of hospital discharge, patient verbalizes knowledge about care of the residual limb and prosthesis and independently returns demonstration of wrapping the residual limb. Patient verbalizes knowledge about indicators of pressure necrosis and irritation from the shrinkage device or prosthesis.

Nursing Interventions

- Assess patient's facility with language; engage an interpreter or provide language-appropriate written materials if necessary.
- For the first 24 hr after surgery, elevate residual limb as prescribed. *This is to reduce edema.* After this period, the lower residual limb should be kept flat when patient is at rest in bed. *This is to reduce risk of flexion contracture.* When patient is in a chair, lower residual limb is elevated. *This is to reduce dependent edema.*
- If molding of residual limb for eventual prosthesis fitting is prescribed, teach application of a shrinkage device such as an elastic wrap or sock. Application of elastic wrap is begun with a recurrent turn over the distal end of the residual limb; then diagonal circumferential turns are made, overlapping to two-thirds the width of the wrap. The shrinkage device should be snug but not too tight *to prevent impeding circulation and healing.* Ensure that all tissue is contained by the elastic wrap; if any tissue is allowed to bulge, proper fitting of prosthesis will be difficult. Rewrapping, combined with careful inspection of residual limb, should be performed q4h.
- Provide extra padding with moleskin or lamb's wool. *This is to prevent irritation to areas that are susceptible to pressure.*
- Teach patient to monitor residual limb for indicators of skin irritations or pressure necrosis caused by shrinkage device or prosthesis, including abrasions, blisters, and hair follicle infection. Explain that if erythema persists after massage, patient should notify health care provider.
- Instruct patient to leave any open areas on residual limb to air for 1-hr periods 4 ×/day. *This is to facilitate healing.*
- Teach a daily routine of skin cleansing with soap and water. Instruct patient to dry residual limb thoroughly before any shrinkage device is applied. The shrinkage device must be changed daily, washed with mild soap and water, and dried thoroughly before reapplication.
- Instruct patient to begin to massage residual limb 3 wk postoperatively. This helps to desensitize the area. Massage will break up adherent scar tissue and prepare skin for stress of prosthesis wear.
- Ensure that patient receives instructions in care of prosthesis by a certified prosthetist-orthotist or nurse expert.

Acute pain or **Chronic pain** related to phantom limb sensation

Desired outcome: Within 24 hr of intervention, patient's subjective perception of pain decreases as documented by pain intensity rating scale.

Nursing Interventions

◆ Ensure adequate pain management before elective surgery. *This is to decrease likelihood that phantom limb sensation will develop.*

◆ Explain that continued sensations often arise postoperatively from amputated part and may be painful, irritating, or simply disconcerting.

◆ Assist in use of a pain intensity rating scale on a scale of 0 (no pain) to 10 (worst pain imaginable). *This is to to evaluate pain and analgesic relief.*

◆ Administer simple analgesics, nonsteroidal antiinflammatory drugs (NSAIDs), opioid analgesics, and adjuncts as prescribed, and reassess their effectiveness in approximately 1 hr using pain intensity rating scale. Although opioids provide effective treatment of incisional pain, they may be ineffective for phantom limb sensation. *This is because they do not alter response of afferent nerves to noxious stimuli.* β-Blockers may be used to control a constant dull ache. *This is because they increase serotonin levels and thus prevent pain transmission to the brain.* Anticonvulsants may be used. *They help control treat stabbing pain.* Tricyclic antidepressants may be used to elevate mood and alleviate insomnia. *They also increase serotonin levels in the brain.* Capsaicin cream may be applied near the surgical wound as a topical analgesic.

◆ Teach patient to use counterirritation. *This is to manage painful sensations.* Transcutaneous electrical nerve stimulation (TENS) may provide effective short-term management of phantom limb sensation. Also consider interventions such as distraction, guided imagery, relaxation, and biofeedback.

◆ Instruct patient to begin to massage residual limb 3 wk postoperatively. *This is to desensitize the area.* After surgical wound healing is complete, vigorous stimulation of end of residual limb may be prescribed. This can be accomplished by hitting the end of the limb with a rolled towel.

◆ Encourage patient to consider use of other modalities, including sympathetic blocking agents, acupuncture, ultrasound, and injection with local anesthetics. *These may decrease phantom limb sensation.*

◆ Explore impact phantom limb pain may have on patient's ability to function on the job or in interpersonal relationships. Refer to a pain clinic for a comprehensive program to manage chronic phantom limb sensation.

◆ If conservative measures are exhausted and phantom limb sensations continue, encourage patient to discuss possible surgical interventions (e.g., cordotomy, deep brain stimulation, spinal cord stimulation, sympathectomy) with health care provider.

Disturbed body image and/or **Ineffective role performance** related to loss of limb

Desired outcome: Within 72 hr of surgery, patient begins to show adaptation to loss of limb and demonstrates interest in resuming role-related responsibilities.

Nursing Interventions

◆ Encourage use of a prosthesis if prescribed immediately after surgery, *to enable patient to be fully ambulatory (and thus "whole").*

◆ Gently encourage patient to look at and touch residual limb and verbalize feelings about the amputation. Show an accepting attitude and encourage significant other to accept patient's new appearance. Provide privacy for patient and significant other to express feelings regarding the amputation.

◆ Assist patient with adapting to loss of limb while maintaining a sense of what is perceived as the normal self. Introduce patient to others who have successfully adapted to a similar amputation. Use teaching aids such as books, pamphlets, audiovisuals, and videotapes. *These help to demonstrate how others have adapted to amputation.*

◆ Discuss ways patient may alter task performance to continue to function in vocational and interpersonal roles.

◆ For patient who continues to have difficulty adapting to the amputation, provide a referral to an appropriate resource person such as a psychologist or psychiatric nurse.

 ### Patient-Family Teaching and Discharge Planning

When providing patient-family teaching, include verbal and written information about the following:

◆ Medications and supplements, including names, dosage, purpose, schedule, precautions, and potential side effects. Also discuss drug/drug, herb/drug, and food/drug interactions.

◆ How and where to purchase necessary supplies and equipment for self-care.

◆ Care of residual limb and prosthesis.

◆ Indicators of wound infection that require medical attention such as swelling, persistent redness, purulent discharge, local warmth, systemic fever, and pain. Suggest use of a small hand mirror if needed to examine incision and residual limb.

◆ Prescribed exercise regimen, including rationale for each exercise, number of repetitions frequency of each.

◆ Ambulation with assistive devices and prosthesis on level and uneven surfaces and on stairs. Patient should demonstrate independence before hospital discharge. For patient with upper extremity amputation, independence with performance of activities of daily living (ADL) should be demonstrated before discharge.

◆ Importance of follow-up care, date of next appointment, and a telephone number to call if questions arise.

◆ Referral to visiting, public health, or home health nurses as necessary for ongoing care after discharge. Also consider referral to appropriate resource person if patient has continued difficulty with grief or body image disturbance.

◆ Referral to community resources, including local amputation support activities. Resources for information include the following organizations:

Amputee Resource Foundation of America: www.amputeeresource.org

National Amputation Foundation: www.nationalamputation.org

❖ ROTATOR CUFF REPAIR

OVERVIEW/PATHOPHYSIOLOGY

Rotator cuff tear is a common cause of pain and disability among adults. The supraspinatus, subscapularis, infraspinatus, and teres minor muscles comprise the rotator cuff, which enables the shoulder to rotate, flex, and extend. A bursa in the subacromial space provides lubrication for rotator cuff function. The repeated overhead shoulder motion that occurs in activities such as racket sports, throwing, and swimming increases the risk for swelling or minor tears. Most tears occur in the supraspinatus muscle, but other parts of the cuff may be involved. Degeneration often begins in the area between the supraspinatus muscle and the coracohumeral ligament because that area is poorly vascularized. Formation of scar tissue then decreases the subacromial space. The resulting impingement syndrome is actually an overuse injury caused by entrapment of soft tissue between the acromion and the head of the humerus. Further repetitive activity leads to rotator cuff bursitis and tendinitis, which may progress to eventual rupture of the rotator cuff.

ASSESSMENT

Signs and symptoms/physical findings: Symptoms of a rotator cuff tear may develop right away after a trauma, such as a lifting injury or a fall on the affected arm. When the tear occurs with an injury, acute pain, a popping feeling (crepitus), and weakness of the arm may be evident. Symptoms may also develop gradually with continued activity, especially overhead movement, or following long-term wear. Pain in the front of the shoulder radiates down the side of the arm. Initially the pain may be mild and be present only with overhead movements, such as reaching or throwing. It may be relieved by over-the-counter (OTC) medication for pain. Eventually the pain becomes noticeable at rest or with no activity at all. There may be pain when lying on the affected side and at night. Patient may be able to abduct the arm to 45-60 degrees but will have difficulty abducting to 60-121 degrees. This is a painful arc because inflamed structures are being impinged on or pinched by the acromion process.

DIAGNOSTIC TESTS

Usually, diagnosis of rotator cuff injury can be made based on clinical findings.

X-ray examination: Not usually needed unless fracture or blunt trauma has occurred. It can be useful in depicting calcific deposits or in ruling out acromioclavicular joint arthritis.

MRI: Provides the best imaging mode for diagnosing rotator cuff abnormalities and also detects early tendinitis.

Arthroscopy: The best diagnostic tool. Clinical findings are also important, but distinction must be made among a complete tear, a partial tear, and a cuff inflammation.

COLLABORATIVE MANAGEMENT

Partial tears and cuff inflammation: Treated conservatively with rest, ice, compression, and elevation (RICE), followed by heat and rest from activity for at least 1 wk. Injections of lidocaine and a corticosteroid may be indicated for pain relief if improvement does not result from conservative treatment. A rehabilitation program is designed to strengthen the rotator cuff complex.

Complete tears: May be directly examined by arthroscopy. Debridement of the subacromial bursa, with resection of the coracoacromial ligament and the inferior acromion, may be performed to increase the subacromial space and prevent recurrence. Larger tears may require open surgical repair. Postoperative care includes pain management, instruction on the use of a shoulder immobilizer, and introduction of a stepped exercise program that often starts with gentle pendulum shoulder movement. Patient is often advised not to perform exercises that stress the supraspinatus.

Pharmacotherapy
Analgesics: For postoperative pain.
Antibiotics: To prevent infection in surgical area.

NURSING DIAGNOSES AND INTERVENTIONS

Acute pain related to surgical repair and rehabilitation therapy
Desired outcomes: Within 1-2 hr of intervention, patient's subjective perception of pain decreases as documented by pain intensity rating scale. Patient demonstrates ability to perform activities of daily living (ADL) with minimal complaints of discomfort.

Nursing Interventions

◆ Assist patient in use of pain intensity rating scale of 0 (no pain) to 10 (worst pain imaginable). *This is to evaluate pain and effectiveness of analgesics.*
◆ Administer simple analgesics, nonsteroidal antiinflammatory drugs (NSAIDs), and opioid analgesics as prescribed, and reassess their effectiveness in approximately 1 hr using pain intensity rating scale.
◆ Advise patient to coordinate time of peak effectiveness of analgesics with periods of exercise or ambulation.
◆ Supplement other pain management strategies with traditional nursing interventions such as back rubs, repositioning, and encouraging patient to verbalize feelings regarding impact of the injury.

Dressing, bathing self-care deficit related to physical limitations secondary to immobilized shoulder
Desired outcome: Within 48 hr of initiation of immobilization, patient demonstrates independence with ADL.

Nursing Interventions

◆ Use assistive devices liberally, especially if surgery is on patient's dominant side. These may include a sock donner, long-handled reacher, and enlarged handles on eating utensils. *This is to maximize independence in self-care.*
◆ As appropriate, use adaptive clothing to accommodate immobilized arm.
◆ Refer to physical therapist (PT) for exercises prescribed.
◆ Ensure that patient receives appropriate treatment as prescribed for pain. *This is because pain management is an essential element for enhancing self-care.*
◆ When needed, teach significant other how to assist patient with self-care activities.

 Patient-Family Teaching and Discharge Planning

When providing patient-family teaching, include verbal and written information about the following:
◆ Medications and supplements, including names, dosage, purpose, schedule, precautions, and potential side effects. Also discuss drug/drug, herb/drug, and food/drug interactions.
◆ Any precautions related to wound care and signs of infection (i.e., persistent redness or pain, swelling or localized warmth, fever, purulent drainage) or other complications of surgery.
◆ Use of prescribed shoulder immobilization device.
◆ Prescribed exercise regimen, including rationale for each exercise, number of repetitions, and frequency of each exercise.
◆ Strategies for dressing and grooming that do not subject the operative site to unnecessary stress before activity prescription has been advanced by the health care provider.
◆ Importance of follow-up care, date of next appointment, and a telephone number to call if questions arise.

❖ BONE GRAFTING

OVERVIEW/PATHOPHYSIOLOGY

A bone graft procedure involves transferring cancellous and cortical bone from one site to another. The bone is typically taken from patient (autograft) or from another human donor (allograft). The most successful results are achieved with autografts, but allografts of donated cadaver bone are widely used for reconstructing serious bone defects. Allograft tissue can be used to fill a traumatic defect with bone chips, or it can be placed at a fracture site to facilitate healing. Depending on patient's condition, allografts occasionally are combined with metal hardware or implants. Spinal fusion currently represents the primary use of allograft.

ASSESSMENT

Signs and symptoms/physical findings: Bone grafting is used to repair bone fractures that are extremely complex, pose a significant health risk to patient, or fail to heal properly. Identification of appropriate candidates for limb salvage surgery through bone grafting is a time-consuming procedure. Patients with diagnosed osteosarcomas, chondrosarcomas, Ewing sarcomas, and other malignancies are likely candidates for allograft surgery as a means of limb salvage. Their prognosis may be poor, but their quality of life may be improved dramatically with this procedure. A potential donor undergoes strict screening that includes physical examination, comprehensive medical history, and social risk review.

DIAGNOSTIC TESTS

X-ray examination: Used to identify bone defects.
Bone scan: Used to rule out osteomyelitis.
Other tests: Donor information is compared against criteria established by the U.S. Public Health Service. In addition, tissue is held in quarantine until microbiologic and blood tests are completed. Tests required by the American Association of Tissue Banks (AATB) and the U.S. Food and Drug Administration include those for infection human immunodeficiency virus (HIV), hepatitis B and C, and syphilis. Determination of blood compatibility between donor and recipient is not necessary except in the case of rhesus (Rh)–negative women of childbearing age.

COLLABORATIVE MANAGEMENT

Bone graft procedure: Procurement of allograft bone is performed under strict aseptic conditions. Femoral heads may be taken from living donors during primary total hip arthroplasty (THA) surgery. Cadaveric bone is procured at the end of a multiorgan retrieval, preferably in a hospital operating room (OR), because freshly harvested and frozen bone is structurally stronger than bone harvested in a mortuary. Bone retrieved in a mortuary may be weakened by the necessary sterilization with irradiation. Cadaveric bones are often long bones or sections of pelvis that cannot be stored in small sealed plastic containers. Instead, larger bones are covered with sterile wraps and sealed in two sterile plastic bags. Before storage, the bone segment is swabbed with a microbiologic culture solution to ensure that contamination in handling has not occurred during retrieval. Packaged bone sections are labeled and identified by number before being sent for quarantine in the freezer of a bone bank. Because blood and bone marrow are removed during processing, allograft tissue is not living bone.

Frozen bone is thawed and reconstituted with sterile fluids. A great deal of time may be spent by the surgeon in preparing the bone for placement into the surgical site. The allograft must be carefully seated to facilitate union of the graft with the recipient's bone. Large areas of bone resection also often require muscle flaps for adequate coverage of the reconstructed limb.

Bone graft replacement: Also available for clinical use to circumvent the need for harvested bone. Bone morphogenetic proteins (BMPs) are capable of inducing any portion of the bone formation cascade.

Postoperative care: Similar to postoperative care provided to any general orthopedic surgical patient, the graft recipient should have regular neurovascular assessments and be watched closely for signs of deep vein thrombosis (DVT). In addition, splints or braces may be prescribed to protect the graft until union occurs. Wound drains may be placed intraoperatively and output closely monitored. The allograft recipient who is also immunosuppressed as a result of chemotherapy and radiation is most susceptible to infection.

Pharmacotherapy

ANALGESICS: For postoperative pain.

ANTIBIOTICS: To prevent infection in surgical area.

NURSING DIAGNOSES AND INTERVENTIONS

Acute pain related to surgical repair and rehabilitation therapy

Desired outcomes: Within 1-2 hr of intervention, patient's subjective perception of pain decreases as documented by pain intensity rating scale. Patient demonstrates ability to perform activities of daily living (ADL) with minimal complaints of discomfort.

Nursing Interventions

◆ Assist patient in use of pain intensity rating scale of 0 (no pain) to 10 (worst pain imaginable). *This is to evaluate pain and effectiveness of analgesics.*
◆ Administer simple analgesics, nonsteroidal antiinflammatory drugs (NSAIDs), and opioid analgesics as prescribed, and reassess their effectiveness in approximately 1 hr using pain intensity rating scale.
◆ Advise patient to coordinate time of peak effectiveness of analgesics with periods of exercise or ambulation.
◆ Supplement other pain management strategies with traditional nursing interventions such as back rubs, repositioning, and encouraging patient to verbalize feelings regarding impact of the injury.

Impaired physical mobility related to musculoskeletal pain and immobilization devices

Desired outcomes: By at least 24 hr before hospital discharge, patient maintains appropriate body alignment with immobilizer in place. Patient verbalizes understanding of use of analgesics and adjunctive methods to decrease pain when performing prescribed exercises or activity.

Nursing Interventions

◆ Teach proper body alignment, most commonly with joints in neutral position. If an orthotic device is used to maintain position, teach application of the device and assessment of areas of excess pressure beneath the device. *This is to prevent the risk of tissue necrosis.* Teach exercises and ROM to do when the device is removed.
◆ Teach patient and significant other active and/or passive ROM of adjacent joints q8h as appropriate.
◆ Instruct patient and significant other in use of analgesics and nonpharmacologic pain management methods.

Patient-Family Teaching and Discharge Planning

◆ When providing patient-family teaching, include verbal and written information about the following:
◆ Medications and supplements, including names, dosage, purpose, schedule, precautions, and potential side effects. Also discuss drug/drug, herb/drug, and food/drug interactions.
◆ Any precautions related to wound care and signs of infection (i.e., persistent redness or pain, swelling or localized warmth, fever, purulent drainage) or other complications of surgery.
◆ Activity restrictions and use of prescribed immobilization device.
◆ Importance of follow-up care, date of next appointment, and telephone number to call if questions arise.
◆ Referral to community resources, including the following organizations:

American Red Cross: www.redcross.org

AlloSource: www.allosource.org

❖ TOTAL HIP ARTHROPLASTY

OVERVIEW/PATHOPHYSIOLOGY

Total hip arthroplasty (THA) involves surgical resection of the hip joint and its replacement with an endoprosthesis. THA may be necessary for conditions such as osteoarthritis (OA), rheumatoid arthritis (RA), Legg-Calvé-Perthes disease, avascular necrosis (AVN) of the hip joint, and benign or malignant bone tumors. Because conservative treatments usually fail to decrease the impact of disease on patient's functional ability, surgery becomes the next best alternative. Arthroscopy, osteotomy, excision, or arthrodesis (joint fusion) may be considered before patient and surgeon choose THA.

THA is more commonly done on older patients, but younger patients with severe disease are also undergoing this procedure. Advanced age is not an absolute contraindication to THA because poor surgical outcomes appear to be related more to comorbidy than to aging alone. Contraindications to surgery include recent or active joint sepsis, arterial impairment or deficit to the extremity, neuropathic joint, and patient's inability to cooperate in postoperative interventions and rehabilitation.

If patient's condition indicates, replacement of only the femoral head can be accomplished with a bipolar or universal endoprosthesis. With THA, however, both femoral and acetabular components are replaced. A typical prosthesis design includes a polyethylene-lined metal cup that fits over a metal femoral component. Metal-on-metal, ceramic-on-polyethylene, and ceramic-on-ceramic components are also used. The ceramic-on-ceramic components show very little wear and have minimal particle debris, thus extending the life of the hip replacement. Components may be secured in place with cement (polymethylmethacrylate [PMMA]), or noncemented components with porous or roughened surfaces may be chosen to enable bony ingrowth. Because cemented components typically allow early weight bearing, they may be ideal for patient whose activities do not place great demand on the joint but who would benefit from early mobility. The noncemented arthroplasty requires early weight-bearing restriction but accepts more strenuous activity after patient's recovery. It is typically used on younger patients. Newer techniques have been developed that allow surgeons to perform hip replacement through two small incisions and with minimal muscle dissection. The surgeon uses x-ray assistance rather than direct visualization to position the replacement hip. This procedure is less invasive, so patient's hospital stay and recuperative period are shorter.

Postoperative complications include infection, breakage, dislocation, and aseptic loosening of components. Risk of dislocation remains high until the periarticular tissues heal around the endoprosthesis (approximately 6 wk). If dislocation occurs once, the potential for recurrence is increased because of stretching of the periarticular tissues. A confirmed dislocation is treated with closed reduction using general anesthesia. Recurrent dislocations may require revision arthroplasty or surgery to tighten periarticular tissues. Patient is also at risk for deep vein thrombosis (DVT).

DIAGNOSTIC TESTS

Routine tests are combined with patient's history and physical findings to confirm the presence of conditions that necessitate THA. Presurgical tests may be determined by patient's history and comorbidity.

X-ray examination: Commonly required, with patient bearing weight for the anteroposterior (AP) view, to enable assessment of bone shape and quality.

COLLABORATIVE MANAGEMENT

Surgical procedure: THA is performed most often using a posterolateral approach. However, the anterolateral approach may be used because of its decreased risk for dislocation. PMMA may be used as a cement to hold the prosthetic components in place, or special porous-coated prostheses may be used to enable bony ingrowth that will fix the device internally. The acetabulum is prepared and the component placed before the intermedullary canal of the femur is reamed to accept the femoral prosthesis. A passive wound drain may be inserted into the deeper layers of the surgical bed; the amount of drainage is monitored during each shift until patient has achieved hemostasis, and then the drain is removed. Wound closure is accomplished with sutures for the inner layers of tissue and staples for the external incision.

Blood replacement: Although THA has resulted in significant postoperative blood loss, improved techniques have decreased surgical time and resulted in less postoperative bleeding. Because of the perceived dangers of disease transmission (e.g., human immunodeficiency virus (HIV) infection, hepatitis, cytomegalovirus infection, Epstein-Barr virus infection, syphilis, malaria) from the general pool of donated blood, transfusion of patient's own previously banked blood (autologous transfusion), which carries no danger of disease transmission, has become the standard of care for blood loss following THA. Perioperative blood salvage with reinfusion is another treatment option. Postoperative collection is also possible via drainage tubes that empty through a filter into a blood salvage canister. Various devices allow collection and infusion of either whole blood or centrifuged, washed RBCs.

Postoperative activity: Following THA using the posterolateral approach, patient may use an abduction wedge to prevent internal rotation and keep the hip in an abducted position. Avoidance of flexion past 90 degrees is required to decrease risk of dislocation. Following THA using an anterolateral approach, patient must avoid external rotation and adduction. For patient with a cemented prosthesis, the surgeon typically prescribes weight bearing as tolerated. Patient is able to become mobile within 1-2 days because of the immediate fixation of the components. Patients with a noncemented prosthesis will have restricted weight bearing for approximately 6 wk until bony ingrowth into the components has been shown on x-ray film.

Pharmacotherapy

Analgesics: For postoperative pain. Postoperative protocols often call for use of patient-controlled analgesia (PCA) in an attempt to achieve more consistent pain management for patients after THA. Epidural analgesia also has become popular as a pain management strategy because it permits adequate pain relief without some of the side effects of IV medications. Within 1-2 days after surgery, patient should be taking oral analgesics. Once hemostasis has been achieved, nonsteroidal antiinflammatory drugs (NSAIDs) may be prescribed for less severe postoperative pain.

Antibiotics: To prevent infection in surgical area. Infection is a serious complication that may necessitate temporary or permanent removal of the prosthesis. If revision surgery is needed at a later time, because of THA infection, appropriate use of vancomycin-impregnated (or tobramycin) cement may be used.

Anticoagulant therapy: Because of increased risk of DVT with THA. Low-molecular-weight heparin is administered by subcutaneous injection, or oral warfarin is prescribed. Unfractionated heparin also may be used for DVT prevention. External modalities such as antiembolism stockings, intermittent pneumatic compression devices, or venous foot pump compression devices may be used. Calf pumping/ankle circle exercises and early mobilization also help to decrease risk for DVT.

Physical therapy (PT) and occupational therapy (OT): PT generally includes a prescription for muscle strengthening exercises and gait training with a walker or crutches to maximize patient's mobility. Exercises also target upper extremities because weakness of these limbs can make walker use difficult. OT focuses on self-care issues such as dressing, bathing, and toileting through use of assistive devices that may include a long-handled reacher and sock donner.

NURSING DIAGNOSES AND INTERVENTIONS

Deficient knowledge related to appropriate activity precautions to decrease risk for dislocation of the operative hip

Desired outcome: At least 24 hr before hospital discharge, patient verbalizes knowledge about the potential for dislocation of the operative hip and activity precautions that decrease risk for dislocation. (The following discussion relates to the posterolateral approach for THA; other approaches require different positional restrictions.)

Nursing Interventions

- Assess patient's facility with language; engage an interpreter or use language-appropriate written materials if necessary.
- During preoperative instruction, advise patient of the potential for postoperative dislocation.
- Show patient an endoprosthesis and describe how it can be dislocated when positional restrictions are not followed (i.e., flexion of the hip past 90 degrees, internal rotation, or adduction).
- During preoperative instruction, explain and demonstrate use of ambulatory aids and activities of daily living (ADL)-assistive devices. *These will enable independence without violating positional restrictions.*
- After surgery, reinforce position restrictions and discuss activities that may violate restrictions, including pivoting on the operative leg, sitting on a toilet seat of regular height, bending over to tie shoelaces, or crossing legs.
- Advise patient of the need for a long-handled shoehorn, sock donner, long-handled reacher, elastic shoelaces, and raised toilet seat. *These will be needed at home after discharge to prevent dislocation during the 6 wk of bone regrowth.*
- Ensure that patient verbalizes and demonstrates understanding of the positional restrictions and can perform ADL independently using appropriate assistive devices. *This is to ensure safety once patient is at home.*
- Instruct patient to report pain in hip, buttock, or thigh or prolonged limp. *These may be indicators of prosthesis loosening.*
- Instruct patient to use an elevated toilet seat. *This is to avoid flexing the hip past 90 degrees which could cause dislocation.*

Risk for peripheral neurovascular dysfunction related to interrupted arterial blood flow secondary to compression from abduction wedge

Desired outcomes: Patient maintains adequate peripheral neurovascular function distal to operative site as evidenced by warmth, normal color, and ability to dorsiflex foot and feel sensations with testing of the area enervated by peroneal nerve. Patient verbalizes knowledge about peripheral neurovascular complications and importance of promptly reporting signs of impairment.

Nursing Interventions

- Perform neurovascular assessment of operative leg at regular intervals along with VS. *This is because pressure from the abductor wedge can interrupt arterial blood flow and compress the peroneal nerve.* Assess the peroneal nerve that runs superficially by the fibular neck. It is assessed by testing sensation in first web space between the great and second toes and by having patient dorsiflex the foot. *Loss of sensation or movement signals impaired peroneal nerve function and must be promptly reported to health care provider.*
- Ensure that patient is aware the importance of promptly reporting alterations in sensation, strength, movement, temperature, and color of operative extremity. *These may signal neurovascular impairment.*
- Encourage patient to perform prescribed exercises. *These will stimulate circulation to distal extremity.*

Ineffective peripheral tissue perfusion (or risk for same) related to possible development of DVT

Desired outcome: Patient demonstrates adequate tissue perfusion in lower extremities, as evidenced by maintenance of normal skin temperature and color and absence of calf pain and/or swelling.

Nursing Interventions

- Encourage patient to perform calf pumping/ankle circle exercises. *This is to decrease risk for thrombus development.*
- Encourage patient to perform prescribed exercises and participate fully in PT program. *This is to decrease risk for thrombus development. Early mobilization also decreases risk of thrombus formation.*
- Discuss use of anticoagulants and other modalities. Encourage patient to wear antiembolic stockings, intermittent pneumatic compression devices, or venous foot pump compression devices whenever in bed or seated on chair. *These are to decrease risk for thrombus formation.*
- Administer anticoagulants as prescribed and monitor results of any associated blood tests, and ensure that health care provider has been informed of laboratory results.
- Promptly report to health care provider patient's complaints of swelling, warmth, or pain/tenderness along vein tracts in lower extremities.

Patient-Family Teaching and Discharge Planning

When providing patient-family teaching, include verbal and written information about the following:

- Medications and supplements, including names, dosage, purpose, schedule, precautions, and potential side effects. Also discuss drug/drug, herb/drug, and food/drug interactions.
- Any precautions related to wound care and signs of infection (i.e., persistent redness or pain, swelling or localized warmth, fever, purulent drainage), or other complications of surgery.
- Need to consult health care provider about possible prophylactic antibiotics before any minor surgical procedure (e.g., dental surgery).
- Activity and weight-bearing restrictions related to surgical approach and choice of prosthesis.
- Use of prescribed immobilization device such as abductor wedge.
- Prescribed exercise regimen, including how exercise is performed, number of repetitions, and frequency of exercise. Ensure that patient independently demonstrates each exercise.
- For ADL and ambulation, ensure that patient demonstrates independence in use of walker/crutches and assistive devices before hospital discharge.
- Assessment of neurovascular status at least 4 ×/day, including need to immediately report to physician symptoms such as numbness and tingling or coolness in extremity.
- Importance of follow-up care, date of next appointment, and a telephone number to call if questions arise.

❖ TOTAL KNEE ARTHROPLASTY

OVERVIEW/PATHOPHYSIOLOGY

Total knee arthroplasty (TKA) involves surgical resection of the knee joint and its replacement with an endoprosthesis. TKA may be necessary for conditions such as osteoarthritis (OA), rheumatoid arthritis (RA), gouty arthritis, hemophilic arthritis, and severe knee trauma. Because conservative treatments have failed to decrease the impact of disease on functional ability in most patients, surgery is the next best alternative. Arthroscopy, osteotomy, excision, or arthrodesis (joint fusion) may be considered before patient and surgeon choose TKA.

Contraindications to surgery include recent or active sepsis in the joint, arterial impairment or deficit in the extremity, neuropathic joint, and inability of patient to cooperate in postoperative interventions and rehabilitation. Infection in the operative joint is a possible complication, with increased risk for patients with diabetes mellitus (DM), immunosuppression, or significant peripheral vascular disease (PVD). Incidence of deep vein thrombosis (DVT) is significant if prophylaxis is not initiated. Risk of dislocation is minimal, but component loosening is a long-term complication that may necessitate revision arthroplasty. A hematoma may form within the tissues after surgery or trauma. A tourniquet is often used during TKA to restrict blood flow in the operative field. The tourniquet may be left in place until wound closure is complete and a dressing applied, so major bleeding may not be noted during surgery. Even when the tourniquet is removed, it is possible that a bleeding vessel may be overlooked or that bleeding will begin later during patient's recovery.

DIAGNOSTIC TESTS

Routine tests are combined with patient's history and physical findings to confirm the presence of conditions that necessitate TKA. Presurgical tests may be determined by patient's history and comorbidity.

Arthroscopy: Useful in confirming extent of joint pathology and in identifying appropriate prosthesis.

X-ray examination: Commonly required, with patient bearing weight to confirm the extent of joint pathology.

COLLABORATIVE MANAGEMENT

Surgical procedure: The surgical approach for TKA is either medial parapatellar or lateral parapatellar. After incision, soft tissue is balanced across the joint to enable trimming of the proximal tibia and distal femur to fit the prosthesis. The trimmed bony surfaces are prepared to accept either cemented or noncemented components, which are chosen according to the demand patient will place on the new joint. The patella is resurfaced with a polyethylene button after ensuring that it will track appropriately during flexion and extension. A passive wound drain may be inserted into deeper layers of the surgical bed; the amount of drainage is monitored during each shift until patient has achieved hemostasis, and then the drain is removed. Wound closure is accomplished with sutures for the inner layers of tissue and staples for the external incision.

Blood replacement: Blood loss during knee surgery may be somewhat controlled via a thigh tourniquet, but postoperative wound drainage may result in need for transfusion. See discussion under "Total Hip Arthroplasty," p. 614.

PT/postoperative activity: Continuous passive movement (CPM) may be prescribed to help patient gain early ROM of operative joint. The CPM machine rests on patient's bed, and the operative extremity is positioned in two slings (one above and one below the knee) in the device. The machine then moves the leg through prescribed ROM in preset timed cycles. For initial application, the CPM machine is set as prescribed at 0-10 degrees of extension and 30-45 degrees of flexion. Daily progression during patient's hospitalization is directed toward achieving 90-110 degrees of flexion. The device should be used at least 6-8 hr daily for optimal benefit. Patient's progress and tolerance of the CPM should be reassessed at regular intervals. Instead of using CPM, some surgeons prescribe early and extended physical therapy (PT) to maximize joint ROM. PT generally includes a prescription for muscle strengthening exercises and for gait training with a walker or crutches to maximize patient's mobility. Exercises also target the upper extremities because weakness of these limbs can make walker use difficult. For patient with a cemented prosthesis, the surgeon usually prescribes weight bearing as tolerated. Patients usually become mobile within 1-2 days because of the immediate fixation of the components. Patients with a noncemented prosthesis will have restricted weight bearing for approximately 6 wk until bony ingrowth into the components has been shown on x-ray film.

Pharmacotherapy

Analgesics: For postoperative pain. Postoperative protocols often call for use of patient-controlled analgesia (PCA) in an attempt to achieve more consistent pain management for patients after TKA. Epidural analgesia also has become popular as a pain management strategy; it permits adequate pain relief without some of the side effects of IV medications. Within 1-2 days after surgery, patient should be taking oral analgesics. Once hemostasis has been achieved, nonsteroidal antiinflammatory drugs (NSAIDs) may be prescribed for less severe postoperative pain.

Antibiotics: To prevent infection in surgical area. Infection is a serious complication that may necessitate temporary or permanent removal of the prosthesis. If revision surgery is needed at a later time, because of TKA infection, appropriate use of vancomycin (or tobramycin)-impregnated cement may be used.

Anticoagulant therapy: Risk of thrombus formation is less for patients following TKA than following total hip arthroplasty (THA). However, anticoagulants are commonly prescribed. Low-molecular-weight heparin is administered by subcutaneous injection, or oral warfarin is prescribed. Unfractionated heparin also may be used for DVT prevention. External modalities such as antiembolism stockings, intermittent pneumatic compression devices, and venous foot pump compression devices typically are used. Calf pumping/ankle circle exercises and early mobilization also help to decrease risk for DVT.

Edema/pain management: A commercial iced knee cuff with automatic ice slush circulator (cryotherapy) may be used to limit edema formation and for pain control.

NURSING DIAGNOSES AND INTERVENTIONS

Risk for deficient fluid volume related to postoperative hemorrhage or hematoma formation

Desired outcome: Within 36 hr of surgery, patient is free of symptoms of excessive bleeding or hematoma formation, as evidenced by maintenance of heart rate (HR), respiratory rate (RR), and BP within patient's normal range, balanced I&O, output from wound drain 50 mL/hr or less, brisk capillary refill (less than 2 sec or consistent with preoperative assessment), peripheral pulses 2+ or more on 0-4+ scale, and warmth and normal color in the operative extremity distal to the surgical site.

Nursing Interventions

- When taking vital signs (VS), monitor drainage from wound drainage system and on surgical dressing. Promptly report to health care provider output from drainage system that exceeds 50 mL/hr. *This may cause a fluid volume deficit.*
- Carefully evaluate patient's VS, subjective complaints, and neurovascular activity. Promptly report to health care provider patient complaints of warmth beneath dressing, sensation of "things crawling" under dressing, increasing pressure or pain, or coolness distal to area of surgery. *These findings may indicate hemorrhage or hematoma formation.*
- Reassess VS at regular intervals for indications of shock or hemorrhage, including hypotension and increasing pulse rate. Promptly report abnormal findings to health care provider.
- Reassess at regular intervals for pallor, decreased posterior tibial or dorsalis pedis pulses, slowed capillary refill, or coolness of distal extremity. *These findings may indicate hemorrhage or hematoma formation.*

◆ If hemorrhage or hematoma formation is suspected, notify health care provider promptly. Prescriptions may include limb elevation or application of elastic wrap to provide direct pressure on site of bleeding.

◆ If patient's VS are indicative of shock related to suspected hemorrhage or hematoma formation and health care provider is unavailable, the surgical area should be exposed by loosening dressing. *This is to enable direct inspection of the area.* Apply direct pressure. *Direct pressure will usually control hemorrhage.* If not, apply a thigh-high BP cuff over sheet wadding. *This will serve as a tourniquet until health care provider arrives for definitive therapy.*

Ineffective peripheral tissue perfusion (or risk for same) related to possible development of DVT
Desired outcome: Patient demonstrates adequate tissue perfusion in lower extremities, as evidenced by maintenance of normal skin temperature and color and absence of calf pain and/or swelling.

Nursing Interventions

◆ Encourage patient to perform prescribed exercises and participate fully in PT program. *This is to decrease risk for thrombus development.* Early mobilization also decreases risk of thrombus formation.

◆ Encourage patient to perform calf pumping/ankle circle exercises. *This is to decrease risk for thrombus development.*

◆ Discuss use of anticoagulants and other modalities. Encourage patient to wear antiembolic stockings, intermittent pneumatic compression devices, or venous foot pump compression devices whenever in bed or seated on chair. *These are to decrease risk for thrombus formation.*

◆ Promptly report to health care provider patient's complaints of swelling, warmth, or pain/tenderness along vein tracts in lower extremities.

Patient-Family Teaching and Discharge Planning

When providing patient-family teaching, include verbal and written information about the following:

◆ Use of CPM machine, if prescribed for home use.

◆ Medications and supplements, including names, dosage, purpose, schedule, precautions, and potential side effects. Also discuss drug/drug, herb/drug, and food/drug interactions.

◆ Any precautions related to wound care and signs of infection (i.e., persistent redness or pain, swelling or localized warmth, fever, purulent drainage), or other complications of surgery.

◆ Need to consult health care provider about possible prophylactic antibiotics before any minor surgical procedure (e.g., dental surgery).

◆ Activity and weight-bearing restrictions.

◆ Prescribed exercise regimen, including how exercise is performed, number of repetitions, and frequency of exercise. Ensure that patient independently demonstrates each exercise.

◆ For activities of daily living (ADL) and ambulation, ensure that patient demonstrates independence in use of walker/crutches and assistive devices before hospital discharge.

◆ Assessment of neurovascular status at least 4 ×/day, including need to report abnormal symptoms to physician.

◆ Importance of follow-up care, date of next appointment, and a telephone number to call if questions arise.

❖❖ UTERINE FIBROIDS

OVERVIEW/PATHOPHYSIOLOGY

Uterine fibroids are the most common tumors of the female pelvis, and they occur in 35%-50% of women, with diagnosis most often between ages 35 and 50 yr. Fibroids are benign neoplasms composed of smooth muscle cells. They range in size from very small to extremely large—more than 100 lb—and are most often multiple. Fibroids are caused by the hormones estrogen and progesterone and other factors. They rarely occur before menarche and usually disappear after menopause. Fibroids are most commonly located in the uterine body, where they are described as submucosal, intramural, or subserosal, depending on their location in the myometrium, They also occur in the cervix and broad ligament. Fibroids are the most common reason for hysterectomy.

ASSESSMENT

Signs and symptoms/physical findings: The patient is asymptomatic in 60%-90% of cases. Menorrhagia, chronic dull backache, dysmenorrhea, pelvic pressure, and dyspareunia can occur. If the tumor is large, abdominal distortion can occur. Depending on location, tumors can cause urinary symptoms (frequency, urgency, incontinence, retention) or gastrointestinal (GI) symptoms (rectal pressure, constipation). Infertility, habitual abortion, or premature labor may also occur. Uterine shape is irregular, and size usually is greater than normal. Determination of size is based on equivalent gestational size for the pregnant uterus. A uterus of greater than 12-wk gestational size is considered large and usually can be palpated on abdominal examination.

DIAGNOSTIC TESTS

Ultrasound: Provides information on uterine volume, number of fibroids, and their location. In addition, the adnexa and abdominal cavity are evaluated for other possible causes of symptoms, such as hydronephrosis of the kidney, ovarian neoplasms, and adenomyosis.

MRI: More accurate than ultrasound, it can differentiate among fibroids, adenomyosis, and solid adnexal masses. However, cost is usually prohibitive.

COLLABORATIVE MANAGEMENT

Most fibroids decrease by 40%-60% at menopause, which is the natural endpoint to their growth.

Gonadotropin-releasing hormone (GnRH) agonists: Decrease anemia and tumor size before surgery and thus allow use of optimal surgical techniques.

Maximum effect is usually seen about 12 wk after start of medication, with an approximately 50% decrease in tumor size. However, regrowth to previous size occurs within 6 mo after discontinuation of these agents. Side effects include those found in hypoestrogenic states (e.g., bone demineralization, hot flashes, mood changes, vaginal dryness).

Hysteroscopic resection: Removes submucous fibroids via a hysteroscope inserted vaginally using electrocautery and laser. Incomplete resection is common.

Endometrial ablation: Destroys submucous fibroids via hysteroscope using either laser or electrosurgical techniques or with balloon technology.

Uterine artery embolization: Uses small injected particles to block the arteries supplying the fibroids, thereby cutting off blood supply and causing the tumors to shrink.

Focused ultrasound surgery: Noninvasive, magnetic resonance imaging (MRI)-guided procedure that removes the fibroids and preserves the uterus.

Myomectomy: Removes tumor surgically via laparascope or laparotomy; preserves fertility but increases the risk of adhesions and uterine rupture during subsequent pregnancy.

Hysterectomy: Surgical removal of the uterus. It can be through a vaginal, abdominal, or laparoscopically assisted vaginal approach.

Total abdominal hysterectomy with bilateral salpingo-oophorectomy (TAH-BSO): For women who desire to decrease risk of ovarian cancer or manage pathology involving the ovaries.

NURSING DIAGNOSES AND INTERVENTIONS

Acute pain related to surgery

Desired outcomes: Within 1 hr of intervention, patient's subjective perception of pain decreases, as documented by pain scale. Objective indicators, such as grimacing, are absent or diminished.

Nursing Interventions

◆ Evaluate for incisional pain as well as referred pain to the shoulders from the diaphragm resulting from accumulation of gas used during the procedure.

◆ Provide back rubs, which are especially helpful for patients who were in the lithotomy position during surgery.

◆ For other interventions, see "Pain," p. 13, in Chapter 1.

Risk for deficient fluid volume related to operative or postoperative bleeding

Desired outcomes: Patient is normovolemic, as evidenced by BP 90/60 mm Hg or greater (or within patient's usual range), heart rate (HR) 60-100 beats per minute (bpm), urinary output 30 mL/hr or greater, respiratory rate (RR) 20 breaths/min or less with normal depth and pattern (eupnea), skin dry and of normal color, and a soft and nondistended abdomen. Patient and significant other verbalize knowledge about signs and symptoms of excessive bleeding and are aware of the need to alert staff promptly if these findings are noted.

Nursing Interventions

◆ Monitor VS q2-4h during first 24 hr. Be alert to indicators of hemorrhage and impending shock: hypotension, increased pulse and respirations, pallor, and diaphoresis.

◆ Assess postoperative bleeding q2-4h by noting amount and quality of drainage on dressings and perineal pads if abdominal approach was used or on perineal pads alone if vaginal approach was used. Normally, postoperative bleeding is minimal. It should be dark in color (or serosanguineous if an abdominal hysterectomy was performed).

- Inspect abdomen for distention, and assess patient for presence of severe abdominal pain; both are indicators of internal bleeding.
- Review complete blood count (CBC) values for evidence of bleeding: decreases in hemoglobin (Hgb) and hematocrit (Hct). Notify health care provider of significant findings. Optimal values are Hct 37% or greater and Hgb 12 g/dL or greater.
- Inform patient and significant other about signs of excessive bleeding and need to alert staff immediately if they occur.

Impaired urinary elimination (oliguria or anuria) related to inadequate intake, obstruction of indwelling catheter, or ureteral ligation
Desired outcome: Within 24 hr of surgery, patient demonstrates a balanced I&O, with urinary output at least 30 mL/hr immediately following surgery.

Nursing Interventions

- Monitor I&O, and document every shift. Notify health care provider if urinary output falls below 30 mL/hr for 2 hr in the presence of adequate intake. Along with low back pain or costovertebral angle tenderness, this sign can indicate ureteral ligation during surgery.
- Ensure patency of indwelling catheter.
- Administer oral or parenteral fluids as prescribed. Ensure totals of 2-3 L/day in nonrestricted patients.
- Assess for bladder distention by inspecting suprapubic area and percussing or palpating bladder.

Grieving related to actual or perceived loss or changes in body image, body function, or role performance secondary to lost reproductive function with hysterectomy
Desired outcomes: Before hospital discharge, patient and significant other express grief, explain meaning of the loss, and communicate concerns with each other. Patient completes self-care activities as her condition improves.

Nursing Interventions

- Anticipate patient's concern about loss of uterus and "loss of womanhood." Provide emotional support and an unhurried atmosphere for patient and significant other to ask questions and express concerns, frustrations, and fears.
- Recognize covert signs of grief that can accompany self-image disturbances: anger, withdrawal, demanding behavior, or inappropriate affect. Clarify patient's coping behaviors to significant other as necessary.
- For additional interventions, see "Psychosocial Support" for **Anticipatory grieving,** p. 36.

 Patient-Family Teaching and Discharge Planning

Provide verbal and written information about the following areas of self-care to patients who have had a hysterectomy:
- Need to report signs of infection to health care provider: incisional swelling, local warmth around incision, fever, redness, purulent drainage, vaginal bleeding, odorous vaginal discharge, incisional or abdominal pain.
- Care of the incision.
- Restriction of activities as directed, such as heavy lifting (more than 10 lb) and sexual intercourse. Advise patient to get maximum amount of rest and avoid fatigue.
- If ovaries were removed, risks and benefits of estrogen therapy and types available and management of symptoms such as hot flashes, weight gain, altered mood, and changes in sexual response.
- Medications, including drug names, dosage, purpose, schedule, precautions, and potential side effects. Also discuss drug/drug, herb/drug, and food/drug interactions.

- Need for follow-up care; confirm date and time of next medical appointment if known.
- Phone numbers to call if questions or concerns arise following hysterectomy. Additional general information can be obtained by contacting the following organization.

Hysterectomy Educational Resources and Services (HERS) Foundation: E-mail: HERSFdn@earthlink.com: www.Hersfoundation.com

❖ PELVIC ORGAN PROLAPSE

OVERVIEW/PATHOPHYSIOLOGY

A pelvic organ prolapse is a downward displacement of the vaginal walls and/or the uterus as a result of weakness of the supporting muscles and ligaments. In severe cases, tissues may protrude from the vaginal opening. In the past, types of prolapse were described by naming the adjacent organ and included such terms as the following: *cystocele,* bulging of the posterior bladder wall into the vagina; *uterine prolapse,* bulging of the uterus through the pelvic floor into the vagina; *rectocele,* protrusion of the rectum into the posterior vagina; and *enterocele,* herniation of the small bowel into the vagina. Now anatomic descriptions of nine specific sites in the vagina with the hymen as the reference point are used to describe prolapse.

The primary cause of pelvic organ prolapse is a vaginal delivery in which pelvic connective tissue is stretched and torn. Other causes include connective tissue disorders, neuromuscular dysfunction, and surgical procedures, as well as conditions that cause repetitive increased abdominal pressure to the pelvic floor such as chronic cough or a long history of straining with constipation.

ASSESSMENT

Symptoms usually do not appear until menopause or later and are not usually consistent with the degree of prolapse.

Signs and symptoms/physical findings: Vary with the involved organs; can include a sensation of vaginal fullness, heaviness, or of bearing down in the pelvis; low backache (more severe by day's end); inability to empty bladder with voiding; urinary frequency, dysuria, stress incontinence, incontinence resulting from urgency, and recurrent cystitis; dyspareunia or lack of sensation with intercourse; bulging at the introitus; continuous urge to have a bowel movement, constipation, difficulty generating pressure to pass stool (intravaginal digital pressure may be needed to facilitate defecation), incontinence of flatus or feces, and presence of hemorrhoids or fecal impaction. Manual pelvic examination reveals a soft mass that bulges into the vagina. The mass increases in size with coughing or straining and can be more apparent when a divided speculum is used. The pelvic examination provides more information when performed with patient standing. As patient bears down, a firm mass can be palpated in the lower vagina. Diagnosis may be aided with insertion of a pessary (i.e., reduced symptoms after insertion increase likelihood that symptoms are related to pelvic organ prolapse).

DIAGNOSTIC TESTS

Urine culture and sensitivity: Check for bladder infection.
Urodynamic evaluation: Involves study of the flow of urine from the bladder through the urethra to differentiate stress incontinence from urgency incontinence. A combination of tests is used, including voiding flow rate, urethral pressure profile, urethroscopy, and cystometrogram.
Defecography: Dynamic rectal examination using radiographic dye and fluoroscopy to identify rectoanal function during defecation and thereby delineate involved structures.

COLLABORATIVE MANAGEMENT

Urinary catheterization: Empties a distended bladder. This is an emergency measure rather than a permanent correction.

Antibiotics: Given if urinary retention results in an infection.

Estrogen therapy: For urogenital symptoms in the postmenopausal woman. It is provided intravaginally in small daily doses as cream, suppository, or ring and used in combination with a progesterone if the uterus is present. For example, a vaginal ring that delivers a small dose of estradiol may be inserted for 90 days.

Kegel isometric exercises: Help with bladder control.

Pessary: A rubber, plastic, or silicone device inserted into the vagina to support pelvic structures. It may be used if there is prolapse of the uterus or if surgery is contraindicated or unwanted by patient.

High-fiber diet: Aids in bowel elimination.

Hysterectomy: Corrects uterine prolapse. It may be performed abdominally or vaginally, although the latter approach is used if other vaginal surgery is also being performed.

Anterior colporrhaphy: Surgical procedure via vaginal approach to suspend the bladder. It involves separating the anterior vaginal wall from the bladder and urethra, excising the redundant thinned vaginal wall, urethropexy (urethral suspension), plicating the bladder neck, and suturing the remaining vagina to provide support for the bladder.

Posterior colporrhaphy: Surgical procedure via vaginal approach to separate the posterior vaginal wall from the rectum, excise redundant vaginal tissue, and rejoin the rectovaginal septum with sutures to reduce the rectal herniation.

Surgical techniques for stress incontinence: Procedures include those that correct anatomic hypermobility, such as retropubic bladder neck suspension operations, needle suspension procedure, tension-free vaginal tape procedures, and some sling procedures. Procedures that correct intrinsic sphincteric weakness or dysfunction include sling operations and periurethral injections. Salvage operations include implantation of an artificial urinary sphincter and urinary diversion.

NURSING DIAGNOSES AND INTERVENTIONS

Constipation related to restriction against straining, low-residue diet, or pain with defecation secondary to surgical procedure

Desired outcomes: After the early postoperative period, patient reports bowel movements within her normal pattern and with minimal discomfort. Patient verbalizes need to alert staff before and after bowel movements and to avoid straining during defecation.

Nursing Interventions

◆ Administer stool softeners or mild laxatives as prescribed. Ensure that patient drinks a full 8-10 oz of water with each dose.

◆ Unless otherwise contraindicated, push fluids to at least 2500 mL/day or more. Explain that good hydration softens stool.

◆ Expect the patient to be on a low-residue diet during early postoperative period to minimize potential for disruption of surgical site. Subsequently consult health care provider about introducing high-residue foods to promote bowel movements.

◆ Instruct patient to avoid straining when having a bowel movement because this can disrupt surgical repair.

◆ Advise patient that defecation may be painful and to alert staff as soon as urge to defecate is felt so that patient can be medicated before the bowel movement.

◆ Avoid use of enemas or rectal tubes, which can disrupt the surgical repair.

◆ Provide sitz baths as a comfort measure after bowel movements.

- Request that patient notify staff after each bowel movement; document accordingly.

Patient-Family Teaching and Discharge Planning

Provide verbal and written information about the following areas of self-care to patients who have had surgery for a pelvic prolapse:
- Medications, including drug names, purpose, dosage, schedule, precautions, potential side effects, and drug/drug, herb/drug, and food/drug interactions.
- Activity restrictions during first 6 wk or as directed, including no heavy lifting (more than 10 lb) or strenuous exercises. Explain importance of abstinence from sexual intercourse for 6 wk or as prescribed if vaginal surgery was performed. Discuss alternate methods of sexual expression. Advise patient that initially coitus may be painful.
- If discharged with a suprapubic catheter, teach need to monitor postvoid residual (PVR) and how to attach tubing to a drainage bag overnight.
- Importance of notifying health care provider of the following indicators of infection: fever; persistent abdominal or rectal pain; local warmth; purulent, foul-smelling vaginal discharge; urinary retention.
- Kegel exercises (see p. 213) to improve sphincter control and aid in defecation.
- Importance of regular bowel elimination pattern to prevent constipation and straining.
- Importance of a high-fiber diet and a fluid intake of at least 2-3 L/day (unless this is contraindicated by a renal, hepatic, or cardiac disorder). High-fiber foods include bran, whole grains, nuts, and raw and coarse vegetables and fruits with skins.
- Importance of follow-up appointments; confirm date and time of next appointment if known.

SECTION TWO ECTOPIC PREGNANCY

OVERVIEW/PATHOPHYSIOLOGY

An ectopic pregnancy is a fertilized ovum implanted outside the uterus. The most common site is the fallopian tube. Less common sites are the peritoneum, ovary, and cervix. In the fallopian tube, the implanted ovum can weaken the tubal wall, which in a few cases results in rupture that can cause bleeding into the peritoneum, a medical emergency. Factors that predispose to ectopic pregnancy include pelvic inflammatory disease, prior fallopian tube surgery, history of infertility, previous ectopic pregnancy, and smoking. If an intrauterine device (IUD) is in use, a resulting pregnancy, although rare, has an increased risk of being ectopic. These factors can affect the structure and function of the fallopian tube and cause a delay in passage of the ovum into the uterus, with a resulting ectopic pregnancy.

ASSESSMENT

Signs and symptoms/physical findings: Indications of pregnancy (i.e., amenorrhea, nausea, fatigue, breast tenderness, urinary frequency), uterine bleeding or spotting, and abdominal pain. Most symptoms appear 6-8 wk after the last menstrual period. The following acute signs and symptoms may develop before or may accompany rupture: mild to moderate vaginal bleeding with unilateral lower abdominal cramping that becomes increasingly sharp and constant, referred shoulder pain caused by irritation of the diaphragm from the pooling of blood in the peritoneum, and falling hematocrit (Hct) and hemoglobin (Hgb) values. These acute mamfestitions necessitate immediate intervention *to prevent loss of blood, which can lead to shock and death.*

Abdominal palpation may reveal lower quadrant tenderness, as well as size and date discrepancy. If ectopic pregnancy is suspected, pelvic examination is deferred *to minimize risk of tubal rupture.*

DIAGNOSTIC TESTS

CBC: May reveal decreased Hgb and Hct and increased leukocyte count.

Serum human chorionic gonadotropin (hCG): Serial levels plateau and then diminish. There are lower than normal levels of serum progesterone and urinary metabolites of serum progesterone.

Ultrasound: May identify pregnancy location via transvaginal probe. Doppler ultrasound using color identifies the direction of blood flow in relationship to the transducer; abnormal flow patterns in the adnexa may enable identification of ectopic pregnancy.

Laparoscopy: Confirms the presence of ectopic pregnancy and enables immediate treatment.

COLLABORATIVE MANAGEMENT

Methotrexate: Given to select patients who are compliant and asymptomatic and have serum hCG levels less than 5000 units/L, tubal size less than 3 cm, and no fetal cardiac activity. Methotrexate is a folic acid antagonist that induces abrupt tubal abortion. It is given in a single dose. Folic acid supplements are discontinued with use of methotrexate.

Rh$_o$(D) immune globulin (RhoGAM): If indicated, is given to Rh-negative mothers after ectopic pregnancy.

Administration of whole blood or packedred cells: Replaces loss if necessary.

Analgesics/opioids: For pain management.

Laparoscopy: Often used for tube-sparing procedures. Salpingectomy (removal of the fallopian tube) also may be performed through the laparoscope if tubal rupture has occurred.

NURSING DIAGNOSES AND INTERVENTIONS

Risk for deficient fluid volume related to bleeding or hemorrhage with ectopic rupture

Desired outcome: Patient is normovolemic, as evidenced by urinary output 30 mL/hr or more, blood pressure (BP) 90/60 mm Hg or greater, respiratory rate (RR) 20 breaths/min or less with normal depth and pattern (eupnea), heart rate (HR) 100 beats per minute (bpm) or less, warm and dry skin, and absent or scant vaginal bleeding.

Nursing Interventions

◆ Assess VS at frequent intervals, and note changes in BP, HR, and RR. Be alert to hypotension, increases in HR and RR, and cool and clammy skin as indicators of impending shock.

◆ Assess amount and quality of vaginal bleeding. Bright red, frank bleeding, along with abnormal vital signs (VS), should be reported to health care provider at once.

◆ Review results of CBC, and note values of Hgb and Hct that are decreased with blood loss. Optimal values are Hct 37% or higher and Hgb 12 g/dL or higher.

◆ Infuse parenteral and blood products as prescribed.

Ineffective role performance related to fetal loss

Desired outcome: Patient verbalizes change in her role as wife or childbearer or verbalizes plans for adaptation.

Nursing Interventions

- Provide emotional support for patient and significant other. Provide time and a supportive atmosphere for patient to feel comfortable with expressing feelings and concerns. Do not minimize patient's feelings of loss. Conversely, if the pregnancy was not desired, recognize the patient may experience feelings of relief or guilt regarding the loss.
- Assist patient in identifying concerns, if present, with role performance as a wife or childbearer. Assist patient in developing plans for adaptation. Provide referral for genetic counseling if genetics was a factor in pregnancy loss.
- Involve social services if needed.

 Patient-Family Teaching and Discharge Planning

Provide verbal and written information about the following areas of self-care to patients who have had an ectopic pregnancy:

- Medications, including drug names, purpose, dosage, schedule, precautions, and potential side effects. Also discuss drug/drug, food/drug, and drug/herb interactions.
- Importance of monitoring vaginal drainage, including amount, color, consistency, and odor and reporting significant findings to health care provider.
- Activity restrictions as directed, including strenuous exercise, housework, and sexual relations.
- Indicators of incisional infection, including persistent redness, swelling, local warmth, fever, purulent discharge, and incisional/abdominal pain.
- Importance of follow-up care and purpose for serial hCG levels (with more conservative treatment) or methotrexate management; confirm time and date of next medical visit if known.

SECTION THREE **BENIGN PROSTATIC HYPERTROPHY**

OVERVIEW/PATHOPHYSIOLOGY

The prostate is an encapsulated gland that surrounds the male urethra below the bladder neck and produces a thin, milky fluid during ejaculation. As a man ages, the prostate gland grows larger. Although the exact cause of enlargement (benign prostatic hypertrophy [BPH]) is unknown, hormonal changes affecting estrogen/androgen balance appear to be involved. This noncancerous enlargement is found in more than 50% of men over age 50 yr and more than 90% of those over age 70 yr. Treatment is given when symptoms of bladder outlet obstruction appear.

ASSESSMENT

Signs and symptoms/physical findings
Chronic indicators: Urinary frequency, hesitancy, urgency, and dribbling or postvoid dribbling; decreased force and caliber of stream; nocturia (several times each night); hematuria. Scores on American Urological Association (AUA) questionnaire are 0-7 (mild), 8-19 (moderate), and 20-35 (severe).
Acute indicators/bladder outlet obstruction: Anuria, nausea, vomiting, severe suprapubic pain, severe and constant urgency, flank pain during micturition. Bladder is distended, with a kettledrum sound heard when percussed. Rectal examination reveals a smooth, firm, symmetric, and elastic enlargement of the prostate.

DIAGNOSTIC TESTS

Urinalysis: Checks for the presence of WBCs, leukocyte esterase, WBC casts, bacteria, and microscopic hematuria.

Urine culture and sensitivity: Verify the presence of an infecting organism, identifies the type of organism, and determines the organism's antibiotic sensitivities. All urine specimens should be sent to the laboratory immediately after they are obtained, or they should be refrigerated if this is not possible (specimens for urine culture should not be refrigerated) because *urine left at room temperature has a greater potential for bacterial growth, turbidity, and alkaline pH, any of which can distort test results.*

Hct and Hgb: Decreased values may signal mild anemia from local bleeding.

BUN/serum creatinine: Evaluate renal and urinary function. BUN can be affected by patient's hydration status, and results must be evaluated accordingly: fluid volume excess reduces BUN levels, whereas fluid volume deficit increases them. Serum creatinine may not be a reliable indicator of renal function in older adults *because of decreased muscle mass and decreased glomerular filtration rate.* Results of this test must be evaluated along with those of urine creatinine clearance, other renal function studies, and patient's age.

Prostate-specific antigen (PSA): Elevated above normal (0-4.0 ng/mL; normal range may increase with age); correlates well with positive digital examination findings. This glycoprotein is produced only by the prostate and reflects prostate size.

Cystoscopy: Visualizes prostate gland, estimates its size, and ascertains the presence of any damage to the bladder wall secondary to an enlarged prostate. Cystoscopy is contraindicated in patients with acute urinary tract infection (UTI) *because of the danger of hematogenic spread of gram-negative bacteria and the development of septic shock.*

Transrectal ultrasound (TRUS): Assesses prostate size and shape via a probe inserted into the rectum.

Maximal urinary flow rate (MUFR): MUFR less than 15 mL/sec indicates significant obstruction to flow.

Postvoid residual (PVR) volume: A normal volume is less than 12 mL; higher volumes signal obstructive process.

COLLABORATIVE MANAGEMENT

Catheterization: Relieves urinary retention. Because of the high incidence of bacteriuria from indwelling catheterization (50% after the first 24 hr), intermittent catheterization is preferred.

Antibiotics and antimicrobial agents: Treat infection if one is present.

α_1-**Adrenergic receptor blockers:** Relieve symptoms of outflow obstruction by acting to relax the bladder neck and prostatic smooth muscle. When beginning therapy, warn patient that these agents may result in orthostatic changes leading to postural dizziness or syncope; advise patient to change positions slowly to avoid dizziness.

5α-Reductase inhibitors: Inhibit conversion of testosterone to the potent androgen dihydrotestosterone (DHT), which is responsible for development of the prostate; can reduce prostate size in a few months up to a year and thus reduce symptoms. When necessary, inform patient that pregnant women should not handle this medication or semen from a man taking this medication *because of adverse effects on the developing fetus.*

Restriction of rapid intake of fluids (particularly alcohol): Can result in episodes of acute urinary retention from loss of bladder tone secondary to rapid distention.

Phytotherapy: Use of plants and plant extracts for medicinal purposes. Mechanisms of action are unknown. Efficacy and safety of these agents have not been tested in scientifically controlled research studies.

Stents: Placement of a small metal coil, via cystoscopy, into the prostatic urethra to maintain a patent urethra for improved urination. This procedure is usually restricted to patients who are at high surgical risk.

Thermotherapy: Use of heat to reduce prostatic overgrowth. Transurethral microwave thermotherapy (TUMT) uses a special urethral catheter introduced into the prostatic urethra. Transrectal hyperthermia (THT) is applied to the prostate through the rectum via a specially designed rectal probe.

Transurethral incision of the prostate (TUIP): Incisions made into the prostatic urethra via cystoscopy to release bladder neck stricture and improve bladder emptying. This procedure is used in symptomatic men with a small prostate (less than 30 g).

Transurethral needle ablation (TUNA) of the prostate: Introduction of a special probe into the prostatic urethra through which heat and low radiofrequency waves are directed to selected prostatic areas. These waves do not injure the prostatic urethra but destroy the underlying prostatic tissue. This is done to relieve outlet obstructive symptoms and is usually an outpatient procedure.

Prostatectomy: Removal of enlarged prostatic tissue.

Transurethral resection of the prostate (TURP): Resection of prostatic tissue via cystoscopy. This is the most common approach, especially in patients who are poor surgical risks. It is done with patient under general or spinal anesthesia.

Suprapubic transvesical prostatectomy/retropubic extravesical prostatectomy/perineal resection: Removal of prostatic tissue via an incision high in the bladder (abdominal approach), a low abdominal incision without entry into the bladder, or an incision between the scrotum and rectum. These procedures are indicated for a large prostate (40 g or greater) that cannot be removed transurethrally. These approaches may be used if large bladder diverticula or calculi exist that can be corrected at the time of surgery, in the presence of a severe urethral stricture, and with orthopedic conditions that contraindicate positioning for other approaches.

Laser prostatectomy: Use of a laser probe, via cystoscopy, to excise overgrown prostatic tissue to widen the urethra and reduce symptoms. Coagulation necrosis of affected tissue sloughs off and is voided with urine over the following weeks.

NURSING DIAGNOSES AND INTERVENTIONS

Risk for deficient fluid volume related to postsurgical bleeding/hemorrhage
Desired outcomes: Patient is normovolemic, as evidenced by balanced I&O; heart rate (HR) 100 beats per minute (bpm) or less (or within patient's normal range); BP 90/60 mm Hg or more (or within patient's normal range); respiratory rate (RR) 20 breaths/min or less; and skin that is warm, dry, and of normal color. Following instruction, patient identifies actions that may result in hemorrhage of the prostatic capsule and participates in interventions to prevent them.

Nursing Interventions

♦ On patient's return from recovery room, monitor VS as patient's condition warrants or per agency protocol. Be alert to increasing pulse, decreasing BP, diaphoresis, pallor, and increasing respirations, which can occur with hemorrhage and impending shock.

♦ Monitor and document I&O q8h. Subtract amount of fluid used with continuous bladder irrigation (CBI) from total output.

♦ Monitor catheter drainage closely for first 24 hr. Watch for dark red drainage that does not lighten to reddish pink or drainage that remains thick in consistency after irrigation; such findings can signal bleeding within the operative site. Drainage should lighten to pink or blood-tinged within 24 hr after surgery.

♦ Be alert to bright red, thick drainage at any time, which can occur with arterial bleeding within the operative site.

♦ Avoid actions that can result in pressure on the prostatic capsule *because they may lead to hemorrhage.* Do not measure temperature rectally or insert tubes or enemas into the rectum. Instruct patient not to strain with bowel movements or sit for long periods. Obtain prescription for and provide stool softeners or cathartics as necessary. Encourage a diet high in fiber, and increase fluid intake *to aid in producing soft stool.*

◆ The surgeon may establish traction on an indwelling urethral catheter that usually has a large (30 mL) balloon, *to help prevent bleeding.* Maintain traction for 4-8 hr after surgery or as directed.

◆ Monitor patient for signs of disseminated intravascular coagulation (DIC), which can result from release of large amounts of tissue thromboplastins during TURP. Watch for active bleeding (dark red) without clots and unusual oozing from all puncture sites. Report significant findings promptly if they occur. For more information, see "Disseminated Intravascular Coagulation," p. 562.

Risk for infection (septic shock) related to invasive procedure (cystoscopy or TURP) resulting in risk of introducing gram-negative bacteria and leading to septic shock

Desired outcome: Patient is free of gram-negative infection, as evidenced by normothermia; urinary output 30 mL/hr or greater; RR 12-20 breaths/min; HR and BP within patient's normal range; no mental status changes; and orientation to person, place, and time (within patient's normal range).

Nursing Interventions

◆ Monitor VS and mentation status at frequent intervals for indicators of the early (warm) stage of septic shock. During first 24 hr after surgery, be alert to temperatures of 38.3°-40.0° C (101°-104° F), which occur in the presence of infection caused by increased metabolic activity and release of pyrogens. Also assess for moderately increased RR and HR and decreased BP. Classic circulatory signs of collapse occur in the late (cold) stage of septic shock, including profoundly decreased BP (because of decreased stroke volume), greatly increased and weakened HR (compensatory mechanism to maintain cardiac output), and decreased RR (because of respiratory center depression). Mental status changes of inappropriate behavior, personality changes, restlessness, increasing lethargy, and disorientation may signal hypoxia caused by decreased cerebral perfusion.

◆ Monitor patient's skin for flushing and warmth, which are early signs of septic shock caused by vasodilation. In the cold stage of septic shock, skin becomes clammy, cool, and pale because of sustained vasoconstriction.

◆ Monitor urinary output for decrease and for increased concentration (normal specific gravity is 1.010-1.030).

◆ Notify health care provider promptly if septic shock is suspected. Prepare for the following if septic shock is confirmed: IV infusion (e.g., lactated Ringer's or normal saline); oxygen administration; specimens for WBC count, arterial blood gas (ABG) values, and electrolyte values; and administration of antibiotics.

◆ Teach indicators of infection and early septic shock to patient, and stress importance of notifying staff promptly.

Excess fluid volume (or risk for same) related to absorption of irrigating fluid during surgery (TURP syndrome)

Large amounts of fluid, commonly plain sterile water, are used to irrigate the bladder during operative cystoscopy to remove blood and tissue to allow visualization of the surgical field. Over time, this fluid may be absorbed through the bladder wall into the systemic circulation.

Desired outcomes: Following surgery, patient is normovolemic, as evidenced by balanced I&O (after subtraction of irrigant from total output); orientation to person, place, and time with no significant changes in mental status; BP and HR within patient's normal range; absence of dysrhythmias; and electrolyte values within normal range. Urinary output is 30 mL/hr or more.

Nursing Interventions

♦ Monitor and record VS. Watch for sudden increases in BP with corresponding decrease in HR. Monitor pulse for dysrhythmias, including irregular rate and skipped beats.

♦ Monitor and record I&O. To determine true amount of urinary output, subtract amount of irrigant (CBI) from total output. Report discrepancies, which can signal fluid retention or loss.

♦ Monitor patient's mental and motor status. Assess for presence of muscle twitching, seizures, and changes in mentation. These are signs of water intoxication and electrolyte imbalance, which can occur within 24 hr after surgery because of the high volumes of fluid used as irrigation.

♦ Monitor electrolyte values, in particular those of Na^+ for evidence of hyponatremia. Normal range for serum Na^+ is 137-147 mEq/L.

♦ Promptly report indications of fluid overload and electrolyte imbalance to health care provider.

Acute pain related to bladder spasms
Desired outcomes: Within 1 hr of intervention, patient's subjective perception of pain decreases, as documented by pain scale. Objective indicators, such as grimacing, are absent or diminished.

Nursing Interventions

♦ Assess and document quality, location, and duration of pain. Have patient rate pain on a scale from 0 (no pain) to 10 (worst pain).

♦ Medicate patient with prescribed analgesics, narcotics, and antispasmodics as appropriate; evaluate and document patient's response, using pain scale. Suppositories (e.g., belladonna and opium [B&O] suppositories) are contraindicated if retropubic prostatectomy was done. Oral anticholinergics, such as oxybutynin, are used instead.

♦ Instruct patient to request analgesic before pain becomes severe.

♦ Provide warm blankets or heating pad to affected area *to increase regional circulation and relax tense muscles.*

♦ Monitor for leakage around catheter, *which can signal presence of bladder spasms.*

♦ If patient has spasms, assure him that they are normal and can occur from irritation of bladder mucosa by the catheter balloon or from a clot that results in backup of urine into the bladder with concomitant irritation of the mucosa. Encourage fluid intake *to help prevent spasms.* If health care provider has prescribed catheter irrigation for removal of clots, follow instructions carefully to prevent discomfort and injury to patient.

♦ Monitor for presence of clots in the tubing. If clots are present for patient with CBI, adjust rate of bladder irrigation to maintain light red urine (with clots). Total output should be greater than the amount of irrigant instilled. If output equals amount of irrigant or patient complains that his bladder is full, the catheter may be clogged with clots. If clots inhibit flow of urine, irrigate catheter by hand according to agency or health care provider's directive.

Risk for impaired skin integrity related to wound drainage from suprapubic or retropubic prostatectomy
Desired outcome: Patient's skin remains nonerythremic and intact.

Nursing Interventions

♦ Monitor incisional dressings frequently during first 24 hr, and change or reinforce as needed. If incision has been made into the bladder, irritation can result from prolonged contact of urine with the skin.

♦ Use Montgomery straps or gauze net (Surginet) rather than tape to secure dressing.

◆ If drainage is copious after drain removal, apply wound drainage or ostomy pouch with skin barrier over the incision. Use pouch with an antireflux valve *to prevent contamination from reflux.*

Sexual dysfunction related to fear of impotence caused by lack of knowledge about postsurgical sexual function
Desired outcome: Following intervention/patient teaching, patient discusses concerns about sexuality and relates accurate information about sexual function.

Nursing Interventions

◆ Assess patient's level of readiness to discuss sexual function; provide opportunities for patient to discuss fears and anxieties.
◆ Assure patient who has had a simple prostatectomy that ability to attain and maintain an erection is unaltered; retrograde ejaculation (backward flow of seminal fluid into the bladder, which is eliminated with next urination) or "dry" ejaculation is likely but probably will end after a few months; ability to achieve orgasm is not affected.
◆ Encourage communication between patient and his significant other.
◆ Be aware of your own feelings about sexuality. If you are uncomfortable discussing sexuality, request that another staff member take responsibility for discussing feelings and concerns with patient.
◆ As indicated, encourage continuation of counseling after hospital discharge. Confer with health care provider and social services to identify appropriate referral.

Constipation (or risk for same) related to postsurgical discomfort or fear of exerting excess pressure on prostatic capsule
Desired outcome: By the third to fourth postoperative day, patient reports presence of a bowel pattern that is normal for him, with minimal pain or straining.

Nursing Interventions

◆ Assess for presence of clots and irrigate the catheter as indicated if a patient states that he needs to have a bowel movement during the first 24 hr after surgery *because he may have clots in the bladder that are creating pressure on the rectum.*
◆ Document the presence or absence and quality of bowel sounds in all four abdominal quadrants.
◆ Gather baseline information on patient's normal bowel pattern and document findings.
◆ Unless contraindicated, encourage patient to drink 2-3 L of fluids on the day after surgery.
◆ Consult health care provider and dietitian about need for increased fiber in patient's diet.
◆ Teach patient to avoid straining when defecating to prevent excess pressure on prostatic capsule.
◆ Encourage patient to ambulate and be as active as possible.
◆ Consult health care provider about use of stool softeners for patient during postoperative period.
◆ See "Prolonged Bed Rest" for **Constipation,** p. 29, for more information.

Urge urinary incontinence related to urethral irritation after removal of urethral catheter
Desired outcome: Patient reports increasing periods of time between voidings by the second postoperative day and regains normal pattern of micturition within 4-6 wk after surgery.

Nursing Interventions

◆ Before removing urethral catheter, explain to patient that he may void in small amounts for first 12 hr after catheter removal because of irritation from the catheter.

◆ Instruct patient to save urine in a urinal for first 24 hr after surgery. Inspect each voiding for color and consistency. First urine specimens can be dark red from passage of old blood. Each successive specimen should be lighter in color.

◆ Note and document time and amount of each voiding. Initially patient may void q15-30min, but the time interval between voidings should increase toward a more normal pattern.

◆ Encourage patient to drink 2.0-3.0 L/day if not contraindicated.

◆ Before hospital discharge, inform patient that dribbling may occur for first 4-6 wk after surgery because of disturbance of the bladder neck and urethra during prostate removal. As muscles strengthen and healing occurs (the urethra reaches normal size and function), dribbling will stop.

◆ Teach patient Kegel exercises (see p. 213) to improve sphincter control.

Acute confusion (or risk for same) related to fluid volume deficit secondary to postsurgical bleeding/hemorrhage, fluid volume excess secondary to absorption of irrigating fluid during surgery, or cerebral hypoxia secondary to infectious process or sepsis

Desired outcomes: Patient's mental status returns to normal for patient within 3 days of treatment. Patient exhibits no evidence of injury as a result of altered mental status.

Nursing Interventions

◆ Assess patient's baseline level of consciousness (LOC) and mental status on admission. Ask patient to perform a three-step task (e.g., "Raise your right hand, place it on your left shoulder, then place right hand by your side."). Test short-term memory by showing patient how to use call light, having patient return the demonstration, then waiting 5 min before having patient demonstrate use of call light again. Inability to remember beyond 5 min indicates poor short-term memory. Document patient's response.

◆ Document patient's actions in behavioral terms. Describe "confused" behavior.

◆ Obtain description of prehospital functional and mental status from sources familiar with patient (e.g., patient's family, friends, personnel at nursing home or residential care facility).

◆ Identify cause of acute confusion. Assess oximetry or request ABG values to determine oxygenation levels, check serum or finger stick glucose to determine glucose levels, and request current serum electrolytes and CBC to ascertain imbalances and/or presence of elevated WBC count as a determinant of infection. Assess hydration status by reviewing I&O records after surgery. Note any imbalances either way; output should match intake. Assess legs for presence of dependent edema, which can signal overhydration with poor venous return. Assess cardiac and lung status for presence of abnormal heart sounds or rhythms and presence of crackles (rales) in lung bases, which can indicate fluid excess. Assess mouth for furrowed tongue and dry mucous membranes, which are signals of fluid deficit.

◆ For oximetry readings 92% or less, anticipate initiation of oxygen therapy to increase oxygenation.

◆ As appropriate, anticipate initiation of antibiotics in the presence of sepsis, diuretics to increase diuresis, and increased fluid intake by mouth or IV infusion to rehydrate patient.

◆ As appropriate, have patient wear glasses and hearing aid, or keep them close to the bedside and within patient's easy reach.

- Keep patient's urinal and other commonly used items within easy reach. If patient has a short-term memory problem, do not expect him to use call light.
- As indicated by mental status, check on patient frequently or every time you pass by the room.
- If indicated, place patient close to nurse's station if possible. Provide environment that is nonstimulating and safe. Provide music, but avoid use of television *because individuals who are acutely confused regarding place and time often think action on television is happening in the room.*
- Attempt to reorient patient to surroundings as needed. Keep clock and calendar at the bedside, and remind patient verbally of date and place.
- Encourage patient or significant other to bring items familiar to patient to provide a foundation for orientation. These items can be simple and include blankets, bedspreads, and pictures of family or pets.
- If patient becomes belligerent, angry, or argumentative while you are attempting to reorient him, *stop this approach.* Do not argue with patient or patient's interpretation of the environment. State, "I can understand why you may (hear, think, see) that."
- If patient displays hostile behavior or misperceives your role (e.g., nurse becomes thief, jailer), leave the room. Return in 15 min. Introduce yourself to patient as though you have never met and begin dialogue anew *because acutely confused patients have poor short-term memory and may not remember previous encounter or that you were involved in that encounter.*
- If patient attempts to leave the hospital, walk with him and attempt distraction. Ask patient to tell you about his destination (e.g., "That sounds like a wonderful place! Tell me about it."). Keep tone pleasant and conversational. Continue walking with patient away from exits and doors around the unit. After a few minutes, attempt to guide patient back to his room.
- If patient has permanent or severe cognitive impairment, check on him frequently and reorient to baseline mental status as indicated. Do not argue with patient about his perception of reality *because a cognitively impaired person may become aggressive and combative.*

Stress urinary incontinence related to temporary loss of muscle tone in urethral sphincter after radical prostatectomy
Desired outcome: Within the 24-hr period before hospital discharge, patient relates understanding of cause of the temporary incontinence and regimen that must be observed to promote bladder control.

Nursing Interventions

- Explain to patient that there is a potential for urinary incontinence after prostatectomy but that it should resolve within 6 mo. Describe reason for the incontinence, and use aids such as anatomic illustrations.
- Encourage patient to maintain fluid intake of at least 2-3 L/day (unless contraindicated by an underlying cardiac dysfunction or other disorder). Explain that *dilute urine is less irritating to prostatic fossa.*
- Instruct patient to avoid fluids that irritate the bladder, such as caffeine-containing drinks. Explain that caffeine has a mild diuretic effect, which would make bladder control even more difficult.
- Establish a bladder routine with patient before hospital discharge (see "Urinary Incontinence," p. 207).
- Teach patient Kegel exercises to enhance sphincter control (see "Urinary Incontinence," p. 213).

- Remind patient to discuss any incontinence problems with health care provider during follow-up examinations.

 Patient-Family Teaching and Discharge Planning

Provide verbal and written information about the following areas of self-care to patients who have had surgery for BPH:

- Medications, including drug names, purpose, dosage, schedule, precautions, and potential side effects. Also discuss drug/drug, herb/drug, and food/drug interactions.
- Necessity of reporting the following indicators of UTI: chills; fever; hematuria; flank, costovertebral angle, suprapubic, low back, buttock, or scrotal pain; cloudy and foul-smelling urine; frequency; urgency; dysuria; and increasing or recurring incontinence.
- Care of incision, if appropriate, including cleansing, dressing changes, and bathing. Advise patient to be aware of indicators of wound infection: persistent redness, increasing pain, edema, increased warmth along incision, or purulent or increased drainage.
- Care of catheters or drains if patient is discharged with them.
- Daily fluid requirement of at least 2-3 L/day in nonrestricted patients.
- Importance of increasing dietary fiber or taking stool softeners *to soften stools and minimize risk of damage to the prostatic capsule by preventing straining with bowel movements.* Caution patient to avoid using suppositories or enemas for treatment of constipation.
- Use of a sofa, reclining chair, or footstool *to promote venous drainage from legs and to distribute weight on the perineum, not the rectum.*
- Avoiding the following activities for the period prescribed: sitting for long periods, heavy lifting (more than 10 lb), and sexual intercourse.
- Kegel exercises *to help regain urinary sphincter control for postoperative dribbling.*
- As appropriate, refer patients with BPH to the following website for information on the problem and its management:

  www.kidney.niddk.nih.gov/kudiseases/pubs/prostateenlargement/

  NIH Publication No. 07-3012, June 2006

- For patients experiencing impotence, provide the following information, as appropriate:

  Impotence Anonymous (IA) (615) 983-6092

SECTION ONE **TRANSFUSION REACTIONS**

OVERVIEW/PATHOPHYSIOLOGY

Transfusion reactions can occur when mismatched blood or blood products (whole blood, fresh or frozen RBCs, washed RBCs, leukocyte-reduced RBCs, platelets, fresh frozen plasma) are administered. Reactions to blood are most commonly the result of human error; therefore, extreme caution is essential with administration of such products. The most common types of transfusion reactions are immunologic and nonimmunologic.

Immunologic reactions

Acute hemolytic reaction: An acute hemolytic reaction to blood is an immune-mediated reaction most commonly caused by ABO incompatibility. The reaction occurs immediately after the infusion of incompatible blood and may be mild or life-threatening. There are four ABO blood types, two of which have RBC antigens and two of which do not (**BOX 11-1**). When a person receives donated blood that does not have a matching antigen, the immune system produces antibodies against the donor erythrocytes and destroys these blood cells by hemolysis. For example, if a person with type A blood receives type B blood, anti-B antibodies will be produced against the type B blood. In severe acute hemolytic reactions, hemoglobin (Hgb) is released when donor erythrocytes are destroyed (hemolyzed), thus leading to renal failure, disseminated intravascular coagulation (DIC), cardiovascular collapse, shock, and death.

Delayed hemolytic reaction: Delayed hemolytic reactions are often mild and may go unnoticed, or they may cause discomfort for the patient. This reaction occurs when the recipient produces antibodies against donor erythrocytes and thus shortens the life of the RBC.

Febrile reaction: A febrile reaction exists when the recipient develops an unexplained fever and chills while receiving or within several hours of receiving a transfusion. Febrile reactions can occur when antibodies in the recipient's blood following a previous transfusion or pregnancy react to leukocytes (WBCs) in the donor blood or from cytokine accumulation that occurs when blood is stored. Febrile reactions cause discomfort to the patient but rarely lead to hypotension or other serious problems because erythrocyte hemolysis does not occur.

Allergic reaction: Allergic reactions to blood can be mild or severe (anaphylaxis). Mild reactions are uncomfortable but not life-threatening. Anaphylactic reactions to blood are rare but life-threatening. They most often occur in persons with hereditary immunoglobulin A (IgA) deficiency. Anaphylaxis is a medical emergency. Without intervention, shock and cardiorespiratory

BOX 11-1   ABO BLOOD GROUPS

BLOOD TYPE	RED CELL ANTIGEN	ANTIBODIES AGAINST
A	A	B
B	B	A
AB	AB	None
0	None	AB

collapse are likely. (See "Type I Hypersensitivity Reaction [Anaphylaxis]," pp. 640.)

Graft-versus-host disease (GHD): Posttransfusion GHD occurs when donor lymphocytes proliferate and reject recipient host cells. The reaction occurs days to weeks following transfusion and damages tissues and organs.

Nonimmunologic reactions

Infectious diseases: Blood, an excellent medium for bacterial growth, may cause disease in recipients especially if blood was contaminated during collection or storage. Platelets, in particular, can harbor bacteria because they must be stored at room temperature. Blood can also transmit diseases from donor to recipient such as human immunodeficiency virus (HIV) infection, hepatitis B and C, malaria, and toxoplasmosis, to name a few. Careful screening of donors and extensive blood testing are the best preventive measures for these transfusion complications.

Circulatory overload: Can occur when blood is infused too rapidly or when fluid is drawn into the intravascular space from osmotic pull.

Other types of transfusion reactions: Possibilities include noncardiac pulmonary edema, hypothermia, iron toxicity, or K^+ imbalance.

ASSESSMENT

Signs and symptoms/physical findings

Acute hemolytic reaction: Chills, fever, pain (along the IV line, back, chest), hypotension, dark urine, uncontrolled bleeding from DIC.

Delayed hemolytic reaction (may occur days to years after transfusion): Fever, jaundice, decreased hematocrit (Hct).

Allergic reaction: Rash, hives, anxiety, cyanosis, pallor, hypotension, cough, dyspnea, wheezing, respiratory arrest.

Infection: Fever, chills, hypotension, vomiting, diarrhea, generally occurring within a few hours of transfusion.

Circulatory overload: Tachycardia, hypertension, dyspnea, crackles and/or wheezing, distended neck veins.

History and risk factors: Previous transfusions, pregnancies, and reactions to transfusions. Before infusing blood or blood products, a thorough history should be obtained from the patient about each of these risk factors.

DIAGNOSTIC TESTS

Blood type and Rhesus (Rh) factor: Identify recipient's blood type based on the proteins on the surface of blood cells and the presence or absence of Rh factor.

Crossmatching: Tests donor and recipient blood for compatibility.

Antibody screen: Determines the presence of antibodies to prevent recipient's antibodies from attacking and destroying transfused donor erythrocytes.

CBC: Decreased Hgb and Hct (acute and delayed hemolytic reactions).

Blood cultures: Identify causative pathogen (febrile reactions).

Oximetry: Assesses oxygenation.

Urinalysis: Determines adequacy of urine output, detects the presence of myoglobinuria, and detects presence of hematuria.

COLLABORATIVE MANAGEMENT

The focus of collaborative management is on prevention of transfusion reactions, as well as on early identification and treatment of specific reaction.

Prevention: Involves identifying patients at risk, confirming compatibility between donor and recipient blood products, and accurate identification of patient receiving the transfusion.

O_2 therapy: Relieves hypoxia and maintains oxygenation; usually given by nasal cannula at 2-4 L/min to maintain O_2 saturation greater than 92%.

IV infusion of normal saline: Keeps vein open for emergency drug and fluid administration.

Pharmacotherapy

Acetaminophen: Controls fever.

Corticosteroids (methylprednisolone): Reduce inflammation.

Diphenhydramine: Antihistamine that prevents mast cell breakdown.

Diuretics: Reduce intravascular fluid volume from circulatory overload and help preserve renal output by increasing renal blood flow.

Epinephrine: Relieves bronchoconstriction.

Morphine: Controls pain.

Calcium chloride or calcium gluconate: Treats symptomatic hypocalcemia.

NURSING DIAGNOSES AND INTERVENTIONS

Risk for or actual ineffective protection related to adverse reactions from blood products secondary to blood product incompatibility or contamination

Desired outcomes: Patient remains free of transfusion reaction. If reaction occurs, patient maintains patent airway and demonstrates absence of wheezing or dyspnea, and VS remain within normal limits for patient.

Nursing Interventions

Before Infusion of Blood Product

◆ Ensure that informed consent has been obtained for infusion in accordance with facility policy.

◆ Obtain history of previous transfusion reactions from patient *to determine whether patient is at risk for another reaction.*

◆ Assess patient's VS and lung sounds *to establish a baseline for later comparison.*

◆ Access vein with a large-bore catheter (18 or 19 gauge) and initiate infusion with normal saline *to prevent damage to RBCs. Normal saline is the only fluid that should be administered with blood products.*

◆ Explain the procedure and reason for the infusion to the patient, *to prevent anxiety.*

◆ Follow facility protocols for obtaining blood from the blood bank and administer within 20-30 min *to minimize the risk for bacterial growth and subsequent infection.*

◆ Premedicate with diphenhydramine or acetaminophen at least a half hour before infusion as prescribed *to foster comfort and minimize risk for allergic reaction.*

◆ Inspect the blood product bag for leaks and verify expiration date. Inspect blood for clots or bubbles. *These indicate possible contamination or outdated product and should not be infused.*

◆ Use only IV administration set with filter specifically designed for infusion of blood or blood products, *to prevent fibrin clots or other matter from infusing into the patient.*

◆ With another registered nurse (RN), verify the physician's order for the infusion, the patient's identity, and carefully check the blood product label against the patient's wristband, *to prevent transfusion reaction as a result of blood product incompatibility.*

During Infusion of Blood Product

◆ Implement standard precautions.

◆ Infuse product slowly over first 15 min, and monitor patient *to detect early signs of reaction.*

◆ Infuse according to type of product and patient's tolerance or according to health care provider's order. Platelets may be infused rapidly, but products such as packed RBCs must be infused more slowly.

◆ Assess VS and lung sounds every 15 min for the first hour following initiation of the infusion and every hour thereafter until the infusion is completed, *to detect changes that may indicate a reaction.*

◆ Monitor for signs of hemolytic or allergic reaction (see signs and symptoms, p. 637).
  • Stop the transfusion.
  • Change IV tubing and keep the IV line open with normal saline solution (0.9% sodium chloride [NaCl]).
  • Notify health care provider.
  • Remain with patient, and monitor VS and lung sounds.
  • Prepare to administer emergency drugs such as epinephrine, antihistamines, or corticosteroids.
  • Obtain a urine sample to send to the laboratory.
  • Return blood tubing, unit of blood or blood product bag, and all identifying documents to the laboratory.

◆ Monitor for signs of circulatory overload (see signs and symptoms, p. 637).
  • Slow the infusion.
  • Place patient in an upright position and administer O_2.
  • Notify health care provider.
  • Stay with patient and prepare to give prescribed medications (diuretics, analgesics).

After Infusion of Blood Product

◆ Instruct patient to report chills, abdominal pain, nausea, vomiting, diarrhea, difficulty breathing, and other signs that indicate a reaction, *to facilitate early treatment.*

◆ Monitor for signs of infectious process (fever, chills, nausea, vomiting).
  • Notify health care provider.
  • Collect blood sample for culture.
  • Return blood bag and tubing to laboratory for culture.
  • Initiate O_2 and prepare to give medications as prescribed (acetaminophen, antibiotics, corticosteroids).

◆ Return blood bag and tubing to laboratory or discard (if no reaction) in accordance with facility policy.

◆ Document the procedure, assessment findings, and reactions according to facility policy.

Acute pain related to tissue inflammation secondary to infection
Desired outcomes: Within 1 hr of intervention, patient's subjective perception of discomfort decreases, as documented by pain scale. Objective indicators, such as grimacing, are absent or diminished.

Nursing Interventions

◆ Devise a pain scale with patient, rating pain from 0 (absent) to 10 (worst pain).

◆ Follow protocol for transfusion reaction, *to minimize reaction and reduce accompanying pain.*

◆ Administer prescribed analgesic as needed and document effectiveness using the pain scale. Encourage patient to request medication before discomfort becomes severe. *Pain is more easily controlled when treated before it becomes severe.*

- Reposition for comfort *to reduce pain.*
- Use nonpharmacologic interventions when possible (e.g., relaxation techniques, guided imagery, distraction). *Distraction may reduce patient's perception of pain.*

Deficient knowledge related to risk factors for transfusion reactions and signs/symptoms of delayed reactions
Desired outcomes: Patient verbalizes knowledge of transfusion reaction risk factors and signs and symptoms that should be reported if they occur.

Nursing Interventions

- Assess patient's facility with language; engage an interpreter or provide language-appropriate written materials if indicated.
- Teach the need for reporting signs and symptoms that indicate delayed hemolytic reaction (fever, jaundice, fatigue from decreased Hct), *to ensure appropriate intervention.*
- Teach patient to always report transfusion reaction *because a previous reaction is a risk factor for future transfusion reactions.*
- Encourage patient to take prescribed antihistamines or analgesics *to facilitate comfort following transfusion reaction.*

 Patient-Family Teaching and Discharge Planning

Include verbal and written information about the following:
- See **Deficient knowledge,** earlier in this section.
- Prescribed medications, including name of medication, dose, schedule, and side effects that must be reported.
- Importance of follow-up care if indicated (e.g., infectious disease process following transfusion, delayed hemolytic reaction).

SECTION TWO # TYPE I HYPERSENSITIVITY REACTION (ANAPHYLAXIS)

OVERVIEW/PATHOPHYSIOLOGY

Immediate hypersensitivity (type I) reactions occur in persons who have been sensitized to a specific antigen. The first contact with the antigen, such as mold or pollen, serves as the sensitizing dose and prompts the activation of T-helper (T_H2) cells. Only genetically predisposed individuals produce these cells. TH2 cells stimulate the production of sensitizing type E immunoglobulins (IgE). Upon subsequent exposure to the same antigen, IgE attaches to mast cells and basophils and causes rapid release of histamine, kinins, and other vasoactive mediators, which are responsible for the manifestations of allergy. *Anaphylaxis* is the most serious of the type I hypersensitivities. *Localized anaphylaxis* is confined to one area of the body, such as the lungs, skin, or nasal passages. *Systemic anaphylaxis* is a severe, widespread hypersensitivity reaction that can result in death without immediate treatment. Latex, drugs (penicillin, aspirin), insect venoms, foods (peanuts) and blood products cause the majority of anaphylactic reactions, which affect between 1% and 3% of the population.

ASSESSMENT

Signs and symptoms/physical findings: The characteristics of anaphylaxis vary depending on the location of the reaction and the degree of antigen exposure.

Mild reactions: Hives, urticaria, angioedema, sneezing, nasal congestion, runny nose, or watery eyes.

Moderate reactions: Bronchoconstriction, cough, increased mucous production, wheezing, chest tightness, dyspnea, nausea, vomiting, diarrhea, dizziness, malaise, and anxiety.

Severe reactions (anaphylactic shock): In addition to moderate symptoms, patients also experience hypotension, tachycardia, throat swelling, cyanosis, pallor, severe apprehension, restlessness, airway compromise, respiratory arrest, coma, and death.

History and risk factors: Previous exposure to known allergens, genetic predisposition (one or both parents with allergies).

DIAGNOSTIC TESTS

Tryptase level: Elevated level differentiates anaphylaxis from other forms of shock. Test should be performed within 4 hr of the event.

Urinary histamine: If present, aids in differentiation between anaphylaxis and other forms of shock.

Radioallergosorbent test (RAST): Measures specific IgE antibodies and is useful in identifying specific antigens.

Cap-RAST: IgE antibody assay more sensitive than RAST.

Skin tests: Intradermal test useful for identifying specific allergens. A very small amount of suspected antigen is injected intradermally. A positive reaction indicates allergy.

Eosinophil count: Elevated during allergic reactions.

ABG values: Monitor for acid-base imbalance.

Pulse oximetry: Monitors for adequacy of oxygenation.

COLLABORATIVE MANAGEMENT

A severe, systemic, anaphylactic reaction (anaphylactic shock) is a medical emergency.

Establish a patent airway: Tracheotomy may be necessary if airway obstruction is severe.

Pharmacotherapy

Epinephrine: First-line treatment for anaphylaxis. Counteracts histamine and temporarily relieves bronchoconstriction and bronchospasms, to facilitate a patent airway. Intramuscular route of administration may be used when IV access is not available. *Intramuscular (IM) dose*: 0.3 to 0.5 mL of 1 : 1000 solution; *IV dose*: 0.5 to 1.0 mg (5 to 10 mL) of 1 : 10,000 solution.

Antihistamines: Prevent action of histamine by competing for histamine receptor sites; do not work immediately.

Corticosteroids: Reduce airway inflammation and help prevent bronchospasms.

Aminophylline: Promotes respiratory tract relaxation and bronchodilation.

O_2 therapy: Increases availability of O_2 in presence of constricted airway.

IV access: Normal saline or other isotonic fluid may be administered at keep open rate to provide IV access for 24 hr following systemic anaphylaxis. The patient is at increased risk for going back into shock for at least 24 hr as medications are excreted.

Implement shock protocol: Per facility policy.

NURSING DIAGNOSIS AND INTERVENTIONS

Ineffective airway clearance related to bronchoconstriction and bronchospasms secondary to allergic reaction

Desired outcomes: A patent airway is achieved and maintained immediately after implementation of emergency measures, as evidenced by clear lung sounds, patient report of ability to breathe with ease, and pulse oximetry reading greater than 95%.

Nursing Interventions

- Assess for patent airway *to detect respiratory compromise.* Anaphylaxis can result in death within a few minutes because of airway obstruction.
- Administer epinephrine per facility protocol. *Opposes histamine and provides temporary bronchodilation to facilitate oxygenation.*
- Elevate head of bed (HOB) and initiate O_2 via a rebreather mask *to maximize ventilation and oxygenation.*
- Encourage slow, deep breathing *to maximize oxygenation and decrease anxiety.*
- Administer bronchodilators and/or corticosteroids as prescribed *to maximize ventilation.*
- Monitor pulse oximetry and ABG values *to detect acid-base balance and evaluate oxygenation.*

Deficient knowledge related to cause of reaction, actions to prevent future reactions, and any needed follow-up care
Desired outcomes: Before discharge, patient verbalizes understanding of cause, clinical manifestations, and emergency treatment for anaphylactic reaction and verbalizes need for informing health care providers of allergies and anaphylactic reaction.

Nursing Interventions

- Teach patient about the allergen and ways to avoid exposure to the allergen (when possible), *to minimize future exposure to the allergen and another anaphylactic reaction.*
- Teach patient and significant other how to detect future reactions if they occur, *to facilitate rapid treatment and reversal of the reaction.*
- Have patient demonstrate self-administration of epinephrine if prescribed, *to ensure correctness of technique and rapid treatment of reaction.*
- Encourage patient to use MedicAlert system (e.g., necklace or bracelet) and inform heath care providers about allergic reactions. *Facilitates communication regarding allergy and avoidance of antigen.*
- Teach patient actions, dosage, schedule, and possible side effects of all prescribed medications, *to ensure accuracy of self-administration of medications.*

Anxiety related to fear of death because of inability to breathe
Desired outcomes: Patient reports decreased fear of the situation, rests quietly, has VS within normal parameters for patient, and demonstrates minimal or no breathing difficulty.

Nursing Interventions

- Reassure patient that you will stay until patient reports ability to breathe with ease or is moved to critical care area. *Reduces patient's fear and thus lowers anxiety.*
- Explain all care and treatments, *to decrease patient's anxiety about the unknown.*
- Carry out functions calmly, *to convey a sense of control over the situation.*
- Encourage slow, deep breathing, *to maximize oxygenation and decrease anxiety.*

Patient-Family Teaching and Discharge Planning

Include verbal and written information about the following:

- Medications, including drug names, rationale for use, dosage schedule, route of administration, precautions and potential side effects, and food/drug, herb/drug, and food/drug interactions.

◆ Where to obtain MedicAlert devices:

MedicAlert Foundation: www.medicalert.org

◆ The importance of recognizing signs and symptoms of anaphylaxis and need for initiating immediate treatment, including self-administration of epinephrine if prescribed.

◆ The importance of avoiding the allergen if known, such as latex, drugs, or foods.

◆ The benefits and risk of allergy testing (if appropriate).

SECTION THREE **ACQUIRED IMMUNODEFICIENCY SYNDROME**

OVERVIEW/PATHOPHYSIOLOGY

Acquired immunodeficiency syndrome (AIDS) is a life-threatening illness caused by the human immunodeficiency virus (HIV). AIDS is an acquired disease characterized by severe immune dysfunction. HIV targets CD4⁺ (helper) T lymphocytes and renders them incapable of augmenting B-lymphocyte production of antibodies. This breakdown of the immune system leaves the patient highly vulnerable to opportunistic infections such as *Pneumocystis jiroveci* (formerly known as *P. carinii*) pneumonia (PCP) or tumors such as Kaposi's sarcoma (KS). According to the Centers for Disease Control and Prevention (CDC), the HIV epidemic in the United States continues to grow, with an estimated 56,300 new HIV infections per year (CDC, 2008). AIDS is the advanced phase of HIV infection. It is a chronic viral disease that covers a wide spectrum of illnesses and symptoms for a variable course of time. There is no classic disease progression (e.g., some individuals proceed from an asymptomatic, seropositive state to AIDS, whereas others may experience symptoms for many years). HIV disease is therefore considered a continuum of infection. The stages of illness are described under "Assessment."

Confirmed routes of transmission of HIV infection are as follows:

◆ *Blood*: Mucocutaneous exposure to blood or other infected body fluids, exposure by sharing of unsterile needles or other drug paraphernalia, unsterile invasive instruments, occupational exposure to needlesticks or sharps, transfusion with contaminated blood.

◆ *Semen:* Exposure during male-to-male or male-to-female sexual activity through contact with infected semen. Anal-receptive sex with an HIV-positive person is the greatest sexual risk factor for exposure to the virus.

◆ *Vaginal fluid:* Exposure during vaginal intercourse.

◆ *Breast milk:* From HIV-infected woman to infant.

◆ *Perinatal transmission:* From HIV-infected, untreated woman to fetus; this can occur during all stages of pregnancy, with the highest rates of transmission during labor and delivery.

Conversion to a seropositive status (development of HIV antibodies) following infection with HIV usually takes between 6 and 8 wk, although antibody response may be absent for 1 yr or more. Therefore, a negative test result does not guarantee absence of infection. Individuals with a recent history of high-risk behavior and a negative HIV antibody test should be retested at 3- and 6-mo intervals for 1 yr and follow the guidelines for safer sex practices (**BOX 11-2**). Anyone with a positive HIV antibody test result is considered infectious and capable of transmitting the virus.

Epidemiologic focus is no longer on groups but on high-risk behaviors. HIV infection transcends all racial, social, sexual, and economic barriers. Primarily, high-risk behaviors are responsible for HIV transmission. To a

BOX 11-2	SAFE SEX GUIDELINES

Safer Sexual Practices
- Social (dry) kissing
- French (wet) kissing
- Hugging
- Massage
- Mutual masturbation
- Body-to-body contact (except mucous membrane areas)
- Activities not involving direct body contact

Sexual Practices of Questionable Safety
- Anal-oral contact (rimming) using a latex barrier
- Anal or vaginal intercourse using latex condoms*
- Fellatio (mouth to penis) without ejaculation
- Cunnilingus (mouth to vaginal area)
- Water sports (enemas, urination)

Unsafe Sex Practices
- Anal or vaginal intercourse without latex condom
- Oral contact with body fluids (semen, urine, feces, vaginal secretions)
- Contact with blood
- Oral-anal contact (rimming)
- Manual anal/vaginal penetration (fisting)
- Sharing of sexual aids or needles

*Petroleum-based lubricants have been shown to increase the risk of condom rupture. Water-based products, such as K-Y Jelly and similar products, are preferred.

minimal extent, health care workers who come into contact with body substances of patients also are at some risk. Understanding and practicing stringent infection control are essential for all health care workers. Review **BOX 11-3** for a discussion of the handling of blood and body fluids for all patients.

Phases of HIV infection (for untreated individuals)

◆ *Acute or primary infection:* Period of rapid viral replication and decrease in blood CD4+ T cells. Infection may produce flulike symptoms, particularly at the time of seroconversion. HIV-1 antibodies are usually negative during this phase.

◆ *Chronic asymptomatic phase:* Long period of time following acute phase in which the patient is free of symptoms or opportunistic infections. This phase may last 10 yr or more and often is characterized by stable levels of virus and CD4+ T cell counts. However, viral replication continues during this phase and causes a gradual increase in viral load and a steady decline in immune fuction.

◆ *Advanced stage, AIDS:* The end phase of HIV infection, leading to death within 2-3 yr. Virus control immune mechanisms fail and result in large amounts of circulating virus and significant destruction of CD4+ T cells. Individuals develop signs and symptoms of infection including wasting and opportunistic viral, bacterial, and fungal infections and neoplasms. Dementia also can occur, characterized by cognitive impairment and mood changes.

ASSESSMENT

The four stages of HIV infection can be categorized as acute infection, asymptomatic infection, symptomatic infection, and AIDS.

Signs and symptoms/physical findings

General: Fever, cachexia, weight loss.

Cutaneous: Herpes zoster or simplex infection, seborrheic or other forms of dermatitis, fungal infections of the skin (moniliasis, candidiasis) or nail beds (onychomycosis), KS lesions, petechiae.

BOX 11-3   SPECIFIC ASSESSMENTS

Sexual History: Key Components

- Focus on sexual "behaviors" rather than on categories or labels.
- Avoid making assumptions about individuals.
- Ask about specific sexual behavior rather than asking general questions.
    - For example, "How many sexual partners have you had?" "In the last 5 years?" "In the last month?"
    - "Do you have sex with men, women, or both?"
    - "When is the last time you had sex while under the influence of drugs or alcohol?"
- Ask nonjudgmentally about traditional and nontraditional sexual practices.
    - "What type of sexual intercourse (vaginal, anal, oral) do you have with your partner?"
- For patient at HIV risk:
    - "When you have intercourse, are you the insertive or receptive partner?

Drug History: Key Components

- Focus on specific drug-using behaviors. Examples of specific questions include the following:
    - "Do you use alcohol or tobacco?" "If so, how much?"
    - "Have you ever injected any kind of drug?"
    - "What drugs do you ingest?" "What drugs do you inject?"
    - "When did you last inject drugs?" "share needles?"
    - "Do you clean your works?" "How do you do this?"
- Avoid making assumptions about individuals, because drug use occurs in all socioeconomic groups.
- Convey a nonjudgmental attitude.

Head/neck: "Cotton-wool" spots visualized on funduscopic examination; oral KS; candidiasis (thrush); hairy leukoplakia; aphthous ulcers; enlarged, hard, and occasionally tender lymph nodes.

Respiratory: Tachypnea, dyspnea, diminished or adventitious breath sounds (crackles [rales], rhonchi, wheezing).

Cardiac: Tachycardia, friction rub, gallops, murmurs.

Gastrointestinal (GI): Enlargement of liver or spleen, diarrhea, constipation, hyperactive bowel sounds, abdominal distention.

Genital/rectal: KS lesions, herpes, candidiasis, fistulas.

Neuromuscular: Flattened affect, apathy, withdrawal, memory deficits, headache, muscle atrophy, speech deficits, gait disorders, generalized weakness, incontinence, neuropathy.

DIAGNOSTIC TESTS

Enzyme-linked immunosorbent assay (ELISA): Tests for HIV antibody and is the initial test for HIV infection. Because it can take up to 6 mo to develop enough antibodies to test positive, the person may test negative even though infected. This is often referred to as the "window period" for HIV infection. Individuals who test negative should be retested in 3 mo to confirm seronegativity. A positive ELISA result with a confirmatory Western blot (WB) signals infection with HIV. In the test, an initially reactive ELISA should be repeated on the same specimen. If one or two repeats are reactive, the confirmatory WB is performed.

WB: A confirmatory test used to detect immune response and production of antibodies against the specific viral proteins of HIV. Typically, the ELISA with a confirmatory WB is used to determine HIV infection.

p24 antigen test: Detects HIV p24 antigen in serum, plasma, and cerebrospinal fluid (CSF) of infected individuals. Its advantage is that it detects viral antigen (HIV p24) early in the course of infection before seroconversion occurs.

Immunofluorescence assay: Tests for HIV antibody and has three distinct advantages over the WB test: more sensitive, less expensive, and less technically demanding.

OraSure test system: Detects immunoglobulin G (IgG) in saliva for determining antibody presence. This noninvasive test consists of placing a specially treated swab between the teeth and gum tissue. Sensitivity and specificity are comparable to those of standard serologic testing.

OraQuick test: Rapid antibody test indicates the presence of HIV antibodies within about 20 min. As with other HIV tests, OraQuick requires confirmation by standard methods. This method of testing is important because many high-risk individuals who are tested often fail to return for test results.

CD4$^+$ cell count: Measures the amount of CD4$^+$ T lymphocytes/mL in the blood. This measurement is a marker for the impact of HIV infection on the immune system. As viral load increases, CD4$^+$ counts decrease because of HIV destruction of these lymphocytes.

Viral load: Measures the amount of free virus in the plasma but not in other areas. Only 3%-4% of the virus is located in the plasma. The remaining 90%+ is located in lymphoid tissues and other blood cells. This measurement is used to determine response of antiretroviral therapy (ART), monitor development of drug resistance, and determine need to change ART.

Viral resistance testing: Measures HIV resistance to specific ART drugs. It is used to determine whether the person is already resistant to a specific agent before initiating treatment. It is also used to assess treatment failure and assist in determining whether new or alternative ART agents should be initiated. There are two different types of resistance testing: (1) genotypic tests, which look for genetic mutations that are linked to drug resistance; and (2) phenotypic tests, which assess which drugs can stop HIV growth in a laboratory setting.

COLLABORATIVE MANAGEMENT

Clinical management of HIV disease includes, but is not limited to, the following:

◆ Early identification of HIV-infected persons for early initiation of care and treatment.

◆ Immediate assessment of clinical status, CD4$^+$ count, and viral load to determine need for ART intervention.

◆ Initiation of ART based on current U.S. Department of Health and Human Services (DHHS) guidelines. There has been a dramatic reduction in HIV-related morbidity and mortality since the introduction of ART. Strict adherence to a combination of ART agents slows viral replication at different points in the life cycle of HIV within the CD4$^+$ cell. Use of combinations of these ART agents reduces the amount of circulating virus (viral load). Reducing viral load has been shown to enable immune system recovery and to slow progression of the disease, with a consequent reduction of symptoms and opportunistic diseases, a prolonged survival time, and improvement in the quality of life.

◆ Linkage with support services to assist with comorbidy factors such as substance abuse, psychiatric illness, homelessness, poverty, or other situations or conditions that may interfere with maintaining care and adherence to treatment.

◆ Ongoing monitoring of and intervention with co-occurring conditions, such as hepatitis, tuberculosis (TB), or sexually transmitted diseases.

◆ HIV drug treatment adherence assessment to determine readiness to take medication and use of a drug regimen that fits the person's lifestyle, schedule, and abilities.

- Ongoing education regarding strict adherence to the ART regimen along with use of reminder tools for timely, scheduled self-administration of medication.
- Anticipatory guidance regarding potential side effects of medication and an intervention plan to treat side effects to prevent nonadherence to medication caused by side effects.
- Development of a comprehensive treatment plan by the patient and treatment team to ensure adaptability to the lifestyle, joint patient-clinician treatment decisions, successful adherence, and treatment response.
- Development of a plan to ensure ongoing follow-up, continued risk reduction, and prevention of HIV transmission to others through safe sex and harm reduction.
- Psychosocial support and guidance, including life planning and career development. A positive attitude by the patient and caregivers is an essential element in the therapeutic plan, but an honest approach to this life-threatening illness is also important.

Recommendations for the treatment of persons with HIV disease are continually evolving. The National Institutes of Health (NIH) updates recommendations for treatment of HIV disease and related conditions based on new research findings, clinical trials, and best practices derived from clinical experiences of HIV experts. The following resources provide the most current information on treatment recommendations for adults and adolescents, children, pregnant women, postexposure prophylaxis, and treatment of opportunistic diseases:

National Institute of Allergy and Infectious Diseases, NIH www.niaid.nih.gov

AIDSinfo, U.S. Department of Health and Human Services (information on HIV/AIDS treatment, prevention, and research): www.hivatis.org, http://www.aids.gov/

AIDSinfo, U.S. Department of Health and Human Services, "Clinical Trials": http:// www.aids.gov/hiv-aids-basics/diagnosed-with-hiv-aids/treatment-options/ first-steps-to-treatment/

HRSA, HIV/AIDS Bureau, U.S. Department of Health and Human Services: www.hab. hrsa.gov

Centers for Disease Control and Prevention (CDC), "HIV/AIDS Prevention" (Guidelines): http://www.cdc.gov/hiv/resources/guidelines/index.htm

NURSING DIAGNOSES AND INTERVENTIONS

Risk for infection related to inadequate secondary defenses of the immune system, malnutrition, or side effects of chemotherapy
Desired outcome: Patient is free of infections, as evidenced by cultures or biopsies.

Nursing Interventions

- Perform a complete physical assessment at least q8h *to identify changes from baseline assessment.*
- Assess for signs of active infection or sepsis at frequent intervals (e.g., increased temperature, increased heart rate (HR), decreased blood pressure [BP], diaphoresis, confusion or mental status changes, decreased level of consciousness [LOC]). *These signs are related to the vasodilator effect of increased body temperature.*
- Assess for changes in breath sounds (crackles and/or wheezing). *Indicate infiltrates from infection or bronchoconstriction from inflammation and/or infection.*
- Assess for indicators of opportunistic infections (e.g., persistent fevers, night sweats, fatigue, involuntary weight loss, persistent and dry cough, persistent diarrhea, headache). See **BOX 11-4** for common opportunistic infections and organisms that infect individuals with HIV disease.

BOX 11-4	COMMON OPPORTUNISTIC INFECTIONS IN HIV DISEASE

Viral
- Cytomegalovirus
- Epstein-Barr
- Hepatitis A, B and C
- Herpes (types 1 and 2)
- Varicella

Protozoal
- *Cryptosporidium enteritidis*
- *Entamoeba histolytica*
- *Giardia lamblia*
- *Pneumocystis jiroveci* (formerly known as *P. carinii*)
- *Toxoplasma gondii*

Fungal
- *Candida*
- *Coccidioides*
- *Cryptococcus*
- *Histoplasma capsulatum*

Bacterial
- *Mycobacterium avium intracellulare* (MAI)
- *Mycobacterium tuberculosis*
- *Neisseria gonorrhoeae*
- *Salmonella*
- *Shigella*
- *Treponema pallidum* (syphilis)

- Monitor laboratory data, especially CBC, differential, erythrocyte sedimentation rate (ESR), and cultures, to evaluate course of infection. Be alert to abnormal results and notify health care provider of significant findings.
- Monitor sites of invasive procedures for erythema, swelling, local warmth, tenderness, and purulent exudate. *These indicate infection.*
- Maintain strict sterile technique for all invasive procedures, *to prevent introduction of new pathogens,* and enforce good handwashing before contact with patient. Inadequate handwashing and/or contamination of access sites or invasive lines is a common source of infection in persons who are immunocompromised. Good handwashing remains the single most important intervention *to minimize the risk of transmitting microorganisms to the patient.*
- Assist patient in maintaining meticulous body hygiene, especially if patient has diarrhea, *to prevent spread of organisms from body secretions into skin breaks.*
- Promote pulmonary toilet by encouraging patient to engage in frequent breathing or incentive spirometry exercises. Use caution when performing postural drainage and chest physiotherapy, if prescribed, *because patient may be too ill to tolerate these activities.*
- Teach patient home care considerations for infection prevention after hospital discharge (see "Patient-Family Teaching and Discharge Planning," p. 655).

Impaired gas exchange related to altered O_2 supply secondary to presence of pulmonary infiltrates, hyperventilation, or sepsis
Desired outcomes: Following treatment/intervention, patient has adequate gas exchange, as evidenced by respiratory rate (RR) 12-20 breaths/min with normal depth and pattern (eupnea) and absence of adventitious sounds, nasal flaring, and other clinical indicators of respiratory dysfunction. By hospital discharge, patient's oximetry demonstrates an O_2 saturation (SaO_2) greater than 92% or arterial blood gas (ABG) results as follows: PaO_2 80 mm Hg or higher; $PaCO_2$ 35-45 mm Hg; pH 7.35-7.45.

Nursing Interventions

- Assess respiratory status q2h during patient's awake period, and note rate, rhythm, depth, and regularity of respirations, use of accessory muscles, flaring of nares, presence of adventitious sounds, cough, changes in color or character of sputum, or cyanosis. *These are signs of respiratory dysfunction.*

♦ Assess O_2 saturation via oximetry if indicated. Report Sao_2 92% or less to health care provider.

♦ Monitor ABG results closely for decreased $Paco_2$ (less than 35 mm Hg) and increased pH (greater than 7.40). *These indicate hyperventilation.*

♦ Monitor for changes in color or character of sputum; obtain sputum for culture and sensitivity as indicated. *Changes in color and character of sputum may indicate the presence of infection.*

♦ Adjust humidified O_2 therapy to attain optimal oxygenation, as determined by ABG values or pulse oximetry. *Humidified O_2 relieves mucous membrane irritation that can predispose patient to coughing spells.*

♦ Provide chest physiotherapy as prescribed *to maintain adequate tidal volume;* encourage deep breathing and use of incentive spirometry at frequent intervals *to encourage lung expansion, help remove excess mucus or fluid from the lungs, and prevent pneumonia.*

♦ Reposition patient q2h *to prevent stasis of lung fluids and resulting pneumonia.*

♦ Group nursing activities, optimally 90-120 min at a time, *to provide patient with uninterrupted rest periods.*

♦ Instruct patient to report changes in cough and dyspnea that increases with exertion.

♦ Administer sedatives and analgesics judiciously *to help prevent or minimize respiratory depression.*

♦ Wear respiratory protection consistent with current CDC and Occupational Safety and Health Administration (OSHA) recommendations when providing care to patients diagnosed with active TB. See "Pulmonary Tuberculosis," p. 80, and "Infection Prevention and Control," p. 743, for more information.

Imbalanced nutrition: less than body requirements related to diarrhea, nausea, and loss of appetite associated with side effects of medications, malabsorption, anorexia, dysphagia, and fatigue
Desired outcomes: By hospital discharge, patient has adequate nutrition, as evidenced by stable weight, serum albumin 3.5-5.5 g/dL, transferrin 180-260 mg/dL, thyroxine-binding prealbumin 20-30 mg/dL, retinol-binding protein 4-5 mg/dL, and a state of N balance or a positive N state. Patient states that nausea and other GI side effects associated with ART are controlled.

Nursing Interventions

♦ Assess nutritional status daily, and note weight, caloric intake, and protein and albumin values. Be alert to progressive weight loss, wasting of muscle tissue, loss of skin tone, and decreases in both total protein and albumin, *to facilitate wound healing and maximize the patient's ability to withstand infection.*

♦ Provide small, frequent, high-caloric, high-protein meals, and allow sufficient time for patient to eat. Offer supplements between feedings. As a rule, these patients are kept in a slightly positive N state (after resolution of the critical phases of this illness) by ensuring daily caloric intake equal to 50 kcal/kg of ideal body weight with an additional 1.5 g of protein per kg (e.g., a man weighing 70 kg should receive 3500 kcal plus 105 g of protein per day), *to facilitate positive N state.*

♦ Discuss potential need for total parenteral nutrition (TPN) with health care provider if patient's caloric intake is insufficient,

♦ Provide supplemental vitamins and minerals as prescribed *to replace deficiencies.*

◆ Provide oral hygiene before and after meals *to minimize anorexia and prevent stomatitis,* which can occur as a side effect of chemotherapy. See "Stomatitis," p. 441, for more information.

◆ Encourage significant other to visit at mealtimes and bring patient's favorite high-caloric, high-protein foods from home *to help prevent patient from feeling socially isolated, which can negatively affect appetite.*

◆ Provide instructions for deep breathing and voluntary swallowing if patient is nauseated, *to decrease stimulation of vomiting center.*

◆ Administer antiemetics as prescribed. Encourage patients to request medication before discomfort becomes severe. *Pain is more readily controlled when treated before it becomes severe.*

◆ If patient is dysphagic, encourage intake of fluids that are high in calories and protein; provide different flavors and textures for variation *to increase intake.*

◆ Deliver isotonic tube feedings as prescribed for patients unable to eat. *Isotonic fluids cause less diarrhea than hypertonic or hypotonic fluids.*

◆ Check placement of gastric tube before each feeding; assess absorption by evaluating amount of residual feeding q4h. Do not deliver feeding if residual is greater than 50-100 mL. Keep head of bed (HOB) elevated 30 degrees while feeding, and position patient in a right side-lying position *to facilitate gastric emptying.*

Diarrhea related to GI infection, chemotherapy, or tube feeding intolerance
Desired outcome: By the time of hospital discharge, patient has formed stools and a bowel elimination pattern that is described as normal by patient.

Nursing Interventions

◆ Maintain accurate I&O records *to monitor changes in fluid volume status.*

◆ Assess number and content of stools. Patients with AIDS may experience severe diarrhea, which may be as much as or greater than 10 L/day.

◆ Assess for signs of hypovolemia, such as cool and clammy skin, increased HR (greater than 100 beats per minute [bpm]), increased RR (greater than 20 breaths/min), and decreased urinary output (less than 30 mL/hr).

◆ Assess for anxiety, confusion, muscle weakness, cramps, dysrhythmias, weak pulse, and decreased BP. *These indicate electrolyte imbalance.*

◆ Monitor stool cultures, *to detect new infectious organisms.*

◆ Implement oral or IV rehydration as prescribed with solutions that contain glucose, sodium bicarbonate (HCO_3^-), K^+, magnesium, and phosphorus when diarrhea is severe, *to replace lost fluids and electrolytes.*

◆ Administer antimotility agents (loperamine or tincture of opium) as prescribed.

◆ Teach patient to avoid large amounts (greater than 300 mg/day) of caffeine, *to prevent increased peristalsis and resulting diarrhea.*

◆ Dilute strength or decrease rate of infusion of tube feedings. *Concentrated solutions pull water into the bowel lumen (solute drag) and may cause or intensify diarrhea.*

◆ Encourage foods high in K^+ (see BOX 4-2, p. 174) and Na^+ (see BOX 4-1, p. 165), *to replace any decrements of these ions.*

◆ Protect anorectal area by keeping it cleansed and using compounds such as zinc oxide, *to prevent or retard skin excoriation.*

Impaired tissue integrity (or risk for same) related to cachexia and malnourishment, diarrhea, side effects of chemotherapy, KS lesions, negative N state, and decreased mobility secondary to arthralgia and fatigue
Desired outcome: At hospital discharge, patient's tissues are intact.

Nursing Interventions

◆ Assess skin integrity, and note temperature, moisture, color, vascularity, texture, lesions, and areas of excoriation or poor wound healing.

◆ Assess KS lesions for location, dissemination, weeping, or significant changes. Note and record presence of herpes lesions, especially those that are perirectal.

◆ Turn and reposition patient q2h or encourage patient to change positions frequently, *to avoid prolonged pressure on dependent body parts, which inhibits circulation and promotes tissue breakdown and ulcer formation.*

◆ Provide pressure relief mattress, as indicated.

◆ Teach patient to use mild, hypoallergenic, nondrying soaps or lanolin-based products for bathing and to pat rather than rub skin to dry it, *to prevent skin breakdown.*

◆ Use lotions and emollients *to soften and relieve itching of dry, flaky skin.*

◆ Use soft sheets on the bed, and avoid wrinkles. If patient is incontinent, use some type of rectal device (e.g., fecal incontinence bags, rectal tube) *to protect skin and prevent perirectal excoriation and skin breakdown.*

◆ Assist patient toward a state of N balance by promoting adequate amounts of protein and carbohydrates *to promote skin and tissue healing* (see discussion under **Imbalanced nutrition** earlier in this section).

◆ Encourage ROM and weight-bearing mobility, when possible, *to increase circulation to skin and tissue*

◆ Encourage the use of a soft-bristled toothbrush *to prevent gum trauma and bleeding.*

Acute pain related to prolonged immobility, side effects of chemotherapy, infections, peripheral neuropathy, and frequent venipunctures
Desired outcomes: Using pain scale, patient rates pain as controlled or decreased within 1 hr of intervention. Nonverbal indicators of discomfort, such as grimacing, are absent or diminished.

Nursing Interventions

◆ Assess location, onset, duration, and factors that precipitate and alleviate patient's pain. With patient, establish a pain scale, rating pain from 0 (no pain) to 10 (worst pain). Use the scale to evaluate degree of pain and to document degree of relief achieved. *Establishes a baseline for later comparison.*

◆ Administer analgesic as prescribed. Encourage patient to request medication before the pain becomes severe. *Pain is more easily controlled when treated before it becomes severe.*

◆ Provide moist heat or cold applications to affected areas (e.g., apply heat to painful joints and cold packs), *to reduce swelling associated with infections or multiple venipunctures. Moist heat promotes vasodilation and relaxation and thus helps relieve pain. Cold causes vasodilation, which reduces swelling and pain.*

◆ Encourage patient to engage in diversional activities as a means of increasing pain tolerance and decreasing pain intensity (e.g., soothing music; quiet conversation; reading; slow, rhythmic breathing, deep breathing, biofeedback, relaxation exercises). *Noninvasive techniques stimulate large-diameter nerve fibers and reduce the patient's awareness of pain (gate control theory).*

◆ Discuss with health care provider the desirability of a capped venous catheter for long-term blood withdrawal if frequent venipunctures are necessary, *to prevent discomfort.*

◆ Administer anticonvulsant agents as prescribed, *to relieve peripheral neuropathy,* if present.

Activity intolerance related to generalized weakness secondary to fluid and electrolyte imbalance, arthralgia, myalgia, dyspnea, fever, pain, hypoxia, and effects of chemotherapy

Desired outcome: Before hospital discharge, patient rates perceived exertion at 3 or less on a scale of 0-10 and exhibits tolerance to activity as evidenced by HR 20 bpm or less over resting HR, RR 20 breaths/min or less, and SBP 20 mm Hg or less over or under resting SBP.

Nursing Interventions

- Assess patient's tolerance to activity by assessing HR, RR, and BP before and immediately after activity, and ask patient to rate his or her perceived exertion. See "Prolonged Bed Rest" for **Activity intolerance,** p. 23.
- Monitor electrolyte levels *to ensure that muscle weakness is not caused by hypokalemia.*
- Monitor oximetry or ABG values and adjust O_2 delivery accordingly *to ensure that patient is oxygenated adequately.*
- Plan adequate (90- to 120-min) rest periods between scheduled activities. Adjust activities as appropriate *to reduce energy expenditures.*
- Encourage regular periods as possible to help prevent cardiac intolerance to activities, which can occur quickly after periods of prolonged inactivity. *Conserves energy and minimizes O_2 consumption.*
- Encourage patient to keep anecdotal notes on factors that exacerbate or relieve signs and symptoms *so these factors can be included in the plan for pain control.*

Anxiety related to threat of death and social isolation

Desired outcome: Following intervention, patient freely expresses feelings and experiences reduced anxiety as evidenced by HR 100 bpm or less, RR 20 breaths/min or less with normal depth and pattern (eupnea), and BP within patient's normal range.

Nursing Interventions

- Monitor for verbal or nonverbal expressions of anxiety: inability to cope, apprehension, guilt for past actions, uncertainty, concerns about rejection and isolation, and suicidal ideation.
- Spend time with patient and encourage expression of feelings and concerns. *Verbalizing fears often reduces anxiety.*
- Support effective coping patterns (e.g., allow patient to cry or talk rather than denying his or her legitimate fears and concerns).
- Provide accurate information about HIV disease, related diagnostic procedures, and emerging treatments, *to prevent misconceptions that may increase anxiety.*

Deficient knowledge related to disease process, prognosis, lifestyle changes, and treatment plan

Desired outcome: Before hospital discharge, patient verbalizes accurate information about the disease process, prognosis, behaviors that increase risk of transmitting the virus to others, and treatment plan.

Nursing Interventions

- Assess patient's facility with language, and engage an interpreter or provide language-appropriate written materials if necessary.
- Assess patient's knowledge about HIV disease, including pathophysiologic changes that will occur, ways the disease is transmitted, necessary

BOX 11-5	FACTORS INFLUENCING HIV TREATMENT ADHERENCE

Patient Characteristics
- Knowledge
- Health beliefs
- Trust in health care system
- Lifestyle
- Social support
- Funding for care

Treatment Regimen
- Number of medications
- Dosing schedule
- Duration of treatment
- Side effects
- Behavior change needed
- Cost of medications

Patient-Provider Relationship
- Communication
- Trust in provider
- Collaboration with provider
- Convenient access to provider
- Consistency of provider
- Support

behavioral changes, treatment regimen, and side effects of treatment, *to correct misinformation and misconceptions.*
- ◆ Involve significant other in the teaching and learning process, *to facilitate accuracy of understanding.*
- ◆ Provide literature that explores myths and realities of HIV disease process, *to facilitate accuracy of understanding.*
- ◆ Teach the importance of the following:
  - Adherence to ART regimens. **BOX 11-5** provides a description of factors that influence HIV treatment adherence. **BOX 11-6** provides strategies to imporve drug treatment adherence. Interruptions in drug treatment can lead to development of viruses resistant to specific ART drugs and may result in future treatment failures. *Maximizes patient compliance with prescribed ART regimen.*
  - Informing sexual partners of HIV condition, modifying high-risk behaviors known to transmit the virus, and the significance and importance of refraining from donating blood.
  - Avoiding use of recreational drugs, which are believed to potentiate the immunosuppressive process and lower resistance to infection.
  - Thoroughly washing fruits and vegetables; thoroughly cooking meats at appropriate temperatures, and avoiding raw eggs, raw fish (sushi), and unpasteurized milk, *to decrease risk of infection from foodborne opportunistic microorganisms.*
  - Limiting contact with persons known to have active infections because of decreased resistance to infection. In addition, pets may harbor various fungal, protozoal, and bacterial organisms in their excrement. Therefore, contact with birdcages, cat litter, and tropical fish tanks should be avoided.
  - Meticulous hygiene, *to prevent spread of any extant or new infectious organisms.*
  - Cleaning damp areas in bathrooms (e.g., shower) with solutions of bleach, thoroughly cleaning refrigerators with soap and water, and disposing of leftover foodstuffs within 2-3 days, *to avoid exposure to fungi.*
  - Limiting participation in social activities, getting maximum amounts of rest, and minimizing physical exertion *to avoid fatigue.*

BOX 11-6	STRATEGIES FOR IMPROVING AND MAINTAINING HIV TREATMENT ADHERENCE

Patient-Directed Strategies

Patient Education
- Names, dosages of drugs
- Frequency, special instructions
- Dealing with missed doses
- Dealing with side effects

Memory Aids
- Calendars, charts
- Pill boxes
- Beepers
- Help with organizing

Provider-Directed Strategies

Psychosocial Support
- Support group
- Realistic goals
- Treatment "buddies"
- Positive reinforcement of adherence

Access to Care
- Convenient clinic hours
- "Check-in" calls from provider
- After hours contact method
- Contact person for timely problem solving

Provider Care
- Enough time to teach
- Cultural sensitivity
- Tailor regimen
- Availability

- ◆ Inform patient of private and community agencies that are available to help with tasks such as handling legal affairs, cooking, housecleaning, and nursing care.
- ◆ Provide patient and significant other with telephone numbers and addresses for HIV support groups, self-help groups, and HIV resources.

Social isolation related to altered state of wellness, societal rejection, loss of support system, feelings of guilt and punishment, fatigue, and changed patterns of sexual expression
Desired outcome: Before hospital discharge, patient communicates and interacts with others.

Nursing Interventions

- ◆ Keep patient and significant other well informed about patient's status and treatment plan. *Honesty promotes therapeutic relationship.*
- ◆ Provide periods of private time for patient to interact with significant other, *to facilitate closeness and communication.*
- ◆ Encourage significant other to share in care of patient.
- ◆ Encourage physical closeness between patient and significant other when feasible.

- Involve patient in unit or group activities as appropriate, *to facilitate social interaction.*
- Provide link with community support services.

Impaired environmental interpretation syndrome related to physiologic changes and impaired judgment secondary to infection, space-occupying lesion in the central nervous system (CNS), or HIV dementia
Desired outcomes: Patient verbalizes orientation to person, place, and time following intervention. Optimally, by hospital discharge, patient correctly completes exercises in logical reasoning, memory, perception, concentration, attention, and sequencing of activities.

Nursing Interventions

- Assess for minor alterations in personality traits that cannot be attributed to other causes, such as stress or medication.
- Assess for signs of dementia, which include a slowing of all cognitive functioning, with problems in the areas of attention, concentration, memory, perception, logical reasoning, and sequencing of activities.
- Encourage patient to report persistent headaches, dizziness, or seizures. *These may signal CNS involvement.*
- Assess for that signs that differ from patient's past medical history *to detect CNS involvement.* Most commonly, the fifth (trigeminal), seventh (facial), and eighth (acoustic) nerves are involved in infectious processes of the CNS.
- Assess for signs of mental aberration, blindness, aphasia, hemiparesis, or ataxia. *These may indicate the presence of a demyelinating disease.*
- Divide activities into small, easily accomplished tasks that can be readily completed, *to decrease anxiety and frustration and prevent exacerbation of confusion.*
- Maintain a stable environment (i.e., do not change location of furniture in room), *to help patient familiarize self with immediate surroundings.*
- Write notes as reminders; encourage use of a calendar for appointments, *to prevent frustration from memory loss.*
- Provide some mechanism (e.g., pillbox) *to ensure that patient takes medications as prescribed.*
- Teach importance of reporting changes in neurologic status (e.g., increasing severity of headaches, blurred vision, gait disturbances, or blackouts). Notify health care provider of all significant findings.

Patient-Family Teaching and Discharge Planning

Patient-family teaching should include information about the disease, treatment plan, and need for follow-up care. Include verbal and written information about the following:

- Principles and importance of maintaining a balanced diet; ways to supplement diet with multivitamins and other food sources, such as high-caloric substances (e.g., Isocal, Ensure).
- Techniques of self-assessment for early signs of infection (e.g., erythema, tenderness, local warmth, swelling, purulent exudate) in all cuts, abrasions, lesions, or open wounds; fever, chills, diarrhea, or other changes from normal.
- Importance of reporting changes in neurologic status (e.g., increasing severity of headaches, blurred vision, gait disturbances, blackouts).
- Care of venous access device if present, including technique for self-administration of TPN or medications (see "Providing Nutritional Support," p. 692); care of gastric tube, and administration of enteral tube feedings if prescribed.

- Prescribed medications, including drug names, dosage, purpose, and potential side effects. Also discuss drug/drug, herb/drug, and food/drug interactions. Instruct patient and significant other in the necessity of taking ART medications as prescribed to avoid viral resistance (especially in the case of protease inhibitors).
- Medical follow-up appointments. Stress the importance of keeping all scheduled appointments and under what circumstances the patient should seek emergency care.
- Advisability of sharing feelings with significant other or within a support group.
- Community hospice or agency that provides home help. This should occur before discharge planning begins, to ensure continuity of care between hospital and home or hospice.
- Phone numbers to call if questions or concerns arise about hospice after discharge. Information for these patients can be obtained by contacting the following:

National Hospice and Palliative Care Organization: www.nhpco.org

OVERVIEW/PATHOPHYSIOLOGY

The term *cancer* refers to several disease entities, all of which have in common the proliferation of abnormal cells. To various degrees, these cells have lost their ability to reproduce in an organized fashion, function normally, and die a natural death (apoptosis). As a result they may develop new functions not characteristic of their site of origin, spread and invade uncontrollably (metastasize), and cause dysfunction and death of other cells.

Cancer continues to be the second leading cause of death in the United States after cardiac disease. It can cause damage and dysfunction at the site of origin or regionally or metastasize and cause problems at more distant body sites. Eventually a malignancy may cause irreversible systemic damage and failure.

SECTION ONE SPECIFIC TYPES OF CANCER

❖ LUNG CANCER

Lung cancer remains the most common cause of cancer death among men and women in the United States. National Cancer Institute statistics indicate that 90% of lung cancer deaths in men and 86% in women may be attributed to smoking cigarettes, cigars or pipes. Secondhand tobacco smoke is responsible for 3400 deaths per year. Other risk factors are hookah smoking, radon exposure, which is the leading cause of lung cancer among nonsmokers, radiation therapy to the chest, and automobile pollution. Despite treatment advances in surgery, chemotherapy, and radiation therapy, the cure rate remains low. Although exposure to certain known carcinogens such as radon and asbestos may cause lung cancer, the greatest number of lung cancer cases is linked to tobacco smoking or exposure to secondhand smoke.

Most cases of lung cancer are classified as small cell or non–small cell cancer, but a small portion of lung cancer cases consists of mesotheliomas, bronchial gland tumors, or carcinoids. The cell type, diagnosed via biopsy and pathologic staging, determines the appropriate treatment. Depending on the stage of lung cancer at presentation, surgery, chemotherapy, and/or radiation therapy may be part of the medical treatment plan. For patients with advanced disease for whom cure is not foreseen, palliative care should be initiated concurrently with other treatment modalities, but actually palliation may be the only truly appropriate treatment course.

Screening: Currently there are no routine recommendations for screening for lung cancer, although the National Lung Screening Trial (NLST) is in progress to evaluate efficacy of routine spiral computed tomography (CT) scanning for individuals at high risk for developing lung cancer. Lung cancer may be diagnosed through routine chest x-ray examination, but diagnosis in early stages is usually incidental when the x-ray study is performed for other reasons. The ACS recommends current smokers be educated that the most important preventive strategy to avoid lung cancer is smoking cessation.

❖ NERVOUS SYSTEM TUMORS

Tumors of the nervous system may be primary or secondary tumors of the central nervous system (CNS), which includes the brain and spinal cord. These tumors are classified according to their cell of origin and graded according to their malignant behavior. Although histologically the tumor may be benign, the enclosed nature of the CNS may result in tumor effects causing significant damage or even death.

The primary CNS tumor, whether benign or malignant, can manifest with interrupted neuronal function, compression of the spinal cord or brain and surrounding vasculature, cerebrospinal fluid (CSF) obstruction with resulting increased intracranial pressure, or degeneration of surrounding tissue. Treatment is initially surgical if the tumor site is accessible. The surgical approach may be conventional open skull, or minimally invasive keyhole surgery via the nose or the eyebrow. For some tumors, complete resection is tantamount to cure. For very aggressive tumors or when residual tumor is present postoperatively, radiation therapy and chemotherapy may be implemented.

Surgical excision of metastatic CNS tumors may be an option, but these tumors are more often treated with radiation therapy, including stereotactic radiosurgery, in which a system of three-dimensional coordinates is used to locate the site for irradiation. Chemotherapy also may be an option for control. **Screening:** Currently there are no recommendations for screening for CNS tumors.

❖ GASTROINTESTINAL MALIGNANCIES

Malignancies of the gastrointestinal (GI) system include carcinomas of the stomach, esophagus, bowel, anus, rectum, pancreas, liver, and gallbladder. Each disease site has its own staging criteria and prognostic factors. Most early-stage tumors of all sites are surgically treated. Many treatment plans now begin with preoperative chemotherapy and/or concurrent radiation therapy in the weeks preceding surgery. This approach may eliminate the need for extensive surgeries, increase the chances for cure, or in the case of the anorectal-sparing approach, eliminate the necessity for a colostomy. Radiation therapy is less common in gastric, colon, and liver tumors because of the toxicities associated with irradiating these areas. Radiofrequency ablation is an interventional radiologic approach that is sometimes successful in managing metastatic liver tumors.

Screening: Currently the colon is the only GI site with recommended screening parameters. Because colon cancers generally develop from colon polyps, the goal of screening for colorectal cancer is now prevention rather than early detection. As a result, a screening method that detects polyps as well as early cancer is preferred. Screening options for persons over age 50 yr with average risk are as follows:

- ◆ *Detection of cancer and polyps:* (1) flexible sigmoidoscopy every 5 yr*, (2) colonoscopy every 10 yr, (3) double-contrast barium enema every 5 yr*, or (4) CT colonography (virtual colonoscopy) every 5 yr*.
- ◆ *Detection of cancer:* (1) annual take-home, muptiple sample fecal occult blood test (FOBT)*; (2) annual take-home, multiple sample fecal immunochemical test (FIT)*; or (3) stool DNA test (sDNA)* (no frequency recommended).

---

*Followed by colonoscopy if positive.

The ACS recommends screening for individuals with average risk starting at 50 yr of age. When family history includes first-degree relatives with colorectal cancer, the ACS recommends that screening begin earlier than age 50 yr.

❖ NEOPLASTIC DISEASES OF THE HEMATOPOIETIC SYSTEM

Hematopoietic system cancers include lymphomas, leukemias, plasma cell disorders, and myeloproliferative disorders.

Lymphomas

Depending on cellular type, *lymphomas* are classified as Hodgkin or non-Hodgkin and are characterized by abnormal proliferation of lymphocytes. In addition to characteristic lymph node enlargement, involvement of other lymphoid organs such as the liver, spleen, and bone marrow does occur. Treatment planning, based on disease stage, usually involves chemotherapy and sometimes radiation therapy for eradication of local disease. Patients with Hodgkin lymphoma may have a chance for cure, whereas patients with certain grades of non-Hodgkin lymphoma may be given treatment to simply prolong survival.

Screening: Currently there is no routine screening recommended for the lymphomas.

Leukemia

Leukemia is the abnormal proliferation and accumulation of WBCs. The clinical presentation of leukemia may be either acute or chronic, depending on cellular characteristics. *Acute leukemia,* characterized by abnormal proliferation of immature WBCs also known as precursor or progenitor cells, is classified by the type of WBC involved. Treatment consists predominantly of chemotherapy and biologic therapy, with radiation therapy for central nervous system (CNS) prophylaxis when indicated.

Chronic leukemia, characterized by abnormal proliferation of mature differentiated WBCs, is typically treated with chemotherapy. Some forms of chronic leukemia may remain indolent for years, a characteristic that delays treatment indefinitely. In both types of leukemia, abnormal cells may interfere with normal production of other WBCs, red blood cells, and platelets. Patients with chronic lymphocytic leukemia may have compromised immunity, resulting in frequent and possibly fatal infections.

Screening: No screening recommendations currently exist for leukemia. Diagnosis usually occurs when presenting symptoms include fever, malaise, bruising or bleeding, infections, adenopathy, hepatosplenomegaly, weight loss, or night sweats, but the disease also may be initially noted on routine complete blood count (CBC). Diagnosis is confirmed with a CBC and peripheral smear and by bone marrow biopsy.

❖ HEAD AND NECK CANCERS

Head and neck cancers include tumors of the tonsils, larynx, pharynx, tongue, and oral cavity. Incidence is greatest in men over age 50 yr, and incidence rates in men are double those in women. By far the greatest risk factors are tobacco consumption through smoking or smokeless tobacco and alcohol consumption.

Screening: Although no formal recommendations regarding screening exist, routine dental examinations are one mechanism by which early detection occurs.

❖ BREAST CANCER

According to the ACS, the incidence of breast cancer continues to rise; the disease occurs in one out of seven women (lifetime risk) in the United States. Several factors must be taken into consideration to determine disease stage and prognosis and to establish a treatment plan upon diagnosis. Tumor differentiation is a prognostic factor, with poorly differentiated tumors boding a worse prognosis. Other factors considered in treatment and prognosis are rate of tumor growth (S-phase), DNA characteristics (ploidy), estrogen and progesterone receptors, other biochemical changes (e.g., HER-2/*neu*), lymph node metastases, and distant metastases. Treatment may include any, all, or a combination of the following: surgery, chemotherapy, radiation therapy, hormonal treatment, and biologic therapy. Metastatic breast cancer, considered a chronic disease in some women, may result in therapy spanning several years.

Screening: The ACS recommends that all women over age 40 yr have an annual mammogram and annual clinical breast examination (CBE) by a clinician. Women between the ages of 20 and 39 yr should have CBE performed by a clinician every 3 yr. Women with a higher than 20% lifetime risk should have an annual mammogram and magnetic resonance imaging (MRI) scan; those with a lifetime risk between 15% and 20% should have an annual mammogram and determine need for an annual MRI scan with their physician.

The ACS no longer recommends routine monthly breast self-examination (BSE). Instead, it recommends educating women regarding potential benefits and limitations of BSE and allows women the choice of whether to perform BSE or not.

❖ GENITOURINARY CANCERS

Renal Cell Carcinoma

Renal cell carcinomas, most predominantly classified as adenocarcinomas with histologic variants, occur in about 2% of all malignant diagnoses. Surgery is nearly always the treatment of choice for early-stage renal cell cancers, and radiation therapy for control of symptoms is usually indicated for more advanced disease. Chemotherapy has a limited role in management of renal cell cancer. Biologic response modifiers are an option for more advanced disease. The incidence of renal cancer is higher in men than in women.

Screening: No screening programs exist to detect renal cell cancer, and the incidence likely would be lowered if the predominance of cigarette smoking could be reduced. Reports of hematuria should be investigated thoroughly. Presentation with any other symptoms compatible with renal cell carcinoma may indicate disease that is more advanced.

Bladder Cancer

Bladder cancer is classified as superficial or invasive. Treatment is chosen based on extent of disease and may include surgery, local or systemic chemotherapy, laser surgery, or radiation. Metastases occur commonly in bone, liver, and lungs. Bladder cancer incidence is higher in men than in women.

Screening: No standards currently exist for screening for bladder cancer; however, survival may depend on prompt evaluation of early symptoms.

Prostate Cancer

Prostate cancer occurs most commonly in men over age 50 yr. Treatment may consist of a combination of interstitial or external beam radiation therapy, chemotherapy, surgery, or hormonal therapy. Choice of treatment is determined in part by the disease stage and cellular histology at diagnosis and by clinician preference. In general, prostate cancers tend to grow slowly and metastasize late, thus enabling most patients to live several years with the disease.

Screening: The ACS does not recommend routine screening for prostate cancer. The ACS does believe that men age 50 yr or older who have an average risk for prostate cancer and a life expectancy of at least 10 yr should be offered digital rectal examination (DRE) and prostate-specific antigen (PSA) testing annually. For men at higher risk such as African-American men and men with a first-degree relative diagnosed before age 65 yr, testing should be offered starting at age 45 yr. For those with even greater risk such as men with a number of first-degree relatives diagnosed before age 65 yr, testing should be offered at age 40 yr. If a man asks his health care provider to make the decision regarding testing, the recommendation is that annual DRE and PSA testing be done.

Testicular Cancer

Testicular cancer occurs most often in men between ages 20 and 40 yr. Tumors are classified as seminomas and nonseminomas, depending on their cellular line of differentiation; many tumors consist of a mixed cellular type. Nonseminomas tend to grow and metastasize more aggressively. Treatment nearly always begins with surgery and, depending on histology, blood tumor markers, and bulk of disease, may be followed by chemotherapy and/or radiation therapy.

Screening: Surgical correction for cryptorchidism is recommended before age 6 yr to significantly reduce the risk of later development of testicular cancer. Screening programs are not routinely conducted, but a routine physical examination should include examination of the testes, which would detect an undescended testicle or mass. Any scrotal mass should be evaluated promptly.

Ovarian Cancer

Ovarian tumors occasionally detected during an annual pelvic examination are more commonly occult until symptoms of advanced disease are present. Treatment is initially surgical, which is a vital step for proper tumor staging. Survival, directly related to proper treatment, can be determined only by proper staging. Chemotherapy is commonly given after surgery.

Endometrial Cancer

Endometrial cancer is usually treated with surgery, followed by radiation therapy in all but the earliest stages. Chemotherapy and hormonal therapy are usually reserved for advanced stages in which a surgical cure is not feasible and invasion of local or more distant tissues has occurred.

Screening: Endometrial biopsy remains the definitive standard to assess for endometrial cancer. Women at high risk for endometrial cancer should consider routine surveillance beginning at age 35 yr, but currently the ACS has no definitive recommendations regarding screening for endometrial cancer.

Cervical Cancer

Cervical cancer is caused by human papillomaviruses (HPVs) spread by sexual contact. With increased screening by Papanicolaou (Pap) test, the incidence of invasive cervical cancer has decreased, whereas the incidence of preinvasive carcinoma in situ (CIS) has increased. Treated early, usually with surgery and sometimes with radiation therapy, cervical cancer is a curable disease. Surgery, chemotherapy, and/or radiation may control disease in stages that are more advanced. A vaccine now is available that provides young female patients with protection against the four types of HPV that cause most cervical cancers.

Screening: The ACS recommends an annual Pap test and pelvic examination for women 3 yr after beginning vaginal intercourse or by age 21 yr. If a liquid-based Pap test is used, women should be screened every 2 yr. If conventional Pap tests are used, screening should be done annually. At or after age 30 yr, women who have had three normal consecutive annual exams may elect to have screening every 2 or 3 yr, as recommended by their health care provider. Alternatively, they may get screened every 3 yr, but not more frequently, with either type of Pap test plus the HPV DNA test. Those with a weakened immune system should continue with annual screening. Women aged 70 yr or older who have had three consecutive normal Pap tests and no abnormal tests in the past 10 yr may elect to discontinue annual Pap tests. Likewise, women with a total hysterectomy, including removal of the cervix, may elect no further Pap tests.

❖ ❖ ❖

SECTION TWO **NURSING CARE**

NURSING DIAGNOSES AND INTERVENTIONS FOR GENERAL CANCER CARE

The following nursing diagnoses, desired outcomes, and interventions relate to generalized cancer care. Those for care specific to chemotherapy, immunotherapy, and radiation therapy are discussed in the following major subsection, beginning on p. 672.

Ineffective breathing pattern related to decreased lung expansion secondary to fluid accumulation in the lungs (pleural effusion)
For desired outcome and interventions, see this nursing diagnosis in "Pleural Effusion," p. 69. Patients at increased risk for pleural effusion are those with malignancies, including lymphoma, leukemia, mesothelioma, lung and breast cancers, and metastasis to the lung from other primary cancers.

Ineffective breathing pattern related to decreased lung expansion secondary to pulmonary fibrosis, cellular damage, and decreased lung capacity (pneumonectomy or lobectomy)
*For desired outcome and interventions, see this nursing diagnosis in "Perioperative Care," p. 5. Some chemotherapeutic agents (**BOX 12-1**) can cause pulmonary toxicity, an inflammatory reaction that results in fibrotic lung changes, cellular damage, and decreased lung capacity. Radiation therapy also can cause pulmonary damage and changes resulting in decreased lung capacity.*

Ineffective breathing pattern related to dyspnea secondary to anemia, pulmonary tumors, pneumonia, pulmonary emboli, pulmonary atelectasis, ascites, radiation, pericardial effusion, superior vena cava syndrome, or hepatomegaly
*For desired outcomes and interventions, see this nursing diagnosis in "Atelectasis," p. 58. See **Impaired gas exchange**, p. 64, in "Pneumonia."*

Constipation related to treatment with certain chemotherapy agents, opioids, tranquilizers, and antidepressants; less than adequate intake of food and fluids because of anorexia, nausea, or dysphagia; hypercalcemia; spinal cord compression; mental status changes; decreased mobility; or colonic disorders
*For desired outcomes and interventions, see "Perioperative Care" for **Constipation**, p. 9; "Prolonged Bed Rest" for **Constipation**, p. 29; and "General Care of Patients with Neurologic Disorders" for **Constipation**, p. 363. Patients with cancer should not go more than 2 days without having a bowel movement. Patients receiving vinca alkaloids are at risk for ileus in addition to constipation. Preventive measures such as use of senna products*

BOX 12-1   CHEMOTHERAPEUTIC DRUGS THAT MAY CAUSE PULMONARY TOXICITY

- Bleomycin
- Busulfan
- Carmustine
- Cyclophosphamide
- Cytarabine
- Fludarabine

- Interferon alfa-2b
- Interleukin-2
- Melphalan
- Methotrexate
- Mitomycin C

or docusate calcium with casanthranol, especially for patients taking opioids, are highly recommended. In addition, all individuals taking opioids should receive a prophylactic bowel regimen.

Diarrhea related to chemotherapeutic agents; biologic agents; antacids containing magnesium; radiation therapy to the abdomen or pelvis; tube feedings; food intolerance; and bowel dysfunction such as tumors, Crohn's disease, ulcerative colitis, and fecal impaction
For desired outcomes and interventions, see "Malabsorption/Maldigestion" for **Diarrhea,** *p. 456; and* **Risk for deficient fluid volume** *related to diarrhea, p. 457; "Ulcerative Colitis" for* **Diarrhea,** *p. 482, and* **Risk for impaired perineal/perianal skin integrity** *related to persistent diarrhea, p. 482; "Caring for Patients with Human Immunodeficiency Virus Disease" for* **Diarrhea,** *p. 650; and "Nutritional Support Modalities" for* **Diarrhea,** *p. 706. For patients receiving chemotherapy with potential to cause diarrhea (e.g., 5-fluorouracil, irinotecan), instruct patient regarding need to have appropriate antidiarrheal medications available and other methods used to combat the effects of diarrhea (fluid replacement, addition of psyllium to the diet to provide bulk to stool, perineal hygiene). Instruct patient to notify health care provider if experiencing more than six loose stools per day.*

Risk for disuse syndrome related to upper extremity immobilization secondary to discomfort, lymphedema, treatment or disease-related injury, or infection after breast surgery
Desired outcomes: Before surgery, patient verbalizes knowledge about importance of and rationale for upper extremity movements and exercises. Upon recovery, patient has full ROM of the upper extremity.

Nursing Interventions

- Consult surgeon before the breast surgery to determine type of surgery anticipated. With the surgeon, develop an individualized exercise plan specific to patient's needs, considering factors of wound healing, suture lines, and extent of surgical procedure.
- Encourage finger, wrist, and elbow movement *to aid circulation and help minimize edema.*
- Elevate extremity as tolerated *to decrease edema.*
- Encourage progressive exercise to regain preoperative ROM and use of affected arm. Have patient use affected arm for personal hygiene and activities of daily living (ADL). Other exercises (e.g., clasping hands behind the head and "walking" fingers up the wall) should be added as soon as patient is ready. After drains and sutures have been removed (usually 7-10 days postoperatively), patient should begin exercises that will enhance external rotation and abduction of the shoulder. Patient should be able to achieve maximum shoulder flexion by touching fingertips together behind her back if patient was capable of performing this activity before surgery.

◆ Patients who have had an axillary dissection involving loss of lymph nodes are at increased risk for infection. To minimize risk of lymphedema and infection, avoid giving injections in, measuring BP on, or taking blood samples from affected arm. Remind patient about lowered resistance to infection and importance of promptly treating any breaks in the skin. To help prevent infection after hospital discharge, advise patient to treat minor injuries with soap and water and to notify health care provider if signs of infection occur.

◆ Advise patient to wear a MedicAlert bracelet that cautions against injections and tests in the involved arm, *to decrease risk of infection.*

◆ *To protect hand and arm from injury,* advise patient to wear a thimble when sewing and a protective glove when gardening or doing chores that require exposure to harsh chemicals such as cleaning fluids. Explain that cutting cuticles should be avoided and lotion should be used to keep the skin soft. An electric razor should be used for shaving the axilla.

Urinary stress incontinence related to loss of muscle tone in the urethral sphincter after radical prostatectomy
Desired outcome: Within the 24-hr period before hospital discharge, patient relates understanding of incontinence cause and suggested regimen to promote bladder control.

Nursing Interventions

◆ Explain to patient that there is potential for permanent urinary incontinence after prostatectomy but that it may resolve within 6 months. Describe the reason for the incontinence, and use aids such as anatomic illustrations.

◆ Encourage patient to maintain adequate fluid intake of at least 2-3 L/day (unless contraindicated), and explain that *dilute urine is less irritating to the prostatic fossa.*

◆ Establish a bladder routine with patient before hospital discharge (see "Urinary Incontinence," p. 207).

◆ Teach patient Kegel exercises *to enhance sphincter control* (see "Urinary Incontinence," p. 213).

◆ Remind patient to discuss any incontinence problems with health care provider during follow-up examinations.

Deficient knowledge related to side effects of antiandrogen therapy or bilateral orchiectomy
Desired outcome: Within the 24-hr period before hospital discharge, patient verbalizes knowledge about the extent and duration of body changes.

Nursing Interventions

◆ Assess patient's facility with language, and engage an interpreter or provide language-appropriate written materials if necessary.

◆ Inform patient of side effects of estrogen therapy and orchiectomy (e.g., breast enlargement, breast tenderness, loss of sexual desire, hot flashes).

◆ For patients taking estrogen therapy, provide instruction about symptoms related to complications of thromboembolic disorders and myocardial infarction, which should be reported to health care provider (e.g., shortness of breath; orthopnea; dyspnea; pedal edema; unilateral leg swelling or pain; left arm, left jaw, or left-sided chest pain).

◆ Provide reassurance that discontinuance of therapy, when it occurs, will result in resolution of most side effects.

◆ If appropriate, explain to patient that before initiating estrogen therapy, health care provider may prescribe radiation therapy to areolae of the breasts *to minimize painful gynecomastia.* However, this procedure will not decrease other side effects.

Deficient knowledge related to purpose, type, and management of venous access device (VAD)

Desired outcome: Within the 24-hr period before hospital discharge, patient and significant other/caregiver verbalize understanding regarding the VAD, including its purpose, appropriate management measures, and reportable complications.

Nursing Interventions

♦ Three types of VADs are generally used: tunneled catheters, nontunneled catheters, and implanted ports.

- *Nontunneled catheters (peripheral or central):* Inserted by venipuncture into the vessel of choice, usually basilic, cephalic, or medial cubital vein, near or at the antecubital area, or jugular or subclavian vein in the upper thorax. A peripherally inserted central catheter (PICC) is an example of a nontunneled catheter. Maintenance involves flushing daily and after each use with normal saline and/or heparinized solution. Sterile dressing and cap changes are necessary. Refer to institutional policies for specific instructions.

- *Tunneled central venous catheters:* Inserted into a central vein with a portion of the catheter tunneled through subcutaneous tissue and exiting the body at a convenient area, usually the chest. A Dacron cuff encircles the catheter about 2 inches from the exiting end of the catheter. Tissue grows into this cuff and helps to prevent catheter dislodgment, as well as decreasing risk of microorganisms migrating along the catheter surface and entering the bloodstream. Single-lumen or multilumen catheters are available. Examples of tunneled central venous catheters include Broviac, Hickman, and Groshong. Maintenance involves flushing per institutional protocol and after each use with saline and/or heparinized saline solution. A sterile dressing change is performed 24 hr after insertion and then every 5 to 7 days until healed. Cap changes are performed using sterile technique. Refer to institutional policies for specific instructions.

- *Implanted venous access ports:* Consist of a catheter attached to a plastic or metal port inserted into a central or peripheral vein and then sutured in place in a surgically created subcutaneous pocket, most commonly on the chest. Venous access ports are completely embedded under the skin and may have single or dual access ports. Access to the port may be from the top or side, depending on port style. Noncoring needles must be used to access the port, to allow the system to reseal when the needle is removed. Do not flush catheter with any syringe smaller than 10 mL because of excess pressures generated by smaller syringes. When removing needle, apply pressure to sides of the port to promote ease of removal and patient comfort. Maintenance involves preparation of the site for access with an antibacterial preparation solution (e.g., povidone-iodine solution), optional local anesthetic, and flushing at least monthly or after each use with normal saline and/or heparinized solution. Refer to institutional policies for specific instructions. Dressings are not required after healing of the insertion site. There is a wide variety of catheter types, and the type of catheter determines the proper flushing solution. Before flushing a catheter, the nurse must be certain of catheter type and recommended flushing solution. Patients should be instructed always to carry the card provided by the manufacturer that identifies the type of catheter and recommended flushing solution.

♦ Determine patient's and caregiver's level of understanding of the VAD's purpose. As appropriate, explain that the device can be used for venipunctures and administration of drugs, fluids, and blood products.

♦ Show a model of the device, and explain insertion procedure. Nontunneled catheters may be inserted at the bedside or in the clinic under local anesthesia. Tunneled central venous catheters and implanted ports are inserted in the operating room with local anesthesia. There may be mild discomfort, similar to a toothache, for 48 hr after the procedure. Reassure patient that discomfort responds readily to pain medication.

◆ If possible, introduce patient and caregiver to another individual who has the device so they may discuss their concerns with someone who has experienced insertion and care of a VAD.

◆ Teach VAD maintenance care. Provide both verbal and written instructions, including educational materials provided by the VAD manufacturer. Have patient or caregiver demonstrate dressing care, flushing technique, and cap-changing routine before hospital discharge. Provide a 24-hr emergency number to call in the event of problems.

◆ Discuss the following potential complications associated with VADs, along with appropriate self-management measures:

- *Infection:* Teach how to check for fever (temperature higher than 38° C [100.4° F]) and how to assess exit site for erythema, swelling, local increased temperature, discomfort, and purulent drainage.

- *Bleeding:* Teach how to apply pressure to the site. Instruct patient and caregiver to notify health care team member if bleeding does not stop in 5 min.

- *Clot in the catheter:* Teach how to flush catheter without using excessive pressure, which could damage or dislodge catheter (particularly an implanted port). If flushing does not dislodge the clot, instruct patient and caregiver to notify health care team member. It is not unusual for small blood clots or fibrin sheaths to develop on the end of the catheter. The most common manifestation of a fibrin sheath is ability to infuse fluids with inability to aspirate blood. Both fibrin sheaths and small blood clots respond readily to urokinase therapy. Instill after obtaining a medical directive and reviewing institutional procedure.

- *Disconnected cap:* Teach how to tape all connections and importance of always carrying hemostats or alligator clamps with padded blades *to prevent catheter from tearing.* Teach measures to take if the cap becomes disconnected.

- *Fractured catheters:* If the patient has an external catheter, teach appropriate method for clamping a fractured catheter and provide the clamps. Instruct patient to seek skilled assistance immediately.

- *Extravasation:* Although this is a relatively rare complication, it can cause severe damage if a chemotherapy agent with vesicant properties is involved. Instruct patient to report pain, burning, and stinging in the chest, clavicle, and port pocket or along the subcutaneous tunnel during drug administration.

Acute pain related to disease process, surgical intervention, or treatment effects
For desired outcome and interventions, see this nursing diagnosis in "Pain," p. 13.

Chronic pain related to direct tumor involvement such as infiltration of tumor into nerves, bones, or hollow viscus; postchemotherapy pain syndromes (peripheral neuropathy, avascular necrosis of femoral or humeral heads, or plexopathy); or postradiation syndrome (plexopathy, radiation myelopathy, radiation-induced enteritis or proctitis, burning perineum syndrome, or osteoradionecrosis)
Desired outcome: Patient participates in a prescribed pain regimen and reports that pain and side effects associated with the prescribed therapy are reduced to level of 3 or less within 1-2 hr of intervention, based on pain assessment tool (e.g., descriptive, numeric [on a scale of 1-10], or visual scale).

BOX 12-2	PHYSIOLOGIC CAUSES OF ACUTE PAIN IN CANCER PATIENTS

- Nerve compression or infiltration of nerves by tumor
- Obstruction of hollow viscera or ductal system by tumor
- Infiltration/obstruction of blood vessels
- Exacerbation of altered body functions unrelated to cancer (e.g., preexisting conditions such as chronic headaches, arthritis)
- Extravasation of vesicant drug
- Mucositis
- Pain preceding appearance of herpes zoster lesions
- Central nervous system neoplasm/metastases (e.g., impending spinal cord compression, intracranial metastases, leptomeningeal metastases)
- Bone pain from metastatic lesions or fractures at sites of metastases
- Tumor infiltration of brachial or lumbar plexus
- Deep vein thrombosis
- Pulmonary embolism

BOX 12-3	PHYSIOLOGIC CAUSES OF CHRONIC PAIN IN CANCER PATIENTS

Tumor unresponsive to therapy
Postsurgical pain (e.g., postmastectomy pain, post–radical neck dissection pain, postthoracotomy pain, phantom pains)
Postchemotherapy pain (peripheral neuropathies, avascular necrosis of femoral or humeral head, plexopathies)
Paraneoplastic syndromes (gynecomastia)
Postradiation pain (plexopathy, radiation myelopathy, radiation-induced enteritis or proctitis, osteoradionecrosis)
Postherpetic neuralgia
Altered body functions (e.g., chronic arthritis, back pain, or any musculoskeletal disorder)
Bone pain (metastatic lesions and fractures)

Nursing Interventions

- *Nociceptive pain* refers to the body's perception of pain and its corresponding response. It begins when tissue is threatened or damaged by mechanical or thermal stimuli that activate the peripheral endings of sensory neurons known as nociceptors. In contrast, *neuropathic pain* is caused by damage to CNS or peripheral nervous system tissue or results from altered processing of pain in the CNS. The resulting pain is chronic, may be difficult to manage, and is often described differently (burning, electric, tingling, numbness, pricking, shooting) from nociceptive pain.
- After patient has undergone a complete medical evaluation for the causes of pain (**BOXES 12-2** and **12-3**) and the most effective strategies for pain relief, review evaluation and pain relief strategies with patient and caregivers *to determine level of understanding*. Empower patient as much as possible to participate in controlling his or her pain.
- *Never* ignore a patient's report of pain; remember that a patient's definition of pain may be different from that of the assessing nurse.
- Ongoing assessment of pain is essential and should occur at frequently scheduled intervals. Promptly report *any* change in pain pattern or new complaints of pain to health care provider.
- Be aware that neuropathic pain may present differently from nociceptive pain. Patients with neuropathic pain may not describe their discomfort as pain; therefore, be sure to question them regarding their level of

"discomfort" or abnormal sensations in addition to your usual pain queries. Include the following in your pain assessments:

- Characteristics (e.g., "burning" or "shooting" often describes nerve pain).
- Location and sites of radiation.
- Onset and duration.
- Severity: Use a pain scale that is comfortable for patient (e.g., descriptive, numeric, or visual scale).
- Aggravating and relieving factors.
- Previous use of strategies that have worked to relieve pain.

◆ Assess patient's and caregiver's attitudes and knowledge about the pain medication regimen. Many patients and their families have fears related to patient's ultimate addiction to narcotics. Dispel any misperceptions about narcotic-induced addiction when chronic pain therapy is necessary.

◆ Pharmacologic management of pain is often the mainstay of treatment of chronic cancer pain. Incorporate the following principles:

- Administer nonopioid and opioid analgesics in the correct dose, at the correct frequency, and via the correct route. Chronic cancer analgesia is often administered orally. If pain is present most of the day, analgesia should be given at scheduled intervals around the clock (ATC), rather than as needed (prn).
- Recognize and treat side effects of opioid analgesia early. Side effects include nausea and vomiting, constipation, sedation, itching, and respiratory depression. The presence of these side effects does not necessarily preclude continued use of the drug.
- Use prescribed adjuvant medications to help increase efficacy of opioids. See Box 1-3, p. 15.
- Monitor for signs and symptoms of tolerance, and when tolerance occurs discuss treatment with health care provider. *Patients with chronic pain often require increasing doses of opioids.* Respiratory depression occurs rarely in these individuals.
- Be aware of the potential for physical dependence in patients taking opioids for a prolonged period. Opioids should not be stopped abruptly but rather tapered slowly in these patients, *to prevent withdrawal discomfort.*
- Evaluate effectiveness of analgesics at regular and frequent intervals after administration, particularly after initial dose.
- Use nonpharmacologic approaches (see Box 1-6, p. 22) when appropriate. See discussion in **Acute pain,** p. 13.

Impaired physical mobility related to musculoskeletal or neuromuscular impairment secondary to bone metastasis or spinal cord compression, pain and discomfort; intolerance to activity, or perceptual or cognitive impairment
For desired outcome and interventions, see this nursing diagnosis in "Osteoarthritis," p. 589, and "Osteomyelitis," p. 571. See discussions on care of patients at risk for pressure ulcers, p. 722.

Sexual dysfunction (erectile dysfunction, body changes, decreased libido, impaired sexual self-concept, infertility secondary to treatment) related to the disease process; psychosocial issues; radiation therapy to the lower abdomen, pelvis, and gonads; chemotherapeutic agents; or surgery
Desired outcome: Following instruction, patient identifies potential treatment side effects on sexual and reproductive function and acceptable methods of contraception during treatment.

Nursing Interventions

◆ Determine patient's readiness to discuss sexual concerns.

◆ Initiate discussion about effects of treatment on sexuality and reproduction. The PLISSIT model provides an excellent framework for discussion. This four-step model includes the following: (1) **P**ermission—give the patient permission to discuss issues of concern; (2) Limited Information—provide patient with information about expected treatment effects on sexual and reproductive function, without going into complete detail; (3) Specific Suggestions—provide suggestions for managing common problems that occur during treatment; and (4) Intensive Therapy—although most individuals can be managed by nurses using the first three steps in this model, some patients may require referral to a counselor expert in sexuality.

◆ Assess the impact of diagnosis and treatment on patient's sexual functioning and self-concept.

◆ If female patient is of childbearing age, inquire if pregnancy is a possibility before treatment is initiated. *Pregnancy will cause a delay in treatment;* therefore, a therapeutic abortion may be recommended if treatment cannot be delayed.

◆ Discuss possibility of decreased sexual response or desire, which may result from side effects of chemotherapy. Encourage patient to maintain open communication with partner about needs and concerns. Explore alternative methods of sexual fulfillment, such as hugging, kissing, talking quietly together, or massage. In the presence of symptoms related to therapy, such interventions as taking a nap before sexual activity or use of pain or antiemetic medication may help decrease symptoms. Other suggestions include using a water-based lubricant for dyspareunia. If fatigue is a problem, consider changing usual time of day for intimacy, or using supine or side-lying positions, which require less energy expenditure.

◆ Discuss possibility of temporary or permanent sterility resulting from treatment. Explore possibility of sperm banking for men before chemotherapy treatment or oophoropexy (surgical displacement of ovaries outside the radiation field) for women undergoing abdominal radiation therapy.

◆ Teach patients importance of contraception during treatment if relevant. Discuss issues related to timing of pregnancy after treatment.

◆ If appropriate, inform patients that healthy offspring have been born from parents who have received radiation therapy or chemotherapy, but long-term effects have not been clearly identified. Suggest that patients receive genetic counseling before attempting pregnancy, as indicated.

◆ For patient undergoing lymphadenectomy for testicular cancer, explain that ejaculatory failure may occur if the sympathetic nerve is damaged, but erection and orgasm will be possible. Explain that if ejaculatory failure does occur, artificial insemination is possible because semen flows back into the urine, from which it can be extracted.

◆ If appropriate, explain that a silicone prosthesis may be placed in the scrotum to achieve a normal appearance after orchiectomy. Consult health care provider about the potential for this procedure.

Impaired skin integrity related to malignant skin lesions
Desired outcome: Following instruction, patient verbalizes measures that promote comfort, preserve skin integrity, and promote competent management of and infection prevention of open wounds.

Individuals with breast, lung, colon, and renal cancers; T-cell lymphoma; melanoma; and extensions of head and neck cancers may be prone to developing skin metastases. These skin metastases often erode, providing challenges to wound care, patient dignity and body image, and odor control. Treatment may include radiation, systemic or local chemotherapy, cryotherapy, or excision.

Nursing Interventions

◆ Identify common sites of cutaneous metastases: anterior chest, abdomen, head (scalp), and neck.

◆ Inspect skin lesions, and document the following: general characteristics, location and distribution, configuration, size, morphologic structure (e.g., nodule, erosion, fissure), drainage (color, amount, character), and odor.

◆ Monitor for indicators of infection: local warmth, swelling, erythema, tenderness, and purulent drainage.
◆ Perform the following skin care for nonulcerating lesions and teach these interventions to the patient and significant other, as indicated:
   • Wash affected area with tepid water and pat dry.
   • Avoid pressure on the area.
   • Apply dry dressing *to protect the area from exposure to irritants and mechanical trauma* (e.g., scratching, abrasion).
   • Apply occlusive dressings, such as Telfa, and use paper tape *to enhance penetration of topical medications.*
   • Teach patient to avoid wearing irritating fabrics, such as wool and corduroy.
◆ Perform skin care for ulcerating lesions and teach these interventions to the patient and significant other, as indicated here:

To cleanse and debride
◆ Use half-strength hydrogen peroxide and normal saline solution for irrigation, followed by a normal saline rinse.
◆ Use cotton swabs or sponges to apply gentle pressure and thereby debride the ulcerated area.
◆ As necessary, if the ulcerated area is susceptible to bleeding, gently irrigate only, using a syringe.
◆ Use soaks (wet dressings) of saline, water, Burow's solution (aluminum acetate), or hydrogen peroxide for debridement. Rinse hydrogen peroxide or aluminum acetate off the skin to avoid causing further skin breakdown.
◆ As necessary, use wet-to-dry dressings for gentle debridement.
◆ See Table 13-9, p. 721, in Chapter 13 for appropriate dressings for wound care.

To prevent and manage local infection
◆ Irrigate and scrub with antibacterial agents, such as acetic acid solution or povidone-iodine.
◆ Collect wound cultures, as prescribed.
◆ Apply topical antibacterial agents (e.g., sulfadiazine cream, bacitracin ointment) to open areas susceptible to infection, as prescribed.
◆ Administer systemic antibiotics, as prescribed.

To maintain hemostasis
◆ For capillary oozing, use silver nitrate sticks for cautery.
◆ For larger surface area bleeding, use oxidized cellulose or pack the wound with Gelfoam or similar product.

To control odor
◆ Cleanse wound and change dressings as often as necessary.
◆ Collect specimens for culture and sensitivity of the wound drainage, as prescribed.
◆ Use antiodor agents (e.g., open a bottle of oil of peppermint or place a tray of activated charcoal) in patient's room.
◆ Collaborate with an enterostomal nurse as needed on wound healing techniques.
◆ See "Providing Nutritional Support," p. 692, "Managing Wound Care," p. 716, and "Infection Prevention and Control," p. 743.

Ineffective tissue perfusion related to interrupted blood flow secondary to pericardial effusion and cardiac tamponade
*For desired outcome and interventions see "Pericarditis" for **Activity intolerance**, p. 124.*
   Causes of pericardial effusion and tamponade may include accumulation of fluid in the pericardial space, tumor, invasion of the mediastinum, pericardial fibrosis, or effusion from radiation therapy. Patients at increased risk include those with leukemia, lymphoma, melanoma, and lung and breast tumors. Pericardial effusion can manifest initially with dyspnea, cough, chest

pain, fever, and edema. As the situation worsens and tamponade develops, orthopnea, cold clammy extremities, poor capillary refill, jugular venous distention (JVD), distant heart sounds, and narrowed pulse pressure may be present.

Ineffective tissue perfusion related to interrupted blood flow secondary to lymphedema
Desired outcome: Following intervention/treatment, patient exhibits adequate peripheral perfusion, as evidenced by peripheral pulse amplitudes greater than 2+ on a 1+-4+ scale, normal skin color, decreasing or stable circumference of edematous site, equal sensation bilaterally, and ability to perform ROM in the involved extremity.
Patient populations at risk include those who have had a radical mastectomy, lymph node dissection (upper and lower extremities), blockage of the lymphatic system from tumor burden, radiation therapy to the lymphatic system, or any combination of these.

Nursing Interventions

- Assess involved extremity for degree of edema, quality of peripheral pulses, color, circumference, sensation, and ROM.
- Assess for signs of infection: tenderness, erythema, and warmth at edematous site.
- Elevate and position involved extremity on a pillow in slight abduction. If surgery has been performed, instruct patient not to perform heavy activity with the affected limb during recovery period.
- Encourage patient to wear loose-fitting clothing.
- Avoid BP readings, venipuncture, IV lines, and vaccinations in affected arm.
- Consult physical therapist (PT) and health care provider about development of exercise plan for ensuring mobility. Suggest use of compression garments or bandages to promote a decrease in mild, chronic lymphedema or use of sequential compression devices for more severe cases of swelling.

Ineffective tissue perfusion related to interrupted venous flow secondary to deep vein thrombosis (DVT)
Desired outcome: Before hospital discharge, patient and/or caregivers competently administer anticoagulant therapy as prescribed and describe reportable signs and symptoms suggestive of progressive coagulopathy.

Nursing Interventions

- Individuals with certain malignancies (especially brain, breast, colon, renal, and lung) are at higher than average risk for DVT. Other possible contributing factors include recent surgery, presence of a VAD, sepsis, obesity, concurrent cardiac disease, and underlying increased coagulability disorders.
- Instruct patient in technique of self-administration of injectable low-molecular-weight heparin (LMWH), if it is prescribed.
- If patient is taking oral anticoagulants, teach dietary modifications with warfarin therapy. *Foods high in vitamin K (antidote to warfarin) may interfere with achievement of therapeutic anticoagulation.* These include green leafy vegetables, avocados, and liver. However, be aware that some prescribers do not restrict dietary intake of vitamin K–containing foods. Instead, patients are instructed to maintain dietary consistency in moderation without large variations, and the warfarin dose is adjusted accordingly. If patients are consistent in their dietary intake, their international normalized ratio (INR) should remain stable and therapeutic.
- *Because DVT may recur*, instruct patient regarding reportable signs and symptoms, such as unilateral edema of a limb with possible associated warmth, erythema, and tenderness. Caution that a sudden increase in shortness of breath with or without chest pain also should be reported immediately because DVT may progress to pulmonary embolism.

NURSING DIAGNOSES AND INTERVENTIONS SPECIFIC TO PATIENTS UNDERGOING CHEMOTHERAPY, IMMUNOTHERAPY, AND RADIATION THERAPY

Activity intolerance related to decreased O_2-carrying capacity of the blood secondary to anemia (caused by some chemotherapeutic drugs, radiation therapy, chronic disease such as renal failure, or surgery), or related to decreased oxygenation secondary to acute or chronic lung changes (e.g., occurring with lobectomy, pneumonectomy, pulmonary fibrosis)

Desired outcome: After treatment, patient rates perceived exertion at 3 or less on a 0-10 scale and exhibits tolerance to activity, as evidenced by respiratory rate (RR) 12-20 breaths/min with normal depth and pattern (eupnea), heart rate (HR) 100 breaths per minute (bpm) or less, and absence of dizziness and headaches.

Nursing Interventions

◆ Advise patient that fatigue and activity intolerance are manifestations of decreased O_2-carrying capacity and can be tempered by various interventions mentioned here.

◆ Stress the importance of good nutrition: vitamin and iron supplements and intake of foods high in iron such as liver and other organ meats, seafood, green vegetables, cereals, nuts, and legumes.

◆ As prescribed, administer erythropoietin for anemia. (Erythropoietin is not effective in patients who are iron-deficient.)

◆ As patient performs activities of daily living (ADL), be alert for signs of activity intolerance and decreased tissue oxygenation: dyspnea on exertion, dizziness, palpitations, headaches, and verbalization of increased exertion level. Ask patient to rate perceived exertion per Borg scale (see "Prolonged Bed Rest" for **Risk for activity intolerance,** p. 24).

◆ Facilitate coordination of care providers *to provide rest periods as needed between care activities*, and allow time for at least 90 min of undisturbed rest per day.

◆ Monitor oximetry and report O_2 saturation at 92% or less. Administer O_2 as prescribed, and encourage deep breathing *to augment O_2 delivery to the tissues.* (See "Asthma" for **Impaired gas exchange,** p. 93.)

◆ Administer blood components as prescribed. Double-check type and cross-match with a colleague per institutional protocol; monitor for and report signs of transfusion reaction.

◆ Encourage gradually increasing activities to tolerance as patient's condition improves. Set mutually agreed upon goals with patient.

Activity intolerance related to fatigue secondary to chemotherapy and radiation therapy and deconditioning secondary to treatment and disease
*For desired outcomes and interventions see" Prolonged Bed Rest" for **Risk for activity intolerance,** p. 23. In addition, note the following interventions.*

Nursing Interventions

◆ Monitor patient for hematologic values consistent with anemia (hemoglobin less than 12 g/dL in women and less than 14 g/dL in men), and consult with health care provider accordingly regarding erythropoietin therapy inasmuch as anemia can contribute to fatigue.

◆ *To promote energy conservation*, assist patient with ADL and teach patient to pace activities and rest when fatigued.

Disturbed body image related to alopecia secondary to radiation therapy to head and neck or administration of certain chemotherapeutic agents

Desired outcome: Patient discusses the effects alopecia may have on self-concept, body image, and social interaction and identifies measures to cope satisfactorily with alopecia.

Nursing Interventions

◆ Discuss potential for hair loss with patient before treatment.
◆ Radiation therapy of 1500-3500 cGy to the head and neck will produce either partial or complete hair loss. Hair loss is usually temporary, and loss onset usually occurs 14-21 days from initiation of treatment. Regrowth begins as early as 2-3 months after final treatment but in some cases may take longer.
  • Radiation therapy of more than 4000 cGy usually results in permanent hair loss.
  • Hair loss associated with chemotherapy is temporary and related to specific agent, dose, and duration of administration. See **BOX 12-4** for common chemotherapeutic agents that may cause alopecia. Inform patient that hair regrowth is often a different texture but usually returns to normal after several months.
◆ Explore impact hair loss has on patient's self-concept, body image, and social interaction.
◆ Recognize that alopecia is an extremely stressful side effect for most patients.
◆ Explain that scalp hypothermia and tourniquet applications during IV chemotherapy have not proved to be effective in minimizing hair loss and are considered controversial and possibly may be contraindicated.
◆ Suggest measures that may help minimize the psychologic impact of hair loss on women, such as cutting the hair short before treatment. Selecting a wig before hair loss occurs enables patient to match color and style of her own hair. Wearing a hair net or turban during hair loss assists with collecting hair as it falls out. Wearing scarves, hats, caps, turbans, makeup, and accessories may enhance self-concept. Wigs are tax deductible and are often reimbursed by insurance companies with an appropriate prescription. Some centers and communities have wig banks that provide used and reconditioned wigs at no cost. The ACS hosts the "Look Good Feel Better" program, which provides women with encouragement and tips for managing body image changes during treatment.
◆ Inform patient that hair loss may occur on body parts other than the head, including axillae, groin, legs, eyelashes, and eyebrows, but hair loss in these areas tends to occur later because it is not usually growing as fast as scalp hair. Facial hair, which helps makeup stay in place, may be lost as well.

BOX 12-4	CHEMOTHERAPEUTIC DRUGS THAT MAY CAUSE ALOPECIA

- Actinomycin D
- Bleomycin
- Cyclophosphamide
- Daunorubicin
- Docetaxel
- Doxorubicin
- Epirubicin
- Etoposide
- Ifosfamide
- Paclitaxel
- Topotecan

◆ Instruct patient to keep head covered *during the summer to minimize sunburn and during the winter to prevent heat loss.*

Risk for infection related to inadequate defenses resulting from myelosuppression secondary to malignancy, chemotherapy, radiation therapy, and/or immunotherapy

Desired outcomes: Patient is free of infection, as evidenced by oral temperature 38° C (100.4° F) or less, BP 90/60 mm Hg or higher, and HR 100 bpm or less. Patient identifies risk factors for infection, verbalizes early signs and symptoms of infection and reports them promptly to health care professional if they occur, and demonstrates appropriate self-care measures to minimize risk of infection.

Nursing Interventions

◆ Before administering chemotherapy, ensure that blood counts and other related laboratory studies are within accepted parameters per institutional policy. See Appendix 2, p. 756, for normal values.
◆ Identify patients at risk for infection by obtaining the absolute neutrophil count (ANC). Calculate ANC by using the following formula:

$$ANC = (\% \text{ of segmented neutrophils} + \% \text{ of bands}) \times \text{total WBC count}$$

- ANC of 15012-2000/mm^3 = No significant risk.
- ANC of 10012-1500/mm^3 = Minimal risk.
- ANC of 5012-1000/mm^3 = Moderate risk. Initiate neutropenic precautions.
- ANC of less than 500/mm^3 = Severe risk. Initiate neutropenic precautions.

◆ Assess each body system thoroughly to determine potential and actual sources of infection.
◆ Avoid invasive procedures when possible.
◆ Monitor VS and temperature q4h. Be alert to temperature of 38° C (100.4° F) or higher, increased HR, decreased BP, and the following clinical signs of infection: tenderness, erythema, warmth, swelling, and drainage at invasive sites; chills; and malaise. Signs of infection may be absent in the presence of neutropenia. A temperature of 38° C (100.4° F) or higher may be the only sign of infection in neutropenic patient.
◆ Use method identified in institutional policy to alert all persons entering patient's room that neutropenic precautions are in effect for patients with ANC 1000/mm^3 or less.
◆ Instruct all persons entering patient's room to wash hands thoroughly, the *most important form of infection prevention.* Current guidelines from the Centers for Disease Control and Prevention (CDC) state that individuals caring for patients at high risk for infection should not wear artificial nails and should consider keeping natural nails less than $\frac{1}{4}$ inch long.
◆ Restrict individuals from entering patient's room who have transmissible illnesses such as colds, influenza, chickenpox, or herpes zoster.
◆ Encourage patient to practice good personal hygiene, including good perineal care after elimination.
◆ Notify health care provider immediately if patient's temperature is higher than 38° C (100.4° F). Administer antibiotic therapy within 1 hr when prescribed for a febrile patient.
◆ Implement an oral care routine *to minimize risk of infection associated with nonintact mucosa.* Teach patient to use a soft-bristle toothbrush after meals and before bed (bristles may be softened further by running them under hot water). Inspect the oral cavity daily, and note the presence of lesions, erythema, or exudate on the tongue or mucous membranes. Individuals with prolonged neutropenia are at risk for fungal, bacterial, and viral infections.

- Encourage coughing, deep breathing, and turning, *to minimize risk of skin breakdown and pneumonia.*
- Avoid use of rectal suppositories, rectal thermometer, or enemas, *to minimize risk of traumatizing the rectal mucosa and thereby increasing risk of infection.* Be aware that patients with prolonged neutropenia are at increased risk for perirectal infection, and monitor accordingly. Caution patient to avoid straining at stool. Suggest use of stool softener.
- Implement measures that maintain skin integrity, and instruct patient accordingly: Use electric shaver rather than razor blade; avoid vaginal douche and tampons; use emery board rather than clipper for nail care; check with health care provider before dental care; avoid all invasive procedures; use antimicrobial skin preparations before injections; change IV sites q48-72h or per protocol.
- Instruct patient to use water-soluble lubricant before sexual intercourse and avoid oral and anal manipulation during sexual activities. Patients should abstain from sexual intercourse during periods of severe neutropenia.
- Avoidance of raw vegetables and fresh fruit to eliminate sources of potential infection for neutropenic patients remains controversial; therefore, follow institutional policy accordingly.
- Be alert to signs of impending sepsis, including subtle changes in mental status: restlessness or irritability; warm and flushed skin; chills, fever, or hypothermia; increased urine output; bounding pulse; tachypnea; and glycosuria. *These symptoms often precede the classic signs of septic shock,* which include cold and clammy skin, thready pulse, decreased BP, and oliguria.
- As prescribed, administer colony-stimulating factors *to minimize risk of myelosuppression associated with chemotherapy*, especially for patients with a history of neutropenic fever.
- See "Infection Prevention and Control," p. 743, for more information.

Ineffective protection related to risk of bleeding/hemorrhage secondary to thrombocytopenia (for all patients receiving chemotherapy and radiation therapy, as well as those with cancers involving the bone marrow)
Desired outcome: Patient is free of signs and symptoms of bleeding, as evidenced by negative occult blood tests, HR 100 bpm or less, and SBP 90 mm Hg or greater.

Nursing Interventions

- Identify platelet counts that place individuals at increased risk for bleeding.
  - Platelets 150,000-300,000/mm^3 = normal risk for bleeding.
  - Platelets less than 50,000/mm^3 = moderate risk for bleeding. Initiate thrombocytopenic precautions.
  - Platelets less than 10,000/mm^3 = severe risk for bleeding. Patient may develop spontaneous hemorrhage.
- Perform a baseline physical assessment, monitoring for evidence of bleeding, including petechiae, ecchymosis, hematuria, hematemesis, tarry or bloody stools, hemoptysis, heavy menses, headaches, somnolence, mental status changes, confusion, and blurred vision. Also, monitor VS every shift, being alert for hypotension and tachycardia. Report SBP higher than 140 mm Hg because patient may be at risk for intracranial bleeding. Avoid use of rectal thermometer, which can cause rectal bleeding (use a tympanic thermometer when available).
- Test all secretions and excretions for occult blood.
- Perform a psychosocial assessment, including patient's past experience with thrombocytopenia; the effect of thrombocytopenia on patient's lifestyle; and changes in patient's work pattern, family relationships, and social activities. Identify learning needs and necessity of skilled care after hospital discharge.

- For patients with platelet count less than 50,000/mm^3, follow institutional policy to alert person's entering room that thrombocytopenia precautions are in effect.
- In the presence of bleeding, begin pad count for heavy menses (discourage use of tampons, which may cause trauma during placement), measure quantity of vomiting and stool, elevate (when possible) and apply direct pressure and ice to site of bleeding (venous access device [VAD], venipuncture), and deliver platelet transfusion as prescribed.
- Initiate oral care at frequent intervals *to promote integrity of gingiva and mucosa.* Advise patient to brush with soft-bristle toothbrush after meals and before bed (hot water run over bristles may soften them further). Avoid oral irrigation tools. In the presence of gum bleeding, teach patient to use sponge-tipped applicator rather than toothbrush, avoid dental floss, and avoid mouthwash with alcohol content. Suggest use of normal saline solution mouthwashes 4×/day and water-based ointment for lubricating lips. Dental care should not be performed until platelet count approaches normal.
- Implement bowel program and check with patient daily for bowel movement. Assess need for stool softeners or psyllium to prevent constipation; encourage adequate hydration (at least 2500 mL/day) and high-fiber foods to promote bowel function; and avoid use of rectal suppositories, enemas, or harsh laxatives to minimize risk of bleeding.
- Implement measures that prevent bleeding. Teach patient to use electric shaver; apply direct pressure and elevate extremity for 3-5 min after injections and venipuncture; and avoid vaginal douche and tampons and constrictive clothing. Alcohol is to be avoided, as are medications that could induce bleeding, such as aspirin or aspirin-containing products, anticoagulants, and nonsteroidal antiinflammatory drugs (NSAIDs). Caution patient to perform gentle nose blowing and use emery board rather than clippers for nail care. Avoid bladder catheterization if possible.
- When appropriate, instruct patient to abstain from sexual intercourse when the platelet count is less than 50,000/mm^3. Otherwise, instruct patient to use water-soluble lubrication during sexual intercourse. Patient should avoid anal intercourse.
- Caution patient to avoid activities that predispose to trauma or injury, and remove hazardous objects or furniture from patient's environment. Assist with ambulating if patient's physical mobility is impaired. When patient's platelet count is less than 20,000/mm^3, teach importance of avoiding activities involving Valsalva's maneuver, which increases intracranial pressure. These activities include moving up in bed, straining at stool, bending at the waist, and lifting heavy objects (more than 10 lb). Suggest bed rest if patient's platelet count is less than 10,000/mm^3.
- Avoid invasive procedures when possible, including intramuscular (IM) injections. Use smaller-gauge needles if punctures are necessary, and apply gentle pressure at puncture site until bleeding stops.
- See "Thrombocytopenia," p. 558.

Risk for injury (to staff, patients, and environment) related to preparation, handling, administration, and disposal of chemotherapeutic agents
Desired outcome: Minimize chemotherapy exposure of staff and environment by proper preparation, handling, administration, and disposal of waste by individuals familiar with these agents.

Nursing Interventions

- Pharmacists or specially trained and supervised personnel should prepare chemotherapy, and nurses familiar with these agents should administer them. Institutional guidelines should be readily available for safe preparation, handling, and potential complications such as spills or individual contact with these drugs. A chemotherapy administration certification course, which includes clinical mentoring, is highly recommended for nurses planning to administer chemotherapeutics.

◆ Implement measures to minimize aerosolization and direct contact with drugs during preparation. Measures include using a biologic safety cabinet (laminar flow hood); an absorbent, plastic-backed pad placed on the work area; latex gloves (powder free and a minimum of 0.007-inch thick); full-length impervious (nonabsorbent) gown with cuffed sleeves and back closure; and goggles. Gloves and gowns should be worn during all handling and disposal of these agents.

◆ Prime IV tubing with diluent rather than with fluid containing the chemotherapy agent.

◆ Use syringes and IV administration sets with Luer-Lok fittings.

◆ When removing the IV administration set, wear latex gloves and wrap sterile gauze around the insertion port to prevent direct or aerosol contact with the drug. Place all needles (that have not been crushed, clipped, or recapped), syringes, drugs, drug containers, and related material in a puncture-proof container that is clearly marked "Biohazardous Waste." Follow this procedure for disposal of immunotherapy waste as well.

◆ Wear latex gloves (and impermeable gown and goggles if splashing is possible) when handling all body excretions for 48 hr after chemotherapy because these drugs are excreted through urine and feces.

◆ Ensure that only specially trained personnel wearing double gloves, eye protection, and an appropriate full-length gown should clean a chemotherapy spill with a spill kit. Absorbent pads are used to absorb liquid, solid waste is picked up with moist absorbent gauze, and glass fragments are collected with a small scoop, never with the hands. The contaminated area is cleansed three times with a detergent solution, and all waste is placed in a biohazard waste container.

◆ *To prevent oral ingestion of the drug*, avoid any activity in which the hand goes to the mouth (e.g., eating, drinking, smoking) in any area in which the drug is prepared or administered.

◆ In the event of skin contact with the drug, wash the affected area with soap and water. Notify health care provider for follow-up care. If eye contact occurs, irrigate the eye with water for 15 min and notify health care provider for follow-up care.

Risk for injury (to staff, other patients, and visitors) related to risk of exposure to sealed sources of radiation, such as cesium-137 (^{137}Cs), iridium-192 (^{192}Ir), iodine-125 (^{125}I), palladium-103 (^{103}Pd), strontium-90 (^{90}Sr), or samarium-153 (^{153}Sm); or unsealed sources of radiation, such as iodine-131 (^{131}I) or phosphorus-32 (^{32}P)

Desired outcome: Staff and visitors verbalize understanding about potential adverse effects of exposure to radiation and measures that must be taken to ensure personal safety.

Nursing Interventions

◆ Most institutions have a radiation safety committee to assist in providing and enforcing guidelines that minimize radiation risks to employees and the environment (committee guidelines should be readily available). The committee approves certain rooms used for patients undergoing radioactive treatment in order to minimize exposure to employees and other patients.

◆ Assign patient a private room (with private bathroom), and place an appropriate radiation precaution sign on patient's chart, door, and identification bracelet. Be aware of appropriate radiation precautions (listed on safety precaution sheet) before beginning care of the patient.

◆ Follow radiologist or agency protocol for visitor restrictions. Visitors should stand 6 ft from the bed and stay no longer than the time specified by precaution sheet.

◆ Pregnant women and children younger than age 18 yr should not enter the room.

◆ To ensure optimal care planning, recognize type and amount of radiation source. Two major principles are time and distance.

  • *Time:* Plan care to minimize amount of time spent in patient's room. Staff members should not spend more than 30 min/shift with patient and should not care for more than two patients with implants at the same time. Staff should perform nondirect care activities in the hall (e.g., opening food containers, preparing food tray, opening medications). Linen should be changed only when it is soiled, rather than routinely, and complete bed baths should be avoided.

  • *Distance:* Maximize distance from implant (e.g., if implant is in patient's prostate, stand at head of bed [HOB]).

◆ Wear gloves when in contact with secretions and excretions of all patients treated with unsealed radiation sources, which are radioactive. Flush toilet at least three times after depositing urine or feces from commode. Urine from individuals with sealed radiation is not radioactive and may be discarded in the usual manner. However, patients with implanted ^{125}I seeds should save all urine so it may be assessed for the presence of seeds.

◆ Save all linen, dressings, and trash from patients with sealed sources of radiation. The safety committee representative will analyze them before discard to ensure seeds have not been misplaced.

◆ Long, disposable forceps and a sealed box should be kept in the room at all times in the event that displaced seeds are found. Caution all staff members to use forceps, never the hands, to pick up seeds.

◆ Use disposable products for all patients with unsealed radiation because they will be radioactive for several days. Cover all articles in the room with paper to prevent contamination.

◆ Attach a radiation badge (dosimeter) before entering room to monitor amount of personal radiation exposure. According to federal regulations, radiation should not exceed 400 mrem/mo. Nurses who care for patients with radiation implants rarely receive this much exposure.

Deficient knowledge related to type of, procedure for, and purpose of radiation implant (internal radiation) and measures for preventing and managing complications

Desired outcome: Before radiation implant is inserted, patient and significant other/caregiver verbalize understanding of implant type and procedure and identify measures for preventing and managing complications.

Nursing Interventions

◆ Assess patient's facility with language, and engage an interpreter or provide language-appropriate written materials if necessary.

◆ Determine patient's and caregiver's level of understanding of the radiation implant. Explain the following, as indicated:

  • *Afterloading:* The implant carrier is inserted in the operating room, and the radioactive source is inserted later.

  • *Preloading:* Radioactive source is implanted with the carrier.

◆ Explain that the implant is used to provide high doses of radiation therapy to one area, thereby sparing normal tissue.

◆ Explain that radiation precautions (see **Risk for injury,** p. 677) are required to protect health care team, other patients, and visitors.

◆ Explain the following assessment guidelines and management interventions for specific types of implants.

Gynecologic implants

◆ Explain that the following may occur: vaginal drainage, bleeding, or tenderness; impaired bowel or urinary elimination; and phlebitis. Instruct patient to report any of these, or associated signs and symptoms.

- Explain that complete bed rest is required *to prevent displacement of implants*. HOB may be elevated to 30-45 degrees, and patient may log roll from side to side. Ensure that a urinary catheter is inserted *to facilitate urinary elimination*. Generally, a bowel cleanout (oral cathartics and/or enemas until clear) is prescribed. A low-residue diet and medications *to prevent bowel elimination* may be prescribed to prevent bowel movements during implant period.
- Teach patient to perform isometric exercises while on bed rest *to minimize risk of contractures or muscle atrophy*.
- Encourage patient to take analgesics routinely for pain or to request analgesic before pain becomes severe.
- Explain importance of and rationale for wearing antiembolism hose and performing calf-pumping and ankle-circling exercises while on bed rest. If prescribed, describe rationale for and use of sequential compression devices or pneumatic foot pumps *to prevent lower extremity venostasis*.
- Explain that ambulation will be increased gradually when bed rest no longer is required (see "Prolonged Bed Rest," p. 23, for guidelines after prolonged immobility).
- Explain that after radiation source has been removed, patient should dilate her vagina either through sexual intercourse or by use of a vaginal dilator *to prevent fibrosis or stenosis*.

Head and neck implants
- After a complete nutritional assessment, discuss measures for nutritional support during the implantation, such as a soft or liquid diet, a high-protein diet, and optimal hydration (more than 2500 mL/day).
- Teach signs and symptoms of infection: fever, pain, swelling, local increased warmth, erythema, and purulent drainage at site of implantation.
- When appropriate, advise need for careful and thorough oral hygiene while implant is in place. When implants are placed within the tongue, palate, or other structures of the buccal cavity, oral hygiene will be specifically prescribed by the health care provider and generally given by the nurse.
- Encourage patient to take analgesics routinely for pain or to request analgesic before pain becomes severe.
- Use humidifier *to aid in maintaining moist mucous membranes*.
- Identify alternative means for communication if patient's speech deteriorates (e.g., cards, Magic Slate, pencil and paper, picture boards). Consult speech therapist as appropriate.

Breast implants
- Teach signs of infection that may appear in the breast: pain, fever, swelling, erythema, warmth, and drainage at insertion site.
- Teach importance of avoiding trauma at implant site and keeping skin clean and dry *to help maintain skin integrity*.
- Encourage patient to take analgesics routinely for pain or to request analgesic before pain becomes severe.

Prostate implants
- Explain need for patient to use a urinal for voiding *so that urinary output can be measured every shift and to enable inspection of urine for presence of radiation seeds*.
- Instruct patient or caregiver to report dysuria, decreasing caliber of stream, difficulty urinating, voiding small amounts, feelings of bladder fullness, or hematuria.
- Inform patient that linen, dressings, and trash will be saved and examined for the presence of seeds.
- Encourage patient to take analgesics routinely for pain or to request analgesic before pain becomes severe.
- Caution that caregiver should limit amount of time spent close to implant site.

Deficient knowledge: Purpose and procedure for external beam radiation therapy, appropriate self-care measures after treatment, and available educational and community resources

Desired outcome: Before external beam radiation therapy is initiated, patient and significant other/caregiver identify its purpose and describe the procedure, appropriate self-care measures, and available educational and community resources.

Nursing Interventions

◆ See first eight interventions under **Deficient knowledge** related to chemotherapy, below.

◆ Provide information about treatment schedule, duration of each treatment, and number of treatments planned.
  - Radiation therapy usually is given 5 days/wk, Monday through Friday.
  - The treatment itself lasts only a few minutes, and the majority of the treatment time is spent preparing patient for treatment. Immobilization devices and shields are positioned before treatment *to ensure proper delivery of radiation and to minimize radiation to surrounding normal tissue.*

◆ Explain that the skin will be marked with pinpoint dots called *tattoos* to facilitate delivery of radiation to the desired area during a process called *simulation.* Tattoos, which are permanent, are used *to ensure precise delivery of the radiation.* However, if gentian violet is used, explain importance of not washing the marks (see **Impaired skin/tissue integrity**, p. 686, for more information). Caution patient that it is important not to use skin lotions, deodorants, or soaps unless approved by the radiation therapy provider.

◆ Discuss side effects that may occur with radiation treatment and appropriate self-care measures. Systemic side effects include fatigue and anorexia; however, the most commonly occurring side effects appear locally (e.g., side effects associated with head and neck radiation include mucositis, xerostomia, altered taste sensation, dental caries, sore throat, hoarseness, dysphagia, headache, and nausea and vomiting). See subsequent nursing diagnoses and interventions for more detail about local side effects.

◆ Skin care includes preventing local irritation by clothing, belts, or collars; avoiding chemical irritants such as alcohol, deodorants, or lotions; avoiding sun exposure of irradiated areas; and avoiding tape application to radiation field.

◆ Provide patient with written materials that list radiation side effects and their management.

◆ Provide information about community resources for transportation to and from the radiation center and for skilled nursing care, as needed.

Deficient knowledge related to chemotherapy and purpose, expected side effects, and potential toxicities related to chemotherapy drugs; appropriate self-care measures for minimizing side effects; and available community and educational resources

Desired outcome: Before the nurse administers specific chemotherapeutic drugs, patient and caregiver verbalize knowledge about potential side effects and toxicities, appropriate self-care measures for minimizing side effects, and available community and educational resources.

Nursing Interventions

◆ Assess patient's facility with language, and engage an interpreter or provide language-appropriate written materials if necessary.

◆ Discuss treatment plan and goals of treatment with patient and significant other.

◆ Establish patient's and caregiver's current level of knowledge about patient's health status, goals of therapy, and expected outcomes.

- Assess patient's and caregiver's cognitive and emotional readiness to learn.
- Recognize barriers to learning, such as ineffective communication, inability to read, neurologic deficit, sensory alterations, fear, anxiety, language barriers, or lack of motivation. Define all terminology as needed. Correct any misconceptions about therapy and expected outcomes. Provide written materials to reinforce information taught. The ACS, National Cancer Institute, pharmaceutical companies, and other organizations publish high-quality patient education materials the nurse may use to complement any verbal teaching.
- Assess patient's and caregiver's learning needs and establish short-term and long-term goals. Identify preferred methods of learning and amount of information they would like to receive. Develop teaching plan based on this information.
- Use individualized verbal and audiovisual strategies to promote learning and enhance understanding. Give simple, direct instructions; reinforce this information often.
- Provide an environment free from distractions and conducive to teaching and learning.
- Discuss drugs patient will receive, including route of administration, duration of treatment, schedule, frequency of laboratory tests, most common side effects and toxicities, follow-up care, and appropriate self-care. Provide both written and verbal information.
- Provide emergency phone numbers for use if patient has any questions or develops a fever or other side effects.
- Identify appropriate community resources to assist with transportation, costs of care, emotional support, and skilled care, as appropriate.

Deficient knowledge related to immunotherapy and its purpose, potential side effects and toxicities, appropriate self-care measures to minimize side effects, and available community and education resources
Desired outcome: Before immunotherapy is administered, the patient and significant other/caregiver verbalize understanding of its purpose, potential side effects and toxicities, appropriate self-care measures to minimize side effects, injection technique and site rotation (if appropriate), and available community and education resources.

Nursing Interventions

- See first eight interventions under **Deficient knowledge: Chemotherapy,** p. 680.
- *Because these patients often give their own injections of interferon,* teach proper technique and site rotation schedule. Teach importance of recording site of injection, time of administration, side effects, self-management of side effects, and any medications taken, as well as proper disposal of needles.
- Teach proper handling and storage of medication (e.g., refrigeration). As appropriate, arrange for community nursing follow-up for additional supervision and instruction.
- Teach importance of being alert to the following side effects of interferon: fever, chills, and flulike symptoms. Suggest that patient take acetaminophen, with health care provider's approval, *to manage these symptoms,* but avoid aspirin and NSAIDs *because they may interrupt action of interferon.*
- Monitor intake, output, and weights closely for hospitalized patients inasmuch as fluid shifts may occur with interleukin-2 (IL-2) treatment.
- Teach patient to monitor and record temperature twice daily and to drink 2000-3000 mL fluid/day. *Because anorexia, taste changes, and weight loss are common side effects of biologic therapies,* information regarding nutritional supplementation should be given early.
- See "Providing Nutritional Support," p. 692.

Imbalanced nutrition: Less than body requirements related to nausea and vomiting or anorexia occurring with chemotherapy, radiation therapy, or disease; fatigue; or taste changes

Desired outcome: At least 24 hr before hospital discharge, patient and caregiver verbalize understanding of basic nutritional principles to prevent further weight loss.

Nursing Interventions

For anorexia
- See "Providing Nutritional Support" for **Imbalanced nutrition,** p. 692.
- Weigh patient daily.
- Assess patient's food likes and dislikes, as well as cultural and religious preferences related to food choices.
- Anorexia may be caused by the pathophysiology of cancer and surgery or side effects of chemotherapy and radiation therapy and should be explained to patient, *to avoid unnecessary anxiety.*
- Teach importance of increasing caloric intake, *to increase energy and minimize weight loss.*
- Teach importance of increasing protein intake, *to facilitate repair and regeneration of cells.*
- Suggest that patient eat several small meals at frequent intervals throughout the day.
- Encourage use of nutritional supplements.
- Megestrol acetate and prednisone may be prescribed for their proven positive influence on appetite stimulation and weight gain in individuals with cancer. Consult patient's health care provider accordingly.

For nausea and vomiting
- Assess patient's pattern of nausea and vomiting: onset, frequency, duration, intensity, and amount and character of emesis. See **BOX 12-5** for a list of antineoplastic agents with emetic action.

BOX 12-5	ANTINEOPLASTIC AGENTS WITH EMETIC ACTION

Mild Emetic Action
- Bleomycin
- Chlorambucil
- Cytarabine*
- Gemcitabine
- Hydroxyurea
- Lomustine
- Melphalan*
- Mercaptopurine
- Paclitaxel
- Tamoxifen
- Thioguanine
- Thiotepa
- Vinblastine
- Vincristine
- Vinorelbine

Moderate Emetic Action
- L-Asparaginase
- Carboplatin
- Daunorubicin
- Docetaxel
- Doxorubicin
- Etoposide (VP-15)
- 5-Fluorouracil (5-FU)
- Flutamide
- Hexamethylmelamine
- Ifosfamide
- Mitomycin
- Mitoxantrone
- Procarbazine
- Topotecan

Severe Emetic Action
Cisplatin*
Cyclophosphamide*
Cytarabine*
Dacarbazine
Dactinomycin
Etoposide*
Interleukin-2*
Mechlorethamine
Melphalan*
Methotrexate*
Mitomycin C
Plicamycin
Streptozocin

*Dose related.

BOX 12-6   COMMON ANTIEMETIC AGENTS

AGENT	GENERIC NAME
Dopamine antagonist	Prochlorperazine
	Metoclopramide
	Droperidol
	Haloperidol
Corticosteroid	Dexamethasone
Antihistamine	Diphenhydramine
Benzodiazepine	Lorazepam
Cannabinoid	Dronabinol
Serotonin antagonist	Granisetron
	Ondansetron
	Dolasetron
	Aprepitant
	Palonosetron

◆ Explain to patient that nausea and vomiting may be side effects of chemotherapy and radiation therapy. (Nausea and vomiting may occur with advanced cancer, bowel obstruction, some medications, and metabolic abnormalities.)

◆ Teach patient to take antiemetic, if prescribed, 1 hr before chemotherapy and to continue to take the drug as prescribed to cover the expected emetogenic period of the chemotherapy agent given. Consider duration of previous nausea and vomiting episodes following chemotherapy when recommending antiemetic administration schedule. Explain that antiemetics are most effective if taken prophylactically or at nausea onset. A list of commonly used antiemetic agents is found in **BOX 12-6**.

◆ Teach patient to eat cold foods or foods served at room temperature *because the odor of hot food may aggravate nausea.*

◆ Suggest intake of clear liquids and bland foods.

◆ Teach patient to avoid sweet, fatty, highly salted, and spicy foods, as well as foods with strong odors, *any of which may increase nausea.*

◆ Minimize stimuli such as smells, sounds, or sights, *all of which may promote nausea.*

◆ Encourage patient to eat sour or mint candy during chemotherapy *to decrease the unpleasant, metallic taste.*

◆ If not contraindicated, teach patient to take oral chemotherapy with antiemetics at bedtime *to minimize incidence of nausea.*

◆ Encourage patient to explore various dietary patterns.
  • Avoid eating or drinking for 1-2 hr before and after chemotherapy.
  • Follow a clear liquid diet for 1-2 hr before and 1-24 hr after chemotherapy.

◆ Avoid contact with food while it is being cooked; avoid being around people who are eating.

◆ Eat small, light meals at frequent intervals (5-6 ×/day).

◆ Suggest that patient sit near an open window to breathe fresh air when feeling nauseated.

◆ Help patient find an appropriate distraction technique (e.g., music, television, reading).

◆ Teach patient to use relaxation techniques, *which may help prevent anticipatory nausea and vomiting.* An example is found in **Health-seeking behaviors:** Relaxation technique effective for stress reduction, p. 106.

◆ Instruct patient to slowly sip clear liquids such as broth, ginger ale, cola, tea, or gelatin; suck on ice chips; and avoid large volumes of water.

For fatigue
◆ If patient is easily fatigued, encourage him or her to eat frequent, small meals and document intake.
◆ Provide foods that are easy to eat.
◆ If patient wears an O_2 device with exertion, encourage wearing it while eating.
◆ Avoid offering meals immediately after exertion.

For taste changes
◆ Suggest that patient try foods not previously enjoyed *because previously enjoyed foods are no longer attractive.*
◆ Encourage good mouth care; assess mucous membrane for thrush, lesions, or mucositis.
◆ Suggest that patient try strongly flavored foods *because patients often report that food tastes like sawdust.*

Impaired oral mucous membrane related to side effects of chemotherapy or biotherapy; radiation therapy to head and neck; ineffective oral hygiene; gingival diseases; poor nutritional status; tumors of the oral cavity and neck; and infection
Desired outcomes: Patient complies with therapeutic regimen within 1 hr of instruction. Patient's oral mucosal condition improves, as evidenced by intact mucous membrane; moist, intact tongue and lips; and absence of pain and lesions.

Nursing Interventions

◆ With myelosuppression, caution patient not to floss teeth or use oral irrigators or a stiff toothbrush.
◆ Be aware that for moderate to severe mucositis, patient may require parenteral analgesics, such as morphine.
◆ Suggest to patients with xerostomia (dryness of the mouth from a lack of normal salivary secretion) caused by radiation therapy that they may benefit from chewing sugarless gum; sucking on sugarless candy, frozen fruit juice pops, or sugar-free Popsicles or taking frequent sips of water. Saliva substitutes are another option, although they are expensive and do not last long.
◆ Close dental follow-up is essential *because the lack of or decrease in salivary fluid predisposes the patient to dental caries.* Fluoride treatment is recommended for these patients.
◆ See "Stomatitis," p. 441, for other interventions.

Impaired swallowing related to mucositis of the oral cavity or esophagus (esophagitis) secondary to radiation therapy to the neck, chest, and upper back; use of chemotherapy agents; obstruction (tumors); or thrush
Desired outcomes: Before food or fluids are given, patient exhibits gag reflex and is free of symptoms of aspiration, as evidenced by RR 12-20 breaths/min with normal depth and pattern (eupnea), normal skin color, and the ability to speak. Following instruction, patient verbalizes early signs and symptoms of esophagitis, alerts health care team as soon as they occur, and identifies measures for maintaining nutrition and comfort.

Nursing Interventions

◆ Monitor patient for evidence of impaired swallowing with concomitant respiratory difficulties.
◆ Teach patient the early signs and symptoms of esophagitis (sensation of lump in the throat with swallowing, difficulty swallowing solid foods, discomfort or pain with swallowing) and stomatitis (generalized burning sensation of oral cavity, white patches on oral mucosa, ulcerations, pain) and the importance of reporting symptoms promptly if they occur.

- Monitor patient's dietary intake and weight, and teach the following guidelines: maintain a high-protein diet; eat foods that are soft and bland; add milk or milk products to the diet *to coat the esophageal lining* (for individuals without excessive mucus production); and add sauces and creams to foods *because they may facilitate swallowing.*
- Ensure adequate fluid intake of at least 2 L/day.
- Implement the following measures that promote comfort, and discuss them with patient accordingly:
  - Use a local anesthetic, as prescribed, *to minimize pain with meals.* Lidocaine 2% and diphenhydramine may be taken by patient via swish and spit or swallow before eating. These anesthetics may decrease patient's gag reflex.
  - Suggest patient sit in an upright position during meals and for 15-30 min after eating.
  - Obtain prescription for analgesics and administer as prescribed. Teach patient importance of taking analgesics before eating or drinking to promote proper nutrition and hydration.
  - Encourage frequent oral care with normal saline and sodium bicarbonate solution (1 teaspoon of each to 1 quart of water).
  - Teach patient to avoid irritants, such as alcohol, tobacco, and alcohol-based commercial mouthwashes.
  - Have suction equipment readily available in the event that patient experiences aspiration. Educate patient about ways to manage oral secretions.
  - Suction mouth prn, using low, continuous/suction equipment.
  - Teach patient to expectorate saliva into tissues, and dispose of it per institutional policy.
- See "Stomatitis" for **Impaired oral mucous membrane**, p. 442, and "Nutritional Support Modalities" for **Risk for impaired swallowing**, p. 707 for desired outcomes and interventions.

Disturbed sensory perceptions related to neuropathies associated with certain chemotherapeutic drugs
Desired outcome: Patient reports early signs and symptoms of ototoxicity and peripheral neuropathy (functional disturbance of the peripheral nervous system), and measures are implemented promptly to minimize these side effects.

Nursing Interventions

- *Because cumulative doses of cisplatin can result in irreversible loss of high-frequency range hearing or tinnitus,* teach patient to report early symptoms of hearing loss. Instruct caregivers to observe for early symptoms inasmuch as they may notice signs before patient does.
- Suggest that patient face speaker and watch speaker's lips during conversation while being aware that background noise may interfere with hearing ability.
- A hearing aid also may be helpful, or it may amplify background noise and worsen speech comprehension; suggest a trial before purchase. In instances of cisplatin-induced hearing loss, refer patient to community resources for hearing-impaired persons. A baseline audiogram may be done before cisplatin administration.
- Monitor patient for development of peripheral neuropathy (see **BOX 12-7** for drugs with the potential to cause neurotoxicity). Numbness and tingling (paresthesias) of fingers and toes occur initially and can progress to difficulty with fine motor skills, such as buttoning shirts or picking up objects. The most severely affected individuals may lose sensation at the hip level and have difficulty with balance and ambulation. Instruct patient to report early signs and symptoms. Suggest consultation with PT or occupational therapist (OT) to assist with maintaining function. Teach patient that the

BOX 12-7	CHEMOTHERAPEUTIC DRUGS THAT MAY CAUSE NEUROTOXICITY

- Asparaginase (mental status changes)
- Cisplatin (ototoxicity, mental status changes, sensory nerve deficits, cranial nerve deficits)
- Cytarabine (sensory nerve deficits, cerebellar impairment)
- Docetaxel (motor and sensory nerve deficits)
- Methotrexate (high dose: mental status changes)
- Oxaliplatin (sensory nerve deficits)
- Paclitaxel (motor and sensory nerve deficits)
- Vinblastine (motor and sensory nerve deficits, autonomic nervous system deficits)
- Vincristine (motor and sensory nerve deficits, autonomic nervous system deficits, cranial nerve deficits)
- Vinorelbine (sensory and autonomic nervous system deficits)

severity of symptoms may abate when treatment is halted; however, recovery may be slow and is usually incomplete.

◆ Patients with neuropathies may experience neuropathic pain, which is often described and treated differently from nociceptive pain. See **Chronic pain,** p. 13, for desired outcomes and interventions.

◆ Patients receiving vinca alkaloids should be monitored for bowel elimination daily, *because they may be at risk for paralytic ileus.* Administer stool softeners, psyllium, or laxatives daily if patient does not have bowel movements at least every other day. Instruct patient to increase dietary fiber and fluid intake.

Impaired skin integrity or Impaired tissue integrity (or risk for same) related to treatment with chemotherapy or biotherapy

Desired outcome: Before chemotherapy, patient identifies potential skin and tissue side effects of chemotherapy and measures that will maintain skin integrity and promote comfort.

Alterations of the skin or nails that occur in conjunction with chemotherapy are a result of destruction of the basal cells of the epidermis (general) or of cellular alterations at the site of chemotherapy administration (local). Reactions are specific to the agent used and vary in onset, severity, and duration. Skin reactions include the following: transient erythema/urticaria, hyperpigmentation, telangiectasis, photosensitivity, hyperkeratosis, acne-like reaction, ulceration, and radiation recall. Fingernails may develop half-moon markings called Beau's lines, *which are clinically insignificant.*

Transient erythema/urticaria: This condition may be generalized or localized at the site of chemotherapy administration. It occurs soon after chemotherapy is administered and disappears in several hours. It is critical to differentiate between local irritation of the vein, flare reaction, or extravasation on the local level and hypersensitivity or beginning anaphylaxis on a general level.

Nursing Interventions

◆ Perform and document a pretreatment assessment of patient's skin for posttreatment comparison.

◆ If it is infusing, halt chemotherapy temporarily until the nature of the reaction can be ascertained.

◆ Assess and document onset, pattern, severity, and duration of the reaction after treatment.

Hyperpigmentation: Caused by increased levels of epidermal melanin-stimulating hormone, hyperpigmentation can occur on the nail beds, oral

BOX 12-8	CHEMOTHERAPEUTIC DRUGS THAT MAY CAUSE HYPERPIGMENTATION

- Bleomycin
- Carmustine
- Cyclophosphamide
- Daunorubicin
- Doxorubicin
- 5-Fluorouracil
- Melphalan

BOX 12-9	CHEMOTHERAPEUTIC DRUGS THAT MAY CAUSE PHOTOSENSITIVITY

- Bleomycin
- Dacarbazine
- Dactinomycin
- Daunomycin
- Doxorubicin
- 5-Fluorouracil
- Methotrexate

*National Cancer Institute Common Toxicity Criteria. http://www.accessdata.fda.gov/scripts/cder/onctools/toxcrit1.cfm 7/9/2007

mucosa, skin, or along veins used for chemotherapy administration. It may be caused by chemotherapeutic agents listed in **BOX 12-8** as well as by vesicant agents listed in Box 12-10. In addition, it can occur with tumors of the pituitary gland.

Nursing Interventions

- ◆ Inform patient before treatment that this reaction is to be expected and may or may not disappear over the first few months when treatment is finished.
- ◆ *Because sunlight may exacerbate hyperpigmentation,* caution patient to wear sunscreen with a high sun protection factor (SPF) and cover exposed areas.

Photosensitivity: This condition is enhanced when skin is exposed to ultraviolet light. Acute sunburn and residual tanning may occur with very short exposure to the sun when receiving certain chemotherapy drugs (see **BOX 12-9** for examples). Photosensitivity can occur during the time the agent is administered, or it can reactivate a skin reaction caused by recent sun exposure before chemotherapy.

Nursing Interventions

- ◆ Assess onset, pattern, severity, and duration of the reaction.
- ◆ Teach patient to avoid exposing skin to the sun. Advise patient to wear protective clothing and use an effective sunscreen (SPF of 15 or higher).
- ◆ Teach patient to treat sunburns with comfort measures such as tepid baths, moisturizing creams, and aloe and to consult health care provider accordingly.

Acne-like reaction: An acne-like reaction manifests as erythema, especially of the face, chest, and upper back, and progresses to papules and pustules, which are characteristic of acne. Reassure patient that the reaction will disappear when treatment is discontinued.

Nursing Interventions

- Suggest use of commercial acne preparations, such as benzoyl peroxide lotion, gel, or cream, to treat blemishes.
- Teach proper skin care.
- Avoid hard scrubbing.
- Avoid use of antibacterial soap *because the removal of nonpathogenic bacteria on the skin results in replacement by pathogens, which are implicated in the genesis of acne.* Use a mild plain soap.
- Avoid use of oil-based cosmetics.

Radiation recall reaction: This reaction occurs when chemotherapy is given after treatment with radiation therapy, and radiation enhancement occurs when radiation and chemotherapy are given concurrently. Both reactions present as erythema, followed by dry desquamation at the radiation site. More severe reactions can progress to vesicle formation and wet desquamation. After the skin heals, it may be permanently hyperpigmented. Teach patient to protect skin at the site of recall reaction as described in the following interventions.

Nursing Interventions

- Assess skin daily during radiation therapy, and observe for radiation effect as well as signs of infection.
- Avoid wearing tight-fitting clothes and harsh fabrics. Avoid excess heat or cold exposure to the area, salt water or chlorinated pools, deodorants, perfumed lotions, cosmetics, and shaving of the area.
- Use mild detergents and soaps.
- For pruritus, use corticosteroid cream (triamcinolone acetonide 0.1%) or prescribed medications such as diphenhydramine.
- Caution patients receiving IL-2 regarding sun exposure, *which may precipitate a reaction similar to radiation recall.*
- See **Impaired skin integrity,** which follows, for wound care.

Dry, pruritic skin: This problem commonly occurs with biologic therapy and should be treated aggressively. It may be accompanied by a rash and eventual desquamation. Teach patient the measures described in the following interventions

Nursing Interventions

- Apply creams and water-based lotions several times a day, and avoid perfumed products.
- Avoid hot bathing water and use only mild soaps.
- Manage pruritus with antipruritic medications such as diphenhydramine or hydroxyzine hydrochloride. Teach patients receiving IL-2 not to use topical steroids, *which may interfere with therapy.*
- See **Impaired skin integrity,** which follows, for wound care.

Impaired skin integrity related to radiation therapy

Desired outcome: Within 24 hr of instruction, patient identifies potential skin reactions and management interventions that will promote comfort and skin integrity.

Nursing Interventions

- Assess the degree and extent of the skin reaction as follows (National Cancer Institute Common Toxicity Criteria):
  - *Grade 1:* Scattered macular or papular rash or erythema that is asymptomatic
  - *Grade 2:* Moderate edema, scattered macular or papular rash or erythema with pruritus or other symptoms
  - *Grade 3:* Generalized symptomatic macular, papular, or vesicular rash
  - *Grade 4:* Exfoliative or ulcerating dermatitis
- Teach patient the following skin care for the treatment field:
  - Cleanse skin gently and in a patting motion, using mild soap, tepid water, and soft cloth. Rinse the area and pat it dry.

- Apply cornstarch, A&D ointment, ointment containing aloe or lanolin, or mild topical steroids as prescribed to skin with grade 2 reaction.
◆ For patients with grade 3 skin reaction, teach the following regimen:
  - Cleanse area with half-strength hydrogen peroxide and normal saline, and use irrigation syringe. Rinse with saline or water and pat dry gently.
  - Use nonadhesive absorbent dressings for draining areas. Be alert to signs and symptoms of infection.
  - To promote healing, use moisture- and vapor-permeable dressings, such as hydrocolloids and hydrogels, on noninfected areas.
◆ For grade 4 reaction, teach the following interventions:
  - Topical antibiotics (e.g., sulfadiazine cream) may be applied to open areas prone to infection.
  - Debride wound of eschar (necessary before healing can occur).
  - After removing eschar (results in yellow wound), keep wound clean to prevent infection. (Wet-to-moist dressings often are used to keep the wound clean.)
  - Collaborate with wound, ostomy, and continence (WOC)/enterostomal therapy (ET) nurse as needed regarding techniques to promote wound healing.
◆ Teach patient potential long-term skin changes associated with radiation, such as altered pigmentation, atrophy, fragility, or ulceration.

Impaired tissue integrity (or risk for same) related to extravasation of vesicant or irritating chemotherapy agents
Desired outcome: Patient's tissue remains intact without evidence of inflammation or tissue damage near the injection site.
*Only nurses experienced in venous access and knowledgeable about chemotherapy should administer vesicant drugs (**BOX 12-10**). It is vital for the nurse to be knowledgeable regarding any vesicant or irritant properties specific to a drug before the drug is administered.*

Nursing Interventions

◆ A new venous access site should be obtained before vesicant administration. Avoid sites where there is increased risk of damage to underlying tendons or nerves, such as the antecubital fossa, wrist, or dorsal surface of the hand.
◆ Assess patency of venous site before and during administration of the drug. Instruct patient to report burning, itching, or pain immediately.
◆ Assess venous access site at frequent intervals. Pain, burning, and stinging are common with extravasation, as are erythema and swelling around needle site. Blood return should not be used as the sole indicator to ascertain that extravasation has not occurred inasmuch as blood return is possible even if extravasation has occurred.

BOX 12-10	VESICANT AGENTS

- Cisplatin*
- Dacarbazine
- Dactinomycin
- Daunorubicin
- Doxorubicin
- Epirubicin
- Etoposide*
- Mechlorethamine
- Mitomycin C
- Vinblastine
- Vincristine
- Vinorelbine

*Concentration related.

- ◆ Keep extravasation kit readily available, along with institutional guidelines for extravasation management.
- ◆ In the event of extravasation, follow these general guidelines:
  - Stop infusion immediately, and aspirate any remaining drug from needle. To do this, first don latex gloves, then attach syringe to the tubing and aspirate the drug.
  - Consult chemotherapy infusion guidelines for specifics regarding management of extravasation of individual drugs.
  - Leave needle in place if using an antidote for the extravasated drug.
  - Do not apply pressure to the site. Apply a sterile occlusive dressing, elevate site, and apply heat or cold as recommended by guidelines.
  - Document incident, and note date, time, needle insertion site, VAD type and size, drug, drug concentration, approximate amount of drug extravasated, patient symptoms, extravasation management, and appearance of the site. Review institutional guidelines regarding necessity of photo documentation. Monitor site at frequent intervals.
  - Provide patient with information about site care and follow-up appointments for evaluation of the extravasation. If appropriate, collaborate with health care provider regarding a plastic surgery consultation.

Impaired urinary elimination related to hemorrhagic cystitis secondary to cyclophosphamide/ifosfamide treatment, oliguria or renal toxicity secondary to cisplatin or high-dose methotrexate administration, renal calculi secondary to hyperuricemia, or dysuria secondary to cystitis
Desired outcomes: Patients receiving cyclophosphamide/ifosfamide test negative for blood in their urine, and patients receiving cisplatin exhibit urinary output of 100 mL/hr or more 1 hr before treatment and 4-12 hr after treatment. Patients with leukemia and lymphomas and those taking methotrexate exhibit urine pH 7.5 or higher.

Nursing Interventions

- ◆ Ensure adequate hydration during treatment and for at least 24 hr after treatment for patient taking cyclophosphamide (Cytoxan), ifosfamide, methotrexate, or cisplatin. Teach patient importance of drinking at least 2-3 L/day. IV hydration also may be required, especially with high-dose chemotherapy.
- ◆ Administer cyclophosphamide early in the day *to minimize retention of metabolites in the bladder during the night.* Encourage patient to urinate every 2 hours during the day and before going to bed. Test urine for presence of blood, and report positive results to health care provider. Monitor I&O q8h during high-dose treatment for 48 hr after treatment. Be alert to decreasing urinary output.
- ◆ Mesna is administered before ifosfamide and then 4 hr and 8 hr after the infusion (or via a continuous infusion), *to minimize risk of hemorrhagic cystitis.* Test all urine for presence of blood *to maintain urine output at approximately 100 mL/hr.* Monitor I&O during infusion and for 24 hr after therapy *to ensure that this level of urinary output is attained.*
- ◆ For patient receiving cisplatin, prehydrate with IV fluid (150-200 mL/hr). Cisplatin can be administered as soon as patient's urine output is 100-150 mL/hr or more. Monitor I&O hourly for 4-12 hr after therapy *to ensure that urine output is maintained at 100-150 mL/hr or more.* Patient may require diuretics to maintain this output. Promote fluid intake to ensure a positive fluid state for at least 24 hr after treatment, especially for patient taking diuretics. Notify health care provider promptly if urine output drops to less than 100 mL/hr. Urine output should be kept at a relatively high level *because nephroticity can occur as a side effect of this treatment.*

- Alkaline urine will enhance excretion of methotrexate and of the uric acid that results from tumor lysis, which is associated with leukemia and lymphoma. Monitor I&O q8h, and watch for decreasing output. Test urine pH with each voiding *to ensure that it is 7.5 or higher*. Sodium bicarbonate and acetazolamide (Diamox) are used *to alkalinize the urine*. Allopurinol prevents uric acid formation and is often administered before chemotherapy for patients with leukemia or lymphoma.

- Hyperuricemia may be caused by chemotherapy treatment for leukemia and lymphoma. The rapid cell lysis and increased excretion of uric acid may result in renal calculi. For more information, see "Ureteral Calculi," p. 199.

- Teach patient signs of cystitis, which can occur secondary to cyclophosphamide and ifosfamide treatment: fever, pain with urination, malodorous or cloudy urine, blood in the urine, and urinary frequency and urgency. Instruct patient to notify health care professional if these signs and symptoms occur.

Care for Patients with Special Needs

SECTION ONE **PROVIDING NUTRITIONAL SUPPORT**

Hospitalized patients are at high risk for developing protein-energy malnutrition. Studies have shown that 40%-50% of hospitalized surgical patients have insufficient nutrient intake. This situation may be seen in surgical patients who are given IV dextrose electrolyte solutions alone for extended periods and in patients kept fasting for diagnostic procedures. If this state persists for more than 10-14 consecutive days in an individual with moderately or severely reduced nutritional stores, that individual should be considered and evaluated for nutritional support. When individuals are well nourished, there are no defined timeframes during which they can be without water or food before addressing artificial replacement. The best markers to use for initiation of water and food in otherwise well-nourished people are magnitude of the injury/insult to the body and amount of time the individual will be unable to resume normal oral intake.

❖ NUTRITIONAL ASSESSMENT

Because no single sensitive and comprehensive nutritional assessment factor exists, multiple sources of information are used, including any of the following: historical data including medical/surgical history, nutritional history, anthropometric data, biochemical analysis of blood and urine, and duration of the disease process.

DIETARY HISTORY

A dietary history is compiled to reveal adequacy of usual and recent food intake. Based on the information obtained, the nurse may identify the need to consult with a registered dietitian for additional interventions. Be alert to excesses or deficiencies of nutrients and any special eating patterns (e.g., various types of vegetarian or prescribed diets), use of fad diets, and excessive supplementation. Include in the care plan anything that impairs adequate selection, preparation, ingestion, digestion, absorption, or excretion of nutrients, as follows:

- Food allergies, food aversions, and use of nutritional supplements (prescribed or over-the-counter [OTC]).
- Any alternative therapies such as use of herbs.
- Any OTC medications.
- Recent unplanned weight loss or gain.

- Chewing or swallowing difficulties. Include questions related to dental care, such as dentures (note presence of dentures; ask about fit of dentures or other problems); missing teeth, no teeth, and/or loose teeth.
- Nausea, vomiting, or pain with eating.
- Altered pattern of elimination (e.g., constipation, diarrhea).
- Chronic disease affecting utilization of nutrients (e.g., malabsorption, pancreatitis, diabetes mellitus [DM]).
- Surgical resection; disease of the gut or accessory organs of digestion (i.e., pancreas, liver, gallbladder).
- Current pregnancy or lactation.
- Use of medications (e.g., laxatives, antacids, antibiotics, antineoplastic drugs) or alcohol. Long-term use of drugs may affect appetite, digestion, or utilization or excretion of nutrients.

SIGNS AND SYMPTOMS/PHYSICAL FINDINGS

Most physical findings are not specific to a particular nutritional deficiency. Compare current assessment findings with past assessments, especially related to the following:

- Loss of muscle and adipose tissue.
- Fit of clothing, rings, and watches. Be aware that assessment of obese patients or individuals who have an excess of fluid accumulation because of body edema may be difficult.
- Temporal wasting in individuals who have ascites or other forms of body edema.
- Work and muscle endurance.
- Ability to maintain activities of daily living (ADL).
- Recent changes in mobility and/or activities.
- Muscle weakness, which may reflect several different deficiencies that may require additional evaluation and tests:
  - Selenium
  - Vitamin D
  - Potassium
  - Magnesium
- Changes in hair, skin, or neuromuscular function.
- Excessive bruising or bleeding, which may reflect vitamin K deficiency.
- Alopecia or seborrheic dermatitis, which can be related to biotin deficiency.
- Scaly dermatitis, which may reflect essential fatty acid deficiency.
- Sores at edges of mouth, palms of hands, and soles of feet, with peeling of skin along with brittle nails, which can result from zinc deficiency.
- Dry and scaling skin, brittle nails, and/or dry hair, which can result from hypocalcemia.

ANTHROPOMETRIC DATA

Height: Used to determine ideal weight and body mass index (BMI). If patient's height is unavailable or impossible to measure, obtain an estimate from family or significant other.

Weight: Used by many to determine nutritional status, but fluctuations may be a result of amputation, dehydration, diuresis, fluid retention (renal failure, edema, third spacing), fluid resuscitation, wound dressings, or clothing. (It is helpful to remember that 1 L of fluid equals approximately 2 lb.) More reliable information may be obtained by asking patient to recall usual weight, weight changes (gains and losses), and timeframe in which these occurred. Unintentional loss in weight of greater than 10% over a 6-mo period is considered significant and may be associated with severe malnutrition. The greater the unintentional weight loss, the more predictive this weight loss may be of mortality.

Most dietitians use the Hamwi "rule of thumb" calculation to determine ideal body weight.

Ideal body weight: Men

> 106 lb for the first 5 ft, then add 6 lb for each inch over 5 ft

> **or**

> 48 kg for the first 1.5 cm, then add 2.7 kg for each 2.54 cm over 1.5 cm

Ideal body weight: Women

> 100 lb for the first 5 ft, then add 5 lb for each inch over 5 ft

> **or**

> 45 kg for the first 1.5 cm, then add 2.3 kg for each 2.54 cm over 1.5 cm

BMI: Used to evaluate the weight of adults. One calculation and one set of standards are applicable to both men and women:

$$BMI\,(kg\,m/m^2) = \frac{Weight}{Height\,(m^2)}$$

BMI values of 19-25 are appropriate for 19-34 yr olds, whereas BMI values of 21-27 are appropriate for individuals older than 35 yr of age. Obesity is defined as BMI greater than 27.5, with severe or morbid obesity greater than 40. A BMI of 16-18.5 is considered mild to moderate malnutrition, whereas a value lower than 16 indicates severe malnutrition.

BIOCHEMICAL DATA

If an individual is ill, these biochemical data are more accurate as predictors of outcome or recovery than as indicators of nutritional state.

Protein status: Evaluated via the following tests, with normal values in parentheses: serum albumin (3.5-5.0 g/dL), transferrin (200-400 mg/dL), and prealbumin (20-30 mg/dL). Normal values may vary somewhat with different laboratory procedures and standards. Albumin and transferrin have relatively long half-lives of 14-20 days and 8-10 days, respectively, whereas prealbumin (a short-phase protein) has a very short half-life of 48-72 hr. If hydration status is normal and anemia is absent, albumin and transferrin levels can be used as baseline indicators of adequacy of protein intake and synthesis. For evidence of response to nutritional therapy, prealbumin values are the most useful when patient has normal renal function.

Iron status: Measurement of RBC size (i.e., mean corpuscular volume [MCV] [normal: 80-95 μm^3]) aids in determining the type of nutrient anemia. In iron-deficiency anemia, RBCs are smaller than normal, whereas in folate or vitamin B_{12} deficiencies, RBCs are larger than normal.

ESTIMATING NUTRITIONAL REQUIREMENTS

The primary goal of nutritional support is to meet the needs for body temperature, metabolic processes, and tissue repair. Having collected all the data, energy needs may be estimated using the following options.

Harris-Benedict equations: Used to determine basal energy expenditure (BEE). The following equations can be used to calculate BEE (weight = weight in kg; height = height in cm; age = age in yr):

BEE (Male)

$$66.5 + (13.8 \times weight) + (5.0 \times height) - (6.8 \times age)$$

BEE (Female)

$$655.1 + (9.6 \times weight) + (1.9 \times height) - (4.7 \times age)$$

Calorie estimation: Prevents overfeeding, and calculates the total calorie intake as follows:

Average nourished patient	25 total calories per kg of body weight
Mildly stressed patient	30 total calories per kg of body weight
Severely stressed patient	35 total calories per kg of body weight
Morbidly obese patient	18 total calories per kg of body weight

Distribution of calories: A relatively normal distribution of calories is adequate. Percentages of total calories from carbohydrates (CHOs), protein, and fat should equal approximately 60%, 15%-20%, and 15%-25%, respectively.

Protein requirements: Usually 0.8-1.5 g/kg/24 hr. (Protein will be restricted if patient has hepatic or renal failure that is not being treated with dialysis.)

$$1 \text{ g protein} = 4.0 \text{ kcal}$$

$$1 \text{ g N} = 6.25 \text{ g protein}$$

CHO requirements: Daily glucose administration of 9-15 g/kg/24 hr is an adequate range. Excess amounts of CHO are not utilized or tolerated. Over-feeding of CHO may lead to hyperglycemia, increased CO_2 production, hypo-phosphatemia, and fluid overload in short-term use or fatty liver syndrome in long-term use.

$$1 \text{ g IV dextrose} = 3.4 \text{ kcal}$$

$$1 \text{ g CHO in food} = 4.0 \text{ kcal}$$

Fat requirements: Fat can be administered in minimal quantities to satisfy needs for essential fatty acids but should not exceed 1 g fat/kg/24 hr because of the potential for suppression of the immune system.

$$1 \text{ g fat} = 9.0 \text{ calories}$$

Special diets for organ-specific pathologic conditions: Commercially available oral supplements and enteral formulas are available for patients with respiratory disease, DM, renal failure, hepatic failure, inflammatory bowel disease, and immune compromise. Well-designed clinical trials may not be available to support the suggested indication.

Vitamin and essential trace mineral requirements: In general, follow the recommended dietary allowances (RDAs) to provide minimum quantities of vitamins, minerals, and essential fatty acids. For specific patients, supplement specific vitamins or minerals needed in increased amounts for existing disease states (e.g., burns: zinc, vitamins A and C; chronic alcohol ingestion: thiamine, folate, vitamin B_{12}).

Fluid requirements: Many factors affect fluid balance. Under usual circumstances, an estimate of fluid needs can be made by providing 1 mL of free water for each calorie provided, or 30-50 mL/kg body weight. Daily loss of water includes approximately 1400 mL in urine (60 mL/hr), 350 mL via respiration, 600 mL as evaporation through skin, and about 200 mL in feces. Fluid losses are 100-150 mL/day for each degree of temperature increase above 37° C. If loss by any of these routes is increased, fluid needs will increase; if loss by any of these routes is impaired, fluid restriction may be necessary. Areas to include in the nursing assessment for fluid requirements are:

◆ I&O: Evaluate that neither one is in excess of the other and for decreases in urine output.
◆ Daily weights: Rapid changes may represent problems with technique or equipment rather than actual changes in body weight. If sudden increases in weight occur, look for imbalances in I&O, occurrence of edema, and dilution of serum electrolytes.
◆ Presence or absence of edema.
◆ Skin turgor: May be helpful in younger patients, but less useful in older adults because of normal changes in skin elasticity that occur with aging.

TABLE 13-1	DESCRIPTIVE TERMS ASSOCIATED WITH TYPES OF ENTERAL FORMULAS
TERM	**DEFINITION**
Isotonic	Formula having an osmolarity of 300 mOsm/L, which is the same as blood Osmotic gradient between the formula and the blood flow within the intestines is equal
Hypertonic	Formula having an osmolarity greater than 300 mOsm/L, usually in the range of 450-600 mOsm/L; osmotic gradient between the formula and the blood flow within the intestines is unequal, and the formula will pull fluid into the intestines during the digestive process
Osmolarity	Referred to as mOsm/L and describes the osmotic gradient between blood and the intestines; normal level found in the blood is300 mOsm/L
Caloric density	Number of calories delivered to patient in each mL of liquid feeding Ranges from 0.5-2 kcal/mL
Modular	Consists of a single nutrient that may be combined with other modules (nutrients) to treat specific deficits (e.g., protein, carbohydrate, or fat) in an individual

❖ NUTRITIONAL SUPPORT MODALITIES

OVERVIEW/PATHOPHYSIOLOGY

Specialized nutritional support refers to provision of an artificial formulation of nutrients via the oral, enteral, or parenteral route for the treatment or prevention of malnutrition. Oral supplements are preferred because they are less invasive, more natural, and less costly, and enteral nutrition is preferred over parenteral.

Terms associated with formulas for oral supplements or enteral delivery: See **TABLE 13-1**.

Nutritional composition: See **TABLE 13-2**.

Types of feeding tubes

Small-bore nasal tubes: Defined as 12F or smaller tube; require abdominal x-ray examination for confirmation of placement. Composition may be polyurethane, silicone, or polyvinyl chloride. Location cannot be verified in the gastrointestinal (GI) tract by auscultation after injecting an air bolus, asking patient to speak, or submerging the tube's proximal tip into a glass of water. Usual length of tube is 36-45 inches, and it may or may not require a stylet for insertion. The physician should determine whether the distal tip ends in the stomach or small intestine. Insertion by a nurse is determined by hospital policy. The tube also may be inserted using fluoroscopy in the radiation or endoscopy department. Because of their diameter and composition, these tubes are easily dislocated proximally in the GI tract without any external signs.

Large-bore nasal tubes: Defined as larger than 12F tube; best practice is x-ray examination for confirmation of placement. Composition is either polyurethane or polyvinyl chloride. Usual length of tube is 36 inches. Stylet is not required for insertion. Insertion may be performed by a nurse.

Gastrostomy tubes: Exit stomach directly through abdominal wall and are usually anchored with either a balloon or a disk on the inside of the stomach. Generally they are 12F or larger. Composition may be polyurethane, silicone, or rubber, and these tubes may contain multiple ports for insertion of air into

TABLE 13-2	NUTRITIONAL COMPOSITION OF ENTERAL FORMULAS AND ORAL SUPPLEMENTS	

COMPONENT	TYPE	DESCRIPTION
Protein	Polymeric	Standard, complete protein nitrogen source
	Hydrolyzed	Reduced into smaller forms to assist with absorption
	Elemental/free amino acids	Simple amino acids that require no further digestion and are ready for absorption
		Usually increases formula osmolarity; bitter taste
Carbohydrate		The most easily digested and absorbed component in enteral formulas; 80% of all carbohydrate is broken down and absorbed as simple glucose in the normal intestine; most commercially available formulas are lactose free
Fat	Long-chain triglycerides	Provide an isotonic, concentrated energy source
	Medium-chain triglycerides	Used for patients with impaired fat digestion and absorption; no stimulation of pancreatic lipase secretion
	Omega-3 fatty acids	Addition of fish oils to improve immune function of the body by producing eicosapentaenoic acid
Fiber		Soy polysaccharide is most commonly added to enteral formulas as a treatment for diarrhea, although its usefulness has not been proven with research; because fiber is absorbed in the large intestine, a patient with an ileostomy would not benefit; formula viscosity increases with fiber, and it should be delivered via an enteral tube 10F or larger with an enteral feeding pump

the balloon, delivery of medications, and the main lumen. Initially a physician in the radiology, endoscopy, or surgery department performs the insertion. When the tube is placed by a physician in the radiology or endoscopy department, the common term used to describe the tube is *percutaneous endoscopic gastrostomy (PEG)*. Reinsertion by a nurse is determined by hospital policy.

Gastrostomy button: Placed into a mature gastrostomy stoma. It fits into the stoma tract flush with the outer abdominal wall. The button contains an antireflux valve to prevent leakage, but gastric samples or residuals usually cannot be obtained via the button.

Jejunostomy tubes: Placed by a physician either surgically or percutaneously (percutaneous endoscopic jejunostomy [PEJ]). Diameter is usually about 12F-18F. Anchoring the tube inside the jejunum presents a problem because a balloon larger than 5 mL may cause bowel obstruction. Confirmation of position requires x-ray examination with contrast. No residuals should be obtained from this tube. If the tube becomes displaced, the entry site into the jejunum will close down rapidly (approximately 20-30 min). Reinsertion by a nurse is determined by hospital policy, but it is not recommended without special training.

Gastrostomy-jejunostomy tubes: Exit stomach directly through the abdominal wall with a small-bore jejunostomy tube placed through the main lumen of the gastrostomy and the distal tip positioned in the jejunum.

BOX 13-1 presents nursing care guidelines for enteral tubes.

Feeding sites

Stomach: Simulates normal GI functions; may be used for bolus, intermittent, or continuous feedings; indicated for patients who have intact gag or cough reflex.

Duodenum, jejunum: Must be used for continuous feedings only, to prevent dumping syndrome and diarrhea. A small-bore diameter tube is recommended.

BOX 13-2 and **TABLE 13-3** present guidelines for administration of enteral products.

❖ TOTAL PARENTERAL NUTRITION

OVERVIEW/PATHOPHYSIOLOGY

Total parenteral nutrition (TPN) provides some or all nutrients by the IV route. TPN is used to provide complete nutrition for patients who cannot receive enteral nutrition or to supplement nutritional needs of patients who are unable to absorb sufficient calories via the GI tract. TPN is more expensive than enteral nutrition and has the potential for causing severe complications more rapidly.

Parenteral solutions: IV solutions are customized combinations of dextrose (CHO), amino acids (protein), IV fat emulsions (fat), electrolytes, vitamins, and trace metals.

CHO: Dextrose provides the bulk of calories and energy needs, with concentrations ranging from 5%-70%. The percentage of dextrose selected is based on the available administration site and patient's volume status. All final mixed solutions that are more than 12.5% dextrose must be administered via central venous catheter (CVC). (If unsure or if information is unavailable on the infusion container related to infusion route, consult with pharmacist or refer to hospital policy.) The average amount of CHO calories delivered is approximately 60% of the total. The more CHO is delivered, the greater is the potential for complications, which include fatty liver syndrome, increased CO_2 production, and hyperglycemia.

Protein: Synthetic crystalline essential and nonessential amino acid formulations are available in concentrations of 3.5%-15%. Special amino acid formulations are available that vary the ratio of essential to nonessential amino acids for specific disorders (e.g., liver, renal disease). The amount of protein delivered depends on patient's renal and hepatic function.

Fat: Intravenous fat emulsion (IVFE) of 10%, 20%, or 30% is an isotonic solution providing essential fatty acids and a source of concentrated calories.

$$10\% \text{ IVFE} = 1.1 \text{ calorie/mL}$$

$$20\% \text{ IVFE} = 2 \text{ calories/mL}$$

$$30\% \text{ IVFE} = 3 \text{ calories/mL}$$

When fats are mixed in the same infusion bag with the CHO and amino acids, the solution is referred to as a *total nutrient admixture* (TNA) or a *3:1 solution* (all three nutrient components in one bag). The IVFE may be given piggyback into the amino acid/dextrose infusion to infuse over 8-12 hr. The amount of IVFE administered may be reduced or removed for patients who have hypertriglyceridemia (e.g., patients receiving antirejection medication following organ transplant, coronary artery disease, pancreatitis, acquired

BOX 13-1   GENERAL NURSING CARE GUIDELINES FOR ENTERAL TUBES

- Best patency is maintained with regular flushing of the tube before and after each medication, before and after each intermittent feeding, and routinely during continuous feedings.
- Flush tube with water using 25-50 mL, depending on physician prescription and patient's underlying medical condition. Dark cola also has been suggested as a potential agent for flushing tubes.
- Because of impurities and bacteria in tap water, sterile water has been suggested for high-risk patients, including infants and older adults, and for any tube feeding that enters the body in the small intestine. (Check agency policy for type of water used to flush enteral feeding tubes in your patient population.)
- If the enteral tube becomes clogged, it is best to identify whether the change in flow was related to formula buildup within the tube or a chemical reaction from medications being administered through the tube. If the tube is clogged with formula, products that have been suggested for declogging it are dark cola, hot water, and pancrease or other commercially available enzymatic medication pushed down the tube, using a push-pull method and correct syringe size recommended by the manufacturer. If the tube has become clogged with medications, hot water may be used via the aforementioned push-pull method. Mechanical devices are also available for declogging a tube, but use may be restricted to trained individuals within the institution. (Check with agency policy for type of declogging recommended in enteral feeding tubes.)
- Always insert smallest-bore tube possible to minimize complications. A large-bore nasogastric tube may be used temporarily in the stomach until a small-bore tube can be placed; a small-bore tube must be inserted if intestinal placement is required for delivery of the formula.
- When anchoring the tube in place, ensure adequate skin protection and observe for pressure on the skin.
- Nasal tubes may result in pressure on the nares if the tube is taped too tightly to the nose. (Check with agency policy for frequency of nasal assessment recommended for nasal enteral feeding tubes.)
- Gastric tubes may result in an increase in reflux or damage to the stoma if the tube is angled and pulled flat against the abdominal wall. Some newer tubes are being designed with an angle to facilitate taping to the abdominal wall.
- If bumpers are used with a gastric tube, check with manufacturer or agency policy to identify whether it is necessary to routinely rotate the bumper around the tube while inspecting the skin daily.
- If bumpers are used with a gastric tube, a dressing may not be necessary and may be avoided under the bumpers to prevent too much pulling on the tube. A dressing under a bumper may cause internal and external anchoring devices to become too tight and may thereby produce some vascular insufficiency to the abdominal wall.
- If inserting a small-bore feeding tube, always verify initial placement in the stomach or small intestine with x-ray film before initiating the feeding.
- Use manufacturer recommendations regarding syringe size when irrigating the tube.
- Verify with pharmacy that medications are appropriate for administration via an enteral feeding tube. Change in route or delivery form may be necessary to maintain medication effects. For example:
  - Time-released medications may have to be changed to a short-acting form because time-released medications should not be crushed.
  - A medication that is absorbed in the stomach may have to be reevaluated when the distal tip of the tube is in the small intestine.
  - Elixirs or suspensions may be suggested because they are easier than a crushed pill to administer through an enteral tube.

BOX 13-2 GENERAL NURSING CARE GUIDELINES FOR ADMINISTRATION OF AN ENTERAL FORMULA

- Perform frequent oral care, especially if the individual is not taking any food by mouth.
- Monitor patient to ensure delivery of prescribed volume and formula type.
- Monitor daily weights.
- Initially, monitor electrolyte values daily until they are stable with appropriate replacements.
- If the individual has a history of glucose intolerance or is taking medications that may cause hyperglycemia, or if an increase in blood glucose is noted on serum electrolyte values, routine monitoring of the glucose should include bedside assessments q4h and treatment appropriate for maintaining glucose within normal limits.
- Monitor I&O q8h. Separate intake of formula from intake of other nutrients or fluids. Keep enteral tube flushing amounts separate from enteral formula intake.
- Administer formula at full strength.
- Use an enteral pump for all continuous administrations of formula.
- If using an open delivery system, do not use formula that has been opened for more than 24 hr. If using a closed delivery system, refer to manufacturer or agency policy for duration of hang time.
- Refer to agency policy regarding checking of residuals.
- Several key points in the delivery of enteral formulas established by Hazard Analysis Critical Control Point (HACCP) developed by the U.S. Department of Agriculture (USDA) and the Food and Drug Administration (FDA) include the following:
  - Train staff to ensure that preparation and sanitation procedures are followed.
  - Perform meticulous handwashing when handling all aspects of the products, including bag, formula, pump and additives.
  - Only hang a volume of formula that will infuse within a designated timeframe. Mark bag indicating how long it should hang.
  - If giving intermittent feedings, flush bag and set with water between feedings. Refer to agency policy for type of water to be used (sterile vs. tap).
  - Clean top of the can, if using one, with alcohol before opening and pouring into enteral bag.
  - Refrigerate and date all opened containers of formula.
  - Dispose of enteral bag, administration set, and syringes q24h.
  - Wear gloves while handling the equipment and products.

TABLE 13-3 ADMINISTRATION OF ENTERAL PRODUCTS

TYPE	DEFINITION	COMPLICATIONS
Bolus	Given by gravity; pushed via syringe	May cause cramping, bloating, nausea, diarrhea, aspiration; not recommended
Intermittent	Administered over 30-60 min via infusion bag; total volume should not exceed 450 mL/feeding	May cause cramping, nausea, bloating, diarrhea, aspiration; may need to ↓ infusion rate to ↓ complications
Continuous	Given at the same infusion rate over 24 hr; may be cycled over 12-24 hr if patient tolerates the volume	May cause cramping, nausea, bloating, diarrhea, aspiration; may need to ↓ infusion rate to ↓ complications

BOX 13-3   GENERAL NURSING CARE GUIDELINES FOR THE ADMINISTRATION OF TOTAL PARENTERAL NUTRITION

- Use a 0.22-μm filter on all solutions containing amino acids and dextrose; use a 1.2-μm filter with all solutions containing amino acids, dextrose, and IVFEs. The purpose of the filter is to reduce infusion of crystals that may form from the interaction between calcium and phosphorus in the admixture. In addition, the 0.22-μm filter removes bacteria that may be in the infusion or IV system.
- Administer all solutions via an IV infusion pump.
- Monitor CVC insertion site for signs and symptoms of infection.
- Maintain sterile, occlusive dressing on central catheter insertion site.
- Refrigerate solution, if it is agency policy, until 30-60 min before administration.
- The total number of calories initiated is determined by a person trained in nutritional therapy (RN, RD, or RPh) and is based on patient's metabolic and nutritional status.
- The infusion may be initiated at full rate.
- Tapering is not necessary for initiation or discontinuation.
- Solution may be administered over 12-24 hr, depending on patient's medical condition.
- IV push administration of D_{50} or infusion of $D_{10}W$ is not required with an interruption in the infusion.
- Monitor for hyperglycemia.
  - Nondiabetic: q6h for 24-48 hr, then discontinue if no signs of glucose intolerance have occurred. If the individual is glucose-intolerant, advance bedside assessment to q4h, and begin administration of sliding scale insulin as prescribed.
  - Diabetic: q4h, with sliding scale regular insulin prescribed; consult with health care provider who specializes in care of the diabetic patient.

CVC, Central venous catheter; D_{50}, 50% dextrose; $D_{50}W$, 50% dextrose in water; *IV,* intravenous; *IVFE,* intravenous fat emulsion; *RD,* registered dietitian; *RN,* registered nurse; *RPh,* registered pharmacist.

immunodeficiency syndrome [AIDS]). Determine whether patient has an egg allergy because long-chain triglycerides in IVFEs may originate from phospholipids in egg yolks. If a patient develops a rash during IVFE infusion, consider an allergy immediately. If the ratio of the protein, CHO, and IVFE in the admixture is not stable, separation of the intravenous fats from the emulsion may occur and is called "cracking" of the solution. The intravenous fats may float on top of the mixture much like an egg yolk floating in the solution or appear as an uneven yellow consistency. In addition, "oiling out" may occur and looks like an oil slick or oil droplets on top of the solution. Return to the pharmacy any solution that appears "different," and do not use it.

BOX 13-3 presents guidelines for administration of TPN.

Selection of administration site

Central venous catheter (CVC): Used for all IV solutions whose final concentration is greater than 12.5% dextrose or a solution with an osmolarity 800 mOsm/L or greater. (If unsure or if information is unavailable on the infusion container related to infusion route, consult with a pharmacist or refer to hospital policy.) CVC use requires a large central vein with the distal tip of the catheter in the superior vena cava. The flow of blood through the large vessels rapidly dilutes hypertonic solutions and decreases the potential for thrombophlebitis.

Peripheral venous catheter: Reserved for individuals with a need for nutritional support for short-term periods, with small nutritional requirements, and for whom CVC access is unavailable. Only a low-osmolarity solution (less than 800 mOsm/L) can be used. To reduce osmolarity of the base solution,

TABLE 13-4	TYPES OF CENTRAL VENOUS CATHETERS USED FOR ADMINISTERING PARENTERAL NUTRITION
CATHETER	**DESCRIPTION**
Temporary	
Multilumen	May have up to 4 lumens; dedicate 1 lumen (preferably distal) for administration of TPN; may be inserted by physician at the bedside
PICC	May be single or dual lumen; may be used for home TPN administration because catheter may remain in place for several months; may be placed by either RN trained in IV catheter insertions or physician (usually radiologist)
Permanent	
Right atrial	Placed by physician, usually surgically, into subclavian or jugular vein with catheter tunneled and exiting from the skin; the catheter usually contains a Dacron cuff from which the catheter exits the vessel; this catheter is associated with the lowest infection rate of all central venous catheters
IVAD	May be placed in either radiology department or OR; designed for repeated access over a long period, thus making repeated venipunctures unnecessary

IV, Intravenous; *IVAD,* implantable venous access device; *OR,* operating room; *PICC,* peripherally inserted central venous catheter; *RN,* registered nurse; *TPN,* total parenteral nutrition.

dilution of the components is usually required. The required large volume limits the type of patients in whom this admixture can be administered. (If unsure or if information is unavailable on the infusion container related to infusion route, consult with a pharmacist or refer to hospital policy.)

See **TABLE 13-4** for types of CVCs used for administration of parenteral nutrition. **TABLE 13-5** presents guidelines for management of catheter complications.

TRANSITIONAL FEEDING

A transition is necessary before discontinuing nutritional support. Reduce the percentage of total calories supplied from enteral nutrition as oral intake increases to 60%-70% of estimated needs. Similarly, patients who have received TPN for more than 2-3 wk may have some mucosal atrophy of the bowel and will need a period of adjustment before the bowel can fully resume its usual functions of digestion and absorption. The best diet advancement includes starting with clear liquids, then advancing to a soft diet. Because these individuals have been ill, the lactase in their stomach has decreased, placing them at higher risk for lactose deficiency; therefore, they should limit or avoid a full liquid diet because of increased incidence of bloating, nausea, and diarrhea associated with lactose deficiency.

NURSING DIAGNOSES AND INTERVENTIONS

(Related primarily to both **Enteral Nutrition** and **Parenteral Nutrition**)
less than body requirements related to inability to ingest, digest, or absorb nutrients
Desired outcome: Patient has adequate nutrition, as evidenced by stabilization of weight at desired level or steady weight gain of $\frac{1}{2}$-1 lb/wk; presence of wound granulation (i.e., pinkish white tissue around wound edges; wound edges approximating together), and absence of infection (see **Risk for infection,** p. 715).

TABLE 13-5	MANAGEMENT OF CATHETER COMPLICATIONS IN PATIENTS RECEIVING PARENTERAL NUTRITION

POTENTIAL COMPLICATION	MANAGEMENT STRATEGY
Infection: insertion site	Maintain occlusive, dry dressing
	Change dressing per institutional policy using sterile technique
	When drainage appears at insertion site, change the dressing immediately
	Culture the drainage prn
	Remember: Patients who are neutropenic will develop redness at catheter insertion site because of their decrease in neutrophils
Infection: bacteremia	Observe temperature curve for signs/symptoms of increase
	Monitor for chills, rigor, tachycardia
	Maintain occlusive, dry dressing; change per institutional policy using sterile technique
	If prescribed, obtain blood cultures: one from catheter and one from a peripheral site to differentiate whether the organism is from the catheter or another site within patient
	Restrict blood drawing from lumen used for TPN administration
	Maintain blood glucose within normal limits
	Change IV caps on each lumen per hospital policy
	Use only Luer-Lok connections
	Have extra skin prep, sterile supplies available for physician during insertion of a temporary catheter
Catheter occlusion	Flush routinely using positive pressure and saline solution before and after each piggyback infusion and blood drawing; if the catheter manufacturer recommends heparin, use a heparinized solution following saline administration; if an individual develops HIT, eliminate all heparin products from IV lines, even in catheters whose manufacturer recommends using heparin
	Maintain IV filter to reduce infusion of any crystals that may have formed during admixture process
	Do not try to push occlusion through the catheter
	Notify physician
Leakage or catheter puncture	Do not insert needles into lumen cap
	Notify physician immediately if this occurs and prepare for changing of catheter (if temporary catheter) or repair of catheter (if right atrial catheter)
Pneumothorax	Position rolled towel under patient's back, parallel to the spine, before physician inserts temporary catheter
	Obtain chest x-ray film after inserting catheter and before using catheter (except in an emergency)
	Listen for breath sounds bilaterally
	Evaluate for onset of acute chest pain that occurred with catheter insertion
	Evaluate for ear pain on the side of attempted insertion
	Assess for dyspnea or shortness of breath
	Remember: The greater the number of attempts for insertion, the greater the chance of a pneumothorax

Continued

TABLE 13-5	MANAGEMENT OF CATHETER COMPLICATIONS IN PATIENTS RECEIVING PARENTERAL NUTRITION—cont'd
POTENTIAL COMPLICATION	**MANAGEMENT STRATEGY**
Air embolism	Examine catheter to determine whether an open port has enabled entry of air into circulatory system
	Clamp catheter if open to air
	Turn patient onto left side with head down and feet up
	Immediately notify physician of this medical emergency after positioning patient correctly
	Administer oxygen as prescribed
CVC thrombosis with upper extremity DVT	Assess any swelling of upper extremities, noting skin color, size of extremity, presence or absence of pulses
	Notify physician of upper extremity size change
	Elevate extremity
	Evaluate need for removal of CVC
	Administer anticoagulation therapy as prescribed
	Monitor laboratory parameters per agency policy to assess results of anticoagulation therapy, if indicated
Pulmonary thromboembolism	Evaluate for presence of pleuritic pain
	Assess for predisposing factors such as surgery, high estrogen states (pregnancy or use of birth control pills), history or presence of malignancy, trauma, immobilization, presence of CVC, heart failure, spinal cord injury, history of previous thromboembolic disease, history of hypercoagulable states, history of hematologic conditions (e.g., polycythemia vera), nephritic syndrome, inflammatory bowel disease
	Assess for dyspnea or shortness of breath, hemoptysis, cough, fever, syncope, and orthopnea
	Encourage use of sequential compression devices when in bed, if medically indicated
	Use antiembolism stockings, if medically indicated
	Encourage ambulation, if medically indicated
	Administer oxygen for hypoxemia
	Administer anticoagulation therapy as prescribed
	Monitor laboratory parameters per agency policy to assess anticoagulation therapy, if indicated
Pulmonary edema	Monitor I&O, daily weights
	Assess for frothy sputum; dyspnea, shortness of breath, cyanosis
	Administer oxygen as prescribed
	Assess need for fluid restriction

CVC, Central venous catheter; *DVT,* deep vein thrombosis; *HIT,* heparin-induced thrombocytopenia; *I&O,* intake and output; *IV,* intravenous; *prn,* as needed; *TPN,* total parenteral nutrition.

Nursing Interventions
For Oral Nutrition

◆ Ensure nutritional screening and assessment of patient within 24 hr of admission; document and reassess weekly.

◆ Position patient in high Fowler's position for eating; assist with preparation of food tray for eating as needed. Involve significant other in meal rituals for companionship.

♦ Assess for food allergies/intolerances, and avoid these foods.
♦ Provide small, frequent feedings of diet compatible with disease state and patient's ability to ingest foods.
♦ Respect food aversions, religious guidelines, and food preferences.
♦ If appropriate, allow family and friends to bring food from home.
♦ Provide liquid nutritional supplements as prescribed. Serve them cold or over ice *to enhance palatability.*
♦ Obtain weight weekly.
♦ Provide psychologic support.
♦ Provide good oral hygiene, including of dentures, if indicated.
♦ Provide food in the consistency that accommodates patient's needs.
♦ Monitor I&O to assess fluid balance trends.

For Enteral or Parenteral Nutrition in an Acute Care Setting

♦ Ensure nutritional screening and assessment within 24 hr of health care provider's directive; document and reassess weekly.
♦ Administer continuous enteral feedings by using a pump at the prescribed rate. Check infused volume and rate q4h.
♦ Administer TPN using a volumetric pump at the prescribed rate. Check infused volume and rate q4h.
♦ Monitor laboratory data every day until stable for TPN and enteral feedings, then at least weekly: electrolytes, blood glucose, blood urea nitrogen (BUN), creatinine, phosphorus, magnesium, and calcium.
♦ Monitor other laboratory data initially and then at least weekly: liver function tests including albumin, triglycerides (if patient at risk—e.g., pancreatitis, transplant antirejection medications, AIDS).
♦ Record I&O carefully, and track fluid balance trends.
♦ Weigh patient initially and daily during an acute illness, then advance to weekly.
♦ Ensure that patient receives prescribed caloric intake.
♦ Assess for fluid imbalance, especially fluid excess, via monitoring for peripheral edema, adventitious breath sounds (especially crackles or rales), and weight.

NURSING DIAGNOSES AND INTERVENTIONS
(Related primarily to **Enteral Nutrition**)

Risk for aspiration related to GI feeding or delayed gastric emptying
Desired outcome: Patient is free of aspiration problems, as evidenced by auscultation of clear lung sounds, VS within normal limits for patient, and no signs of respiratory distress.

Nursing Interventions

♦ Mark tube to determine length exiting from the body. Check this mark to determine tube migration. Secure tubing in place per agency policy; reassess q4h and before each feeding.
♦ Assess respiratory status q4h, including respiratory rate, effort, and adventitious breath sounds.
♦ Monitor temperature q4h; report any parameters as defined by health care provider.
♦ Auscultate bowel sounds q8h. If patient develops high-pitched or absent bowel sounds, abdominal distention, nausea, or vomiting, contact health care provider.
♦ Depending on patient's medical condition, raise head of bed (HOB) 30 degrees or higher, or place patient in a right side-lying position during and for 1 hr after administration of a bolus or intermittent feeding. *These*

positions promote gravity flow from the greater stomach curvature through the pylorus into the duodenum.

◆ Stop the tube feeding ½-1 hr before chest physical therapy or placing patient supine.

◆ Check residuals per agency policy. The best practice is to hold the feeding if residuals are greater than 200 mL from a nasogastric tube (NG) or orogastric tube or greater than 100 mL from a gastrostomy. No residuals or minimal volume should be obtained from a tube placed into the small intestine. Avoid use of formulas that have been tinted with coloring to assess for aspiration. This practice has received a warning from the U.S. Food and Drug Administration (FDA), and such formulas should not be used under any circumstance.

◆ Be aware that there are two syndromes associated with aspiration. Assess for and document the following events to assist health care provider in making the correct differential diagnosis:
  • Regurgitation or vomiting of gastric contents.
  • Aspiration from the oropharynx of saliva and upper airway secretions.

Diarrhea (or risk for same) related to medications, dumping syndrome, bacterial contamination, or formula intolerance
Desired outcome: Patient has formed stools within 2-3 days of intervention.

Nursing Interventions

◆ Assess abdomen and GI status: bowel sounds, distention, cramping, nausea, and frequency of bowel movements.

◆ Remember that liquid intake will normally produce a pasty stool. This is not considered diarrhea.

◆ Ask patient to define diarrhea. Determine patient's normal stool pattern.

◆ Suggest stopping prokinetic medication (e.g., metoclopramide), which stimulates the bowels.

◆ Suggest a review of medications by pharmacy.

◆ Suggest stopping any stool softeners being administered.

◆ Consider giving yogurt or the medication equivalent to replace normal flora removed by antibiotics. *This will clog a small-bore feeding tube*—evaluate route of delivery.

◆ Consider binding bile salts if diarrhea occurs secondary to uncontrolled diabetes mellitus (DM).

◆ Contact pharmacy about elixirs being administered. Most elixirs contain sorbitol, which speeds transit time in the intestines and causes diarrhea. Discuss with health care provider and pharmacist changing form of medication or switching to another medication within the same class.

◆ Collect a stool sample for bacterial culture and sensitivity testing.

◆ Collect a stool sample for ova and parasites.

◆ Collect a stool sample for *Clostridium difficile* toxin. If present, the volume of the daily stool output may exceed 500 mL and will occur whether or not the individual consumes food or enteral products. This type of diarrhea is considered secretory because the fluid is secreted from the intestinal wall and can lead to imbalances in fluid status.

◆ Do not administer an antidiarrheal medication until stool culture is confirmed as negative. Giving this medication when stool culture is positive increases risk for toxic megacolon and bowel perforation.

◆ Maintain optimal hydration.

◆ Record I&O status every shift. Obtain parameters from health care provider for notification of output.

◆ Check weight daily to assess fluid status.

◆ If patient is receiving a bolus feeding, switch to intermittent or continuous feeding.

◆ Follow Hazard Analysis Critical Control Point (HACCP) guidelines for handling of enteral products, feeding tube, and feeding sets (Box 13-2).

- Change all equipment per agency policy.
- Refrigerate all opened products, but discard after 24 hr. Date and time all products.
- Store all unopened products at room temperature (about 70° F), *to prevent clumping of proteins in the container.*
- Use enteral solutions at room temperature for a maximum of 12 hr when using an open delivery system vs. 24-48 hr when using a closed system. Check manufacturer guidelines for specific duration of open container or system hang time.

Nausea (or risk of same) related to underlying medical condition, too rapid infusion of enteral product, food intolerance, or medication administration
Desired outcome: Patient has no nausea with food intake.

Nursing Interventions

- Give antiemetic as prescribed.
- Offer food in small portions, 6 ×/day.
- Give ice chips, chewing gum, or hard candies prn if permitted.
- Suggest patient brush teeth and tongue q8h and prn.
- If odor of food induces nausea, remove it immediately.
- Reduce rate/min of enteral formula infusion. If patient is receiving bolus infusion, change to intermittent or continuous.
- Inspect abdomen for distention and auscultate bowel sounds.
- Monitor for and record flatus and bowel movements.
- Consider prokinetic medication to stimulate GI tract.
- If medically indicated, consider bowel suppository to stimulate intestinal tract.
- Monitor electrolytes, especially potassium (hypokalemia is associated with ileus). **TABLE 13-6** presents potential electrolyte imbalances in enteral and parenteral nutrition.

Constipation related to inadequate fluid and fiber in diet
Desired outcome: Patient states that he or she has had a soft bowel movement within 3-4 days of this diagnosis (or within patient's usual pattern).

Nursing Interventions

- If patient is receiving a formula that contains fiber and is on fluid restriction or receiving large amounts of diuretics, consider changing formula to an isotonic formula without fiber.
- If patient is receiving a formula that contains fiber, assess intake of free water. Optimal water intake is 1 mL/calorie of intake or 30-50 mL/kg body weight.
- Give free water q4h or as prescribed and after each medication.
- If medically indicated, consider a reduction in the amount of narcotic being administered.
- Consider a stool softener, especially if patient regularly uses a laxative at home.

Risk for impaired swallowing related to decreased or absent gag reflex, facial paralysis, mechanical obstruction, fatigue, weight loss, or deceased strength or excursion of muscles involved in mastication
Desired outcome: Before food or fluids are initiated, patient demonstrates adequate cough and gag reflexes and the ability to ingest foods via the phases of swallowing as instructed.

Nursing Interventions

- Assess oral motor function within 24 hr of admission or on patient's progression to oral diet.

TABLE 13-6 POTENTIAL ELECTROLYTE IMBALANCES IN ENTERAL AND PARENTERAL NUTRITION

ELECTROLYTE	IMBALANCE	ETIOLOGY/RISK FACTORS	SIGNS AND SYMPTOMS	PLAN OF CARE
Sodium	Hyponatremia	Gastrointestinal losses	CNS changes	Sodium administration
		Excessive sweating	General exhaustion	Restriction of water
		Excessive water replacement	Dulling of sensorium	Daily weights
		Diuretics	Lethargy	I&O
		Adrenal insufficiency	Muscular twitching	
		SIADH	Focal weakness	
			Hemiparesis	
			Ataxia	
			Convulsions	
			Papilledema	
			Coma	
			Pitting edema	
			Increased severity of symptoms	
	Hypernatremia	Medications:	Thirst	Gradual lowering of serum sodium
		Sodium penicillin	Elevated body temperature	I&O
		Sodium heparin	Tongue dry/swollen	Monitoring of changes in behavior
		Hypertonic tube feedings without adequate water supplements	Disorientation	Monitoring of serum sodium
		Corticosteroids (sodium retention)	Hallucination	
		Deprivation of water	Lethargy	
		Increased insensible water loss	Irritable	
		Watery diarrhea	Focal/grand mal seizures	

		Diabetes insipidus	Elevated serum sodium	Treatment of underlying problem
		Uncontrolled diabetes mellitus	Elevated serum osmolality	
		Heatstroke	Profuse sweating	
		Drowning in sea water		
		Excessive IV administration		
Potassium	Hypokalemia	Gastrointestinal losses from:	Fatigue	Administration of potassium supplementation as one of the following:
		Diarrhea	Nausea/vomiting	Potassium acetate
		Prolonged gastric suction	Muscle weakness	Potassium chloride
		Protracted vomiting	Anorexia	Potassium phosphorus
		Renal losses	Decreased bowel motility	If serum level is not improving or maintaining after replacement therapy is given, check serum magnesium level
		Medications:	Postural hypotension	IV potassium replacement should be limited to 10 mEq/hr; in patients with cardiac dysrhythmias caused by severe potassium depletion, replacement therapy can be increased to 20 mEq/hr with continuous cardiac monitoring
		Diuretics	Digitalis toxicity	
			ECG changes	
		Laxative overuse	Flattened T wave	
		Steroids	Prominent U wave	
		Amphotericin B	Impaired renal concentration ability	
		Insulin	Insulin suppression	
		Sweat losses	Laboratory data	
		Shift into cells with metabolic alkalosis		

Continued

TABLE 13-6   POTENTIAL ELECTROLYTE IMBALANCES IN ENTERAL AND PARENTERAL NUTRITION—cont'd

ELECTROLYTE	IMBALANCE	ETIOLOGY/RISK FACTORS	SIGNS AND SYMPTOMS	PLAN OF CARE
Potassium (cont'd)	Hyperkalemia	Prolonged poor oral intake Magnesium deficiency Pseudohyperkalemia Too tight a tourniquet Too small a needle during blood drawing Blood drawn above IV administration of potassium or from line with potassium infusing Decreased excretion (renal failure) High intake from foods or medications Use of salt substitutes in diet Confusion with home medications Change in renal status with potassium supplementation Presence of metabolic acidosis causing a shift out of the cells DKA Cardiac arrest	Low serum potassium Metabolic alkalosis Low urine osmolality Vague muscular weakness Cardiac dysrhythmias Paresthesias: face, hands, and feet Flaccid muscle paralysis Gastrointestinal symptoms ECG changes: Wide, flat, or no P wave Widening QRS Peaked T wave Elevated serum potassium	Restriction of potassium intake Dialysis Insulin administration Correction of acid-base disorder (potassium decreases by 0.4-1.5 mEq/L for every 0.1 increase in pH)

		Causes	Signs/Symptoms	Treatment
Phosphorus	Hypophosphatemia	Lactic acidosis Glucose administration Refeeding Hyperalimentation Alcoholism DKA Respiratory alkalosis Phosphate binding antacids Recovery from severe burns Vomiting Secretory diarrhea Hypomagnesemia Vitamin D deficiency Catabolic stress	Paresthesias Muscle weakness Muscle pain/tenderness Mental changes Cardiomyopathy Acute respiratory failure Seizures Decreased tissue oxygenation Joint stiffness Low serum phosphorus	Administration of phosphorus prescribed in mmol Available as: Potassium phosphorus Sodium phosphorus
	Hyperphosphatemia	Organ infarction Acute and chronic renal failure Rhabdomyolysis Hypocalcemia Acute metabolic acidosis Acute respiratory acidosis Vitamin D overdose	Metastatic calcification of phosphorus in soft tissues, joints, and arteries Oliguria Corneal haziness Conjunctivitis Papular eruptions Anorexia Nausea Vomiting	Reduction or elimination of source of phosphorus Use of phosphate binders that contain calcium, aluminum, or magnesium to reduce intestinal absorption Avoidance of magnesium-based antacids if renal failure is present Administration of hypotonic saline to provide volume expansion; administration of diuretics after fluids to increase renal excretion of phosphorus

Continued

TABLE 13-6　POTENTIAL ELECTROLYTE IMBALANCES IN ENTERAL AND PARENTERAL NUTRITION—cont'd

ELECTROLYTE	IMBALANCE	ETIOLOGY/RISK FACTORS	SIGNS AND SYMPTOMS	PLAN OF CARE
Phosphorus (cont'd)			Muscle weakness Neuromuscular irritability Hyperreflexia Tetany Tachycardia	
Magnesium	Hypomagnesia	Alcohol withdrawal Refeeding syndrome Gastrointestinal losses: 　Diarrhea 　Suctioning 　Ileostomy 　High-output fistulas 　Laxative overuse 　Steatorrhea Drugs: 　Diuretics 　Insulin Hypercalcemic state Hypophosphatemia SIADH Acute pancreatitis DKA	Neuromuscular changes: 　Muscular weakness 　Tremors 　Tetany 　Tonic clonic seizures 　Focal seizures 　Laryngeal stridor 　Trousseau's sign 　Chvostek's sign 　Choreiform movements 　Difficulty swallowing CNS changes: 　Apathy 　Depression 　Apprehension 　Extreme agitation 　Ataxia 　Vertigo 　Confusional state 　Delirium 　Psychoses 　Audiovisual hallucinations	Monitoring of serum magnesium level Administration of magnesium

	Causes	Signs and Symptoms	Treatment
Hypermagnesemia	Administration of too much magnesium: Milk of Magnesia Magnesium citrate Antacids	Lowered blood pressure Cardiac dysrhythmias and ECG changes: PVCs Supraventricular tachycardia Ventricular fibrillation Prolonged P-R interval Prolonged Q-T interval Widened QRS complex ST depression T wave inversion Peripheral vasodilatation Facial flushing Thirst Nausea/vomiting Lethargy Tetany	Discontinuation of any medications that contain magnesium Renal dialysis
Calcium Hypocalcemia	Surgical hypoparathyroidism Infusion of citrated blood Acute pancreatitis Hyperphosphatemia Inadequate vitamin D Magnesium deficiency Respiratory alkalosis Metabolic alkalosis Chronic renal failure	Trousseau's sign Chvostek's sign ECG changes: Increased Q-T interval Delayed ventricular repolarization Increased ST segment Mental changes Dry, scaling skin	Administration of intravenous calcium: Calcium chloride Calcium gluconate Measurement of ionized calcium level (serum calcium is measured based on amount bound to albumin, which may affect results if albumin is decreased)

Continued

TABLE 13-6	POTENTIAL ELECTROLYTE IMBALANCES IN ENTERAL AND PARENTERAL NUTRITION—cont'd			
ELECTROLYTE	**IMBALANCE**	**ETIOLOGY/RISK FACTORS**	**SIGNS AND SYMPTOMS**	**PLAN OF CARE**
Calcium (cont'd)		Rhabdomyolysis Low serum albumin	Brittle nails Dry hair Cataracts Laryngospasm Airway obstruction Respiratory arrest Seizures	
	Hypercalcemia	Malignant neoplastic disease Hyperparathyroidism Immobilization Thiazide diuretics Alkaline antacids High calcium intake Hyperthyroidism Adrenocortical insufficiency Acromegaly	Neuromuscular changes: Lethargy Mental confusion Muscular weakness Incoordination Anorexia Constipation Decreased pain sensation Decreased vibration sensation Behavior changes: Mental confusion Memory impairment Slurred speech Acute psychotic behavior Coma ECG changes Short Q-T interval	Treatment of underlying disease Forcing of large amounts of IV fluids Low-calcium diet Inorganic phosphate salts Increase in mobilization

CNS, Central nervous system; *DKA,* diabetic ketoacidosis; *ECG,* electrocardiogram; *I&O,* intake and output; *IV,* intravenous; *PVCs,* premature ventricular contractions; *SIADH,* syndrome of inappropriate antidiuretic hormone.

- Assess cough and gag reflexes before the first feeding. If patient is likely to have difficulty with swallowing, liquids will be the most difficult and most likely to be aspirated. Offer semisolid foods and progress to thicker textures as tolerated. Coach patient through phases of ingesting food: opening mouth, inserting food, closing lips, chewing, transferring food from side to side in the mouth and then to the back of the oral cavity, elevating tongue to roof of mouth (hard palate), and swallowing between breaths.
- Order extra sauces, gravies, or liquids if dryness of the oral cavity impairs patient's swallowing ability. Suggest that patient moisten each bite of food with these substances.
- If tolerated, keep patient in high Fowler's position for $\frac{1}{2}$ hr after eating, *to minimize risk of aspiration.*
- Provide mouth care before and after meals and dietary supplements.
- Provide small, frequent meals; *six smaller feedings per day may be more tolerable than three larger feedings.*
- Provide foods at temperatures acceptable to patient.
- Respect food and religious dietary restrictions; honor food preferences whenever possible.
- Provide oral supplements or tube feeding supplements as prescribed. Advise patient of transition status, and praise progress.
- In conjunction with speech, physical, or occupational therapist, assist in retraining or facilitating patient's swallowing.
- Monitor and record intake (via calorie count, daily weight) and output.

NURSING DIAGNOSES AND INTERVENTIONS

(Related primarily to **Parenteral Nutrition**)

Risk for infection related to invasive procedures, malnutrition, and suppression of the immune system
Desired outcome: Patient is free of infection, as evidenced by temperature, pulse, and respirations within patient's normal range and absence of clinical signs of sepsis: erythema, swelling at catheter insertion site, chills, fever, and glucose intolerance.

Nursing Interventions

- Ensure adequate nutritional support based on individual needs; reassess weekly.
- Weekly and as needed (prn), monitor WBC count with differential for values outside the normal range.
- Monitor bedside glucose for values outside the normal range. If the individual is glucose-intolerant, begin q4h bedside assessment and administer sliding scale insulin as prescribed by health care provider *to maintain blood glucose within normal limits.*
- Examine catheter insertion site (if using a transparent dressing) q12h for erythema, swelling, or purulent discharge. If using a gauze dressing, examine site at time of dressing change.
- Use meticulous sterile technique when changing central line dressing, containers, or administration lines. Follow agency policy for central line dressing changes.
- Restrict use of lumen used for administration of TPN, if possible. Avoid drawing blood specimens or other fluids, pressure monitoring, or medication administration, if possible.
- Change all administration sets, as established by Centers for Disease Control and Prevention (CDC).

Risk for imbalanced fluid volume related to failure of regulatory mechanisms, hyperglycemia, medications, fever, infection, fluid administration, or immobility

Desired outcome: Patient's hydration status is adequate, as evidenced by baseline VS, serum glucose less than 200 mg/dL, balanced I&O, 1-2 lb weight gain/wk, and serum electrolytes and WBC count within normal limits.

Nursing Interventions

◆ Assess rate and volume of nutritional support q4h.

◆ Weigh patient daily initially, and advance to weekly.

◆ Monitor I&O q8h or more frequently if medically indicated.

◆ Monitor electrolytes daily, and advance to a minimum of weekly, depending on patient's medical condition.

◆ Monitor for signs of circulatory overload during fluid replacement. Be alert to peripheral edema, bounding pulse, jugular distention, and adventitious lung sounds (especially crackles [rales]).

◆ Provide additional free water to meet individual patient's requirement as medically indicated Monitor for hyperglycemia as follows.

   ● In patient who is not diabetic: q6h for 24-48 hr, then discontinue.

   ● In patient who is glucose-intolerant: q4h, with sliding scale regular insulin prescribed and administered.

   ● In patient who is diabetic: q4h, with sliding scale regular insulin prescribed and administered; consult with a health care provider who specializes in care of patients with DM.

❖ ❖ ❖

SECTION TWO   MANAGING WOUND CARE

A wound is a disruption of tissue integrity caused by trauma, surgery, or an underlying medical disorder. Wound management is directed at preventing infection and deterioration in wound status and promoting healing.

❖ WOUNDS CLOSED BY PRIMARY INTENTION

OVERVIEW/PATHOPHYSIOLOGY

Clean, surgical, or traumatic wounds whose edges are closed with sutures, clips, tissue glue, or sterile tape strips are referred to as *wounds closed by primary intention.* Impairment of healing most commonly manifests as dehiscence, evisceration, or infection.

ASSESSMENT

Normal healing: Warm, reddened, indurated, tender incision line immediately after injury. After 1-2 days, epithelial cells migrate across the incision line and seal the wound. Over time, a pink scar is visible. After 7-9 days, a healing ridge—a palpable accumulation of scar tissue—forms. See **TABLE 13-7**. In patients who undergo cosmetic surgery, the healing ridge is purposely avoided to minimize scar formation. Healing is complete when structural and functional integrity is reestablished.

Impaired healing: Lack of an adequate inflammatory response manifested by absence of initial redness, warmth, and induration or inflammation that persists or occurs after the fifth postinjury day; continued drainage from the incision line 2 days after injury (when no drain is present); absence of a healing ridge by the ninth day after injury; presence of purulent exudate (Table 13-7).

History and risk factors for impaired healing: Very young or very old age, poorly controlled diabetes mellitus (DM), cigarette smoking, use of steroids or other immunosuppressive drugs, obesity, malnourishment, chemotherapy, or radiation therapy.

TABLE 13-7	ASSESSMENT OF HEALING BY PRIMARY INTENTION	
CHARACTERISTIC	**NORMAL FINDINGS**	**ABNORMAL FINDINGS**
Wound edges	Well approximated	Not well approximated
Inflammatory response	Good initial response: redness, warmth, induration, pain	Diminished or no response, or response persists or occurs after day 5
Drainage	None 48 hr after closure	Continues longer than 72 hr after closure
Healing ridge	Present by postoperative day 7-9	None by postoperative day 9; hypertrophic scar or keloid developing

DIAGNOSTIC TESTS

WBC count with differential: Assesses for infection.

Gram stain of drainage: If infection is suspected, identifies offending organism and aids in selection of preliminary antibiotics.

Culture and sensitivity testing of tissue obtained by biopsy or swab: Determine optimal antibiotic. Sample is obtained from clean tissue, not from exudate, pus, or necrotic tissue. Infection is present when there are 105 organisms/g or more from tissue or when there is fever and drainage. In older persons, infection may not be accompanied by fever or pus but rather is manifested only by changes in cognition or functional status that lead to a search for the site of infection.

COLLABORATIVE MANAGEMENT

Application of a sterile dressing in surgery: Protects wound from external contamination and trauma for the first 48 hr postoperatively or provides pressure. Usually, the surgeon changes the initial dressing.

Regular (house) diet: Promotes positive N balance for optimal wound healing.

Multivitamins, especially vitamin C: Promote tissue healing.

Minerals, especially zinc and iron: May be prescribed if patient's serum levels are low.

Supplemental O_2: Empirically, 2-4 L/min in high-risk patients. After injury, wound Po_2 is low, and administration of O_2 may promote healing.

Transdermal sustained O_2 therapy delivered directly to wound via catheter from a "fuel cell" that concentrates O_2 to nearly 100% from ambient air.

Insulin: As needed to control glucose levels (at 125 mg/dL or less) in persons with DM.

Local or systemic antibiotics: Given when infection is present and sometimes used prophylactically.

Incision and drainage: Drain pus when infection is present and localized. These techniques allow healing by secondary intention. The wound may be irrigated with normal saline to remove exudates.

NURSING DIAGNOSES AND INTERVENTIONS

Impaired tissue integrity of wound related to altered blood flow, metabolic disorders (e.g., DM), alterations in fluid volume and nutrition, and medical therapy (chemotherapy, radiation therapy, steroid administration)

Desired outcome: Patient exhibits the following signs of wound healing: well-approximated wound edges; good initial postinjury inflammatory response (erythema, warmth, induration, pain); no inflammatory response past the fifth day after injury; no drainage (without drain present) 48 hr after closure; healing ridge present by postoperative day 7-9.

Nursing Interventions

◆ Assess wound for indications of impaired healing, including absence of a healing ridge, presence of drainage or purulent exudate, and delayed or prolonged inflammatory response. Monitor VS for signs of infection, including elevated temperature and heart rate (HR). Document findings.

◆ Follow sterile technique when changing dressings. If a drain is present, keep it sterile, maintain patency (e.g., empty drainage reservoir and recharge suction on closed drainage systems as needed), and handle it gently *to prevent it from becoming dislodged.* If wound care will be necessary after hospital discharge, teach dressing change procedure to patient and significant other. Most outpatient wound care is done with clean technique.

◆ Maintain blood glucose within normal range for persons with DM by performing serial monitoring of capillary glucose and administering insulin *to keep glucose level 125 mg/dL or less.*

◆ Explain to patient that deep breathing promotes oxygenation, which enhances wound healing. Encourage deep breathing q2h while awake. Splint incision as needed. If indicated, provide incentive spirometry. Stress importance of position changes and activity as tolerated *to promote ventilation.* As indicated, monitor oximetry, report O_2 saturation 92% or less, and consult health care provider about administration of O_2.

◆ Monitor perfusion status by checking BP, HR, and capillary refill time in the tissue adjacent to incision, peripheral pulses as appropriate, moisture of mucous membranes, skin turgor, volume and specific gravity of urine, and I&O.

◆ For nonrestricted patients, ensure a fluid intake of at least 30 mL/kg body weight/day.

◆ *To promote wound healing,* provide a diet with adequate protein, vitamin C, and calories. If patient complains of feeling full with three meals per day, give more frequent small feedings. Encourage between-meal high-protein supplements (e.g., yogurt, milk shakes). Monitor the following for decreased values: serum albumin (less than 3.5 g/dL) and total lymphocyte counts (less than 1800/mm³), and report decreases; consult health care provider about high-protein nutrition supplements.

 Patient-Family Teaching and Discharge Planning

Provide verbal and written information about the following:

◆ Local wound care, including type of equipment necessary, wound care procedure, and therapeutic and negative side effects of topical agents used. Have patient or significant other demonstrate dressing change procedure before hospital discharge.

◆ Signs and symptoms of improvement or deterioration in wound status, including those that necessitate notification of health care provider or clinic (Table 13-7).

◆ Diet that promotes wound healing. Discuss importance of adequate protein and calorie intake. See "Providing Nutritional Support," p. 692. Involve dietitian, patient, and significant other as necessary.

◆ Activities that maximize ventilatory status: a planned regimen for ambulatory patients and deep breathing and turning (at least q2h) for those on bed rest.

◆ Importance of taking multivitamins, antibiotics, and supplements of iron and zinc as prescribed. For all medications to be taken at home, provide the following: drug names, purpose, dosage, schedule, precautions, and potential side effects. Also discuss drug/drug, herb/drug, and food/drug interactions.

◆ Importance of follow-up care with health care provider; confirm time and date of next appointment, if known.

◆ If needed, arrange for a visit by a home health nurse before hospital discharge.

◆ How and where to obtain wound care supplies.

❖ SURGICAL OR TRAUMATIC WOUND HEALING BY SECONDARY INTENTION

OVERVIEW/PATHOPHYSIOLOGY

Wounds healing by secondary intention are those with tissue loss or heavy contamination that form granulation tissue and contract in order to heal. Most often, impairment of healing is caused by contamination and inadequate blood flow, oxygenation, and nutrition.

ASSESSMENT

Normal healing: Initially the wound edges are inflamed, indurated, and tender. At first, granulation tissue on the floor and walls is pink, progressing to a deeper pink and then to a beefy red; wound tissues should be moist. Epithelial cells from the tissue surrounding the wound gradually migrate across the granulation tissue. As healing occurs, the wound edges become pink, the angle between surrounding tissue and the wound becomes less acute, wound contraction occurs, and the wound gets smaller. Occasionally a wound has a tract or sinus that gradually decreases in size as healing occurs. When a drain is in place, volume, color, and odor of the drainage should be evaluated. Timeframe for healing depends on wound size and location and on patient's physical and psychologic status. Healing is complete when structure and function have been reestablished.

Impaired healing: Exudate/slough/necrotic tissue on the floor and walls of the wound. Note distribution, color, odor, volume, and adherence of the exudates/slough/dead tissue and damage to skin surrounding the wound, including disruption, discoloration, swelling, local increased warmth, and increasing pain (**TABLE 13-8**).

History and risk factors for impaired healing: Very young or very old age, poorly controlled DM, cigarette smoking, use of steroids or other immunosuppressive drugs, obesity, malnourishment, radiation therapy, or chemotherapy.

DIAGNOSTIC TESTS

CBC with WBC differential: CBC to assess hematocrit (Hct) level and for presence of severe anemia (less than 25 g/dL). Increased WBC count signals infection, whereas a decrease occurs with immunosuppression. Watch the

TABLE 13-8	ASSESSMENT OF HEALING BY SECONDARY INTENTION	
CHARACTERISTIC	**NORMAL FINDINGS**	**ABNORMAL FINDINGS**
Wound edges	Initially after injury, wound edges inflamed, indurated, and tender; with epithelialization, edges become pink	Initially after injury, decreased inflammatory response or inflammation around wound that continues past day 5 after injury; epithelialization slowed or mechanically disrupted and not continuous around wound
Granulation tissue	Initially avascular and moist, then turns pink; becomes beefy red over time	Tissue remains pale or is excessively dry or moist
Odor	No	Yes
Exudate or necrotic tissue	No	Yes

differential for a shift to the left, which indicates infection. Monitor lymphocyte count (1800/mm^3 or less) and serum albumin (less than 3.5 g/dL) as signs of malnutrition.

Gram stain: Determines characteristics of the offending organism, if present, and aids in selection of preliminary antibiotic.

Tissue biopsy and culture: Determine the presence of infection and the optimal antibiotic, if appropriate.

X-ray examination and bone scan: Determine the presence of osteomyelitis.

COLLABORATIVE MANAGEMENT

Debriding enzymes (e.g., Accuzyme, Santyl [ointments]): Remove necrotic tissue.

Drain: Removes excess tissue fluid or purulent drainage.

Dressings: Keep healthy wound tissue moist or provide antiseptic agent to decrease wound surface bacterial counts (**TABLE 13-9**).

Hydrotherapy: Softens and removes debris mechanically in heavily contaminated wounds.

Irrigation of the wound: Dislodges and removes bacteria and loosens necrotic tissue, foreign bodies, and exudate.

IV fluids: Ensure adequate perfusion for patients unable to take adequate oral fluids.

Negative-pressure therapy: Promotes wound closure by increasing blood flow, decreasing edema, and lowering bacteria count.

Surgical debridement: Removes dead tissue and reduces debris.

Skin graft: Provides coverage of wound with homograft, cultured keratinocytes, or synthetic cells.

Tissue flaps: Used to fill tissue defect and provide wound closure with their own blood supply.

Topical or systemic vitamin A: As needed to reverse adverse effects of steroids on healing. Use is limited to 7-10 days.

Regular diet, supplemental O$_2$, multivitamins and minerals, insulin, and incision and drainage: See discussion in "Wounds Closed by Primary Intention," p. 716.

NURSING DIAGNOSES AND INTERVENTIONS

Impaired tissue integrity of wound related to presence of contaminants, metabolic disorders (e.g., DM), medical therapy (e.g., chemotherapy, radiation therapy), altered perfusion, or malnutrition

Desired outcomes: Patient's wound exhibits the following signs of healing: initially after injury, wound edges are inflamed, indurated, and tender; with epithelialization, edges become pink; granulation tissue develops over time (identified by pink tissue that becomes beefy red); and there is no odor, exudate, or necrotic tissue. Patient or significant other successfully demonstrates wound care procedure before hospital discharge, if appropriate.

Nursing Interventions

- Monitor for the following signs of impaired healing: initially after injury, decreased inflammatory response or inflammatory response that lasts more than 5 days; epithelialization slowed or mechanically disrupted and noncontiguous around the wound; granulation tissue remaining pale or excessively dry or moist; presence of odor, exudate, slough, and/or necrotic tissue.
- *To help prevent contamination,* cleanse drainage or secretions from skin surrounding wound with a mild disinfectant (e.g., soap and water). Do not use friction with cleansing if tissue is friable.
- Cleanse wound with each dressing change using 100-150 mL normal saline or a commercial wound cleanser via a 35-mL syringe and an 18-gauge

TABLE 13-9 DRESSINGS USED FOR WOUND CARE

DRESSING	ADVANTAGES	LIMITATIONS
Moist to moist* (apply and remove moist)	Provides topical moisture; no wound desiccation; removal painless; inexpensive	Needs to be changed while still moist (minimum twice daily); if dries out, must be moistened before removal; removal may be painful
Transparent dressing (e.g., Op-Site, Tegaderm, Bioclusive)	Prevents loss of wound fluid; protects wound from external contamination; protects from friction	Cannot be used with infected, contaminated, or heavily draining wounds
	Causes minimal pain with removal	Some brands should not be used with skin tears because of high adhesive content; skin damage results on removal
Hydrocolloid dressing (e.g., DuoDerm, Restore, Intact)	Maintains moist wound surface while minimizing pooling	Depending on thickness of brand, wound may not be directly assessed without removing dressing; limited absorption
	Easy to apply; causes minimal pain upon removal	
Hydrogel (e.g., Vigilon, Intrasite Gel)	Maintains moist wound surface for 1-2 days, necessitating fewer dressing changes; nonadherent	Maceration on direct contact with normal tissue
	Compatible with topical medications	Minimal absorption of exudates
	Easy to apply with minimal pain upon removal	
Alginates (e.g., Sorbsan)	Physiologic and absorbs large volume; removal painless	Not for use on dry wounds; requires a cover dressing
Foams (e.g., Lyofoam, Allevyn)	Maintains moist wound surface; insulates wound; nonadherent	Not designed for use with wounds with copious drainage
	Some come with vapor-permeable backing	
Hypertonic (e.g., Mesalt)	Noninvasive debridement, reactivates inflammatory process	Not designed for use on dry wounds
Silver (e.g., Arglaes, Acticoat)	Antimicrobial; long life (up to 7 days); effective against MRSA and VRE	More expensive per item
	Easy to apply	

*Dressings are sterile, coarse mesh gauze without cotton fiberfill and are covered with a dry, sterile outer layer to prevent ingress of organisms. When moisture is prescribed, it is provided with a physiologic solution.

MRSA, Methicillin-resistant *Staphylococcus aureus*; *VRE*, vancomycin-resistant *Enterococcus*.

angiocatheter, and follow meticulous infection control procedures (see p. 743).

♦ When topical enzymes are prescribed, use them on necrotic tissue only and follow package directions carefully. Be aware that some agents, such as silver, deactivate the enzymes.

♦ Apply prescribed dressings (Table 13-9), and follow meticulous infection control procedures (see p. 743). Insert dressing into all *tracts to promote gradual closure of those areas.* Ensure good handwashing before and after dressing changes, and dispose of contaminated dressings appropriately.

♦ When a drain is used, maintain its patency, prevent kinking of the tubing, and secure tubing *to prevent the drain from becoming dislodged.* Use sterile technique when caring for drains. With closed drainage systems, empty drainage reservoir and maintain suction as needed.

♦ Teach patient or significant other the prescribed wound care procedure, if indicated.

 Patient-Family Teaching and Discharge Planning

See teaching and discharge planning interventions in "Wounds Closed by Primary Intention," p. 718.

❖ PRESSURE ULCERS

OVERVIEW/PATHOPHYSIOLOGY

Pressure ulcers result from a disruption in tissue integrity and are caused most often by excessive tissue pressure.

ASSESSMENT

High-risk individuals should be identified on admission assessment, with daily assessments during hospitalization that use a standard assessment schema.

Signs and symptoms/physical findings: When pressure ulcers are present, their severity can be staged on a scale of I to IV (**TABLE 13-10**). See also "Surgical or Traumatic Wound Healing by Secondary Intention," p. 719, for other assessment data.

History and risk factors: Old age, decreased mobility, decreased level of consciousness (LOC), impaired sensation, debilitation, incontinence, sepsis/ elevated temperature, or malnutrition.

DIAGNOSTIC TESTS

See "Diagnostic Tests," p. 719, in "Surgical or Traumatic Wound Healing by Secondary Intention."

TABLE 13-10	STAGING OF PRESSURE ULCERS

STAGE	DESCRIPTION
I	Nonblanchable erythema of intact skin; in people with dark skin, discoloration, warmth, edema, induration, or hardness may be seen
II	Partial-thickness skin loss that involves epidermis or dermis or both; seen as an abrasion, blister, or shallow crater
III	Full-thickness skin loss that involves subcutaneous tissue but does not extend through fascia
IV	Full-thickness injury that involves muscle, bone, or supporting structures

COLLABORATIVE MANAGEMENT

Debriding enzymes (e.g., Accuzyme, Santyl [ointments]): Remove necrotic tissue.

Diet: Provides adequate protein and calories to promote positive N balance for rapid wound healing.

Dressings: Keep healthy tissue moist or apply an antiinfective agent (Table 13-9).

Growth factors: Naturally occurring proteins stimulate new cell formation (e.g., platelet-derived growth factor).

Hyperbaric O₂: Used with more challenging wounds to support oxidative processes in healing and control of infection.

Hydrotherapy: Softens and removes debris mechanically.

Supplemental vitamins and minerals: As needed.

Surgical debridement: Removes devitalized tissue with a scalpel or scissors to reduce the amount of debris.

Tissue flaps: Provide wound closure with their own blood supply.

Wound irrigation with antiinfective agents: Reduces contamination.

NURSING DIAGNOSES AND INTERVENTIONS

Impaired tissue integrity (or risk for same) related to excessive tissue pressure

Desired outcomes: Patient's tissue remains intact. Patient or significant other participates in preventive measures and verbalizes understanding of the rationale for these interventions.

Nursing Interventions

- Identify individuals at risk, and systematically assess skin over bony prominences daily; document. Use a standard risk assessment scale such as the Braden scale (see p. 765 for website information).
- Establish and post a position-changing schedule.
- Assist patient with position changes. There is an inverse relationship between pressure and time in ulcer formation; therefore, heavier patients need to change position more frequently. Position changes include turning the bed-bound patient q1-2h and having the wheelchair-bound patient (who is able) perform pushups in the chair q15min (and not less than hourly) *to ensure periodic relief from pressure on the buttocks.* Use pillows, foam wedges, or gel pads *to protect bony prominences from direct pressure.* In addition, patients with history of previous pressure ulcers require pressure-relief measures more frequently. Because high Fowler's position results in increased shearing, use low Fowler's position and alternate supine position with prone and 30-degree elevated side-lying positions.
- For immobile patients, totally relieve pressure on heels by raising them off the bed surface.
- Minimize friction and shear on tissue during activity. Lift rather than drag patient during position changes and transferring; use a draw sheet to facilitate patient movement. Do not massage over bony prominences because this can result in tissue damage.
- Minimize skin exposure to moisture. Cleanse at the time of soiling and at routine intervals. Use moisture barriers and disposable briefs as needed.
- Use a mattress that reduces pressure, such as foam, low air loss, alternating air, gel, or water.
- *To promote blood flow,* encourage patient to maintain or increase current level of activity.

Impaired tissue integrity related to presence of pressure ulcer, with increased risk for further breakdown related to altered circulation and presence of contaminants or irritants (chemical, thermal, or mechanical)

Desired outcomes: Stages I and II show progressive healing over days to weeks; stages III and IV may require months to heal. Following intervention and instruction, patient or significant other verbalizes causes and preventive measures for pressure ulcers and successfully participates in the plan of care to promote healing and prevent further breakdown.

Nursing Interventions

◆ Evaluate stage of pressure ulcer (Table 13-10) and wound status (Table 13-8).
◆ Maintain a moist physiologic environment *to promote tissue repair and minimize contaminants.* Change dressings as needed, and use meticulous infection control procedure (see p. 743).
◆ Be sure patient's skin is kept clean with regular bathing, and be especially conscientious about washing urine and feces from the skin. Soap should be used and then thoroughly rinsed from the skin.
◆ If patient has excessive perspiration, ensure frequent bathing and change bedding as needed.
◆ To absorb moisture and prevent shearing when patient is moved, apply heel and elbow protection as needed.
◆ Teach patient and significant other the importance of and measures for preventing excess pressure as a means of preventing pressure ulcers.
◆ Provide wound care as needed (described under "Surgical or Traumatic Wound Healing by Secondary Intention," p. 719).

 Patient-Family Teaching and Discharge Planning

Provide verbal and written information about the following as appropriate:
◆ Location of local medical supply stores that have pressure-reducing mattresses and wound care supplies.
◆ Planning a schedule for changing patient positions.

❖ ❖ ❖

SECTION THREE   **BURNS**

OVERVIEW/PATHOPHYSIOLOGY

Heat, chemicals, electricity, and radiation may cause burn injury affecting the skin, muscle, or lungs. The degree of injury depends on the type of burn agent and length of exposure to the burn agent. *Superficial* (first-degree) burns involve only the epidermal layer of the skin. *Partial thickness* (second-degree) burns may be superficial or deep. *Superficial partial-thickness* burns affect the upper third of the dermis and cause intense pain. *Deep partial-thickness burns* affect deep layers of the dermis and destroy structures contained within the dermis. *Full-thickness* (third- and fourth-degree) burns destroy the epidermis and dermis and result in the need for skin grafts. *Deep full-thickness burns* damage the subcutaneous layer, muscle, and bone. Inhalation burns occur when smoke, hot air, fumes, or toxic chemicals are inhaled and damage the pulmonary parenchyma. Burns elicit localized and systemic responses. *Localized burn responses* include inflammation, edema, ischemia, and hyperemia. *Systemic burn responses* result from increased capillary permeability secondary to tissue injury and cause edema, hypovolemia (burn shock), tachycardia, pulmonary edema, acute respiratory distress syndrome (ARDS), hypermetabolism, renal and immune compromise, and fluid and electrolyte imbalances. Infection is the most common and most serious complication of extensive burns.

ASSESSMENT

Signs and symptoms/physical findings: *Thermal burns:* Blisters; bullae; white, black, or cherry-red skin color; cyanosis; tachycardia; increased or

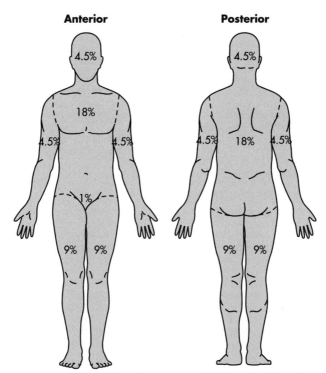

FIGURE 13-1 ◆ The rule of nines. The percentage of body burned can be estimated by adding the % according to this chart. (From Monahan F, Sands J, Neighbors M, Marek J, Green C: *Phipp's Medical-Surgical Nursing: Health and Illness Perspectives*, ed 8, St. Louis, 2007, Mosby).

decreased BP; severe pain to no pain; oliguria; anuria, decreased or absent bowel sounds; respiratory crackles or wheezing; fluid shifts from intravascular to interstitial spaces (24-48 hr after burn) that cause mild to extensive edema, hypovolemia, metabolic acidosis, hyperkalemia, and hypernatremia; fluid shifts back into the intravascular space (48-72 hr) that cause hypokalemia and hyponatremia. In adults, the rule of nines tool (**FIGURE 13-1**) is used to estimate the percentage of total body surface area (TBSA) burned. Modifications are made when this tool is used to estimate TBSA in children less than 10 yr old because of the larger head size relative to the rest of the body. *Chemical burns:* Burning, irritation, pain, numbness, redness at site of contact; dyspnea, cough, dizziness, weakness, hypotension, headache, cardiac dysrhythmias, seizures. *Electrical burns:* May include extensive partial-thickness burns, cardiopulmonary arrest. *Radiation:* Burns on the skin with redness, swelling and peeling; mouth, esophagus, stomach and intestinal ulcers; nausea, vomiting, diarrhea; bleeding from mucous membranes, urinary tract and bowel; weakness, fatigue.

History and risk factors: Recent exposure to heat, chemicals, electricity or radiation.

DIAGNOSTIC TESTS

CBC and differential: Assesses WBC, hemoglobin (Hgb), and hematocrit (Hct). Leukocyte count higher than 12,000 μL, lower than 4000 μL, or more than 10% immature cells indicates a systemic inflammatory response.

Chemistry panel: Detects organ compromise and electrolyte balance.

Arterial blood gases: Assess oxygenation and determine the need for ventilator support.

Serum protein: Determines the extent of protein loss from wound seepage.

Urinalysis: Determines renal compromise.

Serum creatinine and BUN: Determine renal compromise.

Urine myoglobin: Detects destruction of muscle tissue when third-degree burns are present.

Chest x-ray examination: Rules out lung damage, which may not be evident until several days following injury.

Bronchoscopy: Definitive diagnosis of inhalation injury.

Arterial or venous carboxyhemoglobin level: Excludes carbon monoxide poisoning.

Wound cultures: Detect pathologic organism

COLLABORATIVE MANAGEMENT

This careplan primarily pertains to care of the patient with thermal injury treated at an acute care facility. It does not address the care of the severely burned patient. Severely burned patients who meet the American Burn Association criteria for transfer to a pain center should be immediately transferred. Criteria for transfer of severely burned patients may be accessed at http://www.ameriburn.org/ Patients with other types of burns require specialized care. The immediate goals of therapy for patients with thermal burns include minimizing the burn injury, preventing complications and maintaining preburn function. Treatment also focuses on rehabilitation and reintegration of patient back into the family and community. Reconstruction comes later.

Superficial and partial-thickness burns: Many patients are treated on an outpatient basis because such burns are unlikely to become infected. Treatment includes removal of the burn source, cooling the site to dissipate heat, cleaning the wound with soap and water, applying a clean dressing and/or protective antimicrobial agent such as triple antibiotic ointment (neomycin, bacitracin zinc, and polymyxin B sulfate) or Polysporin (polymyxin and bacitracin zinc), and controlling pain with oral analgesics or nonsteroidal antinflammatory drugs (NSAIDs) (e.g., ibuprofen, naproxen) or oral (PO) narcotics (e.g., acetaminophen with codeine or oxycodone). When pain is severe, hospitalization and more intensive pain control therapy are required.

Deep partial-thickness, full-thickness, and deep full-thickness burns: Treatment of severe burns requires hospitalization and occurs in phases:

Emergent phase: 0-48 hr after burn injury. The focus of care is on maintaining a patent airway and body temperature, supporting circulation, controlling pain, preventing fluid and electrolyte imbalance and infection, and providing emotional support.

Acute phase: Begins at the conclusion of resuscitation, which generally occurs about 48-72 hours after the burn has occurred and ends when wounds are covered. The focus of care is on preventing infection, treating wounds, preventing complications (renal failure, septicemia, cardiac compromise, pneumonia), providing continued emotional support, and maintaining function.

Rehabilitation and reintegration phase: Begins a few days before discharge from the hospital and extends throughout the recuperative process. Treatment during this phase involves counseling about reintegration into family and/or work role, controlling chronic pain, addressing sleep disturbances, posttraumatic stress disorder (PTSD), or ability to perform own activities of daily living (ADLs).

Pharmacotherapy

Analgesics

- *Emergent phase:* IV morphine, fentanyl, hydromorphone (Dilaudid). Dosing depends on patient's response to pain management.

- *Acute phase:* IV morphine, fentanyl or PO morphine (Roxanol), hydromorphone (Dilaudid), oxycodone (Percocet). Patient-controlled analgesia is the method of choice for pain control during this burn phase until patient is able to tolerate oral pain medications.
- *Rehabilitative phase:* Mild opioid analgesics such as PO hydromorphone (Dilaudid) transmucosal fentanyl, and NSAIDs with or without narcotics (acetaminophen, ibuprofen). . Pain varies due to neuronal rearrangement and stretch of tissues. NSAIDs are contraindicated in patients with GI tract problems, stress ulcers or clotting disorders.

Topical antiinfective agents

- Silver sulfadiazine: broad-spectrum antibacterial agent; reduces bacterial density and colonization; can burn on application; minimal penetration of eschar.
- Mafenide acetate: broad-spectrum antibacterial agent; painful application; penetrates eschar.
- Cerium nitrate–silver sulfadiazine: antimicrobial; produces wound bacteriostasis better than sulfadiazine alone.
- Acticoat: long-acting, time-released antimicrobial silver.

Anxiolytics: Indicated for anxiety in conjunction with aggressive treatment of pain. *Emergent phase*: IV lorazepam (Ativan), midazolam; *acute phase:* PO lorazepam; *rehabilitation phase*: PO lorazepam.

Tetanus booster: For tetanus prophylaxis if patient has not been immunized or received a booster within the past 5 yr.

Antipruritus medications: Antihistamines (e.g., diphenhydramine, hydroxyzine), colloid and oatmeal baths, PO antiseizure agents (e.g., gabapentin), or PO antiserotonergic agents (e.g., cyproheptadine) may be prescribed to relieve itching associated with burn injury and healing.

Fluid resuscitation: The goal of timely fluid resuscitation is to give the least amount of fluid necessary while at the same time replacing sequestered or lost fluids adequately to maintain organ perfusion.

Ringer's lactate solution (crystalloid solution): Consensus formula: Infuse 2-4 mL/kg/% TBSA burned. Infuse $\frac{1}{2}$ over the first 8 hours and $\frac{1}{2}$ over the next 16 hours during the first 24-hr period of burn injury. Other formulas such as the Parkland, Brooke, Evans, or Army, include crystalloid and colloid infusions over the first and second 24-hr periods.

Thereafter, fluid replacement depends on patient's age, extent and severity of burns, and physiologic status and is directed at maintaining urine output at 0.5-1.0 mL/kg/hr in adults and at 0.5 mL/kg/hr in children.

Colloid solutions and fresh frozen plasma (albumin, dextran, hetastarch [Hespan]): Provide volume and generate oncotic pressure to facilitate movement of fluid back into the intravascular space when given after the first 24 hr following the burn.

Skin grafts: Provide temporary or permanent wound coverage, speed healing, decrease length of recovery, and provide cosmetic and functional benefits. *Autografts* are permanent grafts obtained from patient. Temporary wound coverings include: *allograft (homograft),* which is obtained from a deceased donor, and a *heterograft (xenograft) is* obtained from another species. Skin grafts vary in thickness from epidermal layers (split-thickness grafts) to layers of skin containing subcutaneous tissue (full-thickness grafts). Skin grafts can be meshed or unmeshed.

Dermal replacements (e.g., Integra [artificial skin], AlloDerm [collagen matrix]): Synthetic skin substitutes that cover the wound and provide protection from infection and drying and facilitate tissue regeneration.

Wound debridement: *Mechanical debridement* is the removal of dead tissue (eschar) with wet gauze or instruments. It is generally done at patient's bedside. *Surgical debridement* is performed in the operating room (OR) and involves the surgical removal of dead tissue. *Enzymatic debridement* involves the use of topical enzymes that loosen eschar for easy removal.

Hydrotherapy: Facilitates range of motion and the removal of sloughing eschar, exudates, and topical medications.

Burn center: Patients with severe, extensive burn injuries are best treated in specialized care units with personnel specifically educated to care for burned patients' unique needs.

NURSING DIAGNOSES AND INTERVENTIONS

Risk for infection related to loss of tissue integrity (burns), invasive procedures, nutritional deficits

Desired outcome: Patient is free of infections, as evidenced by absence of fever, chills, and purulent drainage from wounds, as well as negative culture results.

Nursing Interventions

- Assess for signs of active infection or sepsis at frequent intervals (e.g., increased temperature, increased HR, decreased BP, diaphoresis, confusion or mental status changes, decreased level of consciousness (LOC)).
- Monitor laboratory data, especially CBC, differential, and cultures *to detect changes that indicate infection.*
- Monitor burn wounds and IV sites for erythema, swelling, local warmth, tenderness, or purulent exudate. *These indicate infection.*
- Implement strict protective precautions *to decrease the risk for infection.*
- Use standard precautions, wear gloves and maintain aseptic technique when changing dressings or applying topical medications *to prevent introduction of pathogens into the burn wound.*
- Assist ambulatory patient with maintaining meticulous body hygiene *to prevent spread of organisms from body secretions into burn wounds.*
- Promote pulmonary toilet by encouraging patient to engage in frequent breathing or incentive spirometry exercises *to prevent pneumonia from stasis of pulmonary secretions.*
- Perform wound debridement as prescribed *to promote healing and decrease risk for infection.*
- Remove plants or fresh flowers from patient's room *to minimize risk for transmission of microorganisms to patient.*
- Restrict visitors who have upper respiratory or other infections *to minimize risk for transmitting infection to patient.*
- *Panculture patient when body temperature is greater than 101° F to detect presence of microorganisms.*
- Obtain wound cultures as prescribed when exudate is purulent or foul-smelling *to facilitate early detection of wound infection.*

Acute pain related to exposed nerve endings from burn injury

Desired outcomes: Patient's subjective perception of pain decreases within 1 hr of intervention, as documented by a pain scale. Objective indicators, such as grimacing, are absent or diminished.

Nursing Interventions

- Assess and document quality, location, intensity, and duration of pain. Devise a pain scale with patient that ranges from 0 (no pain) to 10 (worst pain). Notify health care provider of sudden and/or severe pain that is unrelieved by pain interventions.
- Implement a systematic and collaborative approach to managing burned patient's pain *because uncontrolled pain affects all aspects of patient's recovery.*
- Medicate patient with prescribed analgesic on a continuous basis during emergent phase *to achieve maximum pain control.*

- Encourage patients on PO analgesics to request medication before it becomes severe. *Pain is more easily controlled when it is treated before it becomes severe.*
- Administer prescribed antipruritus *PO or topical medications as prescribed to minimize itching, which can also be painful.*
- Encourage the use of nonpharmacologic interventions such as music, meditation, relaxation, diversion, or presence *to potentiate pain medication effectiveness and/or reduce pain.*
- Encourage pain medication before dressing changes or wound debridement *to decrease pain during these procedures.*
- Administer prescribed antianxiety medications if necessary *to enhance pain control and reduce anxiety.*

Risk for deficient fluid volume related to changes in vascular permeability and loss of protein from burned tissues
Desired outcome: Patient remains normovolemic or becomes normovolemic within 24-48 hr following burn injury, as evidenced by stable weight, urine output 30-50 mL/hr, moist oral mucous membranes, and HR and BP within normal limits for patient prior to burn injury.

Nursing Interventions

- Monitor I&O, daily weight, and VS closely, and report changes to health care provider. *Detects hypovolemia.*
- Monitor serum electrolytes *to detect changes precipitated by fluid and protein losses.*
- Encourage oral fluids as tolerated *to replace losses from denuded skin.*
- Administer IV fluids as prescribed if patient is unable to tolerate PO fluids, *to prevent hypovolemia.*
- Administer serum albumin as prescribed *to facilitate revascularization of fluids.*

Imbalanced nutrition: less than body requirements related to loss of appetite resulting from pain and/or inability to ingest food/fluids resulting from extensive burn injury
Desired outcomes: Patient has adequate nutrition, as evidenced by stable weight, serum albumin 3.5-5.5 g/dL, transferrin 180-260 mg/dL, thyroxine-binding prealbumin 20-30 mg/dL, retinol-binding protein 4-5 mg/dL, and a state of N balance or a positive N state; verbalizes the need to increase caloric and protein intake when weight loss is present.

Nursing Interventions

- Assess nutritional status daily, and note weight, caloric intake, and protein and albumin values. Be alert to progressive weight loss, wasting of muscle tissue, decreases in both total protein and albumin, and signs of ileus and constipation. *Protein and albumin losses adversely affect wound healing and impair patient's ability to protect self from infection.*
- Monitor daily weights using the same scale *to ensure accuracy and determine whether weight loss or weight gain is occurring.*
- Implement pain control measures as prescribed. *Pain decreases appetite and the desire to eat.*
- Provide small, frequent, high-caloric, high-protein meals, and allow sufficient time for patient to eat. Offer supplements between feedings *to facilitate positive N balance and prevent weight loss.*
- Provide means for enteral feeding if caloric intake is insufficient to meet patient needs *to prevent weight loss resulting from increased metabolic needs.*
- Provide supplemental vitamins and minerals as prescribed *to replace deficiencies.*

- Provide oral hygiene before and after meals *to minimize anorexia.*
- Encourage significant other to visit at mealtimes and bring patient's favorite high-caloric, high-protein foods from home *to facilitate increased intake.*
- Provide instructions for deep breathing and voluntary swallowing if patient is nauseated *to decrease stimulation of vomiting center.*
- Administer antiemetics as prescribed. Encourage patient to request medication before discomfort becomes severe.
- Deliver isotonic tube feedings as prescribed for patients unable to eat. Check placement of gastric tube before each feeding; assess absorption by evaluating amount of residual feeding q4h. Do not deliver feeding if residual is greater than two times the rate of tube feeding/hr. Keep head of bed (HOB) elevated 30 degrees while feeding, and position patient in a right side-lying position. *Isotonic fluids help prevent diarrhea associated with hypertonic or hypotonic fluids. HOB elevation and right side-lying position help facilitate gastric empting.*

Disturbed body image related to altered appearance and/or function from burn injury
Desired outcome: Before discharge, patient will verbalize ways to adapt lifestyle changes from burn injury by managing burn scars, making positive statements about self, and verbalizing positive adjustment to body changes.

Nursing Interventions

- Provide anticipatory counseling about body changes, and include ways for patient to cope with reactions from others, *to prepare patient for reentry into social settings.*
- Assess patient's readiness to view burn injuries and participate in care of wounds, *to evaluate patient's acceptance of body changes.*
- Encourage patient to identify personal strengths, *to help patient focus on self-worth rather than physical changes.*
- Encourage patient to complete the Baird Body Image Assessment Tool or other self-assessment survey, *to determine subjective response to physical changes.*
- Use survey results along with patient statements, *to help patient consider meaning and impact of physical changes.*
- Encourage participation of family and significant other in care, *to facilitate patient's feelings of acceptance by others.*
- Demonstrate positive regard for patient and acceptance of any physical changes from burns, *to demonstrate acceptance.*
- Allow patient to cry and grieve for former appearance and/or function. *Grieving facilitates spiritual and emotional healing.*
- Refer to counseling as needed. *Some patients may need assistance with integrating physical changes in a positive and constructive manner.*
- Encourage patient to join a burn support group, *to facilitate adjustment to postburn changes.*

Deficient knowledge related to care of wounds and/or grafts, pain control, signs and symptoms of infection, and the need for follow-up care and counseling
Desired outcomes: Before discharge, patient verbalizes understanding of prescribed medications, care of dressings, wounds or grafts, signs and symptoms that must be reported, and need for follow-up care and monitoring.

Nursing Interventions

- Assess patient's facility with language; engage an interpreter or provide language-appropriate written materials if necessary.
- Assess patient's knowledge of dressing, wound, or graft care and provide information or clarify as appropriate *to facilitate self-care.*

- Assess patient's understanding of dietary needs to support increased metabolic rate while burns are healing. Assist patient with making appropriate dietary selections *to prevent weight loss or maintain normal weight for patient's height.*
- Teach patient to monitor for changes in wound appearance, fever, and increased or foul-smelling exudate and report them to health care provider. *These indicate infection.*
- Teach patient about methods for controlling chronic pain or itching, including pharmacologic and nonpharmacologic measures, *to facilitate comfort during healing process.*
- Teach patient that it is okay to seek counseling if needed, *to facilitate adjustment to changes in body appearane or function.*

 Patient-Family Teaching and Discharge Planning

Include verbal and written information about the following:
- Medications, including drug names, rationale, dosage, schedule, route of administration, precautions, and potential side effects. Also discuss drug/drug, herb/drug, and food/drug interactions.
- Signs and symptoms that necessitate medical attention, including fever, significant wound changes, weight loss, or changes in urinary patterns.
- Dietary management to promote nutritional and fluid maintenace and prevent weight loss.
- Care of dressings, wounds, or graft and donor sites.
- The availability of community resources and support groups.
- Importance of follow-up care until recovery is complete. Confirm date and time of next appointment.

SECTION FOUR **PALLIATIVE AND END-OF-LIFE CARE**

OVERVIEW/PATHOPHYSIOLOGY

According to the World Health Organization (1990) and the National Consensus Project for Quality Palliative Care (2004), *palliative care* is the active total care of patients whose disease is not responsive to curative treatment. Control of pain and other symptoms and of psychologic, social, and spiritual problems is paramount. The goal of palliative care is achievement of the best quality of life for patients and their families. The following nursing diagnoses relate specifically to issues, outcomes, and interventions that are common across medical diagnoses for patients in the terminal phase of illness.

NURSING DIAGNOSES AND INTERVENTIONS

Deficient knowledge related to choices regarding disease management when cure is unrealistic, including data about advance directives and comfort-focused care

Desired outcome: Patient and family express knowledge about advance directives and complete documents in accordance with state laws within weeks of diagnosis of life-limiting illness or before an acute crisis occurs.

Nursing Interventions

- Assess patient's facility with language; engage an interpreter or provide language-appropriate written materials as necessary.
- Assist patient with identifying an appropriate durable power of attorney for health care (DPOA-HC).
- Discuss role/limitations of the DPOA-HC.

BOX 13-4   FIVE WISHES

- The person I want to make care decisions for me when I can't
- The kind of medical treatment I want or don't want
- How comfortable I want to be
- How I want people to treat me
- What I want my loved ones to know

From *Five wishes* (an advance directive document), available from The Commission on Aging With Dignity, 1-888-5WISHES or www.agingwithdignity.org.

- ◆ Assist patient in completion of advance directive documents. This may also include Five Wishes, a program currently available in most states. (**BOX 13-4** lists topics included in the Five Wishes advance directive document.)
- ◆ Ensure that patient's preferences for hydration and nutrition are addressed specifically in DPOA-HC or Living Will documents as required by state law.
- ◆ Discuss meaning of Do Not Resuscitate (DNR) order and preferences for withholding or withdrawing other life-sustaining therapies.
- ◆ Explain what is meant by Comfort Measures Only (**FIGURE 13-2**).
- ◆ Advise family of need for prompt legal preparations (will, trusts, DPOA-HC).
- ◆ Discuss and document wishes regarding autopsy, organ donation/transplantation, hydration and feeding tubes, use of antibiotics, chemotherapy, radiation therapy, diagnostic procedures, blood transfusions, and IV infusions.
- ◆ Explain process of care related to withholding and/or withdrawing food and fluids.
- ◆ Secure copies of legal documents, and place in patient's medical record.
- ◆ Encourage professional counseling if any of these wishes or preparations cause discord within the family.

Deficient knowledge related to progressive disease process and expectations as death approaches
Desired outcome: Patient and family relate understanding of the palliative care approach to management of disease progression and express preferences for care, care goals, and preferred site of death.

Nursing Interventions

- ◆ Assess patient's facility with language; engage an interpreter or provide language-appropriate written materials as necessary.
- ◆ Educate patient and family about signs and symptoms of disease progression, including appetite loss, changes in respiratory and mental status, and potential for pain to increase in intensity and severity.
- ◆ Describe principles of palliative care to patient and family. For example, "Palliative care is not 'giving up' but rather it focuses on achieving the best possible quality of life for you and your family when the disease is no longer curable."
- ◆ Discuss interventions for managing symptoms as death approaches. For example, "You should not feel that 'there is nothing more to be done' because curative treatment is no longer effective. At this point in your care, aggressive symptom management and ensuring the best quality of life are very active treatments that can be provided." See **BOX 13-5** for a model of nursing diagnoses that relate to a quality of life perspective in palliative care.
- ◆ Refer patients to palliative care or hospice care providers while maintaining relationships with family/primary care physicians, community, and specialist care providers as appropriate *so that patient and family do not feel abandoned as care shifts to a palliative focus.*

Guidelines for Comfort Measures Orders

Discontinue ALL PREVIOUS ORDERS: Assess and reorder existing orders effective for comfort.

Activity: Goal is patient comfort. Activity level and hygiene routine should be based on patient's preference.

Hunger: Goal is to respond to patient's hunger, not to maintain a "normal nutritional intake."

Thirst: Goal is to respond to patient's thirst, which is best accomplished by oral fluids, sips, ice chips, and mouth care per patient desires, not IV hydration.

IV fluids: Goal is to avoid overhydration, which can lead to discomfort from edema, pulmonary and gastric secretions, and urinary incontinence. A small volume of IV fluid may assist with medication metabolism and delirium.

Dyspnea: Respond to the patient's perception of breathlessness rather than "numerical abnormalities" (e.g., oxygen saturation via pulse oximetry). Interventions include medications (e.g., opioids, antianxiety agents, steroids), scopolamine patch, and minimizing IV fluids to decrease secretions; oxygen therapy per nasal cannula prn for patient comfort; avoid face mask.

Fans at Bedside: Fans are available for patient comfort and are often more effective for perception of breathlessness than other interventions.

Elimination: Focus on managing distress from bowel or bladder incontinence. Insert Foley catheter prn, per patient comfort and desire.

Oral Care: Studies show dry mouth is the most common and distressing symptom in conscious patients at end of life. Ice chips and sips of fluid prn; humidify oxygen to minimize oral/nasal drying. Mouth care, every 12 hours and prn; sponge oral mucosa and apply lubricant to lips and oral mucosa.

Skin Care Air Mattress, Pressure Sore Prevention Measures: Per DHMC skin care guidelines. Incontinent care every 2 hours and prn.

Monitoring: Focus monitoring on the patient's symptoms (e.g., pain) and responses to comfort measures.

Psychosocial Consults: Goal is to provide resources and support through the dying process.

Medication for Symptom Management (Scheduled and PRN):

Pain Management: Scheduled and breakthrough; consider PCA/IV/subcutaneous/rectal analgesics.

Dyspnea Management: Consider opioids, scopolamine patch, atropine for secretions.

Anxiety/Agitation Management: Consider combination of lorazepam (Ativan) and haloperidol (Haldol).

Myoclonus: Consider benzodiazepines and/or opioid rotation for myoclonus.

Depression Management: Evaluate for antidepressants or methylphenidate.

Sleep Disturbance Management: Consider diphenhydramine (Benadryl).

Pruritus Management: Consider diphenhydramine (Benadryl) PO/IV

Fever Management: Consider acetaminophen (Tylenol) PO/rectal.

Nausea/Vomiting Management: Consider prochlorperazine (Compazine), metoclopramide; 5-HT3 antagonist PO/IV.

Constipation Management: Consider Narcotic Bowel Orders.

Diarrhea Management: Consider diphenoxylate/atropine (Lomotil) or loperamide (Imodium).

FIGURE 13-2 ◆ Guidelines for comfort measures orders. (Copyright Dartmouth-Hitchcock Medical Center, Lebanon, NH, 2004. May be reproduced for noncommercial purposes.)

BOX 13-5	QUALITY OF LIFE CONSIDERATIONS IN PALLIATIVE CARE

Physical
- Acute confusion
- Acute pain
- Alteration in elimination
- Chronic pain
- Disturbed thought processes
- Fatigue
- Impaired oral mucous membrane: dry mouth (xerostomia)
- Impaired swallowing
- Ineffective airway clearance
- Ineffective breathing pattern (dyspnea)
- Nausea
- Risk for imbalanced fluid volume
- Risk for imbalanced nutrition
- Self-care deficit
- Sleep deficit

Psychologic
- Anxiety
- Death anxiety
- Disturbed body image
- Dysfunctional grieving
- Fear
- Ineffective coping
- Ineffective denial
- Sorrow

Social
- Disabled family coping
- Interrupted family processes
- Risk for caregiver role strain
- Social isolation

Spiritual
- Hopelessness
- Impaired religiosity
- Powerlessness
- Spiritual distress

◆ Understand practical insurance and financial issues related to hospice care vs. home care. For example, Medicare hospice benefits provide a package of services via approved hospice programs (**BOX 13-6**), whereas the regular Medicare plan (Parts A and B) does not cover these services unless patient is homebound. There is a wide variation of reimbursement for hospice and palliative care provided by private insurers and health maintenance organizations (HMOs).

◆ Provide alternatives to calling for emergency care (i.e., calling 911) when death is imminent, such as calling the hospice or palliative care team for a home visit and/or symptom management suggestions.

◆ Keep patient and family informed about any changes in the treatment plan.

Chronic pain related to progressive disease state, immobility, obstructions, organ failure, or neuropathy

Desired outcomes: Within 4 hr of this nursing diagnosis, patient expresses or exhibits acceptable level of physical comfort with minimal side effects from analgesics. Family assists patient with maintaining, responding to, and titrating analgesia as patient's condition changes.

BOX 13-6	BENEFITS/REQUIRED SERVICES UNDER MEDICARE HOSPICE BENEFIT PLAN

- Pain- or symptom-control medications
- Coverage for non-homebound patients
- No deductibles/copayments
- Inpatient respite care
- Continuous RN care in the home during periods of crisis
- Counseling in the home (for patient and family)
- Homemakers
- Bereavement services
- Trained volunteers
- Continuity of care between inpatient and home settings

Nursing Interventions

♦ Distinguish between physical pain and suffering. Although this distinction can be difficult, consider the cause of distress to be other than physical suffering if rapid, appropriate titration of analgesics does not relieve distress. In this case, sedation may be the only means to relieve suffering.
♦ Assess regularly and use behavioral cues (Box 1-1) for patient unable to communicate.
♦ Allow patient to define a balance between discomfort and analgesics.
♦ Realize that many symptoms (e.g., dry mouth) cause discomfort and are managed in ways other than by use of analgesics.
♦ Address addiction concerns of patient and family. Remind them that pain is an appropriate indication for use of opioids and that under these circumstances patients are not "addicted" to medications.
♦ Address fears of respiratory depression from increasing opioid use.
♦ Realize that most patients will be receiving opioid analgesics at the end of life and that decreasing (LOC) and respirations are expected as part of the dying process and are not a toxicity of opioids.
♦ Implement nonpharmacologic treatments of pain, for example, massage and soft music.
♦ Discuss with health care provider the need to stop medications that are no longer necessary or that require a different route. Most patients are unable to take medications orally during the last days or hours of life.
♦ Consider using a comfort care flow sheet rather than a VS sheet to record patient comfort. (An example is shown in "Palliative Care for Advanced Disease Pathway [PCAD] Unit Reference Manual—Patient Care Flow Sheet, 2004" [website]: www.stoppain.org.)
♦ Recognize that The Joint Commission (TJC) standards call for "optimizing comfort and dignity" for patients dying in a hospital.
♦ See "Pain," p. 13, for more information.

Ineffective breathing pattern (dyspnea) related to progression of disease process and/or anxiety
Desired outcome: Within 1 hr of this nursing diagnosis, patient states that he or she does not perceive difficulty with breathing.

Nursing Interventions

♦ Assess patient's perception of dyspnea, and use this perception to guide treatment interventions. Recognize that objective parameters may not coincide with patient's perception of dyspnea (e.g., patient may have low O_2 saturation as measured by pulse oximetry but not feel dyspneic, and vice versa).
♦ Assess for treatable causes, such as anemia, heart failure, pleural effusion, ascites, pneumonia. Consider least invasive interventions first (e.g.,

antibiotics, steroids, diuretics) *to relieve underlying pathology causing dyspnea.* Carefully evaluate risk/benefit of more invasive techniques such as thoracentesis, paracentesis, radiation therapy. Consider imminence of death and whether invasive therapies will have time to offer relief or simply cause undue discomfort during the dying process.

♦ Advise family that although breathing changes are common and distressing, they are manageable.

♦ Maintain room at cool temperature to minimize feelings of suffocation. Place cool cloth on patient's face or forehead as indicated.

♦ Administer O_2 by nasal cannula only if this offers subjective relief of dyspnea. Use lowest flow rate possible and offer humidification if technically possible. Avoid face mask, which is usually uncomfortable and can interfere with patient's ability to communicate with significant others.

♦ Administer morphine or other opioid regularly by available route *to relieve dyspnea.* The oral route (pills or elixir) is preferred, but if this is not possible, use the rectal, sublingual, nebulized, subcutaneous, or IV route.

♦ Place fan close to patient's face; realize that the face contains baroreceptors that respond to air movement and can effectively relieve perception of dyspnea.

♦ Position patient with head and upper body elevated.

♦ Suggest sleeping in chair, if needed.

♦ Administer nebulized bronchodilators, steroids, and/or opioids *to relieve dyspnea.*

♦ Teach relaxation breathing techniques to patient and family.

♦ Encourage physical touch or massage *as a calming technique.*

♦ Consider need for pharmacologic management of anxiety (e.g., use of anxiolytics) *to alleviate fear and perception of breathlessness.*

♦ Discuss principle of "double effect" of medications. For example, explain to patient and family that some medicines may relieve symptoms but at the expense of the unintended side effect of sedation or hastened death. Elicit patient preferences and values about alertness vs. sedation or discomfort if both goals cannot be achieved. Honor patient's choices for symptom management.

Ineffective airway clearance related to increased pulmonary secretions and congestion secondary to diminishing LOC as death approaches
Desired outcomes: Patient does not show signs of struggle or discomfort when "death rattle" is present. The family expresses understanding that these noisy respirations are more distressing to them than to the (unconscious) patient.

Nursing Interventions

♦ Explain etiology of the noisy breathing: It is a result of secretions in the upper airway in patients who are too weak to cough effectively.

♦ Assure family and significant others that patient's breathing, although noisy, is peaceful and unlabored.

♦ Attempt to position patient laterally and recumbent, rather than supine, *to maintain as patent an airway as possible.*

♦ Use O_2 only if it enables patient to have unlabored respirations.

♦ Avoid suctioning, other than in the oral cavity, inasmuch as this intervention will likely increase, not decrease, secretions.

♦ Maintain patient in a relatively dehydrated *state to minimize accumulation of pulmonary secretions.*

♦ If death rattle persists despite dehydration, administer anticholinergics via the least invasive route. Recognize that these agents are much more effective when administered early in the onset of this symptom. Effective agents include scopolamine patch, glycopyrrolate (IV, subcutaneous, PO), atropine, and hyoscine butylbromide.

♦ Reassure family that patients are often unaware of discomfort at this point.

BOX 13-7	RISK FACTORS FOR DELIRIUM IN TERMINAL ILLNESS

- Impending death
- Advanced age
- Severity of illness
- Limitation of physical mobility
- Social isolation
- Reduced sensory acuity (vision, hearing)
- Underlying neurologic degeneration or injury
- Seizures
- Brain tumor, abscess, hemorrhage
- Fever or hypothermia
- Hypoxia
- Severe anemia
- Infections
- Dehydration
- Metabolic imbalances
- Low serum albumin
- Polypharmacy
- Drug withdrawal (e.g., benzodiazepines, alcohol, opiates)
- Exposure to certain drugs
  - High-dose opiates, especially meperidine
  - Anticholinergic agents (e.g., antihistamines)
  - Corticosteroids
  - Antiemetics
  - Psychostimulants
  - Sedatives-hypnotics
  - Alcohol and drugs of abuse

From Shuster JL Jr: Delirium, confusion, and agitation at the end of life, *J Palliat Med* 1(2):177-186, 1998.

Disturbed thought processes related to delirium, related to disease progression, infection, altered metabolic state, or symptom management side effects
Desired outcomes: Reversible etiologies of delirium are treated within hours of onset. When delirium is irreversible, agitation is reduced or minimized.

Nursing Interventions

- Recognize etiologies of delirium in the terminally ill (**BOX 13-7**).
- Assess for common treatable causes: brain metastasis, steroids, opioid toxicity, anticholinergics, benzodiazepines, withdrawal from drug/ethanol (ETOH), unrelieved pain, itching, constipation, urinary retention, infection, hepatic encephalopathy, hypoglycemia or hyperglycemia, hypoxia, hypercalcemia, dehydration.
- Treat potentially reversible causes. Correct metabolic abnormalities, empty bladder, relieve constipation, and provide gentle hydration.
- As prescribed, decrease or eliminate medications that are not directed at comfort.
- Maintain a quiet, well-lit environment.
- Assess whether gentle massage is appropriate as a calming measure.
- Encourage family to provide comforting items from patient's home, such as a favorite pillow or blanket.
- Role model soft-spoken language and remind family that patient likely maintains sense of hearing even when other senses are impaired.
- Encourage family to touch patient.
- Ensure patient's physical safety, for example, with padded side rails, bed in low position.

BOX 13-8	CRITICAL ISSUES IN FAMILY COUNSELING REGARDING DELIRIUM CHARACTERISTICS

- Delirium can be rapid onset and short term duration (if reversible)
- Patient's cognition can fluctuate
- Polypharmacy may be a possible cause (e.g., opioids, benzodiazepines)
- It may be a distressing experience for the patient
- Family may have difficulty communicating with the patient
- A calm, comforting, compassionate approach may help soothe the patient
- Overall goals of care should be determined while identifying effective delirium treatment (advance directives and family input are key while patient lacks decision-making capacity)

Modified from Kuebler K, Heidrich D, Vena C, English N: Delirium, confusion, and agitation. In Ferrell B, Coyle N, editors: *Textbook of palliative nursing*, ed 2, New York, 2006, Oxford University Press.

- ◆ Avoid physical restraints. Use patient companion or other environmental safety measures (e.g., bed alarms).
- ◆ Administer medication to manage delirium and control agitation; many drugs are used but there is little evidence to support their effectiveness; low-dose haloperidol appears to work best and with fewest side effects.
- ◆ Reorient patient frequently. Have large-faced clocks and calendars within sight.
- ◆ Counsel family about the distressing effects of patient's delirium according to issues that are involved (**BOX 13-8**). Reassure family that communication is still possible via familiar voices, soothing words, or massage.
- ◆ Advise family that delirium may signal imminent death.
- ◆ Consider sedation if this is consistent with patient and family preferences and values. Avoid use of phrase "terminal sedation" and instead use "sedation in imminently dying" *because the former implies sedation to end patient's life rather than intent of sedation for alleviation of symptom distress in patient who is dying.*
- ◆ Realize that it is usually unrealistic to discontinue opioids for pain in a dying patient. However, if the current opioid regimen is believed to be the cause of delirium, a different opioid in an equianalgesic dose may provide pain relief without delirium. For example, hydromorphone and oxycodone may be less deliriogenic than morphine.

Risk for imbalanced fluid volume related to dehydration or edema, related to inability to regulate fluid I&O secondary to disease progression

Desired outcomes: Patient's desires for fluid intake are determined by subjective feelings of thirst. Patient receives hydration according to stated preferences. Hydration goals are realistic with appropriate end-points such as correction of a metabolic disorder that results in enhanced subjective well-being.

Nursing Interventions

- ◆ Do not attempt to manage perception of dry mouth by achieving normal hydration *because this perception is often the result of mouth breathing or other causes that are not responsive to hydration.*
- ◆ Maintain oral care *to minimize discomfort of dry mouth* (xerostomia).
- ◆ Be aware of signs and symptoms of uncomfortable fluid overload (e.g., peripheral edema, urinary incontinence, pleural effusion, ascites, pulmonary congestion, enhanced "death rattle").
- ◆ Address issue of nutrition/feeding tubes on advance directive.
- ◆ Advise family that it is normal to eat and drink less at the end of life.
- ◆ Encourage family not to insist that patient eat.

- Recognize cultural/ethnic implications of food and eating.
- Reassure family that dehydration results in a peaceful, painless death.
- Administer rectal acetaminophen regularly to reduce discomforts of dehydration-related fever.
- If family wishes to continue oral feedings, encourage frequent meals, small portions, use of small plates, and companionship during meals.
- Prepare soft, easily swallowed foods such as soup, milk shake, yogurt, custard, or ice cream.
- Prepare foods away from patient's sight or smell.
- Provide fluids that contain electrolytes.
- Administer IV fluids if patient or family so request.
- Advise family to expect urine to become scant and dark.

Impaired oral mucous membrane related to dry mouth/xerostomia, related to reduced saliva, mouth breathing, oral infections, mucositis, and/or dehydration
Desired outcomes: Patient's oral mucous membrane becomes moist. Patient does not report or exhibit discomfort from dry mouth.

Nursing Interventions

- Recognize that IV fluids and interventions directed at normal hydration status rarely relieve dry mouth. Instead, encourage topical interventions.
- Use a misting spray bottle with saline *to moisten oral mucous membrane.*
- Use emollients on lips.
- Encourage family to assist with mouth care.
- If patient is on O_2, add humidifier.
- Rule out oral thrush and herpes; treat if necessary.
- Encourage fluid intake via frequent sips of water, Popsicles, or ice chips.
- Encourage intake of soups, sauces, gravies, ice cream, and frozen yogurt in patients able to eat.
- Avoid drying substances such as caffeine, alcohol, and alcohol-based products (e.g., mouthwash, cough syrups).
- Offer spray bottle filled with water and a few drops of vegetable oil *to keep mucous membranes moist.*
- Suggest use of lemon drops or other sour candy if patient can tolerate without aspiration.
- Administer saliva substitutes.
- Encourage good dental hygiene (soft-bristled toothbrush, regular brushing, and flossing).

Risk for imbalanced nutrition: less than body requirements related to anorexia, nausea and vomiting, cachexia, intestinal obstruction, impaired swallowing, and aspiration risk secondary to disease progression
Desired outcomes: Patient does not report presence of hunger. Family honors patient's wishes regarding artificial nutrition.

Nursing Interventions

- Recognize that many families see food as an expression of love and will become distressed when patient is no longer able to have a "normal" nutritional intake. Remind family that eating will not reverse the underlying disease state.
- Identify other ways family can express love.
- Help patient and family to understand that a normal nutritional status is unrealistic as the disease progresses and the body no longer processes ingested nutrients. Loss of interest in food is normal near death.
- Explain that artificial nutrition such as parenteral nutrition does not relieve feelings of hunger if present, nor does it prolong survival in a terminal state. The body only takes in what it needs.

- Oral nutrition is the method of choice for patients who can swallow and who have intact GI systems. Enteral routes include nasogastric, gastrostomy, and jejunostomy tubes. However, these routes can result in harm if the GI system cannot absorb and digest nutrients. If appropriate, obtain a nutritional consult *to determine the most digestible feedings, given patient's underlying disease.*
- Avoid giving commercial nutritional supplements *because they likely will suppress patient's appetite and may be unpalatable.* Giving supplements may result in inability to ingest foods patient likes and enjoys.

Fear related to life-threatening condition, pain, the unknown (death), and patient's concern that he or she will be forgotten
Desired outcomes: Patient's fears are acknowledged and addressed. Patient states that fear has been lessened.

Nursing Interventions

- Distinguish between anxiety (a state of apprehension and dread whose source patient cannot identify) and fear (which often has a realistic, definable cause). Identify appropriate interventions (see nursing diagnosis **Death anxiety**, following).
- Reassure patient that pain and other discomforts will be managed.
- Identify and address family's fears and concerns. Keep family informed of physical symptoms to expect as death approaches (e.g., changes in breathing, decreased LOC, coolness and mottling of skin).
- If appropriate, encourage patient and family to seek support from pastoral counselors in addressing religious beliefs about the meaning of suffering, death, and afterlife.
- Assist patient and family with creating videos or audios and scrapbooks for recalled memories.
- Encourage patient to use this time to create a legacy. For example, see "A Legacy to Remember" (website) at www.alegacytoremember.com.

Death anxiety related to impending death, fear of unmanaged physical symptoms, and fear of unknown
Desired outcomes: Patient states (or exhibits) that he or she is free of physical discomforts and emotional distress. Family members verbalize understanding of the dying process.

Nursing Interventions

- Provide aggressive symptom management of physical discomforts before attempting to assess anxiety.
- Explore patient's feelings and perceptions of anticipatory grief.
- Assess whether patient has insight about physical manifestations of anxiety (e.g., racing heart, sweating, feeling flushed, wheezing). Help patient recognize these symptoms early and use a preemptive strategy *to minimize escalation.*
- Allow patient and family to express fears and anxieties related to previous experiences with the dying.
- Listen carefully to stories *to anticipate special needs during current death event.* For instance, if family members tell you they feel guilty about not saying "I love you" before the death of another individual, encourage them to say or write down what they most want the dying patient to know, even if patient is not conscious.
- Review age-appropriate guidelines for child participation in care and presence with dying family member, and encourage family to allow children to be present consistent with these guidelines.
- Ask about content of bad dreams or nightmares.

◆ Encourage patient to share impressions of what happens after death. Obtain referrals to or guidance of specific religious counselors *to support patient through anxiety regarding this issue.*

◆ Encourage use of relaxation techniques such as imagery, progressive muscle relaxation, and relaxation breathing.

◆ Administer anxiolytics as appropriate.

◆ Refer to interventions listed under other nursing diagnoses in this section and in "Psychosocial Support," p. 31.

Powerlessness related to actual debility and inability to carry out normal role functions
Desired outcome: Patient makes choices for end-of-life care.

Nursing Interventions

◆ Reinforce use of patient's advance directives and advance care planning activities in guiding care.

◆ Remind patient and family of their continuing ability to make choices involving end-of-life care. Some examples include patient's right to choose whether to eat or drink, have certain care procedures performed, have or decline treatments, and actualize preferences around site of dying (e.g., home vs. institution).

◆ Encourage open communication with family. Suggest resources that facilitate conversations within the family. An example: Byock I: *The four things that matter MOST: a book about living,* New York, 2004, Free Press.

Spiritual distress related to religious, cultural, and existential beliefs about dying
Desired outcome: Patient states that he or she has ability to connect with spiritual/pastoral counselors to discuss issues of spirituality, existential concerns, and their meanings.

Nursing Interventions

◆ Support patient's religious customs around end-of-life issues.

◆ Offer to pray with patient and family if appropriate.

◆ Remember that being "spiritual" is not necessarily synonymous with being "religious."

◆ Ask patient what has brought his or her life satisfaction, joy, and sorrow.

◆ Include priest/minister/rabbi as integral member of caregiving team.

◆ Assist family in creation of rituals (e.g., letting go, remembering, forgiving).

◆ Suggest planning of funeral/memorial service, music, readings.

Risk for caregiver role strain related to multiple demands on family members and resources when caring for dying loved one
Desired outcome: Caregivers are assisted with providing care, given respite, and reassured that they are doing a good job.

Nursing Interventions

◆ Identify available resources (e.g., hospice, friends, community, church members) to assist with caregiving in patient's and family members' preferred site of death.

◆ Recognize that there may be a lack of insurance funding for many activities of care (e.g., childcare, transportation, housekeeping) and other worries caregivers may have regarding loss of time from work, loss of savings, and loss of income of ill family member.

◆ Remind caregivers of their own health care needs. Encourage family to take breaks for meals, relaxation, and attention to family members who are not ill, especially young children.

- Suggest counseling and other psychosocial support resources that assist family with maintaining integrity and avoiding conflict during the strain of illness.
- Offer family members unrestricted access to patient as death approaches but also encourage them to take frequent rest periods.
- If family members are unable to be present for a period, provide phone numbers so that they can stay in contact with staff.

Anticipatory grieving related to impending loss of loved one

Desired outcome: Family and significant others identify and express feelings appropriately and demonstrate balancing caregiving with their own physical and emotional respite needs.

Nursing Interventions

- Recognize that anger is often substituted for grief.
- Assist family with recalling successful past coping strategies.
- Encourage grieving and expression of feelings by patient, family, and staff.
- Be available to listen, and respect the need to use denial occasionally as an effective coping mechanism.
- Appreciate the value of anticipatory grieving.
- Give family permission to express ambivalence about impending death. For instance, "Many people in your circumstance don't want to lose their loved one, yet they wish for the suffering to be over. I wonder if you've had feelings like these?"
- Permit silences—don't try to say something meaningful or profound.
- Offer locks of hair and other tangible mementos to survivors.
- Notify other health care providers (e.g., primary care provider, surgeon, ambulatory care nurses) of patient's death so that they can express their sympathy to family.
- Permit family to stay with patient after death *to say goodbye and express grief.*
- Arrange bereavement follow-up for family members. For example, inform them about availability of bereavement groups, books on grieving, and available counseling resources.
- Consider making a bereavement phone call or sending a sympathy card.
- Recommend judicious use of anxiolytics or sedatives for acutely grieving survivors.
- Provide phone numbers or concrete information *to assist family in beginning process of identifying funeral plans.*

Infection Prevention and Control

For several decades, infection prevention and control efforts have focused on the use of barriers (e.g., gloves, gowns, masks) to interrupt transmission of organisms among and between patients and health care workers. These barriers are a major component of various systems of transmission precautions.

SYSTEMS OF TRANSMISSION PRECAUTIONS

Many different systems of transmission precautions have been used in hospitals over the years and are commonly called *isolation precautions.* These recommendations are updated periodically, with the most recent revision (2007) by the Centers for Disease Control and Prevention (CDC) intended to reflect evidence-based practices and current knowledge. The purpose of these techniques and procedures is to interrupt transmission of organisms by adhering to five guiding principles: (1) to provide infection control recommendations for all components of the health care delivery system, including hospitals, long-term care facilities, ambulatory care, and home care and hospice; (2) to reaffirm Standard Precautions as the foundation for preventing transmission during patient care in all health care settings; (3) to reaffirm the importance of implementing transmission-based precautions based on clinical presentation or syndrome and likely pathogens until the infectious etiology has been determined; (4) to provide epidemiologically sound and, whenever possible, evidence-based recommendations; and (5) to provide a unified infection control approach to multidrug-resistant organisms (MDROs). The 2007 guideline contains two tiers of precautions (**Table A-1**): Standard Precautions, which are designed for the care of all patients in any health care setting, regardless of diagnosis or presumed infection status, and Transmission-Based Precautions, which are used for patients known to be or suspected of being infected or colonized with epidemiologically important pathogens that can be transmitted by airborne or droplet transmission or by contact with dry skin or contaminated surfaces. A new type of Transmission-Based Precautions also has been added, the Protective Environment, which is specifically for patients undergoing hematopoietic stem cell transplantation (HSCT), who are at particular risk for infections with airborne fungi.

The 2007 guideline replaces the 1996 guideline for isolation precautions in hospitals. The 1996 Standard Precautions system synthesized the major features of Universal Precautions and Body Substance Isolation and applied to the following: (1) blood; (2) all body fluids, secretions, and excretions, except sweat, regardless of whether they contain visible blood; (3) nonintact skin; and (4) mucous membranes. In addition, Standard Precautions were designed to reduce risks of transmission of microorganisms from both recognized and unrecognized sources of infectious agents. The 2007 guideline continues these same principles of Standard Precautions and applies them to a broader range of situations and care settings. The 1996 Transmission-Based

Text continued on page 755.

TABLE A-1 | RECOMMENDATIONS FOR ISOLATION PRECAUTIONS IN HEALTH CARE SETTINGS, 2007

	STANDARD PRECAUTIONS	TRANSMISSION-BASED PRECAUTIONS: AIRBORNE INFECTION ISOLATION	TRANSMISSION-BASED PRECAUTIONS: DROPLET	TRANSMISSION-BASED PRECAUTIONS: CONTACT	TRANSMISSION-BASED PRECAUTIONS: PROTECTIVE ENVIRONMENT
When to Use	For care of all patients in all health care settings	For patients known or suspected to be infected with microorganisms transmitted from person to person by airborne droplet nuclei that remain suspended in the air and that can be dispersed widely by air currents	For patients known or suspected to be infected with microorganisms transmitted by respiratory droplets (more than 5 μm in size) generated by patient when coughing, sneezing, talking, or during performance of cough-inducing procedures	For patients with known or suspected infections or evidence of syndromes that represent increased risk for contact transmission, including colonization or infection with MDROs according to recommendations in the CDC Isolation Guideline (2007)	For patients undergoing allogeneic HSCT to minimize fungal spore counts in the air; specific requirements for the Protective Environment were defined by the CDC in 2000* and updated in 2007
Hand Hygiene 1. When hands are visibly dirty or contaminated with proteinaceous material or visibly soiled with blood or other body fluids, wash hands with either a	Decontaminate hands in the following circumstances: before having direct contact with patients; after contact with blood, body fluids or excretions, mucous membranes, nonintact skin, or				

nonantimicrobial soap and water or an antimicrobial soap and water

2. If hands are not visibly soiled, use an alcohol-based hand rub for routinely decontaminating hands in all other clinical situations; alternatively, wash hands with an antimicrobial soap and water

wound dressings; after contact with a patient's intact skin (e.g., when taking a pulse or blood pressure or lifting a patient); if hands will be moving from a contaminated body site to a clean body site; after contact with inanimate objects in the immediate vicinity of the patient; after removing gloves

Gloves

Wear gloves when it can be reasonably anticipated that contact with blood or other potentially infectious materials, mucous membranes, nonintact skin, or potentially contaminated intact skin could occur

Wear gloves with fit and durability appropriate to the task; wear disposable medical

Wear gloves as indicated according to Standard Precautions and whenever touching patient's intact skin or surfaces and articles in close proximity to patient (e.g., medical equipment or bed rails); don gloves upon entry into the room

Continued

TABLE A-1   RECOMMENDATIONS FOR ISOLATION PRECAUTIONS IN HEALTH CARE SETTINGS, 2007—cont'd

STANDARD PRECAUTIONS	TRANSMISSION-BASED PRECAUTIONS: AIRBORNE INFECTION ISOLATION	TRANSMISSION-BASED PRECAUTIONS: DROPLET	TRANSMISSION-BASED PRECAUTIONS: CONTACT	TRANSMISSION-BASED PRECAUTIONS: PROTECTIVE ENVIRONMENT
examination gloves for providing direct patient care; wear disposable medical examination gloves or reusable utility gloves for cleaning the environment or medical equipment Remove gloves after contact with patient and/or surrounding environment (including medical equipment, and use proper technique to prevent hand contamination; do not wear same pair of gloves for care of more than one patient; change gloves during patient care if hands will move from a contaminated body site to a clean body site				

Continued

Mouth, Nose, Eye, and Respiratory Protection	Wear a mask and eye protection or a face shield to protect mucous membranes of eyes, nose, and mouth during procedures and patient care activities that are likely to generate splashes or sprays of blood, body fluids, secretions, and excretions; select masks, goggles, face shields, and combinations of each according to the task performed	Restrict susceptible health care personnel from entering rooms of patients known or suspected to have measles (rubeola), varicella (chickenpox), zoster, or smallpox if other immune health care personnel are available; wear fit-tested NIOSH-approved N95 or higher PR for respiratory protection when entering room or home of a patient when the following diseases are suspected or confirmed: infectious pulmonary or laryngeal tuberculosis or draining tuberculous skin lesions; smallpox, SARS, avian influenza	Wear a mask for close patient contact (e.g., within 3 ft); use of eye protection should follow pathogen-specific recommendations in the CDC Isolation Guideline (2007)	During periods of construction, to prevent inhalation of respirable particles that could contain infectious spores, provide respiratory protection (e.g., N95 PR) to patients who are medically fit enough to tolerate a PR when they are required to leave the Protective Environment; ensure that patients are instructed on PR use; in the absence of construction, the CDC makes no recommendation for use of when leaving the Protective Environment
Respiratory Hygiene/ Cough Etiquette	Educate staff on importance of source control measures to contain respiratory secretions and prevent droplet and fomite			

TABLE A-1 RECOMMENDATIONS FOR ISOLATION PRECAUTIONS IN HEALTH CARE SETTINGS, 2007—cont'd

STANDARD PRECAUTIONS	TRANSMISSION-BASED PRECAUTIONS: AIRBORNE INFECTION ISOLATION	TRANSMISSION-BASED PRECAUTIONS: DROPLET	TRANSMISSION-BASED PRECAUTIONS: CONTACT	TRANSMISSION-BASED PRECAUTIONS: PROTECTIVE ENVIRONMENT
transmission of respiratory pathogens, especially during seasonal outbreaks of viral respiratory tract infections Post signs in ambulatory and impatient settings with instructions to patients and other persons to inform them to cover mouth/nose when coughing or sneezing, use and dispose of tissues, and perform hand hygiene after hands have been in contact with respiratory secretions; the health care facility should provide tissues and no-touch receptacles for disposal				

of used tissues as well as conveniently located dispensers of alcohol-based hand rubs, and where sinks are available, supplies for handwashing; although this is most important during periods of increased rates of respiratory infections in the community, some facilities may find it logistically easier to institute these recommendations year-round as a standard practice

Gowns

Wear a gown or other PPE attire that is appropriate to the task, to protect skin and prevent soiling of clothing during procedures and patient care activities when contact with blood, body fluids, secretions, or excretions is anticipated

Wear a gown whenever anticipating that clothing will have direct contact with patient or potentially contaminated environmental surfaces or items in patient's room; don gown upon entry into the room

Continued

TABLE A-1	RECOMMENDATIONS FOR ISOLATION PRECAUTIONS IN HEALTH CARE SETTINGS, 2007—cont'd				
	STANDARD PRECAUTIONS	TRANSMISSION-BASED PRECAUTIONS: AIRBORNE INFECTION ISOLATION	TRANSMISSION-BASED PRECAUTIONS: DROPLET	TRANSMISSION-BASED PRECAUTIONS: CONTACT	TRANSMISSION-BASED PRECAUTIONS: PROTECTIVE ENVIRONMENT
	Wear a gown for direct patient contact if patient has uncontained secretions or excretions Remove gown and other PPE attire and perform hand hygiene before leaving patient's environment			Remove gown and perform hand hygiene before leaving patient's environment; after gown removal, ensure that clothing and skin do not contact potentially contaminated environmental surfaces to avoid transfer of microorganisms to other patients or environmental surfaces	
Patient Placement	Include the potential for transmission of infectious agents when making patient placement decisions	In acute care hospitals or residential settings, place patient in a single-patient AIIR that has been constructed in accordance with current guidelines; keep AIIR door closed when not	In acute care settings, place patient in a single-patient room when available; if single-patient rooms are in short supply, prioritize patients who have excessive cough and	In acute care settings, place patients who may require Contact Precautions in a single-patient room when available; if single-patient rooms are in short supply,	

Continued

required for entry and exit; if appropriate AIIR room is not available, consult facility's ICP for alternatives

Discontinue Airborne Precautions after signs and symptoms have resolved or according to pathogen-specific recommendations in the CDC Isolation Guideline (2007)

sputum production for single-patient room placement because of their risk of transmission; avoid placing patients who require Droplet Precautions in same room with patients who are at increased risk for infection or adverse outcomes associated with infection (e.g., immunocompromised status or anticipated prolonged length of stay); place together (cohort) in same room patients who are infected with same organism or otherwise are suitable roommates; in other situations or care settings, consult facility's ICP for alternatives

prioritize patients with conditions that may facilitate transmission (e.g., uncontained drainage, stool incontinence) for single-patient room placement; place together (cohort) in same room patients who are infected or colonized with the same pathogen and are suitable roommates; ensure that patients are physically separated (i.e., more than 3 ft) from each other; draw privacy curtain between beds to minimize opportunity for direct contact; change protective attire and perform hand hygiene between patients; for patient placement in other situations or care settings, consult facility's ICP

TABLE A-1   RECOMMENDATIONS FOR ISOLATION PRECAUTIONS IN HEALTH CARE SETTINGS, 2007—cont'd

	STANDARD PRECAUTIONS	TRANSMISSION-BASED PRECAUTIONS: AIRBORNE INFECTION ISOLATION	TRANSMISSION-BASED PRECAUTIONS: DROPLET	TRANSMISSION-BASED PRECAUTIONS: CONTACT	TRANSMISSION-BASED PRECAUTIONS: PROTECTIVE ENVIRONMENT
Patient Transport		In inpatient and residential settings, limit movement and transport of patients who require Airborne Precautions to medically necessary purposes; If transport or movement outside AIIR is necessary, instruct patient to wear a mask; instruct patients who cannot tolerate wearing masks because of medical conditions to observe Respiratory Hygiene/Cough Etiquette procedures; discontinue Airborne Precautions after signs and symptoms have resolved or according to pathogen-specific	Limit movement and transport of patient to medically necessary purposes; instruct patient to wear a mask and follow Respiratory Hygiene/Cough Etiquette during transport; no mask is required for persons who are transporting patient; discontinue Droplet Precautions after signs and symptoms have resolved or according to pathogen-specific recommendations in the CDC Isolation Guideline (2007)	Limit movement and transport of patients; if transport is required, ensure that infected or colonized areas of the patient are contained and covered; remove contaminated PPE and perform hand hygiene before transporting patient on Contact Precautions; don clean PPE to handle patient when transport destination has been reached	

		recommendations in the CDC Isolation Guideline (2007)	
Patient Care Equipment	Follow established policies and procedures for containing, transporting, and handling patient care equipment that may be contaminated with blood or body fluids; always clean patient care equipment to remove organic material before disinfection and sterilization procedures are used		Manage patient care equipment according to Standard Precautions; use disposable patient care items (e.g., blood pressure cuffs) whenever possible or implement patient-dedicated use of noncritical equipment to avoid sharing among patients; if use of common equipment or items is unavoidable, clean and disinfect these items before use on another patient
Care of the Environment	Follow established policies and procedures for cleaning and maintaining environmental surfaces as appropriate for level of patient contact and degree of soiling		Ensure that rooms of patients on Contact Precautions are given cleaning priority with a focus on frequent (e.g., at least daily) cleaning and disinfection of

Continued

TABLE A-1 RECOMMENDATIONS FOR ISOLATION PRECAUTIONS IN HEALTH CARE SETTINGS, 2007—cont'd

	STANDARD PRECAUTIONS	TRANSMISSION-BASED PRECAUTIONS: AIRBORNE INFECTION ISOLATION	TRANSMISSION-BASED PRECAUTIONS: DROPLET	TRANSMISSION-BASED PRECAUTIONS: CONTACT	TRANSMISSION-BASED PRECAUTIONS: PROTECTIVE ENVIRONMENT
				high-touch surfaces (e.g., bed rails, bedside commodes, faucet handles, doorknobs, carts, charts) and equipment in immediate vicinity of patient	
Textiles, Laundry	Handle used textiles and fabrics with minimum agitation to avoid contamination of air, surfaces, and persons				
Workers' Safety	Adhere to federal and state requirements for protection of health care personnel from exposure to bloodborne pathogens				

Modified from Siegel JD, Rhinehart E, Jackson M, Chiarello L, Health Care Infection Control Practices Advisory Committee: 2007 Guideline for isolation precautions: preventing transmission of infectious agents in health care settings (website): http://www.cdc.gov/ncidod/dhqp/pdf/guidelines/Isolation2007.pdf.

PR, particulate respirator; *SARS,* severe acute respiratory syndrome.

Precautions were designed for patients documented to be or suspected of being infected or colonized with organisms transmitted by the airborne route, by droplets, and by contact when extra precautions were necessary to interrupt transmission. As always, the CDC offers hospitals and other types of health care settings the option of modifying the recommendations according to their needs and circumstances and as directed by federal, state, or local regulations. For example, the Bloodborne Pathogens Standard of the Occupational Safety and Health Administration (2001) is still operable, and all facilities are required to comply with its provisions. The CDC's 2007 Standard Precautions incorporate all requirements of the OSHA Bloodborne Pathogens Standard.

TRANSMISSION PRECAUTIONS FOR PATIENTS WITH PULMONARY OR LARYNGEAL TUBERCULOSIS

Airborne Infection Isolation Precautions are for persons diagnosed with or suspected of having pulmonary or laryngeal tuberculosis (TB), which can be transmitted to others via the airborne route. These guidelines focus on early identification and treatment of persons with a diagnosis or suspected diagnosis of active TB. In addition, the CDC defined requirements for special ventilation and use of respiratory protection masks that provide better filtration and a tighter fit than those achievable with standard surgical masks. Masks of this type are called particulate respirators (PRs), and the specific type of PR for TB protection is called an N95 respirator. This type of respiratory protection is also appropriate for susceptible persons caring for patients known to have or suspected of having measles (rubeola), varicella (chickenpox), or smallpox. Of course, the best protection for any of the vaccine-preventable infectious diseases is for all caregivers to be immunized; then respiratory protection masks are not necessary.

MANAGEMENT OF DEVICES AND PROCEDURES TO REDUCE RISK OF NOSOCOMIAL INFECTION

Use of barriers is but one of many strategies that can reduce the risk of nosocomial infection among patients and personnel. In fact, studies from the CDC show that significant gains can be made in reducing infection risks by focusing on the management of devices and procedures commonly used in patient care. For example, many patients need intravascular devices that deliver therapeutic medications, but these patients are put at risk for site infections and bacteremias when these devices are used. It is well known that rotating the access site at appropriate intervals reduces these risks to the patient, and catheter materials that are more "vein friendly" also reduce trauma to the vascular system. In addition, use of needles to deliver medications and fluids to patients through these intravascular devices can put the health care worker at risk for puncture injury. Needleless or needle-free IV access devices are used to access line ports so that it is not necessary to use needles once the intravascular catheter has entered the vascular system. Thus the use of newer and safer intravascular devices and procedures can benefit both the patient and the health care worker by reducing their risk of health care–associated infection.

Research studies of interventions to reduce health care–associated infection risks are published in general and specialty journals and presented at professional meetings each year. Infection control professionals (ICPs) and hospital epidemiologists use these studies to make recommendations about changes in nursing and medical practice. The Joint Commission (TJC) requires that all accredited facilities have on staff a person qualified to provide infection surveillance, prevention, and control services. The national associations for these professionals are the Association for Professionals in Infection Control and Epidemiology, Inc. (APIC), which publishes the *American Journal of Infection Control,* and the Society for Healthcare Epidemiology of America (SHEA), which publishes the journal *Infection Control and Hospital Epidemiology.*

References

Occupational Safety and Health Administration (OSHA), Department of Labor: Occupational exposure to bloodborne pathogens; needlesticks and other sharp injuries: Final rule, *Fed Regist* 66:5318-5325, 2001.

Siegel JD, Rhinehart E, Jackson M, Chiarello L, Health Care Infection Control Practices Advisory Committee: 2007 Guideline for isolation precautions: preventing transmission of infectious agents in health care settings (website): http://www.cdc.gov/ncidod/dhqp/pdf/guidelines/Isolation2007.pdf. Accessed February 2, 2010. (Also available in *Am J Infect Control* 35(10 suppl 2):S65-S164, 2007.)

Need-to-Know
Laboratory Values

TABLE A-2	THE VALUES GIVEN BELOW ARE THOSE SPECIFIED FOR THE NURSE TO KNOW IN THE 2010 DETAILED NCLEX-RN TEST PLAN

	ADULT NORMAL VALUES* (TRADITIONAL U.S.)	SI ADULT NORMAL VALUES* (INTERNATIONAL SYSTEM)
Alanine aminotransferase (ALT)	4-36 units/L	
Albumin (blood)	3.5-5.0 g/dL	35-50 g/L
Ammonia	10-80 mcg/dL	6-47 µmol/L
Aspartate aminotransferase (AST)	0-35 units/L	0-0.58 µ Kat/L
Bicarbonate (HCO_3^-)	21-28 mEq/L	21-28 mEq/L
Bilirubin	Total: 0.3-1.0 mg/dL	Total: 5.1-17 µmol/L
Blood gases, arterial		
O_2 saturation (Sao_2)	95%-100%	95%-100%
Pco_2	35-45 mm Hg	35-45 mm Hg
pH	7.35-7.45	7.35-7.45
Po_2	80-100 mm Hg	80-100 mm Hg
BUN	10-20 mg/dL	3.6-7.1 mmol/L
Calcium (Ca)	9.0-10.5 mg/dL	2.25-2.75 mmol/L
Cholesterol		
Total	Less than 200 mg/dL	Less than 5.20 mmol/L
HDL	Male: more than 45 mg/dL	More than 0.75 mmol/L
	Female: more than	More than 0.91 mmol/L
LDL	55 mg/dL	Less than 3.37 mmol/L
	60-180 mg/dL	
Creatinine	Male: 0.6-1.2 mg/dL	50-110 µmol/L
	Female: 0.5-1.1 mg/dL	
Erythrocyte sedimentation rate (ESR)	Male: 0-15 mm/hr	
	Female: 0-20 mm/hr	
Glucose		
Fasting	70-110 mg/dL	Less than 6.1 mmol/L
Random	200 mg/dL or less	
Glycosylated hemoglobin (glycohemoglobin [HbA_{1c}])	Nondiabetic: 4%-5.9%	0.040-0.066
	Good diabetic control: less than 7%	
	Fair diabetic control: 8%-9%	
	Poor diabetic control: more than 9%	

Continued

TABLE A-2	THE VALUES GIVEN BELOW ARE THOSE SPECIFIED FOR THE NURSE TO KNOW IN THE 2010 DETAILED NCLEX-RN TEST PLAN—cont'd

	ADULT NORMAL VALUES* (TRADITIONAL U.S.)	SI ADULT NORMAL VALUES* (INTERNATIONAL SYSTEM)
Hematocrit (Hct)	Male: 42%-52%	Male: 0.42-0.52 volume fraction
	Female: 37%-47%	Female: 0.37-0.49 volume fraction
Hemoglobin (Hgb)	Male: 14-18 g/dL	Male: 8.7-11.2 mmol/L
	Female: 12-16 g/dL	Female: 7.4-9.9 mmol/L
Ionized calcium (Ca^{++})	4.5-56 mg/dL	1.05-1.3 mmol/L
Magnesium	1.3-2.1 mEq/L	0.65-1.05 mmol/L
Partial thromboplastin time (PTT)	60-70 sec	
Activated partial thromboplastin time (APTT)	30-40 sec	
On anticoagulant therapy	1.5-2.5 × control value in sec	
pH, urine	4.6-8.0	
Phosphate	3.0-4.5 mg/dL; 1.7-2.6 mEq/L	0.97-1.45 mmol/L
Platelets	150,000-400,000/mm^3	150-400 × 10^9/L
Potassium ($K^?$)	3.5-5.0 mEq/L	3.5-5.0 mmol/L
Protein (total blood)	6.4-8.3 g/dL	64-83 g/L
Protein, urine		
Random	None or up to 8 mg/dL	
24 hr	50-80 mg at rest More than 250 mg with exercise	
Prothrombin time (PT)	11-12.5 sec	INR: 0.8-1.1
Red blood cell (RBC) count	Male: 4.7-6.1 × 10^6/μL	Male: 4.7-6.1 × 10^{12}/L
	Female: 4.2-5.4 × 10^6/μL	Female: 4.2-5.4 × 10^{12}/L
Sodium (Na^{++})	136-145 mEq/L	136-145 mmol/L
Specific gravity, urine	1.005-1.030	
Therapeutic drug levels (serum)		
Digoxin	0.625-0.25 mg/da	
Lithium	600-1800 mg/da	
White blood cell (WBC) count	5000-10,000/mm^3	5-10 × 10^9/L
Basophils	0.5%-1.0%	0-0.3 × 10^9/L
Eosinophils	1%-4%	0-0.7 × 10^9/L
Lymphocytes	20%-40%	1-4 × 10^9/L
Monocytes	2%-8%	0-1 × 10^9/L
Neutrophils	55%-70%	2.5-7.5 10^9/L

Values from Pagana KD, TJ Pagana: *Mosby's diagnostic and laboratory test reference*, ed 9, St Louis, 2009, Mosby.
*Normal values may vary significantly with different laboratory methods of testing.
INR, International normalized ratio.

Heart and Breath Sounds

TABLE A-3	ASSESSING HEART SOUNDS					
PATIENT SOUND	AUSCULTATION SITE	TIMING	PITCH	CLINICAL OCCURRENCE		END-PIECE/ POSITION
S_1 (M_1, T_1)	Apex	Beginning of systole	High	Closing of mitral and tricuspid valves; normal sound		Diaphragm/ patient supine
S_1 split	Apex	Beginning of systole	High	Ventricles contracting at different times because of electrical or mechanical problems (e.g., a longer time span between M_1 and T_1 caused by right bundle-branch heart block or reversal [T_1 M_1] caused by mitral stenosis)		Same as S_1
S_2 (A_2 P_2)	A_2 at second ICS, RSB; P_2 at second ICS, LSB	End of systole	High	Closing of aortic and pulmonic valves; normal sound		Diaphragm/ patient supine
S_2 physiologic split	Second ICS, LSB	End of systole	High	Accentuated by inspiration; disappears on expiration; sound that corresponds with the respiratory cycle caused by normal delay in closure of pulmonic valve during inspiration; accentuated during exercise or in individuals with thin chest walls; heard most often in children and young adults		Same as S_2
S_2 persistent (wide) split	Second ICS, LSB	End of systole	High	Heard throughout the respiratory cycle; caused by late closure of pulmonic valve or early closure of aortic valve; occurs in atrial septal defect, right ventricular failure, pulmonic stenosis, hypertension, or right bundle branch block		Same as S_2
S_2 paradoxic (reversed) split (P_2 A_2)	Second ICS, LSB	End of systole	High	Because of delayed left ventricular systole, the aortic valve closes after the pulmonic valve rather than before it (normally during expiration the two sounds merge); causes may include left bundle branch heart block, aortic stenosis, severe left ventricular failure, MI, and severe hypertension		Same as S_2
S_2 fixed split	Second ICS, LSB	End of systole	High	Heard with equal intensity during inspiration and expiration because of split of pulmonic and aortic components, which are unaffected by blood volume or respiratory changes; may be heard in pulmonary stenosis or atrial septal defect		Same as S_2
S_3 (ventricular gallop)	Apex	Early diastole just after S_2	Dull, low	Early and rapid filling of ventricle, as in early ventricular failure, heart failure; common in children, during last trimester of pregnancy, and possibly in healthy adults older than 50 yr of age		Bell/patient in left lateral or supine position
S_4 (atrial gallop)	Apex	Late in diastole	Low	Atrium filling against increased resistance of stiff ventricle, as in heart failure, coronary artery disease, cardiomyopathy, pulmonary artery hypertension, ventricular failure; may be normal in infants, children, and athletes		Same as S_3

ICS, Intercostal space; *LSB*, left sternal border; *MI*, myocardial infarction; *RSB*, right sternal border.

TABLE A-4	COMMONLY OCCURRING HEART MURMURS				
TYPE	TIMING	PITCH	QUALITY	AUSCULTATION SITE	RADIATION
Pulmonic stenosis	Systolic ejection	Medium-high	Harsh	Second ICS, LSB	Toward left shoulder, back
Aortic stenosis	Midsystolic	Medium-high	Harsh	Second ICS, RSB	Toward carotid arteries
Ventricular septal defect	Late systolic	High	Blowing	Fourth ICS, LSB	Toward RSB
Mitral insufficiency	Holosystolic	High	Blowing	Fifth or sixth ICS, left MCL	Toward left axilla
Tricuspid insufficiency	Holosystolic	High	Blowing	Fourth ICS, LSB	Toward apex
Aortic insufficiency	Early diastolic	High	Blowing	Second ICS, RSB	Toward sternum
Pulmonary insufficiency	Early diastolic	High	Blowing	Second ICS, LSB	Toward sternum
Mitral stenosis	Mid-late diastolic	Low	Rumbling	Fifth ICS, left MCL	Usually none
Tricuspid stenosis	Mid-late diastolic	Low	Rumbling	Fourth ICS, LSB	Usually none

ICS, Intercostal space; *LSB*, left sternal border; *MCL*, midclavicular line; *RSB*, right sternal border.

TABLE A-5	ASSESSING NORMAL BREATH SOUNDS		
TYPE	**NORMAL SITE**	**DURATION**	**CHARACTERISTICS**
Vesicular	Peripheral lung	I greater than E	Soft and swishing sounds; abnormal if heard over the large airways
Bronchial	Trachea and bronchi	E greater than I	Louder, coarser, and of longer duration than vesicular; abnormal if heard over peripheral lung
Bronchovesicular	Sternal border of major bronchi	E = I	Moderate in pitch and intensity; abnormal if heard over peripheral lung

E, Expiration; *I*, inspiration.

TABLE A-6	ASSESSING ADVENTITIOUS BREATH SOUNDS		
TYPE	**WAVEFORM**	**CHARACTERISTICS**	**POSSIBLE CLINICAL CONDITION**
Coarse crackle		Discontinuous, explosive, interrupted; loud; low in pitch	Pulmonary edema; pneumonia in resolution stage
Fine crackle		Discontinuous, explosive, interrupted; less loud than coarse crackles, lower in pitch, and of shorter duration	Interstitial lung disease; heart failure; atelectasis
Wheeze		Continuous, of long duration, high-pitched, musical, hissing	Narrowing of airway; bronchial asthma; COPD
Rhonchus		Continuous, of long duration, low-pitched, snoring	Production of sputum (usually cleared or lessened by coughing or suctioning)
Pleural friction rub		Grating, rasping noise	Rubbing together of inflamed parietal linings; loss of normal pleural lubrication

COPD, Chronic obstructive pulmonary disease.

TABLE A-7   ASSESSING RESPIRATORY PATTERNS

TYPE	WAVEFORM	CHARACTERISTICS	POSSIBLE CLINICAL CONDITION
Eupnea		Normal rate and rhythm for adults and teenagers (12-20 breaths/min)	Normal pattern while awake
Bradypnea		Decreased rate (less than 12 breaths/min); regular rhythm	Normal sleep pattern; opiate or alcohol use; tumor; metabolic disorder
Tachypnea		Rapid rate (more than 20 breaths/min); hypoventilation or hyperventilation	Fever; restrictive respiratory disorders; pulmonary emboli
Hyperpnea		Depth of respirations greater than normal	Meeting increased metabolic demand (e.g., sepsis, MODS, SIRS, and exercise)
Apnea		Cessation of breathing; may be intermittent	Intermittent with CNS disturbances or drug intoxication; obstructed airway; respiratory arrest if it persists
Kussmaul's		Deep, rapid (more than 20 breaths/min), sighing, labored	Renal failure, DKA, sepsis, shock
Cheyne-Stokes		Alternating patterns of apnea (10-20 sec) with periods of deep and rapid breathing; lesions located bilaterally and deep within cerebral hemispheres	Heart failure; opiate or hypnotic overdose, thyrotoxicosis, dissecting aneurysm, subarachnoid hemorrhage, IICP, aortic valve disorders; may be normal in older adults during sleep
Central neurogenic hyperventilation		Rapid (more than 20 breaths/min), deep, regular; lesions of midbrain or upper pons thought to be source of pattern	Primary injury (ischemia, infarction, space-occupying lesion); secondary injury (IICP, metabolic disorders, drug overdose)
Apneustic		Deep, prolonged inspiration, followed by 20- to 30-sec pause and short expiration; lesion located in lower pons	Anoxia, meningitis, basilar artery occlusion
Cluster		Irregular breaths occurring in clusters with periods of apnea; overall pattern irregular; lesion located in lower pons or upper medulla	Primary and secondary injury as mentioned may produce this respiratory pattern
Ataxic (Biot's)		Irregular deep or shallow breaths; no discernible pattern; lesion located in medulla	Primary and secondary injury as mentioned may produce this respiratory pattern

CNS, Central nervous system; DKA, diabetic ketoacidosis; IICP, increased intracranial pressure; MODS, multiple organ dysfunction syndrome; SIRS, systemic inflammatory response syndrome.

Selected Bibliography

A legacy to remember (website): www.alegacytoremember.com.

Ackley BJ, Ladwig GB: *Nursing diagnosis handbook*, ed 8, St Louis, 2008, Mosby.

Agency for Health Care Policy and Research: *Clinical practice guideline: management of cancer pain*, AHCPR Pub. No. 94-0592, Rockville, Md, 1994, Agency for Health Care Policy and Research, U.S. Department of Health and Human Services.

Aidridge C: Knee replacement surgery, *Nurs Stand* 22(38):59-69, 2008.

Akinpelu D, Gonzalez JM: *Treadmill and pharmacologic stress testing* (updated May 8, 2009), eMedicine for WebMD (website): http://emedicine-medscape. com/article/160772. Accessed February 11, 2010.

Albert RK, Spiro SG, Jett JR: *Clinical respiratory medicine*, ed 3, St Louis, 2008, Mosby.

American Association of Clinical Endocrinologists/American Association of Endocrine Surgeons (AACE/AAES) Task Force on Primary Hyperparathyroidism: American Association of Clinical Endocrinologists and American Association of Endocrine Surgeons position statement on the diagnosis and management of primary hyperparathyroidism, *J Endocr Pract* 11(1):49-54, 2005.

American Association of Critical-Care Nurses: *Practice alert: verification of feeding tube placement*, May, 2005.

American Cancer Society: *Cancer facts & figures 2009*, Atlanta, 2009, American Cancer Society.

American Cancer Society: *A cancer source book for nurses*, ed 8, Sudbury, Mass, 2004, Jones & Bartlett.

American College of Cardiology/American Heart Association (ACC/AHA): *2007 focused update of the ACC/AHA/SCAI 2005 guideline update for percutaneous coronary intervention: a report of the American College of Cardiology/American Heart Association Task Force on Practice Guidelines* (website): http:// www.guideline.gov/summary/summary.aspx?doc_id=12193&nbr=6290&ss=6 &xl=999. Accessed February 11, 2010.

American College of Rheumatology: Estimates of the prevalence of arthritis and other rheumatic conditions in the United States (January 2008), *Arthritis Rheum* 58:1, pp 15-25, DOI 10.1002/art.23177.

American College of Sports Medicine: *ACSM's guidelines for exercise testing and prescription*, ed 8, Philadelphia, 2009, Lippincott Williams & Wilkins.

American Pain Society: *Principles of analgesic use in the treatment of acute and cancer pain*, ed 6, Glenview, Ill, 2008, American Pain Society.

American Pharmaceutical Association, Semla TP, Beizer JL, Higbee MD, eds: *Geriatric dosage handbook*, ed 15, Hudson, Ohio, 2009, Lexi-Comp.

American Urological Association (AUA) Practice Guidelines Committee: AUA Guideline on management of benign prostatic hyperplasia, *J Urol* 175:815, 2006.

American Urological Health Foundation: *Neurogenic bladder* (website): http://www.urologyhealth.org/adult/index.cfm?cat=03&topic=109. Accessed February 11, 2010.

Anand MK, Routes JM: *Hypersensitivity reactions, immediate*, eMedicine.com (website): http://emedicine.medscape.com/article/136217-overview. Accessed February 11, 2010.

American Heart Association: *Heart attack and angina statistics: final 2005 statistics* (website): americanheart.org/presenter.jhtml?identifier=4591. Accessed February 11, 2010.

American Nephrology Nurses Association (ANNA), Chronic Kidney Disease Special Interest Group: *Chronic kidney disease fact sheet* (website): http://www.annanurse.org/download/reference/practice/ckd_fact.pdf. Accessed February 11, 2010.

American Nephrology Nurses Association (ANNA), Transplantation Special Interest Group: *Transplantation fact sheet* (website): http://www.annanurse.org/download/reference/practice/transplant.pdf. Accessed February 11, 2010.

Anness E, Tirone K: Evaluating the neurologic status of unconscious patients, *Am Nurse Today* 4(4):8-10, 2009.

Anthonisen N: Chronic obstructive pulmonary disease. In Goldman L et al, eds: *Cecil medicine,* ed 23, Philadelphia, 2007, Saunders.

Aschenbrenner DS: A new drug for Crohn's disease, *Am J Nurs* 108(8):33-34, 2008.

Aschenbrenner DS: A new treatment for moderate-to-severe Crohn's disease, *Am J Nurs* 108(5):65-65, 2008.

Aschenbrenner DS: A drug for irritable bowel syndrome with constipation is approved, *Am J Nurs* 108(10):79-79, 2008.

Avis A: Reflexology improved urinary symptoms in multiple sclerosis but was not effective for other outcomes in various conditions, *Evid Based Nurs* 11(4):112, 2008.

Aydin N, Karaöz S: Nutritional assessment of patients before gastrointestinal surgery and nurses' approach to this issue, *J Clin Nurs* 17(5):608-617, 2008.

Bacigalupo A, Passweg J: Diagnosis and treatment of acquired aplastic anemia, *Hematol Oncol Clin North Am* 23(2):159-170, 2009.

Balasubramanian A, Flareau B, Sourbeer JJ: Syndrome of inappropriate antidiuretic hormone secretion, *Hosp Physician* 43(4):33-36, 39, 2007.

Barakzai MD, Gregory J, Fraser D: The effect of culture on symptom reporting: Hispanics and irritable bowel syndrome, *J Am Acad Nurs Pract* 19(5):261-267, 2007.

Bell A, Leader M, Lloyd H: Care of pin sites, *Nurs Stand* 22(33):44-48, 2008.

Bentzen H, Bergland A, Forsen L: Risk of hip fractures in soft protected, hard protected, and unprotected falls, *Injury Prev* 14(5):306-310, 2008.

Berger AM, Shuster JL, Von Roenn JH, eds: *Principles and practice of palliative care and supportive oncology*, ed 3, Philadelphia, 2006, Lippincott Williams & Wilkins.

Bickel K, Arnold R: *Fast fact and concept #109: death rattle and oral secretions*, ed 2, 2008 End-of-Life/Palliative Education Resource Center (website): http://www.eperc.mcw.edu/fastFact/ff_109.htm. Accessed February 11, 2010.

Blakemore S: Toolkit for falls service, *Nurs Older People* 20(10):7-7, 2008.

Blasier MG: Pharmacologic management of multiple sclerosis, *Urol Nur* 28(3):217-219, 2008.

Boekhorst S, et al: Group living homes for older people with dementia: the effects of psychological distress of informal caregivers, *Aging Ment Health* 12(6):761-768, 2008.

Boland MR, Heck C: Acute exercise-induced bilateral thigh compartment syndrome, *Orthopedics* 32(3):218, 2009.

Bolesta S, Roslund B: Elevated hepatic transaminases associated with telithromycin therapy: a case report and literature review, *Am J Health Syst Pharm* 65(1):37-41, 2008.

Borg GA: Psychophysical bases of perceived exertion, *Med Sci Sports Exerc* 14(5):377-381, 1982.

Braden Scale for Predicting Pressure Sore Risk (website): http://www.bradenscale.com

Brown-Guttovz H: About irritable bowel syndrome, *Nursing* 38(2):28-28, 2008.

Burbage G: Detecting and managing rheumatoid arthritis, *Pract Nurs* 19(1):26-30, 2008.

Burgess A: An overview of pancreatic neuroendocrine tumours, *Nurs Stand* 23(8):35-40, 2008.

Burns A et al: Safety and efficacy of galantamine (Reminyl) in severe Alzheimer's disease (the SERAD study: a randomized, placebo-controlled, double-blind trial), *Lancet Neurol* 8(1):39-47, 2009.

Busari OA, Adeyemi AO: Cryptococcal meningitis in AIDS, *Int J Infect Dis* 7(1):1-1, 2009.

Burkitt P: Alzheimer's disease, *Nurs Stand* 23(8):59-59, 2008.

Campigotto MJ et al: Desmopressin (dDAVP) incident signals the need for enhanced monitoring protocols, *Dynamics* 19(3):34-36, 2008.

Carabello BA: Valvular heart disease. In Goldman L et al, eds: *Cecil medicine,* ed 23, Philadelphia, 2007, Saunders.

Carroll P: Exploring chest drain options, *RN* 63(10):50-54, 2000.

Cashin R et al: Acute renal failure, gastrointestinal bleeding, and cardiac arrhythmia after administration of arsenic trioxide for acute promyelocytic leukemia, *Am J Health Syst Pharm* 65(10):941-946, 2008.

Centers for Disease Control and Prevention: Guidelines for preventing the transmission of *Mycobacterium tuberculosis* in health-care settings, *MMWR Morb Mortal Wkly Rep* 54(RR-17):1-141, 2005.

Centers for Disease Control and Prevention, Health Resources and Services Administration (HRSA), National Institutes of Health (NIH), HIV Medicine Association of the Infectious Diseases Society of America, HIV Prevention in Clinical Care Working Group: Recommendation for incorporating human immunodeficiency virus (HIV) prevention into the medical care of persons living with HIV, *Clin Infect Dis* 38(1):104-121, 2004.

Celli BR, MacNee W: ATS/ERS Task Force: Standards for the diagnosis and treatment of patients with COPD: a summary of the ATS/ERS position paper, *Eur Respir J* 23(6):932-946, 2004.

Centers for Disease Control and Prevention: Incorporating HIV prevention into the medical care of persons living with HIV: recommendations of CDC, Health Resources and Services Administration, the National Institutes of Health, and the HIV Medicine Association of the Infectious Diseases Society of America, *MMWR Morb Mortal Wkly Rep* 52(12):1-24, 2003.

Centers for Disease Control and Prevention: *Advancing HIV prevention: progress summary April 2003-September 2005 (*website): http://www.cdc.gov/hiv/topics/prev_prog/AHP/resources/factsheets/progress_2005.htm. Accessed February 11, 2010.

Centers for Disease Control and Prevention: *New HIV incidence estimates: CDC responds, 2008* (website): http://www.cdc.gov/hiv/topics/surveillance/resources/factsheets/pdf/response.pdf. Accessed February 11, 2010.

Centers for Disease Control and Prevention: Revised surveillance case definitions for HIV infection among adults, adolescents, and children aged <18 months and for HIV infection and AIDS among children aged 18 months to <13 years: United States, 2008, *MMWR Morb Mortal Wkly Rep* 57(RR10):1-8.

Center for Disease Control and Prevention: Guidelines for the Prevention and Treatment of Opportunistic Infections among HIV-exposed and HIV-infected children: recommendations from CDC, the National Institutes of Health, the HIV Medicine Association of the Infectious Diseases Society of America, the

Pediatric Infectious Diseases Society, and the American Academy of Pediatrics. *MMWR*, 2009 Sep 4;58(RR-11):1-166, website: http://www.ncbi.nlm.nih.gov/pubmed/19730409

Charbonneau C et al: A retrospective study of cholinesterase inhibitors for Alzheimer's disease: cerebrovascular disease as a predictor of patient outcomes, *Curr Med Res Opin* 24(11):3287-3294, 2008.

Chen J, Trombetta D, Fernandez H: Palliative management of Parkinson disease: focus on nonmotor, distressing symptoms, *J Pharm Pract* 21(4):262-272, 2008.

Chernecky CC, Murphy-Ende K: *Acute care oncology nursing*, ed 2, St Louis, 2009, Saunders.

Cook LS: Learning about blood component therapy, *Nursing* 39(4):30-33, 2009.

Copstead-Kirkhorn LE, Banasik JL: *Pathophysiology*, ed 4, St Louis, 2010, Saunders.

Cornell P: Management of patients with rheumatoid arthritis, *Nurs Stand* 22(4):51-57, 2007.

Corser W, Xu Y: Facilitating patients' diabetes self-management: a primary care intervention framework, *J Nurs Care Qual* 24(2):172-178, 2009.

Cotterill N et al: A patient-centered approach to developing a comprehensive symptom and quality of life assessment of anal incontinence, *Dis Colon Rectum* 51(1):82-87, 2008.

Coutre S: *Heparin-induced thrombocytopenia*, UpToDate (website): www.uptodate.com. Accessed February 11, 2010.

Cowen J, Powderly WG: *Infectious diseases*, ed 2, St Louis, 2004, Mosby.

Criqui MH: Epidemiology of cardiovascular disease. In Goldman L et al, eds: *Cecil medicine*, ed 23, Philadelphia, 2007, Saunders.

Cronin E: Colostomies and the use of colostomy appliances, *Br J Nurs* 17(17 suppl):S12-S19, 2008.

Dalrymple J, Bullock I: Diagnosis and management of irritable bowel syndrome in adults in primary care: summary of NICE guidance, *BMJ* 336(7643):556-558, 2008.

D'Arcy YM: Keep your patient safe during PCA, *Nursing* 38(1):50-55, 2008.

D'Arcy YM: Avoid the dangers of opioid therapy, *Am Nurse Today* 4(5):18-21, 2009.

Dartinger T: Dying from dementia: a patient's journey, *BMJ* 337(7675):931-933, 2008.

David-Raoudi M et al: Role of chondroitin sulfate increases hyaluronan production by human synoviocytes through differential regulation of hyaluronan synthases, *Arthritis Rheum* 60(3):760-770, 2009.

Davis C: Putting pain in perspective, *Nurs Stand* 22(50):20-21, 2008.

Day ML: Fracture in the field, *Nursing* 38(6):72-72, 2008.

DeBeer K, et al: Diabetic ketoacidosis and hyperglycaemic hyperosmolar syndrome: clinical guidelines, *Nurs Crit Care* 13(1):5-11, 2008.

Dementia, *Curr Med Lit Neurol* 24(1):12-17, 2008.

Department of Pain Medicine & Palliative Care, Beth Israel Medical Center: *StopPain* (website): www.stoppain.org. Accessed February 11, 2010.

DeWalt D: *Infective endocarditis* (website): www.med.unc.edu/medicine/web/endocarditis.htm. Accessed February 11, 2010.

Drazen JM: Asthma. In Goldman L et al, eds: *Cecil medicine*, ed 23, Philadelphia, 2007, Saunders.

Drew BG et al: High-density lipoprotein modulates glucose metabolism in patients with type 2 diabetes mellitus, *Circulation* 119(15):2103-2111, 2009.

Durner E, Rea RS: Preventing stress related mucosal disease in the intensive care unit, *Int J Adv Nurs Pract* 8(1):4-4, 2007.

Earhart M: The identification and treatment of toxic megacolon secondary to pseudomembranous colitis, *Dimens Crit Care Nurs* 27(6):249-254, 2008.

Edmondson D, Schiech L: Esophageal cancer: a tough pill to swallow, *Nursing* 38(4):44-51, 2008.

Ervin RB: Prevalence of metabolic syndrome among adults 20 years of age and over, by sex, age, race and ethnicity, and body mass index: United States, 2003–2006, *National Health Statistics Report* (online serial), no 13, May 5, 2009: http://www.cdc.gov/nchs/data/nhsr/nhsr013.pdf. Accessed February 11, 2010.

Fagley MU: Taking charge of seizure activity, *Nursing* 37(9):42-47, 2007.

Fahey VA: *Vascular nursing*, ed 4, St Louis, 2004, Saunders.

Failed efforts to thwart Alzheimer's disease raise questions, *Harv Med Health Lett* 25(8):1-3, 2009.

Falcone T, Hurd WW: *Clinical reproductive medicine and surgery*, Philadelphia, 2009, Mosby.

Favard L, Bacle G, Berhoet J: Rotator cuff repair, *Joint Bone Spine* 74(6):551-557, 2007.

Ferri FF: *Ferri's 2009 clinical advisor: instant diagnosis and treatment*, St Louis, 2009, Mosby.

Fitzgerald MA: Fight fatigue by evaluating thyroid function, *Pract Nurs* 33(12):6-7, 2008.

Five Wishes, an advance directive document available from The Commission on Aging with Dignity:1-888-5-WISHES or (website): www.agingwithdignity.org. Accessed February 11, 2010.

Forbes A, While A, Mathes L: Informal carer activities, carer burden and health status in multiple sclerosis, *Clin Rehabil* 21(6):563-575, 2007.

Fox KA: Management of acute coronary syndromes: an update, *Heart* 90(6):698-706, 2004.

Fracture risk linked to hospitalization, *Nursing* 38(11):25-25, 2008.

Franchini M, Lippi G, Manzato F: Recent acquisitions in the pathophysiology, diagnosis and treatment of disseminated intravascular coagulation, *Thromb J* 4(4):1477-1486, 2006.

Francis CW: Prophylaxis for thromboembolism in hospitalized medical patients, *N Engl J Med* 356:1438-1444, 2007.

Funnell MM, Weiss MA: Empowering patients with diabetes: find out about a different approach to helping patients take charge of this chronic disease, *Nursing* 39(3):34-37, 2009.

Gadler T: Knee injuries, *Adv Emerg Nurs* 29(3):189-197, 2007.

Galat DD et al: Surgical treatment of early wound complications following primary total knee arthroplasty, *J Bone Joint Surg Am* 91A(1):48-54, 2009.

Gall C et al: Patient satisfaction and health-related quality of life after treatment for colon cancer, *Dis Colon Rectum* 50(6):801-809, 2007.

Garrick V et al: Successful implementation of a nurse-led teaching programme to independently administer subcutaneous methotrexate in the community setting to children with Crohn's disease, *Aliment Pharmacol Ther* 29(1):90-96, 2009.

Geetha D: *Glomerulonephritis, poststreptococcal*, eMedicine.com (website): http://emedicine.medscape.com/article/240337-overview. Accessed February 11, 2010.

Gharahbaghian L et al: Central diabetes insipidus misdiagnosed as acute gastroen-teritis in a pediatric patient, *J Can Assoc Emerg Physician* 10(5):488-492, 2008.

Gideon C: Amebic colitis, *Int J Adv Nurs Pract* 9(2):3-3, 2008.

Gioe TJ et al: Can patients help with long-term total knee arthroplasty surveillance? Comparison of the American Knee Society score self-report and surgeon assess-ment, *Rheumatology* 48(2):160-160, 2009.

Global Initiative for Chronic Obstructive Lung Disease (GOLD): *Executive summary: global strategy for the diagnosis, management, and prevention of COPD, updated 2009* (website): www.goldcopd.com. Accessed February 11, 2010.

Goldman L et al, eds: *Cecil medicine*, ed 23, Philadelphia, 2007, Saunders.

Gray-Vickery P: The people behind the statistics, *Alzheimer's Care Today* 9(4):217-218, 2008.

Griffing GT, Odeke S, Nagelberg SB: *Addison disease: treatment and medication*, eMedicine from WebMD, September 29, 2009 (website): http://emedicine.medscape.com/article/116467-treatment. Accessed February 11, 2010.

Griffith HR et al: Cognitive functioning over 3 years in community dwelling for older adults with chronic partial epilepsy, *Epilepsy Res* 74(2/3):91-96, 2007.

Gutierrez C, Blanchard DG: Diastolic heart failure: challenges of diagnosis and treatment, *Am Fam Physician* 69:2609, 2004.

Hanks G et al, eds: *Oxford textbook of palliative medicine*, ed 4, New York, 2009, Oxford University Press.

Hawkins R, Grunberg S: Chemotherapy-induced nausea and vomiting: challenges and opportunities for improved patient outcomes, *Clin J Oncol Nurs* 13(1):54-64, 2009.

Held-Warmkessel J: Responding to 4 gastrointestinal complications in cancer patients, *Nursing* 38(7):32-39, 2008.

Henn RF et al: Patient's preoperative expectations predict the outcome of rotator cuff repair, *J Bone Joint Surg* 89(9):1913-1919, 2007.

Herndon DN: *Burn care*, St Louis, 2007, Saunders.

Herr KA et al: Evaluation of the Faces Pain Scale for use with the elderly, *Clin J Pain* 14(1):29-38, 1998.

Hertuig V: Daily stress and gastrointestinal symptoms in women with irritable bowel syndrome, *Nurs Res* 56(6):399-406, 2007.

Higgins S: Outlining and defining the role of the epilepsy specialist nurse, *Br J Nurs* 17(3):154-157, 2008.

Hill J: Reducing the risk of complications associated with diabetes, *Nurs Stand* 23(25):49-55, 2009.

Hochman JS et al: Coronary intervention for persistent occlusion after myocardial infarction, *N Engl J Med* 355:2395, 2007.

Hogan DB et al: Diagnosis and treatment of dementia: approach to management of mild to moderate dementia, *CMAJ* 179(8):787-793, 2008.

Hu G et al: Botulinum toxin (Dysport) treatment of the spastic gastrocnemius muscle in children with cerebral palsy: a randomized trial comparing two injection volumes, *Clin Rehabil* 23(1):64-71, 2009.

Hunter DJ, Le Graverand MPH, Eckstein F: Radiologic markers of osteoarthritis progression, *Curr Opin Rheumatol* 21(2):110-117, 2009.

Hurley MV, Walsh NE: Effectiveness and clinical applicability of integrated rehabilitation programs for knee osteoarthritis, *Curr Opin Rheumatol* 21(2):171-176, 2009.

Ilyas M, Tolaymat A: Changing epidemiology of acute post-streptococcal glomerulonephritis in Northeast Florida: a comparative study, *Pediatr Nephrol* 23(7):1101-1106, 2008.

In the clinic: Dementia, *Ann Intern Med* 148(7):1-16, 2008.

Institute for Safe Medication Practices: Safety issues with patient-controlled analgesia. Part I: how errors occur, *ISMP Medication Safety Alert* 8(14), 2003 (serial online): www.ismp.org.

Institute for Safe Medication Practices: Safety issues with patient-controlled analgesia. Part II: how to prevent error, *ISMP Medication Safety Alert* 8(15), 2003 (serial online): www.ismp.org.

Institute for Safe Medication Practices: Safety issues with patient-controlled analgesia. Part I, *ISMP Medication Safety Alert Nurse Advise—ERR* 3(1), 2003 (serial online): www.ismp.org.

Institute for Safe Medication Practices: Safety issues with patient-controlled analgesia. Part II, *ISMP Medication Safety Alert Nurse Advise—ERR* 3(2), 2003 (serial online): www.ismp.org.

Jacobson AF et al: Patients' perspectives on total knee replacement, *Am J Nurs* 108(5):54-63, 2008.

Jarrett ME et al: Relationship of SERT polymorphisms to depressive and anxiety symptoms in irritable bowel syndrome, *Biol Res Nurs* 9(2):161-169, 2007.

Jimenez CC: Recognizing and managing diabetes-related emergencies, *Athl Ther Today* (2):6-10, 32-3, 64, 2004.

Johnston CS, White AM, Kent SM: Preliminary evidence that regular vinegar ingestion favorably influences hemoglobin A1c values in individuals with type 2 diabetes mellitus, *Diabetes Res Clin Pract* 84(2):e15-e17, 2009.

Karnath BM, Karnath BM: Signs of hyperandrogenism in women, *Hosp Physician* 44(10):25-30, 2008.

Karnath BM, Ojo OB, Karnath BM: Cushing's syndrome, *Hosp Physician* 44(4):25-29, 2008.

Katz SD: Mechanisms and treatment of anemia in chronic heart failure, *Congest Heart Fail* 10(5):243-247, 2004.

Kavoussi LR et al, eds: *Campbell-Walsh urology*, vol 2, ed 9, Philadelphia, 2007, Saunders.

KDOQI clinical practice guideline and clinical practice recommendations for anemia in chronic kidney disease: 2007 update of hemoglobin target. *Am J Kidney Dis* 2007 Sep;50(3):471-530.

KDOQI clinical practice guidelines and clinical practice recommendations for diabetes and chronic kidney disease. *Am J Kidney Dis* 2007 Feb;49(2 Suppl 2):S12-154.

KDOQI clinical practice guidelines and clinical practice recommendations for peritoneal dialysis adequacy: update 2006. *Am J Kidney Dis* 2006 Jul;48 Suppl 1:S98-129.

Kim EJ, Buschmann MT: Reliability and validity of the FACES pain scale with older adults. *Int J Nurs Stud* 43(4):447-456, 2006 May.

Klauer KM: (2009, December 16). *Adrenal insufficiency and adrenal crisis: treatment and medication, eMedicine from WebMD* (website): http://emedicine.medscape.com/article/765753-treatment. Accessed February 11, 2010.

Kliger AS: Frequent nocturnal hemodialysis: a step forward? *JAMA* 298:1331, 2007.

Kosashvili Y et al: Digital versus conventional templating techniques in preoperative planning for total hip arthroplasty, *Can J Surg* 52(1):6-11, 2009.

Koul PB: Diabetic ketoacidosis: a current appraisal of pathophysiology and management, *Clin Pediatr* 48(2):135-144, 2009.

Kring DL, Crane PB: Factors affecting quality of life in persons on hemodialysis, *Nephrol Nurs J* 36(1):15-25, 55, 2009.

Krost WS, Mistovich JJ, Limmer DD: Beyond the basics: crush injuries and compartment syndrome, *EMS Mag* 37(2):67-73, 2008.

Kruger S et al: Neuroleptic-induced parkinsonism is associated with olfactory dysfunction, *J Neurol* 255(10):1574-1579, 2008.

Kusuma B, Schultz TK, Perazella MA: Acute disseminated intravascular coagulation, *Hosp Physician* 45(3):35-40, 2009.

Lahl M, Fisher VL, Laschinger K: Ewing's sarcoma family of tumors: an overview from diagnosis to survivorship, *Clin J Oncol Nurs* 12(1):89-97, 2008.

Langsang RS: *Bladder management*, eMedicine.com (website): http://emedicine.medscape.com/article/321273-overview

Larkin P et al: The management of constipation in palliative care: clinical practice recommendations, *Palliat Med* 22(7):796-807, 2008.

Larson K, VanBuskirk S: Stabilizing hemoglobin levels: what's new in IV iron and anemia management, *Nephrol Nurs J* 35(5):493-502, 2008.

Latham CL, Calvillo E: Predictors of successful diabetes management in low-income Hispanic people, *West J Nurs Res* 31(3):364-388, 2009.

Laustsen G et al: Drug approvals: '08 in review, *Nurs Pract* 34(2):25-35, 2009.

Lee D et al: Treatment fatigue in multiple sclerosis: a systematic review of the literature, *Int J Nurs Pract* 14(2):81-93, 2008.

Lee MS, Lam OP, Ernst E: Effectiveness of tai chi for Parkinson's disease: a critical review, *Parkinsonism Relat Disord* 14(8):589-594, 2008.

Lee RY, Colville JM, Schuberth JM: Acute compartment syndrome of the leg with avulsion of the peroneus longus muscle: a case report, *J Foot Ankle Surg* 48(3):365-367, 2009.

Lehne RA: *Pharmacology for nursing care,* ed 7, St Louis, 2010, Mosby.

Lehne RA: *Pharmacology for nursing care,* ed 6, St Louis, 2007, Mosby.

Leng SX et al: Inadvertent self-healing in desperate times, *Lancet* 370(9596):1458-1458, 2007.

Leopold SS: Minimally invasive total knee arthroplasty for osteoarthritis, *N Engl J Med* 360(17):1749-1758, 2009.

Levin A et al: Guidelines for the management of chronic renal disease, *CMAJ* 179(11):1154-1162, 2008.

Levin B et al: Screening and surveillance for the early detection of colorectal cancer and adenomatous polyps, 2008: a joint guideline from the American Cancer Society, the US Multi-Society Task Force on Colorectal Cancer, and the American College of Radiology. Published online March 5, 2008, *CA Cancer J Clin* 58, 2008.

Levodopa/benserazide/olanzapine, *Reactions Wkly* (1229):18, 2008.

Liapis K et al: Syndrome of inappropriate secretion of antidiuretic hormone associated with imatinib, *Ann Pharmacother* 42(12):1882-1886, 2008.

Limper AH: Overview of pneumonia. In Goldman L et al, eds: *Cecil medicine,* ed 23, Philadelphia, 2007, Saunders.

Ling-Ling L: A multifactorial intervention did not prevent falls or fractures in elderly patients during short hospital stays, *Evid Based Nurs* 11(4):120, 2008.

Lip G, Tse H: Management of atrial fibrillation, *Lancet* 370:604, 2007.

Liu, KD, Chertow, GM: Dialysis in the treatment of renal failure. In: Fauci AS, et al, eds: *Harrison's principles of internal medicine,* ed 17, New York, 2008, McGraw-Hill.

Long HJ et al: Prevention, diagnosis, and treatment of cervical cancer, *Mayo Clin Proc* 82(12):1556-1574, 2007.

Lucas B: Preparing patients for hip and knee replacement surgery, *Nurs Stand* 22(2):50-56, 2007.

Lucas B: Total hip and knee replacement: preoperative nursing management, *Br J Nurs* 17(21):1346-1351, 2008.

Lucas B: Total hip and knee replacement: postoperative nursing management, *Br J Nurs* 17(22):1410-1414, 2008.

Mack G: Joint replacement rehab: a team approach to recovery, *Nurs Homes* 56(8):52-54, 2007.

Madden J: Managing patients with resistant rheumatoid arthritis, *Nurs Stand* 22(43):51-58, 60, 2008.

Malanga GA, Ramirez-del Toro JA: Common injuries of the foot and ankle in the child and adolescent athlete, *Phys Med Rehabil Clin North Am* 19(2):347-371, 2008.

Malhotra A: Low tidal volume ventilation in acute respiratory distress syndrome, *N Engl J Med* 357:1113, 2007.

Malik A et al: Acute compartment syndrome: a life and limb threatening surgical emergency, *J Periop Pract* 19(5):137-142, 2009.

Manning WJ: Pericardial disease. In Goldman L et al, eds: *Cecil medicine,* ed 23, Philadelphia, 2007, Saunders.

Marino J et al: Continuous lumbar plexus block for postoperative pain control after total hip arthroplasty, *J Bone Joint Surg Am* 91A(1):29-37, 2009.

Marsh L, Sweeney J: Nurses' knowledge of constipation in people with learning disabilities, *Br J Nurs* 17(4): S11-S16, 2008.

Martinelli L et al: Learning and consolidation of visuo-motor adaption in Parkinson's disease, *Parkinsonism Relat Disord* 15(1):6-11, 2009.

Massie BM: Heart failure: pathophysiology and diagnosis. In Goldman L et al, eds: *Cecil medicine,* ed 23, Philadelphia, 2007, Saunders.

Matsumoto AK, Bathon J, Bingham CO: *Rheumatoid arthritis treatment,* Johns Hopkins Arthritis Center (website): http://www.hopkins-arthritis.org/arthritis-info/rheumatoid-arthritis/rheum_treat.html#tcell. Accessed February 11, 2010.

Mavrakis AN, Tritos NA: Diabetes insipidus with deficient thirst: report of a patient and review of the literature, *Am J Kidney Dis* 51(5):851-859, 2008.

Max MB: Pain. In Goldman L et al, eds: *Cecil medicine*, ed 23, Philadelphia, 2007, Saunders.

Mayo Clinic: *Hyperthyroidism (overactive thyroid): tests and diagnosis*, Mayo-Clinic.com (website): http://www.mayoclinic.com/health/hyperthyroidism/DS00344/DSECTION=tests-and-diagnosis. Accessed February 11, 2010.

Mayo Clinic: *Hypoparathyroidism: tests and diagnosis*, MayoClinic.com (website): http://www.mayoclinic.com/health/hypoparathyroidism/DS00952/DSECTION=tests-and-diagnosis. Accessed February 11, 2010.

Mayo Clinic: *Hypoparathyroidism: treatments and drugs*, MayoClinic.com (website): http://www.mayoclinic.com/health/hypoparathyroidism/DS00952/DSECTION=treatments-and-drugs. Accessed February 11, 2010.

Mayo Clinic: *Polycythemia vera*, MayoClinic.com (website): http://www.mayoclinic.com/health/polycythemia-vera/DS00919. Accessed February 11, 2010.

Mayo Clinic: *Sickle cell anemia: treatment and medications*, MayoClinic.com (website): MayoClinic.com: http://www.mayoclinic.com/health/sickle-cell-anemia/DS00324/DSECTION=treatments-and-drugs. Accessed February 11, 2010.

Mayrand MH et al: Human papillomavirus DNA versus Papanicolaou screening tests for cervical cancer, *N Engl J Med* 357:1579-1588, 2007.

Mazer M, Chen E: Is subcutaneous administration of rapid-acting insulin as effective as intravenous insulin for treating diabetic ketoacidosis? *Ann Emerg Med* 53(2):259-263, 2009.

McAdams-Jones D: Reversing SIADH: when the feedback mechanism for antidiuretic hormone fails, counter with a quick response, *Am Nurse Today* 3(9):40, 2008.

McCaffrey DD et al: Acute compartment syndrome of the anterior thigh in the absence of fracture secondary to sporting trauma, *J Trauma* 66(4):1238-1242, 2009.

McCance KL, Huether SE: *Pathophysiology: the biologic basis for disease in adults and children*, ed 5, St Louis, 2006, Mosby.

Mccrea G et al: Self-report measures to evaluate constipation, *Aliment Pharmacol Ther* 27(8):638-648, 2008.

McMurray JJV, Pfeffer MA: Heart failure: management and prognosis. In Goldman L et al, eds: *Cecil medicine*, ed 23, Philadelphia, 2007, Saunders.

Medline Plus: *Acute adrenal crisis*, National Library of Medicine and National Institutes of Health (website): http://www.nlm.nih.gov/medlineplus/ency/article/000357.htm. Accessed February 11, 2010.

Medline Plus: *Primary hyperparathyroidism*, National Library of Medicine and National Institutes of Health (website): http://www.nlm.nih.gov/medlineplus/ency/article/000384.htm. Accessed February 11, 2010.

MEDTEP Update archive: *Acute pain management*, Agency for Healthcare Research and Quality (website): http://www.ahrq.gov/clinic/medtep/acute.htm. Accessed February 11, 2010.

Mendelssohn DC et al: Elevated levels of serum creatinine: recommendations for management and referral, *CMAJ* (online journal): http://www.pubmedcentral.nih.gov/articlerender.fcgi?artid=1230545. Accessed February 11, 2010.

Merkle D, McDonald DD: Use of recommended osteoarthritis pain treatment by older adults, *J Adv Nurs* 65(4):828-835, 2009.

Metheny M: Preventing respiratory complications of tube feedings: evidence-based practice. *Am J Crit Care* 15(4):360-369, 2006.

Miller EA, Schneider LS, Rosenheck RA: Assessing the relationship between health utilities, quality of life, and health services use in Alzheimer's disease, *Int J Geriatr Psychiatry* 24(1):96-105, 2009.

Mitchell M: Hip and knee replacement surgery, *Nurs Stand* 22(38):59-59, 2008.

Mitka M: Hemoglobin A1c poised to become preferred test for diagnosing diabetes, *JAMA* 301(15):1528, 2009.

Monahan FD: *Mosby's expert physical exam handbook: rapid inpatient and outpatient assessments*, ed 3, St Louis, 2009, Mosby.

Monahan FD et al: *Phipp's medical-surgical nursing: health and illness perspectives*, ed 8, St Louis, 2007, Mosby.

Moore K: Knee replacement, *Am J Nurs* 108(10):14-14, 2008.

Moore T: Diabetic emergencies in adults, *Nurs Stand* 18(46):45-52, 54, 2004.

Morrison RD et al: A novel interdisciplinary analgesic program reduces pain and improves function in older adults after orthopedic surgery, *J Am Geriatr Soc* 57(1):1-10, 2009.

Morse K et al: Arthroscopic versus mini-open rotator cuff repair, *Am J Sports Med* 36(9):1824-1828, 2008.

Mortimer KJ et al: Oral and inhaled corticosteroids and adrenal insufficiency: a case control study, *Thorax* 61(5):405–408, 2006.

Motta R, Carvalho M: Management of bladder dysfunction in multiple sclerosis patients: the nurse's point of view, *Neurol Sci* 29(suppl 4):356-359, 2008.

Mozaffarian D et al: Lifestyle risk factors and new-onset diabetes mellitus in older adults: the cardiovascular health study, *Arch Intern Med* 169(8):798-807, 2009.

Mueller C et al: Use of B-type natriuretic peptide in the evaluation and management of acute dyspnea, *N Engl J Med* 350(7):647-654, 2004.

Munn Z: Care delivery and self-management strategies for adults with epilepsy, *J Adv Nurs* 64(5):455-456, 2008.

Myrianthefs PM et al: Nosocomial pneumonia, *Crit Care Nurs Q* 27(3):241-257, 2004.

Naal FD et al: Habitual physical activity and sports participation after total ankle arthroplasty, *Am J Sports Med* 37(1):95-102, 2009.

Napier DE, Bass SS: Postoperative benefits of intrathecal injection for patients undergoing total knee arthroplasty, *Orthop Nurs* 26(6):374-378, 2008.

National Adrenal Disease Foundation (NADF): *Addison's disease: the facts you need to know* (website): http://www.nadf.us/diseases/addisons.htm#what. Accessed February 11, 2010.

National Comprehensive Cancer Network: *NCCN clinical practice guidelines in oncology* (website): http://www.nccn.org/professionals/physician_gls/f_guidelines.asp. Accessed February 11, 2010.

National Consensus Project for Quality Palliative Care (NCP): *National Consensus Project* (website): www.nationalconsensusproject.org. Accessed February 11, 2010.

National Endocrine and Metabolic Diseases Information Service: Hyperthyroidism (website): http://www.endocrine.niddk.nih.gov/pubs/Hyperthyroidism. Accessed February 11, 2010.

National Heart, Lung and Blood Institute: *Seventh report of the Joint National Committee on prevention, detection, evaluation, and treatment of high blood pressure (JNC 7)*, Pub No. 04-5230, Washington, DC, 2003, National Heart, Lung and Blood Institute, Department of Health and Human Services, National Institutes of Health. Also available (website): www.nhlbi.nih.gov/guidelines/hypertension/jnc7full.htm. Accessed February 11, 2010.

National Heart, Lung and Blood Institute: *What is aplastic anemia?* (website): http://www.nhlbi.nih.gov/health/dci/Diseases/aplastic/aplastic_whatis.html. Accessed February 11, 2010.

National Heart, Lung and Blood Institute, ARDS Clinical Trials Network: Efficacy and safety of corticosteroids for persistent acute respiratory distress syndrome, *N Engl J Med* 354:1671, 2006.

National Institute for Occupational Safety and Health: *Preventing occupational exposure to antineoplastic and other hazardous drugs in health care settings* (website): http://www.cdc.gov/niosh/docs/2004-165/#sum. Accessed February 11, 2010.

National Institute of Diabetes and Digestive and Kidney Diseases: *Adrenal insufficiency and Addison's disease* (website): http://www.endocrine.niddk.nih.gov/pubs/addison/addison.htm. Accessed February 11, 2010.

National Institute of Diabetes and Digestive and Kidney Diseases: *Urinary retention* (website): http://www.kidney.niddk.nih.gov/Kudiseases/pubs/pdf/UrinaryRetention.pdf. Accessed February 11, 2010.

National Institute of Diabetes and Digestive and Kidney Diseases: *Nerve disease and bladder control* (website): http://kidney.niddk.nih.gov/Kudiseases/pubs/nervedisease/index.htm. Accessed February 11, 2010.

National Institute of Diabetes and Digestive and Kidney Diseases: *Treatment methods for kidney failure: hemodialysis* (website): http://www.kidney.niddk.nih.gov/Kudiseases/pubs/hemodialysis. Accessed February 11, 2010.

National Institute of Medical Sciences: *Burn fact sheet*, National Institutes of Health (website): http://www.nigms.nih.gov/Publications/Factsheet_Burns.htm Accessed February 17, 2010.

National Institutes of Health: *Pain management fact sheet*, August 2007 (website): www.NINR.nih.gov/NR/rdonlyres/DC0351A6-7029-4FED-BEEA-7. Accessed May 12, 2009.

National Kidney Foundation (NKF): Kidney stones (website): http://www.kidney.org/atoz/content/kidneystones.cfm. Accessed February 17, 2010.

National Kidney and Urologic Diseases Information Clearinghouse (NKUDIC): NIH Publication No. 08–4132, *Urinary incontinence in women* (website): http://www.kidney.niddk.nih.gov/kudiseases/pubs/uiwomen/index.htm. Accessed February 11, 2010.

National Kidney Disease Education Program (NKDEP): *Health professionals GRF calculators* (website): http://www.nkdep.nih.gov/professionals/gfr_calculators/index.htm. Accessed February 11, 2010.

National Kidney Foundation: *Hemodialysis* (website): http://www.kidney.org/atoz/content/hemodialysis.cfm. Accessed February 17, 2010.

National Kidney Foundation: *Chronic kidney disease (CDK)* (website): http://www.kidney.org/kidneydisease/ckd/index.cfm. Accessed February 11, 2010.

National Kidney Foundation: *KDOQI clinical practice guidelines and clinical practice recommendations for anemia in chronic kidney disease* (website): http://www.kidney.org/professionals/kdoqi/guidelines_anemia/pdf/AnemiaInCKD.pdf. Accessed February 11, 2010.

National Kidney Foundation: *KDOQI clinical practice guidelines for chronic kidney disease: evaluation, classification, and stratification* (website): http://www.kidney.org/professionals/kdoqi/guidelines_ckd/toc.htm. Accessed February 11, 2010.

Naucler P et al: Human papilloma virus and Papanicolaou tests to screen for cervical cancer, *N Engl J Med* 357:1589-1597, 2007.

Naue U, Kroll T: "The demented other": identity and difference in dementia, *Nurs Philos* 10(1):26-33, 2009.

Nettina SM, ed: *The Lippincott manual of nursing practice*, ed 8, Philadelphia, 2009, Lippincott Williams & Wilkins.

Newman MF, Fleisher LA, Fink MP: *Perioperative medicine: managing for outcome*, Philadelphia, 2008, Saunders.

Newton EJ, Love J: Acute complications of extremity trauma, *Emerg Med Clin North Am* 25(3):751-761, 2007.

Niu J et al: Is obesity a risk factor for progressive radiographic knee osteoarthritis? *Arthritis Rheum* 61(3):329-335, 2009.

North American Nursing Diagnosis Association: *Nursing diagnosis: definitions and classification 2009-2011,* Oxford: United Kingdom, NANDA International.

Oliver S: Best practice in the treatment of patients with rheumatoid arthritis, *Nurs Stand* 21(42):47-56, 58, 60, 2007.

Oncology Nursing Society, Itano JK, Taoka KN: *Core curriculum for oncology nursing*, ed 4, Philadelphia, 2005, Saunders.

Opperwall B: Asthma, allergy, and upper airway disease, *Nurs Clin North Am* 38(4):697-711, 2003.

Orin RJ, Swan KG, Tan V: Acute forearm compartment syndrome secondary to local arterial injury after penetrating trauma, *J Trauma* 66(4):989-993, 2009.

Owens BB: A review of primary hyperparathyroidism, *J Infus Nurs* 32(2):87-92, 2009.

Pach R, Orzel-Nowak A, Scully T: Ludwik Rydygier: contributor to modern surgery, *Gastric Cancer* 11(4):187-191, 2008.

Pain VM, Strandhoy JW, Assimis DG: Pathophysiology of urinary tract obstruction. In *Palliative and end-of-life care: clinical practice guidelines*, ed. 2, St Louis, 2006, Mosby.

Panel on the Treatment of Pressure Ulcers: *Treatment of pressure ulcers: clinical practice guideline*, No. 15, Pub No. 95-0652, Rockville, Md, 1994, U.S. Department of Health and Human Services, Agency for Health Care Policy Research.

Paul L et al: The effect of functional electrical stimulation on the physiological cost of gait in people with multiple sclerosis, *Mult Scler* 14(7):954-961, 2008.

Pedersen SJ et al: A comprehensive hip fracture program reduces complication rates and mortality, *J Am Geriatr Soc* 56(10):1831-1838, 2008.

Penny K et al: An examination of subgroup classification in irritable bowel syndrome patients over time: a prospective study, *Int J Nurs Stud* 45(12):1715-1720, 2008.

People with bowel disorders look for additional therapies, *Nurs Stand* 23(19):16, 2009.

Pereira K, Brown AJ: Postpartum thyroiditis: not just a worn out mom, *J Nurs Pract* 4(3):175-182, 184, 2008.

Physician's desk reference, ed 62, Montvale, NJ, 2008, Thomson Healthcare.

Pivonello R et al: Cushing's syndrome, *Endocrinol Metabol Clin North Am* 37(1):135-149, 2008.

Poaton K, Frucht S: Movement disorder emergencies, *J Neurol* 255(suppl 4):2-13, 2008.

Pua YH et al: Association of physical performance with muscle strength and hip range of motion in hip osteoarthritis, *Arthritis Rheum* 61(4):442-450, 2009.

Quigley PA et al: Reducing serious injury from falls in two veterans' hospital medical-surgical units, *J Nurs Care Qual* 24(1):33-41, 2009.

Rackley R et al: *Neurogenic bladder*, eMedicine.com (website): http://emedicine. medscape.com/article/453539-overview. Accessed February 11, 2010.

Raisbeck E: Understanding thyroid disease, *Pract Nurs* 37(1):34-36, 2009.

Raj DS: Role of interleukin-6 in anemia of chronic disease, *Semin Arthritis Rheum* 38(5):282-288, 2009.

Ramirez EG: Management of calcaneus fractures in emergency care, *Adv Emerg Nurs J* 30(3):201-208, 2008.

Renella R, Wood WG: The congenital dyserythropoietic anemias, *Hematol Oncol Clin North Am* 23(2):283-306, 2009.

Resources, *Primary Health Care* 18(7):5, 2008.

Riepe MW, Ibach B: Neurological and psychiatric practitioners' views on Alzheimer's disease and treatment thereof, *Dement Geriatr Cogn Disord* 26(6):541-546, 2008.

Robertson S et al: High incidence of renal failure requiring short-term dialysis: a prospective observational study, *Oxford Journals* (online journal): http:// qjmed.oxfordjournals.org/cgi/content/full/95/9/585. Accessed February 11, 2010.

Rodbard HW et al: AACE Diabetes Mellitus Clinical Practice Guidelines Task Force: American Association of Clinical Endocrinologists medical guidelines for clinical practice for the management of diabetes mellitus, *Endocr Pract* 13(suppl 1):1-68, 2007.

Rombeau JL: Enteral nutrition. In Goldman L et al, eds: *Cecil medicine,* ed 23, Philadelphia, 2007, Saunders.

Rosen J: The syndrome of inappropriate antidiuretic hormone, *Long-Term Care Interface* 8(5):37-38, 2007.

Ruffing V: Advances in rheumatoid arthritis treatment: infusion nurse perspectives, *Johns Hopkins Adv Stud Nurs* 2:24-25, 2008.

Ruffolo DC: Pulmonary embolism: intervene quickly to halt the great masquerader, *Adv Nurs Pract* 12(6):30-34, 2004.

Rutherford RB: *Vascular surgery*, ed 6, Philadelphia, 2005, Saunders.

Sankri-Tarbichi AG, Saydain G: A patient with Cushing syndrome and reduced lung volumes, *J Respir Dis* 29(7):281-284, 2008.

Santana-Sosa E et al: Exercise training is beneficial for Alzheimer's patients, *Int J Sports Med* 29(10):845-850, 2008.

Saslow D et al, for the American Cancer Society Breast Cancer Advisory Group: American Cancer Society guidelines for breast screening with MRI as an adjunct to mammography, *CA Cancer J Clin* 57:75-89, 2007.

Scharf JL et al: Thyroidectomy for Grave's disease: a case-control study, *Ann Otol Rhinol Laryngol* 115(12):902-907, 2006.

Scott A: Acting on screening results: a guide to treating malnutrition in the community, *Br J Commun Nurs* 13(10):450-456, 2008.

Senneville E et al: Outcome of diabetic foot osteomyelitis treated non-surgically, *Diabetes Care* 31(4):637-642, 2008.

Serebrisky D, Nazarian EB, Connolly H: *Inhalation injury* (website): http:// emedicine.medscape.com/article/1002413-overview. Accessed February 11, 2010.

Sergot, PB, Nelson, LS: Hyperosmolar hyperglycemic state, eMedicine. (website): http://emedicine.medscape.com/article/766804-overview. Accessed February 17, 2010.

Seventh Report of the Joint National Committee (JNC 7) on prevention, detection, evaluation and treatment of high blood pressure, *JAMA* 289:2560, 2003.

Shukla PC, Sheridan RL: *Initial evaluation and treatment of the burn patient*, eMedicine (website): http://emedicine.medscape.com/article/435402-overview. Accessed February 11, 2010.

Shumaker T, Cotton A: Issues in renal nutrition: focus on nutritional care for nephrology patients, *Nephrol Nurs J* 36(1):65-66, 2009.

Sickle Cell Disease Association of America: *What is sickle cell disease?* (website): http://www.sicklecelldisease.org/about_scd/index.phtml. Accessed February 11, 2010.

Sidor MI et al: *Burns, thermal: differential diagnoses and workup*, eMedicine.com (website): http://emedicine.medscape.com/article/926015-diagnosis. Accessed February 11, 2010.

Siegel JD, Rhinehart E, Jackson M, Chiarello L, and the Healthcare Infection Control Practices Advisory Committee: 2007 Guideline for Isolation Precautions: Preventing Transmission of Infectious Agents in Healthcare Settings (website): http://www.cdc.gov/ncidod/dhqp/pdf/isolation2007.pdf

Silva OE, Stefano Z: *Breast cancer: a practical guide*, ed 3, Philadelphia, 2005, Saunders.

Silver J, Naveh-Many T: Phosphate and the parathyroid, *Kidney Int* 75(9):898-905, 2009.

Simon Foundation for Continence: *About incontinence* (website): http://www.simonfoundation.org/About_Incontinence.html. Accessed February 11, 2010.

Singisetti K: Postoperative acute compartment syndrome in the nonoperated "well leg": implications to orthopaedic nursing, *Orthop Nurs* 28(2):91-95, 2009.

Smith HS: *Current therapy in pain*, Philadelphia, 2009, Saunders.

Smith, SC et al: AHA/ACC Guidelines for secondary prevention for patients with coronary and other arteriosclerotic vascular disease: 2006 update, *Circulation* 113:2363, 2006.

Snow V et al: Management of venous thromboembolism: a clinical practice guideline from the American College of Physicians and the American Academy of Family Physicians, *Ann Intern Med* 146:204-210, 2007.

Spaak J et al: Long-term bed rest–induced reductions in stroke volume during rest and exercise: cardiac dysfunction vs. volume depletion, *J Appl Physiol* 98(2):648-654, 2005.

Spratto G, Woods L: *PDR nurse's drug handbook 2009 edition*, Clifton Park, NJ, 2009, Thompson Delmar Learning.

Squizzato A, Romualdi E, Middeldorp S: Antiplatelet drugs for polycythaemia vera and essential thrombocythaemia, *Cochrane Database Syst Rev* 2:CD006503, 2008.

Sreeja I et al: Comparison of burden between family caregivers of patients having schizophrenia and epilepsy, *Int J Epidemiol* 6(2):2-2, 2009.

Steen S et al: Predictive factors for early postoperative hypocalcemia after surgery for primary hyperparathyroidism, *Univ Med Cent Proc* 22(2):124-127, 2009.

Stewart PM: The adrenal cortex. In Kronenberg H et al, eds: *Williams textbook of endocrinology,* ed 11, Philadelphia, 2008, Saunders.

Strauss JF, Barbieri RL, eds: *Yen and Jaffe's reproductive endocrinology*, ed 6, Philadelphia, 2009, Saunders.

Straznicky NE et al: Weight loss may reverse blunted sympathetic neural responsiveness to glucose ingestion in obese subjects with metabolic syndrome, *Diabetes* 58(5):126-132, 2009.

Sturdy, D: Why we all need to be worried about the impact of falling, *Nurs Older People* 20(5):13-13, 2008.

Swearingen P: *All-in-one care planning resource,* ed 2, St Louis, 2008, Mosby.

Sweiss NJ, Hushaw LL: Biologic agents for rheumatoid arthritis: 2008 and beyond. *J Infus Nurs* 32(1 suppl):S4-S17, 2009.

Takahashi PY: Pressure ulcers and prognosis: candid conversations about healing and death, *Geriatrics* 63(11):6-9, 2008.

Tapson VF: Pulmonary embolism. In Goldman L et al, eds: *Cecil medicine,* ed 23, Philadelphia, 2007, Saunders.

Tarassoff C: A reflection on hospice, *J Palliat Med* 12(1):91-91, 2009.

Taylor C: Supporting the carers of individuals affected by colorectal cancer, *Br J Nurs* 17(4):226-230, 2008.

The Joint Commission: *Ambulatory care national patient safety goals* (website): www.jointcommission.org.

The Joint Commission: *Patient's rights standard Ri.2.80* (website): www.jointcommission.org.

The Joint Commission: *Universal protocol for preventing wrong site, wrong procedure, wrong person surgery* (website): www.jointcommission.org.

Theroux P: Angina pectoris. In Goldman L et al, eds: *Cecil medicine*, ed 23, Philadelphia, 2007, Saunders.

Thomas A et al: Recommendations for the treatment of knee osteoarthritis, using various therapy techniques, based on categorizations of a literature review, *J Geriatr Phys Ther* 32(1):33-38, 2009.

Thomassian BD: Nurses can be "diabetes detectives," *Nurs Spectr (Wash DC)* 17(25):14-16, 2007.

Thorogood N, Baldeweg S: Pituitary disorders: an overview for the general physician, *Br J Hosp Med (Lond)* 69(10):597, 2008.

Torpy J: Cardiac stress testing, *JAMA* 300(15):1836, 2008.

Tukker A, Visscher T, Picavet H: Overweight and health problems of the lower extremities: osteoarthritis, pain and disability, *Public Health Nutr* 12(3):359-368, 2009.

Ullrich S, McCutcheon H: Nursing practice and oral fluid intake of older people with dementia, *J Clin Nurs* 17(21):2910-2919, 2008.

University of Virginia Health System: *Neurogenic bladder* (website): http://www.healthsystem.virginia.edu/uvahealth/adult_urology/neurblad.cfm#. Accessed February 11, 2010.

Urden LD, Stacy KM, Lough ME: *Thelan's critical care nursing: diagnosis and management*, ed 5, St Louis, 2006, Mosby.

Vallenga D et al: Improving decision-making in caring for people with epilepsy and intellectual disability: an action research project, *J Adv Nurs* 61(3):261-272, 2008.

Van Doorn PA, Ruts L, Jacobs BC: Clinical features, pathogenesis, and treatment of Guillain-Barre syndrome, *Lancet Neurol* 7(10):939-950, 2008.

Victor RG: Arterial hypertension. In Goldman L et al, eds: *Cecil medicine,* ed 23, Philadelphia, 2007, Saunders.

Vouganti S, Maniam P: *Hydronephrosis and hydroureter,* eMedicine.com (website): http://emedicine.medscape.com/article/436259-overview. Accessed February 11, 2010.

Wang DS, Terashi T: Laparoscopic adrenalectomy, *Urol Clin North Am* 35(3):351-363, 2008.

Warrington G: Compartment syndrome: a case of increased pressure, *Nurs BC* 41(1):27-28, 2009.

Watanabe Y et al: Two cases of type 1 diabetic women with diabetic ketoacidosis presenting as alkalaemia, *Diabetes Res Clin Pract* 83(2):e54-e57, 2009.

Wells M: Managing urinary incontinence with BioDerm external continence device, *Br J Nurs* 17(9): s24-s29, 2008.

Wexler R, Aukerman G: Nonpharmacologic strategies for managing hypertension, *Am Fam Physician* 73(11):1953, 2006.

Whiteing NL: Fractures: pathophysiology, treatment and nursing care, *Nurs Stand* 23(2):49-57, 2008.

Wilkins RL, Dexter JR, Heuer AJ: *Clinical assessment in respiratory care,* ed 6, St Louis 2010, Mosby.

Wilmer A, Van den Berghe G: Parenteral nutrition. In Goldman L et al, eds: *Cecil medicine,* ed 23, Philadelphia, 2007, Saunders.

Wilt TS et al: Systematic review: comparative effectiveness and harms of treatments for clinically localized prostate cancer, *Ann Intern Med* 148:435-448, 2008.

Wing S: Pleural effusion: nursing care challenge in the elderly, *Geriatr Nurs* 25(6):348-352, 2004.

Wolters EC, vander Werf YD, van den Heubel OA: Parkinson's disease–related disorders in the impulsive-compulsive spectrum, *J Neurol* 255(suppl 5):48-56, 2008.

Woods SL et al: *Cardiac nursing,* ed 5, Philadelphia, 2004, Lippincott Williams & Wilkins.

World Health Organization: *Palliative care: what is it?* (website), Geneva, 1990, World Health Organization: www.who.int/hiv/topics/palliative/. Accessed March, 2009.

Wright E: Neurovascular impairment and compartment syndrome, *Paediatr Nurs* 21(3):26-29, 2009.

Yokochi M: Reevaluation of levodopa therapy for the treatment of advanced Parkinson's disease, *Parkinsonism Relat Disord* 15(suppl 1):S25-S25, 2009.

ABBREVIATIONS USED IN THIS MANUAL

α: alpha
AA: Alcoholics Anonymous
AAA: abdominal aortic aneurysm
ABG: arterial blood gas
ABI: ankle-brachial index
ACBaE: air contrast barium enema
ACC: American College of Cardiology
ACE: angiotensin-converting enzyme
ACL: anterior cruciate ligament
ACLS: advanced cardiac life support
ACS: American Cancer Society; acute coronary syndrome
ACT: activated clotting time
ACTH: adrenocorticotropic hormone
AD: autonomic dysreflexia
ADA: American Diabetes Association
ADH: antidiuretic hormone
ADHF: acute decompensated heart failure
ADL: activities of daily living
ADR: artificial disk replacement
AED: automated external defibrillator
AEH: antiembolism hose
AFB: acid-fast bacillus
AHA: American Heart Association
AHCPR: Agency for Health Care Policy and Research
AHG: antihemophilic globulin
AHRQ: Agency for Healthcare Research and Quality
AIDS: acquired immunodeficiency syndrome
AII: airborne-infection isolation
ALT: alanine aminotransferase
ALZ: Alzheimer's disease
AMI: acute myocardial infarction
ANAC: Association of Nurses in AIDS Care
ANC: absolute neutrophil count
ANS: autonomic nervous system
4-AP: 4-aminopyridine
AP: anteroposterior
ARB: angiotensin receptor blocker
ARDS: acute respiratory distress syndrome
ARF: acute respiratory failure
ART: antiretroviral therapy
ASA: acetylsalicylic acid (aspirin)
5-ASA: 5-aminosalicylic acid
ASIA: American Spinal Injury Association
AST: aspartate aminotransferase

ATC: around-the-clock
ATG: antithymocyte globulin
ATN: acute tubular necrosis
AUA: American Urological Association
A-V: atrioventricular
AVM: arteriovenous malformation

β: beta
BBB: bundle branch block
BCNU: bleomycin and carmustine
BEE: basal energy expenditure
bid: twice per day
BiPAP: bilevel positive airway pressure
BMI: body mass index
BMPR2: bone morphogenetic protein receptor type II
BMT: bone marrow transplantation
BNP: brain natriuretic peptide
BOLD: blood oxygen level dependent
BP: blood pressure
BPEG: British Pacing and Electrophysiology Group
BPH: benign prostatic hypertrophy
bpm: beats per minute
BPS: behavioral pain scale
BR: buffered regular
BSE: breast self-examination
BUN: blood urea nitrogen
BWSTT: body weight–supported treadmill training

C: Celsius
Ca/Ca₂⁺/Ca⁺⁺: calcium
CABG: coronary artery bypass grafting
CAD: coronary artery disease
cal: calorie
CAPD: continuous ambulatory peritoneal dialysis
CBC: complete blood count
CBE: clinical breast examination
CBF: cerebral blood flow
CBI: continuous bladder irrigation
CCB: calcium channel blocker
CCPD: continuous cycling peritoneal dialysis
CCU: coronary care unit
CD: Crohn's disease
CDC: Centers for Disease Control and Prevention
CDE: common duct exploration
CEA: carcinoembryonic antigen
cGy: centigray
CHO: carbohydrate
CIAT: constraint-induced aphasia therapy
CIE: counterimmunoelectro-phoresis
CIS: carcinoma in situ
CK: creatine kinase

CKD: chronic kidney disease
CK-MB: creatine kinase, myocardial bound
Cl/Cl⁻: chloride
cm: centimeter
CMV: cytomegalovirus
CNS: central nervous system
CO₂: carbon dioxide
COMT: catechol O-methyltransferase
COPD: chronic obstructive pulmonary disease
COX: cyclooxygenase
CPAP: continuous positive airway pressure
CPK: creatine phosphokinase (as in former use)
CPK-MB: creatine phosphokinase with MB isoenzymes (as in former use)
CPM: continuous passive movement
CPP: cerebral perfusion pressure
CPR: cardiopulmonary resuscitation
CPZ: chlorpromazine
CrCl: creatinine clearance
CRP: C-reactive protein
CRT: cardiac resynchronization therapy
CSF: cerebrospinal fluid
CSII: continuous subcutaneous insulin infusion
CT: computed tomography
CVA: cerebrovascular accident
CVC: central venous catheter
CVP: central venous pressure
CVVHDF: continuous venovenous hemodiafiltration

D₅₀: 50% dextrose
D₅1/2NS: 5% dextrose in half-normal saline
D₅NS: 5% dextrose in normal saline
D₅W: 5% dextrose in water
D₁₀W: 10% dextrose in water
DAI: diffuse axonal injury
DBP: diastolic blood pressure
DCM: dilated cardiomyopathy
DDAVP: desmopressin (i.e., 1-desamino-8-D-arginine vasopressin)
DEXA: dual energy x-ray absorptiometry
DHHS: U.S. Department of Health and Human Services
DHT: dihydrotachysterol
DI: diabetes insipidus
DIC: disseminated intravascular coagulation
DIP: distal interphalangeal
DJD: degenerative joint disease
DKA: diabetic ketoacidosis
dL: deciliter
DM: diabetes mellitus

DMARD: disease-modifying antirheumatic drug
DNA: deoxyribonucleic acid
DNR: do not resuscitate
DOE: dyspnea on exertion
DOT: directly observed therapy
DPL: diagnostic peritoneal lavage
DPOA-HC: durable power of attorney for health care
DRE: digital rectal examination
DSA: digital subtraction angiography
DTP: distal interphalangeal
DTR: deep tendon reflex
DVT: deep vein thrombosis

e.g.: for example
EBV: Epstein-Barr virus
ECG: electrocardiogram
ED: emergency department
EEG: electroencephalogram
EF: ejection fraction
EGD: esophagogastroduodenoscopy
ELISA: enzyme-linked immunosorbent assay
EMG: electromyography
EMT: emergency medical technician
EP: evoked potential
EPA: eicosapentaenoic acid
EPO: erythropoietin
ERCP: endoscopic retrograde cholangiopancreatography
ESR: erythrocyte sedimentation rate
ESRD: end-stage renal disease
ESWL: extracorporeal shock wave lithotripsy
ET: endotracheal
ETOH: ethanol

F: Fahrenheit; French (catheter size)
FAP: familial adenomatous polyposis
FAST: Focused Assessment Sonogram for Trauma
FDA: U.S. Food and Drug Administration
FDG: ^{18}F-fluorodeoxyglucose
FDOPA: 6-^{18}F-fluoro-L-dopa
FDP: fibrin degradation product
FES: functional electrical stimulation
FEV$_1$: forced expiratory volume in 1 sec
FEV$_2$: forced expiratory volume in 2 sec
FEV$_3$: forced expiratory volume in 3 sec
FFA: free fatty acid
FIo$_2$: fraction of inspired oxygen
FIT: fecal immunochemical test
FLAIR: fluid-attenuated inversion recovery
fMRI: functional MRI
FOBT: fecal occult blood test
FSP: fibrin split product
ft: foot; feet
FTI: free thyroxine index

5-FU: 5-fluorouracil
FVC: forced vital capacity

γ: gamma
g: gram
G6PD: glucose-6-phosphate dehydrogenase
GABA: γ-aminobutyric acid
GBS: Guillain-Barré syndrome
GCS: Glasgow Coma Scale
Gd: gadolinium
GDC: Guglielmi detachable cord
GDM: gestational diabetes mellitus
GDNF: glial cell line–derived neurotrophic factor
GE: gastroesophageal
GERD: gastroesophageal reflux disease
GFR: glomerular filtration rate
GGT: γ-glutamyl transpeptidase
GHD: graft-versus-host disease
GI: gastrointestinal
GIG: Gluten Intolerance Group of North America
GN: glomerulonephritis
GnRH: gonadotropin-releasing hormone
GOT: glutamic oxaloacetic transaminase
GPR: global postural reeducation
GU: genitourinary

h: hour (also hr)
H$_2$O: water
HACCP: hazard analysis and critical control point system
HAV: hepatitis A virus
HbA$_{1C}$: glycosylated hemoglobin
HBcAg: hepatitis B core antigen
HBIG: hepatitis B immune globulin
HbS: hemoglobin S, sickle-cell hemoglobin
HBsAg: hepatitis B surface antigen
HBV: hepatitis B virus
hCG: human chorionic gonadotropin
HCO$_3$/HCO$_3^-$: bicarbonate
Hct: hematocrit
HCV: hepatitis C virus
HDL: high-density lipoprotein
HDV: hepatitis D virus
HERS: Hysterectomy Educational Resources and Services
HEV: hepatitis E virus
HF: heart failure
Hgb: hemoglobin
HGV: hepatitis G virus
HHHT: hypervolemic, hypertensive, hemodilution therapy
HHNK: hyperosmolar hyperglycemic nonketotic (syndrome)
HIDA: hepatoaminodiacetic acid

HIT: heparin-induced thrombocytopenia
HIV: human immunodeficiency virus
HLA: human leukocyte antigen
HMG-CoA: 3-hydroxy-3-methylglutaryl coenzyme A
HMO: health maintenance organization
HO: heterotopic ossification
HOB: head of bed
HPV: human papillomavirus
HR: heart rate
hr: hour (also h)
HRSA: Health Resources and Services Administration
HSCT: hematopoietic stem cell transplantation
HTLV-I: human T-cell leukemia virus I
HTN: hypertension
H$^+$: hydrogen ions

I&O: intake and output
i.e.: that is
IA: Impotents Anonymous
IBD: inflammatory bowel disease
ICD: implantable cardioverter-defibrillator
ICP: intracranial pressure
ICU: intensive care unit
ID: identification
IDET: intradiskal electrothermal treatment
IE: infective endocarditis
IFG: impaired fasting glucose
IgA: immunoglobulin A
IgE: immunoglobulin E
IgG: immunoglobulin G
IgM: immunoglobulin M
IGT: impaired glucose tolerance
IICP: increased intracranial pressure
IL-2: interleukin-2
IM: intramuscular
INH: isoniazid
INR: international normalized ratio (used to monitor oral anticoagulant therapy)
IPAA: ileal pouch anal anastomosis
IPD: intermittent peritoneal dialysis
IPPB: intermittent positive-pressure breathing
ISI: International Sensitivity Index
ISMP: Institute for Safe Medication Practices
ITP: idiopathic thrombocytopenic purpura
IUD: intrauterine device
IV: intravenous
IVAD: implantable venous access device
IVFE: intravenous fat emulsion
IVP: intravenous pyelogram
IVUS: intravascular ultrasound

JDRF: Juvenile Diabetes Research Foundation International
JVD: jugular venous distension

K/K⁺: potassium
KCl: potassium chloride
kcal: kilocalorie
kg: kilogram
KS: Kaposi's sarcoma
KUB: kidney, ureter, bladder

L: liter; lumbar
lb: pound
LDH: lactate dehydrogenase
LDL: low-density lipoprotein
LE: lower extremities
LES: lower esophageal sphincter
LLQ: left lower quadrant
LMN: lower motor neuron
LMWH: low-molecular-weight heparin
LOC: level of consciousness
LP: lumbar puncture
LPA: latex particle agglutination
LTBI: latent tuberculosis infection
LUQ: left upper quadrant
LV: left ventricular
LVEF: left ventricular ejection fraction

μ: micro-
μL: microliter
μm: micrometer
m: meter
MAC: Mycobacterium avium complex
MAO: monoamine oxidase
MAP: mean arterial pressure
MCHC: mean corpuscular hemoglobin concentration
MCP: metacarpophalangeal
MCT: medium-chain triglyceride
MCV: mean corpuscular volume
MDCT: multidetector computed tomography
MDR: multidrug resistant
MDRD: modification of diet in renal disease
MEG: magnetoencephalography
mEq: milliequivalent
Mg/Mg₂⁺/Mg⁺⁺: magnesium
mg: milligram
MI: myocardial infarction
min: minute
mL: milliliter
mm Hg: millimeters of mercury
mm: millimeter
MMSE: Mini-Mental State Exam
mo: month
MODY: maturity-onset diabetes of the young
mOsm: milliosmole
6-MP: mercaptopurine
MPTP: 1-methyl-4-phenyl-1,2,3,6-tetrahydropyridine (heroin-like substance)
MR: magnetic resonance; mitral regurgitation

MR-CP: magnetic resonance cholangiopancreatography
MRA: magnetic resonance angiography
MRI: magnetic resonance imaging
MRSA: methicillin-resistant Staphylococcus aureus
MS: multiple sclerosis
MSH: melanocyte-stimulating hormone
MSI: magnetic source imaging
MTP: metatarsophalangeal
MTX: methotrexate
MUFR: maximal urinary flow rate
MUGA scan: multiple-gated acquisition scan
mV: millivolt

N: nitrogen
Na/Na⁺: sodium
NAA: N-acetylaspartate; nucleic acid amplification
NaCl: sodium chloride
NASPE: North American Society for Pacing and Electrophysiology
NCV: nerve conduction velocity
NDIC: National Diabetes Information Clearinghouse
ng: nanogram
NG: nasogastric
NIAMS: National Institute of Arthritis and Musculoskeletal and Skin Diseases
NIH: National Institutes of Health
NIHSS: National Institute of Health Stroke Scale
NINDS: National Institute of Neurological Disorders and Stroke
NIPPV: noninvasive positive-pressure ventilation
NKDEP: National Kidney Disease Education Program
NLST: National Lung Screening Trial
NMDA: N-methyl-D-aspartate
NPH: neutral protamine Hagedorn
NPO: nothing by mouth (Latin, nil per os)
NRS: numerical rating scale
NSAID: nonsteroidal antiinflammatory drug
NSCIA: National Spinal Cord Injury Association
NSTEMI: non–ST-elevation myocardial infarction
NTG: nitroglycerin
NYHA: New York Heart Association

O₂: oxygen
OA: osteoarthritis
OGTT: oral glucose tolerance test
OR: operating room
ORIF: open reduction with internal fixation
OSA: obstructive sleep apnea

OSHA: Occupational Safety and Health Administration
OT: occupational therapist/therapy
OTC: over-the-counter
oz: ounce

PA: pulmonary artery
Paco₂: partial pressure of dissolved carbon dioxide in arterial blood
PACU: postanesthesia care unit
PAD: peripheral arterial disease
PAH: Pulmonary Arterial Hypertension
PAINAD: pain assessment in advanced dementia
Pao₂: partial pressure of dissolved oxygen in arterial blood
Pap: Papanicolaou
PBC: primary biliary cirrhosis
PbtO₂: brain tissue oxygen tension
PCA: patient-controlled analgesia
PCAD: Palliative Care for Advanced Disease Pathway
PCEA: patient-controlled epidural anesthesia
PCI: percutaneous coronary intervention
PCV7: pneumococcal conjugate vaccine
PCWP: pulmonary capillary wedge pressure
PD: Parkinson's disease
PDR: Physicians' Desk Reference
PE: phenytoin equivalent; pulmonary embolus
PEEP: positive end expiratory pressure
PEFR: peak expiratory flow rate
PEG: percutaneous endoscopic gastrostomy
PEJ: percutaneous endoscopic jejunostomy
PEP: positive expiratory pressure
PET: positron emission tomography
PFT: pulmonary function test
pH: hydrogen ion concentration
PICC: peripherally inserted central catheter
PIGD: postural instability and gait disturbance
PIP: proximal interphalangeal
PJC: premature junctional contraction
PLISSIT: permission, limited information, specific suggestions, intensive therapy
PMI: point of maximal impulse
PNF: proprioceptive neuromuscular facilitation